Neonatal Nutrition and Metabolism

Neonatal nutrition has a pivotal role in normal child development and is of even greater importance in the sick or premature neonate. This substantially revised and updated new edition includes a comprehensive account of the basic science, metabolism, and nutritional requirements of the neonate, and a greatly expanded number of chapters dealing in depth with clinical issues ranging from intrauterine growth restriction, intravenous feeding, nutritional therapies for inborn errors of metabolism, and care of the neonatal surgical patient. Evolving from these scientific and clinical aspects, the volume highlights the important long-term effects of fetal and neonatal growth on health in later life. In addition, there are very practical chapters on methods and techniques for assessing nutritional status, body composition, and evaluating metabolic function. Written by an authoritative, international team of contributors, this will be an essential source of scientific knowledge and clinical reference.

Dr. Patti J. Thureen and Dr. William W. Hay Jr. are at the Department of Pediatrics, University of Colorado Health Sciences Center, Denver, Colorado.

Neonatal Nutrition and Metabolism

Second Edition

Edited by

Patti J. Thureen
William W. Hay Jr.

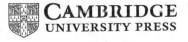

CAMBRIDGE UNIVERSITY PRESS
Cambridge, New York, Melbourne, Madrid, Cape Town,
Singapore, São Paulo, Delhi, Mexico City

Cambridge University Press
The Edinburgh Building, Cambridge CB2 8RU, UK

Published in the United States of America by Cambridge University Press, New York

www.cambridge.org
Information on this title: www.cambridge.org/9781107411791

First published 1999 by Mosby Year Book
Second edition published 2006 by Cambridge University Press
First paperback edition 2012

A catalogue record for this publication is available from the British Library

ISBN 978-0-521-82455-2 Hardback
ISBN 978-1-107-41179-1 Paperback

Patti Thureen: To my very caring and supportive family – Ken, Alex and Christina.

Bill Hay: To Judy, Emily and Bill, and Andy, who make everything I do worthwhile.

Contents

Contributors

John E. E. van Aerde
Stollery Children's Hospital
8440-114 Street
Edmonton
Alberta
Canada, T6G 2B7

Diane M. Anderson
Section of Neonatology
Department of Pediatrics
Baylor College of Medicine
6621 Fannin Street
MC WT 6–104
Houston, TX 77030, USA

Stephanie A. Atkinson
Department of Pediatrics
HSC 3V42
McMaster University
1200 Main St. West
Hamilton, ON
Canada L8N 3Z5

James S. Barry
University of Colorado Health Sciences Center
The Children's Hospital
1056 East 9th Ave
Box B070
Denver, CO 80218, USA

Stephen Baumgart
Division of Neonatology
Department of Pediatrics
State University of New York at Stony Brook
Health Sciences Center T11–060
Stony Brook
NY 1794-8111, USA

Hilton Bernstein
Department of Pediatrics
University of Florida
1600 SW Archer Road
Room HD-513
PO Box 100296
Gainesville, FL 32610, USA

Laurie Bernstein
Department of Pediatrics
The Children's Hospital
1056 East 9th Ave
B300
Denver, CO 80218, USA

Carol Lynn Berseth
Mead Johnson Nutritionals
2400 Lloyd Expressway
Evansville
IN 47721, USA

Frank H. Bloomfield
Liggins Institute
University of Auckland
Private Bag 92019
Auckland
New Zealand

J. Brennan
The Hospital for Sick Children
555 University Avenue
Toronto
Ontario
Canada

Michael S. Caplan
Department of Pediatrics
2650 Ridge Ave
Evanston
IL 60201, USA

Jane Carver
Department of Pediatrics
University of South Florida College of Medicine
17 Davis Blvd.
Suite 200
Tampa
FL 33606, USA

Irene Cetin
Department of Obstetrics and Gynaecology
University of Milan
Milan, Italy

Richard J. Cooke
Department of Pediatrics
University of Tennessee Newborn Center
853 Jefferson Avenue
Room 201
Memphis
Tennessee 38163, USA

Richard M. Cowett
CIGNA Insurance
Pittsburgh, USA

Scott C. Denne
Department of Pediatrics
RR208
Indiana School of Medicine
702 Barnhill Dr.
Indianapolis IN 46202-5210, USA

Sherin U. Devaskar
Division of Neonatology and Developmental Biology
Department of Pediatrics
David Geffen School of Medicine at UCLA
10833 Le Conte Avenue
Room B-2-377
Los Angeles
CA 90095-1752, USA

Simon Eaton
Senior Lecturer in Biochemistry

Kenneth J. Ellis
USDA/ARS Children's Nutrition Research Center
1100 Bates St.
Houston
TX 77030, USA

Camille Fung
Division of Neonatology and Developmental Biology
Department of Pediatrics
David Geffen School of Medicine at UCLA
10833 Le Conte Avenue
Room B-2-377
Los Angeles
CA 90095-1752, USA

Michael K. Georgieff
Department of Pediatrics
University of Minnesota School of Medicine
Box 39 UMHC
420 Delaware Street SE
Minneapolis
MN 55455, USA

Johannes B. van Goudoever
Erasmus MC/Sophia Children's Hospital
Division of Neonatology
Department of Pediatrics
Dr. Molewaterplein 60
3015 GJ Rotterdam
The Netherlands

Frank R. Greer
Department of Pediatrics and Nutritional Sciences
University of Wisconsin
Madison
and Perinatal Center
Meriter Hospital
202 S. Park St.
Madison
WI 53715, USA

Maureen Hack
Rainbow Babies and Children's Hospital
University Hospitals of Cleveland
11,100 Euclid Ave
Cleveland
OH 44106, USA

K. Michael Hambidge
University of Colorado Health Sciences Center
C225, 4200 East 9th Ave
Denver, CO 80262, USA

Margit Hamosh
9410 Balfour Court
Bethesda
MD 20814, USA

Jane E. Harding
Liggins Institute
University of Auckland
Private Bag 92019
Auckland
New Zealand

Jane M. Hawdon
Neonatal Unit
University College London Hospitals
Huntley Street
London WC1E 6AU, UK

William W. Hay Jr.
University of Colorado Health Sciences Center
Department of Pediatrics
Division of Perinatal Medicine
Perinatal Research Center
PO Box 6508
F441, Aurora
Colorado 80045, USA

Morey Haymond
5-1000 CNRC 7072
Children's Nutrition Research Center
Baylor School of Medicine

William C. Heird
Department of Pediatrics
Children's Nutrition Research Center
Room 8066
Baylor College of Medicine
1100 Bates St.
Houston
TX 77030-2600, USA

Ying Huang
University of Florida
Department of Pediatrics
Division of Neonatology
Children's Hospital of Fudan University
Shanghai
China

Oussama Itani
Michigan State University and Kalamazoo Center of
Medical Studies
and Borgess Medical Center
1521 Gull Road
Kalamazoo
MI 49048, USA

Sudarshan Rao Jadcherla
Columbus Children's Hospital
700 Children's Drive
Columbus
OH 43205, USA

Tamas Jilling
Department of Pediatrics
2650 Ridge Ave
Evanston
IL 60201, USA

Sudha Kashyap
Department of Pediatrics
College of Physicians and Surgeons
Columbia University
630 West 168th St.
New York
NY 10032, USA

C. Lawrence Kien
Gastroenterology and Nutrition Division
Department of Pediatrics
Children's Hospital
Room 3.240
301 University Blvd.
Galveston
TX 77555-0352, USA

Sean W. Limesand
University of Colorado Health Sciences Center
Department of Pediatrics
Division of Perinatal Medicine
Perinatal Research Center
PO Box 6508
F441, Aurora
Colorado 80045, USA

Amy Mackey
Department of Pediatrics
University of Florida
1600 SW Archer Road
Room HD-513
PO Box 100296
Gainesville
FL 32610, USA

Jane E. McGowan
Division of Neonatology
The Johns Hopkins Hospital
600 N Wolfe St.
CMSC 210
Baltimore
MD 21287, USA

James L. McManaman
Department of Obstetrics and Gyneco
University of Colorado School of Medi
University of Colorado Health Science
Box C240
Room 3802
4200 E. Ninth Avenue
Denver
CO 80262, USA

Michael Narvey
Stollery Children's Hospital
8440-114 Street
Edmonton
Alberta
Canada, T6G 2B7

Josef Neu
Department of Pediatrics
University of Florida
1600 SW Archer Road
Room HD-513
PO Box 100296
Gainesville
FL 32610, USA

Margaret C. Neville
Departments of Physiology and Biophysics
and Department of Obstetrics and Gynecol
University of Colorado School of Medicine
University of Colorado Health Sciences Cent
Box C240
Room 3802
4200 E. Ninth Avenue
Denver, CO 80262, USA

Deborah L. O'Connor
The Hospital for Sick Children
555 University Avenue
Toronto
Ontario
Canada

Mulchand S. Patel
Department of Biochemistry
School of Medicine
State University of New York at Buffalo
Buffalo
NY 14214, USA

Preface to the second edition

Preterm infants between 500 and 1000 g birth weight are surviving at increased rates. Most of their body growth and the associated development of functional capacity, therefore, take place outside of the uterus. Nutrition to support this growth and development must be provided by intravenous and enteral routes rather than by the placenta.

Many advances in intravenous and enteral nutrition of preterm infants have been developed over the past several years since the first edition of *Neonatal Nutrition and Metabolism*, but the increased survival at lower birth weights, advanced degree of immaturity, and increased dependence on extrauterine nutrition of these unique infants are providing renewed interest in the absolute importance of postnatal nutrition. Furthermore, the diminishing frequency and severity of other disorders in these infants means that their many adverse long-term outcomes cannot be blamed solely, or even primarily, on the consequences of other morbidities. Growth and development of sensitive organs, particularly the brain, clearly are dependent on unique, though variable, mixes of specific nutrients, provided at optimal rates and by safe and efficacious routes. There also is abundant evidence from animal experiments and human observational studies that prolonged undernutrition during critical periods of development (between 22–40 weeks postconceptional age for humans) adversely affects long-term growth and neurodevelopmental and neurocognitive outcomes. Despite the advances in nutrition of these infants, therefore, we now are at a new threshold of determining which specific nutrients should be provided to these infants, at what rates, in what mixtures, and by what means, to optimize their growth and development.

This Second Edition is expanded to include the many recent advances in fetal and neonatal nutrition and metabolism. There also is increased focus on selected fundamental aspects of nutrition of very preterm infants.

A second purpose is to recognize that much still is not known about optimal nutrition of the very preterm infant and that many controversies exist in this field. New research, therefore, must be developed to further optimize nutrition, growth, and developmental outcomes of this vulnerable population of newborn infants. We hope this book will provide, therefore, both up to date information for the clinicians and scientists in this field and the stimulation to pursue new research to resolve the problems that still exist.

New Co-Editor: Lastly, but far from least, the field of Neonatal Nutrition and Metabolism has grown larger and more complicated and rightfully, therefore, a book of this magnitude has needed considerably more help. To meet this need, Dr. Patti Thureen has joined as Co-Editor. Dr. Thureen is an established and well-recognized expert in neonatal nutrition and metabolism. She has brought to the book a large fund of knowledge, unique insights into design and content of individual chapters and topics, and a personal commitment that involved long hours of hard work. Her commitment and efforts have made this Second Edition possible.

Acknowledgments

A lot of people helped produce this book, but we should like to specifically thank Alison Gilman and Tiffany Brown who provided secretarial and editorial assistance.

Our mentors, Frederick C. Battaglia and Giacomo Meschia, are retired but still at work as Professors Emeritus, continuing to provide advice, insight, guidance, and above all, inspiration.

Peter Silver's encouragement, support, and patience kept us going – he and all the leadership and staff at Cambridge University Press are really what made this book possible.

Beyond that, our authors deserve all the credit.

Dr. Hay is supported by NIH Grant MO1 RR00069, General Clinical Research Centers Program, National Centers for Research Resources.

Dr. Thureen is supported by NIH grant K24 RR018358 and NIH Grant MO1 RR00069, General Clinical Research Centers Program, National Centers for Research Resources.

Abbreviations

1,25(OH)2D	1,25 dihydroxyvitamin D
25-OHD	25-hydroxyvitamin D
3-MH	3-methylhistidine
AEDF	absent end-diastolic flow
ATP	adenosine triphosphate
ADP	adenosine-5-diphosphate
AAPCON	American Academy of Pediatric Committee on Nutrition
ACE	angiotensin converting enzyme
AEC	apical endocytic complex
AGA	appropriate-for-gestational-age
AA	arachidonic acid
ARC	arcuate
AVP	arginine vasopressin
ANP	atrial natriuretic peptide
ADHD	attention deficit-hyperactivity disorder
BM	basal membrane
b-FGF	basic-fibroblast growth factor
BSDL	bile salt dependent lipase
BIA	bioelectrical impedance analysis
BIS	bioelectrical impedance spectroscopy
BUN	blood urea nitrogen
BMC	bone mineral mass
BSAP	bone-specific alkaline phosphatase
BAER	brainstem auditory evoked response
BCAA	branched-chain amino acids
BMUS	British Medical Ultrasound Society
BPD	broncho-pulmonary dysplasia
BBM	brush border membrane
CT	calcitonin
VCO$_2$	carbon dioxide production
CEL	carboxyl ester lipase
CBF	cerebral blood flow
CV	coefficients of variation
CDL	colipase-dependent lipase

CF	complementary foods
CHD	congenital heart disease
CNMD	congenital neuromuscular diseases
CPAP	continuous positive airway pressure
CbfaI	core binding factor alpha-I
ICTP	C-propeptide of type I collagen
CHL	crown-heel length
PICP	C-terminal propeptide type I
CREB	cyclic AMP binding protein
cytC	cytochrome C
CLD	cytoplasmic lipid droplets
DSPC	desaturated phosphatidylcholine
DIT	diet-induced thermogenesis
	docosahexaenoic acid
DLW	doubly labeled
	down-regulates
DEXA	dual-energy x-ray absorptiometry
DGR	duodeno-gastric reflux
DGER	duodeno-gastroesophageal reflux
EDF	end-diastolic flow
EI	energy intake
EGF	epidermal growth factor
EFSUMB	European Federation of Societies for Ultrasound in Medicine and Biology
ECW	extracellular water
FHH	familial hypocalciuric hypercalcemia
FIHP	familial isolated hyperparathyroidism
FM	fat mass
FABP	fatty-acid binding protein
FFA	free fatty acids
GIP	gastric inhibitor peptide
GER	gastroesophageal reflux
GIR	gastrointestinal reflux
GDM	gestational diabetes mellitus
GFR	glomerular filtration rate
GNG	gluconeogenesis
GLUT	glucose transporters
G6P	glucose-6-phosphatase
GSHPx	glutathione peroxidase
GP	glycogen phosphorylase
GS	glycogen synthase
GH	growth hormone
GALT	gut-associated lymphoid tissue
HPT-JT	hyperparathyroidism-jaw tumor syndrome
HPS	hyperprostaglandin E syndrome
IIβ-HSD2	IIβ-hydroxysteroid dehydrogenase 2 in utero
IDM	infants of diabetic mothers
IGFBP	insulin-like growth factor binding protein

IGF-I, II	insulin-like growth factors
ICAM-I	intracellular adhesion molecule-I
ICW	intracellular water
IUGR	intrauterine growth restriction
IVN	intravenous nutrition
IVA	isovaleric acid
KHL	knee-heel length
LDH	lactate dehydrogenase
LGG	lactobacillus GG
LMP	last monthly period
LM	lean mass
LA	linoleic acid
LES	lower esophageal sphincter
MSUD	maple syrup urine disease
MVM	maternal microvillous membrane
MCFA	medium-chain fatty acids
MBDP	metabolic bone disease in premature infants
MeAIB	methylaminoisobutyric acid
MFG	milk fat globules
mOsm	milliosmoles
MCTs	monocarboxylase transporters
MSY-I	mouse Y box protein I
MAdCAM-1	mucosal addressin adhesion molecule-1
MEN1	multiple endocrine neoplasia type 1
NAC	N-acetylcysteine
NEC	necrotizing enterocolitis
NBS	neonatal Bartter syndrome
NGF	nerve growth factor
NPY	neuropeptide Y
NEFA	nonesterified fatty acids
VO_2	oxygen consumption
PO_2	oxygen partial pressure
PP	pancreatic polypeptide
PTH	parathyroid hormone
PTHrP	parathyroid hormone related peptide
PDA	patent ductus arteriosus
PVL	periventricular leukomalacia
PIVH	periventricular-intraventricular hemorrhage
PNDM	permanent neonatal diabetes
PPHN	persistent pulmonary hypertension
PP	Peyer's patches
PC	phosphatidylcholine
PG	phosphatidylglycerol
PEPCK	phosphoenolpyruvate carboxykinase
CaBP	placental calcium binding protein
PLGF	placental growth factor
PAF	platelet-activating factor
PARP	poly (ADP)-ribosylating protein

PMN	polymorphonuclear neutrophils	TCIRG1	T cell immune regulator gene 1
PUFA	polyunsaturated fatty acids	TOBEC	total body electric conductivity
PS	population spike	TBW	total body weight
PMA	postmenstrual age	TEE	total energy expenditure
PGR	postnatal growth retardation	TIBC	total iron-binding capacity (plasma)
POMC	pro-opiomelanocortin	TPN	total parental nutrition
PGE2	prostaglandin E2	TGF-beta	transforming growth factor-beta
PDHC	pyruvate dehydrogenase complex	TLESR	transient lower esophageal sphincter relaxation
QUS	quantitative ultrasound		
RANK	receptor to activated NFKappaB	TCA	tricarboxylic acid
RANKL	receptor to activated NFKappaB ligand	TGs	triglycerides
RDI	recommended dietary intakes	TNF	tumor necrosis factor
rCGU	regional cerebral glucose utilization	IDDM	Type I insulin dependent diabetes mellitus
RDR	relative dose response		
RQ	respiratory quotient	UPD	uniparental disomies
RBP	retinol binding protein	UES	upper esophageal sphincter
sIgA	secretory immunoglobulin A	LL/M	urinary lactulose:mannitol
SBS	short bowel syndrome	VEGF	vascular endothelial growth factor
SCFA	short chain fatty acids	VIP	vasoactive intestinal peptide
SGA	small-for-gestational-age	VLDL	very low-density lipoproteins
SER	smooth endoplasmic reticulum	VLBWI	very-low birth weight infant
EDTA	sodium ethylene diamine tetra acetic acid	WFUMB	World Federation of Ultrasound in Medicine and Biology
SDA	specific dynamic action	ALA	α-linolenic acid
SOD	superoxide dismutase	OHB	β-hydroxybutyrate

Fetal nutrition

Frank H. Bloomfield and Jane E. Harding

Liggins Institute, University of Auckland, Auckland, New Zealand

Fetal nutrients are derived largely from the mother, and fetal nutrition is thus closely related to maternal nutrition. However, it is important to appreciate that maternal nutrition is not the same as fetal nutrition. Firstly, the mother has her own nutrient demands which may be in conflict with those of the fetus. For example, pregnant adolescent sheep deliver smaller fetuses, especially when the ewes are very well nourished and therefore growing well, and the growth restriction appears to be predominantly secondary to reduced placental growth.[1–3] Human adolescents also tend to give birth to lighter infants, and birth weight has been reported to be less in offspring of adolescents with a higher dietary sugar intake.[4,5] Secondly, the fetus lies at the end of a long supply line which can be impaired at many points. Nutrients are used by the fetus predominantly for growth and metabolism, with little energy expenditure on other processes such as thermoregulation, movement and digestion. Fetal nutrients are in fact the main drivers of fetal growth, with genetic factors playing a much smaller role. Indeed, the genetic regulation of fetal growth itself appears to be under nutritional regulation, with levels of all the major hormones involved in fetal growth being regulated by circulating nutrient levels. The placenta is also a very metabolically active organ with its own nutrient demands and metabolic pathways. The demands of the fetus and placenta must be in close harmony, particularly in situations where the nutrient supply is precarious, as if the placenta is starved of nutrients and fails the fetus will also not survive. Therefore, in extreme cases the placenta may even consume substrates provided by the fetus. This chapter will attempt to describe the physiology of fetal nutrient supply as we currently understand it, and to relate some aspects of fetal nutrition to clinical data.

The influence of maternal nutrition on fetal nutrient supply

The associations between maternal prepregnancy weight, pregnancy weight gain and birth weight are well known. Birth weight increases with increasing maternal prepregnancy size,[6] and has also been associated with maternal weight gain in pregnancy, particularly with increases in maternal fat mass.[7] Similarly, poor maternal weight gain in all trimesters of pregnancy has been associated with lower birth weight,[8–10] although there is some disagreement about which period of pregnancy is most crucial. Customized growth charts have been developed which take into account maternal height, weight, parity and ethnic group,[11] which may assist in the detection of babies that are not growing appropriately.[12,13] However, these factors account for, at best, 15% of the variability in fetal growth,[14] with the best predictor of birth weight being the mother's own growth in utero. This is true in both developed and developing nations.[14,15]

The fact that less than 15% of the variability in birth weight is accounted for by markers of maternal nutrition before and during pregnancy may explain why maternal nutrient supplementation during pregnancy has little effect on birth weight. A meta-analysis of studies of maternal balanced protein/energy supplementation does demonstrate a reduction in the incidence of small-for-gestation-age (SGA) babies, but not a significant effect on birth weight.[16] However there is increasing evidence that some aspects of maternal diet may have stronger effects on birth weight. High protein supplements during pregnancy actually had a negative effect on birth weight.[17] A study from Southampton found that placental and fetal weights

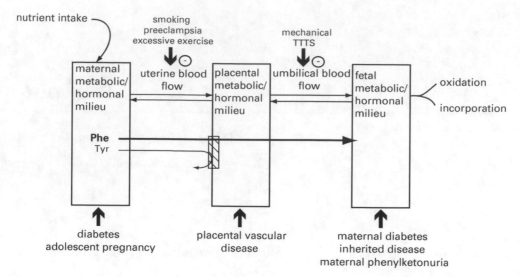

Figure 1.1. The fetal supply line. Nutrients ingested by the mother must pass along a supply line before being utilized by the fetus. The amount of any given nutrient finally utilized by the fetus for growth or metabolism may be affected at any point along this supply line. A few examples are given. Phe = phenylalanine, Tyr = tyrosine, TTTS = twin-twin transfusion syndrome.

were related to the balance of energy obtained from protein and carbohydrate at different times in pregnancy, with high carbohydrate intake in early pregnancy being related to smaller placentae and lower birth weights, and higher protein intake in late pregnancy being related to increased birth weights.[18] This study, and others, have also reported that as many as 40% of pregnant women fail to reach the recommended daily intake for many nutrients.[18–20] Another recent study from the UK found no association between the intake of any macronutrient and birth weight,[21] but a significant, although small, increase in birth weight with increasing vitamin C intake. The potential role of micronutrients in fetal growth is also supported by a recent study in rural Nepal which demonstrated an increase in birth weight with folic acid and iron supplementation and with supplementation with multiple micronutrients.[22] Rural Indian women who consumed more green vegetables and milk, rich sources of several micronutrients including folate, also gave birth to bigger babies.[22] Thus although total maternal energy consumption may have little effect on size at birth, the balance of macronutrients and the micronutrient content of the mother's diet may have an important influence on the nutrition of her baby.

One explanation for the lack of effect of maternal dietary supplementation may be the fact that the fetus lies at the end of a long "supply line" involving maternal metabolic and hormonal status, uterine and umbilical blood flows, placental size and transport capacity and the fetal metabolic and hormonal status. Maternal nutrient

supply to the fetus may be affected at any point along this supply line, for example by placental disease, variations in uterine blood flow (e.g. smoking) etc., thus influencing fetal nutrition (Figure 1.1). An alternative, or additional, explanation may be that certain micronutrients are deficient, or borderline deficient. If one particular micronutrient is supplemented, this may simply lead to the next most marginal nutrient becoming limiting, so that there is little overall effect on fetal growth. Analogous situations may occur in conditions of excess of certain nutrients, e.g. phenylalanine in phenylketonuria, when the high amounts of phenylalanine may saturate placental amino acid transporters and prevent transport of other essential amino acids such as tyrosine and tryptophan (Figure 1.1).[23,24] Another example may be diets high in methionine, which requires glycine for detoxification via transulphuration. Excess methionine in a diet already marginal in glycine may lead to glycine availability to the fetus becoming limiting.[25]

The potential role of folate has been mentioned above. Folate cannot be synthesized by humans, yet is an essential vitamin for many cellular processes including the recycling of methionine and homocysteine, steps in the formation of purines and pyrimidines, and for the formation of glycine from serine. Intake of green leafy vegetables, a rich source of folate, has been found to be strongly associated with birth weight in a rural Indian community.[26] Erythrocyte folate concentrations were also independently associated with birth weight and with intake of green leafy vegetables in this study. It has also been proposed that the intrauterine growth restriction (IUGR) seen in millions of low birth weight babies born to mothers infected with malaria may be, in part, due to disturbances within the folate pathway.[27] Malaria increases folate demand secondary to hemolysis and to a functional folate deficiency caused in part by hyperhomocysteinaemia and also the coexisting deficiency of other vitamins such as B_{12}. A secondary effect of folate deficiency, or of functional disruption of the folate cycle, is glycine deficiency. Glycine is considered to be a conditionally essential amino acid for the fetus and neonate.[28] During growth demands for glycine are high, and it is used in many metabolic processes essential for growth such as purine and porphyrin synthesis, interconversion with serine and also for the production of the free radical scavenger glutathione from α-glutamylcysteine. Glycine is also necessary for the detoxification of excess methionine. Up to 90% of fetal glycine is produced from serine by the placenta, and folate is essential for this interconversion.[29–31] Urinary excretion of 5-L-oxoproline has been used as a measure of glycine insufficiency.[32] 5-L-oxoprolinuria increases throughout pregnancy, and has been found to be higher in women with a poorer diet compared with better-nourished women,[33] suggesting that glycine may be relatively deficient in pregnant women.

Another amino acid that has received attention recently is taurine, the most abundant free amino acid in the body. Taurine is involved in cholesterol degradation, is a neurotransmitter, an osmoregulator and an antioxidant. Reduced activity of placental taurine transporters has been reported following maternal undernutrition and in IUGR in rats.[34,35] Recent interest, however, has focussed upon the role of taurine in pancreatic beta cell development. Rats fed a low protein diet have reduced circulating taurine levels, as do their fetuses.[36,37] Pups from mothers fed a low protein diet have reduced β cell mass and reduced islet area, and this persists into adult life. Supplementation of the mothers' drinking water with 2.5% taurine reversed the IUGR, restored a normal balance of proliferation and apoptosis in pancreatic islets[38] and restored insulin secretion *in vitro* to normal.[36] Furthermore, fetal plasma insulin levels were significantly correlated with fetal taurine concentrations.[37]

Fetal nutrition before placentation is established

Nutrient transfer to the fetus via the placenta in the second and third trimesters is relatively well understood in comparison to fetal nutrient supply in the first trimester. The human blastocyst implants at a relatively early stage and the developing conceptus is enveloped by the superficial layer of the endometrium by day 10 after fertilization.[39]

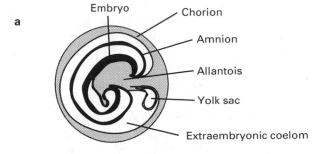

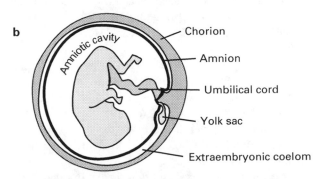

Figure 1.2. Demonstration of the changes in formation of the extraembryonic membranes and fluid cavities over the first 3 months of gestation.

Trophoblast then rapidly invades the vascular network of the endometrium. It has been proposed that maternal blood flows through the developing placenta during the third week, thus establishing the beginnings of hemotrophic nutrition to the embryo.[39,40] However, recent *in vivo* data suggest that significant maternal blood flow through the intervillous spaces may not occur much before the end of the first trimester. The finding of an increase in oxygen tension in the placenta between 10 and 12 weeks of gestation[41–43] may support this hypothesis, although it is still contentious.[44]

Until the placenta does develop sufficiently for hemotrophic nutrition to be established, the developing embryo must be supplied by histiotrophic nutrition. Human trophoblast is highly phagocytic, and has been shown to endocytose maternal erythrocytes and proteins.[45] It has been proposed that this nutrition is supplied via the uterine glands via the fetal fluid compartments.[46] These glandular secretions contain glycogen, glycoproteins and lipids.[45,47] During the first trimester the embryo is surrounded by two fluid-filled cavities, the amniotic sac and the extraembryonic coelom (Figure 1.2a). The allantoic cavity is very small in the human, in contrast to other species such as the cow, pig and sheep, and the secondary yolk sac is devoid of any yolk. As the amniotic sac increases in size the extraembryonic coelom is progressively obliterated and the fluid reabsorbed (Figure 1.2b). Amino acid concentrations have been measured in the extraembryonic coelom, and are significantly higher than amniotic concentrations, suggesting passive diffusion from extraembryonic coelomic fluid to amniotic fluid. Jauniaux *et al.* propose that the fetal fluid compartments, including the secondary yolk sac, may provide a means for nutrient supply to the developing fetus from the uterine glands.[48] Data from studies in the cow and pig also suggest that amino acids may be concentrated in the allantoic fluid of those species, thereby acting both as a potential source of nutrients and as a possible storage place for waste.[49,50]

During this early phase of development, the nutrient requirements of the developing conceptus are very small and are unlikely to ever place a demand upon maternal nutrition that cannot be met. Yet recent intriguing data suggest that nutritional factors during this period of development determine the rate of fetal growth for the rest of gestation, and may also determine the length of gestation. *In vitro* culture of animal embryos for the first few days of pregnancy in media supplemented with human serum results in fetal overgrowth in sheep, goats and cows.[51] In humans, birth weight in donor egg pregnancies is more closely related to the body weight of the recipient rather than the donor.[52] Further evidence of the setting of the fetal growth trajectory early in pregnancy comes from the observation that the growth of twins is different from that of singletons from very early in gestation. Postmortem[53] and ultrasound studies[54] show that growth of twins diverges from that of singletons as early as 8 weeks gestation. Reduction of fetal number in early gestation in higher-order pregnancies does not alter the fetal growth trajectory, nor abolish the risk of prematurity and IUGR.[55-59] Furthermore, there is a significant relationship between birth weight, gestation length and the original number of fetuses.[56,58] Bovine twins are also smaller than singletons from early in gestation.[60] These data strongly suggest that the growth of twins is fundamentally different from that of singletons, and is not merely restricted by fetal space or nutrient supply in late gestation. The mechanism by which growth in twins is regulated differently from so early in gestation is not known.

We have recently demonstrated that the growth trajectory of singleton fetuses can also be set very early in gestation. In sheep subjected to a modest nutrient restriction around the time of conception, fetal growth rate measured in late gestation was significantly less than that in fetuses of ewes that were well nourished throughout.[61] Furthermore, this brief and relatively minor period of undernutrition resulted in preterm birth in half of the undernourished ewes.[62] Whether these changes are the result of hormonal or nutritional signals from the mother to the developing embryo is not clear, but alterations in both individual amino acids and maternal hormonal profiles can be demonstrated.[63-65]

In summary, the nutritional environment of the developing embryo is obviously of great importance, yet there are few data on the route of nutrient supply or on the nutrient requirements during the first trimester.

Fetal nutrition after placentation is established

The main fetal substrates for oxidative metabolism are glucose, lactate and amino acids, with free fatty acids also crossing the placenta in variable amounts (Table 1.1) (Figure 1.3).[66] The amounts of these substrates taken up by the fetus can be calculated in experimental paradigms, such as the sheep, using the Fick principle. Blood flow is measured using the diffusion of an inert substance (such as ethanol, deuterium, tritiated water or antipyrine) across the placenta during steady state.[67-69] As these substances are essentially inert, their loss due to metabolism, accumulation etc. is minimal (usually < 5%) and can usually be ignored. Once blood flow is determined, substrate uptakes can be calculated from arteriovenous differences across the maternal and fetal sides of the placenta. The technique can be further refined using radioactively labeled tracers to determine substrate utilization.[70] The potential contribution of each metabolite to total fetal oxidation can be calculated by comparing the amounts of the metabolite consumed with the amount of oxygen consumed, and taking into account the moles of oxygen required for the complete oxidation of one mole of substrate (the constant, k). Thus, the substrate:oxygen quotient = $(k \times \Delta\text{substrate}) / \Delta\text{oxygen}$, where Δ represents the arterio-venous concentration difference across the organ/fetus/uteroplacental unit. However, it is important to remember that this quotient gives the *maximum* possible contribution of the substrate in question to oxidative metabolism, as it does not allow for carbon incorporation into tissue.

Oxygen consumption

Fetal oxygen consumption varies little between mammalian species and is about 300 μmol Kg$^{-1} \cdot$min^{-1}.[71] The fetal carcass (skeleton, muscle and skin) accounts for approximately 50% of fetal oxygen consumption, although the heart utilizes the most oxygen per unit weight.[71,72]

Table 1.1. Nutrient transfer by the placenta

Substrate	Mechanism	Transporters	Regulation of fetal uptake
Glucose	Facilitated diffusion	GLUT-1 and 3	Concentration gradient Uterine and umbilical blood flow Insulin, IGF-I Placental metabolism
Lactate	Active transport	Proton-dependent, Na$^+$ independent lactate transporter	Bi-directional Placental metabolism IGF-I
Amino acids	Active transport	Many different amino acid transporters	Concentration gradient Uterine and umbilical blood flow Insulin, IGF-I and -II Placental metabolism
Fatty acids	Facilitated diffusion	Fatty acid binding protein	Concentration gradient Uterine and umbilical blood flow Hormones? Placental metabolism
Oxygen	Simple diffusion	-	Blood flow Extraction fraction by tissues Redistribution of blood flow Prior exposure to episodes of reduced oxygen tension

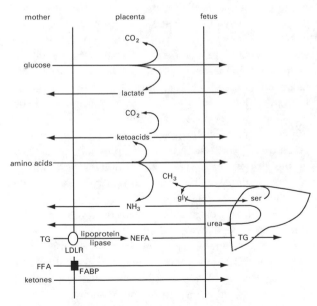

Figure 1.3 Placental transfer and metabolism of nutrients. CO_2 = carbon dioxide, NH_3 = ammonia, ser = serine, gly = glycine, CH_3 = methyl group, TG = triglyceride, LDLR = low density lipoprotein receptor, NEFA = non-esterified fatty acid, FFA = free fatty acid, FABP = fatty acid binding protein.

Oxygen consumption remains fairly constant with changes in nutritional state and with hyperoxia,[73] although consumption can be increased by provision of excess nutrients such as glucose or amino acids,[74] or by increased levels of metabolic hormones such as thyroxine.[75] Hypothyroidism reduces fetal oxygen consumption,[76,77] but in sheep there is little reduction in oxygen consumption if glucose supply is restricted by fasting the ewe.[74] Fetal oxygen supply is determined by maternal oxygenation, and thence by uterine and umbilical blood flows. The fetus operates at the upper end of the cardiac function curve and thus has limited capacity for increasing tissue oxygen supply by increasing cardiac output. However, the fetus can adapt to a limitation in oxygen supply by extracting more oxygen from hemoglobin,[78,79] increasing oxygen-carrying capacity by increasing hemoglobin and by making cardiovascular adaptations. Studies in sheep have demonstrated that when fetal oxygen supply is reduced below a critical level, there is redistribution of cardiac output away from "non-essential" organs, such as the carcass, to essential organs, such as the brain.[80,81] Ultrasound studies in humans suggest that similar changes occur.[82,83] If oxygen deprivation is severe or prolonged, fetal oxygen consumption falls and becomes proportional to oxygen delivery.[69,84] Interestingly, it appears that the fetal response to an acute episode of hypoxemia in late gestation can be altered by the presence of an earlier insult. Fetal sheep exposed to reversible umbilical cord compression which reduced umbilical blood flow by 30% for 3 days then failed to increase oxygen and glucose extraction and blood lactate levels in response to a later acute hypoxemic insult.[85] Gardner *et al.* propose that this adaptation may be a protective mechanism against elevated lactate levels during hypoxic stress.

Glucose metabolism

Glucose is the major fetal oxidative substrate in utero. Glucose crosses the placenta by facilitated diffusion down a concentration gradient from mother to fetus. Thus fetal glucose concentration is always directly related to but lower than that of the mother, although the ratio of maternal:fetal glucose concentrations varies between species. In humans, fetal glucose concentrations are 60–70% of maternal levels, and the glucose:oxygen quotient is about 0.8. In sheep, fetal levels are only 25–30% of maternal levels, and the glucose:oxygen quotient is about 0.55.

In the ovine fetus glucose utilization is between 20–40 $\mu mol\,Kg^{-1}\cdot min^{-1}$, but this can double when extra glucose is provided experimentally, demonstrating that utilization is probably limited by supply rather than by the capacity of the fetus to metabolize glucose. Although the glucose:oxygen quotient in mammals varies between 0.5 and 0.8, not all the glucose entering the fetal circulation is oxidized.[86] The amount that is oxidized increases with increasing glucose concentration, suggesting that when glucose is in plentiful supply, other substrates are spared from oxidation. Non-oxidized glucose is used in other metabolic pathways. Thus glucose oxidation only accounts for about 30% of oxygen consumption in the sheep fetus.[86] In late gestation the fetal liver is capable of gluconeogenesis from substrates such as lactate and alanine,[87,88] but it appears that the contribution of endogenous gluconeogenesis to fetal glucose supply is normally negligible.[25,88,89]

The supply of glucose across the placenta appears to be limited by its diffusion characteristics rather than by blood flow. The main factors affecting these diffusion characteristics are the transplacental concentration gradient, placental utilization of glucose and capacity of the glucose transporters (GLUT) to transport the substrate. In the sheep, placental glucose transfer capacity increases 10-fold over the second half of pregnancy, maintaining glucose supply to the fetus as the fetus grows. This increase arises in part due to an increase in placental transfer capacity, presumably due to the increase in numbers of glucose transporters,[90–92] and in part to a fall in fetal glucose concentration, thus increasing the maternal–fetal glucose concentration gradient.[93] A similar fall in fetal glucose concentrations in late gestation, with an increase in the maternal–fetal glucose concentration gradient has been reported in human pregnancies.[94] The placenta has a high metabolic rate of its own, and extracts 60–75% of the glucose taken up from the uterine artery for its own metabolism. Thus placental glucose uptake has an important influence on fetal glucose supply (see below). If uterine glucose supply from the mother is reduced by decreasing uterine blood flow, the placenta may even take up glucose from the fetus to maintain its own metabolic requirements.[95] Some of the glucose taken up by the placenta is recycled to the fetus as lactate or fructose, but as placental glucose uptake increases with further reductions in uterine blood flow there is a net loss of glucose from the fetus to the placenta.

The transport of glucose across the placenta is mediated by glucose transporters. At least six different glucose transporters are now known, and several members of the GLUT family have been described in the human placenta, although only GLUT-1 is found in the syncytium.[96] In the rat and the sheep, both GLUT-1 and GLUT-3 are present in the placenta,[90–92,97,98] and the levels of both increase with increasing gestation.[90–92] However, in the sheep GLUT-1 expression peaks at around 120 days (term = 145 days) whereas GLUT-3 expression continues to increase until term.[90] In the rat placenta GLUT-3 expression is polarized to the maternal microvillous membrane (MVM), whereas GLUT-1 is expressed on both the MVM and the fetal-facing basal membrane (BM).[97] In the human, the distribution of GLUT-1 in syncytium is also asymmetric, with higher concentrations on the MVM than the BM. When combined with the greater surface area of the MVM (the maternal facing membrane) compared with the BM (the fetal facing membrane), it is likely that GLUT-1 density on the BM is the determinant for the rate of placental glucose transport.[99] GLUT-1 concentrations in the MVM of the human placenta do not appear to increase with increasing gestation.[100,101] However, GLUT-1 expression and activity in the BM increase significantly in later gestation.[101] Placental glucose transport also increases in late gestation.

The regulation of glucose transporter levels has been studied in several tissues, although there is little work specifically looking at regulation in the placenta. In the sheep, hypoglycemia down-regulates placental GLUT-1 levels. Hyperglycemia initially up-regulates placental GLUT-1 levels, although with chronic hyperglycemia there is subsequently a decline in levels.[102] No changes in placental GLUT 1 levels were seen in streptozotocin-induced diabetic rats, although hypoglycemia together with hypoxia following uterine artery ligation resulted in a 50% fall in GLUT-1 levels.[102] In the human, placental

GLUT-1 levels appear to be inversely related to high glucose concentrations,[103,104] although other data suggest that variations in glucose concentration within the physiological range do not affect GLUT-1 levels.[105] In both human and animal IUGR no change in placental GLUT-1 levels have been seen,[101,106] although down-regulation of GLUT-3 has been reported in the placentae from undernourished rats.[107] In diabetic pregnancies a substantial increase in GLUT-1 levels on the BM has been reported with no change in MVM GLUT-1 levels.[108,109] Placental glucose transport was increased by between 40 and 60%. It has been proposed that this up-regulation in BM GLUT-1 levels and consequent glucose transport may be involved in macrosomic growth of the fetus in diabetic pregnancies.[96]

In other tissues, such as brain and muscle, glucose transporters are up-regulated by IGF-I.[110–113] Insulin also upregulates membrane translocation of both GLUT-1 and GLUT-3 in brain and myotubules.[111,112] The regulation of the glucose transporters by insulin and IGF-I has not been well studied in placental tissue.

Lactate metabolism

Lactate is also an important fuel for the fetus. In ruminants, such as the sheep and cow, the fetal lactate:oxygen quotient is between 0.25 and 0.4, compared with only 0.1 for the human.[71] Endogenous production of lactate by the fetus is high even in unstressed fetuses, and most of this is derived from glucose, although some is derived from other carbon sources. The major site of lactate production in the fetus is the carcass, and lactate release from here may provide fuel for other fetal organs in times of substrate deprivation.[114]

The placenta is also a major source of fetal lactate. A significant proportion of placental glucose utilization in sheep is directed towards lactate production which, in late gestation, is released into both the uterine and umbilical circulations.[115,116] Most of the lactate taken up by the sheep fetus is oxidized to CO_2, and this CO_2 contributes substantially to total fetal CO_2 production.[117] However some lactate is incorporated into fetal tissue, including hepatic glycogen, non-essential amino acids and lipids.[118] Thus, the lactate:oxygen quotient underestimates the proportion of fetal oxygen consumption that is accounted for by lactate oxidation.[71] Lactate utilization by the fetus may increase substantially in the face of undernutrition.[119]

Lactate concentrations in the fetus are higher than in the mother, and fetal pH is lower. Both the MVM and the BM of the placenta express proton-dependent, sodium-independent lactate transporters.[1,5,120–122] These transporters appear to be reversible, allowing transport of lactate

in either direction.[120] Thus, lactate can be provided to the fetus as a fuel, or removed should lactate accumulate in the fetus posing a risk to tissues.

Amino acid metabolism

Amino acids are utilized by the fetus for protein synthesis and for oxidation, and certain amino acids are also essential components of pathways such as purine and pyrimidine synthesis. Essential amino acids must be derived from maternal circulating amino acids, whereas non-essential amino acids could be derived either from de novo synthesis by the fetus, from transplacental transfer or via placental synthesis. As well as the traditionally accepted essential amino acids, arginine is regarded as conditionally essential in the fetus. Total amino-nitrogen concentrations in the fetus are higher than in the mother, and concentrations in the placenta for some amino acids are higher than in either the maternal or fetal circulations.

Calculations of uterine and umbilical uptakes of amino acids in the sheep using the Fick principle[123] have demonstrated large uptakes of most basic and neutral amino acids by both the placenta[124] and fetus.[125] Uteroplacental amino acid uptake provides nitrogen in excess of amounts required by the fetus for protein accretion, and the difference is accounted for by ammonia production by the placenta.[124,126] The ammonia produced is released into both the maternal and fetal circulations, where it is converted into urea by the fetal liver.[127] Most of the ammonia is produced by placental metabolism of the branched chain amino acids leucine, isoleucine and valine.[128] Both ovine[129,130] and human placentae[131] have high branched chain amino acids (BCAA) amino transaminase activities, and significant amounts of the products of BCAA deamination, the branched-chain alpha-keto acids, are released from the ovine placenta into maternal and fetal circulations.[132,133] The role of placental metabolism of BCAA may include oxidation as an energy source, conversion to glutamate by transamination and to make nitrogen available for purine synthesis. The proportion of amino acids utilized by the placenta for oxidation increases as glucose availability falls, and in severe conditions BCAA and glutamate may be extracted from the fetal circulation for consumption by the placenta.[130,134]

Amino acids are transported across the placenta by active transport. Many different classes of amino acid transporter have now been described in the placenta[135] and are present on both the MVM and the BM.[136] Experiments on isolated human placental cotyledons have demonstrated that the placenta can take up amino acids from both the maternal and fetal circulations against a concentration gradient.[137] Thus the amino acid transporters on the MVM probably have a more important effect on net transfer of amino acids from mother to fetus.

Placental levels of amino acid transporters are related to fetal amino acid concentrations and thus to fetal nutrition. For example, levels of the system A amino acid transporter have been related to anthropometric measurements at birth,[138] but it is not clear if down-regulation of amino acid transporters follows a reduced growth trajectory, or if the reduced growth is secondary to lower levels of amino acid transporters.[139] MVM levels and activity of both system A transporters[140–144] and β-amino acid transporters[35] are reduced in IUGR, and the activity of the system A transporter is associated with the severity of the IUGR.[140] Oxygenation of the uteroplacental unit has also been correlated with levels of system A and cationic amino acid transporter activity.[145,146] Transplacental transfer of the BCAA leucine has been studied in sheep with IUGR induced by heat stress using tracer techniques.[147] Net uterine uptake, uteroplacental utilization, flux from placenta to fetus and direct maternal–fetal flux were all reduced in IUGR animals.

Further good evidence for a direct role of the amino acid transporters in fetal nutrition and thus growth comes from studies in mice with deletion of a placental-specific transcript (P0) of the *Igf2* gene.[148] Placental growth was restricted from embryonic day 12 (E12), but the transfer of ^{14}C-methylaminoisobutyric acid (MeAIB) per gram of placenta was significantly increased compared with wild type until E16, resulting in transfer of identical amounts of ^{14}C-MeAIB across the placenta. At this time (E16) fetal weight was also not different between mutant and wild type mice. By E19 the increase in transfer of ^{14}C-MeAIB per gram placenta was reduced and therefore, when combined with the reduced placental size, total transfer was also reduced by 26%. By E19 fetal weight in mutants was reduced by 22% compared with wild type.[148]

In addition to amino acid transfer, the placenta is also involved in metabolism of amino acids. The most notable examples of placental amino acid metabolism are the glycine-serine and glutamine-glutamate placenta-hepatic shuttles. These appear to be mechanisms by which nitrogen and carbon can be shuttled between the placenta and fetal liver.[29] In sheep, there is very little umbilical uptake of serine, with almost all fetal serine arising from hepatic production from placental glycine.[149] Serine derived from the fetal pool is used within the placenta for glycine production, some of which is then returned to the fetal circulation. The net effect of such cycling is the transfer of methyl groups derived from glycine oxidation within the liver to the placenta.[149,150]

The ovine placenta takes up glutamate from the fetal circulation,[126] and also forms glutamate by oxidizing branch chain amino acids taken up from the maternal circulation.[151] Amidation of glutamate produces glutamine, which is released into the fetal circulation.[152] Some of the glutamine delivered to the fetus from the placenta is converted back to glutamate by the fetal liver, which is the main source of glutamate consumed by the placenta.[152] Thus a glutamate-glutamine shuttle is established, promoting glutamate amidation by the placenta and allowing hepatic utilization of the amide group of glutamine. This amide group, together with glycine and methylene tetrahydrofolate (derived from the conversion of serine to glycine) can be used for purine synthesis.

Fatty acid metabolism

The human baby is born with a large proportion of fat, and fat deposition increases exponentially with gestational age. Near term the accretion rate is ~7 g day^{-1}.[153] Early in gestation, the fetus derives most of the fatty acids from the mother, but as gestation progresses there is increased de novo synthesis.[74,154,155] Fatty acids are required by the fetus for membrane formation, as precursors of compounds such as prostaglandins, and as a source of energy. All fatty acids can be used as an energy source, but the structural functions are largely performed by the polyunsaturated fatty acids (PUFA). Humans cannot synthesize the ω3 and ω6 fatty acids, and these essential fatty acids must therefore be provided by the mother. Intrauterine requirements for ω3 and ω6 fatty acids in late gestation have been calculated to be approximately 400 and 50 mgKg^{-1} · day^{-1} respectively.[154] In tissues such as the brain, almost half of the lipid content is comprised of long chain polyunsaturated fatty acids (LCPUFA) such as arachidonic acid (AA) and docosahexanoic acid (DHA). The percentage of fatty acids in fetal circulation composed of LCPUFA is higher than in the mother,[156] despite the fact that the human placenta lacks Δ5- and Δ6-desaturase activity and is therefore unable to convert γ-linolenic acid (18:3, ω6) into AA (20:4, ω6).[157] The placenta must therefore be able to extract LCPUFA from the maternal circulation and deliver them to the fetus.

Free fatty acids (FFA) can directly cross the placenta, probably via facilitated membrane translocation involving a plasma membrane fatty acid-binding protein (FABP). There appears to be a specific placental FABP that has higher affinities and binding capacities for AA and DHA compared with FABPs in other tissues.[120,158,159] Placental FABP are found on both the MVM and the BM. Transport of FFA across the placenta via FABP is ATP dependent at the MVM and ATP and Na$^+$ dependent at the BM,[160] but appears to occur predominantly as facilitated transport down a concentration gradient. However, FFA represents a very small amount of PUFA in the maternal circulation, as most are esterified and associated with lipoproteins (VLDL and LDL). Unlike FFAs, triglycerides (TG) and glycerol are not able to cross the placenta in any significant amount.[161] Transfer of LCPUFA from mother to fetus therefore involves placental uptake and metabolism of maternal lipoproteins and TGs. The MVM of trophoblast expresses receptors for both VLDL and LDL,[162–164] enabling uptake of circulating maternal lipoproteins into the placenta. The TG are then hydrolyzed by lipoprotein lipase and the FFA diffuse into the fetal circulation, from where they are taken up by the fetal liver and re-esterified into TG before being released back into the circulation.

In other species TG also do not cross the placenta in any appreciable quantities, and most of the fetal FFA are derived from hydrolysis and re-esterification.[154,157,165–167] The ovine placenta does express increasing levels of Δ6-desaturase during late gestation,[156,168,169] suggesting that there may be some placental synthesis of AA by the ovine placenta, although there is no direct transfer of TG from mother to fetus.[167]

Fetal growth factors and fetal nutrition

Hormones involved in fetal growth are nutritionally regulated in the fetus and also regulate substrate uptake and metabolism. The major fetal growth factors are the insulin-like growth factors (IGF)-I and II, with insulin having a passive role in fetal growth. The roles of other hormones such as growth hormone (GH), placental lactogen, leptin and ghrelin are as yet less clear.

Insulin levels in the fetus are clearly regulated by fetal nutrient supply. Fetal glucose infusion stimulates insulin secretion by the fetus,[170,171] and insulin and glucose concentrations were closely correlated in studies of different nutritional regimens in the sheep.[172] Amino acids appear to potentiate glucose-induced insulin release.[173,174] In turn, insulin stimulates glucose and amino acid uptake into fetal tissues. Fetal pancreatectomy, to prevent fetal insulin secretion, results in impaired fetal growth.[175] However, infusion of high doses of insulin restores growth only to the rate of that in controls, demonstrating that insulin itself cannot stimulate fetal growth in the absence of additional nutrient supply. In diabetic pregnancies the fetus is exposed to increased concentrations of maternal glucose. As placental transfer of glucose occurs down the maternal–fetal concentration gradient, fetal glucose concentrations

are also increased. Fetal insulin release and circulating insulin concentrations are increased in response to the elevated glucose concentrations, and the combination of increased insulin and substrate results in increased fetal growth.

In prenatal life the IGFs are critical in the regulation of fetal growth, acting in both paracrine and endocrine fashion. Direct evidence for the role of IGF-I in fetal growth comes from experiments in mice using homologous recombination of defective IGF-I or IGF type 1 receptor genes to produce animals homozygous for these defects.[176] Less direct evidence is provided by the finding in all species studied that birth-weight correlates with cord blood IGF-I concentrations.[177–179] In babies, levels of IGF-I in umbilical cord blood and blood obtained in utero by fetal blood sampling are reduced in IUGR.[180–183] A case report of partial deletion of the IGF-I gene in a boy with severe IUGR is definitive evidence in the human for the role of IGF-I in fetal growth.[184] Deletion of the IGF type 1 receptor gene has also been reported to result in IUGR, with a Silver–Russell phenotype.[185]

The IGFs are anabolic hormones, and in fetal life circulating levels of these important growth-regulating hormones are regulated by fetal nutrient supply. In fetal sheep IGF-I, IGF-II and IGFBP-3 levels fall with severe maternal undernutrition while IGFBP-1 and -2 levels rise.[186,187] Replacement of glucose or insulin restores fetal IGF-I levels within 24 hours.[188,189] Circulating maternal IGF-I levels in pregnancy are also partly regulated by nutritional status, and maternal IGF-I levels also influence birth weight.[190] In pregnant rats IGF-I concentrations were correlated with changes in nitrogen balance.[191]

In turn, IGF-I regulates fetal nutrient uptake. In fetal sheep IGF-I infusion reduces fetal protein breakdown, increases fetal glucose uptake and appears to alter nutrient distribution between fetus and placenta to enhance fetal nutrient availability.[192,193] IGF-I infusion is also anabolic, increasing the fractional protein synthetic rate,[194] and increasing the conversion of serine to glycine, which would increase the availability of one-carbon groups for biosynthesis.[195] Chronic IGF-I infusion alters placental glucose transfer and placental clearance of MeAIB.[196] Recent evidence from sheep studies suggests that growth-restricted fetuses may be resistant to some of the anabolic effects of IGF-I.[159,193,197]

IGF-II is thought to be most important in embryonic and early gestational growth,[198] acting as an embryonic growth factor by activating cell cycle entry/progression.[199] IGF-II is first expressed in the placenta by 18 days gestation in the human,[200] and is highly expressed in proliferative cytotrophoblasts of the first trimester placenta, acting as a placental growth factor.[201] Recently Constância *et al.* have demonstrated in mice that deletion from the *Igf2* gene of a transcript (P0) that is specifically expressed in the labyrinthine trophoblast of the placenta results in reduced growth of the placenta that occurs before fetal growth restriction.[148] Interestingly, placental transport of methylaminoisobutyric acid (MeAIB, a non-metabolizable analog of amino acids utilizing the system A amino acid transporter) is initially up-regulated in these mice. When this up-regulation fails, fetal growth restriction ensues. Passive permeability of the mutant placenta is also decreased. The temporal separation of placental from fetal growth restriction in this P0 knockout is distinct from the contemporaneous growth restriction of both that occurs in the *Igf-II(p-)* knockout,[198] leading the authors to propose that fetal IGF-II may signal to the placenta to up-regulate amino acid transport.[202] There are many other imprinted genes, some of which are also expressed in the placenta. In general, paternally expressed imprinted genes, such as *Igf2*, *Peg1*, *Peg3*, and insulin enhance fetal growth, whereas maternally expressed genes, such as *Igf2r* and *H19* suppress fetal growth.[203–205] This has led Reik *et al.* to propose that imprinted genes may be involved in the regulation of the balance of fetal nutrient demand and maternal nutrient supply.[202]

Growth hormone levels are also nutritionally regulated, with maternal and fetal GH levels rising in response to undernutrition.[206] It is increasingly becoming apparent that GH does have a role in fetal growth and anabolic metabolism, although the extent of this role is still not clear. GH receptors (GHR) are present in a large number of fetal tissues[207] and GHR/BP mRNA has been shown to co-localize with IGF-I mRNA in the rat fetus.[208] Congenital GH deficiency is associated with a reduction in length at birth,[209] and hypophysectomized fetal lambs supplemented with thyroxine (to abolish the effects of hypothyroidism) have shorter limbs and long bones[210] and reduced IGF-I levels.[211] IGF-II levels were unaffected. Recent data from Bauer *et al.* provide the first evidence that GH supplementation in fetuses can influence IGF-I levels in utero. A 10-day pulsatile infusion of GH to growth-restricted ovine fetuses resulted in an increase in IGF-I levels and an increase in liver and thymus weight.[212] Placental lactate production and fetal lactate uptake were also increased in this study.

Thyroid hormones are also involved in regulating fetal metabolism and thus growth. The metabolic action of thyroxine is mainly via stimulation of oxygen utilization by fetal tissues.[213] This appears to be a general increase in oxidative metabolism, rather than in glucose oxidation alone.[76] Thyroid hormones are reduced, and thyroid stimulating hormone increased (TSH), in fetuses with impaired substrate supply, suggesting that these hormones are also nutritionally regulated in utero.[214]

The role of other hormones that are involved in postnatal nutrition and growth, such as leptin and ghrelin, are beginning to receive more attention in the fetus.[215] Both leptin and ghrelin are expressed in the placenta[216–218] and both can be nutritionally regulated.[218–221] The precise role of these hormones, and other nutritionally regulated hormones such as placental lactogen, remains to be elucidated, but a recurring theme for hormones that are also expressed in the placenta is the possibility that they may play a role in nutrient partitioning between mother and fetus.

Thus there is a close and reciprocal relationship between many of the fetal hormones involved in fetal growth (and thus the utilization of fetal nutrients) and the fetal nutrient supply. Furthermore, there appears to be input from the maternal hormonal milieu on nutrient supply, and the placenta, which is exposed to both maternal and fetal hormonal and nutrient influences, itself produces many of the hormones involved in fetal growth.

The placenta and fetal nutrition

Once the placental circulation is established the fetus receives nutrients via the placenta. The placenta grows throughout gestation, but not in constant proportion to the fetus, comprising 85% of the combined fetal/placental weight at 8 weeks and only 12% at 38 weeks in human pregnancy. However, placental function continues to develop in the second half of gestation with increases in surface area for exchange, transfer capability and diffusion permeability. In mid-gestation in the sheep, when the placenta weighs twice as much as the fetus, the placenta consumes more than 80% of the glucose and oxygen taken up by the uterus.[222] Even in late gestation, when the fetus weighs five times more than the placenta, the placenta still consumes more than half of the glucose and oxygen delivered via the uterine circulation.[95, 115, 134] Thus, under normal conditions the placenta has a greater oxygen and glucose consumption per unit weight than the fetus.

Response of the fetus to a reduction in substrate supply

Most of the information on fetal metabolic responses to alterations in substrate supply is derived from studies in the sheep.

A brief maternal fast has little effect on fetal oxygen or amino acid consumption.[223] With more prolonged fasting the concentrations of BCAA increase,[224] the fetal–maternal urea gradient increases,[225] and there is efflux of glutamine and alanine from the fetal hind limb (representative of carcass),[224] all suggesting increased protein catabolism. Mellor *et al.* have shown that fetal growth rate slows during maternal fasting, and that this is reversible with short periods of fasting but becomes irreversible if fasting is prolonged.[226,227] We have shown that the change in fetal growth rate in late gestation in response to maternal nutritional deprivation depends upon prior growth rate. Fetuses that were growing quickly slowed their growth in response to maternal undernutrition, whereas those that were growing more slowly did not.[228] The fetal growth rate in late gestation is in turn determined by the level of nutrition around the time of conception. Ewes that were undernourished around the time of conception have fetuses that grow more slowly in late gestation,[61,229] and thus peri-conceptional nutrition determines the fetal growth response to a later nutritional insult.[229] Interestingly, fetuses whose mothers were exposed to undernutrition around the time of conception and which fail to reduce growth in response to fasting in late gestation maintain steady arterial oxygen levels, whereas fetuses not exposed to peri-conceptional undernutrition demonstrate a rise in arterial oxygenation in response to fasting in late gestation.[230] Presumably this occurs because fetal growth slows and oxidative metabolism is reduced, thus reducing oxygen consumption. Thus fetal growth and metabolic responses to nutritional or hypoxemic insults in late gestation can be altered by previous experience of the fetus. These adaptations are probably protective in fetal life, for example by setting a reduced growth trajectory to ensure that fetal demand does not outstrip the nutrient supply in late gestation or by down-regulating lactate production and/or release in response to hypoxia. However, these fetal adaptations may permanently reset fetal metabolism and homeostasis resulting in the phenomenon known as fetal programming, which may have consequences far into postnatal life. The topic of fetal programming in response to nutritional stimuli is beyond the scope of this chapter, but there are several reviews which can be consulted.[231]

Paraplacental routes of nutrition

It is becoming increasingly clear that the late-gestation fetus has access not only to nutrients obtained via the placenta, but also to an additional source of nutri-

ent reserves in the form of the fetal fluid compartments. Amniotic fluid is constituted largely from fetal urine production,[232,233] with contributions from lung fluid,[234] nasopharyngeal secretions and intra- and transmembranous fluid fluxes.[235,236] Amniotic fluid contains proteins and carbohydrates, as well as meconium particles, squames and other "debris". Amino acid concentrations in amniotic fluid have been reported in several species as well as in the human.[49,237–241] Broadly speaking, concentrations are similar to those found in fetal plasma.[237,239] Pitkin and Reynolds calculated that amniotic fluid could provide between 10 and 15% of the nitrogen requirements of the late gestation human fetus.[242] They proposed that swallowing and absorption of proteins in fetal life may represent an important physiological mechanism for preparing the fetus for extrauterine life.

From mid-gestation until term, amniotic fluid volume varies little and averages 780 mL. Post-term, volumes decrease so that by 43 weeks the average volume is only 400 mL. In sheep, amniotic fluid volume at term averages 300–500 mL, about half of its maximal volume.[233] Human fetuses begin to ingest amniotic fluid early in gestation, although it is not until the third trimester that appreciable volumes are involved. By term the fetus swallows about 700 mL of amniotic fluid per day.[234,243] Studies with radiolabeled proteins and red blood cells have determined that the late-gestation fetus turns over between 60 and 100% of the amniotic fluid volume in every 24 hours.[234,242,244,245] The inclusion of dead fetuses in two of these studies[244,245] has confirmed that 80–100% of the protein turnover is via fetal swallowing. Although a large proportion of amniotic fluid volume is thought to come from the fetus, various studies have suggested that a significant proportion of the protein content is maternally derived, with concentrations of albumin, IgE, transferrin, orosomucoid and Gc-globulin suggesting passive filtration from maternal serum.[244,246–248] However, some proteins, such as alpha$_1$-fetoprotein and IgG, are fetally derived.[244,247]

There is evidence that not only water, but also macromolecules, are absorbed across the fetal gut lumen and indeed, the anatomical development of the fetal gastrointestinal tract would be consistent with the gut having an active role in fetal life. In late gestation an apical endocytic complex (AEC) develops in the enterocyte villi that allows transfer of relatively large macromolecules from the luminal to the systemic surface.[249] In sheep and humans this capability has disappeared by birth and the gut has mature morphology. Ligation of the jejunum has been shown to delay disappearance of the AEC,[250] and its disappearance is also delayed in IUGR.[251] However, in the rat this complex persists until weaning, allowing the transfer of large immunoglobulins from maternal milk into the systemic circulation.

As long ago as 1972 Gitlin *et al.* demonstrated that large radiolabeled proteins, including hormones and immunoglobulins, injected into the amniotic cavity of human fetuses were absorbed by the digestive tract.[244] Animal experiments later confirmed that these proteins could be used for tissue accretion.[242,252] We have also recently demonstrated that in the late-gestation fetal sheep the gut takes up glutamine from the circulation (with a glutamine:oxygen quotient of 0.65) and releases citrulline into the portal circulation, suggesting that at least some parts of the urea cycle are functional in fetal enterocytes.[237] Fetal urea production by enterocytes has also been reported in pigs.[253]

As well as the AEC potentially contributing to gut uptake of swallowed proteins, the fetal gut brush border enzymes are also functional in utero. All the hydrolases (lactase, sucrase, maltase, isomaltase and trehalase) are found in the gastrointestinal tract from early in gestation (10 weeks in the human, and 50 days in the sheep).[254–257] By 14 weeks in the human activities of sucrase, maltase and isomaltase are equivalent to those in postnatal life.[254,256] Trehalase activity does not peak until between 11 and 23 weeks.[254] From about 19 weeks activities decrease again until just before term.[255] At this time there is a rapid increase in enzyme activity and lactase activity also increases to term levels.[255] This prenatal rise in enzyme activity appears to be related to the glucocorticoid surge.[258,259] Leucine aminopeptidase and alkaline phosphatase activity have been detected from as early as 7 weeks gestation and increase with gestation age.[249]

When various simple carbohydrates were instilled as a bolus into the duodenum of normally growing fetal sheep, fetal serum glucose levels rose, showing that not only were nutrients absorbed via the gastrointestinal tract, but that the mucosa had functioning enzymic apparatus capable of digesting disaccharides.[260] This has also been demonstrated in isolated brush border membrane vesicles prepared from human mid-gestational fetal jejunum.[261] Similarly, bolus intraduodenal administration of amino acids to the fetal sheep resulted in a rise in serum α-aminonitrogen levels over the following 2 hours.[262]

Intra-gastric infusion of amino acids over a 2-hour period also led to increased fetal blood α-aminonitrogen levels, with the intestinal uptake calculated to represent 13% of the infusion rate or 45% of the umbilical uptake. As there was no concomitant reduction in umbilical uptake, this resulted in a net nutrient gain for the fetus.[263] In contrast, when a similar infusion of glucose was given, the umbilical uptake of glucose decreased in proportion to the infusion rate and

to the rise in fetal blood concentrations, thus limiting the amount of extra nutrients that reached the fetus.

Improved fetal growth has been demonstrated in rabbit fetuses receiving amniotic supplementation with dextrose.[264] Furthermore, there was a trend for animals receiving more concentrated dextrose solutions plus amino acids to have better growth than those receiving fewer calories. However, there appeared to be a maximum concentration of additives (in the case of dextrose, 20%) and a maximum volume that could be infused into amniotic fluid before ill effects were seen in the fetus.[265]

There are case reports in the literature of amniotic amino acid supplementation to human fetuses, both in normal term fetuses in an attempt to demonstrate fetal uptake,[266] and in fetuses in which a diagnosis of severe fetoplacental insufficiency has been made.[267–269] Massobrio *et al.* reported on five fetuses who received between 1 and 8 injections of a commercially available amino acid mixture via transabdominal intra-amniotic injections at 24–72 hour intervals. Two of the five fetuses died, the other three were reported to have done well. In two of the cases the authors describe an increase in biparietal diameter on ultrasound assessment that was contemporaneous with the onset of therapy, but there is little other evidence of improved fetal growth.[267]

Finally, there is some evidence that nutrients from amniotic fluid may reach the systemic circulation via routes other than the gastrointestinal tract. Elegant studies immersing isolated lengths of umbilical cord in solutions of amino acids have demonstrated absorption of amino acids across the cord within 10 minutes.[270] Infusion of glucose and amino acids outside intact membranes also results in increased concentrations within the amniotic fluid.[271] Thus nutrients administered into amniotic fluid may not need to be swallowed to be available for fetal metabolism.

These data suggest that in late gestation the fetal gastrointestinal tract is functional, is able to absorb and metabolize nutrients and can transport them to the systemic circulation where they may be incorporated into growing tissues. If, however, ingestion of amniotic fluid is an important source of fetal nutrition in the human fetus, then we would expect that fetuses with impaired swallowing may have impaired growth. There is evidence that this is indeed the case. Babies born with gut atresias have significantly lower birth weights than controls.[272–276] Babies with upper gut atresias also tend to be smaller than those with lower gut atresias, again suggesting a role for at least the upper gut in fetal growth.[276] Furthermore, the effects of gut atresia on birth weight appear to be greater in term than in preterm babies.[277–279] Finally, fetuses with a poorly functioning gut, such as those with gastroschisis,[280,281] are also commonly of low birth weight, suggesting that both the ability to ingest amniotic fluid and a normally functioning gut are important for fetal growth in late gestation, when the fetus may be reaching the limits of its vascular nutrient supply line.

Amniotic fluid also contains growth factors such as epidermal growth factor (EGF),[282] IGFs[283,284] and their binding proteins, especially IGFBP-1.[285] Although the role and sites of action of the IGFs in amniotic fluid is unknown, it is known that the membranes express functional high-affinity IGF-I receptors.[286] More importantly for the purposes of this discussion, the fetal gut expresses both EGF and IGF receptors from early in gestation.[287,288] Both of these hormones are trophic for the fetal gut and act synergistically.[286–290] Indeed, elegant experiments in fetal sheep have demonstrated that fetal ingestion of amniotic fluid is essential for normal development of the gastrointestinal tract in utero. Fetal sheep underwent experimental esophageal ligation at 60–65 days gestation. At 120 days gestation half of the fetuses underwent a second surgical procedure in which the patency of the esophagus was restored.[291] At postmortem at 136 days gestation, intestinal histology in the group of animals that underwent the second operation approached those of fetuses who had only undergone a sham ligation, confirming that swallowed amniotic fluid is indeed trophic for the fetal gut. An experiment by Kimble et al. in which low doses of IGF-I alone were infused beyond an esophageal atresia in fetal sheep, with restoration of gastrointestinal weight, morphology and fetal weight, suggests that IGF-I in amniotic fluid is an important contributor to that trophic effect.[292]

Uptake of swallowed EGF and IGF-I into the portal circulation, and thence into the systemic circulation, has also been demonstrated in fetal sheep.[282,293] Administration of low doses of IGF-I into the amniotic fluid of late-gestation growth restricted fetal sheep has been shown to increase gut growth[251] and to up-regulate expression of IGF1R mRNA in the gut, whilst down-regulating IGF-I mRNA expression in the liver, muscle and placenta,[294] demonstrating systemic effects of amniotic hormones. Thus hormones and growth factors from amniotic fluid are essential for the normal development of the fetal gastrointestinal tract, and may make an important, but as yet largely undefined, contribution to fetal nutrition and growth regulation.

Acknowledgments

The authors would like to acknowledge the scientific contributions of Drs Mark Oliver, Peter Gluckman, Ellen Jensen, Michael Bauer and Paul Hawkins to the work from this laboratory referred to in this review. We would also like to acknowledge the Health Research Council of New Zealand, the New Zealand Lottery Grants Board and the Wellcome Trust for funding support.

REFERENCES

1 Wallace, J. C., Bourke, D. A., Aitken, R. P., Milne, S. M., Hay, W. W. Jr. Placental glucose transport in growth-restricted pregnancies induced by overnourishing adolescent sheep. *J. Physiol.* 2003;**547**:85–94.

2 Wallace, J. M., Bourke, D. A., Aitken, R. P., Leitch, N., Hay, W. W. Jr. Blood flows and nutrient uptakes in growth-restricted pregnancies induced by overnourishing adolescent sheep. *Am. J. Physiol. Regul. Integr. Comp. Physiol.* 2002;**282**:R1027–36.

3 Wallace, J. M., Bourke, D. A., Aitken R. P., et al. Relationship between nutritionally-mediated placental growth restriction and fetal growth, body composition and endocrine status during late gestation in adolescent sheep. *Placenta* 2000;**21**:100–8.

4 Lenders, C. M., Hediger, M. L., Scholl, T. O. et al. Gestational age and infant size at birth are associated with dietary sugar intake among pregnant adolescents. *J. Nutr.* 1997;**127**:1113–1117.

5 Lenders, C. M., McElrath, T. F., Scholl, T. O. Nutrition in adolescent pregnancy. *Curr. Opin. Pediatr.* 2000;**12**:1–296.

6 Kirchengast, S., Hartmann, B. Maternal prepregnancy weight status and pregnancy weight gain as major determinants for newborn weight and size. *Ann. Hum. Biol.* 1998;**25**:17–28.

7 Villar, J., Cogswell, M., Kestler, E. et al. Effect of fat and fat-free mass deposition during pregnancy on birth weight. *Am. J. Obstet. Gynecol.* 1992;**167**:1344–52.

8 Brown, J. M., Murtaugh, M. A., Jacobs, D. R. Jr, Margellos, H. C. Variation in newborn size according to pregnancy weight change by trimester. *Am. J. Clin. Nutr.* 2002;**76**:205–9.

9 Strauss, R. S., Dietz, W. H. Low maternal weight gain in the second or third trimester increases the risk for intrauterine growth retardation. *J. Nutr.* 1992;**167**:1344–52.

10 Abrams, B., Selvin, S. Maternal weight gain pattern and birth weight. *Obstet. Gynecol.* 1995;**86**:163–9.

11 Gardosi, J., Chang, A., Kaylan B., Sahota, D., Symonds, E. M. Customised antenatal growth charts. *Lancet* 1992;**339**:283–7.

12 Mongelli, M., Gardosi, J. Reduction of false-positive diagnosis of fetal growth restriction by application of customised fetal growth standards. *Obstet. Gynecol.* 1996;**88**(5):844–8.

13 Gardosi, J., Francis, A. Controlled trial of fundal height measurement plotted on customised antenatal growth charts. *Br. J. Obstet. Gynaecol.* 1999;**106**:309–17.

14 Hennessy, E., Alberman, E. Intergenerational influences affecting birth outcome. II. Preterm delivery and gestational age in the children of the 1958 British birth cohort. *Paediatr. Perinat. Epidemiol.* 1998;**12**:61–75.

15 Ramakrishnan, U., Martorell, R., Schroeder, D. G., Flores, R. Role of intergenerational effects on linear growth. *J. Nutr.* 1999 Feb;**129**(2S Suppl):544S–9S.

16 Kramer, M. S. Balanced protein/energy supplementation in pregnancy (Cochrane review). *The Cochrane Library*. Oxford: Update Software; 2003.

17 Kramer, M. S. High protein supplementation in pregnancy (Cochrane review). *The Cochrane Library*. Oxford: Update Software; 2003.

18 Godfrey, K., Robinson, S., Barker D. J. P., Osmond, C., Cox, V. Maternal nutrition in early and late pregnancy in relation to placental and fetal growth. *Br. Med. J.* 1996;**312**:410–14.

19 Schofield, C., Steward, J., Wheeler, E. The diets of pregnant and post-pregnant women in different social groups in London and Edinburgh: calcium, iron, retinol, ascorbic acid and folic acid. *Br. J. Nutr.* 1989;**62**:363–77.

20 Rogers, I., Emmett, P. Diet during pregnancy in a population of pregnant women in South West England. ALSPAC Study Team. Avon Longitudinal Study of Pregnancy and Childhood. *Eur. J. Clin. Nutr.* 1998;**52**:246–50.

21 Mathews, F., Yudkin, P., Neil, A. Influence of maternal nutrition on outcome of pregnancy: prospective cohort study. *Br. Med. J.* 1999;**319**:339–43.

22 Christian, P., Khatry, S. K., Pradhan, E. K. *et al.* Effects of alternative maternal micronutrient supplements on low birth weight in rural Nepal: double blind randomised community trial. *Br. Med. J.* 2003;**326**:571–6.

23 Kudo, Y., Boyd, C. A. Placental tyrosine transport and maternal phenylketonuria. *Acta Paediatr*, 1996;**85**:109–10.

24 Kudo, Y., Boyd, C. A. Transport of amino acids by the human placenta: predicted effects thereon of maternal hyperphenylalaninaemia. *J. Inherit. Metab. Dis.* 1990;**13**:617–26.

25 Meakins, T. S., Persaud, C., Jackson, A. A. Dietary supplementation with L-methionine impairs the utilization of urea-nitrogen and increases 5-L-oxoprolinuria in normal women consuming a low protein diet. *J. Nutr.* 1998;**128**: 720–27.

26 Rao, S., Yajnik, C. S., Kanade, A., Fall, C. H. *et al.* Intake of micronutrient-rich foods in rural Indian mothers is associated with the size of their babies at birth: Pune Maternal Nutrition Study. *J. Nutr.* 2001;**131**:1217–24.

27 Brabin, B. J., Alexander Fletcher, K., Brown, N. Do disturbances within the folate pathway contribute to low birth weight in malaria? *Trends Parasitol.* 2003;**19**:39–43.

28 Jackson, A. A. The glycine story. *Eur. J. Clin. Nutr.* 1991;**45**:59–65.

29 Christensen, H. N. Amino acid nutrition across the placenta. *Nutr. Rev.* 1992;**50**(1):13–24.

30 Cetin, I., Marconi, A. M., Baggiani, A. M. *et al. In vivo* placental transport of glycine and leucine in human pregnancies. *Pediatr. Res.* 1995;**37**:571–5.

31 Paolini, C. L., Marconi, A. M., Ronzoni, S. *et al.* Placental transport of leucine, phenylalanine, glycine, and proline in intrauterine growth-restricted pregnancies. *J. Clin. Endocrinol. Metab.* 2001;**86**:5427–32.

32 Jackson, A. A., Badaloo, A. V., Forrester, T., Hibbert, J. M., Persaud, C. Urinary excretion of 5-oxoproline (pyroglutamic aciduria) as an index of glycine insufficiency in normal man. *Br. J. Nutr.* 1987;**58**:207–14.

33 Jackson, A. A., Persaud, C., Werkmeister, G. *et al.* Comparison of urinary 5-L-oxoproline (L-pyroglutamate) during normal pregnancy in women in England and Jamaica. *Br. J. Nutr.* 1997;**77**:183–96.

34 Malandro, M. S., Beveridge, M. J., Kilberg, M. S., Novak, D. A. Effect of low-protein diet-induced intrauterine growth retardation on rat placental amino acid transport. *Am. J. Physiol.* 1996;**271**:C295–303.

35 Norberg, S., Powell, T. L., Jansson, T. Intrauterine growth restriction is associated with a reduced activity of placental taurine transporters. *Pediatr. Res.* 1998;**44**:233–8.

36 Cherif, H., Reusens, B., Ahn, M. T., Hoet, J. J., Remacle, C. Effects of taurine on the insulin secretion of rat fetal islets from dams fed a low-protein diet. *J. Endocrinol.* 1998;**159**:341–8.

37 Bertin, E., Gangnerau, M. N., Bellon, G. *et al.* Development of beta-cell mass in fetuses of rats deprived of protein and/or energy in last trimester of pregnancy. *Am. J. Physiol. Regul. Integr. Comp. Physiol.* 2002;**283**:R623–30.

38 Boujendar, S., Reusens, B., Merezak, S. *et al.* Taurine supplementation to a low protein diet during foetal and early postnatal life restores a normal proliferation and apoptosis of rat pancreatic islets. *Diabetologia.* 2002;**45**(6):856–866.

39 Carlson, B. M. Extraembryonic membranes and placenta. In Carlson, B. M., ed. *Patten's Foundations of Embryology*. New York: McGraw-Hill Inc.; 1996:255–90.

40 Larsen, W. J. *Human Embryology*. New York: Churchill-Livingstone; 2003

41 Rodesch, F., Simon, P., Donner, C., Jauniaux, E. Oxygen measurements in endometrial and trophoblastic tissues during early pregnancy. *Obstet. Gynecol.* 1992;**80**:283–5.

42 Jauniaux, E., Watson, A. L., Burton, G. J. Evaluation of respiratory gases and acid-base gradients in fetal fluids and uteroplacental tissue between 7 and 16 weeks. *Am. J. Obstet. Gynecol.* 2001;**184**:998–1003.

43 Jauniaux, E., Watson, A. L., Hempstock, J. *et al.* Onset of maternal arterial blood flow and placental oxidative stress; a possible factor in human early pregnancy failure. *Am. J. Pathol.* 2000;**157**:2111–22.

44 Kurjak, A., Kupesic, S., Hafner, T. *et al.* Conflicting data on intervillous circulation in early pregnancy. *J. Perinat. Med.* 1997;**25**:225–36.

45 Bell, S. C. Secretory endometrial/decidual proteins and their function in early pregnancy. *J. Reprod. Fertil.* 1988;**36**: 109–25.

46 Burton, G. J., Watson, A. L., Hempstock, J., Skepper, J. N., Jauniaux, E. Uterine glands provide histiotrophic nutrition for the human fetus during the first trimester of pregnancy. *J. Clin. Endocrinol. Metab.* 2002;**87**:2954–9.

47 Boyd, J. D. Glycogen in early human implantation sites. *Mem. Soc. Endocrinol.* 1959;**6**:26–34.

48 Burton, G. J., Hempstock, J., Jauniaux, E. Nutrition of the human fetus during the first trimester – a review. *Placenta* 2001;**22**:S70–6.

49 Baetz, A. L., Hubbert, W. T., Graham, C. K. Developmental changes of free amino acids in bovine fetal fluids with gestational age and the interrelationships between the amino acid concentrations in the fluid compartments. *J. Reprod. Fertil.* 1975;**44**:437.

50 Stanier, M. W. Transfer of radioactive water, urea and glycine between maternal and foetal body fluids in rabbits and pigs. *J. Physiol.* 1965;**178**:127–40.

51 Walker, S. K., Hartwich, K. M., Robinson, J. S., Seamark, R. F. Influences of in vitro culture of embryos on the normality of development. In Lauria, A., Gandolfi, F., eds. *Gametes: Development and Function.* Serono Symposium; 1998:457–84.

52 Brooks, A. A., Johnson, M. R., Steer, P. J., Pawson, M. E., Abdalla, H. I. Birth weight: nature or nurture? *Early Hum. Dev.* 1995;**42**:29–35.

53 Iffy, L., Lavenhar, M. A., Jakobovits, A., Kaminetzky, H. A. The rate of early intrauterine growth in twin gestation. *Am. J. Obstet. Gynecol.* 1983;**146**:970–2.

54 Leveno, K. J., Santos-Ramos, R., Duenhoelter, J. H., Reisch, J. S., Whalley, P. J. Sonar cephalometry in twins: a table of biparietal diameters for normal twin fetuses and a comparison with singletons. *Am. J. Obstet. Gynecol.* 1979;**135**:727–30.

55 Alexander, J. M., Hammond, K. R., Steinkampf, M. P. Multifetal reduction of high-order multiple pregnancy: comparison of obstetrical outcome with nonreduced twin gestations. *Fertil. Steril.* 1995;**64**:1201–3.

56 Groutz, A., Yovel, I., Amit, A. *et al.* Pregnancy outcome after multifetal pregnancy reduction to twins compared with spontaneously conceived twins. *Hum. Reprod.* 1996;**11**:1334–6.

57 Fasouliotis, S. J., Schenker, J. G. Multifetal pregnancy reduction: a review of the world results for the period 1993–1996. *Eur. J. Obstet. Gynecol. Reprod. Biol.* 1997;**75**:183–90.

58 Depp, R., Macones, G. A., Rosenn, M. F. *et al.* Multifetal pregnancy reduction: evaluation of fetal growth in the remaining twins. *Am. J. Obstet. Gynecol.* 1996;**174**:1233–8.

59 Yaron, Y., Johnson, K. D., Bryant-Greenwood, P. K. *et al.* Selective termination and elective reduction in twin pregnancies: 10 years experience at a single centre. *Hum. Reprod.* 1998;**13**:2301–4.

60 Bertolini, M., Mason, J. B., Beam, S. W. *et al.* Morphology and morphometry of in vivo- and in vitro-produced bovine concepti from early pregnancy to term and association with high birth weights. *Theriogenology* 2002;**58**:973–94.

61 Oliver, M. H., Hawkins, P., Harding, J. E. Periconceptional undernutrition alters growth trajectory, endocrine and metabolic responses to fasting in late gestation fetal sheep. *Pediatr. Res.* 2005;**57**:591–8.

62 Bloomfield, F. H., Oliver, M. H., Hawkins, P. *et al.* A periconceptional nutritional origin for non-infectious preterm birth. *Science* 2003;**300**:606.

63 Oliver, M. H., Hawkins, P., Breier, B. *et al.* Maternal undernutrition during the periconceptual period increases plasma taurine levels and insulin response to glucose but not arginine in the late gestational fetal sheep. *Endocrinology,* 2001;**142**:4576–9.

64 van Zijl, P. L., Oliver, M. H., Harding, J. E. Periconceptual undernutrition in sheep leads to longterm changes in maternal amino acid concentrations. *Proceedings of the 6th Annual Congress of the Perinatal Society of Australia and New Zealand,* Parramatta, NSW. 2002; P190 (Abstr.).

65 Bloomfield, F. H., Oliver, M. H., Hawkins, P. *et al.* Periconceptional undernutrition in sheep accelerates maturation of the fetal hypothalamic-pituitary-adrenal axis in late gestation. *Endocrinology* 2004;**145**:4278–85.

66 Battaglia, F. C., Meschia, G. Principal substrates of fetal metabolism. *Phys. Rev.* 1978;**58**:499–527.

67 Rudolph, A. M., Heymann, M. A. Validation of the antipyrine method for measuring fetal umbilical blood flow. *Circ. Res.* 1967;**21**:185–90.

68 Crenshaw, C., Huckabee, W. E., Curet, L. B., Mann, L., Barron, D. H. A method for the estimation of the umbilical blood flow in unstressed sheep and goats with some results of its application. *Q. J. Exp. Physiol.* 1968;**53**:65–75.

69 Wilkening, R. B., Meschia, G. Fetal oxygen uptake, oxygenation, and acid-base balance as a function of uterine blood flow. *Am. J. Physiol.* 1983;**244**:H749–55.

70 Wolfe, R. R. *Tracers in Metabolic Research. Radioisotope and Stable Isotope / Mass Spectrometry Methods.* New York: Alan R. Liss, Inc; 1984.

71 Fowden, A. L. Fetal metabolism and energy balance. In Thorburn, G. D., Harding, R., eds. *Textbook of Fetal Physiology.* Oxford: Oxford University Press; 1994:70–82.

72 Fisher, D. J., Heymann, M. A., Rudolph, A. M. Myocardial oxygen and carbohydrate consumption in fetal lambs *in utero* and in adult sheep. *Am. J. Physiol.* 1980;**238**:H399–405.

73 Owens, J. A., Falconer, J., Robinson, J. S. Effects of maternal hyperoxia on fetal metabolism in experimental intrauterine growth retardation. *Proceedings of the Third Congress of the Australian Perinatal Society,* Parramatta, NSW. 1985; C2–2 (Abstr.).

74 Hay, W. W. Jr, DiGiacomo, J. E., Mezharich, H. K., Hirst, K., Zerbe, G. Effects of glucose and insulin on fetal glucose oxidation and oxygen consumption. *Am. J. Physiol.* 1989;**256**:E704–13.

75 Lorijn, R. H., Nelson, J. C., Longho, L. D. Induced fetal hyperthyroidism: cardiac output and oxygen consumption. *Am. J. Physiol.* 1980;**239**: H302–7.

76 Fowden, A. L., Silver, M. The effects of thyroid hormones on oxygen and glucose metabolism in the sheep fetus during late gestation. *J. Physiol.* 1995;**482**:202–13.

77 Fowden, A. L., Mapstone, J., Forhead, A. J. Regulation of gluconeogenesis by thyroid hormones in fetal sheep during late gestation. *J. Endocrinol.* 2001;**170**:461–9.

78 Owens, J. A., Falconer, J., Robinson, J. S. Effect of restriction of placental growth on oxygen delivery to and consumption

by the pregnant uterus and fetus. *J. Dev. Physiol.* 1987;**9**:137–50.

79 Bard, H., Fouron, J.-C., Prosmanne, J., Gagnon, J. Effect of hypoxemia on fetal hemoglobin synthesis during late gestation. *Pediatr. Res.* 1992;**31**:483–485.

80 Bocking, A. D., Gagnon, R., White, S. E. Circulatory responses to prolonged hypoxemia in fetal sheep. *Am. J. Obstet. Gynecol.* 1988;**159**:1418–24.

81 Itskovitz, J., LaGamma, E. F., Rudolph, A. M. Effects of cord compression on fetal blood flow distribution and O_2 delivery. *Am. J. Physiol.* 1987;**252**:H100–9.

82 Al-Ghazali, W., Chita, S. K., Chapman, M. G., *et al.* Evidence of a redistribution of cardiac output in asymmetrical growth retardation. *Br. J. Obstet. Gynaecol.* 1989;**96**:697–704.

83 Divon, M. Y. Doppler blood flow studies and fetal growth retardation. In Divon, M. Y., ed. *Abnormal Fetal Growth.* New York: Elsevier; 1991:147–62.

84 Itzkovitz, J., LaGamma, E. F., Rudolph, A. M. The effect of reducing umbilical blood flow on fetal oxygenation. *Am. J. Obstet. Gynecol.* 1983;**148**(7):813–18.

85 Gardner, D. S., Giussani, D. A., Fowden, A. L. Hind limb glucose and lactate metabolism during umbilical cord compression and acute hypoxemia in the late gestation ovine fetus. *Am. J. Physiol. Regul. Integr. Comp. Physiol.* 2003;**284**:R954–64.

86 Hay, W. W. Jr, Myers, S. A., Sparks, J. W. *et al.* Glucose and lactate oxidation rates in the fetal lamb. *Proc. Soc. Exp. Biol. Med.* 1983;**173**:553–63.

87 Prior, R. L., Christenson, R. K. Gluconeogenesis from alanine *in vivo* by the ovine fetus and lamb. *Am. J. Physiol.* 1977;**233**:E462–68.

88 Gleason, C. A., Rudolph, A. M. Gluconeogenesis by the fetal sheep liver in vivo. *J. Dev. Physiol.* 1985;**7**:185–94.

89 Teng, C., Battaglia, F. C., Meschia, G., Narkewicz, M. R., Wilkening, R. B. Fetal hepatic and umbilical uptakes of glucogenic substrates during a glucagon-somatostatin infusion. *Am. J. Physiol.* 2002;**282**:E542–50.

90 Currie, M. J., Bassett, N. S., Gluckman, P. D. Ovine glucose transporter-1 and -3: cDNA partial sequences and developmental gene expression in the placenta. *Placenta* 1997;**18**:393–401.

91 Ehrhardt, R. A., Bell, A. W. Developmental increases in glucose transporter concentration in the sheep placenta. *Am. J. Physiol.* 1997;**272**:R1132–41.

92 Zhou, J., Bondy, C. Placental glucose transporter gene expression and metabolism in the rat. *J. Clin. Invest.* 1993;**91**:845–52.

93 Molina, R. D., Meschia, G., Battaglia, F. C., Hay, W. W. Jr. Gestational maturation of placental glucose transfer capacity in sheep. *Am. J. Physiol.* 1991;**261**:R697–704.

94 Marconi, A. M., Paolini, C. L., Buscaglia, M. *et al.* The impact of gestational age and fetal growth on the maternal-fetal glucose concentration difference. *Obstet. Gynecol.* 1996;**87**:937–42.

95 Gu, W., Jones, C. T., Harding, J. E. Metabolism of glucose by fetus and placenta of sheep. The effects of normal fluctuations in uterine blood flow. *J. Dev. Physiol.* 1987;**9**:369–89.

96 Illsley, N. P. Glucose transporters in the human placenta. *Placenta* 2000;**21**:14–22.

97 Shin, B. C., Fujikura, K., Suzuki, T., Tanaka, S., Takata, K. Glucose transporter GLUT3 in rat placental barrier: a possible machinery for the transplacental transfer of glucose. *Endocrinology* 1997;**138**(9):3997–4004.

98 Takata, K., Kasahara, T., Kasahara, M., Ezaki, O., Hirano, H. Immunolocalization of glucose transporter GLUT1 in the rat placental barrier: possible role of GLUT1 and the gap junction in the transport of glucose across the placental barrier. *Cell Tissue Res* 1994;**276**:411–18.

99 Baumann, M. U., Deborde, S., Illsley, N. P. Placental glucose transfer and fetal growth. *Endocrine* 2002;**19**:13–22.

100 Jansson, T., Cowley, E. A., Illsley, N. P. Cellular localization of glucose transporter messenger RNA in human placenta. *Reprod. Fertil. Dev.* 1995;**7**:1425–30.

101 Jansson, T., Wennergren, M., Illsley, N. P. Glucose transporter expression and distribution in the human placenta throughout gestation and in intrauterine growth retardation. *J. Clin. Endocrinol. Metab.* 1993;**77**:1554–62.

102 Das, U. G., Sadiq, F., Soares, M. J., Hay, W. W. Jr, Devaskar, S. U. Time-dependent physiological regulation of rodent and ovine placental glucose transporter (GLUT-1) protein. *Am. J. Physiol.* 1998;**274**:R339–47.

103 Gordon, M. C., Zimmerman, P. D., Landon, M. B., Gabbe, S. G., Kniss, D. A. Insulin and glucose modulate glucose transporter messenger ribonucleic acid expression and glucose uptake in trophoblasts isolated from first-trimester chorionic villi. *Am. J. Obstet. Gynecol.* 1995;**173**:1089–97.

104 Hahn, T., Barth, S., Weiss, U., Mosgoeller, W., Desoye, G. Sustained hyperglycemia in vitro down-regulates the GLUT1 glucose transporter system of cultured human placental trophoblast: a mechanism to protect fetal development? *FASEB J.*, 1998;**12**:1221–31.

105 Illsley, N. P., Sellers, M. C., Wright, R. L. Glycemic regulation of glucose transporter expression and activity in the human placenta. *Placenta* 1998;**19**:517–24.

106 Reid, G. J., Lane, R. H., Flozak, A. S., Simmons, R. A. Placental expression of glucose transporter proteins 1 and 3 in growth-restricted fetal rats. *Am. J. Obstet. Gynecol.* 1999;**180**:1017–23.

107 Lesage, J., Hahn, D., Leonhardt, M. *et al.* Maternal undernutrition during late gestation-induced intrauterine growth restriction in the rat is associated with impaired placental GLUT3 expression, but does not correlate with endogenous corticosterone levels. *J. Endocrinol.* 2002;**174**:37–43.

108 Gaither, K., Quraishi, A. N., Illsley, N. P. Diabetes alters the expression and activity of the human placental GLUT1 glucose transporter. *J. Clin. Endocrinol. Metab.* 1999;**84**:695–701.

109 Jansson, T., Wennergren, M., Powell, T. L. Placental glucose transport and GLUT 1 expression in insulin-dependent diabetes. *Am. J. Obstet. Gynecol.* 1999;**180**:163–8.

110 Fladeby, C., Skar, R., Serck-Hanssen, G. Distinct regulation of glucose transport and GLUT1/GLUT3 transporters by glucose deprivation and IGF-I in chromaffin cells. *Biochim. Biophys. Acta.* 2003;**1593**:201–8.

111 Maher, F., Harrison, L. C. Stabilization of glucose transporter mRNA by insulin/IGF-I and glucose deprivation. *Biochem. Biophys. Res. Comm.* 1990;**171**:210–5.

112 Wilson, C. M., Mitsumoto, Y., Maher, F., Klip, A. Regulation of cell surface GLUT1, GLUT3 and GLUT4 by insulin and IGF-1 in L6 myotubes. *FEBS Lett.* 1995;**368**:19–22.

113 Simmons, R. A., Flozak, A. S., Ogata, E. S. The effect of insulin and insulin-like growth factor-I on glucose transport in normal and small for gestational age fetal rats. *Endocrinology* 1993;**133**:1361–8.

114 Harding, J. E., Charlton, V. E., Evans, P. C. Effects of beta-hydroxybutyrate infusion on hind limb metabolism in fetal sheep. *Am. J. Obstet. Gynecol.* 1992;**166**:671–6.

115 Sparks, J. W., Hay, W. W., Meschia, G., Battaglia, F. C. Partition of maternal nutrients to the placenta and fetus in the sheep. *Eur. J. Obstet. Gynaecol.* 1983;**14**:331–40.

116 Battaglia, F. C., Meschia, G. *An Introduction to Fetal Physiology.* Orlando: Academic Press; 1986.

117 McGowan, J. E., Aldoretta, P. W., Hay, W. W. Jr. Contribution of fructose and lactate produced in placenta to calculation of fetal glucose oxidation rate. *Am. J. Physiol.* 1995;**269**:E834–9.

118 Carter, B. S., Moores, R. R. Jr, Teng, C., Meschia, G., Battaglia, F. C. Main routes of plasma lactate carbon disposal in the midgestation fetal lamb. *Biol. Neonate* 1995;**67**:295–300.

119 Harding, J. E., Johnston, B. M. Nutrition and fetal growth. *Reprod. Fertil. Dev.*, 1995;**7**:539–47.

120 Alonso de la Torre, S. R., Serrano, M. A., Alvarado, F., Medina, J. M. Carrier-mediated L-lactate transport in brush-border membrane vesicles from rat placenta during late gestation. *Biochem. J.* 1991;**278** (Pt 2):535–41.

121 Alonso de la Torre, S. R., Serrano, M. A., Caropaton, T., Medina, J. M. Proton gradient-dependent active transport of L-lactate in basal plasma membrane vesicles isolated from syncytiotrophoblast human placenta. *Biochem. Soc. Trans.* 1991;**19**:409S.

122 Inuyama, M., Ushigome, F., Emoto, A. *et al.* Characteristics of L-lactic acid transport in basal membrane vesicles of human placental syncytiotrophoblast. *Am. J. Physiol. Cell Physiol.* 2002;**283**:C822–30.

123 Meschia, G., Battaglia, F. C., Hay, W. W., Sparks, J. W. Utilization of substrates by the ovine placenta *in vivo. Fed. Proc.* 1980;**39**:245–9.

124 Holzman, I. R., Lemons, J. A., Meschia, G., Battaglia, F. C. Uterine uptake of amino acids and glutamine-glutamate balance across the placenta of the pregnant ewe. *J. Dev. Physiol.* 1979;**1**:137–49.

125 Lemons, J. A., Adcock, E. W. I., Jones, M. D. Jr *et al.* Umbilical uptake of amino acids in the unstressed fetal lamb. *J. Clin. Invest.* 1976;**58**:1428–34.

126 Holzman, I. R., Lemons, J. A., Meschia, G., Battaglia, F. C. Ammonia production by the pregnant uterus. *Proc. Soc. Exp. Biol. Med.* 1977;**156**:27–30.

127 Gresham, E. L., James, E. J., Battaglia, F. C., Makowski, E. L., Meschia, G. Production and excretion of urea by the fetal lamb. *Pediatrics* 1972;**50**:372–9.

128 Jozwik, M., Teng, C., Meschia, G., Battaglia, F. C. Contribution of branched-chain amino acids to uteroplacental ammonia production in sheep. *Biol. Reprod.* 1999;**61**:792–6.

129 Goodwin, G. W., Gibboney, W., Paxton, R., Harris, R. A., Lemons, J. A. Activities of branched-chain amino acid transferase and branched-chain 2-oxo acid dehydrogenase complex in tissues of maternal and fetal sheep. *Biochem. J.* 1987;**242**:305–8.

130 Liechty, E. A., Kelley, J., Lemons, J. A. Effect of fasting on uteroplacental amino acid metabolism in the pregnant sheep. *Biol. Neonate* 1991;**60**:207–14.

131 Jaroszewicz, L., Józwik, M., Jaroszewicz, K. The activity of aminotransferases in human placenta in early pregnancy. *Biochem. Med. Metab. Biol.* 1971;**5**:436–9.

132 Smeaton, T. C., Owens, J. A., Kind, K. L., Robinson, J. S. The placenta releases branched-chain keto acids into the umbilical and uterine circulations in the pregnant sheep. *J. Dev. Physiol.* 1989;**12**:95–9.

133 Loy, G. L., Quick, A. N., Hay, W. W. Jr *et al.* Fetoplacental deamination and decarboxylation of leucine. *Am. J. Physiol.* 1990;**259**:E492–7.

134 Owens, J. A, Owens, P. C., Robinson, J. S. Experimental fetal growth retardation: metabolic and endocrine aspects. In: Gluckman, P. D., Johnston, B. M., Nathanielsz, P. W., eds. *Advances in Fetal Physiology: Reviews in Honour of G. C. Liggins.* Ithaca: Perinatology Press; 1989:263–86.

135 Regnault, T. R., de Vrijer, B., Battaglia, F. C. Transport and metabolism of amino acids in placenta. *Endocrine* 2002;**19**:23–41.

136 Moe, A. J. Placental amino acid transport. *Am. J. Physiol.* 1995;**268**:C1321–31.

137 Yudilevich, D., Sweiry, J. Transport of amino acids in the placenta. *Biochim. Biophys. Acta.* 1985;**822**:169–201.

138 Harrington, B., Glazier, J., D'Souza, S., Sibley, C. System A amino acid transporter activity in human placental microvillous membrane vesicles in relation to various anthropometric measurements in appropriate and small for gestational age babies. *Pediatr. Res.* 1999;**45**(6):810–814.

139 Godfrey, K. M., Matthews, N., Glazier, J. *et al.* Neutral amino acid uptake by the microvillous plasma membrane of the human placenta is inversely related to fetal size at birth in normal pregnancy. *J. Clin. Endocrinol. Metab.* 1998;**83**:3320–6.

140 Glazier, J. D., Cetin, I., Perugino, G. *et al.* Association between the activity of the system A amino acid transporter in the microvillous plasma membrane of the human placenta and severity of fetal compromise in intrauterine growth restriction. *Pediatr. Res.* 1997;**42**(4):514–19.

141 Dicke, J., Henderson, G. Placental amino acid uptake in normal and complicated pregnancies. *Am. J. Med. Sci.* 1988;**295**:223–7.

142 Mahendran, D., Donnai, P., Glazier, J. D. *et al.* Amino acid (System A) transporter activity in microvillous membrane vesicles from the placentas of appropriate and small for gestational age babies. *Pediatr. Res.* 1993;**34**:661–5.

143 Jansson, T., Persson, E. Placental transfer of glucose and amino acids in intrauterine growth retardation: studies with substrate analogs in the awake guinea pig. *Pediatr. Res.* 1990;**28**:203–8.

144 Jansson, T., Ylven, K., Wennergren, M., Powell, T. L. Glucose transport and system A activity in syncytiotrophoblast microvillous and basal plasma membranes in intrauterine growth restriction. *Placenta* 2002;**23**:392–9.

145 Nelson, D. M., Smith, S. D., Furesz, T. C. *et al.* Hypoxia reduces expression and function of system A amino acid transporters in cultured term human trophoblasts. *Am. J. Physiol. Cell. Physiol.* 2003;**284**:C310–15.

146 Radaelli, T., Cetin, I., Ayuk, P. T. *et al.* Cationic amino acid transporter activity in the syncytiotrophoblast microvillous plasma membrane and oxygenation of the uteroplacental unit. *Placenta* 2002;**23**:S69–74.

147 Ross, J. C., Fennessey, P. V., Wilkening, R. B., Battaglia, F. C., Meschia, G. Placental transport and fetal utilization of leucine in a model of fetal growth retardation. *Am. J. Physiol.* 1996;**270**:E491–503.

148 Constância, M., Hemberger, M., Hughes, J. *et al.* Placental-specific IGF-II is a major modulator of placental and fetal growth. *Nature* 2002;**417**:945–8.

149 Moores, R. R. Jr, Rietberg, C. C., Battaglia, F. C., Fennessey, P. V., Meschia, G. Metabolism and transport of maternal serine by the ovine placenta: glycine production and absence of serine transport into the fetus. *Pediatr. Res.* 1993;**53**:590–4.

150 Cetin, I., Fennessey, P., Sparks, J. W., Meschia, G., Battaglia, F. C. Fetal serine fluxes across fetal liver, hindlimb and placenta in late gestation. *Am. J. Physiol.* 1992;**263**:E786–93.

151 Moores, R. R. Jr, Vaughn, P. R., Battaglia, F. C. *et al.* Glutamate metabolism in the fetus and placenta of late-gestation sheep. *Am. J. Physiol.* 1994;**267**:R89–96.

152 Chung, M., Teng, C., Timmerman, M., Meschia, G., Battaglia, F. C. Production and utilization of amino acids by ovine placenta in vivo. *Am. J. Physiol.* 1998;**274**:E13–22.

153 Widdowson, E. M. Growth and composition of the fetus and newborn. In: Assali, N. S., ed. *The Biology of Gestation*. New York: Academic Press; 1968:1–49.

154 Van Aerde, J. E., Feldman, M., Clandinin, M. T. Accretion of lipid in the fetus and newborn. In Polin, R. A., Fox, W. W., eds. *Fetal and Neonatal Physiology*. Philadelphia: W. B. Saunders Co.; 1998:458–77.

155 Dunlop, M., Court, J. M. Lipogenesis in developing human adipose tissue. *Early Hum. Dev.* 1978;**2**:123–30.

156 Innis, S. M. Essential fatty acids in growth and development. *Prog. Lipid Res.* 1991;**30**:39–103.

157 Kuhn, D. C., Crawford, M. Placental essential fatty acid transport and prostaglandin synthesis. *Prog. Lipid. Res.* 1986;**25**:345–53.

158 Campbell, F. M., Bush, P. G., Veerkamp, J. H., Dutta-Roy, A. K. Detection and cellular localization of plasma membrane-associated and cytoplasmic fatty acid-binding proteins in human placenta. *Placenta* 1998;**19**:409–15.

159 Campbell, F. M., Gordon, M. J., Dutta-Roy, A. K. Placental membrane fatty acid-binding protein preferentially binds arachidonic and docosahexaenoic acids. *Life. Sci.* 1998;**63**:235–40.

160 Lafond, J., Moukdar, F., Rioux, A. *et al.* Implication of ATP and sodium in arachidonic acid incorporation by placental syncytiotrophoblast brush border and basal plasma membranes in the human. *Placenta* 2000;**21**:661–9.

161 Herrera, E., Bonet, B., Lasunción, M. A. Maternal-fetal transfer of lipid metabolites. In: Polin, R. A., Fox, W. W., eds. *Fetal and Neonatal Physiology*. Philadelphia: W. B. Saunders Co.; 1998:447–58.

162 Albrecht, E. D., Babischkin, J. S., Koos, R. D., Pepe, G. J. Developmental increase in low density lipoprotein receptor messenger ribonucleic acid levels in placental syncytiotrophoblasts during baboon pregnancy. *Endocrinology* 1995;**136**:5540–6.

163 Overbergh, L., Lorent, K., Torrekens, S., Van Leuven, F., Van den Berghe, H. Expression of mouse alpha-macroglobulins, lipoprotein receptor-related protein, LDL receptor, apolipoprotein E, and lipoprotein lipase in pregnancy. *J. Lipid Res.* 1995;**36**:1774–86.

164 Alonso de la Torre, S. R., Serrano, M. A., Medina, J. M. Carrier-mediated beta-D-hydroxybutyrate transport in brush-border membrane vesicles from rat placenta. *Pediatr. Res.* 1992;**32**:317–23.

165 Ravel, D., Chambaz, J., Pepin, D., Manier, M. C., Bereziat, G. Essential fatty acid interconversion during gestation in the rat. *Biochim. Biophys. Acta.* 1985;**833**:161–4.

166 Thulin, A. J., Allee, G. L., Harmon, D. L., Davis, D. L. Uteroplacental transfer of octanoic, palmitic and linoleic acids during late gestation in gilts. *J. Anim. Sci.* 1989;**67**:738–45.

167 Elphick, M. C., Hull, D., Pipkin, F. B. The transfer of fatty acids across the sheep placenta. *J. Dev. Physiol.* 1979;**1**:31–45.

168 Shand, J. H., Noble, R. C. The metabolism of 18:0 and 18:2(n-6) by the ovine placenta at 120 and 150 days of gestation. *Lipids* 1981;**16**:68–71.

169 Shand, J. H., Noble, R. C. Delta 9- and delta 6-desaturase activities of the ovine placenta and their role in the supply of fatty acids to the fetus. *Biol. Neonate* 1979;**36**:298–304.

170 Fowden, A. L. The role of insulin in fetal growth. *Early Hum. Dev.* 1992;**29**(1–3):177–81.

171 Bassett, J. M., Thorburn, G. D. The regulation of insulin secretion by the ovine fetus *in utero. J. Endocrinol.* 1971;**50**:59–74.

172 Bassett, J. M., Madill, D. The influence of maternal nutrition on plasma hormone and metabolite concentrations of foetal lambs. *J. Endocrinol.* 1974;**61**:465–77.

173 Kervran, A., Randon, J. Development of insulin release by fetal rat pancreas *in vitro*: effects of glucose, amino acids, and theophylline. *Diabetes* 1980;**29**(9):673–8.

174 Kervran, A., Randon, J., Girard, J. R. Dynamics of glucose-induced plasma insulin increase in the rat fetus at different stages of gestation. Effects of maternal hypothermia and fetal decapitation. *Biol. Neonate* 1979;**35**(5–6):242–8.

175 Fowden, A. L., Hughes, P., Comline, R. S. The effects of insulin on the growth rate of the sheep fetus during late gestation. *Q. J. Exp. Physiol.* 1989;**74**(5):703–14.

176 Liu, J.-P., Baker, J., Perkins, A. S., Robinson, E. J., Efstratiadis, A. Mice carrying null mutations of the genes encoding insulin-like growth factor I (IGF-I) and type 1 IGF receptor (IGF1r). *Cell* 1993;**75**:59–72.

177 Gluckman, P. D., Brinsmead, M. W. Somatomedin in cord blood: relationship to gestational age and birth size. *J. Clin. Endocrinol. Metab.* 1976;**43**:1378–81.

178 Verhaeghe, J., Van Bree, R., Van Herck, E. *et al.* C-peptide, insulin-like growth factors I and II, and insulin-like growth factor binding protein-1 in umbilical cord serum: correlations with birth weight. *Am. J. Obstet. Gynecol.* 1993;**169**:89–97.

179 Bennett, A., Wilson, D. M., Liu, F. *et al.* Levels of insulin-like growth factors I and II in human cord blood. *J. Clin. Endocrinol. Metab.* 1983;**57**:609–12.

180 Lassarre, C., Hardouin, S., Daffos, F. *et al.* Serum insulin-like growth factors and insulin-like growth factor binding proteins in the human fetus. Relationships with growth in normal subjects and in subjects with intrauterine growth retardation. *Pediatr. Res.* 1991;**29**:219–25.

181 Gluckman, P. D., Johnson-Barrett, J. J., Butler, J. D., Edgar, B. W., Gunn, T. R. Studies of insulin-like growth factor-I and -II by specific radioligand assays in umbilical cord blood. *Clin. Endocrinol.* 1983;**19**:405–13.

182 Leger, J., Noel, M., Limal, J. M., Czernichow, P. Growth factors and intrauterine growth retardation. II. Serum growth hormone, insulin-like growth factor (IGF) I, and IGF-binding protein 3 levels in children with intrauterine growth retardation compared with normal control subjects: prospective study from birth to two years of age. *Pediatr. Res.* 1996;**40**(1):101–7.

183 Guidice, L. C., de Zegher, F., Gargosky, S. E. *et al.* Insulin-like growth factors and their binding proteins in the term and preterm human fetus and neonate with normal and extremes of intrauterine growth. *J. Clin. Endocrinol. Metab.* 1995;**80**:1548–55.

184 Woods, K. A., Camacho-Hubner, C., Savage, M. O., Clark, A. J. Intrauterine growth and postnatal growth failure associated with deletion of the insulin-like growth factor I gene. *N. Engl. J. Med.* 1996;**335**:1363–7.

185 Tamura, T., Tohma, T., Ohta, T. *et al.* Ring chromosome 15 involving deletion of the insulin-like growth factor 1 receptor gene in a patient with features of Silver–Russell syndrome. *Clin. Dysmorphol.* 1993;**2**:106–13.

186 Gallaher, B. W., Breier, B. H., Oliver, M. H., Harding, J. E., Gluckman, P. D. Ontogenic differences in the nutritional regulation of circulating IGF binding proteins in sheep plasma. *Acta. Endocrinol.* 1992;**126**:49–54.

187 Gallaher, B. W., Oliver, M. H., Eichhorn, K. *et al.* Circulating insulin-like growth factor I/mannose-6-phosphate receptor and insulin-like growth factor binding proteins in fetal sheep plasma are regulated by glucose and insulin. *Eur. J. Endocrinol.* 1994;**131**(4):398–404.

188 Oliver, M. H., Harding, J. E., Breier, B. H., Evans, P. C., Gluckman, P. D. Glucose but not amino acids regulates plasma insulin-like growth factor (IGF)-I concentrations in fetal sheep. *Pediatr. Res.* 1993;**34**:62–5.

189 Oliver, M. H., Harding, J. E., Breier, B. H., Gluckman, P. D. Fetal insulin-like growth factor (IGF)-I and IGF-II are regulated differently by glucose or insulin in the sheep fetus. *Reprod. Fertil. Dev.* 1996;**8**(1):167–72.

190 Boyne, M. S., Thame, M., Bennett, F. I. *et al.* The relationship among circulating insulin-like growth factor (IGF)-I, IGF-binding proteins-1 and -2, and birth anthropometry: a prospective study. *J. Clin. Endocrinol. Metab.* 2003;**88**:1687–91.

191 Nagako, S., Funakoshi, T., Ueda, Y., Maruo, T. Regulation of circulating levels of IGF-I in pregnant rats: changes in nitrogen balance correspond with changes in serum IGF-I concentrations. *J. Endocrinol.* 1999;**163**:373–7.

192 Harding, J. E., Liu, L., Evans, P. C. Circulating IGF-I influences nutrient partitioning between fetus and placenta in sheep. *Growth. Regul.* 1994;**4**(Suppl 1):73 (Abstr.).

193 Jensen, E. C., Harding, J. E., Bauer, M. K., Gluckman, P. D. Metabolic effects of IGF-I in the growth retarded fetal sheep. *J. Endocrinol.* 1999;**161**:485–94.

194 Shen, W., Wisniowski, P., Ahmed, L. *et al.* Protein anabolic effects of insulin and IGF-I in the ovine fetus. *Am. J. Physiol. Endocrinol. Metab.* 2003;**284**:E748–56.

195 Jensen, E. C., van Zijl, P., Evans, P. C., Harding, J. E. The effect of IGF-I on serine metabolism in fetal sheep. *J. Endocrinol.* 2000;**165**:261–9.

196 Bloomfield, F. H., van Zijl, P. L., Bauer, M. K., Harding, J. E. A chronic low dose infusion of IGF-I alters placental function but does not affect fetal growth. *Reprod. Fertil. Dev.* 2002;**14**:393–400.

197 Sohlstrom, A., Fernberg, P., Owens, J. A., Owens, P. C. Maternal nutrition affects the ability of treatment with IGF-I and IGF-II to increase growth of the placenta and fetus, in guinea pigs. *Growth Horm. IGF Res.* 2001;**11**:392–8.

198 Baker, J., Liu, J.-P., Robinson, E. J., Efstratiadis, A. Role of insulin-like growth factors in embryonic and postnatal growth. *Cell* 1993;**75**:79–82.

199 Ohlsson, R., Holmgren, L., Glaser, A., Szpecht, A., Pfeifer-Ohlsson, S. Insulin-like growth factor 2 and short-range stimulatory loops in control of human placental growth. *EMBO J,* 1989;**8**(7):1993–9.

200 Brice, A. L., Cheetham, J. E., Bolton, N., Hill, N. C. W., Schofield, P. N. Temporal changes in the expression of the insulin-like growth factor II gene associated with tissue maturation in the human fetus. *Development* 1989;**106**:543–54.

201 Ohlsson, R., Larsson, E., Nilsson, O., Wahlstrom, T., Sundstrom, P. Blastocyst implantation precedes induction of insulin-like growth factor II gene expression in human trophoblasts. *Development* 1989;**106**(3):555–9.

202 Reik, W., Constância, M., Fowden, A. *et al.* Regulation of supply and demand for maternal nutrients in mammals by imprinted genes. *J. Physiol.* 2003;**547**:35–44.

203 Reik, W., Walter, J. Genomic imprinting: parental influence on the genome. *Nat. Rev. Genet.* 2001;**2**:21–32.

204 Tycko, B., Morison, I. M. Physiological functions of imprinted genes. *J. Cell. Physiol.* 2002;**192**:245–58.

205 Li, L., Keverne, E. B., Aparicio, S. A. *et al.* Regulation of maternal behavior and offspring growth by paternally expressed Peg3. *Science* 1999;**284**:330–3.

206 Bauer, M. K., Breier, B. H., Harding, J. E., Veldhuis, J. D., Gluckman, P. D. The fetal somatotrophic axis during long term maternal undernutrition in sheep: evidence for nutritional regulation in utero. *Endocrinology* 1995;**136**(3):1250–7.

207 Klempt, M., Bingham, B., Breier, B. J., Baumbach, W. R., Gluckman, P. D. Tissue distribution and ontogeny of growth hormone receptor messenger ribonucleic acid and ligand binding to hepatic tissue in the midgestation sheep fetus. *Endocrinology* 1993;**132**:1071–7.

208 Edmondson, S. R., Werther, G. A., Russell, A. *et al.* Localization of growth hormone receptor/binding protein messenger ribonucleic acid (mRNA) during rat fetal development: relationship to insulin-like growth factor-I mRNA. *Endocrinology* 1995;**136**:4602–9.

209 Gluckman, P. D., Gunn, A. J., Wray, A. *et al.* Congenital idiopathic growth hormone deficiency is associated with prenatal and early postnatal growth failure. *J. Pediatr.* 1992;**121**:920–3.

210 Mesiano, S., Young, I. R., Baxter, R. C. *et al.* Effect of hypophysectomy with and without thyroxine replacement on growth and circulating concentrations of insulin-like growth factors I and II in the fetal lamb. *Endocrinology* 1987;**120**:1821–30.

211 Mesiano, S., Young, I. R., Hay, A. W., Browne, C. A., Thorburn, G. D. Hypophysectomy of the fetal lamb leads to a fall in the plasma concentration of insulin like growth factor I (IGF-I) but not IGF-II. *Endocrinology* 1989;**124**:1485–91.

212 Bauer, M. K., Breier, B. H., Bloomfield, F. H. *et al.* Chronic pulsatile infusion of growth hormone to growth-restricted fetal sheep increases circulating fetal insulin-like growth factor-I levels but not fetal growth. *J. Endocrinol.* 2003;**177**:83–92.

213 Fowden, A. L. Endocrine regulation of fetal growth. *Reprod. Fertil. Dev.* 1995;**7**:351–63.

214 Thorpe-Beeston, J. G., Nicolaides, K. H. Fetal thyroid function. *Fetal. Diagn. Ther.* 1993;**8**:60–72.

215 Sagawa, N., Yura, S., Itoh, H. *et al.* Possible role of placental leptin in pregnancy: a review. *Endocrine* 2002;**19**:65–71.

216 Zhao, J., Kunz, T. H., Tumba, N. *et al.* Comparative Analysis of Expression and Secretion of Placental Leptin in Mammals. *Am. J. Physiol. Regul. Integr. Comp. Physiol.* 2003;**285**:R438–46.

217 Masuzaki, H., Ogawa, Y., Sagawa, N. *et al.* Nonadipose tissue production of leptin: leptin as a novel placenta-derived hormone in humans. *Nat. Med.* 1997;**3**:1029–33.

218 Gualillo, O., Caminos, J., Blanco, M. *et al.* Ghrelin, a novel placental-derived hormone. *Endocrinology* 2001;**142**:788–94.

219 Thomas, L., Wallace, J. M., Aitken, R. P. *et al.* Circulating leptin during ovine pregnancy in relation to maternal nutrition, body composition and pregnancy outcome. *J. Endocrinol.* 2001;**169**:465–76.

220 Wang, J., Liu, R., Liu, L. *et al.* The effect of leptin on Lep expression is tissue-specific and nutritionally regulated. *Nat. Med.* 1999;**5**:895–9.

221 Devaskar, S. U., Anthony, R., Hay, W. Jr. Ontogeny and insulin regulation of fetal ovine white adipose tissue leptin expression. *Am. J. Physiol. Regul. Integr. Comp. Physiol.* 2002;**282**:R431–8.

222 Bell, A. W., Kennaugh, J. M., Battaglia, F. C., Makowski, E. L., Meschia, G. Metabolic and circulatory studies of fetal lambs at mid gestation. *Am. J. Physiol.* 1986;**250**:E538–44.

223 Lemons, J. A., Reyman, D., Schreiner, R. L. Fetal and maternal amino acid concentrations during fasting in the ewe. *J. Ped. Gastroenterol. Nutr.* 1984;**3**:249–55.

224 Liechty, E. A., Lemons, J. A. Changes in ovine fetal hindlimb amino acid metabolism during maternal fasting. *Am. J. Physiol.* 1984;**246**:E430–5.

225 Schreiner, R. L., Lemons, J. A., Gresham, E. L. Metabolic and hormonal response to chronic maternal fasting in the ewe. *Ann. Nutr. Metab.* 1981;**25**:38–47.

226 Mellor, D. J., Matheson, I. C. Daily changes in the curved crown-rump length of individual sheep fetuses during the last 60 days of pregnancy and effects of different levels of maternal nutrition. *Q. J. Exp. Physiol.* 1979;**64**:119–31.

227 Mellor, D. J., Murray, L. Effects on the rate of increase in fetal girth of refeeding ewes after short periods of severe undernutrition during late pregnancy. *Res. Vet. Sci.* 1982;**32**:377–82.

228 Harding, J. E. Prior growth rate determines the fetal growth response to acute maternal undernutrition in fetal sheep of late gestation. *Prenat. Neonat. Med.* 1997;**2**:300–9.

229 Harding, J. E. Periconceptual nutrition determines the fetal growth response to acute maternal undernutrition in fetal sheep of late gestation. *Prenat. Neonat. Med.* 1997;**2**:310–19.

230 Oliver, M. H., Hawkins, P., Harding, J. E. Periconceptional undernutrition alters growth trajectory, endocrine and metabolic responses to fasting in late gestation fetal sheep. *Pediatr. Res.* 2005;**57**:591–8.

231 Harding, J. E. The nutritional basis of the fetal origins of adult disease. *Int. J. Epidemiol.* 2001;**30**:15–23.

232 Brace, R. A. Amniotic fluid volume and its relation to fetal fluid balance: a review of experimental data. *Semin. Perinatol.* 1986;**10**:130–12.

233 Brace, R. A. Fetal fluid balance. In Thorburn, G. D., Harding, R., eds. *Textbook of Fetal Physiology.* Oxford: Oxford University Press; 1994:205–18.

234 Harding, R., Bocking, A. D., Sigger, J. N., Wickham, P. J. D. Composition and volume of fluid swallowed by fetal sheep. *Q. J. Exp. Physiol.* 1984;**69**:487–95.

235 Daneshmand, S. S., Cheung, C. Y., Brace, R. A. Regulation of amniotic fluid volume by intramembranous absorption in sheep: Role of passive permeability and vascular endothelial growth factor. *Am. J. Obstet. Gynecol.* 2003;**188**:786–93.

236 Gilbert, W. M., Brace, R. A. The missing link in amniotic fluid volume regulation: intramembranous absorption. *Obstet. Gynecol.* 1989;**74**:748–54.

237 Bloomfield, F. H., van Zijl, P. L., Bauer, M. K., Harding, J. E. Effects of intrauterine growth restriction and intra-amniotic insulin-like growth factor-I treatment on blood and amniotic fluid concentrations and on fetal gut uptake of amino acids in late gestation ovine fetuses. *J. Pediatr. Gastroenterol. Nutr.* 2002;**35**:287–97.

238 Wu, G., Bazer, F. W., Tou, W. Developmental changes of free amino acid concentrations in fetal fluids of pigs. *J. Nutr.* 1995;**125**:2859–68.

239 A'Zary, E., Saifer, A., Schneck, L. The free amino acids in maternal and fetal extracellular fluids collected during early pregnancy. *Am. J. Obstet. Gynecol.* 1973;**116**:854–66.

240 Levy, H. L., Montag, P. P. Free amino acids in human amniotic fluid. A quantitative study by ion-exchange chromatography. *Pediatr. Res.* 1969;**3**:113–20.

241 Mesavage, W. C., Suchy, S. F., Weiner, D. L. *et al.* Amino acids in amniotic fluid in the second trimester of gestation. *Pediatr. Res.* 1985;**19**:1021–24.

242 Pitkin, R. M., Reynolds, W. A. Fetal ingestion and metabolism of amniotic fluid protein. *Am. J. Obstet. Gynecol.* 1975;**123**(4):356–61.

243 Pritchard, J. A. Deglutition by normal and anencephalic fetuses. *Obstet. Gynecol.* 1965;**25**:289–97.

244 Gitlin, D., Kumate, J., Morales, C., Noriega, L., Arévalo, N. The turnover of amniotic fluid protein in the human conceptus. *Am. J. Obstet. Gynecol.* 1972;**113**(5):632–45.

245 Tomoda, S., Brace, R. A., Longo, L. D. Amniotic fluid volume and fetal swallowing rate in sheep. *Am. J. Physiol.* 1985;**249**:R133–8.

246 Abbas, T. M., Tovey, J. E. Proteins of the liquor amnii. *Br. Med. J.* 1960;**2**:476–9.

247 Johnson, A. M., Umansky, I., Alper, C. A., Everett, C., Greenspan, G. Amniotic fluid proteins: maternal and fetal contributions. *J. Pediatr.* 1974;**84**:588–93.

248 Jones, C. A., Warner, J. A., Warner, J. O. Fetal swallowing of IgE. *Lancet* 1998;**351**:1859.

249 Trahair, J. F., Harding, R. Development of the gastrointestinal tract. In: Thorburn, G. D., Harding, R., eds. *Textbook of Fetal Physiology.* Oxford: Oxford University Press; 1994: 219–35.

250 Trahair, J. F., Sangild, P. T. Systemic and luminal influences on the perinatal development of the gut. *Equine. Vet. J.* 1997;Suppl. **24**:40–50.

251 Bloomfield, F. H., Bauer, M. K., van Zijl, P. L., Gluckman, P. D., Harding, J. E. Amniotic IGF-I supplements improve gut growth but reduce circulating IGF-I in growth-restricted fetal sheep. *Am. J. Physiol. Endocrinol. Metab.* 2002;**282**:E259–69.

252 Phillips, J. D., Fonkalsrud, E. W., Mirzayan, A. *et al.* Uptake and distribution of continuously infused intraamniotic nutrients in fetal rabbits. *J. Pediatr. Surg.* 1991;**24**(4):374–80.

253 Wu, G. Urea synthesis in enterocytes of developing pigs. *Biochem. J.* 1995;**312**:717–23.

254 Dahlqvist, A., Lindberg, T. Development of the intestinal disaccharidase and alkaline phosphatase activities in the human fetus. *Clin. Sci.* 1966;**30**:517–28.

255 Antonowicz, I., Chang, S. K., Grand, R. J. Development and distribution of lysosomal enzymes and disaccharidases in human fetal intestine. *Gastroenterology* 1974;**67**:51–8.

256 Trahair, J. F., Harding, R. Development of structure and function of the alimentary tract in fetal sheep. In Nathanielsz, P. W., ed. *Animal Models in Fetal Medicine.* New York: Perinatology Press; 1987:1–36.

257 Antonowicz, A., Milunsky, A., Lebenthal, E., Schwachman, H. Disaccharidase and lysosomal enzyme activities in amniotic fluid, intestinal mucosa and meconium. *Biol. Neonate* 1977;**32**:280–9.

258 Sangild, P. T., Elnif, J. Intestinal hydrolytic activity in young mink (*Mustela vison*) develops slowly postnatally and exhibits late sensitivity to glucocorticoids. *J. Nutr.* 1996;**126**:2061–8.

259 Sangild, P. T., Sjöström, H., Norén, O., Fowden, A. L., Silver, M. The prenatal development and glucocorticoid control of brush-border hydrolases in the pig small intestine. *Pediatr. Res.* 1995;**37**:207–12.

260 Charlton, V., Rudolph, A. M. Digestion and absorption of carbohydrates by the fetal lamb *in utero. Pediatr. Res.* 1979;**13**:1018–23.

261 Iioka, H., Moriyama, I. S., Hino, K., Itani, Y., Ichijo, M. Absorption of D-glucose by the small intestine of the human fetus. *Nippon Sanka Fujinka Gakkai Zasshi* 1987;**39**:347–51.

262 Charlton, V., Reis, B. Response of the chronically catheterized fetal lamb to intestinal administration of amino acids. *Clin. Res.* 1980;**28**:121A (Abstr.).

263 Charlton, V. E., Reis, B. L. Effects of gastric nutritional supplementation on fetal umbilical uptake of nutrients. *Am. J. Physiol.* 1981;**241**:E178–85.

264 Mulvihill, S. J., Albert, A., Synn, A., Fonkalsrud, E. W. In utero supplemental fetal feeding in an animal model: effects on fetal growth and development. *Surgery* 1985;**98**(3):500–5.

265 Harrison, M. R., Villa, R. L. Trans-amniotic fetal feeding I. Development of an animal model: continuous amniotic infusion in rabbits. *J. Pediatr. Surg.* 1982;**17**(4):376–80.

266 Xing, A., Wan, B., Zeng, W. Biochemical effects of maternal intravenous and intra-amniotic infusion of amino-acids on fetal blood. *Hua Xi Yi Ke Da Xue Xue Bao* 1994;**25**:98–102.

267 Massobrio, M., Margaria, E., Campogrande, M., Badini Confalonieri, F., Bocci, A. Treatment of severe feto-placental insufficiency by means of intraamniotic injection of amino acids. In Salvadori, B., ed. *Therapy of Feto-Placental Insufficiency.* Berlin: Springer-Verlag; 1975:296–301.

268 Renaud, R., Kirschtetter, L., Köhl, C. *et al.* Amino-acid intra-amniotic injections. In Persianinov, L. S., Chervakova, T. V., Presl, J., eds. *Recent Progress in Obstetrics and Gynaecology.* Amsterdam: Excerpta Medica; 1974:234–56.

269 Renaud, R., Vincendon, G., Koehl, C. *et al.* Fetal malnutrition. Preliminary results of intra-amniotic perfusions and injections of amino acids. *J. Gynecol. Obstet. Biol. Reprod. (Paris).* 1972;**1**:596–7.

270 Saling, E., Dudenhausen, W., Kynast, G. Basic investigations about intra-amniotic compensatory nutrition of the malnourished fetus. In Persianinov, L. S., Chervakova, T. V., Presl, J., eds.

Recent Progress in Obstetrics and Gynaecology. Amsterdam: Excerpta Medica; 1974:227–33.

271 Saling, E., Kynast, G. A new way for the paraplacental supply of substances to the fetus. *J. Perinatol. Med. Suppl.* 1981;**1**:144–6.

272 Noccioli, B., Pampaloni, F., Fiorini, P. *et al.* Esophageal atresia with distal tracheo-esophageal fistula. Evolution of the treatment in the period of 1955–2000 at the Anna Meyer Children's Hospital of Florence. *Minerva. Pediatr.*, 2002;**54**:131–8.

273 Sparey, C., Jawaheer, G., Barrett, A. M., Robson, S. C. Esophageal atresia in the Northern Region Congenital Anomaly Survey, 1985–1997: prenatal diagnosis and outcome. *Am. J. Obstet. Gynecol.* 2000;**182**:427–31.

274 Martinez-Frias, M. L., Castilla, E. E., Bermejo, E., Prieto, L., Orioli, I. M. Isolated small intestinal atresias in Latin America and Spain: epidemiological analysis. *Am. J. Med. Genet.* 2000;**93**:355–9.

275 Abramovich, D. R. Interrelation of fetus and amniotic fluid. *Obstet. Gynecol. Ann.* 1981;**10**:27–43.

276 Cozzi, F., Wilkinson, A. W. Intrauterine growth rate in relation to anorectal and oesophageal anomalies. *Arch. Dis. Child.* 1969;**44**(233):59–62.

277 Blakelock, R., Upadhyay, V., Kimble, R. *et al.* Is a normally functioning gastrointestinal tract necessary for normal growth in late gestation? *Pediatr. Surg. Int.* 1998;**13**(1):17–20.

278 Surana, R. P. P. Small intestinal atresia: effect on fetal nutrition. *J. Pediatr. Surg.* 1994;**29**:1250–2.

279 Surana, R., Puri, P. Small intestinal atresia: effect on fetal nutrition. *J. Pediatr. Surg.* 1994;**29**:1250–2.

280 Blakelock, R. T., Upadhyay, V., Pease, P. W., Harding, J. E. Are babies with gastroschisis small for gestational age? *Pediatr. Surg. Int.* 1997;**12**:580–2.

281 Raynor, B. D., Richards, D. Growth retardation in fetuses with gastroschisis. *J. Ultrasound. Med.* 1997;**16**:13–16.

282 Weaver, L. T., Gonnella, P. A., Israel, E. J., Walker, W. A. Uptake and transport of epidermal growth factor by the small intestinal epithelium of the fetal rat. *Gastroenterology* 1990;**98**:828–37.

283 Bala, R. M., Wright, C., Bardai, A., Smith, G. R. Somatomedin Bioactivity in serum and amniotic fluid during pregnancy. *J. Clin. Endocrinol. Metab.* 1978;**46**(4):649–52.

284 Merimee, T. J., Grant, M., Tyson, J. E. Insulin-like growth factors in amniotic fluid. *J. Clin. Endocrinol. Metab.* 1984;**59**(4):752–5.

285 Wathen, N. C., Egembah, S., Campbell, D. J., Farkas, A., Chard, T. Levels of insulin-like growth factor-binding protein-I increase rapidly in amniotic fluid from 11 to 16 weeks of pregnancy. *J. Endocrinol.* 1993;**137**:R1–4.

286 Kniss, D. A., Zimmerman, P. D., Su, H.-C. *et al.* Expression of functional insulin-like growth factor-I receptors by human amnion cells. *Am. J. Obstet. Gynecol.* 1993;**169**(3):632–40.

287 Han, V. K. M., Lund, P. K., Lee, D. C., D'Ercole, A. J. Expression of somatomedin/insulin-like growth factor messenger ribonucleic acids in the human fetus: identification, characterisation, and tissue distribution. *J. Clin. Endocrinol. Metab.* 1988;**66**:422–9.

288 Weaver, L. T., Walker, A. W. Epidermal growth factor and the developing human gut. *Gastroenterology* 1988;**94**:845–7.

289 Read, L. C., Howarth, G. S., Lemmey, A. B. *et al.* The gastrointestinal tract: a most sensitive target for IGF-I. *Proc. Nutr. Soc. NZ.* 1992;**17**:136–42.

290 Simmons, J. G., Hoyt, E. C., Westwick, J. K. *et al.* Insulin-like growth factor-I and epidermal growth factor interact to regulate growth and gene expression in IEC-6 intestinal epithelial cells. *Mol. Endocrinol.* 1995;**9**:1157–65.

291 Trahair, J. F., Harding, R. Restitution of swallowing in the fetal sheep restores intestinal growth after midgestation esophageal ligation. *J. Ped. Gastroenterol. Nutr.* 1995;**20**:156–61.

292 Kimble, R. M., Breier, B. H., Gluckman, P. D., Harding, J. E. Enteral IGF-I enhances fetal growth and gastrointestinal development in oesophageal ligated fetal sheep. *J. Endocrinol.* 1999;**162**:227–35.

293 Bloomfield, F. H., Breier, B. H., Harding, J. E. The fate of ^{125}I-IGF-I administered into the amniotic fluid of late gestation sheep. *Pediatr. Res.* 2002;**51**:361–9.

294 Shaikh, S., Bloomfield, F. H., Bauer, M. K., Phua, H. H., Gilmour, R. S., Harding, J. E. Amniotic IGF-I supplementation of growth-restricted fetal sheep alters IGF-I and IGF receptor type 1 mRNA levels in placenta and fetal tissues. *J. Endocrinol.* 2005;**186**(1):145–55.

Determinants of intrauterine growth

John W. Sparks[1] and Irene Cetin[2]

[1]Department of Pediatrics, University of Texas Medical School, Houston, Texas
[2]Clinica Ostetrica e Ginecologica, Universita degli Studi di Milano, Ospedale San Paolo, Milano, Italy

Size matters

When considering outcomes of pregnancy, size at birth is among the most important characteristics of a successful pregnancy. In addition to duration of pregnancy and the qualitative development of the fetus, the anthropometric size of a newborn baby is of considerable significance. Long before the relatively modern concept of gestational age was well understood, medical personnel recognized and recorded the size, particularly the weight, of newborn babies, and both mortality and morbidity were correlated to birth size. This persists even today, with terms such as "Low Birth Weight" infants, which do not incorporate the concept of duration of pregnancy, as an important descriptor in the public health arena. Similarly, among the first questions asked by parents, is "How much does my baby weigh?," a reflection of the importance of size in the common understanding of pregnancy.

As a practical issue, clinicians pay most attention to weight, length and head circumference, in part because both scales and rulers are easily available and accurate. Weight is particularly emphasized, in part because the measurement of weight is particularly insensitive to interobserver measurement error. Other measures, such as surface area, BMI and weights raised to various powers (e.g. $wt^{0.75}$, wt^2, $wt/length^2$) are also in common use, but require more difficult calculation or measurement. The close attention paid to weight is more a reflection of convenience, than biological importance, as other measures may more closely relate to matters of biological importance. For example, drug doses may be better related to surface area than weight.

Intrauterine growth

Over the course of pregnancy, the developing fetus must change qualitatively, in the development and maturation of internal organs, and quantitatively, in increasing fetal size and weight. Fetal growth represents the increase in size over time. The qualitative development and quantitative growth occur simultaneously, and clinicians often merge the two concepts. However, with abnormalities of fetal growth, such as Intrauterine Growth Restriction or a diabetic pregnancy producing a macrosomic infant, the distinctions between maturation and size become evident. Birthweight is a final outcome of a number of factors that influence fetal growth during pregnancy. These factors may induce long-term adaptations in an individual through a process that has been defined as "fetal programming".[1] Based on this hypothesis, some critical periods are hypothesized to exist during fetal life, when altered expression of a number of genes would bear lifelong consequences.

Perinatal growth, especially in case of intrauterine growth restriction (IUGR), has pronounced effects on neonatal and adult health.[2–4] For this reason, the identification of factors playing a role on normal and altered fetal growth can be useful for preventing measures.

Definitions of normal and abnormal intrauterine growth

In the past, normal intrauterine growth has been defined as a normal birth weight, length and head circumference, based on cross sectional data obtained at birth in a given population. These cross-sectional data on birth

Neonatal Nutrition and Metabolism. Second Edition, ed. P. Thureen and W. Hay. Published by Cambridge University Press.
© Cambridge University Press 2006.

size have been widely plotted against duration of pregnancy as "Intrauterine Growth Curves," and are sometimes adjusted for maternal parity, gestational age and neonatal gender. The most widely used population standards for birthweight were obtained before the routine use of ultrasound scanning,[5–7] and are thus based entirely on maternal dates.

One of the most important problems of birthweight curves is the estimation of gestational age. While "age" is fundamentally measured in units of time, accurate timing may be difficult in many pregnancies. Traditionally, gestational age is dated from the first day of the last normal menstrual period, and this dating may be difficult in women who do not have regular menses. Moreover, the concept of gestational age developed before the modern understanding of reproductive biology. Gestational age does not begin timing at conception, which is not normally timed with accuracy, and thus differs from the concept of postconceptional age.

For these reasons and others, many have held that menstrual history is an unreliable indicator of gestational age. Investigators have sought alternative ways of assessing the duration of pregnancy, using as a surrogate for time (age), direct and ultrasonographic measurement in well-timed pregnancies.[8] In the last decade birthweight curves have been obtained from pregnancies dated by ultrasonography,[9,10] showing higher term birthweights and reduced flattening of the birthweight curve at term than those pregnancies dated from menstrual history alone. These data show that ultrasound correction of gestational age leads to a more linear curve of birthweight, probably better describing the biology of human fetal growth.

Birthweight has been generally used as a surrogate for longitudinal growth. However, it has been suggested that different patterns of growth exist for fetal length and weight growth, probably due to differences in the growth curves of lean and fat mass. Lean mass has been associated with linear growth and peak velocity in the first stages of pregnancy, while a significant exponential increase in fetal body fat mass has been observed during the third trimester both at delivery[11] and in utero by longitudinal ultrasound evaluation of fetal fat and lean mass.[12]

Much attention has been given to the diagnosis of Intrauterine Growth Restriction. From a conceptual point of view, growth implies serial measurements of size over time, and restriction of growth implies less rapid increase in size than expected. Physicians presented with a single static measure of size at birth frequently struggle to distinguish restriction in growth from constitutionally small size. Thus a baby's weight at birth may be low, but more information is needed to determine if growth has been restricted,

or if the low birthweight can be reasonably explained by physiologic factors such as gestational age, parity and gender, or by other non-physiologic factors, such as smoking, malnutrition or altitude.

Intrauterine growth restriction is defined as a reduction from the physiological growth rate. It is commonly due to fetal malnutrition, among many other causes. The ultrasound diagnosis of IUGR is based on multiple ultrasound records evidencing an abdominal circumference $<10°$ centile or a reduction of growth during the second part of the pregnancy,[13,14] thus demonstrating restriction in growth by longitudinal measure. This definition provides a tool to distinguish IUGR from SGA (small for gestational-age) babies, nevertheless the correct definition and classification criteria of IUGR is still a challenge. IUGR is primarily determined by a restriction of fetal growth rate during pregnancy, and a low birth weight does not always imply an IUGR condition. At present, no therapies for fetuses showing an abnormal rate of growth are available and the correct timing of delivery remains the best medical approach for this condition.[15]

On the other extreme, some babies undergo excess intrauterine growth, so their birthweight exceeds the normal ranges. Definitions of this condition at birth have been macrosomia or large-for-gestational age (LGA) if birthweight exceeds 4000 grams, thus placing birthweight in relation to gestational age. Also this condition can be diagnosed in utero by ultrasound based on multiple records showing an increasing abdominal circumference, but the intrauterine pattern of growth has never been included in a more strict definition, although many authors now refer to it as "excess fetal growth." In this situation increased fetal fat mass has been reported at the level of the abdominal wall.[16] Decreases in maternal insulin sensitivity with advancing gestation lead to an increase in glucose and nutrient supply to the feto-placental unit[17] and in some cases this can result in a condition of gestational glucose intolerance known as gestational diabetes. The increased fetal growth in these cases results from the combined effects of this excess of nutrients and the permissive environment of fetal hyperinsulinemia.[18]

Determinants of intrauterine growth

Normal intrauterine growth depends on the genetic potential of an individual, modulated by environmental factors including maternal health and nutrition. There is increasing evidence to support the conclusion that genes interact in a complex way resulting in fetal growth and that genes promoting fetal growth can be altered in cases of impaired fetal growth. The complex interactions between genetic growth potential, the ability of the maternal-placental system to transfer nutrients to the fetus and the endocrine environment determine whether the fetus will follow its growth curve during intrauterine life.

Before considering the role of genes and nutrition in fetal growth, it is appropriate to address the epidemiological factors that show the strongest correlations with birthweight. Although there is obviously a genetic control of fetal growth, the contribution due to maternal and paternal genes, race and sex of the baby seems to account for less than 20% of the variance of weight at birth.[19]

Interestingly, birthweights after oocyte donation are more related to anthropometric parameters of the pregnant mother than to those of the oocyte donor.[20]

The paternal contribution to fetal growth seems limited to fetal lean mass. Fetal gender is related to differences in weight and also in body composition, with higher amounts of lean mass in boys compared with girls, and no differences in fat mass.[21,22] Taken together, these observations would suggest that genetic factors affect the growth of fetal lean mass, while factors that influence the intrauterine environment better correlate with fetal fat mass deposition.

Genomic imprinting and epigenetic mechanisms

In the last few years, a new concept has developed in genetics, that some genes are imprinted by their parental origin and do not follow the Mendelian expectation of inheritance. Genomic imprinting is characterized by monoallelic maternal or paternal expression, while the allele that is silenced is called "imprinted." More than 40 imprinted genes have been described in the murine and human species.[23] Numerous studies have provided evidence that an adequate balance of maternal and paternal imprinted genes is required for placental implant and fetal growth, as well as being involved in cell proliferation, some neurobehavioral processes and cancer.[24,25] The role of imprinted genes in fetal growth and its alterations related to genetic changes affecting their expression has been the subject of a recent review.[26] A genetic conflict hypothesis has been advanced by Moore and Haig[27] to explain the meaning of mammalian genetic imprinting. This hypothesis is based on the evidence that most maternal expressed genes act as growth suppressors whereas paternal expressed genes are growth promoters, so that the father tends to promote growth, while the mother controls the fetal demand for nutrients. It is obvious that an imbalance in these attitudes would alter fetal growth as for example in uniparental disomies (UPD), i.e. a chromosome pair originating from one parent only. UPDs of a number of chromosomes have been associated with specific phenotypes, as is the case of maternal UPD7, which is reported in 7% of cases of Silver–Russell syndrome, with pre- and postnatal growth impairment. The candidate imprinted genes in these cases are PEG1/MEST, that codify for an α/β hydrolase involved in fetal growth. Table 2.1 summarizes the reported human chromosome UPDs (for a more detailed review see Miozzo and Simoni, 2002).[26]

The relevance of imprinting mechanisms has been recently highlighted in pregnancies conceived by assisted reproductive technologies (ART).[28] A higher incidence of syndromes related to imprinted genes has been reported in babies born from ART pregnancies. These pregnancies have also been associated with poorer pregnancy outcomes, i.e. low birthweight and prematurity, even in singletons.[29] Potential epigenetic risks related to the manipulation of gametes and embryos in these pregnancies is becoming a matter of debate.[30,31] In particular, evidence has been produced that in vitro culture would have effects not only on the expression of genes, but also on the methylation of parentally imprinted genes. Thus these procedures could be able to strongly influence fetal and placental growth and development.

Nutrition

From a nutritional point of view, the fetus depends upon the maternal supply of nutrients through the placenta into the umbilical circulation. Pregnancy represents a three compartment model, with the mother, placenta and fetus each presenting their own metabolism while interacting with each other. Glucose, amino acids and fatty acids represent the most important nutrients in fetal life, both for tissue deposition and as fuels for oxidative purposes.

It has long been known that both maternal prepregnancy weight and weight gain independently influence newborn weight.[32] However, there is considerable experimental evidence suggesting that in late gestation fetal growth is controlled by both maternal and placental factors.[33] It is difficult to estimate the relative influence of these two compartments in determining the rate of intrauterine fetal growth. In the model of intrauterine growth restriction, maternal characteristics do not seem to be determinants of fetal growth rate, whereas it is generally accepted that the major constraining factor is the ability of the utero-placental unit to supply oxygen and nutrients to the fetus.[34] Rather, in gestational diabetes, excess fetal growth seems to be deriving from the increased availability of maternal nutrients. The increased fetal fat mass in these cases results from the combined effects of this excess of nutrients and the permissive environment of fetal hyperinsulinemia.[35] Furthermore, the increase in fetal fat mass is associated with increased leptin levels in fetuses of mothers with gestational diabetes.[16]

Table 2.1. Reported human chromosome uniparental disomies (UPDs)

Chromosome	UPD	Phenotypic effect
1	Maternal	No effect
	Paternal	No effect
2	Maternal	Pre- and postnatal growth impairment (controversial, maybe related to trisomic cell line in the placenta)
4	Maternal	Pre- and postnatal growth impairment (controversial, maybe related to trisomic cell line in the placenta)
6	Maternal	Intrauterine growth restriction (1 case)
	Paternal	Transient neonatal diabetes mellitus
7	Maternal	Silver–Russell syndrome, pre- and postnatal growth impairment
9	Maternal	No effect
11	Paternal (mosaic)	Beckwith–Wiedemann syndrome
13	Maternal	No effect
	Paternal	No effect
14	Maternal	Low birth weight, small hands, precocious puberty and hypotonia
	Paternal	Polyhydramnios, facial and skeletal anomalies
15	Maternal	Prader–Willi syndrome, low birth weight, severe hypotonia and feeding difficulties
	Paternal	Angelman syndrome, severe mental retardation
16	Maternal	Growth retardation (controversial, maybe related to trisomic cell line in the placenta)
	Paternal	No effect
20	Maternal	Pre- and postnatal growth impairment
21	Maternal	No effect
	Paternal	No effect
22	Maternal	No effect

Maternal

Many studies have sought to link maternal nutrition and metabolism to fetal growth. This relationship has been demonstrated for maternal glucose metabolism as pointed out by the association between maternal indexes of insulin resistance like maternal prepregnancy weight and maternal weight increase [21] and fetal growth.[21]

Maternal nutritional status is also an important factor. The effect of maternal undernutrition during the Dutch famine was different depending on whether occurring during the first or the third trimester.[36] In recent years, a number of studies have also suggested that maternal nutrition in both quantitative and qualitative terms may have long-term effects in increasing the risk of diseases in adult life, and that the effects are different depending on the gestational age of occurrence.[37–39]

Recently, a Danish study has demonstrated that maternal intake of long chain n-3 fatty acids in amounts above 2 g a day may delay spontaneous delivery and prevent recurrence of preterm delivery, whereas low consumption of fish seems to be a strong risk factor for preterm delivery and low birth weight.[40]

Moreover, pregnancy is a period of rapid growth and cell differentiation, when both the mother and the fetus are very susceptible to alterations in dietary supply of nutrients which are usually marginal. The role of micronutrients is essential at every stage in fetal growth and development, but difficult to investigate due to the many interactions between them. Some micronutrients are essential for signaling (like retinoic acid), others as stabilizing factors in enzymes and transcription factors (like zinc) or as central components of catalytic processes (like copper and iron).[41] Iron deficiency, besides being associated with maternal anemia and increased risk of maternal hemorrhage, has been related to an increased placenta/fetal weight ratio, a predictor of cardiovascular disease in adulthood.[42] Amongst vitamins, the fat-soluble vitamins play an important role for their antioxidant capacity, protecting cells against damage induced by free radicals. There is a complex interaction between n-3 and n-6 fatty acids and fat-soluble vitamins. An excess intake of polyunsaturated fatty acids (PUFA) has been shown to reduce antioxidant capacity.[43] The hyperlipidemia characteristic of normal pregnancy during late gestation is associated with enhanced LDL oxidation rate, although this effect is counteracted by increased oxidative resistance.[44] The latter probably occurs thanks to the enhanced level of vitamin E, although other antioxidant vitamins, like β-carotene and vitamin

A remain respectively stable or decreased during normal pregnancy.[44]

The role of maternal nutrition has also been recently investigated in relation to maternal immunity during pregnancy. Deficiencies of micronutrients like iron and vitamin A in animal models alter the profile of cytokines in the placenta, shifting the equilibrium towards pro-inflammatory cytokines.[45,46] This imbalance at the maternal–fetal interface may directly or indirectly reduce the ability of the placenta to grow and function.

Placental function

The fundamental role of the placenta in ensuring normal fetal growth has been recognized both with respect to its function in the feto-maternal transfer of nutrients, and also regarding its metabolic and endocrine effects on the regulation of maternal and fetal metabolism. Placental function in regard to nutrient transfer has been investigated both in vitro and in vivo in human pregnancies. Moreover, a great bulk of our current knowledge derives from studies performed in the chronically catheterized pregnant sheep. These studies all point to the fact that nutrients are transferred to the fetus by the placenta through complex mechanisms involving transport systems present on the trophoblast microvillous and basal membrane and on the endothelial membrane of the fetal capillaries. Moreover, extensive placental metabolism has been demonstrated. Therefore, although the maternal concentration is the main determinant of fetal glucose, amino acid and fatty acid concentrations, the placenta acts to determine the composition of the fetal diet.

Placental function varies through pregnancy so that while at mid gestation the placenta utilizes half of oxygen and glucose uptake and transfers the rest to the fetal circulation, the proportion transferred to the fetus increases with progressing gestation.[47,48] In part, these changes are related to a large increase in the fetal/placental mass ratio during gestation. Moreover, functional maturation of the placenta occurs progressively over gestation, including significant increases in total placental surface area and decreased thickness,[49] allowing increased nutrient transport to meet the needs of advancing fetal growth. In addition, significant changes have been observed in the activity of placental transport systems and in their regulation.[50,51]

Fetal nutrition

During the last decade, a number of studies have expanded our knowledge on fetal nutrition by exploiting the possibility of obtaining fetal blood in utero by fetal blood sampling. This relatively noninvasive procedure has allowed the study of the placental supply of nutrients and the hormonal status of the fetus during the second half of pregnancy.[52] By this means it has been possible to determine the relationship between fetal and maternal glucose concentration from 18 weeks to term.[53] In human pregnancies fetal glucose concentration depends on both maternal glucose concentration and gestational age. In contrast, for most amino acids no significant changes have been observed at different gestational ages,[54] with a significant relationship between fetal and maternal concentrations. However, studies performed in human pregnancies in vivo by infusing stable isotopes in the maternal circulation have demonstrated that for non-essential amino acids, fetal concentrations are in most part obtained by production within the placenta, from metabolically related amino acids. For glycine and serine and for glutamate and glutamine this is part of an interorgan cycle between placenta and fetal liver (see two recent reviews).[55,56]

During the third trimester intrauterine growth of the fetus is accompanied by a large deposition of fat tissue.[11] Fetal fat content increases from 0.7–3.1 at 25 weeks to 10.2–16.1 g 100 g^{-1} weight at term.[57] The brain content of LC-PUFAs (arachidonic acid [20:4 *n-6*, AA] and docosahexaenoic acid [22:6 *n-3*, DHA]) increases progressively during brain organogenesis.[58] The incorporation of preformed arachidonic acid (AA) and docosahexaenoic acid (DHA) into the developing brain is selective and more than ten times faster than incorporation via the biosynthetic routes from linoleic (LA) and α-linolenic acid (α-LA).[59,60]

Essential fatty acids of the *n-3* and *n-6* series are mainly provided to the placenta by nonesterified fatty acids derived from triglycerides by lipoproteins of maternal adipose tissue and liver.[61,62] The percent composition of essential fatty acids and LC-PUFA has been reported as significantly different in fetal than in maternal blood, indicating an important role of the placenta in handling the fatty acid supply to the fetus.[63,64]

Although the fatty acid mix delivered to the fetus is largely determined by the fatty acid composition of the maternal blood, the placenta is able to preferentially transfer AA and DHA to the fetus, which is carried out by means of the combination of several mechanisms, as recently reviewed.[65] Fetal fatty acid plasma composition could also be influenced by fatty acid metabolism in placental and fetal tissues, but human placental tissue shows no activity of both the Δ6- and Δ5-desaturases,[66] and although LC-PUFA synthesis from EFA precursors has been demonstrated to occur in preterm infants as early as 26 wk gestation,[67] other reports have estimated that the contribution of endogenous synthesis to the total plasma LC-PUFA pool in term neonates is small.[68,69]

Hormones

The hormonal regulation of fetal growth during intrauterine life has not been completely understood, but it seems quite clear that the main hormones involved are produced within the placenta. Studies in the model of the dually perfused placenta have shown that the release of placentally produced hormones can be directed proportionally more towards the maternal or the fetal circulation,[70] suggesting a compartmentalization within the placenta. In human pregnancies, significant *in utero* relationships have been reported between fetal weight and circulating levels of hormones involved in growth regulation such as insulin-like growth factor-I (IGF-I),[71] placental growth hormone[72] and leptin.[16]

Insulin-like growth factors (IGFs) are among the most important hormones involved in fetal growth, as they are genetically old peptides that induce cell proliferation and differentiation together with DNA synthesis. Moreover, they increase glucose and amino acid uptake, while simultaneously inhibiting protein breakdown.[73] These effects have been associated with a significant relationship between umbilical venous IGF-I and birthweight.[74] Furthermore, IGF-I receptors are found at high concentrations early in gestation[75] and fetal tissues are highly sensitive to IGF-I stimulation. Although GH is the main regulator of IGF-I synthesis postnatally, however, fetal tissues are relatively deficient in GH receptors suggesting that this hormone is of minor importance during intrauterine development.

A significant role of the IGF system in the implantation phase has also been recently hypothesized. A growing body of literature provides evidence that IGF factors and their binding proteins interact at the maternal–fetal interface during trophoblast invasion and decidualization.[76–78] Crossey *et al.*[79] have recently demonstrated a role of decidual IGFBP-1 in placental growth and morphogenesis in the IGFBP-1 knock-out mice.

The endocrine unit of the placenta produces also a specific growth hormone, placental growth hormone (PGH), which has been characterized in the last 15 years[80] and is the product of the GH-V gene expressed in the syncytiotrophoblast. The secretion of PGH is important in the control of maternal IGF-1 levels. Placental growth hormone secretion in the maternal circulation has been shown to be significantly reduced in pregnancies with fetal growth restriction and this is concomitant with the changes in IGF1, thus supporting a critical role for placental GH and IGF-1 in determining fetal growth.[72]

In the last few years, considerable attention has also been given to the role of leptin as a potential regulator of intrauterine growth. Leptin is a recently described circulating polypeptide hormone, the product of the *ob* gene which is expressed by adipocytes.[81] In humans, circulating levels of leptin are significantly correlated with body fat content and body mass index (BMI), with significantly higher concentrations in females than in males.[82,83]

Leptin levels have been measured in blood from the umbilical cord of newborns and a significant relationship has been reported with fetal weight,[84,85] fetal BMI [86,16] and fetal fat mass.[16] Placental production has also been demonstrated in vitro by detection of *ob* gene expression in placental tissues.[87] Moreover, a study in the dually perfused placenta produced evidence that most of the leptin produced by the placenta is released into the maternal circulation, but compared with other placental hormones such as chorionic gonadotropin and placental lactogen, a considerably higher proportion of leptin is released into the fetal circulation.[70]

Concluding remarks

During human pregnancy, fetal growth is modulated by metabolic and endocrine factors that interact between the maternal, placental and fetal compartment in a complex manner. Moreover, a number of genetic factors, in particular imprinted genes, influence fetal and placental growth and their balance is necessary for the promotion of fetal growth under a controlled nutrient environment. Alterations in patterns of fetal growth can be determined by nutritional, endocrine and genetic factors.

REFERENCES

1 Barker, D. P. G., Gluckman, P. D., Godfrey, K. M., *et al.* Fetal nutrition and cardiovascular disease in adult life. *Lancet* 1993b;**341**:938–41.

2 Allan, W. C., Riviello, J. J. Jr. Perinatal cerebrovascular disease in the neonate. Parenchimal ischemic lesions in term and preterm infants. *Ped. Clin. N. Amer.* 1992;**39**:621–50.

3 Barker, D. J. The fetal and infant origins of adult disease. *Br. Med. J.* 1990;**301**:1111.

4 Barker, D. J. The intrauterine origins of cardiovascular disease. *Acta Pediatr. Suppl.* 1993a;**82**:93–9.

5 Lubchenco, L. O., Hansman, C., Dressler, M., Boyd, E. Intrauterine growth as estimated from liveborn birth-weight data at 24 to 42 weeks of gestation. *Pediatrics* 1963;**32**:793–800.

6 Thomson, A. M., Billewicz, W. Z., Hytten, F. E. The assessment of fetal growth. *J. Obstet. Gynaecol. Br. Commonw.* 1968;**75**:903–16.

7 Yudkin, P. L., Aboualfa, M., Eyre, J. A., Redman, C. W. G., Wilkinson, A. R. New birthweight and head circumference centiles for gestational ages 24 to 42 weeks. *Early Hum. Dev.* 1987;**15**: 45–52.

8 Geirrson, R. T., Busby-Earle, R. M. C. Certain dates may not provide a reliable estimate of gestational age. *Br. J. Obstet. Gynaecol.* 1991;**98**:108–9.

9 Wilcox, M. A., Gardosi, J., Mongelli, M., Ray, C., Johnson, I. R. Birthweight from pregnancies dated by ultrasonography in a multicultural British population. *Br. Med. J.* 1993;**307**:588–91.

10 Hindmarsh, P. C., Geary, M. P. P., Rodeck, C. H., Kingdom, J. C., Cole, T. J. Intrauterine growth and its relationship to size and shape at birth. *Pediatr. Res.* 2002;**52**:263–8.

11 Enzi, G., Zanardo, V., Caretta, F., Inelmen, E. M., Rubaltelli, F. Intrauterine growth and adipose tissue development. *Am. J. Clin. Nutr.* 1981;**34**:1785–90.

12 Bernstein, I. M., Goran, M. I., Amini, S. B., Catalano, P. M. Differential growth of fetal tissues during the second half of pregnancy. *Am. J. Obstet. Gynaecol.* 1997;**176**:28–32.

13 Nicolini, U., Ferrazzi, E., Molla, R., *et al.* Accuracy of an average ultrasonic laboratory in measurements of fetal biparietal diameter, head circumference and abdominal circumference. *J. Perinat. Med.* 1986;**14**:101–7.

14 Ferrazzi, E., Todros, T., Groli, C., *et al.* Fitting growth curves to head and abdomen measurements of the fetus: a multicentric study. *J. Clin. Ultrasound* 1987;**15**:95–105.

15 Pardi, G., Cetin, I., Marconi, A. M. *et al.* Diagnostic value of blood sampling in fetuses with growth retardation. *New Engl. J. Med.* 1993;**328**:692–6.

16 Cetin, I., Morpurgo, P. S., Radaelli, T. *et al.* Fetal plasma leptin concentration: relationship with different intrauterine growth patterns from 19 weeks to term. *Pediatr. Res.* 2000;**48**:646–51.

17 Catalano, P. M., Tyzbir, E. D., Wolfe, R. R. *et al.* Carbohydrate metabolism during pregnancy in control subjects and women with gestational diabetes. *Am. J. Physiol.* 1993;**264**:E60–7.

18 Kalkhoff, R. K. Impact of maternal fuels and nutritional state on fetal growth. *Diabetes* 1991;**40**:61–5.

19 Carrera, J. M., Devasa, R., Carrera, M. *et al.* Regulating factors. In Kurjak, A., ed. *Textbook of Perinatal Medicine.* London: Parthenon; 1998:1132–9.

20 Brooks, A. A., Johnson, M. R., Steer, P. J., Pawson, M. E., Abdalla, H. I. Birthweight: nature or nurture? *Early Hum. Dev.* 1995;**42**:29–35.

21 Catalano, P. M., Drago, N. M., Amini, S. B. Factors affecting fetal growth and body composition. *Am. J. Obstet. Gynaecol.* 1995;**172**:1459–63.

22 Catalano, P. M., Thomas, A. J., Huston, L. P., Fung, C. M. Effects of maternal metabolism on fetal growth and body composition. *Diabetes Care* 1998;**21**:B85–90.

23 Morison, I. M., Paton, C. J., Cleverley, S. D. The imprinted gene and parent-of-origin effect data base. *Nucleic Acids Res* 2001;**29**:275–6.

24 Falls, J. G., Pulford, D. J., Wylie, A. A., Jirtle, R. L. Genomic imprinting: implications for human disease. *Am. J. Pathol.* 1999;**15**:635–47.

25 Tilghman, S. M. The sins of the father and mother: genomic imprinting in mammalian development. *Cell.* 1999;**96**: 185–93.

26 Miozzo, M., Simoni, G. The role of imprinted genes in fetal growth. *Biol. Neonate* 2002;**81**:217–28.

27 Moore, T., Haig, D. Genomic imprinting in mammalian development: a parental tug-of-war. *Trends Genet.* 1991;**7**:45–9.

28 Gosden, R., Trasler, J., Lucifero, D., Faddy, M. Rare congenital disorders, imprinted genes and assisted reproductive technology. *Lancet* 2003;**361**:1975–7.

29 Schieve, L. A., Meikle, S. F., Ferre, C. *et al.* Low and very low birth weight in infants conceived with use of assisted reproductive technology. *New Engl. J. Med.* 2002;**346**:731–7.

30 De Rycke, M., Liebaers, I., van Steirteghem, A. Epigenetic risks related to assisted reproductive technologies. Risk analysis and epigenetic inheritance. *Hum. Reprod.* 2002;**17**:2487–94.

31 Thompson, J. G., Kind, K. L., Roberts, C. T., Robertson, S. A., Robinson, J. S. Epigenetic risks related to assisted reproductive technologies. Short and long-term consequences for health of children conceived through assisted reproduction technology: more reason for caution? *Hum. Reprod.* 2002;**17**:2783–6.

32 Eastman, N. J., Jackson, E. Weight relationships in pregnancy. I. The bearing of maternal weight gain and pre-pregnancy weight on birth weight in full term pregnancies. *Obstet. Gynecol. Surv.* 1968;**23**:1003–25.

33 Gluckman, P. D., Breier, B. H., Oliver, M., Harding, J., Bassett, N. Fetal growth in late gestation – a constrained pattern of growth. *Acta Paediatr. Scand. Suppl.* 1990;**367**:105–10.

34 Pardi, G., Marconi, A. M., Cetin, I. Placental–fetal interrelationship in IUGR fetuses – a review. *Placenta* 2002;**23**:S136–41.

35 Kalkhoff, R. K. Impact of maternal fuels and nutritional state on fetal growth. *Diabetes* 1991;**40**, Suppl. 2:61–5.

36 Stein, Z., Susser, M. The Dutch famine, 1944/45 and reproductive process. Effects of six indices at birth. *Pediatr. Res.* 1975;**9**:70–6.

37 Lumey, L. H., Ravelli, A. C. J., Wiessing, L. G. *et al.* The Dutch famine birth cohort study: design, validation of exposure, and selected characteristics of subjects after 43 years follow up. *Paediatr. Perinat. Epidemiol.* 1993;**7**:354–67.

38 Lumey, L. H., Stein, Z. A., Ravelli, A. C. J. Timing of prenatal starvation in women and birth weight in their first and second born offspring: the Dutch famine birth cohort study. *Eur. J. Obstet. Gynecol. Reprod. Biol.* 1995;**61**:23–30.

39 Lumey, L. H. Compensatory placental growth after restricted maternal nutrition in early pregnancy. *Placenta* 1998;**19**:105–11.

40 Olsen, S. F., Secher, N. J. Low consumption of seafood in early pregnancy as a risk factor for preterm delivery: prospective cohort study. *Br. Med. J.* 2002;**324**:447–50.

41 McArdle, H. J., Ashworth, C. J. Micronutrients in fetal growth and development. *Br. Med. Bull.* 1999;**55**:499–510.

42 Barker, D. J. *Fetal and Infant Origins of Adult Disease.* London: BMJ Press; 1992.

43 Cho S.-H., Choi, Y. Lipid peroxidation and antioxidant status is affected by different vitamin E levels when feeding fish oil. *Lipids* 1994;**29**:47–52.

44 De Vriese, S. R., Dhont, M., Christophe, A. B. Oxidative stability of low density lipoproteins and vitamin E levels increase in maternal blood during normal pregnancy. *Lipids* 2001;**36**:361–6.

45 Antipatis, C., Ashworth, C. J., Riley, S. C. *et al.* Vitamin A deficiency during rat pregnancy alters placental TNF-α signalling and apoptosis. *Am. J. Reprod. Immunol.* 2002;**47**:151–8.

46 Gambling, L., Charania, Z., Hannah, L. *et al.* Effect of iron deficiency on placental cytokine expression and fetal growth in the pregnant rat. *Biol. Reprod.* 2002;**66**:516–23.

47 Bell, A. W., Kennaugh, J. M., Battaglia, F. C., Makowski, E. L., Meschia, G. Metabolic and circulatory studies of the fetal lamb at mid gestation. *Am. J. Physiol.* 1986;**250**:E538–44.

48 Sparks, J. W., Hay, W. W. Jr, Meschia, G., Battaglia, F. C. Partition of maternal nutrients to the placenta and fetus in the sheep. *Eur. J. Obstet. Gynec. Reprod. Biol.* 1983;**14**:331–40.

49 Kaufmann, P., Scheffen, I. Placental development. In Polin, R. A., Fox, W. W., eds. *Fetal and Neonatal Physiology.* Philadelphia, PA: W. B. Saunders; 1998:59.

50 Illsley, N. P. Glucose transporters in the human placenta. *Placenta* 2000;**21**:14–22.

51 Jansson, T. Amino acid transporters in the human placenta. *Pediatr. Res.* 2001;**9**:141–7.

52 Marconi, A. M., Cetin, I., Buscaglia, M., Pardi, G. Midgestation cord sampling: what have we learned. *Placenta* 1992;**13**:115–22.

53 Marconi, A. M., Paolini, C., Buscaglia, M. *et al.* The impact of gestational age and of fetal growth upon the maternal-fetal glucose concentration difference. *Obstet. Gynecol.* 1996;**7**:937–42.

54 Cetin, I., Ronzoni, S., Marconi, A. M. *et al.* Maternal concentrations and fetal-maternal concentration differences of plasma amino acids in normal (AGA) and intrauterine growth restricted pregnancies. *Am. J. Obstet. Gynaecol.* 1996;**174**:1575–83.

55 Cetin, I. Amino acid interconversions in the fetal-placental unit: the animal model and human studies in vivo. *Pediatr. Res.* 2001;**49**:148–54.

56 Battaglia, F. C., Regnault, T. R. H. Placental transport and metabolism of amino acids. *Placenta* 2001;**22**:145–61.

57 Sparks, J. W., Ross, J. C., Cetin, I. Intrauterine growth and nutrition. In Polin, R. A., Fox, W. W., eds. *Fetal and Neonatal Physiology.* Philadelphia, PA: W. B. Saunders; 1998:267–89.

58 Crawford, M. A., Hassam, A. G., Williams, G. Essential fatty acids and fetal brain growth. *Lancet* 1976;**1**:452–3.

59 Sinclair, A. J. Long chain polyunsaturated FAs in the mammalian brain. *Proc. Nutr. Soc.* 1975;**34**:287–91.

60 Greiner, R. C., Winter, J., Nathanielsz, P. W., Brenna, J. T. Brain docosahexaenoate accretion in fetal baboons: bioequivalence of dietary alpha-linolenic and docosahexaenoic acids. *Pediatr. Res.* 1997;**42**:826–34.

61 Dunlop, M., Court, J. M. Lipogenesis in developing human adipose tissue. *Early Hum. Dev.* 1978;**2**:123–30.

62 Herrera, E. Implications of dietary fatty acids during pregnancy on placental, fetal and postnatal development. A Review. *Placenta* 2002;**23**:S9–19.

63 Hendrickse, W., Stammers, J. P., Hull, D. The transfer of free fatty acids across the human placenta. *Br. J. Obstet. Gynaecol.* 1985;**92**:945–52.

64 Koletzko, B., Muller, J. Cis- and trans-isomeric fatty acids in plasma lipids of newborn infants and their mothers. *Biol. Neonate* 1990;**57**:172–8.

65 Haggarty, P. Placental regulation of fatty acid delivery and its effect on fetal growth – a review. *Placenta* 2002;**23**:S28–38.

66 Chambaz, J., Ravel, D., Manier, M. C. *et al.* Essential fatty acids interconversion in the human fetal liver. *Biol. Neonate* 1985;**47**:136–40.

67 Uauy, R., Mena, P., Wegher, B., Nieto, S., Salemn, Jr. Long chain polyunsaturated fatty acid formation in neonates: effect of gestational age and intrauterine growth. *Pediatr. Res.* 2000;**47**:127–35.

68 Demmelmair, H. R. U., Behrendt, E., Sauerwald, T., Koletzko, B. Estimation of arachidonic acid synthesis in full term neonates using natural variation of ^{13}C-abundance. *J. Pediatr. Gastroent. Nutr.* 1995;**21**:31–6.

69 Szitanyi, P., Koletzko, B., Mydlilova, A., Demmelmair, H. Metabolism of ^{13}C-labeled linoleic acid in newborn infants during the first week of life. *Pediatr. Res.* 1999;**45**:669–73.

70 Linnemann, K., Malek, A., Sager, R. *et al.* Leptin production and release in the dually in vitro perfused human placenta. *J. Clin. Endocrinol. Metab.* 2000;**85**:4298–301.

71 Giudice, L. C., De Zegher, F., Gargosky, S. E. *et al.* Insulin-like growth factors and their binding proteins in the term and preterm human fetus and neonate with normal and extremes of intrauterine growth. *J. Clin. Endocrinol. Metab.* 1995;**80**:1548–55.

72 McIntyre, H. D., Serek, R., Crane, D. I. *et al.* Placental growth hormone (GH), GH-binding protein, and insulin-like growth factor axis in normal, growth-retarded, and diabetic pregnancies: correlations with fetal growth. *J. Clin. Endocrinol. Metab.* 2000;**85**:1143–50.

73 Wang, H. S., Chard, T. The role of insulin-like growth factor-I and insulin-like growth factor-binding protein-I in the control of human fetal growth. *J. Endocrinol.* 1992;**133**:149–59.

74 Ashton, I. K., Zapf, J., Einschenk, I., MacKenzie, I. Z. Insulin-like growth factor (IGF) I and II in human fetal plasma and relationship to gestational age and foetal size during midpregnancy. *Acta Endocrinol.* 1985;**110**:558–63.

75 Sara, V. T., Hall, K., Misaki, M. *et al.* Ontogenesis of somatomedin and insulin receptors in the human fetus. *J. Clin. Invest.* 1983;**71**:1084–94.

76 Han, V. K., Bassett, N., Walton, J., Challis, J. R. The expression of insulin-like growth factor (IGF) and IGF-binding protein (IGFBP) genes in the human placenta and membranes: evidence for IGF-IGFBP interactions at the feto-maternal interface. *J. Clin. Endocrinol. Metab.* 1996;**8**:2680–93.

77 Han, V. K., Carter, A. M. Spatial and temporal patterns of expression of messenger RNA for insulin-like growth factors and their binding proteins in the placenta of man and laboratory animals. *Placenta* 2000;**21**:289–305.

78 Nayak, N. R., Giudice, L. C. Comparative biology of the IGF system in endometrium, decidua, and placenta, and clinical implications for foetal growth and implantation disorders. *Placenta* 2003;**24**:281–96.

79 Crossey, P. A., Pillai, C. C., Miell, J. P. Altered placental development and intrauterine growth restriction in IGF binding protein-1 transgenic mouse. *J. Clin. Invest.* 2002;**110**:411–8.

80 Alsat, E., Guibourdenche, J., Couturier, A., Evain-Brion, D. Physiological role of human placental growth hormone. *Mol. Cell Endocrinol.* 1998;**140**:121–7.

81 Zhang, Y., Proneca, R., Maffei, M. Positional cloning of the mouse obese gene and its human homologue. *Nature* 1995;**372**:425–32.

82 Kennedy, A., Gettys, T. W., Wason, P. *et al.* The metabolic significance of leptin in humans: gender-based differences in relationship to adiposity, insulin sensitivity and energy expenditure. *J. Clin. Endocrinol. Metab.* 1997;**82**:1293–300.

83 Saad, M. F., Damani, S., Gingerich, R. L. *et al.* Sexual dimorphism in plasma leptin concentration. *J. Clin. Endocrinol. Metab.* 1997;**82**:579–84.

84 Schubring, C., Kiess, W., Englaro, P. *et al.* Levels of leptin in maternal serum, amniotic fluid, and arterial and venous cord blood: relation to neonatal and placental weight. *J. Clin. Endocrinol. Metab.* 1997;**82**:1480–83.

85 Koistinen, H. A., Koivisto, V. A., Andersson, S. *et al.* Leptin concentration in cord blood correlates with intrauterine growth. *J. Clin. Endocrinol. Metab.* 1997;**82**:3328–30.

86 Shekawat, P. S., Garland, J. S., Shivpuri, C. *et al.* Neonatal cord blood leptin: its relationship to birth weight, body mass index, maternal diabetes, and steroids. *Pediatr. Res.* 1998;**43**:338–43.

87 Masuzaki, H., Ogawa, Y., Sagawa, N. *et al.* Nonadipose tissue production of leptin: leptin as a novel placenta-derived hormone in humans. *Nat. Med.* 1997;**241**:1029–33.

3

Aspects of fetoplacental nutrition in intrauterine growth restriction and macrosomia

Timothy R. H. Regnault, Sean W. Limesand and William W. Hay, Jr.

Perinatal Research Center, University of Colorado Health Sciences Center, Aurora, Colorado

Introduction

Newborn birth weights have been steadily increasing throughout much of the developed world.[1-3] However, the numbers of the two extremes, small fetuses that have suffered some form of intrauterine growth restriction (IUGR) and large or macrosomic fetuses, remain constant, and within some populations are actually increasing.[1,3-6] IUGR and large-for-gestational-age (LGA) fetuses and newborns are at increased risk for fetal and neonatal morbidity and mortality.[7,8] IUGR is an important and relatively common problem in obstetrics, which may represent impaired placental insufficiency and associated placental nutrient transport function. In developed countries, 3–7% of newborns are classified as IUGR,[9] the causes of which include, but are not limited to, maternal malnutrition, maternal hypertension and idiopathic placental insufficiency. These fetuses are at increased risk of hypoxia, hypoglycemia and acidemia and also spontaneous preterm delivery.[8,10-12] Interest in IUGR has increased recently by retrospective epidemiological, clinical follow-up and animal studies,[13,14] that indicate increased susceptibility to adulthood metabolic disorders such as obesity, insulin resistance, type 2 diabetes mellitus and cardiovascular disease, particularly hypertension, in IUGR offspring.[15-18] Furthermore, follow-up studies of infants who displayed abnormal umbilical artery Doppler flow velocity waveforms, commonly associated with IUGR, have demonstrated a lower IQ at 3 and 5 years of age.[5,19] At the other end of the spectrum, the number of macrosomic, LGA births among certain minorities, delivered at term or ≥ 41 weeks, has increased.[1] These fetuses are defined in a newborn as having a birth weight above the 90th percentile for gestational age or a birth weight greater than 4000 grams at term.[3,20,21] These infants have been exposed to an altered in utero environment in which nutrient supply is in excess of requirements. Macrosomic fetuses and newborns have increased risks of neonatal morbidity primarily associated with metabolic complications of maternal diabetes mellitus during pregnancy; they also are at increased risk of birth injuries as a result of their excessive size. Similar to IUGR infants, those born LGA and macrosomic, particularly those that are offspring of diabetic mothers, have later life complications of obesity, insulin resistance, diabetes and cardiovascular disease. This chapter will provide an overview of IUGR and macrosomia dealing with aspects of placental development, fetal nutrition and the potential for adverse later life outcomes.

Intrauterine growth restriction (IUGR)

The period of fetal growth lasts from the end of embryogenesis at week eight of gestation until birth. During this period fetal size increases by hypertrophy and hyperplasia. Cellular differentiation within organs, however, may still occur throughout gestation. Under normal conditions, fetal growth follows its genetic potential, unless the mother is unusually small for the species and limits fetal growth by a variety of factors considered collectively to represent "maternal constraint."[22]

Historically those infants weighing less than two standard deviations below the mean of a population, born at the

Neonatal Nutrition and Metabolism. Second Edition, ed. P. Thureen and W. Hay. Published by Cambridge University Press.
© Cambridge University Press 2006.

same estimated gestational age or for a given gestational age, were considered IUGR. In Western countries these infants generally weigh less than 2500 g and are not part of the natural biological diversity that one would expect, but rather represent a group of fetuses that has undergone some form of in utero insult from placental insufficiency that produces a suboptimal nutrient supply in utero and consequently a restriction of fetal growth. Many terms, based upon fetal weight, are used to describe these variations in fetal growth. For example, human newborns are classified as having normal birth weight (2500–4000 grams), low birth weight (less than 2500 grams), very low birth weight (less than 1500 grams), or extremely low birth weight (less than 1000 grams). However, classification by birth weight alone says little about fetal growth rate and whether infants were restricted in utero because of difficulty in estimating gestation age, preterm delivery or the small, but normal infant.

Cross-sectional growth curves have been developed from anthropometric measurements in populations of newborn infants at different gestational ages. Such curves have been used to estimate whether growth of an individual fetus or newborn is within or outside of the normal range of fetal growth for a given population, which is defined as between the 10th and 90th percentile, although what the curves actually show is simply how big a given fetus or newborn is relative to others at any given gestational age. Fetuses and newborn infants who are between the 10th and 90th percentiles for weight vs. gestational age are considered appropriate-for-gestational-age (AGA). Those who are <10th percentile are considered small-for-gestational-age (SGA), and those who are >90th percentile are considered large-for-gestational-age (LGA). Each curve is based on local populations with variable composition of maternal age, parity, socio-economic status, race, ethnic background, body size, degree of obesity or thinness, health, pregnancy-related problems and nutrition, as well as the number of fetuses per mother, the number of infants included in the study and how well measurements of body size and gestational age were made.

Over the past three decades there have been many refinements to the birth weight/gestational age charts and their use in defining mortality rates and specific morbidities associated with different weight/age classifications. Predominant among these changes is the widespread use of ultrasonographic fetal biometry, which has removed the sole reliance on birth weight measurements in relation to gestational age.[23] The continuing developments in ultrasonographic measurements of head and abdominal circumference together with femur length and umbilical blood flow measurements[24–26] and in utero fetal blood sampling[27,28] now allow clinicians to more accurately identify fetuses that have unique pathophysiology and might benefit from increased antenatal surveillance to determine when to intervene by delivery. Additionally, IUGR induced by placental insufficiency can be detected indirectly by measuring umbilical artery Doppler flow velocity waveforms, which reflect changes in blood flow through the placental vascular bed and corresponding changes observed in umbilical artery blood flow.[9,29,30] The growth of an individual fetus that is examined by ultrasound at different gestational ages can be better correlated with expected fetal growth rates than from cross-sectional, population-based fetal growth curves. Therefore serial ultrasound measurements of fetal growth, in humans or in experimental animals, also can more accurately determine how environmental factors can inhibit (for example, maternal undernutrition globally or hypoglycemia specifically) or enhance (for example, maternal overnutrition globally or hyperglycemia specifically) fetal growth.

Growth rates in utero and IUGR

Mathematical analyses of various fetal growth curves have been used to determine growth rates over relatively short gestational periods or at discrete gestational ages. For example, the data used in the Lubchenco growth curves can be approximated by a simple exponential function showing fetal weight increasing at about 15 g kg^{-1} day^{-1}.[31–33] This rate will vary considerably from the smallest to the largest infants, but among different populations there are only small differences among growth curves of 1–2%. Composite pictures of human fetal growth have been derived from neonatal anthropometric measurements at birth. Mean percentiles among growth curves differ by ±5%, accounted for largely by factors such as suboptimal pregnancy dating, adverse maternal and/or fetal medical and obstetric complications of pregnancy, diet, race, ethnicity, socioeconomic status and altitude differences.[34] Neonatal-derived fetal weight curves appear as sigmoidal functions of weight versus gestational age. In studies that have accounted for many of the factors that can affect fetal growth and fetal size, fetal weight gain appears to be a linear function of gestational age through to term (about 12–15 g kg^{-1} day^{-1}.[35,36] with only slight increases for males versus females and for maternal obesity.[37] The fetal weight change (the rate of weight gain per kg body weight per day) is relatively linear at about 1.5% per day from about 24 to 37 weeks, but tapers off to a plateau between 37 and 42 weeks and may decrease after 43 weeks. These rates of gain in the last third of pregnancy are accomplished through a caloric intake of approximately $100 \, \mathrm{kcal \, kg^{-1} \cdot day^{-1}}$ of which over 90% is deposited as fetal fat at term.[38,39]

Further chemical composition studies of normal human infants have been accomplished. Sparks has reviewed data from 15 studies accounting for 207 infants, and nonfat dry weight and nitrogen content show a linear relationship with fetal weight and an exponential relationship with gestational age.[38] Thus, nonfat dry weight and nitrogen content for a given fetus also can be compared with the "average" fetus. When these comparisons are made, larger fetuses grow faster than smaller fetuses at similar gestational ages, and protein accretion follows accordingly. The growth pattern of an IUGR fetus is reduced in cases of placental insufficiency. The peak growth velocity of a fetus is generally thought to occur at approximately week 32 with the average fetus depositing approximately 200 grams per week. While specific IUGR growth data are scarce, a smaller fetus on the 10th percentile is estimated to accumulate weight at approximately 80% of the normal rate (160 grams per week), and as gestation advances, an IUGR fetus can be expected to accumulate only 640 grams between weeks 37 and 41 in contrast to the normally developing fetus that will deposit upwards of 800 grams.[36,40]

Symmetrical and asymmetrical IUGR

Intrauterine growth restriction can be divided into "symmetrical IUGR" and "asymmetrical IUGR." Symmetrical IUGR, often associated with genetic or congenital problems such as infection, involves a proportional reduction in growth of soft tissue (muscle, fat, organs), length and head circumference. Asymmetrical IUGR refers to a fetal growth pattern in which brain growth is relatively spared in relation to weight and length of the fetus. Asymmetrical IUGR is commonly associated with forms of uteroplacental insufficiency [41,42] in which the fetuses are hypoxic and hypoglycemic and display decreased subcutaneous fat, reduced abdominal circumference and disproportionately large heads. Additionally, the response to the growth insult often involves changes in fetal circulation, including a redistribution of fetal cardiac output to the brain, heart, and adrenals and proportionately decreased umbilical blood flow.[28,43–45] Definable subgroups exist within this group of fetuses with characteristic physiologic changes that are related to the severity of the IUGR.[27,46,47] For example umbilical artery velocimetry and fetal heart rate monitoring have been combined to demonstrate that approximately two-thirds of IUGR infants display an increased umbilical arterial pulsatility index (blood flow pulsatility increases as downstream vascular resistance increases), with 50% of these fetuses having an increased fetal heart

rate. Some of these fetuses did not have increased umbilical arterial velocimetry indices or heart rates were still classified as IUGR and not just SGA, as they still had reduced umbilical blood flow rates per fetal weight.[27]

Many of the IUGR infants with decreased umbilical blood flow also have a reported increased fraction of umbilical blood flow entering the ductus venous, associated with a decreased total umbilical blood flow and hepatic perfusion rate.[46] These studies indicate that hypoperfusion of fetal hepatic tissue results in reduced liver mass and possibly hepatic function. This weight reduction together with a relative increase in brain mass increases the brain/liver weight and size ratio. These increased indices together with reduced fat deposition result in a reduced Ponderal index (weight, grams / [length, cm]^3), a key index of asymmetrical IUGR.

Development of IUGR placental vasculature

Development of the placental vascular bed and placental exchange area are regulated by a number of growth factors, particularly the vascular endothelial growth factor (VEGF) growth factor family.[41,42,48,49] The interactions between oxygen partial pressure (PO_2), vascular cell types, and the regulation of cellular responses, such as growth factor and receptor expression, lead to the development of a low-resistance placental vascular network via placental angiogenesis. The local oxygen environment plays a large role in the development of placental vasculature. Three distinct types of hypoxia occur within the fetoplacental unit that uniquely affect placental angiogenesis,[48] and possibly produce specific alterations in placental nutrient transfer capacity.

Oxygen and angiogenic placental vascular development

Oxygen has a major role in oxidative metabolism, both within the placenta and fetus. It also plays a major role in the development of the placental vasculature and its functional characteristics. Placental blood vessel development is divided into two phases, branching and nonbranching angiogenesis. Branching angiogenesis occurs during the early phases of gestation under relatively hypoxic conditions and is responsible for the expansion of the preexisting vascular bed. This process appears to be driven by VEGF. Nonbranching angiogenesis, in contrast, promotes the elongation of preexisting capillary loops and occurs later in gestation under the influence of placental growth factor (PlGF).[50] The balance of action of these two growth factors throughout gestation is responsible for the formation of the normal placental vasculature. Recently, a number of different villous morphologies have been documented in association with altered states of placental oxygenation. For example, the villous structure observed from IUGR placentas that develop under maternal hypoxia, as in pregnancy at altitude, are characterized by increased branching angiogenesis and a reduced vascular impedance.[51,52] In contrast, those placentas with severe IUGR, characterized by severely increased umbilical artery vascular impedance and absent end-diastolic flow (AEDF), are associated with a predominance of nonbranching angiogenesis.[48,49] There are two alternative pathways by which these IUGR villous structures develop. Villous development with excessive branching-type angiogenesis as a result of elevated VEGF concentrations in relation to PlGF occurs in situations of intraplacental hypoxia. In contrast, nonbranching angiogenesis becomes the dominant form of angiogenesis when there is an increase in the intraplacental oxygen concentration and PlGF dominates.[50,52] The interactions between oxygen partial pressure (PO_2), vascular cell types, and the regulation of cellular responses, such as growth factor and receptor expression, lead to the development of a low resistance placental vascular network in normal pregnancies. Postulated changes in the angiogenic development of placentas, brought on by alterations in uteroplacenta) oxygen tension, may be associated with three different hypoxic IUGR outcomes, pre-placental hypoxia, uteroplacental hypoxia (with preeclampsia), and post-placental hypoxia (with severe IUGR).[48,52]

Pre-placental hypoxia

In pregnancies at altitude, maternal hypoxemic hypoxia results in pre-placental hypoxia that includes intervillous blood hypoxia,[53] and results in subsequent fetal hypoxia.[48] The growth restriction of these fetuses also is characterized by an increased head circumference to body weight ratio, reflecting asymmetric IUGR.[54] This brain-sparing effect occurs in conjunction with alterations in fetal cardiac blood circulation leading to relatively greater brain-blood flow than lower body blood flow.[55] High altitude pregnancies have low umbilical artery flow impedance values suggestive of increases in villous capillary diameter[48,52] from increased branching angiogenesis,[41] likely as a result of a greater VEGF/PlGF ratio. In addition, decreases in uterine artery flow resistance, possibly due to improved trophoblast invasion, may represent a compensatory mechanism in response to reduced oxygen tension at altitude[56] though these differences are not observed at altitudes less than 1600 meters.[57] Where changes in flow are observed, thinner tissue layers are observed within the placenta, leading to an improved diffusion capacity,[58] possibly related to increases in villous capillary diameter.[59,60]

Uteroplacental hypoxia and preeclampsia

Chronic hypertension and preeclampsia increase the risk of IUGR.[61–63] Preeclampsia represents an etiologically heterogeneous condition with two general groups of fetuses. One occurs in mothers with preeclampsia early in pregnancy and displays asymmetrical fetal growth restriction associated with impaired placental perfusion and nutrient (including oxygen) transport function. The other occurs in late gestation preeclampsia pregnancies and displays normal fetal weight indices.[64] In preeclampsia associated with IUGR, despite normal maternal oxygenation, the placental vasculature and fetal circulations are hypoxic and often associated with inadequate trophoblast invasion leading to reduced intraplacental oxygen pressure. Expression of IGF-II and IGFBP-1 at the maternal interface are altered in the preeclamptic placenta.[65] Specifically, IGFBP-1 levels are decreased with severe preeclampsia, suggesting that the altered expression may play a role in the development of this placental type.[65] Both pre-placental and uteroplacental hypoxia are associated with increased placental angiogenesis leading to the development of reduced capillary impedance within the fetal placental vasculature.[41,50] This altered development of the placenta in pregnancies complicated by severe preeclampsia is characterized by diminished arborization of the terminal villi; uteroplacental ischemia probably is the dominant cause.[66] Preeclampsia without IUGR displays little effect on placental weight or composition.[67]

Vascular changes associated with preeclampsia have been linked to possible changes in placental 11β-hydroxysteroid dehydrogenase 2 expression and activity as a result of abnormal oxygen tensions within the vasculature.[68] Placental 11β-HSD2 activity is oxygen dependent, and its activity is impaired in preeclampsia with reduced trophoblast invasion of the maternal arteries associated with areas of hypoxia within the placenta.[68–70] This impairment could result in an increase in maternally derived cortisol in the placenta, which may contribute to altered placental development through increased placental apoptosis[71] and possible adverse fetal development.[68,71] The activation of the Renin-Angiotensin system also is altered in the fetoplacental unit in preeclampsia; angiotensin-converting activity is increased in the venous endothelial cells, leading to related changes in the fetal circulation.[72]

Post-placental hypoxia and severe IUGR

The most severe IUGR fetuses develop with relatively marked fetal hypoxia occurring in conjunction with normal maternal and placental oxygenation.[41,48,73] Severe early-onset IUGR with absent umbilical end-diastolic flow (EDF), however, is associated with increased intra-placental oxygen pressure, or relative "placental hyperoxia."[52,74] In this situation, placental angiogenesis is diminished, resulting in increased vascular impedance; the fetus then is deprived of oxygen because of markedly reduced umbilical blood flow.[75] Reduced vascularization of the intermediate and terminal villi leads to increased fetoplacental impedance, as measured by reduced or absent EDF in the umbilical arteries of human and sheep IUGR pregnancies.[30,76,77] Progressive embolization of the sheep placenta can replicate absent end diastolic velocity as observed in severely growth-restricted human fetuses.[30,77–79] Stereological and plastic cast studies and scanning electron microscope techniques indicate that increased placental vascular impedance is associated with a global reduction in vascularity, not just reduction of small arteries and arterioles.[74,75,80]

Alterations in placental nutrient transfer in IUGR

Changes in the capacity of the placenta to transport oxygen and nutrients to the fetus play major roles in the development of IUGR, both in human and experimental IUGR.[48,67,81–84] As pregnancy advances, the increasing nutrient demands of the developing conceptus (uterus plus fetus plus placenta) must be met through appropriate increases in placental nutrient transport. This enhanced performance is facilitated by increases in placental perfusion, total membrane surface area for transplacental diffusion, and transporters for specific nutrients.[85–87] Both passive and facilitated diffusion of compounds occur in the placenta, representing transfer of substances that is energy independent, moving across the membranes down a maternal-fetal gradient. The exchange of gases, such as oxygen, represents a good example of passive diffusion, where an oxygen gradient across a membrane drives its transcellular diffusion from a high partial pressure region to a lower one. This movement requires no transport systems and movement occurs according to the pressure or concentration gradient across the membrane and the diffusion capacity of the substance, which is based on its solubility in lipid vs. water. In contrast, facilitated diffusion of substances such as glucose involves transport down a concentration gradient using specific transporters; in this case, transfer is concentration dependent, but the substance involved moves more rapidly across the membrane than it would by diffusion alone.

The increasing oxygen requirements of the placenta and fetus as pregnancy advances are met through increases in uterine perfusion (blood flow) and the diffusion capacity of the placenta for oxygen. The relationship between blood flow, placental oxygen consumption, and the diffusion capacity of the placenta leads to the development of the transplacental PO_2 gradient.[88] Increases in uterine blood flow and uterine venous PO_2 in IUGR cases[89] indicate that such conditions involve reduced oxygen diffusion capacity of the IUGR placenta. As a result of this decrease in placental oxygen-diffusing capacity, a compensatory increase of the PO_2 gradient develops which allows oxygen transfer from mother to fetus to continue at normal rates per unit of tissue,[73] although the capacity for this increase in gradient to maintain oxygen transfer in situations of severe IUGR clearly becomes limited.

As pregnancy advances the placental exchange surface area increases, which is associated with a decrease in the thickness of the placental membrane, further facilitating diffusion.[60,90] It is interesting to note that between week 16 of pregnancy and term, human fetal weight increases approximately 20-fold, whereas the peripheral villous surface area increases only 10-fold.[91] Thus, the microvilli density on trophoblast cells cannot explain the exponential fetal growth occurring over this time period, suggesting that fetal growth is supported not by changes in villous surface area alone, but by changes in nutrient (glucose and amino acid) transporter capacity. IUGR placentas have decreased total villous surface area,[60,67,81,83,92,93] indicating that morphometric changes in vascularization contribute to the overall reduction in placental diffusional transport capacity.[67] Experimental models have supported these observations. For example, in transgenic mice in which the placental-specific *Igf*2 gene has been deleted, placental surface area and thickness are increased, significantly reducing the theoretical diffusion capacity of these placentas.[83,94] Thus, both decreased surface area for diffusional exchange for compounds such as oxygen and reductions in the number of specific nutrient transporters and their activities contribute to the global reduction in nutrient transport in IUGR pregnancies.

Glucose transporters and IUGR

Glucose is the principal metabolic fuel for the fetus, and the supply of glucose is an important determinant of fetal growth. Human and animal IUGR pregnancies exhibit fetal hypoglycemia,[10,12,95–102] though reports from glucose transporter density studies in IUGR pregnancies from human [99,100] and rat [101] placentas indicate that transporter density is not altered during IUGR indicating that the reduced glucose transport capacity experienced in IUGR pregnancies is independent of transporter density. However, since several placental structural abnormalities occur in IUGR pregnancies, such as reduced villous number, diameter, and surface area,[67,74,103] total transport capacity may be reduced even if transporter density is unaltered.[97,102]

Maternal glucose is transported into the placental trophoblast cells and subsequently into the fetal circulation via facilitative diffusion.[104,105] A family of structurally related facilitative glucose transporter (GLUT) proteins has been described.[106,107] Several GLUT transporters have been found in the term human placenta.[97,99,108–111] Two primary isoforms of the hexose transporter family (GLUT1 and GLUT3) have been detected in placental trophoblast cells in human,[99,108,109] sheep,[112,113] and mouse.[114] In pregnant sheep, both GLUT1 and GLUT3 are expressed by trophoblast cells of the placenta[113,115,116]; GLUT1 is expressed on both the basal and apical aspects of the chorionic epithelium, whereas GLUT3 appears to be localized to the maternal facing apical microvillous surface.[116] Conversely, in the human, GLUT3 has only been immunolocalized in fetal placental epithelium although mRNA for both transporters could be detected in trophoblast.[117] The expression of both GLUT1 and GLUT3 can be altered by diabetes,[118,119] hypoxia,[120] glucocorticoids[117] and hypothyroxinemia.[121] Therefore, the metabolic environment of the placenta, which is altered in IUGR pregnancies, controls expression of both transporters.

Pregnant sheep have been used to study in vivo placental glucose transport into placental and fetal tissues and are used as models for physiological studies of IUGR.[97,122] Investigations in normal pregnant sheep have demonstrated a gestational-dependent decline in placental GLUT1 protein concentrations with a reciprocal increase in GLUT3 protein.[112,113] As with the human placenta, ovine maternal and fetal hyper- and hypoglycemic states alter expression of both GLUT1 and GLUT3.[115,116] Even though the ratio of maternal to fetal glucose concentration increases in late gestation in the pregnant IUGR sheep model, hypoglycemia still occurs as a result of reduced glucose transport capacity of the placenta.[97] This may indicate a reduction in expression of one or both of the glucose transporters. In fact, in vivo studies have shown that GLUT 1 and GLUT3 decrease in response to hypoglycemia, with a greater reduction in GLUT1 compared with GLUT3. This may allow for preferential glucose uptake by the placenta under chronically low glucose conditions due to greater abundance of the higher affinity GLUT3 transporter. Recently, a third member of the glucose transporter family (GLUT8) has been detected in the ovine placenta.[98] Messenger RNA and protein concentrations for GLUT8 were decreased at 135 days gestational age in ovine IUGR placenta compared with normal control placentas, perhaps indicating a role for GLUT8 in mediating glucose uptake within the placenta and transport to the fetus and, when diminished, contributing to placental glucose transport deficiency in IUGR.

Placental amino acid transporter and IUGR

Placental transport of amino acids has been extensively reviewed.[82,84,123] In studies comparing normal and IUGR placentas total villous surface area is reduced,[67,81,92,93] indicating that morphometric changes contribute to the overall reduction in placental amino acid transport capacity. While this might lead to reduced fetal plasma amino acid concentrations, reports of changes in fetal amino acid concentrations are varied.[124–127] Despite these differences, impaired amino acid transport capacity is characteristic of IUGR placentas. Studies in human IUGR demonstrate that System A is impaired.[128–130] System A is a sodium-dependent, unidirectional transporter with a characteristic affinity for N-methylated substances; its activity has been demonstrated in both microvillous and basal membranes[131–133] and is increased as an adaptation to cellular depletion of amino acid substrates, similar to that described for System X_{AG}^- and the anionic amino acid transport system.[134,135] An in vitro study using microvillous membrane vesicles from the placentas of AGA and SGA neonates demonstrated markedly lower (by 63%) activity of the System A transporters in the SGA compared with the AGA membrane vesicles,[128] indicating a positive association between fetal growth and System A activity. Additionally, reduced V_{max} values for the SGA fetuses suggests that there is a reduction in System A transporter per unit mass of placental tissue.[130] More recent studies have shown that the decrease in System A activity is associated only with those IUGR fetuses displaying abnormal pulsatility indices.[129]

Studies of maternal protein deprivation in rats have demonstrated a down-regulation of placental amino acid transport, specifically System A as well as Systems X_{AG}^- and y^+.[128,136] Inhibition of System A transport in rat pregnancies has been purported to affect fetal weight, demonstrating a role for System A transport in fetal growth.[137] The latter two transport systems, the X_{AG}^- and y^+, are different from System A in their sodium dependence and substrate preference. The sodium/potassium dependent X_{AG}^- system is located within both the microvillous and basal plasma membranes.[136,138–143] This system may mediate the concentrative uptake of anionic amino acids from the maternal and fetal circulations into the placenta. Five cDNAs encoding proteins capable of mediating this high-affinity placental sodium-coupled transport have been reported and three of these have been cloned from both rat and human placenta: excitatory amino acid transport (EAAT)-1 (GLAST1), EAAT-2 (GLT1) and EAAT-3 (EAAC1).[141,142,144]

EAAT-1 and EAAT-3 have been detected in human placental tissue,[145,146] while these two and EAAT-2 have been detected in rat placenta tissues.[141,147] The basal membrane activity of EAAT-1 is reduced in an IUGR rat model, which could impact placental glutamate uptake from the fetal circulation,[136] indicating an important role for this transport system in fetal development. Additionally, recent studies in the sheep model of maternal hyperthermia-induced IUGR have shown reduced fetal plasma glutamate concentrations and a reduced umbilical glutamate coefficient of extraction, highlighting possible alterations in both the fetal liver and placenta X_{AG}^- system in IUGR.[148]

The y^+ transport system, however, is a sodium-independent low affinity, electrogenic high-capacity system, which transports cationic amino acids such as arginine, lysine and ornithine. It is considered to be the major cationic transport system in placental tissues,[149–151] localized to the microvillous membrane[136,149,152,153] and possibly to the basal membranes.[154] The microvillous membrane activities of System y^+ and y^+L are not altered in human IUGR,[155,156] though basal membrane transport of lysine is reduced as represented by reduced fetal lysine uptake and a reduced V_{max} for the y^+L system.[156] System y^+L is a cationic amino acid transporter and is a low-capacity, high-affinity system that exchanges cationic amino acids for neutral amino acids in the presence of sodium; its activity is localized to both the microvillous membrane and basal membrane.[149,152,156,157] This transporter system in the basal membrane is the major supply route of cationic amino acids to the fetus through the uptake of neutral amino acids from the fetal circulation in exchange for cationic amino acids from the placenta.[149] Reductions in the uptake of leucine in both microvillous and basal membrane preparations of IUGR placentas highlight possible alterations in the L transport system.[156] These changes in basal membrane transport properties could be an important adaptive response by the trophoblast, limiting the back-flux of amino acids from the fetal circulation into the placenta. In vivo studies in a sheep model of IUGR have shown reduced back-flux of leucine and threonine from the fetal circulation to the placenta, indicating diminished basal membrane amino acid transport function.[158,159] Studies of human IUGR demonstrate a significant reduction in transplacental flux of essential amino acids such as leucine and phenylalanine.[127] The magnitude of the reduction in leucine transport correlates with the clinical severity of IUGR based on fetal arterial velocimetry and fetal heart rate data,[27] similar to the reports for decreased system A data.[129]

The β-amino acid taurine, which uses the System β transport system, also is decreased in concentration and transport capacity in IUGR placentas. Taurine is necessary for many essential developmental processes in the fetus, particularly for skeletal muscle, heart, and eye. Studies have demonstrated that this β transport system is a sodium-dependent transporter, found on both membranes.[160–166] The β transporter for taurine has exhibited activity in placenta microvillous membrane and basal membrane vesicles,[160–165] though basal membrane activity is only approximately 6% of that in the microvillous membrane.[163] In recent studies concerning IUGR vesicle preparations, the transporter expression was unaltered on the microvillous membranes, suggesting transporter activity may be reduced in IUGR, potentially through changes in NO concentrations.[166]

Macrosomia

Macrosomia is defined in a newborn as a birth weight above the 90th percentile for gestational age or a birth weight greater than 4000 grams at term.[20,21] Macrosomia is characteristic of infants of diabetic mothers (IDMs) whose mothers had diabetes mellitus with hyperglycemia during pregnancy. The diabetes can be long standing, but the most common group of IDMs occurs in women with gestational diabetes mellitus (GDM), which complicates 3–5% of all pregnancies. The risk of macrosomia is consistent across all classes of diabetes,[40] primarily reflecting the degree and duration of maternal hyperglycemia and hypertriglyceridemia from inadequately controlled diabetes. Maternal hyperglycemia results in fetal hyperglycemia and subsequently hyperinsulinemia,[167] while the hypertriglyceridemia contributes to excess fat deposition in the fetus. Macrosomia also may occur in infants from nondiabetic mothers, although often these women have undiagnosed gestational diabetes or have relatively high plasma glucose concentrations from eating an excessively high carbohydrate diet.[168] The macrosomic fetus, in addition to increased fetal mass, displays abnormally high adipose tissue composition, resulting in an increased ponderal index.[21,169,170]

Human fetal insulin secretion in response to glucose has been controversial because of variable tissue or organ culture methods used among studies. However, in vivo administration of glucose to the pregnant mother has been noted to increase fetal insulin concentration in normal fetuses at 26–33 weeks' gestation.[171] Furthermore, in utero fetal insulin secretion has been described for the rat[172] and sheep.[173] Glucose stimulated insulin secretion increases in mildly hyperglycemic (+ 0.5 mM) fetal sheep that also have multiple daily hyperglycemic episodes, much like pregnant women with GDM. In contrast, severe hyperglycemia in either sheep[174] or rat[175] reduces insulin secretion responsiveness, and in the rat and human also results in fetal growth restriction.[176] These observations indicate that moderately controlled diabetes during pregnancy can result in a hypersensitive β-cell population. Hyperglycemic episodes in these cases likely enhance fetal growth by pulsatile stimulation of fetal insulin gene expression leading to increased fetal insulin secretion,[177] its augmentation of fetal fat deposition, and thus, macrosomia. In contrast, severe, overt diabetes can limit fetal β-cell function and, in turn, reduce fetal growth.

Traditionally it has been thought that a macrosomic fetal growth pattern was not apparent until the beginning of the last or third trimester of pregnancy. Earlier reports in fact indicated that deviations of the fetal abdominal circumference become detectable between 30–32 weeks' gestation, as a result of increasing abdominal adipose deposition.[40,169,178] These and other studies investigating fetal head size and femur length did not document significant changes in these parameters when compared with fetuses from nondiabetic mothers.[178,179] More recent reports, however, have shown significantly greater abdominal circumference measurements in IDM macrosomic fetuses as early as 18 weeks' gestation, with the difference becoming more pronounced in the third trimester.[180,181]

Placental development and function in diabetic pregnancy

In studies of trophoblast villi and intervillous pores of placentas from well-controlled diabetes mellitus, no significant differences are detected between control and diabetic placentas.[182] Thus, placental development is preserved by good glycemic control regardless of diabetic grouping. Placental function is not adversely affected in these placentas, supporting the growth of large fetuses.[183] Furthermore, Doppler flow studies suggest that hyperglycemia per se does not adversely affect uteroplacental blood flow of a pregnant diabetic woman,[184,185] indicating that the increased supply of nutrients to the fetus is not affected by flow changes in placental perfusion.

Maternal hyperglycemia results in elevated fetal glucose concentrations, which in turn stimulate fetal insulin production and secretion, promoting accelerated fetal growth.[186] Accelerated fetal growth has been associated with increased GLUT1 in the trophoblast in type 1

diabetes,[187] but not in gestational diabetes mellitus.[188] Furthermore, the GLUT3 transporter isoform is sensitive to ambient glucose concentrations, increasing in expression in hyperglycemic states observed in diabetic pregnancies. In vivo studies have demonstrated that maternal hyperglycemia induces a fourfold increase in placental GLUT3 mRNA and protein expressions, perhaps thereby enhancing glucose supply to the fetoplacental unit.[189] An additional interesting observation of the human diabetic placenta is the development of increased glycogen deposition, probably occurring after fetal glycogen stores in liver and muscle are filled.[168] Placental glycogen deposition may initially modulate glucose supply to the fetus, thereby "protecting" the fetus from excessive hyperglycemia.

Amino acids also contribute essential substrates of nitrogen and carbon for fetal growth. Amino acids promote pancreatic growth and development and are potent stimulators of insulin secretion, contributing to the direct effect of amino acids on fetal protein accretion and growth. Placental transport capacity for amino acids is variable in diabetic pregnancies. System A has been reported as being reduced.[190,191] More recent studies, however, indicate that diabetes in pregnancy is associated with an increased system A activity in the maternal facing membrane of the trophoblast, independent of fetal overgrowth, though System A activity is not changed in normal pregnancies with LGA fetuses.[192] Leucine transport also is increased in pregnancies complicated by diabetes. Thus, the increases in System A activity contribute to increased uptake of several essential amino acids, contributing to increased amino acid metabolism and growth in the placenta as well as the fetus.[192]

The hormonal environment associated with macrosomia

Most macrosomia occurs in fetuses of diabetic mothers. In these fetuses, maternal hyperglycemia produces fetal hyperglycemia, which in turn promotes fetal insulin production and secretion. The resulting fetal hyperinsulinemia is responsible for increased fuel utilization and growth.[193,194] In pregnant diabetic women, poor maternal glucose control resulting in hyperglycemia predicts fetal macrosomia, and during the second and third trimesters of pregnancy, postprandial maternal plasma glucose concentrations show a strong, positive relationship with birth weight.[40] In addition, studies of macrosomic newborns have shown strong correlations between fetal plasma insulin, glucose and amniotic C-peptide concentrations, and fetal body fat content. These findings indicate that excessive fetal fat deposition is the result of glucose-driven elevated fetal insulin concentrations. Of additional interest are separate findings reporting strong correlations between maternal C-peptide levels and in utero fetal growth,[195] as well as between maternal serum triglycerides in late gestation and newborn weight.[196] Maternal fasting triglyceride levels are significantly increased during weeks 24–32 of gestation and are positively correlated with newborn weight. Those patients with fasting triglyceride concentrations above the 75th percentile are at significant risk for producing an LGA fetus, independently of maternal BMI, weight gain, and plasma glucose levels.[196]

Both insulin-like growth factor I and II [IGF-I and IGF-II] concentrations are increased in cord blood and amniotic fluid samples collected from macrosomic newborns [197,198] and IGF-I concentrations are strongly correlated with birth weight.[199] Also, the IGF binding protein, IGFBP-1, demonstrates a strongly negative correlation with birth weight and is significantly reduced in macrosomic newborns.[198] Leptin is another hormone recently associated with fetal macrosomia, it is secreted primarily from adipose tissue,[200] but also from the placenta of several species.[199–205] The expression and secretion of fetal leptin are directly related to fatel body fat content (adipose tissue mass and adipocyte size),[206] indicating that its production is related to fetal nutritional state. Several investigators have reported that umbilical cord leptin is highly associated with fetal macrosomia.[199,207] The leptin gene appears to be regulated by factors such as insulin; thus maternal hyperglycemia and hypertriglyceridemia directly contribute to fetal hyperleptinemia in the presence of fetal hyperinsulinemia.[208]

REFERENCES

1 Ananth, C. V., Wen, S. W. Trends in fetal growth among singleton gestations in the United States and Canada, 1985 through 1998. *Semin. Perinato.* 2002;**26**:260–7.

2 Ananth, C. V., Demissie, K., Kramer, M. S., Vintzileos, A. M. Small-for-gestational-age births among black and white women: temporal trends in the United States. *Am. J. Public Health* 2003;**93**:577–9.

3 Shelley-Jones, D. C., Beischer, N. A., Sheedy, M. T., Walstab, J. E. Excessive birth weight and maternal glucose tolerance – a 19-year review. *Aust. N. Z. J. Obstet. Gynaecol.* 1992;**32**:318–24.

4 Martin, J. A., Hamilton, B. E., Ventura, S. J. Births: preliminary data for 2000. *Natl Vital Stat Rep* 2001;**49**:1–20.

5 Scherjon, S., Briet, J., Oosting, H., Kok, J. The discrepancy betweens maturation of visual-evoked potentials and cognitive outcome at five years in very preterm infants with and without hemodynamic signs of fetal brain-sparing. *Pediatrics* 2000;**105**:385–391.

6 Ventura, S. J., Martin, J. A., Curtin, S. C., Menacker, F., Hamilton, B. E. Births: final data for 1999. *Natl Vital Stat. Rep.* 2001;**49**:1–100.

7 Mondestin, M. A., Ananth, C. V., Smulian, J. C., Vintzileos, A. M. Birth weight and fetal death in the United States: the effect of maternal diabetes during pregnancy. *Am. J. Obstet. Gynecol.* 2002;**187**:922–26.

8 Lackman, F., Capewell, V., Richardson, B., daSilva, O., Gagnon, R. The risks of spontaneous preterm delivery and perinatal mortality in relation to size at birth according to fetal versus neonatal growth standards. *Am. J. Obstet. Gynecol.* 2001;**184**:946–53.

9 Ghidini, A. Idiopathic fetal growth restriction: a pathophysiologic approach. *Obstet. Gynecol. Surv.* 1996;**51**:376–82.

10 Economides, D. L., Nicolaides, K. H., Campbell, S. Relation between maternal-to-fetal blood glucose gradient and uterine and umbilical Doppler blood flow measurements. *Br. J. of Obstet. Gynaecol.* 1990;**97**:543–44.

11 Marconi, A. M., Cetin, I., Ferrazzi, E. *et al.* Lactate metabolism in normal and growth-retarded human fetuses. *Pediatr. Res.* 1990;**28**:652–6.

12 Marconi, A. M., Paolini, C., Buscaglia, M. *et al.* The impact of gestational age and fetal growth on the maternal-fetal glucose concentration difference. *Obstet.Gynecol.* 1996;**87**:937–42.

13 Barker, D. J. The fetal origins of coronary heart disease. *Acta Paediatrica* 1997; (Suppl.) **422**:78–82.

14 Vickers, M. H., Breier, B. H., Cutfield, W. S., Hofman, P. L., Gluckman, P. D. Fetal origins of hyperphagia, obesity, and hypertension and postnatal amplification by hypercaloric nutrition. *Am. J. Physiol. Endocrino. Metab.* 2000;**279**:E83–87.

15 Barker, D. J., Hales, C. N., Fall, C. H. *et al.* Type 2 (non-insulin-dependent) diabetes mellitus, hypertension and hyperlipidaemia (syndrome X): relation to reduced fetal growth. *Diabetologia* 1993;**36**:62–7.

16 Barker, D. J. Fetal programming of coronary heart disease. *Trends Endocrinol. Metab.* 2002;**13**:364–8.

17 Barker, D. J. Intrauterine programming of adult disease. *Molec. Med. Today* 1995;**1**:418–23.

18 Roseboom, T. J., van der Meulen, J. H., Osmond, C. *et al.* Coronary heart disease after prenatal exposure to the Dutch famine, 1944–45. *Heart* 2000;**84**:595–8.

19 Scherjon, S. A., Oosting, H., Smolders-DeHaas, H., Zondervan, H. A., Kok, J. H. Neurodevelopmental outcome at three years of age after fetal 'brain-sparing'. *Early Hum. Dev.* 1998;**52**:67–79.

20 Buchanan, T. A., Metzger, B. E., Freinkel, N., Bergman, R. N. Insulin sensitivity and β-cell responsiveness to glucose during late pregnancy in lean and moderately obese women with normal glucose tolerance or mild gestational diabetes. *Am. J. Obstet. Gynecol.* 1990;**162**:1008–14.

21 Ventura, S. J., Martin, J. A., Curtin, S. C., Mathews, T. J. Births: final data for 1997. *Natl Vital Stat. Rep.* 1999;**47**:1–96.

22 Gluckman, P. D., Morel, P. C., Ambler, G. R. *et al.* Elevating maternal insulin-like growth factor-I in mice and rats alters the pattern of fetal growth by removing maternal constraint. *J. Endocrinol.* 1992;**134**:R1–3.

23 Battaglia, F. C. Clinical studies linking fetal velocimetry, blood flow and placental transport in pregnancies complicated by intrauterine growth retardation (IUGR). *Trans. Am. Clin. Climatol. Assoc.* 2003;**114**:305–13.

24 Arbeille, P. Fetal arterial Doppler-IUGR and hypoxia. *Eur. J. Obstet. Gynecol. Reprod. Biol.* 1997;**75**:51–3.

25 Detti, L., Akiyama, M., Mari, G. Doppler blood flow in obstetrics. *Curr. Opin. Obstet. Gynecol.* 2002;**14**:587–93.

26 Krampl, E., Lees, C., Bland, J. M. *et al.* Fetal Doppler velocimetry at high altitude. *Ultrasound Obstet. Gynecol.* 2001;**18**:329–34.

27 Pardi, G., Cetin, I., Marconi, A. M. *et al.* Diagnostic value of blood sampling in fetuses with growth retardation. *N. Eng. J. Med.* 1993;**328**:692–6.

28 Rigano, S., Bozzo, M., Ferrazzi, E. *et al.* Early and persistent reduction in umbilical vein blood flow in the growth-restricted fetus: a longitudinal study. *Am. J. Obstet. Gynecol.* 2001;**185**:834–8.

29 Trudinger, B. J., Giles, W. B., Cook, C. M., Bombardieri, J. Collins, L. Fetal umbilical artery flow velocity waveforms and placental resistance: clinical significance. *Br. J. Obstet. Gynaecol.* 1985;**92**:23–30.

30 Gagnon, R., Johnston, L., Murotsuki, J. Fetal placental embolization in the late-gestation ovine fetus: alterations in umbilical blood flow and fetal heart rate patterns. *Am. J. Obstet. Gynecol.* 1996;**175**:63–72.

31 Lubchenco, L. O., Hansman, C., Dressler, M., Boyd, E. Intrauterine growth as estimated from liveborn birth-weight data at 24 to 42 weeks of gestation. *Pediatrics* 1963;**32**:793–800.

32 Lubchenco, L. O., Horner, F. A., Reed, L. H. *et al.* Sequelae of premature birth. Evaluation of premature infants of low birth weights at ten years of age. *Am. J. Dis. Child.* 1963;**106**:101–15.

33 Battaglia, F. C., Lubchenco, L. O. A practical classification of newborn infants by weight and gestational age. *J. Pediatr.* 1967;**71**:159–63.

34 Metcoff, J. Fetal growth and maternal nutrition. In Falkner, F., Tanner, J. M., eds. *Human Growth*. New York, NY: Plenum Press; 1985: 333–88.

35 Williams, R. L., Creasy, R. K., Cunningham, G. C. *et al.* Fetal growth and perinatal viability in California. *Obstet. Gynecol.* 1982;**59**:624–32.

36 Williams, R. L., Chen, P. M. Identifying the sources of the recent decline in perinatal mortality rates in California. *N. Eng. J. Med.* 1982;**306**:207–14.

37 Nahum, G. G., Stanislaw, H., Huffaker, B. J. Fetal weight gain at term: linear with minimal dependence on maternal obesity. *Am. J. Obstet. Gynecol.* 1995;**172**:1387–94.

38 Sparks, J. W. Human intrauterine growth and nutrient accretion. *Semin. Perinatol.* 1984;**8**:74–93.

39 Sparks, J. W., Girard, J. R., Battaglia, F. C. An estimate of the caloric requirements of the human fetus. *Biol. Neonate* 1980;**38**:113–19.

40 Moore, T. R. Fetal growth in diabetic pregnancy. *Clin. Obstet. Gynecol.* 1997;**40**:771–86.

41 Ong, S., Lash, G., Baker, P. N. Angiogenesis and placental growth in normal and compromised pregnancies. *Best Pract. Res. Clin. Obstet. Gynaecol.* 2000;**14**:969–80.

42 Regnault, T. R. H., Galan, H. L., Parker, T. A., Anthony, R. V. Placental development in normal and compromised pregnancies – a review. *Placenta* 2002;**23**(Suppl. A, Trophoblast Research 16):S119–29.

43 Wladimiroff, J. W., vd Wijngaard, J. A., Degani, S. *et al.* Cerebral and umbilical arterial blood flow velocity waveforms in normal and growth-retarded pregnancies. *Obstet. Gynecol.* 1987;**69**:705–9.

44 Wladimiroff, J. W. A review of the etiology, diagnostic techniques and management of IUGR, and the clinical application of Doppler in the assessment of placental blood flow. *J. Perinat. Med.* 1991;**19**:11–13.

45 Wladimiroff, J. W., Stewart, P. A., Groenenberg, I. A. Fetal Doppler studies in normal and complicated pregnancies. *J. Perinat. Med.* 1991;**19** (Suppl. 1):288–92.

46 Tchirikov, M., Rybakowski, C., Huneke, B., Schroder, H. J. Blood flow through the ductus venosus in singleton and multifetal pregnancies and in fetuses with intrauterine growth retardation. *Am. J. Obstet. Gynecol.* 1998;**178**:943–9.

47 Jansson, T., Ylven, K., Wennergren, M., Powell, T. L. Glucose transport and system A activity in syncytiotrophoblast microvillous and basal plasma membranes in intrauterine growth restriction. *Placenta* 2002;**23**:392–9.

48 Kingdom, J., Huppertz, B., Seaward, G., Kaufmann, P. Development of the placental villous tree and its consequences for fetal growth. *Eur. J. Obstet. Gynecol. Reprod. Biol.* 2000;**92**:35–43.

49 Ahmed, A., Perkins, J. Angiogenesis and intrauterine growth restriction. *Best Pract. Res. Clin. Obstet. Gynaecol.* 2000;**14**:981–98.

50 Benirschke, K., Kaufmann, P. Architecture of normal villous trees. *Pathology of the Human Placenta*. London: Springer Verlag, 2000:116–54.

51 Ali, K. Z., Burton, G. J., Morad, N., Ali, M. E. Does hypercapillarization influence the branching pattern of terminal villi in the human placenta at high altitude? *Placenta* 1996;**17**:677–82.

52 Kingdom, J. C. P., Kaufmann, P. Oxygen and placental villous development – origins of fetal hypoxia. *Placenta* 1997;**18**:613–21.

53 Zamudio, S., Moore, L. G. Altitude and fetal growth: current knowledge and future directions. *Ultrasound Obstet. Gynecol.* 2000;**16**:6–8.

54 Giussani, D. A., Phillips, P. S., Anstee, S., Barker, D. J. Effects of altitude versus economic status on birth weight and body shape at birth. *Pediatr. Res.* 2001;**49**:490–4.

55 Garcia, F. C., Stiffel, V. M., Gilbert, R. D. Effects of long-term high-altitude hypoxia on isolated fetal ovine coronary arteries. *J. Soc. Gynecol. Invest.* 2000;**7**:211–17.

56 Krampl, E., Lees, C., Bland, J. M. *et al.* Fetal biometry at 4300 m compared to sea level in Peru. *Ultrasound Obstet. Gynecol.* 2000;**16**:9–18.

57 Galan, H. L., Rigano, S., Chyu, J. *et al.* Comparison of low- and high-altitude Doppler velocimetry in the peripheral and central circulations of normal fetuses. *Am. J. Obstet. Gynecol.* 2000;**183**:1158–61.

58 Mayhew, T. M. Thinning of the intervascular tissue layers of the human placenta is an adaptive response to passive diffusion in vivo and may help to predict the origins of fetal hypoxia. *Eur. J. Obstet. Gynecol. Reprod. Biol.* 1998;**81**:101–9.

59 Espinoza, J., Sebire, N. J., McAuliffe, F., Krampl, E., Nicolaides, K. H. Placental villus morphology in relation to maternal hypoxia at high altitude. *Placenta* 2001;**22**:606–8.

60 Zhang, E. G., Burton, G. J., Smith, S. K., Charnock-Jones, D. S. Placental vessel adaptation during gestation and to high altitude: changes in diameter and perivascular cell coverage. *Placenta* 2002;**23**:751–62.

61 Xiong, X., Mayes, D., Demianczuk, N. *et al.* Impact of pregnancy-induced hypertension on fetal growth. *Am. J. Obstet. Gynecol.* 1999;**180**(1 Pt 1):207–13.

62 Eskenazi, B., Fenster, L., Sidney, S., Elkin, E. P. Fetal growth retardation in infants of multiparous and nulliparous women with preeclampsia. *Am. J. Obstet. Gynecol.* 1993;**169**:1112–18.

63 Lenfant, C. Working group report on high blood pressure in pregnancy. *J. Clin. Hypertens. (Greenwich)* 2001;**3**:75–88.

64 Rasmussen, S., Irgens, L. M. Fetal growth and body proportion in preeclampsia. *Obstet. Gynecol.* 2003;**101**:575–83.

65 Gratton, R. J., Asano, H., Han, V. K. The regional expression of insulin-like growth factor II (IGF-II) and insulin-like growth factor binding protein-1 (IGFBP-1) in the placentae of women with pre-eclampsia. *Placenta* 2002;**23**:303–10.

66 Teasdale, F. Histomorphometry of the human placenta in pre-eclampsia associated with severe intrauterine growth retardation. *Placenta* 1987;**8**:119–28.

67 Mayhew, T. M., Ohadike, C., Baker, P. N. *et al.* Stereological investigation of placental morphology in pregnancies complicated by pre-eclampsia with and without intrauterine growth restriction. *Placenta* 2003;**24**:219–26.

68 Alfaidy, N., Gupta, S., DeMarco, C., Caniggia, I., Challis, J. R. Oxygen regulation of placental 11 beta-hydroxysteroid dehydrogenase 2: physiological and pathological implications. *J. Clin. Endocrinol. Metab.* 2002;**87**:4797–805.

69 Challier, J. C., Carbillon, L., Kacemi, A. *et al.* Characterization of first trimester human fetal placental vessels using immunocytochemical markers. *Cell Mol. Biol. (Noisy-le-grand)* 2001;**47** Online Pub:OL79–OL87.

70 Carbillon, L., Perrot, N., Uzan, M., Uzan, S. Doppler ultrasonography and implantation: a critical review. *Fetal Diagn. Ther.* 2001;**16**:327–32.

71 Waddell, B. J., Hisheh, S., Dharmarajan, A. M., Burton, P. J. Apoptosis in rat placenta is zone-dependent and stimulated by glucocorticoids. *Biol. Reprod.* 2000;**63**:1913–17.

72 Ito, M., Itakura, A., Ohno, Y. *et al.* Possible activation of the renin-angiotensin system in the feto-placental unit in preeclampsia. *J. Clin. Endocrinol. Metab.* 2002;**87**:1871–78.

73 Regnault, T. R. H., de Vrijer, B., Galan, H. L. *et al.* The relationship between transplacental O_2 diffusion and placental expression of PlGF, VEGF and their receptors in a placental insufficiency model of fetal growth restriction. *J. Physiol.* 2003;**550**:641–56.

74 Krebs, C., Macara, L. M., Leiser, R. *et al.* Intrauterine growth restriction with absent end-diastolic flow velocity in the umbilical artery is associated with maldevelopment of the placental terminal villous tree. *Am. J. Obstet. Gynecol.* 1996;**175**:1534–42.

75 Jackson, M. R., Walsh, A. J., Morrow, R. J. *et al.* Reduced placental villous tree elaboration in small-for-gestational-age pregnancies: relationship with umbilical artery Doppler waveforms. *Am. J. Obstet. Gynecol.* 1995;**172**:518–25.

76 Giles, W. B., Trudinger, B. J., Baird, P. J. Fetal umbilical artery flow velocity waveforms and placental resistance: pathological correlation. *Br. J. Obstet. Gynaecol.* 1985;**92**:31–8.

77 Trudinger, B. J., Stevens, D., Connelly, A. *et al.* Umbilical artery flow velocity waveforms and placental resistance: the effects of embolization of the umbilical circulation. *Am. J. Obstet. Gynecol.* 1987;**157**:1443–8.

78 Gagnon, R. Placental insufficiency and its consequences. *Eur. J. Obstet. Gynecol. Reprod. Biol.* 2003;**110** (Suppl. 1):S99–107.

79 Morrow, R. J., Adamson, S. L., Bull, S. B., Ritchie, J. W. Effect of placental embolization on the umbilical arterial velocity waveform in fetal sheep. *Am. J. Obstet. Gynecol.* 1989;**161**:1055–60.

80 Macara, L., Kingdom, J. C., Kohnen, G. *et al.* Elaboration of stem villous vessels in growth restricted pregnancies with abnormal umbilical artery Doppler waveforms. *Br. J. Obstet. Gynaecol.* 1995;**102**:807–12.

81 Ansari, T., Fenlon, S., Pasha, S. *et al.* Morphometric assessment of the oxygen diffusion conductance in placentae from pregnancies complicated by intra-uterine growth restriction. *Placenta* 2003;**24**:618–26.

82 Jansson, T. Amino acid transporters in the human placenta. *Pediatr. Res.* 2001;**49**:141–7.

83 Sibley, C. P., Coan, P. M., Ferguson-Smith, A. C. *et al.* Placental-specific insulin-like growth factor 2 (Igf2) regulates the diffusional exchange characteristics of the mouse placenta. *Proc. Natl. Acad. Sci. USA* 2004;**101**:8204–8.

84 Regnault, T. R. H., de Vrijer, B., Battaglia, F. C. Transport and metabolism of amino acids in placenta. *Endocrine* 2003;**19**:23–41.

85 Meschia, G., Cotter, J. R., Breathnach, C. S., Barron, D. H. The diffusibility of oxygen across the sheep placenta. *Q. J. Exper. Physiol. Cognate Med. Sci.* 1965;**50**:466–80.

86 Meschia, G., Battaglia, F. C., Bruns, P. D. Theoretical and experimental study of transplacental diffusion. *J. Appl. Physiol.* 1967;**22**:1171–8.

87 Mayhew, T. M., Jackson, M. R., Haas, J. D. Microscopical morphology of the human placenta and its effects on oxygen diffusion: a morphometric model. *Placenta* 1986;**7**:121–31.

88 Wilkening, R. B., Meschia, G. Effect of occluding one umbilical artery on placental oxygen transport. *Am. J. Physiol.* 1991;**260**:H1319–25.

89 Pardi, G., Cetin, I., Marconi, A. M. *et al.* Venous drainage of the human uterus: respiratory gas studies in normal and fetal growth-retarded pregnancies. *Am. J. Obstet. Gynecol.* 1992;**166**:699–706.

90 Jackson, M. R., Mayhew, T. M., Boyd, P. A. Quantitative description of the elaboration and maturation of villi from 10 weeks of gestation to term. *Placenta* 1992;**13**:357–70.

91 Teasdale, F., Jean-Jacques, G. Morphometric evaluation of the microvillous surface enlargement factor in the human placenta from mid-gestation to term. *Placenta* 1985;**6**:375–81.

92 Woods, D. L., Malan, A. F., Heese, H. D. Placental size of small-for-gestational-age infants at term. *Early Hum. Dev.* 1982;**7**:11–15.

93 Woods, D. L., Rip, M. R. Placental villous surface area of light-for-dates infants at term. *Early Hum. Dev.* 1987;**15**:113–17.

94 Constancia, M., Hemberger, M., Hughes, J. *et al.* Placental-specific IGF-II is a major modulator of placental and fetal growth. *Nature* 2002;**417**:945–8.

95 Economides, D. L., Nicolaides, K. H. Blood glucose and oxygen tension levels in small-for-gestational-age fetuses. *Am. J. Obstet. Gynecol.* 1989;**160**:385–9.

96 Nieto-Diaz, A., Villar, J., Matorras-Weinig, R., Valenzuela-Ruiz, P. Intrauterine growth retardation at term: association between anthropometric and endocrine parameters. *Acta Obstetric. Gynecolog. Scand.* 1996;**75**:127–31.

97 Thureen, P. J., Trembler, K. A., Meschia, G., Makowski, E. L., Wilkening, R. B. Placental glucose transport in heat-induced fetal growth retardation. *Am. J. Physiol.* 1992;**263**:R578–85.

98 Limesand, S. W., Regnault, T. R., Hay, W. W., J.r. Characterization of glucose transporter 8 (GLUT8) in the ovine placenta of normal and growth restricted fetuses. *Placenta* 2004;**25**: 70–7.

99 Jansson, T., Wennergren, M., Illsley, N. P. Glucose transporter protein expression in human placenta throughout gestation and in intrauterine growth retardation. *J. Clin. Endocrinol. Metab.* 1993;**77**:1554–62.

100 Kainulainen, H., Jarvinen, T., Heinonen, P. K. Placental glucose transporters in fetal intrauterine growth retardation and macrosomia. *Gynecol. Obstet. Invest.* 1997;**44**:89–92.

101 Reid, G. J., Lane, R. H., Flozak, A. S., Simmons, R. A. Placental expression of glucose transporter proteins 1 and 3 in growth-restricted fetal rats. *Am. J. Obstet. Gynecol.* 1999;**180**:1017–23.

102 Wallace, J. M., Bourke, D. A., Aitken, R. P., Milne, J. S., Hay, W. W., Jr. Placental glucose transport in growth-restricted pregnancies induced by overnourishing adolescent sheep. *J. Physiol.* 2003;**547**:85–94.

103 Teasdale, F., Jean-Jacques, G. Intrauterine growth retardation: morphometry of the microvillous membrane of the human placenta. *Placenta* 1988;**9**:47–55.

104 Hay, W. W., J., Meznarich, H. K. Effect of maternal glucose concentration on uteroplacental glucose concentration and transfer in pregnant sheep. *Proc. Soc. Exper. Biol. Med.* 1989;**190**:63–9.

105 Molina, R. D., Meschia, G., Battaglia, F. C., Hay, W. W. J. Gestational maturation of placental glucose transfer capacity in sheep. *Am. J. Physiol.* 1991;**261**:R697–704.

106 Joost, H. G., Bell, G. I., Best, J. D. *et al.* Nomenclature of the GLUT/SLC2A family of sugar/polyol transport facilitators. *Am. J. Physiol. Endocrinol. Metab.* 2002;**282**:E974–6.

107 Mueckler, M. Facilitative glucose transporters. *Eur. J. Biochem.* 1994;**219**:713–25.

108 Barros, L. F., Yudilevich, D. L., Jarvis, S. M., Beaumont, N., Baldwin, S. A. Quantitation and immunolocalization of glucose transporters in the human placenta. *Placenta* 1995;**16**:623–33.

109 Hauguel-De Mouzon, S., Challier, J. C., Kacemi, A. *et al.* The GLUT3 glucose transporter isoform is differentially expressed within human placental cell types. *J. Clin. Endocrinol. Metab.* 1997;**82**:2689–94.

110 Xing, A. Y., Challier, J. C., Lepercq, J. *et al.* Unexpected expression of glucose transporter 4 in villous stromal cells of human placenta. *J. Clin. Endocrinol. Metab.* 1998;**83**:4097–101.

111 Gude, N. M., Stevenson, J. L., Rogers, S. *et al.* GLUT12 expression in human placenta in first trimester and term. *Placenta* 2003;**24**:566–70.

112 Currie, M. J., Bassett, N. S., Gluckman, P. D. Ovine glucose transporter-1 and -3: cDNA partial sequences and developmental gene expression in the placenta. *Placenta* 1997;**18**:393–401.

113 Ehrhardt, R. A., Bell, A. W. Developmental increases in glucose transporter concentration in the sheep placenta. *Am. J. Physiol.* 1997;**273**:R1132–41.

114 Devaskar, S. U., Devaskar, U. P., Schroeder, R. E. *et al.* Expression of genes involved in placental glucose uptake and transport in the nonobese diabetic mouse pregnancy. *Am. J. Obstet. Gynecol.* 1994;**171**:1316–23.

115 Das, U. G., Sadiq, H. F., Soares, M. J., Hay, W. W. J., Devaskar, S. U. Time-dependent physiological regulation of rodent and ovine placental glucose transporter (GLUT-1) protein. *Am. J. Physiol.* 1998;**274**:R339–47.

116 Das, U. G., He, J., Ehrhardt, R. A., Hay, W. W., Jr, Devaskar, S. U. Time-dependent physiological regulation of ovine placental GLUT-3 glucose transporter protein. *Am. J. Physiol. Regula. Integrat. Comparat. Physiol.* 2000;**279**:R2252–61.

117 Hahn, T., Barth, S., Graf, R. *et al.* Placental glucose transporter expression is regulated by glucocorticoids. *J. Clin. Endocrinol. Metab.* 1999;**84**:1445–52.

118 Gaither, K., Quraishi, A. N., Illsley, N. P. Diabetes alters the expression and activity of the human placental GLUT1 glucose transporter. *J. Clin. Endocrinol. Metab.* 1999;**84**:695–701.

119 Sciullo, E., Cardellini, G., Baroni, M. G. *et al.* Glucose transporter (Glut1, Glut3) mRNA in human placenta of diabetic and non-diabetic pregnancies. *Early Pregnancy* 1997;**3**:172–82.

120 Esterman, A., Greco, M. A., Mitani, Y. *et al.* The effect of hypoxia on human trophoblast in culture: morphology, glucose transport and metabolism. *Placenta* 1997;**18**:129–36.

121 Pickard, M. R., Sinha, A. K., Ogilvie, L. M. *et al.* Maternal hypothyroxinemia influences glucose transporter expression in fetal brain and placenta. *J. Endocrinol.* 1999;**163**:385–94.

122 DiGiacomo, J. E., Hay, W. W. Jr. Placental-fetal glucose exchange and placental glucose consumption in pregnant sheep. *Am. J. Physiol.* 1990;**258**:E360–7.

123 Kudo, Y., Boyd, C. A. Human placental amino acid transporter genes: expression and function. *Reproduction* 2002;**124**:593–600.

124 Cetin, I., Ronzoni, S., Marconi, A. M. *et al.* Maternal concentrations and fetal-maternal concentration differences of plasma amino acids in normal and intrauterine growth-restricted pregnancies. *Am. J. Obstet. Gynecol.* 1996;**174**:1575–83.

125 Economides, D. L., Nicolaides, K. H., Gahl, W. A., Bernardini, I., Evans, M. I. Plasma amino acids in appropriate- and small-for-gestational-age fetuses. *Am. J. Obstet. Gynecol.* 1989;**161**:1219–27.

126 Cetin, I., Marconi, A. M., Bozzetti, P. *et al.* Umbilical amino acid concentrations in appropriate and small for gestational age infants: a biochemical difference present in utero. *Am. J. Obstet. Gynecol.* 1988;**158**:120–6.

127 Paolini, C. L., Marconi, A. M., Ronzoni, S. *et al.* Placental transport of leucine, phenylalanine, glycine, and proline in intrauterine growth-restricted pregnancies. *J. Clin. Endocrinol. Metab.* 2001;**86**:5427–32.

128 Dicke, J. M., Henderson, G. I. Placental amino acid uptake in normal and complicated pregnancies. *Am. J. Med. Sci.* 1988;**295**:223–7.

129 Glazier, J. D., Cetin, I., Perugino, G. *et al.* Association between the activity of the system A amino acid transporter in the microvillous plasma membrane of the human placenta and severity of fetal compromise in intrauterine growth restriction. *Pediatr. Res.* 1997;**42**:514–9.

130 Mahendran, D., Donnai, P., Glazier, J. D. *et al.* Amino acid (system A) transporter activity in microvillous membrane vesicles from the placentas of appropriate and small for gestational age babies. *Pediatr. Res.* 1993;**34**:661–5.

131 Johnson, L. W., Smith, C. H. Neutral amino acid transport systems of microvillous membrane of human placenta. *Am. J. Physiol.* 1988;**254**:C773–80.

132 Hoeltzli, S. D., Smith, C. H. Alanine transport systems in isolated basal plasma membrane of human placenta. *Am. J. Physiol.* 1989;**256**:C630–7.

133 Novak, D. A., Beveridge, M. J., Malandro, M., Seo, J. Ontogeny of amino acid transport system A in rat placenta. *Placenta* 1996;**17**:643–51.

134 Low, S. Y., Rennie, M. J., Taylor, P. M. Sodium-dependent glutamate transport in cultured rat myotubes increases after glutamine deprivation. *FASEB J.* 1994;**8**:127–31.

135 Taylor, P. M., Kaur, S., Mackenzie, B., Peter, G. J. Amino-acid-dependent modulation of amino acid transport in *Xenopus laevis* oocytes. *J. Exper. Biol.* 1996;**199**:923–31.

136 Malandro, M. S., Beveridge, M. J., Novak, D. A., Kilberg, M. S. Rat placental amino acid transport after protein-deprivation-induced intrauterine growth retardation. *Biochem. Soc. Trans.* 1996;**24**:839–43.

137 Cramer, S., Beveridge, M., Kilberg, M., Novak, D. Physiological importance of system A-mediated amino acid transport to rat fetal development. *Am. J. Physiol. Cell Physiol.* 2002;**282**:C153–60.

138 Hoeltzli, S. D., Kelley, L. K., Moe, A. J., Smith, C. H. Anionic amino acid transport systems in isolated basal plasma membrane of human placenta. *Am. J. Physiol.* 1990;**259**:C47–55.

139 Malandro, M. S., Beveridge, M. J., Kilberg, M. S., Novak, D. A. Effect of low-protein diet-induced intrauterine growth retardation on rat placental amino acid transport. *Am. J. Physiol.* 1996;**271**:C295–303.

140 Moe, A., Smith, C. Anionic amino acid uptake by microvillous membrane vesicles from human placenta. *Am. J. Physiol.* 1989;**257**:C1005–11.

141 Novak, D., Quiggle, F., Artime, C., Beveridge, M. Regulation of glutamate transport and transport proteins in a placental cell line. *Am. J. Physiol. Cell Physiol.* 2001;**281**:C1014–22.

142 Novak, D. A., Beveridge, M. J. Glutamine transport in human and rat placenta. *Placenta* 1997;**18**:379–86.

143 Matthews, J. C., Beveridge, M. J., Malandro, M. S. *et al.* Activity and protein localization of multiple glutamate transporters in gestation day 14 vs. day 20 rat placenta. *Am. J. Physiol.* 1998;**274**:C603–14.

144 Dancis, J., Money, W. L., Springer, D., Levitz, M. Transport of amino acids by placenta. *Am. J. Obstet. Gynecol.* 1968;**101**:820–9.

145 Fairman, W. A., Vandenberg, R. J., Arriza, J. L., Kavanaugh, M. P., Amara, S. G. An excitatory amino-acid transporter with properties of a ligand-gated chloride channel. *Nature* 1995;**375**:599–603.

146 Nakayama, T., Kawakami, H., Tanaka, K., Nakamura, S. Expression of three glutamate transporter subtype mRNAs in human brain regions and peripheral tissues. *Molec. Brain Res.* 1996;**36**:189–92.

147 Matthews, J. C., Beveridge, M. J., Dialynas, E. *et al.* Placental anionic and cationic amino acid transporter expression in growth hormone overexpressing and null IGF-II or null IGF-I receptor mice. *Placenta* 1999;**20**:639–50.

148 Regnault, T. R. H., de Vrijer, B., Trembler, K. A. *et al.* The umbilical uptake of glutamate in IUGR pregnancies. *J. Perinatal Med.* 2001;**29**:546.

149 Ayuk, P. T., Sibley, C., Donnai, P., D'Souza, S., Glazier, J. Development and polarization of cationic amino acid transporters and regulators in the human placenta. *Am. J. Physiol.* 2000;**278**:c1162–71.

150 Kamath, S. G., Furesz, T. C., Way, B. A., Smith, C. H. Identification of three cationic amino acid transporters in placental trophoblast: cloning, expression, and characterization of hCAT-1. *J. Membrane Biol.* 1999;**171**:55–62.

151 Malandro, M. S., Beveridge, M. J., Kilberg, M. S., Novak, D. A. Effect of low-protein diet-induced intrauterine growth retardation on rat placental amino acid transport. *Am. J. Physiol.* 1996;**271**:C295–303.

152 Eleno, N., Deves, R., Boyd, C. A. Membrane potential dependence of the kinetics of cationic amino acid transport systems in human placenta. *J. Physiol.* 1994;**479**:291–300.

153 Malandro, M. S., Beveridge, M. J., Kilberg, M. S., Novak, D. A. Ontogeny of cationic amino acid transport systems in rat placenta. *Am. J. Physiol.* 1994;**267**:C804–11.

154 Furesz, T. C., Moe, A. J., Smith, C. H. Two cationic amino acid transport systems in human placental basal plasma membranes. *Am. J. Physiol.* 1991;**261**:C246–52.

155 Ayuk, P. T., Theophanous, D., D'Souza, S. W., Sibley, C., Glazier, J. D. L-Arginine transport by the microvillous plasma membrane of the syncytiotrophoblast from human placenta in relation to nitric oxide production: Effects of gestation, preclampsia, and intrauterine growth restriction. *J. Clin. Endocrinol. Metab.* 2002;**87**:747–51.

156 Jansson, T., Scholtbach, V., Powell, T. L. Placental transport of leucine and lysine is reduced in intrauterine growth restriction. *Pediatr. Res.* 1998;**44**:532–7.

157 Furesz, T. C., Moe, A. J., Smith, C. H. Lysine uptake by human placental microvillous membrane: comparison of system y+ with basal membrane. *Am. J. Physiol.* 1995;**268**:C755–61.

158 Bell, A. W., Wilkening, R. B., Meschia, G. Some aspects of placental function in chronically heat-stressed ewes. *J. Dev. Physiol.* 1987;**9**:17–29.

159 Bell, A. W., McBride, B. W., Slepetis, R., Early, R. J., Currie, W. B. Chronic heat stress and prenatal development in sheep: I. Conceptus growth and maternal plasma hormones and metabolites. *J. Animal Sci.* 1989;**67**:3289–99.

160 Karl, P. I., Fisher, S. E. Taurine transport by microvillous membrane vesicles and the perfused cotyledon of the human placenta. *Am. J. Physiol.* 1990;**258**:C443–51.

161 Miyamoto, Y., Balkovetz, D. F., Leibach, F. H., Mahesh, V. B., Ganapathy, V. Na+ + Cl− − gradient-driven, high-affinity, uphill transport of taurine in human placental brush-border membrane vesicles. *FEBS Letters* 1988;**231**:263–7.

162 Moyer, M. S., Insler, N., Dumaswala, R. The role of chloride in taurine transport across the human placental brush-border membrane. *Biochim. Biophys. Acta* 1992;**1109**:74–80.

163 Norberg, S., Powell, T. L., Jansson, T. Intrauterine growth restriction is associated with a reduced activity of placental taurine transporters. *Pediatr. Res.* 1998;**44**:233–8.

164 Kulanthaivel, P., Leibach, F. H., Mahesh, V. B., Ganapathy, V. Tyrosine residues are essential for the activity of the human placental taurine transporter. *Biochim. Biophys. Acta* 1989;**985**:139–46.

165 Kulanthaivel, P., Cool, D. R., Ramamoorthy, S. *et al.* Transport of taurine and its regulation by protein kinase C in the JAR human placental choriocarcinoma cell line. *Biochem. J.* 1991;**277**:53–8.

166 Roos, S., Powell, T. L., Jansson, T. The human placental taurine transporter in uncomplicated and IUGR pregnancies: cellular localization, protein expression and regulation. *Am. J. Physiol. Regul. Integr. Comp. Physiol.* 2004;**287**:R886–93.

167 Jimenez-Moleon, J. J., Bueno-Cavanillas, A., Luna-del-Castillo, J. D. *et al.* Impact of different levels of carbohydrate intolerance on neonatal outcomes classically associated with gestational diabetes mellitus. *Eur. J. Obstet. Gynecol. Reprod. Biol.* 2002;**102**:36–41.

168 Desoye, G., Korgun, E. T., Ghaffari-Tabrizi, N., Hahn, T. Is fetal macrosomia in adequately controlled diabetic women the result of a placental defect? – a hypothesis. *J. Maternal-Fetal Neonat. Med.* 2002;**11**:258–61.

169 Ogata, E. S., Sabbagha, R., Metzger, B. E. *et al.* Serial ultrasonography to assess evolving fetal macrosomia. Studies in 23 pregnant diabetic women. *J. Am. Med. Assoc.* 1980;**243**:2405–8.

170 Bernstein, I. M., Goran, M. I., Copeland, K. C. Maternal insulin sensitivity and cord blood peptides: relationships to neonatal size at birth. *Obstet. Gynecol.* 1997;**90**:780–3.

171 Nicolini, U., Hubinont, C., Santolaya, J. *et al.* Maternal-fetal glucose gradient in normal pregnancies and in pregnancies complicated by alloimmunization and fetal growth retardation. *Am. J. Obstet. Gynecol.* 1989;**161**:924–7.

172 Kervran, A., Girard, J. R. Glucose-induced increase of plasma insulin in the rat foetus in utero. *J. Endocrinol.* 1974;**62**:545–51.

173 Aldoretta, P. W., Carver, T. D., Hay, W. W., Jr. Maturation of glucose-stimulated insulin secretion in fetal sheep. *Biol. Neonate* 1998;**73**:375–86.

174 Carver, T. D., Anderson, S. M., Aldoretta, P. W., Hay, W. W., Jr. Effect of low-level basal plus marked "pulsatile" hyperglycemia on insulin secretion in fetal sheep. *Am. J. Physiol.* 1996;**271**:E865–71.

175 Bihoreau, M. T., Ktorza, A., Kervran, A., Picon, L. Effect of gestational hyperglycemia on insulin secretion in vivo and in vitro by fetal rat pancreas. *Am. J. Physiol.* 1986;**251**:E86–91.

176 Eriksson, U. J., Styrud, J. Congenital malformations in diabetic pregnancy: the clinical relevance of experimental animal studies. *Acta Paediatr. Scand. Suppl.* 1985;**320**:72–8.

177 Lepercq, J., Taupin, P., Dubois-Laforgue, D. *et al.* Heterogeneity of fetal growth in type 1 diabetic pregnancy. *Diabetes Metab.* 2001;**27**:339–44.

178 Landon, M. B., Mintz, M. C., Gabbe, S. G. Sonographic evaluation of fetal abdominal growth: predictor of the large-for-gestational-age infant in pregnancies complicated by diabetes mellitus. *Am. J. Obstet. Gynecol.* 1989;**160**:115–21.

179 Reece, E. A., Winn, H. N., Smikle, C. *et al.* Sonographic assessment of growth of the fetal head in diabetic pregnancies compared with normal gestations. *Am. J. Perinatol.* 1990;**7**:18–22.

180 Wong, S. F., Chan, F. Y., Oats, J. J., McIntyre, D. H. Fetal growth spurt and pregestational diabetic pregnancy. *Diabetes Care* 2002;**25**:1681–4.

181 Wong, S. F., Chan, F. Y., Cincotta, R. B., Oats, J. J., McIntyre, H. D. Routine ultrasound screening in diabetic pregnancies. *Ultrasound Obstet. Gynecol.* 2002;**19**:171–6.

182 Mayhew, T. M., Sisley, I. Quantitative studies on the villi, trophoblast and intervillous pores of placentae from women with well-controlled diabetes mellitus. *Placenta* 1998;**19**:371–7.

183 Teasdale, F., Jean-Jacques, G. Morphometry of the microvillous membrane of the human placenta in maternal diabetes mellitus. *Placenta* 1986;**7**:81–8.

184 Salvesen, D. R., Higueras, M. T., Mansur, C. A. *et al.* Placental and fetal Doppler velocimetry in pregnancies complicated by maternal diabetes mellitus. *Am. J. Obstet. Gynecol.* 1993;**168**:645–52.

185 Fadda, G. M., D'Antona, D., Ambrosini, G. *et al.* Placental and fetal pulsatility indices in gestational diabetes mellitus. *J. Reprod. Med.* 2001;**46**:365–70.

186 Pedersen, J. Weight and length at birth of infants of diabetic mothers. *Acta Endocrinol. (Copenh.)* 1954;**16**:330–42.

187 Jansson, T., Wennergren, M., Powell, T. L. Placental glucose transport and GLUT 1 expression in insulin-dependent diabetes. *Am. J. Obstet. Gynecol.* 1999;**180**:163–8.

188 Jansson, T., Ekstrand, Y., Wennergren, M., Powell, T. L. Placental glucose transport in gestational diabetes mellitus. *Am. J. Obstet. Gynecol.* 2001;**184**:111–6.

189 Boileau, P., Mrejen, C., Girard, J., Hauguel-de, M. S. Overexpression of GLUT3 placental glucose transporter in diabetic rats. *J. Clin. Invest.* 1995;**96**:309–17.

190 Godfrey, K. M., Matthews, N., Glazier, J. *et al.* Neutral amino acid uptake by the microvillous plasma membrane of the human placenta is inversely related to fetal size at birth in normal pregnancy. *J. Clin. Endocrinol. Metab.* 1998;**83**:3320–6.

191 Kuruvilla, A. G., D'Souza, S. W., Glazier, J. D. *et al.* Altered activity of the system A amino acid transporter in microvillous membrane vesicles from placentas of macrosomic babies born to diabetic women. *J. Clin. Invest.* 1994;**94**:689–95.

192 Jansson, T., Ekstrand, Y., Bjorn, C., Wennergren, M., Powell, T. L. Alterations in the activity of placental amino acid transporters in pregnancies complicated by diabetes. *Diabetes* 2002;**51**:2214–9.

193 Pedersen, J. Diabetes and pregnancy; blood sugar of newborn infants during fasting and glucose administration. *Nord. Med.* 1952;**47**:1049.

194 Pedersen, J. Course of diabetes during pregnancy. *Acta Endocrinol. (Copenh.)* 1952;**9**:342–64.

195 Valensise, H., Larciprete, G., Vasapollo, B. *et al.* C-peptide and insulin levels at 24–30 weeks' gestation: an increased risk of adverse pregnancy outcomes? *Eur. J. Obstet. Gynecol. Reprod. Biol.* 2002;**103**:130–5.

196 Kitajima, M., Oka, S., Yasuhi, I. *et al.* Maternal serum triglyceride at 24–32 weeks' gestation and newborn weight in nondiabetic women with positive diabetic screens. *Obstet. Gynecol.* 2001;**97**:776–80.

197 Delmis, J., Drazancic, A., Ivanisevic, M., Suchanek, E. Glucose, insulin, HGH and IGF-I levels in maternal serum, amniotic fluid and umbilical venous serum: a comparison between late normal pregnancy and pregnancies complicated with diabetes and fetal growth retardation. *J. Perinat. Med.* 1992;**20**:47–56.

198 Verhaeghe, J., van Bree, R., Van Herck, E. *et al.* C-peptide, insulin-like growth factors I and II, and insulin-like growth factor binding protein-1 in umbilical cord serum: correlations with birth weight. *Am. J. Obstet. Gynecol.* 1993;**169**:89–97.

199 Wiznitzer, A., Furman, B., Zuili, I. *et al.* Cord leptin level and fetal macrosomia. *Obstet. Gynecol.* 2000;**96**:707–13.

200 Margetic, S., Gazzola, C., Pegg, G. G., Hill, R. A. Leptin: a review of its peripheral actions and interactions. *Int. J. Obesity Related Metab. Disord. J. Int. Assoc. Study Obesity* 2002;**26**:1407–33.

201 Masuzaki, H., Ogawa, Y., Sagawa, N. *et al.* Nonadipose tissue production of leptin – leptin as a novel placenta-derived hormone in humans. *Nature Medicine* 1997;**3**:1029–33.

202 Holness, M. J., Munns, M. J., Sugden, M. C. Current concepts concerning the role of leptin in reproductive function. *Mol. Cellul. Endocrinol.* 1999;**157**:11–20.

203 Ashworth, C. J., Hoggard, N., Thomas, L. *et al.* Placental leptin. *Rev. Reprod.* 2000;**5**:18–24.

204 Eckert, J. E., Gatford, K. L., Luxford, B. G., Campbell, R. G., Owens, P. C. Leptin expression in offspring is programmed by nutrition in pregnancy. *J. Endocrinol.* 2000;**165**:R1–6.

205 Jaquet, D., Leger, J., Levy-Marchal, C., Oury, J. F., Czernichow, P. Ontogeny of leptin in human fetuses and newborns: effect of intrauterine growth retardation on serum leptin concentrations. *J. Clin. Endocrinol. Metabol.* 1998;**83**:1243–6.

206 Considine, R. V., Sinha, M. K., Heiman, M. L. *et al.* Serum immunoreactive-leptin concentrations in normal-weight and obese humans. *N. Eng. J. Med.* 1996;**334**:292–5.

207 Tamura, T., Goldenberg, R. L., Johnston, K. E., Cliver, S. P. Serum leptin concentrations during pregnancy and their relationship to fetal growth. *Obstet. Gynecol.* 1998;**91**:389–95.

208 Devaskar, S. U., Anthony, R., Hay, W. W., Jr. Ontogeny and insulin regulation of fetal ovine white adipose tissue leptin expression. *Am. J. Physiol. Regulatory Integrative Comp. Physiol.* 2002;**282**:R431–8.

4

Postnatal growth in preterm infants

Richard J. Cooke

Department of Pediatrics, University of Tennessee Newborn Center, Memphis, Tennessee

Introduction

The fundamental principle in providing nutritional support is to ensure that intake meets requirements thereby ensuring that inadequate intake is not rate-limiting on outcome. However, translating principles into practice is not simple in the preterm, particularly the very-low birth weight infant (VLBWI).

It takes time to establish adequate dietary intakes in the immature infant, and infants become malnourished during initial hospital stay.[1,2] Yet, recommended dietary intakes (RDI) are based on needs for maintenance and normal growth,[3,4] but no allowance is made for 'catch-up' growth, a critical consideration in the preterm infant.[2,5] Accurate and reproducible measures of outcome also are not fully agreed upon.

Any discussion on postnatal growth in preterm infants, therefore, tends to raise more questions than answers. It is recommended that once birth weight has been regained, growth parallels that of the fetus at the same gestational age.[3,4] But what is acceptable early weight loss? Is fetal growth an appropriate reference for postnatal growth? How should growth be assessed? In this chapter, these issues will be discussed, as will a few studies examining postnatal growth in this high-risk population.

Early weight loss

The importance of early weight loss cannot be underestimated. This is illustrated in Figure 4.1. A 27-week gestation 1007 g infant who regains birth weight by the end of the second week and then grows at a rate which parallels that

in utero will weigh ~541 g less than the intrauterine fetus at 37-week gestation. If this infant takes 3 weeks to regain birth weight, then this infant will weigh ~750 g less than the fetus at 37 weeks.

For a more complete discussion on fluid balance in the preterm infant, the reader is directed to the excellent review of Brace.[6] Term infants lose ~5–10% of their body weight during the first week of life. This is thought to reflect a loss of fluid as total water decreases from ~75 to ~65%. Because fractional body water is greater, it is thought that weight loss is likely to be greater in the preterm infant.[6] To examine this issue, fluid intake, nutrient intake and changes in body weight were prospectively examined in a group of preterm infants (n = 54) during the first 2 weeks of life.[7] Study infants were clinically stable, not ventilator- or oxygen-dependent and had achieved a minimal enteral intake of 80 kcal kg^{-1} day^{-1} by 14 days of age. A summary of the results is presented in Table 4.1. Although fluid intake and fractional weight loss were greater, no differences were detected in energy intakes, absolute weight loss or time to regain birth weight in the more immature infants. These data suggest that the otherwise normal preterm infant should also be able to regain birth weight by the end of the second week of life.

In another study of weight loss after birth in preterm infants, Bauer et al. measured body weight, total body water (TBW), nutrient intake and nitrogen balance in eight preterm infants (birth weight = 1060 g) during the first 2 weeks of life.[8] The results are presented in Table 4.2. Infants lost weight during the first 3 days but regained birth weight by ~9 days of age. Changes in weight closely paralleled that in TBW, while energy intakes increased from 26 to 94 kcal kg^{-1} day^{-1} between days 1 and 9.

Neonatal Nutrition and Metabolism. Second Edition, ed. P. Thureen and W. Hay. Published by Cambridge University Press.
© Cambridge University Press 2006.

Table 4.1. Infants of Cooke et al.[7]

Group	A	B	C
Birth weight (g)	883 ± 74	1142 ± 72	1353 ± 47
Gestation (w)	28 ± 1.6	31 ± 1.5	32 ± 1.3
Intake (0–6 days of age)			
1. ml kg^{-1} day^{-1*}	152 ± 39	127 ± 25	125 ± 23
2. cal kg^{-1} day^{-1}	47 ± 34	46 ± 13	47 ± 20
Weight loss			
1. g	102 ± 57	86 ± 63	108 ± 71
2. % of birth weight*	12 ± 7	8 ± 6	8 ± 5
3. Day (max loss)	6 ± 2.1	6 ± 1.4	5 ± 2.2
Regain birth weight (days)	12 ± 5	13 ± 3	12 ± 5

*p < To .05 for differences between A versus B/C.

Table 4.2. Data in study infants of Bauer et al.[8]

Study day	1	3	9
Body weight (g)	1057 ± 213	978 ± 202	1037 ± 201
Total body weight (g)	831 ± 179	735 ± 133	813 ± 141
Intake (kg^{-1} day^{-1})			
Energy intake (kcal)	26 ± 7	57 ± 13	94 ± 15
Protein intake (g)	1.0 ± 0.1	2.4 ± 0.7	3.9 ± 1.2
Urinary protein (g)	0.18	0.49	0.39
Protein retention (g)	0.8	1.8	3.2

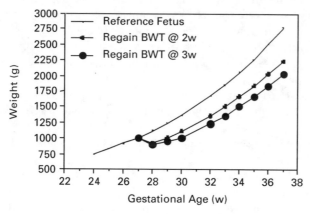

Figure 4.1. Weight of the reference fetus compared with that of a 27 week (w) gestational age infant who regains birth weight (BWT) by 2 and 3 weeks of age.

Estimations of minimal energy requirements vary from 45–60 kcal kg^{-1} day^{-1}.[9] In the first study, energy intake averaged 47 kcal kg^{-1} day^{-1} during the first week of life.[7] In the second study, energy intake increased from 26 ± 7 to 57 ± 13 between days 1 and 3.[8] In both studies, intake did not meet minimal requirements during the few days and barely met requirements during the first week of life. The possibility that catabolism contributed to weight loss cannot be excluded.

Bauer et al. suggested that because nitrogen balance was positive on days 1 and 3, inadequate nutrition did not contribute to changes in body weight.[8] However, urine was collected on pre-weighed diapers and urine nitrogen losses (~0.2–0.5 g kg^{-1} day^{-1}) were less than might have been expected (1–1.5 g kg^{-1} day^{-1}).[10] Since urine rapidly evaporates from diapers,[11] urine output and, therefore, protein losses may have been underestimated giving the erroneous impression of positive nitrogen balance. This is particularly likely on day 1 when energy intake was only 26 kcal kg^{-1} day^{-1}.

For all studies examining early weight loss a singular pattern emerges.[1,2,7,8,12,13] It takes time to establish minimal energy requirements, particularly in the sick, unstable VLBWI. It is, therefore, difficult to disentangle the effects of inadequate intake and catabolism from simple fluid shifts and problematic to determine what is "normal" and what is not.

Fetal growth reference standards

For a more complete review the reader is directed to the excellent treatise of Sparks et al.[14,15] Fetal growth may be assessed using intrauterine ultrasound or body size at different gestational ages. Ultrasound has been used to serially evaluate fetal growth, but the measurement error remains too high and the statistics too complex to readily interpret these curves.[16–18]

The classic growth curves have been created using birth weight at different gestational ages.[19–21] These curves make certain assumptions. It is assumed that cross-sectional data can be used to construct velocity curves. This is questionable. It is assumed that a single growth curve exists for all infants. This is unlikely. Differences in gestational age may explain much of the variability in weight but size at birth is also affected by maternal (e.g. race, socio-economic, and clinical and nutritional status)[22] and fetal (e.g. gender)[23] factors.

Construction of these curves presupposes that gestational age was accurately measured and that gestation and birth weight were independent variables. For the classic studies, gestational age was determined using dating; i.e. the first day of the last monthly period (LMP) or postnatal examination of physical and neurological characteristics.[19–21] If LMP agreed closely with postnatal exam, then LMP was used. If LMP and postnatal exam did not agree, the latter was used.

However, bleeding during the first trimester may be confused with the last menstrual period. In effect, gestational age may be underestimated and weight for age erroneously high.[24–26] If postnatal examination was used to determine gestation then gestation and weight were not truly independent variables.

Estimation of gestation based upon LMP is valid to within 2–4 weeks, while that using the postnatal examination has a standard deviation of 1–2 weeks. A significant variation, therefore, may exist on the x-axis as well as the y-axis. If so, it may lead to a systematic underestimate of true slopes along the y-axis and growth rate will tend to be underestimated.

Most disconcerting is the idea that infants delivering prematurely are "normal" and size at birth represents "optimal" growth. In term infants, fetal growth shows a rapid, consistent increase during the third trimester until 37 weeks, growth "faltering" before birth, and then "catch-up" growth soon after birth. This has led to the suggestion that growth after 37 weeks is in some way restricted and that mean birth weight is less than "optimal", even in the normal term infant.[27]

Such an effect may be even greater in the preterm infant. Fifty percent of preterm labors are associated with placental insufficiency.[28] At the same time, fetal weight assessed by ultrasound is consistently greater than birth weight.[16,29,30–32] Greisen et al., using serial ultrasound measurements, calculated that up to 40% of infants born at 28–30 weeks of gestation are small-for-gestational-age.[31] These data suggest that mean birth weight in preterm infants is not normal, never mind "optimal".

Sparks et al. have observed that across several studies birth weights differed by less than 10% at any given gestational age.[19,26,33,34] These authors calculated a growth rate of 1.5% or 15 g kg^{-1} day^{-1} for the data of Lubchenco et al. and 1.45% or 14.5 g kg^{-1} day^{-1} for the data of Usher and McLean.[14,19,20] The American Academy of Pediatric Committee on Nutrition (AAPCON), therefore, recommended a target growth rate of 15 g kg^{-1} day^{-1}.[3]

Recent studies suggest that fetal growth rates might be greater. Arbuckle et al. reported a fetal weight of ~1000 g at 27 weeks, which had increased to 2318 g at 34 weeks gestation, giving a growth rate ~17 g kg^{-1} day^{-1}.[23] Alexander et al. reported a median weight of 1035 g at 27 weeks increasing to 2667 at 34 weeks giving a growth rate of ~20 g kg^{-1} day^{-1}.[35]

In a comprehensive review, Klein et al. concluded that target growth rates should be closer to 20 g kg^{-1} day^{-1}.[4] Because of concerns about overfeeding and obesity, target growth rates of 17 g day^{-1} between 24–27 weeks and

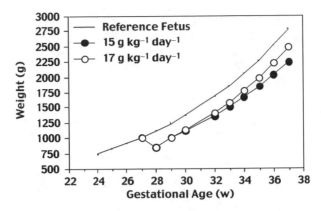

Figure 4.2. Weight of the reference fetus compared to that of a 27 week gestational age infant who regains birth weight by 2 weeks of age and then gains weight at a rate of 15 and 17 g kg^{-1} day^{-1}.

16–17 g kg^{-1} day^{-1} between 27 and 34 weeks gestation were recommended.[4] A 1007 g infant who is delivered at 26 weeks, regains body weight at 28 weeks and then grows at a rate of 17 g kg^{-1} day^{-1} will be ~240 g heavier than an infant who gains 15 g kg^{-1} day^{-1} but still weighs ~300 g less than the intrauterine fetus (Figure 4.2). Is this difference important?

Fetal growth remains the best reference for postnatal growth in the preterm infant. Yet, size at birth is likely to be less than "optimal", while gestational age may not always be accurately measured. Uncritical use of these curves, therefore, may systematically underestimate true growth potential in these infants.

Assessment of growth

Crown-heel length and weight gain

Change in linear growth is generally regarded as the best measure of assessing adequacy of dietary intake[36,37] but it is difficult to measure crown-heel length (CHL) in a precise and reproducible fashion.[38,39] Measurement of knee-heel length (KHL) has, therefore, been advocated.[40–43]

Griffin et al. prospectively took paired measurements of CHL and KHL in a group of thriving preterm infants.[44] KHL was not linearly related to CHL. For consecutive determinations, the coefficients of variation (CVs) were 0.30 (CHL) and 1.25% (KHL), equivalent to 95% CI of ±2.5 (CHL) and ±9 days (KHL) linear growth, respectively.[44] These data suggest that KHL determinations are neither an accurate nor a more sensitive indicator of total linear growth in preterm infants.

Body weight can be measured accurately and reproducibly.[45] It is, therefore, recommended that

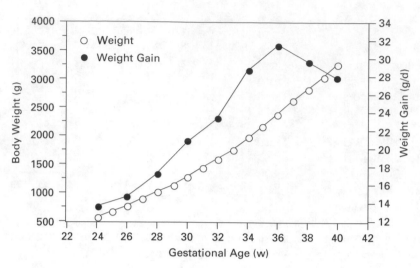

Figure 4.3. A comparison of total fetal body weight and weight gain. Weight gain decreases between 36 weeks and term without a perceptible effect on body weight.

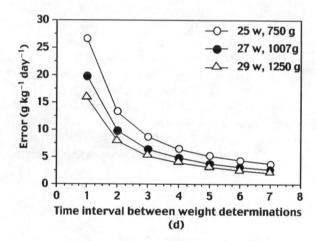

Figure 4.4. Error in weight gain assessment plotted as a function of time interval (days) between weight measurements and body weight. As time interval and body weight decrease, the measurement error increases.

body weight be determined and plotted weekly against a reference curve and the pattern tracked over time.[3,4] This approach, while practical and simple, may not be a sensitive way of detecting growth faltering.[39] This is illustrated for the fetus in Figure 4.3. Weight gain decreases significantly between 36 weeks and term but this is not perceptible when plotting weight for age.

Weight gain is, therefore, recommended.[3,4] Most scales are accurate to $\pm$ 10 g, but scales must be recalibrated on a regular basis. Even so, these errors may occur and be additive. A 27-week infant weighing 1007 g at 2 weeks, who gains

a rate of 1.5% day^{-1} will weigh $\sim$1118 g at 3 weeks of age, a gain of 15.9 g day^{-1}. If an error of +10 g was made at 2 weeks (i.e. infant weighed 1017 g), and an error -10 g at 3 weeks (i.e., infant weight 1108 g), then the rate of gain is 13 g day^{-1}, an error of $\sim$2.9 g day^{-1}.

Yet, preterm infants are weighed more often than once a week. In Figure 4.4, the error is plotted as a function of frequency. In the 1007 g infant, the potential error increases from 2.9 to 20 g kg^{-1} day^{-1} as frequency increases from weekly to daily, an error that is inversely proportional to body weight.

Another consideration is the timing of weighing in reference to feeding. A 1250 g infant fed an enteral intake of 120 kcal kg^{-1} day^{-1} will receive $\sim$188 ml kg^{-1} day^{-1} of a 24 kcal oz^{-1} formula or $\sim$16 ml per feed every 2 hours. If the infant is weighed after feeds on one occasion (+16 g) and before feeds on the next occasion, then growth rate may be erroneously interpreted. Similar errors may be incurred when urination and defecation are considered.

Yet, body weight must be determined frequently to ensure that adequate intakes are maintained. An infant with a baseline weight of 1250 g is prescribed an intake of 120 kcal kg^{-1} day^{-1}. Assuming that the infant is growing appropriately; i.e. 1.5% day^{-1}, then the infant will weigh $\sim$1269 g one day later. Averaged weight for the intervening 24 hours is 1260 g and averaged intake $\sim$119 kcal kg^{-1} day^{-1}, rather a small difference.

Yet, as the time interval between weighing increases so might the deficit. This is illustrated in Figure 4.5. If the 1250 g infant were not weighed for 2 days but grew appropriately, then averaged weight is 1269 g and intake $\sim$118 kcal

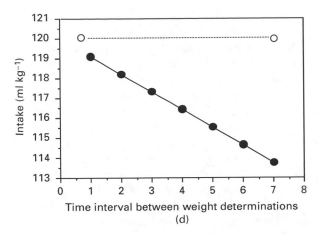

Figure 4.5. Intake plotted as a function of time interval (days) between weight measurements. As the time interval increases, averaged intake decreases.

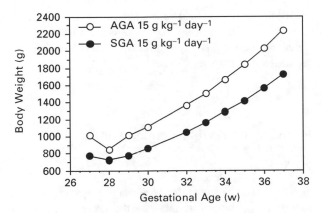

Figure 4.6. Body weight plotted as function of gestation in an average-for-gestational-age (AGA) and small-for-gestational age (SGA) 27 week infant who gains at 15 g kg^{-1} day^{-1}. The discrepancy in weight increases as gestation advances.

kg^{-1} day^{-1}. If the infant were not weighed for 3 days, intake decreases to ~117 kcal kg^{-1} day^{-1}. Appropriate growth is unlikely as intake decreases, but the retrospective way intake is prescribed ensures that the infant is consistently fed less rather than more.

An additional consideration is the interval between weight determination and intake adjustment. It is rare that weight determination is immediately followed by adjustment in nutrient intake. There is always a time lag, further reducing averaged intake. Feedings may also be interrupted for variable periods, while infants may regurgitate or vomit. In both scenarios, intake is not always readjusted to recoup the deficit.

Finally, weight gain may be expressed on a body weight (g kg^{-1} day^{-1}) or absolute (g day^{-1}) basis. Sparks *et al.* suggested that if intake is expressed on a body weight basis then so should weight gain.[15] A comparison of the two is revealing. This is illustrated in Figure 4.6. A 27-week, 1007 g AGA who regains birth weight at 2 weeks of age and then gains at a rate of 15 g kg^{-1} day^{-1} will weigh ~2200 g at 37 weeks. A 27-week, 778 g SGA infant who does exactly the same will weigh ~1700 at 37 weeks, 500 g less.

Collectively, these data raise many questions. How often should infants be weighed? Is plotting weight for age against a fetal growth curve a sensitive means of assessing growth? What constitutes adequate weight gain? Further studies are needed to examine these issues.

Body composition

It is recommended that composition of weight gain in the preterm infant approximates that of the fetus at the same postconceptional age.[3] The advent of dual emission x-ray absorptiometry (DEXA) now makes it possible to measure body composition in a relatively easy and noninvasive fashion. However, the accuracy of DEXA has been questioned because a small error in lean mass (LM) may translate into a large error in fat mass (FM) determination.[46–48] Recent data suggest improved accuracy and precision with updated software.[46,49]

To examine accuracy, body composition was serially determined in a group of preterm infants[51] and the results compared with the reference infant of Fomon *et al.*[52] Significant differences were detected in LM, FM and bone mineral mass (BMC) between the preterm girls and boys, but compared with the reference girl or boy the patterns of growth were similar.[51]

At the same age, LM was less but FM and % FM were similar in the preterm and reference girl and boy. At the same weight, LM was similar but FM was slightly greater in the preterm (continuous) than the reference infant (interrupted line; Figure 4.7). DEXA, therefore, may tend to overestimate FM but the differences appear small.

Such was not true for BMC. These data are presented in Table 4.3. At term, BMC was ~49.3 or 16.7 g of calcium because hydroxyapatite is 34% calcium by weight. This is significantly less than the reference infant at 31.2 g. As age and weight increased, so did BMC calcium. By 12 months, BMC calcium was 65.5 g, significantly greater than the reference infant.

A reduced BMC calcium at term is consistent with the idea that the skeleton is poorly mineralized, and pixels containing bone were counted as LM because the

Table 4.3. Data in study infants of Cooke *et al.*[51]

Age	Weight (g)	BMC (g)	BM Ca (g)	Reference Infant
Term	3530	49.3	16.7	31.2
3 months	6323	104.9	35.7	33.5
6 months	7877	140.6	47.8	37.5
12 months	9920	192.7	65.5	47.4

BMC, bone mineral mass; BM Ca, bone mineral calcium.

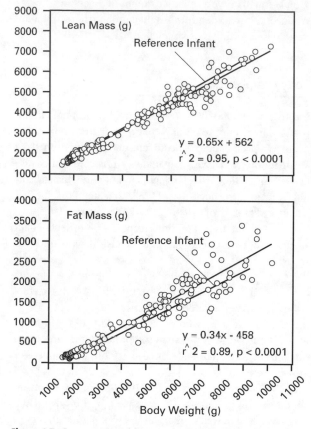

Figure 4.7. Lean mass and fat mass in the reference infant girl compared with the study preterm infants. Lean mass is a little greater and fat mass a little less in the reference infant.

attenuation coefficients are similar.[47] Increased BMC as weight increased is consistent with the idea that DEXA-derived total BMC is affected by body size; i.e. as antero-posterior thickness increases so does BMC.[47,53] Whatever, DEXA does not appear to measure total body mineral mass accurately in the preterm infant.

Nonetheless, the precision of DEXA is excellent. Brunton *et al.* have noted a CV of 0.7% and 4.0% for LM and FM in piglets.[50] Braillon *et al.* have reported a CV of 1.2 and 2.4% in measuring femoral BM in preterm infants and lumbar spine in term infants.[54] Cooke *et al.* have noted a CV of 0.36 and 0.67 in FM and % FM determination.[51]

Two prospective controlled trials have been conducted using DEXA to examine the effects of diet on body composition in preterm infants. Pieltain *et al.* compared weight gain composition in preterm infants fed either human milk (n = 20) or those fed a preterm infant formula (n = 34) during initial hospital stay.[55] Over the 3-week study period, infants fed human milk had a lower weight gain (16 ± 2.2 < 20 ± 3.2 g kg^{-1} day^{-1}), fat gain (3.3 ± 1.3 < 5.1 ± 1.9 g kg^{-1} day^{-1}) and BMC gain (214 ± 64 < 289 ± 99 mg kg^{-1} day^{-1}) than those fed the preterm formula. These authors calculated that with 20 infants per group, the minimal detectable significant difference was 160 g, 86 g and 4.1 g for LM, FM and BM, respectively. Cooke *et al.* compared body composition in preterm infants fed either a term or preterm infant formula after hospital discharge until 6 months corrected age.[51] Although significant differences were detected between the sexes, increased LM, FM and BMC were detected in infants fed the preterm formula. Both these studies suggest that DEXA is precise enough to detect differences in body composition in preterm infants fed different dietary regimens.

Postnatal growth in the preterm infant

Predischarge growth

Several studies have examined postnatal growth in preterm infants during initial hospital stay. Wilson *et al.* randomized VLBWI to either an aggressive or standard parenteral and enteral feeding regimen. Infants fed the aggressive regimen had greater nutrient intakes and grew better.[13] Yet, energy intakes in both groups (0–3 days ∼52, 4–7 days ∼85, 8–42 days ∼90 kcal kg^{-1} day^{-1}) were substantially less than that recommended, and the incidence of postnatal growth retardation (PGR) was high in both groups at the end of the study (aggressive ∼60%; standard 80%).

In an observational study in preterm infants (weight <1300 g), Carlson *et al.* noted that energy intakes averaged 75 ± 12 (0–14 days), 99 ± 12 (15–35 days) and ∼110 ± 15 (36 days to term) kcal kg^{-1} day^{-1}.[1] At these intakes weight gain averaged 13.0, 13.8 and 11.6 g kg^{-1} day^{-1}, respectively, less than that in utero.

In a large multicenter study, it was noted that postnatal growth rates were substantially less than in utero.[12] Intake was not measured but chronic lung disease, intracranial hemorrhage, necrotizing enterocolitis and late-onset sepsis were noted to be high-risk factors for PGR. In this study, all VLBWI developed PGR at hospital discharge.

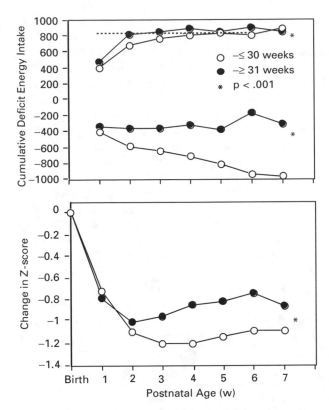

Figure 4.8. Energy intake, cumulative energy deficit and growth in preterm infants in the first 7 weeks of life. Energy intake was less, cumulative energy deficit was greater and fall in Z-score was greater in pre term infants. • 30 weeks gestation.

Embleton *et al.* prospectively examined nutrient intake and growth in preterm infants (weight $\leq$1750 g) over a 6-month period.[2] Daily nutrient deficit was calculated by subtracting recommended energy (120 kcal kg^{-1} day^{-1}) and protein (3.0 g kg^{-1} day^{-1}) from actual intake. Daily deficit was then summed to calculate cumulative deficit. Body weight was converted to standard deviation or z-scores. Z-score at birth was subtracted from that at given postnatal age to determine the degree of PGR. The results are presented in Figure 4.8. Only energy intakes are presented, but protein intakes followed the same pattern. Recommended dietary intakes (RDIs) were rarely achieved during early life. By the end of the first week, the cumulative energy deficit was 406 $\pm$ 92 and 335 $\pm$ 86 kcal kg^{-1} in infants $\leq$30 weeks and those at $\geq$31 weeks gestation. At 5 weeks, the deficit had increased to 013 $\pm$ 542 kcal kg^{-1} day^{-1} in infants <30 weeks but remained unchanged in those at $\geq$31 weeks. Z-scores for weight fell in both groups of infants; the more immature the infant, the greater the decrease. Forty-five percent of the variation in PGR was related to that in cumulative energy and protein deficit.

Clark *et al.* also examined postnatal growth in preterm infants ($\leq$34-week gestation) in a large multicenter study. Intake was not measured but it was noted that as gestational age and birth weight decreased the frequency of PGR increased exponentially. Ventilatory status on days 1 and 28, the development of necrotizing enterocolitis and exposure to steroids were noted to be high-risk factors for PGR.

These data indicate that it takes time to establish RDIs, and that PGR is inevitable during initial hospital stay. In studies where intake was not measured, PGR was related to poorer clinical outcomes. This is not surprising. In the infant with a complicated clinical course, it takes longer to establish RDIs and once established, RDIs are rarely maintained throughout the infant's hospital stay. Requirements are also not well defined and are likely to differ from the clinically stable infant.

Whatever, this raises an important issue. Preterm infants invariably accumulate a nutrient deficit. Yet, RDIs are based on needs for maintenance and normal growth. At the same time, infants are fed up to, but not beyond, current RDIs. As long as these practices continue, these infants will always be underfed during initial hospital stay and growth retarded when they are discharged home.

Post-discharge growth

Many studies have examined post-discharge growth in preterm infants.[57-63] Although some "catch-up" growth has been observed, preterm infants do not grow as well as their term counterparts. The reasons for this are several.

Current in-hospital feeding practices ensure that preterm infants are malnourished and growth-retarded at initial hospital discharge. A "critical epoch" of growth may, therefore, have been missed. Preterm infants also have greater morbidity than term infants during the first year of life, further confusing the issue.[64-68]

Until relatively recently, little attention had been paid to nutritional factors in the genesis of this problem. For most early studies, infants were fed either a term infant formula or human milk after hospital discharge. Both feeding regimens are designed to meet nutritional needs of the term rather than the rapidly growing preterm infant. Infants in these studies may have been, at least, partly underfed during the first year of life.

Lucas *et al.* randomized preterm infants (n =16 per group) to be fed either a term or nutrient-enriched infant formula after hospital discharge. Those fed the nutrient-enriched formula grew better[69] and had better bone mineralization at 3 and 9 months corrected age.[70] However, Chan *et al.* were unable to show any differences in growth between preterm infants fed a term and those fed either a

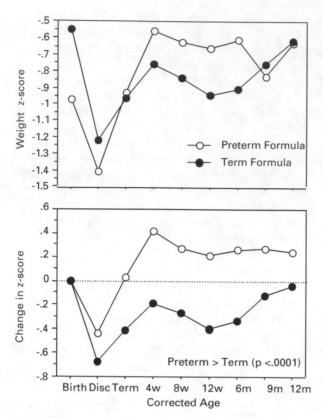

Figure 4.9. Z-scores and changes in z-scores in preterm infant girls fed the preterm and term infant formulas. Changes in z-scores were greater in girls fed the preterm formula. Disc, discharge; w, weeks; m, months.

nutrient-enriched or preterm infant formula after hospital discharge.[71]

Our group randomized otherwise "normal" preterm ($\leq$ 1750 g birth weight, $\leq$ 34 weeks gestation) infants to one of three feeding groups: group A were fed a preterm infant formula (energy: 80 kcal per 100 ml^{-1}; protein: 2.2 g per 100 ml^{-1}) between discharge and 6 m, group B were fed a term formula between discharge and 6 m (energy: 66 kcal/100 ml^{-1}; protein: 1.4 g per 100 ml^{-1}), group C were fed a preterm (discharge to term) and a term formula (term to 6 months).[72]

Initial analyses indicated that boys fed the preterm formula grew faster than boys fed the term formula,[72] with increased growth primarily reflecting increased lean mass accretion.[51] Initial analyses did not detect a difference in growth between girls fed the preterm and term formula. However, a subsequent analysis when data were converted to z-scores was revealing. These results are presented in Figure 4.9. At birth and the beginning of the study, girls fed the preterm formula had lower z-scores than girls fed the term formula. At the end of the study, z-scores were identical in both groups. Expressed as change from birth, girls

fed the preterm formula had greater z-scores than those fed the term formula, suggesting they also benefited. This is consistent with the recent observations of Carver *et al.* where feeding a nutrient-enriched formula after hospital discharge was also associated with better growth.[73]

In the studies of Lucas *et al.*, Chan *et al.* and Carver *et al.*, the nutrient-enriched formulas were fed to 9, 3 and 6 months corrected-age infants, respectively, a time when complementary foods (CF) are fed. In our study, it was hypothesized that if nutrient intake more adequately met requirements, then infants would be satisfied longer and CF introduced later. However, the timing of introduction of CF varied widely across treatment groups, and no differences were detected in age between infants fed the preterm and those fed the term formula (66 ± 34 v. 61 ± 29 days corrected age). It is recommended that CF be introduced after 4 months corrected age. Infants were, therefore, stratified into those who were fed CF before and after 4 months. A trend was observed. Infants who were fed CF earlier were heavier and longer than those who were fed CF later (Figure 4.10). Interestingly, these differences began to appear

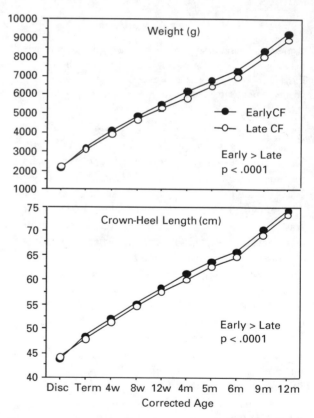

Figure 4.10. Body weight and crown-heel length in infants who were fed complementary foods (CF) early and late. Weight and length were greater in those fed early CF. Disc, discharge; w, weeks; m, months.

between term and 4 weeks corrected age, somewhat earlier than the average age of introduction of CF. This raises the possibility that infants who were fed CF early were inherently different from those who are fed CF later. The timing of introduction of CF, therefore, may be an important confounding variable when examining growth in these high-risk infants during the first year of life.

Conclusions

Issues pertaining to postnatal growth in preterm infants continue to raise more questions than answers. Further studies are needed to differentiate the effects of inadequate intake from simple fluid shifts during early life, and to better define what is normal and what is not.

The use of fetal growth curves as a reference for postnatal growth is questionable. If the weight of an infant delivered prematurely is consistently less than the infant who remains in utero, then fetal growth curves may underestimate "true" postnatal growth potential in these infants. Further studies must better define "optimum" growth rates in these infants.

Serial evaluation of weight gain is recommended to assess adequacy of intake. Yet, accurate and reproducible measurements of body weight are difficult to achieve in the clinical arena. Given the retrospective way in which intake is prescribed, and the problems in accurately measuring weight, intake might be better based on "expected" rather than actual weight and weight gain reviewed on a weekly rather than a daily basis.

It is highly unlikely that RDIs will be achieved during the first 7–10 days of life. It is also unlikely that RDIs will be consistently maintained throughout initial hospital stay. Attention must be paid to the cumulative nutrient deficits and the importance of recouping these deficits. Feeding must be tailored to meeting needs for "catch-up" as well as maintenance and "normal" growth.

Recent attention has focused on the role of nutrient-enriched formulas in feeding preterm infants after initial hospital discharge. Although growth is improved, further studies are needed that better define optimal composition and duration of feeding of such formulas. Attention must also focus on the nature and timing of introduction of complementary foods fed to these high-risk infants.

REFERENCES

1 Carlson, S. J., Ziegler, E. E. Nutrient intakes and growth of very low birth weight infants. *J. Perinatol.* 1998a;**18**:252–8.

2 Embleton, N. E., Pang, N., Cooke, R. J. Postnatal malnutrition and growth retardation: an inevitable consequence of current recommendations in preterm infants? *Pediatrics* 2001;**107**: 270–3.

3 AAPCON. Nutritional needs of preterm infants. In Kleinman, R. E., ed. *Pediatric Nutrition Handbook*. Elk Groove Village, IL: American Academy of Pediatrics; 1998:55–88.

4 Klein, C. J. Nutrient requirements for preterm infant formulas. *J. Nutr.* 2002:**132**:1395S–577S.

5 Kashyap, S., Heird, W. C. Protein requirements of low birth weight, very low birth weight, and small for gestational age infants. In Raiha, N., ed. *Protein Metabolism during Infancy*. New York, NY: Raven Press; 1994:133–51.

6 Brace, R. A. Fluid distribution in the fetus and neonate. In Poland, R. A., Fox, W. W., eds. *Fetal and Neonatal Physiology*. Philadelphia, PA: WB Saunders; 1998:1703–13.

7 Cooke, R. J., Ford, A., Werkman, S., Conner, C., Watson, D. Postnatal growth in infants born between 700 and 1500 g. *J. Pediatr. Gastroenterol. Nutr.* 1993;**16**:130–5.

8 Bauer, K., Bovermann, G., Roithmaier, A. *et al.* Body composition, nutrition, and fluid balance during the first two weeks of life in preterm neonates weighing less than 1500 grams. *J. Pediatr.* 1991;**118**:615–20.

9 Putet, G. Energy. In Tsang, R. C., Lucas, A., Uauy, R., Zlotkin, S., eds. *Nutritional Needs of Preterm Infants: Scientific Basis and Practical Guidelines*. Baltimore, MD: Williams & Wilkins; 1993:15–28.

10 Anderson, T. L., Muttart, C. R., Bieber, M. A., Nicholson, J. F., Heird, W. C. A controlled trial of glucose versus glucose and amino acids in premature infants. *J. Pediatr.* 1979;**94**: 947–51.

11 Cooke, R. J., Werkman, S., Watson, D. Urine output measurement in premature infants. *Pediatrics* 1989;**83**:116–18.

12 Ehrenkranz, R. A., Younes, N., Lemons, J. A., *et al.* Longitudinal growth of hospitalized very low birth weight infants. *Pediatrics* 1999;**104**:280–9.

13 Wilson, D. C., Cairns, P., Halliday, H. L. *et al.* Randomised controlled trial of an aggressive nutritional regimen in sick very low birthweight infants. *Arch. Dis. Child. Fetal Neonatal Ed.* 1997;**77**:F4–11.

14 Sparks, J. W. Human intrauterine growth and nutrient accretion. *Semin Perinatol.* 1984;**8**:74–93.

15 Sparks, J. W., Ross, J. C., Cetin, I. Intrauterine growth and nutrition. In Polin, R. A., Fox, W. W., eds. *Fetal and Neonatology Physiology*. 2nd edn. Philadelphia, PA: WB Saunders Co; 1998:267–89.

16 Gallivan, S., Robson, S. C., Chang, T. C., Vaughan, J., Spencer, J. A. An investigation of fetal growth using serial ultrasound data. *Ultrasound Obstet. Gynecol.* 1993;**3**:109–14.

17 Chang, T. C., Robson, S. C., Spencer, J. A., Gallivan, S. Ultrasonic fetal weight estimation: analysis of inter- and intra-observer variability. *J. Clin. Ultrasound* 1993;**21**:515–19.

18 Robson, S. C., Gallivan, S., Walkinshaw, S. A., Vaughan, J., Rodeck, C. H. Ultrasonic estimation of fetal weight: use of targeted formulas in small for gestational age fetuses. *Obstet. Gynecol.* 1993;**82**:359–64.

19 Lubchenco, L. O. Intrauterine growth as estimated from live-born birth-weight data at 24 to 42 weeks of gestation. *Pediatrics* 1963;**32**:793–800.

20 Usher, R., McLean, F. Intrauterine growth of live-born Caucasian infants at sea level: standards obtained from measurements in 7 dimensions of infants born between 25 and 44 weeks of gestation. *J. Pediatr.* 1969;**74**:901–10.

21 Gruenwald, P. Growth of the human fetus. I. Normal growth and its variation. *Am. J. Obstet. Gynecol.* 1966;**94**:1112–19.

22 Thompson, J. M., Clark, P. M., Robinson, E. *et al.* Risk factors for small-for-gestational-age babies: The Auckland Birthweight Collaborative Study. *J. Paediatr. Child Health* 2001;**37**:369–75.

23 Arbuckle, T. E., Wilkins, R., Sherman, G. J. Birth weight percentiles by gestational age in Canada. *Obstet. Gynecol.* 1993;**81**:39–48.

24 Battaglia, F. C., Frazier, T. M., Hellegers, A. E. Birth weight, gestational age, and pregnancy out-come, with special reference to high birth weight-low gestational age infant. *Pediatrics* 1966;**37**:417–22.

25 Berg, A. T., Bracken, M. B. Measuring gestational age: an uncertain proposition. *Br. J. Obstet. Gynaecol.* 1992;**99**:280–2.

26 Naeye, R. L., Dixon, J. B. Distortions in fetal growth standards. *Pediatr. Res.* 1978;**12**:987–91.

27 Briend, A. Normal fetal growth regulation: nutritional aspects. In Gracey, M. G., Falkner, F., eds. *Nutritional Needs and Assessment of Normal Growth.* New York, NY: Raven Press; 1985:1–21.

28 Fedrick, J., Adelstein, P. Factors associated with low birth weight of infants delivered at term. *Br. J. Obstet. Gynaecol.* 1978;**85**:1–7.

29 Larsen, T., Greisen, G., Petersen, S. Prediction of birth weight by ultrasound-estimated fetal weight: a comparison between single and repeated estimates. *Eur. J. Obstet. Gynecol. Reprod. Biol.* 1995;**60**:37–40.

30 Larsen, T., Petersen, S., Greisen, G., Larsen, J. F. Normal fetal growth evaluated by longitudinal ultrasound examinations. *Early Hum. Dev.* 1990;**24**:37–45.

31 Greisen, G. Estimation of fetal weight by ultrasound. *Horm. Res.* 1992;**38**:208–10.

32 Thomson, A. M., Billewicz, W. Z., Hytten, F. E. The assessment of fetal growth. *J. Obstet. Gynaecol. Br. Commonw.* 1968;**75**:903–16.

33 Babson, S. G., Behrman, R. E., Lessel, R. Fetal growth. Liveborn birth weights for gestational age of white middle class infants. *Pediatrics* 1970;**45**:937–44.

34 Brenner, W. E., Edelman, D. A., Hendricks, C. H. A standard of fetal growth for the United States of America. *Am. J. Obstet. Gynecol.* 1976;**126**:555–64.

35 Alexander, G. R., Himes, J. H., Kaufman, R. B., Mor, J., Kogan, M. A United States national reference for fetal growth. *Obstet. Gynecol.* 1996;**87**:163–8.

36 Babson, S. G., Bramhall, J. L. Diet and growth in the premature infant. The effect of different dietary intakes of ash-electrolyte and protein on weight gain and linear growth. *J. Pediatr.* 1969;**74**:890–900.

37 Davies, D. P. Physical growth from fetus to early childhood. In Dobbing, J., ed. *Scientific Foundation of Paediatrics.* London: William Heinemann; 1981:303–30.

38 Lucas, A. Enteral nutrition. In Tsang, R., Lucas, A., Uauy, R., Zlotkin, S., eds. *Nutritional Needs of the Preterm Infant: Scientific Basis and Practical Guidelines.* Pawling, NY: Caduceus Medical Publishers, Inc. for Williams & Wilkins; 1993:209–23.

39 Fomon, S. Size and growth. In Fomon, S., ed. *Nutrition of Normal Infants.* 2nd edn. St Louis, MO: Mosby; 1993:36–84.

40 Hermanussen, M. Knemometry, a new tool for the investigation of growth. A review. *Eur. J. Pediatr.* 1988;**147**:350–5.

41 Davies, H. A., Pickering, M., Wales, J. K. A portable knemometer: a technique for assessment of short-term growth. *Ann. Hum. Biol.* 1996;**23**:149–57.

42 Gibson, A. T., Pearse, R. G., Wales, J. K. Knemometry and the assessment of growth in premature babies. *Arch. Dis. Child.* 1993;**69**:498–504.

43 Wales, J. K., Milner, R. D. Knemometry in assessment of linear growth. *Arch. Dis. Child.* 1987;**62**:166–71.

44 Griffin, I. J., Pang, N. M., Perring, J., Cooke, R. J. Knee-heel length measurement in healthy preterm infants. *Arch. Dis. Child. Fetal Neonatal Edn* 1999;**81**:F50–5.

45 Katrine, K. F. Anthropometric assessment. In Groh-Wargo, S., Thompson, M., Cox, J., eds. *Nutritional Care for High-Risk Newborns.* 3rd edn. Chicago, IL: Precept Press; 2000:11–22.

46 Brunton, J. A., Bayley, H. S., Atkinson, S. A. Validation and application of dual-energy x-ray absorptiometry to measure bone mass and body composition in small infants. *Am. J. Clin. Nutr.* 1993;**58**:839–45.

47 Roubenoff, R., Kehayias, J. J., Dawson-Hughes, B., Heymsfield, S. B. Use of dual-energy x-ray absorptiometry in body-composition studies: Not yet a 'gold standard'. *Am. J. Clin. Nutr.* 1993;**58**:589–91.

48 Tothill, P., Roubenoff, R., Kehayias, J. J., Dawson Hughes, B., Heymsfield, S. B. Limitations of dual-energy x-ray absorptiometry (1). *Am. J. Clin. Nutr.* 1995;**61**:398–400.

49 Picaud, J. C., Rigo, J., Nyamugabo, K., Milet, J., Senterre, J. Evaluation of dual-energy X-ray absorptiometry for body-composition assessment in piglets and term human neonates. *Am. J. Clin. Nutr.* 1996;**63**:157–63.

50 Brunton, J. A., Weiler, H. A., Atkinson, S. A. Improvement in the accuracy of dual energy x-ray absorptiometry for whole body and regional analysis of body composition: validation using piglets and methodologic considerations in infants. *Pediatr. Res.* 1997;**41**:590–6.

51 Cooke, R. J., Rawlings, D. J., McCormick, K. *et al.* Body composition of preterm infants during infancy. *Arch. Dis. Child. Fetal Neonatal Edn.* 1999;**80**:F188–91.

52 Fomon, S., Haschke, F., Ziegler, E., Nelson, S. Body composition of reference children from birth to age 10 years. *Am. J. Clin. Nutr.* 1982;**35**:1169–75.

53 Hannan, W. J., Cowen, S. J., Wrate, R. M., Barton, J. Improved prediction of bone mineral content and density. *Arch. Dis. Child.* 1995;**72**:147–9.

54 Braillon, P. M., Salle, B. L., Brunet, J. *et al.* Dual energy x-ray absorptiometry measurement of bone mineral content in newborns: validation of the technique. *Pediatr. Res.* 1992;**32**:77–80.

55 Pieltain, C., De Curtis, M., Gerard, P., Rigo, J. Weight gain composition in preterm infants with dual energy X-ray absorptiometry. *Pediatr. Res.* 2001;**49**:120–4.

56 Cooke, R. J., McCormick, K., Griffin, I. J. *et al*. Feeding preterm infants after hospital discharge: effect of diet on body composition. *Pediatr Res*. 1999;**46**:461–4.

57 Ernst, J. A., Bull, M. J., Rickard, K. A., Brady, M. S., Lemons, J. A. Growth outcome and feeding practices of the very low birth weight infant (less than 1500 grams) within the first year of life. *J. Pediatr*. 1990;**117**:S156–6.

58 Casey, P. H., Kraemer, H. C., Bernbaum, J. *et al*. Growth patterns of low birth weight preterm infants: a longitudinal analysis of a large, varied sample. *J. Pediatr*. 1990;**117**:298–307.

59 Fitzhardinge, P. M., Inwood, S. Long-term growth in small-for-date children. *Acta Paediatr. Scand. Suppl*. 1989;**349**:27–34.

60 Fenton, T. R., McMillan, D. D., Sauve, R. S. Nutrition and growth analysis of very low birth weight infants. *Pediatrics* 1990;**86**:378–83.

61 Kitchen, W. H., Doyle, L. W., Ford, G. W., Callanan, C. Very low birth weight and growth to age 8 years. I: Weight and height. *Am. J. Dis. Child*. 1992;**146**:40–5.

62 Kitchen, W. H., Doyle, L. W., Ford, G. W. *et al*. Very low birth weight and growth to age 8 years. II: Head dimensions and intelligence. *Am. J. Dis. Child*. 1992;**146**:46–50.

63 Ross, G., Lipper, E. G., Auld, P. A. Growth achievement of very low birth weight premature children at school age. *J. Pediatr*. 1990;**117**:307–9.

64 McCormick, M. C., Shapiro, S., Starfield, B. H. Rehospitalization in the first year of life for high-risk survivors. *Pediatrics* 1980;**66**:991–9.

65 Hack, M., Caron, B., Rivers, A., Fanaroff, A. A. The very low birth weight infant: the broader spectrum of morbidity during infancy and early childhood. *J. Dev. Behav. Pediatr*. 1983;**4**: 243–9.

66 Navas, L., Wang, E., de Carvalho, V., Robinson, J. Improved outcome of respiratory syncytial virus infection in a high-risk hospitalized population of Canadian children. Pediatric Investigators Collaborative Network on Infections in Canada. *J. Pediatr*. 1992;**121**:348–54.

67 Thomas, M., Bedford-Russel, A., Sharland, M. Hospitalisation of RSV infection in ex-preterm infants – implications for RSV immune globulin. *Arch. Dis. Child*. 2000;**83**:122–7.

68 Wang, E., Law, B., Stephens, D. Pediatric Investigators Collaborative Network on Infections in Canada (PICNIC) prospective study of risk factors and outcomes in patients hospitalised with respiratory syncytial viral lower respiratory tract infection. *J. Pediatr*. 1995;**126**:212–19.

69 Lucas, A., Bishop, N. J., King, F. J., Cole, T. J. Randomised trial of nutrition for preterm infants after discharge. *Arch. Dis. Child*. 1992;**67**:324–7.

70 Bishop, N. J., King, F. J., Lucas, A. Increased bone mineral content of preterm infants fed with a nutrient enriched formula after discharge from hospital. *Arch. Dis. Child*. 1993;**68**: 573–8.

71 Chan, G. M., Borschel, M. W., Jacobs, J. R. Effects of human milk or formula feeding on the growth, behavior, and protein status of preterm infants discharged from the newborn intensive care unit. *Am. J. Clin. Nutr*. 1994;**60**:710–16.

72 Cooke, R. J., Griffin, I. J., McCormick, K., *et al*. Feeding preterm infants after hospital discharge: Effect of dietary manipulation on nutrient intake and growth. *Pediatr. Res*. 1998;**43**: 355–60.

73 Carver, J. D., Wu, P. Y., Hall, R. T., *et al*. Growth of preterm infants fed nutrient-enriched or term formula after hospital discharge. *Pediatrics* 2001;**107**:683–9.

5

Thermal regulation and effects on nutrient substrate metabolism

Jane Hawdon

Neonatal Unit, University College London Hospitals, London, UK

One of the most stimulating and rewarding aspects for many clinicians practicing neonatology is the application of basic physiological principles to the understanding of disease processes and to determining optimal management. This is particularly true in the area of thermal regulation. Those who carried out the early and pioneering work were also pioneers in neonatal physiology. Their work was of immeasurable value in reducing neonatal mortality and morbidity, and has informed subsequent technological advances. The current generation of practicing neonatologists has been fortunate enough to be taught by these "masters" and learn from their works. It is our responsibility to hand on to our juniors enthusiasm and respect for the application of physiology to neonatal care.

This chapter covers normal physiological changes, the challenges to these, the impact of disturbed thermal regulation, and therapeutic strategies.

Changes in the thermal environment at birth

Fetal temperature rises and falls with maternal temperature and is maintained at 0.5 °C above that of the mother.[1] Fetal heat loss is via the placenta and amniotic fluid.

At birth, a fall in body temperature is physiological; indeed stimulation of peripheral thermal receptors is a trigger for spontaneous breathing.[2] The usual rectal temperature of the newborn baby is 36.5–37.0 °C with skin temperature 0.5 °C below this.

Physiological responses first described 40 years ago are triggered by the postnatal fall in temperature resulting in heat conservation and heat production.[3,4] Unlike adults, the neonatal physiological responses to cold are more influenced by skin temperature than core temperature and the cutaneous thermal receptors are most sensitive in the trigeminal area of the face.[5] Therefore, even when a baby is well wrapped and has a normal core temperature, cold stimulation of the face, e.g. via air flow, will result in triggering of thermal responses. The responses to stimulation of thermal receptors emanate from the thermal control center in the hypothalamus.

A neutral thermal environment has been defined for the neonate as "that environment (usually a range of air temperatures in an incubator or an abdominal skin temperature under a radiant warmer) in which the infant, when quiet or asleep, is not required to increase heat production above 'resting levels' to maintain body temperature."[6–8] Within this range of temperatures, the infant is neither gaining nor losing heat, metabolic rate and oxygen consumption are minimal, and the core-skin temperature gradient is low. Above this range, the neonate is expending energy to dissipate heat and below this range there is energy expenditure to generate heat; at extreme low temperature, metabolic rate again falls as enzyme systems shut down (see below).

The range of temperatures for the thermal neutral environment in the neonate is 32–34 °C (a higher temperature and wider range than for adults whose range is 25–30 °C) and is higher in the preterm infant.[8] The range is wider in a clothed subject, i.e. when clothed the subject "tolerates" both lower and higher temperatures.[1] It is likely that in the very preterm baby evaporative heat loss is so great that it is almost impossible to achieve a thermal neutral environment. For these babies, Sauer et al.[8,9] proposed that the aim should be to maintain an ambient temperature at which the core temperature of the infant is 36.7–37.3 °C, and the core

Neonatal Nutrition and Metabolism. Second Edition, ed. P. Thureen and W. Hay. Published by Cambridge University Press.
© Cambridge University Press 2006.

and mean skin temperatures are changing less than 0.2 and 0.3 °C hour^{-1} respectively.

Thermal changes

After delivery, there are many factors which challenge and influence the baby's ability to maintain control of body temperature. Heat loss is first through passage of heat from the blood to the external surface of the skin, and then by loss from the skin.

Heat loss from blood to skin is influenced by blood flow and by tissue insulation (fat). A neonate, even well grown and at full term, has less insulating fat than an adult, and the growth-retarded or preterm infant will have even less.

Considering routes of heat loss from the surface of the skin, compared with older infants, children and adults, neonates have a high radiant and convective heat loss because of their relatively high surface area:mass ratio and small radius of curvature of body surfaces. Of particular note is the high head size:body size ratio (the head constitutes one-fifth of the total surface area), which results in most circumstances in a high exposed:unexposed skin ratio. This is of relevance as metabolic rate and heat production by the brain accounts for 55% of total heat production.[10]

Evaporative heat losses are also higher because skin permeability is high and after birth the baby's skin and hair have a covering of amniotic fluid. These losses continue to be particularly high in the extremely preterm baby with very thin skin. Water loss through the skin may be up to 120 ml kg^{-1} day^{-1} if measures are not taken to reduce this, resulting in equivalent heat loss of 72 kcal kg^{-1} day^{-1}.[11,12] Evaporative losses are greater if inspired or surrounding gas is of low humidity and, paradoxically, are increased by placing the baby under a radiant warmer.[13,14] Like convective losses, they are higher if air temperature is low or if there is high air flow. There are also evaporative heat losses from the lung during breathing or assisted ventilation.

In addition, some environmental factors, especially in the delivery room and neonatal unit, contribute to heat loss – conductive via cold surfaces, convective via fans or air conditioning, evaporative if bathed and radiant if environmental temperature is low.

Less likely, is the risk that a baby may become overheated if placed near radiant heat sources, such as direct sunlight, radiant warmers, phototherapy units. The baby's ability to lose excess heat by radiation is additionally compromised if a baby is over wrapped.

The baby's response to becoming cold

The first protective response to cold stress is of peripheral vasoconstriction.[15] Subsequently mechanisms to generate heat are required. The neonate has a limited ability to generate heat by physical movement (involuntary shivering or increased voluntary activity) and to retain heat by adopting a flexed posture.[1]

Metabolic means of generating energy (non-shivering thermogenesis) are of greater importance. These metabolic processes are under hormonal and autonomic control. The stimulation of cutaneous cold receptors triggers noradrenaline release, from the adrenal medulla and by the sympathetic nervous system within brown fat. Noradrenaline stimulates the systemic and brown fat metabolic changes described below. In addition thyroxine has the same action, by direct lipolytic effect and by enhancing the effect of noradrenaline.[16–18] Corticosteroids are also likely to play a role, which may include release of carbohydrate for metabolism.[19] A chemically mediated response to separation of the placenta to enhance non-shivering thermogenesis has been described.[17] It is also likely that there are local mediators as increased oxygen delivery to brown fat also stimulates nonshivering thermogenesis.[17]

Many studies have confirmed an increased metabolic rate in response to cold stress (up to double that of baseline) resulting in heat production.[3,4] Noradrenaline stimulates lipase, which releases fatty acids from adipose tissue stores and oxidation of these fatty acids to produce heat.[5] The resulting increase in oxygen consumption (calorimetry) has been used in many studies as a measurement of metabolic rate and neonatal responses to the thermal environment, and has informed practical and technical developments in this important aspect of neonatology.

The value of this increased metabolic rate is limited as it results in high oxygen demand and the breakdown of substrates, which would be better used for growth and storage. If a neonate is dependent upon increased metabolic rate for thermal control, he will not grow and gain weight.[20]

However, the neonate is unique in its capacity for non-shivering thermogenesis, a process that occurs in brown fat. Brown fat constitutes up to 7% of birthweight and is stored in the thoracic trunk, especially around the scapulae. There are additional stores around some of the abdominal organs. Lipolysis in brown fat is at a rate three times greater than in white adipose tissue.[5]

The mechanisms by which brown fat metabolism generates heat are summarized in Table 5.1.[5,21]

Table 5.1. Mechanisms of heat production by brown adipose tissue[5]

	Mechanism		
1	2	3	4

Step

1	Noradrenaline stimulates adenyl cyclase	Noradrenaline stimulates adenyl cyclase	Noradrenaline/thyroxine disrupt sodium pump	Noradrenaline/thyroxine uncouple oxidative phosphorylation
2	Conversion ATP to cAMP	Conversion ATP to cAMP	Activation ATP to restore pump	Heat rather than ATP generated
3	Activates lipase	Activates lipase	Heat production	
4	Reformation triglycerides	Oxidation and resynthesis fatty acids		
5	Heat production	Heat production		

The baby's response to heat

The initial response is vasodilatation to increase heat loss through the skin. Subsequently a term neonate will sweat, to allow increased evaporative heat loss.[22] This response is less effective than that of an adult, and is minimal in preterm babies, whose evaporative losses are actually transdermal (and uncontrolled) rather than via sweating.[23]

Cold Injury

Risk factors

All neonates are susceptible to becoming too cold, but some have additional risk factors. As outlined above, preterm babies are particularly vulnerable because they have reduced or absent fat stores, very high surface area:body mass ratio and very permeable skin. In addition, many undergo frequent or prolonged procedures, which result in their being outside of their ideal thermal environment.

Babies who are full term but have undergone intrauterine growth retardation (IUGR) also have an even greater surface area:body mass ratio and virtually absent insulating fat stores. Animal studies have demonstrated a marked reduction in brown fat mass after IUGR, and the same may be true of human IUGR babies.[24]

Studies of neonatal rats have demonstrated that intrauterine alcohol exposure is associated with postnatal thermoregulatory difficulties, but there are no reported equivalent studies or clinical concerns in human neonates.[25]

Infants who have congenital abnormalities, inborn errors of metabolism and postnatal complications are also at increased risk. These conditions include:

- neurological abnormalities and conditions that affect movement, so that the baby is highly dependent upon nonshivering thermogenesis
- maternal benzodiazepine sedation
- those that are associated with reduced skin covering e.g. gastroschisis, spina bifida
- structural brain abnormalities associated with hypothalamic abnormalities
- thyroid insufficiency or deficiency
- untreated cardiorespiratory problems, resulting in insufficient circulating oxygen to meet metabolic demands.
- hypoglycemia, resulting in reduced substrate for nonshivering thermogenesis and in the extreme, neurological abnormalities
- infection – reduced body temperature is a more common presenting sign in the neonate than pyrexia.[5,26]

Clinical signs and sequelae

It has been recognized since the nineteenth century that babies who become cold after delivery, especially at preterm gestations, do not grow well and have a higher mortality.[20,27–31] Recent publications of outcomes after preterm delivery have confirmed that low body temperature in the hours after delivery is an independent risk factor for respiratory distress syndrome. Even with current neonatal interventions, hypothermia is found more often in babies who die than babies who survive.[32,33]

Initially, the clinical signs will be of vasoconstriction, the motor response and the noradrenaline-induced response to cold stress – tachycardia, peripheral vasoconstriction, increased activity, shivering. Subsequently if the cold stress continues, the clinical signs will be of "metabolic shutdown" and responses designed to conserve energy. Finally energy failure will occur, with impaired function of all organs.[5]

As with many other neonatal complications, the clinical signs of hypothermia are nonspecific and may be shared with the underlying abnormality. Signs that may occur are pallor, reduced movement and level of consciousness, poor feeding and poor weight gain. Therefore, it is important not to attribute the clinical signs in a cold baby to hypothermia alone, but at the same time to investigate for underlying or coexisting complications such as infection or hypoglycemia.

Extreme cold stress will result in a heightened metabolic response to cold, which may become exhausted by substrate deficiency. There are theoretical reasons, backed up by anecdotal accounts, why cold babies could become hypoglycemic if substrate stores become depleted.[5] There is no doubt that glycogen stores will be rapidly depleted by catecholamine-induced glycogenolysis. However, even in fasted infants, part of the catabolic response is to release gluconeogenic precursors from fat and muscle so that glucose production may continue.[34,35] There is no direct evidence that the gluconeogenic pathway fails in hypothermia. It is not clear from published literature whether hypoglycemia and hypothermia are epi-phenomena in a sick baby, or whether this is a causal relationship (and, if so, which is cause and which is effect).

Some information is available from experimental studies of therapeutic cooling (see below). Findings from animal studies vary. In one, cooling to a body temperature of 30 °C and 32 °C resulted in a greater contribution of glucose to metabolism. Measured rates of glucose production and glucose utilization increased in parallel, so there was no change in blood glucose concentration.[36] Another study suggested that infused glucose requirements are increased during hypothermia.[37]

It is likely that most neonates who are not receiving infused glucose are able to achieve increased glucose delivery when required via glycogenolysis then gluconeogenesis. A clinical study of mild therapeutic hypothermia did not report hypoglycemia.[38] In a cross-sectional study of 578 neonates in Nepal, it was demonstrated that hypothermia was not a risk factor for development of hypoglycemia, after correcting for other confounders.[39] However, in the same cohort, hypothermia and low infant thyroxine level were independently associated with failure to mount a ketone body response to hypoglycemia.[40]

Again, in theory, the increased metabolic demand could result in oxygen demand outweighing supply so that tissue hypoxia and lactic acidosis results. There is no published evidence that hypoxia occurs as a direct result of the metabolic response to hypothermia. However, if cold stress impairs control of breathing, respiratory insufficiency itself may result in hypoxia. Respiratory insufficiency and reduced tissue perfusion are the most likely etiology for the lactic acidosis seen in hypothermia.[41]

There are anecdotal reports that hypothermia causes surfactant deficiency, but the mechanism for this has not been described.[5] It is possible that this is mediated via the lactic acidosis that develops.

Clinical studies of therapeutic cooling vary as to whether blood clotting abnormalities are a feature.[42–45] These differences are likely to be related to the prevalence of coagulation abnormalities after hypoxic-ischemic injury and may not be directly related to hypothermia. Results from larger randomized controlled trials should resolve this.

Pathological associations with over-heating

There is increasing evidence that maternal and fetal hyperthermia is associated with an adverse fetal and neonatal outcome, even after correcting for the effects of any concurrent infection.

Hyperthermia in early pregnancy was the first described teratogen, and is associated with neural tube defects, limb disruptions and anencephaly.[46–49] This has resulted in advice to pregnant women regarding avoiding hot baths and saunas, and has raised concerns regarding safety of diagnostic ultrasound.[50] However, the World Federation of Ultrasound in Medicine and Biology (WFUMB),[51] European Federation of Societies for Ultrasound in Medicine and Biology (EFSUMB),[52] and the British Medical Ultrasound Society (BMUS)[53] have reviewed the evidence and produced guidelines for use in diagnostic ultrasound, which protect patients (including fetuses), from excessive or dangerous exposure.

Intrapartum fever is associated with an increased risk for need for neonatal resuscitation and with neonatal encephalopathy, even after correcting for other intrapartum risk factors.[54,55] This may be through maternal hemodynamic changes, the associated increase in fetal temperature or inflammatory mediators. There has been concern regarding overheating of the fetus during labour and delivery in a birthing pool, and high water temperatures are associated with fetal tachycardia.[56]

Overheating of the neonate is usually "iatrogenic." Dehydration, withdrawal from opiate drugs, and rare conditions such as hypothalamic disorders, also result in increased body temperature. Neonatal infection more often results in hypothermia than hyperthermia.

Clearly if a baby is exposed to an excessive heat source for an excessive period of time there is a risk of thermal burn. This has secondary implications in terms of prevention of infection, fluid balance, and thermal control as all of these processes are dependent on intact skin covering. Long-term scarring of the skin may also result. Very rarely, but with devastating consequences, the lungs may be injured by excessively hot inspired gas.

Just as with hypothermia, hyperthermia places metabolic demands upon a baby with increased oxygen consumption and diverting fuels from growth and storage. In addition, the associated cardiovascular changes, e.g. tachycardia and vasodilatation, may precipitate cardiovascular collapse in a vulnerable baby. Dehydration is another potential complication. Severe neonatal hyperthermia may also result in fits, disseminated intravascular coagulation, and renal and hepatic failure.[1]

In older infants, and some neonates, over-wrapping and high body temperature is considered a risk for sudden infant death ("cot death").[57]

Therefore, it is essential to prevent neonatal body temperature rising above normal.

Clinical interventions

There are basic interventions to prevent vulnerable babies from becoming cold, or for rewarming babies who have become cold. An understanding of the routes of heat loss will ensure that this is minimized by each route (Table 5.2). These principles have been incorporated into strategies for neonatal care and equipment design throughout the history of neonatology.

In addition, there are circumstances when additional measures prove more effective or when the thermal environment is manipulated for possible therapeutic potential.

Basic measures

Although basic technology to keep babies warm has been available for over a century, there was a prolonged period in the history of neonatology ("the hands-off years") when it was considered inadvisable to "force the body temperature of small infants to the supposedly normal range".[31]

Design technology has introduced sophisticated methods of monitoring baby and environmental temperature and adjusting via servo control.[58] It is difficult to monitor core temperature on the neonate as the most approximate measure, rectal temperature, has practical and risk-related limitations, e.g. cross-infection, trauma, parental acceptability. Axillary temperature may be used as another approximate measure, but requires sufficiently long contact with the thermometer, again there being practical limitations in the sick (or squirming) baby. A thermometer

Table 5.2. Strategies to prevent heat loss

Route	Intervention
Conduction	Avoid contact with cold surfaces e.g. wrap X-ray plates
	Pre-warmed bedding and clothing
	Pre-warmed, low conductivity mattress
Convection	Adequate external air temperature (32–36 °C)
	Clothing, especially hat
	Minimal air flows e.g. from fans, air conditioning
	Enclosed environment e.g. incubator, transport incubator
	Minimize opening of incubator portholes
	Warmed ambient and inspired gases
Evaporation	Dry wet babies
	Wipe dry and avoid pooling of cleaning solutions
	High air temperature
	Clothing, especially hat
	Minimal air flows e.g. from fans, air conditioning
	Warmed ambient and inspired gases
	Humidified ambient gases – incubator or under polythene
	Humidified inspired gases
Radiation	Position babies away from cool external walls and surfaces
	Heat shields
	Double-walled incubator

measuring core temperature via the ear drum has been developed, but its accuracy is questionable and widespread use has not been adopted.[59,60] Skin temperature recording, via surface probes has the advantage of simplicity, but also of being a sensitive indicator of external thermal challenge. Skin temperature falls earlier and to a greater degree during cold stress.[5] In order to avoid spuriously high readings (and therefore the risk of allowing the baby to become cold), the probes should be protected (via reflecting material) from radiant heat sources and should not be placed over brown adipose tissue sites, or areas of inflamed or broken skin. If placed too peripherally or on vasoconstricted skin, the baby's body temperature may be underestimated and there may be excess heat delivery and overheating of the baby.

In a servo-controlled thermal environment, it is important to take into account incubator or radiant warmer temperature when assessing the baby. The baby may be recorded as having a "normal" temperature but at the same time an excessively high incubator temperature would imply difficulty for the baby in maintaining thermal control, or an excessively low incubator temperature may imply a masked neonatal pyrexial state. As disordered thermal control (in either direction) is a marker of neonatal infection, failure to take into account incubator temperature may lead to a delay in diagnosis and treatment.

It should be noted that a normal body temperature does not guarantee thermal stability. The baby may be maintaining body temperature via the mechanisms listed above and these mechanisms may themselves have negative consequences, e.g. for growth. Or the baby may be reaching the limit of his capacity to generate heat with imminent de-compensation. Therefore, it is important to put in place measures that minimize thermal challenge to the neonate.

Drying and clothing the neonate reduce heat loss of all types. Adding a hat of high insulating material is of particular importance as the head is a major focus of heat generation and heat loss (see above). [10,61,62] Clothing and hats will block radiant heat so reduce the effectiveness of a radiant warmer.

For over a century, small infants have been nursed in incubators with heat delivered by convection of warmed air.[31] The walls of the incubator allow entry of light, which is converted to heat when absorbed by the baby's skin. However, short wave heat energy cannot leave the incubator, thus preserving heat in the incubator. The insulating effect of a double-walled incubator reduces the temperature gradient across the incubator wall, thus reducing heat loss from incubator to external environment and, in turn, heat loss from the baby to incubator environment.[1,63,64]

Infants may also be nursed under radiant heaters, which have the advantage of access to the baby.[1] However, convective and evaporative losses are greater than in an incubator. Convective losses may be minimized by use of a plastic heat shield with the ends closed by polythene or by "bubble wrap". However, these in turn reduce radiant heat gain as radiant heat does not pass through these materials. An alternative, in common use, is to make a polythene "tent", under which the infant is nursed.

Finally, for the larger and stable preterm baby, an open cot with a water-filled electrically heated mattress or a preheated gel-filled mattress is often sufficient to maintain thermal control.[1] There are also mattresses available that are heated by a crystallization reaction, which is useful in a transport setting.[65]

The recognition of the requirement for humidified ambient and inspired gases has been of particular benefit to the care of preterm babies, in terms of both thermal control and fluid balance. These babies are now normally nursed in 100% ambient humidity until the skin keratinizes, and at this humidity evaporative losses are minimal.[9,66] This is achieved in an incubator by control of humidified gas. If the baby is under a radiant warmer, warmed, humidified air is delivered to the baby nursed under polythene or a heat shield with polythene wrapped around the ends.[67] To optimize radiant heat gain, polythene sheeting is preferable to a heat shield. The aim is to achieve high humidity so that there is "rain out" on the incubator or polythene surface. Inspired gases, especially delivered by assisted ventilation must be warmed and humidified.

There is no universally agreed strategy for rewarming the baby who has become hypothermic.[1,5] The rate of rewarming may need to be slowed if the baby shows evidence of cardiovascular compromise during rewarming. Complications associated with hypothermia, such as respiratory distress, blood clotting abnormalities, feeding difficulties and hypoglycemia should be detected and treated.

The corollary to preventing cold stress is to avoid thermal injury to the baby. The baby should not be placed in contact with or close to hot surfaces. As radiant heat uptake is independent of ambient temperature, it should be noted that a baby may become over-heated in an incubator, despite a normal incubator temperature.

Kangaroo care

For decades it has been recognized that kangaroo care (skin to skin contact), with the baby nursed on the mother's chest, has immense benefits, particularly for thermal stability, establishment of maternal lactation and for psychological well-being.[68,69] The practice arose in developing countries where access to incubators may be limited. A recent Cochrane database systematic review concluded that in developing countries, when compared with conventional neonatal care, kangaroo care reduces the risk of nosocomial infection and severe illness, and increases rates of exclusive breast-feeding and maternal satisfaction.[70] There is also evidence that kangaroo care accelerates autonomic and neurobehavioral maturation, which in turn improve parenting outcome.[71,72] For healthy term infants, the practice is associated with reduced crying behavior, and more rapid resolution of negative base excess and a higher blood glucose after delivery, when compared with babies kept in cots.[73]

Studies have demonstrated this method of caring for babies does not pose a cold stress.[74] However, a note of caution is introduced by one study, demonstrating that a marked increase in body temperature associated with skin to skin contact is associated with increased frequency of bradycardia and hypoxemia. Therefore, it is recommended that for small and vulnerable babies, temperature and cardiorespiratory monitoring should continue during skin to skin contact.[75]

With this proviso, kangaroo care should be recommended as an integral aspect of neonatal care, even for extremely preterm babies.

Polythene bags

Although not a new invention, it has become popular practice to place newborn preterm babies in polythene bags or wrapping immediately after delivery.[30,76,77] This is most effective at extremely preterm gestations (<28 weeks) and may be associated with decreased mortality.[77] However, anecdotal accounts now exist of babies becoming overheated by this method, which may itself cause harm. Therefore, there must be careful audit by neonatal units that introduce the practice.

Cooling as a cerebro-protective strategy

For decades, body cooling has been an important strategy to protect heart and brain during pediatric cardiac surgery necessitating circulatory arrest.[78,79] It has also been introduced as an experimental strategy in neonates receiving ECMO.[43]

More recently, studies on neonatal animals have demonstrated a cerebro-protective effect of cooling shortly after a hypoxic-ischemic insult.[80,81] Clinical trials of selective head cooling and whole body cooling have been carried out and further trials continue.[82]

Whilst definitive outcome data are awaited, these trials have added further information regarding the cardiovascular and metabolic effects of cooling.[83] Mild hypothermia to 34.0–35.0 °C produces moderate reduction in heart rate and blood pressure, but without cardiovascular compromise. However, the strategy is associated with increased inspired oxygen requirements.[83] Another study confirms no significant clinical sequelae, including no increased risk of hypoglycemia, when babies are cooled to 34.5–35.0 °C.[38] A study using the piglet model cooled to 35.0 °C describes no increased risk of organ damage, although during hypothermia there were increased oxygen and glucose requirements.[37] Increased glucose requirements have not been found by other groups using a similar model (J.S. Wyatt, personal communication).

Although therapeutic cooling appears to be safe and to carry no risks additional to those of the underlying disorder, it should only be carried out by experienced professionals in an intensive care setting with availability of appropriate monitoring and laboratory support.[84]

Summary

Robertson eloquently describes the history of knowledge of neonatal thermal control and its applications, pointing out the errors that occurred in the early "hands-off years" of neonatal practice.[31] It is essential that those caring for neonates continue to receive basic teaching of the physiology of the neonate so that this may be applied to practice and to an understanding of the advanced technology now in common use. Less "technological" methods, e.g. polythene wrapping and kangaroo care, still have a role, but must still be treated with respect so as not to introduce risk. Finally, there must be initiatives to ensure international understanding of the importance of thermal regulation.[85] The basic physiological needs of the neonate must be understood and met, prior to introducing advanced technologies and treatments.

Acknowledgements

Dr. Topun Austin for figures.

Mr. Raj Dave, for information about ultrasound.

Dr. Edmund Hey, for teaching and inspiring.

REFERENCES

1 Rutter, N. Temperature control and its disorders. In Robertson, N. R. C., Rennie, J. M., eds. *Textbook of Neonatology*. Edinburgh: Churchill Livingstone; 1999.

2 Harned, H. S., Herrington, R. T., Ferreiro, J. I. The effects of immersion and temperature on respiration in newborn lambs. *Pediatrics* 1970;**45**:598–602.

3 Adamsons, K., Gandy, G. M., James, L. S. The influence of thermal factors upon oxygen consumption of the newborn human infant. *J. Pediatr.* 1965;**66**:495–508.

4 Bruck, K. Temperature regulation in the newborn infant. *Biol. Neonate.* 1961;**3**:65–119.

5 Blackburn, S. T., Loper, D. L. Thermoregulation. In Blackburn, S. T., Loper, D. L., eds. *Maternal, Fetal and Neonatal Physiology: a Clinical Perspective*. Philadelphia, PA: W. B. Saunders; 1992:677–97.

6 Hey, E. N., Katz, G. The optimum thermal environment for naked babies. *Arch. Dis. Child.* 1970;**45**:328–34.

7 Hey, E. Thermal neutrality. *Br. Med. Bull.* 1975;**31**:69–74.

8 Sauer, P. J., Dane, H. J., Visser, H. K. A. New standards for neutral thermal environment of healthy very low birth weight infants in week one of life. *Arch. Dis. Child.* 1984;**59**:18–22.

9 Sauer, P. J., Dane, H. J., Visser, H. K. A. Influences of variations in ambient humidity on insensible water loss and thermoneutral environment of low birthweight infants. *Acta Paediatr. Scand.* 1984;**73**:615–19.

10 Rowe, M. I., Weinberg, G., Andrews, W. Reduction of neonatal heat loss by an insulated head cover. *J. Pediatr. Surg.* 1983;**18**:909–13.

11 Fanaroff, A. A., Wald, M., Gruber, H. S., Klaus, M. H. Insensible water loss in low birth weight infants. *Pediatrics* 1972;**50**:236–45.

12 Rutter, N., Hull, D. Water loss from the skin of term and preterm babies. *Arch. Dis. Child.* 1979;**54**:858–68.

13 Baumgart, S. Partitioning of heat losses and heat gains in premature newborn infants under radiant warmers. *Pediatrics* 1985;**75**:89–99.

14 Jones, R. W., Rochefort, M. J., Baum, J. D. Increased insensible water loss in newborn infants nursed under radiant heaters. *Br. Med. J.* 1976;**2**:1347–50.

15 Hey, E. N., Katz, G. The range of thermal insulation in the tissues of the newborn baby. *J. Physiol.* 1970;**207**:667–81.

16 Polk, D. H., Callegari, C. C., Newnham, J. *et al.* Effect of fetal thyroidectomy on newborn thermogenesis in lambs. *Pediatr. Res.* 1987;**21**:453–7.

17 Gunn, T. R., Gluckman, P. D. The endocrine control of the onset of thermogenesis at birth. *Bailieres Clin. Endocrinol. Metab.* 1989;**3**:869–86.

18 Marchini, G., Persson, B., Jonsson, N., Marcus, C. Influence of body temperature on thyrotrophic hormone release and lipolysis in the newborn infant. *Acta Paediatr.* 1995;**84**:1284–8.

19 Deavers, D. R., Musacchia, X. J. The function of glucocorticoids in thermogenesis. *Fed. Proc.* 1979;**38**:2177–81.

20 Glass, L., Silverman, W. A., Sinclair, J. C. Effect of thermal environment on cold resistance and growth of small infants after the first week of life. *Pediatrics* 1968;**41**:1033–46.

21 Davis, V. The structure and function of brown adipose tissue in the neonate. *J. Obstet. Gynecol. Neonatal Nurs.* 1980;**9**:368–72.

22 Hey, E. N., Katz, G. Evaporative water loss in the newborn baby. *J. Physiol.* 1969;**200**:605–19.

23 Foster, K. G., Hey, E. N., Katz, G. The response of sweat glands of the newborn baby to thermal stimuli and to intradermal acetylcholine. *J. Physiol.* 1969;**203**:13–29.

24 Cogneville, A. M., Cividino, N., Tordet-Caridroit, C. Lipid composition of brown adipose tissue as related to nutrition during the neonatal period in hypotrophic rats. *J. Nutr.* 1975;**105**:982–8.

25 Zimmerberg, B. Thermoregulatory deficits following prenatal alcohol exposure: structural correlates. *Alcohol* 1989;**6**:389–93.

26 Blakelok, R. T., Harding, J. E., Kolbe, A., Pease, P. W. Gastroschisis: can the morbidity be avoided? *Pediatr. Surg. Int.* 1997;**12**:276–82.

27 Silverman, W. A., Fertig, J. W., Berger, A. P. The influence of the thermal environment upon survival of newly born premature infants. *Pediatrics* 158;**22**:876–86.

28 Beutow, K. C., Klein, S. W. Effects of maintenance of "normal" skin temperature on survival of infants of low birthweight. *Pediatrics* 1964;**34**:163–70.

29 Glass, L., Lala, R. V., Jaiswal, V., Nigam, S. K. Effect of thermal environment and caloric intake on head growth of low birthweight infants during the late neonatal period. *Arch. Dis. Child.* 1975;**50**:571–3.

30 Narendran, V., Hoath, S. B. Thermal management of the low birth weight infants: a cornerstone of neonatology. *J. Pediatr.* 1999;**134**:529–31.

31 Robertson, A. F. Reflections on errors in neonatology: I. The "hands-off" years, 1920–1950. *J. Perinatol.* 2003;**23**:48–55.

32 Costeloe, K., Hennessy, E., Gibson, A. T., Marlow, N., Wilkinson, A. R. The EPICure study: outcomes to discharge from hospital for infants born at the threshold of viability. *Pediatrics* 2000;**106**:659–71.

33 CESDI. Project 27/28. An enquiry into quality of care and its effect on the survival of babies born at 27–28 weeks. Confidential Enquiry into Stillbirths and Deaths, UK. 2003. Available at: *http://www.cemach.org.uk*

34 Schultz, K., Soltesz, G., Molnar, D., Mestyan, J. Effect of hypothermia on plasma metabolites in preterm newborn infants with particular reference to plasma free amino acids. *Biol. Neonate.* 1979;**36**:220–4.

35 Deshpande, S., Hawdon, J. M., Ward Platt, M. P., Aynsley-Green, A. Metabolic adaptation to extrauterine life. In Rodeck, C. H., Whittle, M. J., eds. *Fetal Medicine: Basic Science and Clinical Practice.* London: Churchill Livingstone; 1999:1059–69.

36 Hetenyi, G. Jr, Cowan, J. S. Effect of cooling on the glucoregulation of anesthetized and non-anesthetized newborn dogs. *Biol. Neonate* 1981;**40**:9–20.

37 Satas, S., Loberg, E. M., Porter, H. *et al.* Effect of global hypoxia-ischemia followed by 24h of mild hypothermia on organ pathology and biochemistry in a newborn pig survival model. *Biol. Neonate* 2003;**83**:146–56.

38 Battin, M. R., Penrice, J., Gunn, T. R., Gunn, A. R. Treatment of term infants with head cooling and mild systemic hypothermia (35 °C and 34.5 °C) after perinatal asphyxia. *Pediatrics* 2003;**111**:244–51.

39 Pal, D. K., Manandhar, D. S., Rajbhandari, S. *et al.* Neonatal hypoglycemia in Nepal. 1. Prevalence and risk factors. *Arch. Dis. Child.* 2000;**82**:46–51.

40 de L' Costello, A. M., Pal, D. K., Manandhar, D. S. *et al.* Neonatal hypoglycaemia in Nepal. 2. Availability of alternative fuels. *Arch. Dis. Child.* 2000;**82**:52–8.

41 Stayer, S. A., Steven, J. M., Nicolson, S. C. *et al.* The metabolic effects of surface cooling neonates prior to cardiac surgery. *Anesth. Analg.* 1994;**79**:834–9.

42 Azzopardi, D., Robertson, N. J., Cowan, F. M. *et al.* Pilot study of treatment with whole body hypothermia for neonatal encephalopathy. *Pediatrics* 2000;**106**:684–94.

43 Ichiba, S., Killer, H. M., Firmin, R. K. *et al.* Pilot investigation of hypothermia in neonates receiving extracorporeal membrane oxygenation. *Arch. Dis. Child.* 2003;**88**:128–33.

44 Debillon, T., Daoud, P., Durand, P., *et al.* Whole-body cooling after perinatal asphyxia: a pilot study in term neonates. *Dev. Med. Child. Neurol.* 2003;**45**:17–23.

45 Compagnoni, G., Pogliani, L., Lista, G. *et al.* Hypothermia reduces neurological damage in asphyxiated newborn infants. *Biol. Neonate* 2002;**82**:222–7.

46 Sasaki, J., Yamaguchi, A., Nabeshima, Y. *et al.* Exercise at high temperature causes maternal hyperthermia and fetal anomalies. *Teratology* 1995;**51**:233–6.

47 Graham, J. M. Jr, Edwards, M. J. Teratogen update: gestational effects of maternal hyperthermia due to febrile illness and resultant patterns of defects in humans. *Teratology* 1998;**58**:209–21.

48 Martinez-Frias, M. L., Garcia Mazario, M. J., Caldas, C. F. *et al.* High maternal fever during gestation and severe congenital limb disruptions. *Am. J. Med. Genet.* 2001;**98**:201–3.

49 Chambers, C. D., Johnson, K. A., Dick, L. M., Felix, R. J., Jones, K. L. Maternal fever and birth outcome: a prospective study. *Teratology* 1998;**58**:251–7.

50 Miller, M. W., Nyborg, W. L., Dewey, W. C. *et al.* Hyperthermic teratogenicity, thermal dose and diagnostic ultrasound during pregnancy: implications of new standards on tissue heating. *J. Hyperthermia* 2002;**18**:361–84.

51 World Federation of Ultrasound in Medicine and Biology. Available at: http://www.wfumb.org.

52 European Federation of Societies for Ultrasound in Medicine and Biology. Available at http://www.efsumb.org.

53 British Medical Ultrasound Society. Guidelines for the use of diagnostic ultrasound equipment. *BMUS Bulletin.* Aug. 2000;29–33.

54 Lieberman, E., Lang, J., Richardson, D. K. *et al.* Intrapartum maternal fever and neonatal outcome. *Pediatrics* 2000;**105**:8–13.

55 Impey, L., Greenwood, C., MacQuillan, K., Reynolds, M., Sheil, O. Fever in labour and neonatal encephalopathy: a prospective study. *Br. J. Obstet. Gynaecol.* 2001;**108**:594–7.

56 Deans, A. C., Steer, P. J. Labour and birth in water. Temperature of pool is important. *Br. Med. J..* 1995;**11**:390–1.

57 Fleming, P. J., Azaz, Y., Wigfield, R. Development of thermoregulation in infancy: possible implications for SIDS. *J. Clin. Pathol.* 1992;**45**:S17–19.

58 Sinclair, J. C. Servo-control for maintaining abdominal skin temperature at 36 °C in low birth weight infants. *Cochrane Database Syst Rev.* 2002;CD001074.

59 Johnson, K. J., Bhatia, P., Bell, E. F. Infrared thermometry of newborn infants. *Pediatrics* 1991;**87**:34–8.

60 Craig, J. V., Lancaster, G. A., Taylor, S., Williamson, P. R., Smyth, R. L. Infrared ear thermometry compared with rectal thermometry in children: a systematic review. *Lancet* 2002;**360**: 603–9.

61 Stothers, J. K. Head insulation and heat loss in the newborn. *Arch. Dis. Child.* 1981;**56**:530–4.

62 Marks, K. H., Devenyi, A. G., Bello, M. E. *et al.* Thermal head wrap for infants. *J. Pediatr.* 1985;**107**:956–9.

63 Marks, K. H., Lee, C. A., Bolan, C. D. Jr, Maisels, M. J. Oxygen consumption and temperature control of premature infants in a double wall incubator. *Pediatrics* 1981;**68**:93–8.

64 Yeh, T. F., Voora, S., Lilien, L. D. *et al.* Oxygen consumption and insensible water loss in premature infants in single versus double-walled incubators. *J. Pediatr.* 1980;**97**:967–71.

65 Nielsen, H., Jung, A., Atherton, S. Evaluation of the Porta-Warm mattress as a source of heat for neonatal transport. *Pediatrics* 1976;**58**:500–54.

66 Sulyok, E., Jequier, E., Ryser, G. Effect of relative humidity on the thermal balance of the newborn infant. *Biol. Neonate* 1982;**21**:210–18.

67 Baumgart, S., Engle, W. D., Fox, W. W., Polin, R. A. Effect of heat shielding on convection and evaporation, and radiant heat transfer in the premature infant. *J. Pediatr.* 1981;**97**:948–56.

68 Whitelaw, A. Kangaroo baby care: just a nice experience or an important advance for preterm infants. *Pediatrics* 1990;**85**:604–5.

69 Charpak, N., Ruiz-Pelaez, J. G., Figueroa de Calume, Z. Current knowledge of Kangaroo Mother intervention. *Curr. Opin. Pediatr.* 1996;**8**:108–12.

70 Conde-Agudelo, A., Diaz-Rossello, J. L., Belizan, J. M. Kangaroo mother care to reduce morbidity and mortality in low birth-weight infants. *Cochrane Database Syst Rev.* 2003:CD002771

71 Feldman, R., Eidelman, A. I. Skin-to-skin contact (Kangaroo Care) accelerates autonomic and neurobehavioural maturation in preterm infants. *Dev. Med. Child. Neurol.* 2003;**45**:274–81.

72 Feldman, R., Eidelman, A. I., Sirota, L., Weller, A. Comparison of skin-to-skin (kangaroo) and traditional care: parenting outcomes and preterm infant development. *Pediatrics* 2002;**110**:16–26.

73 Christensson, K., Siles, C., Moreno, L. *et al.* Temperature, metabolic adaptation and crying in healthy full-term newborns cared for skin-to-skin or in a cot. *Acta Paediatr.* 1992;**81**:488–49.

74 Bauer, K., Uhrig, C., Sperling, P. *et al.* Body temperatures and oxygen consumption during skin-to-skin (kangaroo) care of preterm infants weighing less than 1500 grams. *J. Pediatr.* 1997;**130**:240–4.

75 Bohnhorst, B., Heyne, T., Peter, C. S., Poets, C. F. Skin-to-skin (kangaroo) care, respiratory control, and thermoregulation. *J. Pediatr.* 2001;**138**:193–217.

76 Besch, N. J., Perlstein, P. H., Edwards, N. K., Keenan, W. J., Sutherland, J. M. The transparent baby bag: a shield against heat loss. *N. Engl. J. Med.* 1971;**284**:121–4.

77 Vohra, S., Frent, G., Campbell, V., Abbott, M., Whyte, R., Effect of polythene occlusive skin wrapping on heat loss in very low birth weight infants at delivery: a randomized trial. *J. Pediatr.* 1999;**134**:547–51.

78 Harden, A., Pampiglione, G., Waterston, D. J. Circulatory arrest during hypothermia in cardiac surgery: an EEG study in children. *Br. Med. J.* 1966;**2**:1105–8.

79 Kirkham, F. J. Recognition and prevention of neurological complications in pediatric cardiac surgery. *Pediatr. Cardiol.* 1998;**19**:331–45.

80 Thoresen, M., Penrice, J., Lorek, A. *et al.* Mild hypothermia after severe transient hypoxia-ischaemia ameliorates delayed cerebral energy failure in the newborn piglet. *Pediatr. Res.* 1995;**37**:667–70.

81 Gunn, A. J., Gunn, T. R., Gunning, M. I., Williams, C. E., Gluckman, P. D. Neuroprotection with prolonged head cooling started before postischemic seizures in fetal sheep. *Pediatrics* 1998;**102**:1098–116.

82 Whitelaw, A., Thoresen, M. Clinical trials of treatments after perinatal asphyxia. *Curr. Opin. Pediatr.* 2002;**14**:664–8.

83 Thoresen, M., Whitelaw, A. Cardiovascular changes during mild therapeutic hypothermia and rewarming in neonates with hypoxic-ischaemic encephalopathy. *Pediatrics* 2000;**106**:92–9.

84 Thoresen, M. Cooling the newborn after asphyxia – physiological and experimental background and its clinical use. *Semin. Neonatol.* 2000;**5**:61–73.

85 Dragovich, D., Tamburlini, G., Alisjahbana, A. *et al.* Thermal control of the newborn: knowledge and practice of health professionals in seven countries. *Acta Paediatr.* 1997;**86**:645–50.

6

Development and physiology of the gastrointestinal tract

Carol Lynn Berseth

Mead Johnson Nutritionals, Evansville, Indiana

When the gut evaginates and the cloacal and oral membranes rupture, the interface between amniotic fluid and the fetus is established. This interface serves as a conduit for the transfer of nutrients that are external to the fetus and the neonate. The aboral movement of amniotic fluid occurs as early as 18 weeks' gestation, and up to 450 ml of amniotic fluid move aborally through the intestine by term. While the intrauterine environment is sterile, the introduction of feedings presents a major challenge to host defense. Thus, the neonatal intestine is a digestive organ as well as an important component of the immune system. Both aspects of intestinal function will be reviewed in this chapter.

Digestion and absorption

Mucosal differentiation

During the second and third trimesters of pregnancy, growth and maturation of the gastrointestinal tract occur in preparation for postnatal life. The timing of structural and functional maturation is summarized in Tables 6.1 and 6.2. The gut lengthens to 250–300 cm by term, and gastric capacity is about 30 mL. During the second trimester, the glycocalyx appears, and the brush border is structurally well defined. Superficial glands are present in the pharyngeal and esophageal mucosa by 20 weeks and squamous cells by 28 weeks. Mucous and lingual lipases are also secreted. Endocrine, chief, mucus and parietal cells appear in the stomach by 12 weeks; by 16 weeks, these cells actively secrete hydrochloric acid, intrinsic factor, pepsin, gastrin and mucus. Although acid secretion is present shortly after birth in preterm and term infants, it is approximately 10% of that seen in adults.[1]

Endocrine cells are well established, and granules containing gastrin, secretin, cholecystokinin, motilin, serotonin, somatostatin and substance P are present by 12–18 weeks. Gastrin, secretin, motilin and gastrin inhibitory polypeptide are localized to duodenum and jejunum, whereas enteroglucagon, neurotensin, somatostatin and vasoactive intestinal polypeptide are distributed throughout the intestines. Brush-border membrane function remains immature during the third trimester. Alpha-glucosidases, dipeptidases and sucrase are functional by the end of the second trimester, but lactase activity at 24 weeks is less than 25% of that seen at term[2] and maltase activities are 50–75% of those found in term infants.[2,3] The abrupt rise in lactase activity that occurs from 32–34 weeks' gestation coincides with an increase in lactase mRNA, implying that its delay in appearance is due to transcriptional control.[4]

Sucrase-isomaltase exists in a single high molecular-weight form.[5] Glucoamylase, which is responsible for absorption of starches and glucose polymers, is present by the end of the second trimester with activities approximately half that found at term.[2] Other brush-border peptidases, including alpha-glutamyl transpeptidase, aminopeptidase, oligoaminopeptidase, dipeptidyl-aminopeptidase IV and carboxypeptidase are present by the end of the second trimester. Thus, active glucose transport occurs by 10 weeks[6] and amino acid uptake by 12 weeks.[7]

Gastrointestinal hormones and peptides

Numerous regulatory gut peptides are produced in the gastrointestinal tract. As in adults, they may be true hormones

Neonatal Nutrition and Metabolism. Second Edition, ed. P. Thureen and W. Hay. Published by Cambridge University Press.
© Cambridge University Press 2006.

Table 6.1. Structural maturation of the gastrointestinal tract

Esophagus	
Superficial glands develop	20 weeks
Squamous cells appear	28 weeks
Stomach	
Gastric glands form	14 weeks
Pylorus and fundus defined	14 weeks
Small intestine	
Crypt/villus appear	14 weeks
Lymph nodes appear	14 weeks
Intestinal peptides and hormones appear	14 weeks
Neurotransmitters appear	12 weeks
Myenteric plexus present	14 weeks
Colon	
Diameter decreases	20 weeks
Villi disappear	20 weeks
Pancreas	
Differentiation of exocrine and endocrine tissue	14 weeks
Liver	
Lobule formation	11 weeks

Table 6.2. Functional maturation of the gastrointestinal tract

Sucking	32 weeks
Gastric secretion	20 weeks
Pancreatic zymogen	20 weeks
Bile acid secretion	22 weeks
Intestinal transport of amino acids	14 weeks
Intestinal glucose transport	18 weeks
Intestinal fatty acid absorption	24 weeks

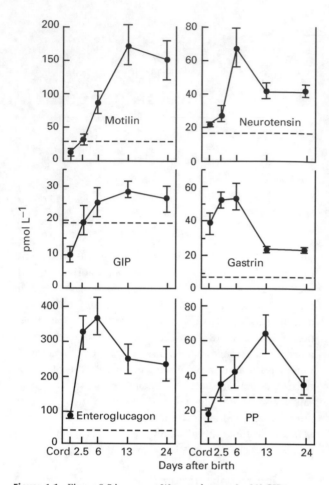

Figure 6.1. Figure 3.5 in current Weaver chapter. [p. 81] GIP gastric inhibitac peptide; pp, pancreatic polypeptide.

(e.g. gastrin, cholecystokinin, motilin, pancreatic polypeptide and somatostatin), while others have paracrine or neurocrine function (e.g. gastric inhibitory polypeptide, bombesin, vasoactive intestinal polypeptide, neurotensin, enteroglucagon and peptide YY). All of these peptides are identified to be present in the fetal intestine by the end of the first trimester. Some of these hormones are released in response to feeding.[8] However, their releases are limited in the newborn compared with the adult (Figure 6.1).[9,10]

Pancreas and liver

Differentiation of the endocrine and exocrine structure of the pancreas is present by 14 weeks. Amylase is present by 16 weeks, and trypsin, lipase and amylase are secreted into the duodenum by 31 weeks.[11] Concentrations of these enzymes are lower in preterm than term infants and, in turn, are significantly lower in term infants than children. Postnatally, trypsin increases in concentration, followed by chymotrypsin, carboxypeptidase, lipase and amylase (Figure 6.2).[12]

Hepatic lobules and bile canaliculi are present by 6 weeks; bile acids are synthesized by 12–14 weeks and they are actively secreted by 22 weeks. Bile acid synthesis is decreased in the preterm infant compared with the term infant, which, in turn, is approximately half of that seen in adults, as is bile acid pool size (Figure 6.1).[13] Hepatic hydroxylation is not fully developed in the fetus and there is a decreased cholic acid: deoxycholic acid ratio. The active ileal transport mechanism of bile salts is present but immature (Figure 6.2).[14]

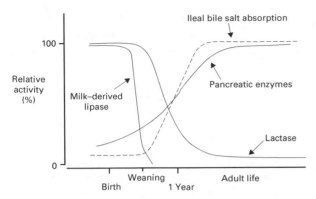

Figure 6.2. Diagramatic representation of the major changes in digestive function in the fetus, newborn and child. Reproduced with permission.[69]

Digestion of carbohydrates

Although lactose is the predominant source of carbohydrate in breast milk and formulas for term infants, some preterm formulas also contain glucose polymers. Despite having relatively low levels of lactase activity, preterm infants display normal growth when they are fed lactose-containing milk and formula.[15] The relative absence of lactase activity may permit the conversion of malabsorbed lactose by colonic bacteria to volatile organic acids, which are subsequently absorbed.[16] Because pancreatic amylase levels are quite low, glucose polymers are likely hydrolyzed by salivary amylase or absorbed directly at the mucosal level via mucosal glucoamylase (Figure 6.2).[17]

Digestion of lipids

Fat provides 50% of the caloric intake of the newborn. Fats are emulsified and hydrolyzed to form free fatty acids and monoglycerides by the action of bile acids and lipases, both of which are limited in presence and function in the preterm infant. Additional alternate mechanisms for fat hydrolysis appear to be present in the newborn. Lingual lipases and gastric lipases are present by 26 weeks' gestation. Additional lipases are also present in breast milk. Preterm formulas contain medium-chain triglycerides which do not require micellar formation for absorption. Although the absorption of fats is not nearly as efficient as carbohydrates and proteins, absorption is sufficient to permit growth and uptake of fat-soluble vitamins.

Digestion of protein

Although proteins contribute less than 10% of ingested calories, they are essential for normal somatic growth and

maturation. In the upper intestine, pancreatic proteases are fairly efficient in splitting peptides to oligopeptides and amino acids. Most of the brush border and cytosolic peptidases are well developed in the preterm infant and the peptide transport system is efficient. In addition, macromolecules can be actively taken up by pinocytosis by the neonatal intestine,[18] and preterm infants have been demonstrated to absorb intact lactoferrin.[19] As a result, preterm infants exhibit increased intestinal permeability that resolves with advancing gestational age,[20] as shown in Figure 6.3.

The role of nutrients

There have been concerns that preterm infants have limited capacity to process carbohydrates, fats and proteins.

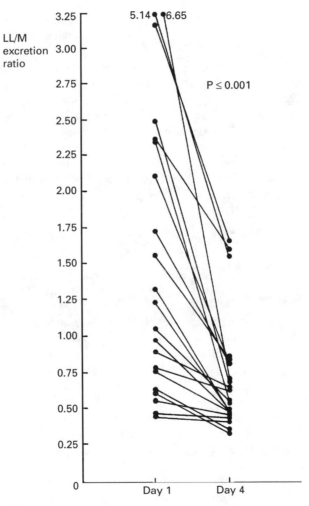

Figure 6.3. Figure 3.2 in current Weaver chapter. [p. 78] LL/M, urinary lactulose:mannitol.

Hence, preterm formulas contain glucose polymers and medium chain triglycerides. Recently, investigators have shown that preterm infants fed formula pretreated with lactase experience a modest increase in weight gain 10 days after the initiation of feeding; however this advantage was not maintained by day 14.[21] Another investigator has shown that preterm infants given formula containing hydrolyzed protein reach full feeding volumes approximately 2 days sooner than infants given routine preterm formula.[22] Although there are concerns that hydrolyzed formulas may fail to provide adequate nutrition,[23] Szajewska *et al.*[24] have shown that they may provide adequate growth.

Alternatively, the introduction of enteral feedings may hasten maturation of digestion and absorption. Infants given small enteral feedings have been shown to regain birth weight sooner, establish full feeding volumes sooner, release gastrointestinal hormones better, produce more gastric acid and have more mature motor patterns than infants who remain unfed.[1,9,25,26] Moreover, these infants fail to incur a higher incidence of necrotizing enterocolitis.[27]

There is an emerging consensus that early nutrition and growth "program" the infant for adult health and disease. Very low birth weights and very heavy birth weights have been associated with higher risk for cardiovascular mortality in adults.[28] Small size at birth has also been associated with an increased risk for adolescent hypertension[29] and glucose intolerance.[30] The ingestion of breast milk appears to have a protective effect against childhood obesity,[31] adolescent hypertension,[32] and type 2 diabetes among Pima Indians.[33]

Host defenses

Gut flora

The gut is sterile in utero, but colonization begins at birth. The pattern of bacterial growth reflects the maternal and neonatal environment and enteric bacteria colonize the human infant in an oral-to-anal direction.[34] In healthy infants, aerobic organisms appear within a few hours. Anaerobic organisms are present by 24 hours and increase in number over the first 3 weeks.[35] Stools of breast milk-fed infants have a predominance of *Bifidobacterium*, whereas stools of formula-fed infants have a predominance of *Escherichia coli* and Klebsiella.[36]

Because the gut is in continuity with the neonatal environment, it is constantly exposed to antigens and bacteria that have potential to gain access to the intestinal lumen.

The newborn has a complex series of host defenses that are immune and nonimmune in nature. The nonimmune system is also called the innate immune system as it responds in a nonspecific fashion. The immune system is comprised of specific humoral and cellular responses that are activated in response to specific antigens.

The innate immune system

The innate immune system constitutes the first line of host defense in the neonate and it prevents many antigens and organisms from reaching the intestinal mucosa. The components of the innate system include physical barriers, cells and chemical barriers.

First, intestinal motility is an important factor in moving nutrients aborally so that they do not have time to establish colonization in the lumen of the gut. As described in the section on motor function, the migrating motor complex, which is responsible for propelling luminal contents forward through the small intestine, is often absent in the preterm infant.[9,37] As a result, overall intestinal transit times are delayed in the preterm infant.[38,39]

The release of gastric acid and pancreaticobiliary secretions also are important components of the innate system. These secretions inhibit bacterial growth and activate proteolysis, which alters antigen structure. There are concerns that withholding enteral feedings in preterm infants results in a decreased release of these secretions and, thus, may impair an important function of host defense in the preterm infant. Hyman *et al.*[1] have confirmed that basal and maximal gastric acid production is significantly lower in unfed infants and rates of infection are higher among infants whose gastric acid production is suppressed by H_2 blockers.[40]

Another physical barrier is created by mucus, which contains mucins, glycoproteins, inmunoglobulins, glycolipids and albumin. These constituents form a protective gel over the surface of the intestine. Mucus presents a slippery surface that propels antigens forward and inhibits the diffusion of large molecules.

Cells that provide innate immune defense include epithelial cells, goblet cells, M cells and subepithelial cells (Figure 6.4). The intestinal epithelial cells are closely approximated to one another by a series of tight junctions. These junctions permit the physiologic passage of fluids and electrolytes while preventing the passage of larger proteins. In addition, microvilli form a physical barrier that prevents or retards the cellular penetration of large macromolecules and charged particles. M cells are epithelial cells that lack well-developed microvilli; the absence of

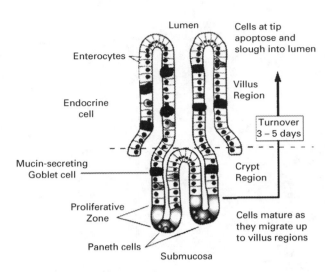

Lumen

Cells at tip apoptose and slough into lumen

Enterocytes

Endocrine cell

Mucin-secreting Goblet cell

Proliferative Zone

Paneth cells

Submucosa

Villus Region

Turnover 3 – 5 days

Crypt Region

Cells mature as they migrate up to villus regions

- Intestinal absorptive epithelium (9 weeks)
- Paneth cells (11–12 weeks)
- Goblet cells (8 –10 weeks)
- Enteroendocrine cells (9 –11 weeks)
- M-cells (17 weeks)
- Intraepithelial lymphocytes (8 weeks)
- Dendritic cells (19 weeks)

Figure 6.4. Schematic representation of the epithelial cells that provide a barrier function in the gastrointestinal tract. (Kindly provided by Dr. Josef Neu.)

this physiological barrier permits macromolecular transport. M cells are found in follicles that overlie lymphoid tissue and their function is to deliver foreign antigens and microorganisms to the lymphoid tissue. Goblet cells are interspersed among the epithelial cells and they secrete mucus.

Subepitheleal cells include follicular dendritic cells, Peyer's patches and mast cells. Dendritic cells, which are located in the subepithelium, extend appendages up into the intestinal lumen, likened to a submarine with a periscope. These cells "sample" the luminal environment and transport antigens to the T and B cells which reside in the subepithelial layer below. Peyer's patches, which are clusters of lymphoid tissue, are present by 19 weeks' gestation and become more abundant in number between 24 and 40 weeks' gestation.[41] Mast cells play an important role in regulating intestinal permeability and in defending against parasitic infection.

The immune system

The immune system of host defense is composed of cellular components and secretory components. T cells, B cells and macrophages are present in the fetal intestine by 20 weeks' gestation (Figure 6.5). Lymphocytes proliferate in response to a mitogen as early as 12 weeks, but antigenic stimulation of lymphoid tissues cannot be demonstrated until 46 weeks. The newborn intestine has few IgA-producing plasma cells and plasma immunoglobulin

A (IgA) is relatively low in the newborn. When preterm infants are fed exogenous protein they are unable to form antibodies.[42]

A variety of soluble proteins that regulate growth and differentiation of lymphocytes are called *cytokines* and include the interleukins, tumor necrosis factors, interferon and platelet-activating factor. These cytokines play important roles in stimulating chemotaxis of neutrophils, promoting IgA expression and stimulating epithelial cell proliferation after mucosal injury. When cultured fetal enterocytes (18–21 weeks) are stimulated by the general chemotoxin lipopolysaccharide, they release significantly greater amounts of the proinflammatory cytokine Il-8,[43] suggesting that there may be an imbalance of release of pro- and anti-inflammatory cytokines in response to a stimulus in the preterm infant.

The role of nutrients in host defense

A number of host defense functions appear to be mediated by enteral nutrients. Among those that have been recently studied are glutamine, arginine, long-chain fatty acids, nucleotides and prebiotics. Although not nutrients, per se, probiotics will also be reviewed.

Glutamine plays an important role in maintaining epithelial cell integrity, cell growth and inflammatory responses. In the face of glutamine depletion intestinal cell growth is retarded[44] and small intestinal interepithelial junctional integrity is impaired.[45] Neonatal rats fed

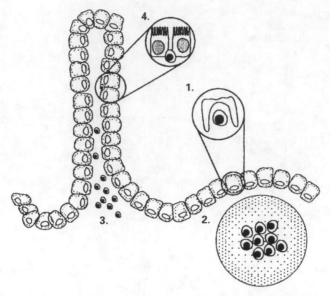

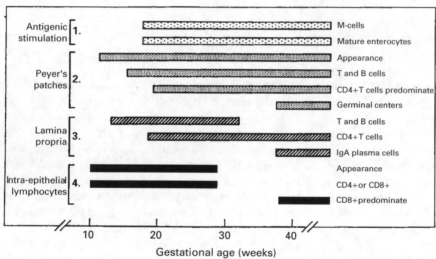

Figure 6.5. Ontogeny of the human mucosal immune system. The major components of the mucosal immune system are shown. The respective developmental time points for key components are highlighted. Note germinal center in Peyer's patches. IgA plasma cell in the lamina propria and predominant CD8$^+$ intraepithelial lymphocytes do not appear until the perinatal and neonatal periods. Reproduced with permission.[70]

a diet that is glutamine deficient exhibit increases in bacterial translocation.[46] Preterm infants given glutamine supplementation had a lower incidence of sepsis compared with infants given no supplementation.[47]

Arginine plays an important role in immune function, wound healing and growth. Plasma concentrations of arginine are lower among preterm infants who subsequently develop NEC than those who do not.[48,49] Arginine supplementation has been shown to reduce severity of NEC in piglets[50] and in human infants.[51]

Long-chain fatty acids play an important role in growth, mental development and inflammatory response. The incidence of NEC and sepsis was significantly reduced in neonatal rats fed formula containing DHA and ARA for 72 hours,[52] but recent prospective trials using DHA and ARA supplemented formulas have failed to show a difference in the incidence of NEC or sepsis among infants fed formulas with and without DHA and ARA supplementation for a month or longer.[53,54] Another study demonstrated that formulas supplemented with egg phospholipid reduced the occurrence of NEC but not sepsis.[55] Nucleotides may enhance antibody responses. Although some infant formulas are now supplemented with nucleotides, no large clinical trials have been performed to date in preterm infants.

Prebiotics are defined to be nondigestible substrates that preferentially enhance the growth of nonpathogenic organisms. For example, breast milk contains galacto-oligosaccharides, which favor the growth of Bifidobacteria. Fructo-oligosaccharides increase bifidobacterial counts and colonic metabolic activity in adults.[56]

In a recent study, preterm infants fed preterm formula containing an oligosaccharide mixture containing galacto-oligosaccharides and fructo-oligosaccharides for 28 days experienced greater fecal colonization with bifidobacteria, higher stool frequency and softer stool consistency than infants fed unsupplemented preterm formula, but comparable with that seen in a breast milk-fed reference group.[57] However, other clinical outcomes have yet to be assessed in clinical trials.

Probiotics are live organisms that can compete with and overgrow pathogenic organisms. Researchers have speculated that colonizing the gut with these less pathogenic bacteria may reduce the incidence of sepsis and necrotizing enterocolitis. In an animal model, oral administration of bifidobacteria reduced the incidence of necrotizing enterocolitis (NEC).[58] Attention has focussed largely on lactobacillus GG (LGG) in children.[59,60,61] However, the bowel flora of infants fed breast milk contains a predominance of bifidobacteria,[36] and several probiotics have been studied in preterm infants. Investigators have recently shown that the oral administration of bifidobacteria,[62] nonpathogenic *E. coli*[63,64] and LGG[65,66] can successfully result in colonization of these organisms in the preterm intestine. Colonization may be inhibited, however, when infants are given antibiotics[65] or indomethacin.[67] Hoyos recently demonstrated that the incidence of necrotizing enterocolitis was lower in preterm infants given daily LGG.[68] However, a randomized, prospective trial has not yet confirmed these findings.

REFERENCES

1 Hyman, P. E., Feldman, E. J., Ament, M. E., Byrne, W. J., Euler, A. R. Effect of enteral feeding on the maintenance of gastric acid secretory function. *Gastroenterology* 1983;**84**:341–5.

2 Antonowicz, I., Chang, S. K., Grand, R. J. Development and distribution of liposomal enzymes and disaccharidases in human fetal intestine. *Gastroenterology* 1974;**67**:51–8.

3 Auricchio, S., Rubino, A., Mürset, G. Intestinal glycosidase activities in the human embryo, fetus and newborn. *Pediatrics* 1965;**3S**:944–54.

4 Villa, M., Ménard, D., Semenza, G., Mantei, N. Expression of the lactase enzymatic activity and mRNA in human fetal jejunum. *FEBS Lett.* 1992;**301**:202–6.

5 Triadou, N., Zweibaum, A. Maturation of sucrase-isomaltase complex in human fetal small and large intestine during gestation. *Pediatr. Res.* 1985;**19**:136–8.

6 Jirsova, V., Koldovsky O., Heringova, A. *et al.* The development of the functions of the small intestine of the human fetus. *Biol. Neonate* 1996;**9**:44–9.

7 Levin, R. J., Koldovsky, O., Hoskova, J., Jirsova, V., Uher, J. Electrical activity across human foetal small intestine associated with absorption processes. *Gut* 1968;**9**:206–13.

8 Berseth, C. L., Nordyke, C. K., Valdes, M. G., Furlow, B. L., Go, V. L. W. Responses of gastrointestinal peptides and motor activity to milk and water feedings in preterm and term infants. *Pediatr. Res.* 1992;**31**:587–90.

9 Berseth, C. L. Effect of early feeding on maturation of the preterm infant's small intestine. *J. Pediatr.* 1992;**120**:947–53.

10 Lucas, A., Bloom, S. R., Aynsley-Green, A. Development of gut hormone responses to feeding in neonates. *Arch. Dis. Child.* 1980;**55**:678–82.

11 Zoppi, G., Andreotti, G., Pajno-Ferrara, F., Njai, D. M., Gaburro, D. Exocrine pancreas function in premature and term infants. *Pediatr. Res.* 1972;**6**:880–6.

12 Lebenthal, E., Lee, P. C. Development of functional responses in human exocrine pancreas. *Pediatrics* 1980;**66**:556–60.

13 Watkins, J. B., Szczepanik, P., Gould, J. B., Klein, P., Lester, R. Bile metabolism in the premature infant: preliminary observations of pool size and synthesis rate following prenatal administration of dexamethasone and phenobarbital. *Gastroenterology* 1975;**69**:706–13.

14 Heubi, J. E., Balistreri, W. F. Bile salt metabolism in infants and children after protracted diarrhea. *Pediatr. Res.* 1980;**14**:943–6.

15 MacLean, W. C. Jr, Fink, B. B. Lactase malabsorption by premature infants: Magnitude and clinical significance. *J. Pediatr.* 1980;**97**:383–8.

16 Potter, G. D., Lester, R. The developing colon and nutrition. *J. Pediatr. Gastroenterol. Nutr.* 1984;**3**:485–7.

17 Kerzner, B., Sloan, H. R., Haase, G., McClung, H. J., Ailabouni, A. H. The jejunal absorption of glucose oligomers in the absence of pancreatic enzymes. *Pediatr. Res.* 1981;**15**:250–3.

18 Walker, W. A. Antigen handling by the gut. *Arch. Dis. Child.* 1978;**53**:527–31.

19 Hutchens, T. W., Henry, J. F., Yip, T. T. *et al.* Origin of intact lactoferrin and its DNA-binding fragments found in the urine of human milk fed preterm infants: evaluation by stable isotope enrichment. *Pediatr. Res.* 1991;**29**:243–50.

20 Weaver, L. T., Laker, M. F., Nelson, R. Intestinal permeability in the newborn. *Arch. Dis. Child.* 1984;**59**:236–41.

21 Erasmus, H. D., Ludwig-Auser, H. M., Paterson, P. G., Sun, D., Sankaran, K. Enhanced weight gain in preterm infants

receiving lactase-treated feeds: a randomized, double-blind, controlled trial. *J. Pediatr.* 2002;**141**:532–7.

22 Mihatsch, W. A., Franz, A. R., Hogel, J., Pohlandt, F. Hydrolyzed protein accelerates feeding advancement in very low birth weight infants. *Pediatrics* 2002;**110**:1199–203.

23 Rigo, J., Salle, B. L., Picaud, J. C., Putet, G., Sonterre, J. Nutritional evaluation of protein hydrolysate formulas. *Eur. J. Clin. Nutr.* 1995;**49**:S26–38.

24 Szajewska, H., Albrecht, P., Stoitiska, B. *et al.* Extensive and partial protein hydrolysate preterm formulas: the effect on growth rate, protein metabolism indices and plasma amino acid concentrations. *J. Pediatr. Gastroenterol. Nutr.* 2001;**32**:303–9.

25 Slagle, T. A., Gross, S. J. Effect of early low-volume enteral substrate on subsequent feeding tolerance in very low birth weight infants. *J. Pediatr.* 1988;**113**:526–31.

26 Meetze, W. H., Valentine, C., McGuigan, J. E., *et al.* Gastrointestinal priming prior to full enteral nutrition in very low birth weight infants. *J. Pediatr. Gastroenterol. Nutr.* 1992;**15**;163–70.

27 Tyson, J. E., Kennedy, K. A. Minimal enteral nutrition for promoting feeding tolerance and preventing morbidity in parenterally fed infants. *Cochrane Database Syst Rev.* 2000;**2**:CD000504.

28 Barker, D. J., Osmond, C., Simmonds, S. J., Wield, G. A. The relation of small head circumference and thinness at birth to death from cardiovascular disease in adult life. *Br. Med. J.* 1993;**306**:422–6.

29 Nilsson, P. M., Ostergren, P. O., Nyberg, P., Soderstrom, M., Alleback, P. Low birth weight is associated with elevated systolic blood pressure in adolescence: a prospective study of a birth cohort of 149,378 Swedish boys. *J. Hypertens.* 1997;**15**:1627–31.

30 Hales, C. N., Barker, D. J., Clark, P. M. *et al.* Fetal and infant growth and impaired glucose tolerance at age 64. *Br. Med. J.* 1991;**303**:1019–22.

31 Von Kries, R., Koletzko, B., Sauerwald, T. *et al.* Breastfeeding and obesity: cross sectional study. *Br. Med. J.* 1999;**319**:147–50.

32 Singhal, A., Cole, T. J., Lucas, A. Early nutrition in preterm infants and later blood pressure: two cohorts after randomised trials. *Lancet* 2001;**357**:413–19.

33 Pettit, D. J., Forman, M. R., Hanson, R. L. Breastfeeding and incidence of non-insulin-dependent diabetes mellitus in Pima Indians. *Lancet* 1997;**350**:166–8.

34 Rotimi, V. O., Duerden, B. The development of anaerobic fecal flora in healthy newborn infants. *J. Pediatr.* 1977;**91**:298–301.

35 Cooperstock, M. S., Zedd, A. J. Intestinal flora of infants. In Hentgis, D., ed. *Human Intestinal Microflora in Health and Disease.* New York, NY: Academic Press; 1983:79.

36 Harmsen, H. J., Wildeboer-Veloo, A. C., Raangs, G. C. *et al.* Analysis of intestinal flora development in breast fed and formula fed infants by molecular identification methods. *J. Pediatr. Gastroenterol. Nutr.* 2000;**30**:61–7.

37 Amarnath, R. P., Berseth, C. L., Malagelada, J.-R. *et al.* Postnatal maturation of small intestinal motility in preterm and term infants. *J. Gastrointestin. Motil.* 1989;**1**:138–43.

38 Berseth, C. L., Bisquera, J. A., Paje, V. U. Prolonging small feeding volumes early in life decreases the incidence of NEC in very low birth weight infants. *Pediatrics* 2003;**111**:529–34.

39 Baker-Wills, E., Berseth, C. L. Antenatal steroids enhance maturation of small intestinal motor activity in preterm infants. *Pediatr. Res.* 1996;**39**:193A.

40 Beck-Sague, C. M., Azimi, P., Fonseca, S. N., *et al.* Bloodstream infections in neonatal intensive care unit patients: results of a multicenter study. *Pediatr. Infect. Dis. J.* 1994;**13**:1110–16.

41 Cornes, J. S. Number, size and distribution of Peyer's patches in the human small intestine. *Gut* 1965;**6**:225–33.

42 Rieger, C. H., Rothberg, R. M. Development of the capacity to produce specific antibody to an ingested food antigen in the premature infant. *J. Pediatr.* 1975;**87**:515–18.

43 Nanthakumar, N. N., Fusunyan, R. D., Sanderson, I., Walker, W. A. Inflammation in the developing human intestine: a possible pathophysiologic contribution to necrotizing enterocolitis. *Proc. Natl. Acad. Sci. USA.* 2000;**97**:6043–8.

44 He, Y., Sanderson, I. R., Walker, W. A. Uptake, transport and metabolism of exogenous nucleosides in intestinal epithelial cell cultures. *J. Nutr.* 1994;**124**:1942–9.

45 Weiss, M. D., DeMarco, V., Strauss, D. M. *et al.* Glutamine synthetase: a key enzyme for intestinal epithelial differentiation. *JPEN.* 1999;**23**:140–6.

46 Neu, J. Glutamine deprivation: effect on the small intestinal barrier. *FASEB* J. 2001;**15**:A294.

47 Neu, J., Roig, J. C., Meetze, W. H. *et al.* Enteral glutamine supplementation for very low birth weight infants decreases morbidity. *J. Pediatr.* 1997;**131**:691–9.

48 Becker, R. M., Wu, G., Galanko, J. A. *et al.* Reduced serum amino acid concentrations in infants with necrotizing enterocolitis. *J. Pediatr.* 2000;**137**:785–93.

49 Zamora, S. A., Amin, H. J., McMillan, D. D. *et al.* Plasma L-arginine concentrations in premature infants with necrotizing enterocolitis. *J. Pediatr.* 1997;**131**:226–32.

50 Di Lorenzo, C., Flores, A. F., Hyman, P. E. Age-related changes in colon motility. *J. Pediatr.* 1995;**127**:593–6.

51 Amin, H. J., Zamora, S. A., McMillan, D. D., *et al.* Arginine supplementation prevents necrotizing enterocolitis in the premature infant. *J. Pediatr.* 2002;**140**:425–31.

52 Caplan, M. S., Russell, T., Xiao, Y. *et al.* Effect of polyunsaturated acid (PUFA) supplementation on intestinal inflammation and necrotizing enterocolitis (NEC) in a neonatal rat model. *Pediatr. Res.* 2001;**49**:647–52.

53 O'Connor, D. L., Hall, R., Adamkin, D. *et al.* Growth and development in preterm infants fed long-chain polyunsaturated fatty acids: a prospective, randomized controlled trial. *Pediatrics* 2001;**108**:359–71.

54 Clandinin, M. T., VanAerde, J., Antonson, D. *et al.* Formulas with docosahexaenoic (DHA) and arachidonic acid (ARA) promote better growth and development scores in very-low-birth-weight infants (VLBW). *Pediatr. Res.* 2002;**51**:187A–8A.

55 Carlson, S. E., Montalto, M. B., Ponder, D. L. *et al.* Lower incidence of necrotizing enterocolitis in infants fed a preterm formula with egg phospholipids. *Pediatr. Res.* 1998;**44**:491–8.

56 Gibson, G. R., Beatty, E. R., Wang, X., Cummings, J. H. Selective stimulation of bifidobacteria in the human colon by oligofructose and insulin. *Gastroenterology* 1995;**108**:975–82.

57 Boehm, G., Lidestri, M., Casetta, P. *et al.* Supplementation of a bovine milk formula with an oligosaccharide mixture increases counts of faecal bifidobacteria in preterm infants. *Arch. Dis. Child. Fetal Neonatal Ed.* 2002;**86**:F178–81.

58 Caplan, M. S., Miller-Catchpole, R., Kaup, S. *et al.* Bifidobacterial supplementation reduces the incidence of necrotizing enterocolitis in a neonatal rat model. *Gastroenterology* 1999;**117**:577–83.

59 Vanderhoof, J. A., Whitney, D. B., Antonson, D. L. *et al.* Lactobacillus GG in the prevention of antibiotic-associated diarrhea in children. *J. Pediatr.* 1999;**135**:564–8.

60 Arvola, T., Laiho, K., Torkkeli, S. *et al.* Prophylactic Lactobacillus GG reduces antibiotic-associated diarrhea in children with respiratory infections: a randomized study. *Pediatrics* 1999;**104**:e64.

61 Oberhelman, R. A., Gilman, R. H., Sheen, P. *et al.* A placebo-controlled trial of Lactobacillus GG to prevent diarrhea in undernourished Peruvian children. *J. Pediatr.* 1999;**134**:15–20.

62 Bennet, R., Nord, C. E., Zetterstrom, R. Transient colonization of the gut of newborn infants by orally administered bifidobacteria and lactobacilli. *Acta Paediatr.* 1992;**81**:784–7.

63 Lari, A. R., Gold, F., Borderon, J. C., Laugier, J., Lafont, J.-P. Implantation and in vivo antagonistic effects of antibiotic-susceptible *Escherichia coli* strains administered to premature newborns. *Biol. Neonate* 1990;**58**:73–8.

64 Cukrowaska, B., Lodinova-Zadnikova, R., Enders, C. *et al.* Specific proliferative and antibody responses of premature infants to intestinal colonization with nonpathogenic probiotic *E. coli* strain Nissle 1918. *Scand. J. Immunol.* 2002;**55**:204–9.

65 Agarwal, R., Sharma, N., Chaudhry, R. *et al.* Effects of oral Lactobacilllus GG on enteric microflora in low-birth-weight neonates. *J. Pediatr. Gastroenterol. Nutr.* 2003;**36**:397–402.

66 Millar, M. R., Bacon, C., Smith, S. L., Walker, V., Hall, M. A. Enteral feeding of premature infants with Lactobacillus GG. *Arch. Dis. Child.* 1993;**69**:483–7.

67 Gotteland, M., Cruchet, S., Verbeke, S. Effect of Lactobacillus ingestion on the gastrointestinal mucosal barrier alterations induced by indomethacin in humans. *Aliment. Pharmacol. Ther.* 2001;**15**:11–17.

68 Hoyos, A. B. Reduced incidence of necrotizing enterocolitis associated with enteral administration of *Lactobacillus acidophilus* and *Bifidobacterium infantis* to neonates in an intensive care unit. *Int. J. Infect. Dis.* 1999;**3**:197–202.

69 Turnberg, L. A., Riley, S. A. Digestion and absorption of nutrients and vitamins. In Sleisenger, M. H., ed. *Gastrointestinal Disease: Pathophysiology, Diagnosis, Management.* 5th edn. Philadelphia, PA: W.B. Saunders; 1993:978.

70 Insoft, R. M., Sanderson, I. R., Walker, W. A. Development of immune function in the intestine and its role in neonatal diseases. *Pediatr. Clin. N. Am.* 1996;**43**:551–71.

7

Metabolic programming as a consequence of the nutritional environment during fetal and the immediate postnatal periods

Mulchand S. Patel and Malathi Srinivasan

Department of Biochemistry, State University of New York at Buffalo, Buffalo, NY

Normal fetal/neonatal development

Although the early development of living creatures is primarily governed by genetic instructions acquired at the time of conception, the expression of these genetic codes is influenced by the environmental conditions under which the organism develops. Fetal and neonatal growth in mammals is therefore a complex process regulated by interactions between the genome and the environment. The quality and quantity of nutrition during such critical periods of development play pivotal roles in the regulation of growth.

Acquisition of metabolic capacities and their adaptations in early life are influenced by three critical periods: (i) fetal development during gestation, (ii) an abrupt fetal-postnatal transition occurring at birth and (iii) a gradual postnatal-weaning transition occurring when the mammal begins to consume solid food.[1] Rapid changes in enzyme activities occur in response to the nature of the available nutrients during these periods under normal development.[1] As an example of this phenomenon, Figure 7.1 depicts the appearance of enzyme clusters related to carbohydrate and lipid metabolism that appear in the rat liver during fetal, suckling and weaning phases of development in response to the nature of the diet encountered during these periods of life. During fetal life the nutrition of the fetus is determined by the supply of substrates (principally glucose) via the placenta and hepatic metabolic activity in the late phase of gestation is characterized primarily at the level of glycogen synthesis (for example, glycogen synthase for storage of nutrients) in preparation for life immediately after birth (Figure 7.1A; Cluster I). At birth the continuous maternal supply of nutrients ceases and the mode,

composition and frequency of the feed are drastically modified, as breast milk becomes the only source of nutrition during the suckling period. Rat milk is a high fat-low carbohydrate diet and the transition from maternal supply of nutrients to breast milk is accompanied by rapid metabolic adaptations in carbohydrate metabolism to maintain glucose homeostasis in the newborn (Figure 7.1A; Cluster II).[1] This phase is characterized by the appearance of gluconeogenic enzymes (for example, PEP carboxykinase) in response to the high fat content of rat milk (Figure 7.1A; Cluster II). At the time of weaning the nature of the diet once again undergoes a change from high fat in rat milk to high carbohydrate in chow diet (in the case of rat) and is accompanied by the appearance of a different set of enzymes (enzymes involved in lipogenesis, for example malic enzyme, and glucose utilization (for example glucokinase) in the liver to counter the changes in the quality of nutrition (Figure 7.1A; Cluster III). In most mammals, the prenatal-postnatal transition and the suckling-weaning transition are accompanied by important adaptations in carbohydrate metabolism due to the change in the quality and quantity of the type of nutrients. This suggests that even normal development demands metabolic adaptations in target tissues but such adaptations are part of the process of maturation during early periods of life. An altered nutritional environment during such periods induces abnormal metabolic adaptations. For example, we have observed that when rat milk is replaced by a high carbohydrate (HC) milk formula during the suckling period, the cluster III enzymes (for e.g., glucokinase and malic enzyme) appear precociously in the liver and cluster II enzymes (for example, PEP carboxykinase) are significantly reduced in the liver (Figure 7.1B) suggesting that adaptations during development

Neonatal Nutrition and Metabolism. Second Edition, ed. P. Thureen and W. Hay. Published by Cambridge University Press.
© Cambridge University Press 2006.

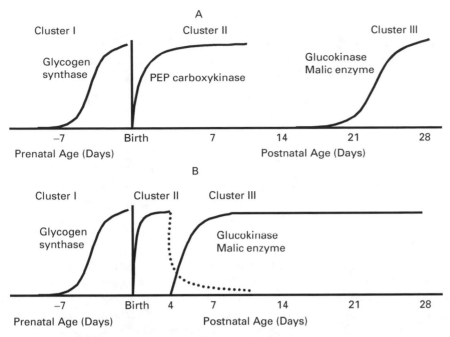

Figure 7.1. An illustration of the cluster of enzymes with respect to carbohydrate and lipid metabolism that appear in rat liver during the fetal (Cluster I), suckling (Cluster II), and the immediate postnatal (Cluster III) periods. Panel A depicts the clusters in a normal rat and Panel B shows the alterations in the appearance of these clusters when the diet presented in the suckling period is switched from rat milk to a high carbohydrate milk formula.

correspond to the nutritional environment encountered during such periods.[2]

Metabolic programming due to altered early life nutritional experiences

Metabolic programming is the phenomenon by which a nutritional stress/stimuli experienced during early periods of life overlapping with the critical window of organogenesis of target tissues permanently alters the physiology and metabolism of the organism.[3] The consequences of this phenomenon are observed much later in life in the absence of the stress/stimuli that initiated these responses.[3] In addition to genetics, nature has provided the organism with the advantage of plasticity, which enables the operation of "biological switches" in response to different environmental triggers resulting in adaptations in target tissues. An example of such an environmental trigger is nutrition at critical periods of development. Metabolic programming provides survival advantages for the present but such adaptations become unfavorable for health in adulthood as the responses to environmental influences encountered later in life are altered due to these early life adaptations.

Conventional wisdom suggests that the onset of the inter-associated metabolic diseases such as obesity, cardiovascular diseases, hypertension, type 2 diabetes, etc., in middle age is linked to the genetic background of the individual which could be exasperated by lifestyle factors. In the recent past, a series of provocative epidemiological findings have indicated that in addition to genetics, environmental factors in early life also substantially contribute to disease risk later in life. An indication for this association was suggested as early as 1934 when Kermack et al.[4] showed that although people survived the neonatal period, the year in which they died appeared to have some relationship to the year in which they were born and suggested that this association was due to the maternal environment to which they were exposed during their fetal development. The "fetal origins hypothesis" subsequently proposed by Barker after analysis of human epidemiological data suggests that in humans a compromised maternal-fetal nutrient supply due to malnutrition in the pregnant female results in developmental adaptations in the fetus that permanently alter the structure, physiology and metabolism of target organs in the fetus thereby priming the individual for the onset of metabolic diseases such as type 2 diabetes, cardiovascular diseases, hypertension, etc. later in adulthood.[5,6] Data from over 20 epidemiological studies carried out in several geographical locations worldwide confirm the association between restricted fetal growth and the development of metabolic diseases later on in life.[7] The postulated mechanism for this association is afforded by the thrifty phenotype hypothesis which suggests that the developing fetus makes adaptations in response to a malnourished pregnancy in order to allow near-normal development of the brain whereas the growth of other organs like liver, muscle, pancreas, etc. are compromised.[8] Such fetal adaptations aid survival when food supply is poor or intermittent but later in adult life when food supply is adequate or abundant become detrimental to health.[8]

Although evidence from human epidemiological studies strongly supports the fetal origins of adult-onset pathological conditions, there are intrinsic difficulties in long-term retrospective human studies. Animal models pertaining to an altered nutrition during fetal life demonstrate the unique role of early life nutritional experiences for the onset of pathological situations later in life. Hence animal models are useful tools to examine specific aspects revealed by human epidemiological evidence and also to explore mechanistic pathways related to the contribution of early life nutritional experiences to metabolic programming and adult-onset diseases. A number of animal models have been developed mainly to examine the role of fetal nutritional experiences and in utero programming of adult-onset diseases; models for the role of postnatal nutrition have also been examined. Several species including rat, mouse, guinea pig, sheep and nonhuman primates have been used and in addition to the role of nutrition, pharmacological, genetic and surgical manipulations have also been employed to mimic the human situation. Rat is an extensively used experimental animal and there is abundant literature on metabolic programming due to altered fetal and neonatal dietary experiences in rat models. For these reasons, we will restrict our discussion to mainly such studies in this chapter. This will include models for low protein, caloric restriction and diabetes during pregnancy and under- or overnourishment in the immediate postnatal period. The consequences of caloric redistribution (from fat to high carbohydrate) in the immediate postnatal life as occurs in the high carbohydrate (HC) rat model will also be discussed.

Animal models for fetal programming

In this section metabolic programming in rat models due to malnutrition during the period of fetal development induced by either maternal protein deficiency or total caloric restriction will be briefly discussed. The imme-

diate and long-term consequences of fetal development in the altered intrauterine environment due to a diabetic pregnancy will also be discussed. The results from studies on fetal programming by nutritional modifications in the mother are briefly summarized in Table 7.1. The reader is referred to recent reviews on these topics for detailed accounts.[9–12]

Maternal protein restriction

The immediate and permanent consequences of maternal malnutrition due to a low protein diet during gestation and lactation for the progeny have been extensively studied in the rat as a model mimicking the mammalian malnourished environment resulting in an altered fetal development. These results will be discussed in this section under the headings (i) immediate effects observed in fetal and neonatal life and (ii) persistent effects observed in adult life. The important outcomes of such a pregnancy for the progeny are consolidated in Table 7.1.

Immediate effects observed in fetal and neonatal life

The immediate consequences of the low protein dietary regimen are observed in the pregnant dams as well as in their fetuses (refer to Table 7.1). Pregnant rats fed a 8% protein (low protein; LP) diet maintain similar weight gain up to gestation day 18 compared with pregnant rats fed a 20% protein diet (control diet).[13] From day 19 of gestation up to parturition the LP group of pregnant rats weigh less than control rats.[13] The effects of the low protein diet on plasma constituents are apparent even on gestation day 4–5 when the plasma insulin levels and amino acid contents are significantly reduced in the LP pregnant rats compared to controls.[14] These authors showed that in the LP group pre-implanted embryos (up to 4.5 days of age) have reduced cell numbers indicating cellular differences very early in gestation probably due to slower rate of proliferation of cells.[14] The offspring born to LP mothers are approximately 20% lighter 2 days after birth.[13] The difference in body weights increases in the offspring if the nursing dam continues to be fed the LP diet.[13,15]

Several studies have shown that the structural development and function of pancreatic islets are compromised in the fetuses of the LP diet-fed female rats. Such changes include reduced β cell proliferation, islet size and islet vascularization.[16] Additionally, the insulin secretory capacity of such islets in response to various secretagogues in vitro is significantly reduced.[17,18] The progeny of LP diet-fed dams during gestation and lactation have reduced numbers of pancreatic β cells and increased

Table 7.1. Summary of the consequences of an altered nutritional experience during fetal development

Nutritional experience	References
Maternal protein restriction	
Immediate effects	
Reduced birth weight	13
Depressed insulin secretory response; reduced islet size, islet proliferation and islet vascularization	16–18
Malformation of hypothalamic nuclei	23
Persistent effects	
Increased whole body insulin sensitivity in young adults	15
Glucagon resistance, reduced hepatic glucose output, increased insulin receptor content in liver	29
Decreased activity and gene expression of glucokinase and increased activity and gene expression of PEPCK in liver	29,30
Increased insulin receptor expression, glucose uptake and GLUT4 protein in skeletal muscle	31
Increased glucose utilization, and expression of insulin receptors in mesenteric adipocytes	15,33,34
Impaired suppression of isoprenaline-stimulated rates of lipolysis by insulin in isolated adipocytes	28,34,35
Hypertension, renal defects	36–40
Impaired glucose tolerance at 15 months of age and frank diabetes by 17 months of age	7,32,43,44
Global caloric restriction	
50% caloric restriction	
Impaired islet development, glucose intolerance and insulinopenia	49,50
30% caloric restriction	
Hypertension, hyperphagia, increased fasting insulin, adult-onset obesity	51,52
Pregnancy complicated with diabetes	
Mild diabetes	
Fetal β cell hypertrophy and hyperplasia; increased response to a glucose stimulus by fetal islets	55,56
Decreased insulin secretory response to a glucose stimulus in adulthood	58
Impaired glucose tolerance in adulthood	58–61
Severe diabetes	
Fetal growth retardation results in microsomic pups which remain small in adulthood	55
Over stimulation of fetal β cells due to fetal hyperglycemia	55
Islets depleted of insulin, degranulated and unresponsive to a glucose stimulus	55
Onset of insulin resistance in liver, muscle, and adipose tissue in adulthood	64,65
Increase in β cell mass in adulthood due to increased number of smaller islets and augmented response to a glucose stimulus by adult islets	55,57

number of α cells.[19] In neonatal life the islets from LP dams show an altered cellular development due to an increased rate of apoptosis and decreased rate of proliferation.[20] Although pancreatic duodenal homeobox transcription factor-1 (PDX-1) mRNA levels are not altered, the protein content of PDX-1 is significantly reduced in 28-day-old progeny of LP dams.[21]

On postnatal day 3 the LP diet progeny demonstrate reduced cerebral cortex blood vessel density, lower DNA concentrations in the forebrain and higher DNA concentrations in the cerebellum suggesting that although brain development is protected at the expense of the development of other organs, functional alterations are still evident in the brain.[22] Additional changes in the brain include malformation of hypothalamic nuclei in the offspring of LP dams.[23] Expression of hepatic acetyl-CoA carboxylase and

fatty acid synthase genes is increased two-fold in weanling rats exposed to a LP intrauterine environment suggesting programming of gene expression during this period in a manner favoring fat synthesis thereby predisposing these offspring to adult-onset clinical complications.[24] Although insulin secretory ability is affected in fetal islets of offspring of LP dams, at three weeks after weaning the LP diet offspring demonstrate increased sensitivity to insulin in target tissues and have better glucose tolerance than controls.[25] In addition, they have a greater number of insulin receptors in the adipose tissue.[25]

Persistent effects observed in adult life

Functional studies related to whole body insulin sensitivity and insulin action in target tissues (liver, skeletal muscle and adipose tissue) carried out mostly in young adults in the LP offspring indicate significant differences compared with age-matched controls (Table 7.1). The results from such studies demonstrate an altered programming of metabolic responses in these tissues due to fetal development in the LP dam. In hyperinsulinemic clamp studies it was shown that increased rates of glucose infusion are required to maintain euglycemia, suggesting increased whole body insulin sensitivity.[15] In keeping with the observed increase in insulin sensitivity these animals have decreased plasma triglyceride levels.[26,27] Additionally, even in the fed-state plasma adrenaline and noradrenaline are increased suggesting that in these rats basal metabolism operates as it would in a starved normal rat.[8,28]

The offspring of LP dams demonstrate significant changes in liver, skeletal muscle and adipose tissues in adulthood. Altered zonation and enzyme activity including a reduction in glucokinase and an increase in phosphoenolpyruvate carboxy-kinase activities are observed in livers of LP progeny.[29] Parallel changes are evident in the mRNA levels of glucokinase and phosphoenolpyruvate carboxykinase.[30] Additionally, in vitro perfusion studies in hepatocytes indicate glucagon resistance due to the reduced ability of glucagon to stimulate glucose output and decreased hepatic glucagon receptor expression.[29] The expression of insulin receptors is significantly increased in the livers of LP progeny.[29] In the tibialis anterior muscle an increased expression of insulin receptor and an increase in insulin-stimulated glucose uptake are observed which likely contribute to the improvement in glucose tolerance observed in young adult progeny of LP dams.[31,32] Mesenteric adipocytes from LP offspring demonstrate enhanced glucose utilization under euglycemic-hyperinsulinemic conditions and increased expression of insulin receptors in epididymal and intra-abdominal adipose tissues.[15,33,34] Despite an increase in the number of insulin receptors, adipocytes from LP offspring show resistance to the antilipolytic activity of insulin.[25] Consistent with this observation, isolated adipocytes from such rats demonstrate increased β-adrenergic receptor expression.[34,35] Alterations in the expression and activity of the insulin-signaling components in the adipose tissue may be responsible for the observed resistance to the antilipolytic action of insulin. In support of this proposition it was shown that adipocytes isolated from LP progeny have significantly increased expression and activity in both basal and insulin-stimulated conditions for insulin receptor substrate-1-associated phosphatidylinositol 3-kinase and protein kinase B.[33] The observed functional alterations in the insulin-sensitive peripheral tissues in the LP adult progeny are probably intermediate events prior to the onset of overt diabetes.

An association between fetal development in a protein-malnourished dam and onset of hypertension later in life has been implicated (Table 7.1). A diet containing 9% protein supplemented with methionine when fed to pregnant rats consistently produced hypertension in the progeny, although an 8% protein diet without methionine supplementation did not produce hypertension in the offspring in adulthood. This occurrence has been attributed to impairment in nephrogenesis, a hyperactive renin-angiotensin system and an early exposure to increased concentrations of glucocorticoids.[36–40]

The other significant observations in adulthood of LP progeny include the following. Female progeny of LP diet-fed mothers demonstrated reduced pancreatic and specifically islet blood flow.[41] Pancreatic insulin and amylin contents were reduced in such animals while glucagon content was increased.[42] In the cerebral cortex of the brain the reduced vascularization observed in neonatal rats continued to be evident even in adulthood.[22] Male progeny born to LP diet-fed rats and suckled by normal foster mothers demonstrated initial growth restriction followed by rapid catch-up growth and premature death in adulthood.[32] With respect to glucose tolerance, although in middle age there appears to be no difference in the glucose tolerance between LP progeny and age-matched controls, by 15–16 months of age there is a rapid deterioration in the glucose tolerance of the offspring of the LP group such that they had significantly higher blood glucose concentrations at certain time points in the intraperitoneal glucose-tolerance test compared with controls.[7,32,43] By 17 months overt hyperglycemia is evident in these rats.[44] These higher plasma glucose concentrations were associated with hyperinsulinemia in male offspring and hypoinsulinemia in female offspring, suggesting insulin resistance in the former and insulin deficiency in the latter.[9] Although the exact mechanisms by which a low protein pregnancy primes the progeny for later onset of diseases are not clearly understood at present, it appears that the early structural and functional changes observed in target organs are important for this phenomenon.

Global caloric restriction

Although maternal protein malnutrition during fetal and neonatal development is the most extensively studied model for intrauterine growth retardation, other nutritional models to achieve the same end have also been explored. One such model involves total caloric restriction to the dam during pregnancy induced by either reducing the amount of food available or by uterine arterial ligation to reduce nutrient availability to the fetuses. Only results from food restriction will be discussed here.

Reducing maternal food intake during pregnancy to 50% of that consumed by normal controls results in perinatal growth retardation (Table 7.1).[45–47] The effects on the progeny depend on the window of gestation when the total caloric restriction is applied. Offspring of rats fed 50% of the caloric intake during the last trimester of pregnancy do not depict any defects in glucose tolerance, glucose utilization or glucose production.[48] Increasing the period of maternal malnutrition from day 15 of pregnancy to the time of weaning of the pups results in impaired pancreatic development and glucose intolerance and insulinopenia at one year of age (Table 7.1).[49,50] Severe maternal food restriction (30% of that of controls) results in hypertension, hyperphagia, increased fasting insulin and leptin levels and obesity in adult offspring (Table 7.1).[51,52] These studies emphasize the importance of adequate nutrition not only for normal development of the fetus but also for good health in adulthood.

Pregnancy complicated with diabetes

There is evidence that a diabetic intrauterine environment has long-term consequences for the progeny. In the human, due to increased transport of glucose and other nutrients in a diabetic pregnancy, fetal macrosomia has been frequently observed.[53,54] However, in a severe diabetic intrauterine environment complicated with vasculopathy and nephropathy, intrauterine growth retardation could be present.[55] Animal models have been developed to mimic the human scenario and results from such studies are briefly summarized in Table 7.1. Intrauterine development in a mild diabetic pregnancy (plasma glucose levels increased by 20%) results in hypertrophy and hyperplasia of the pancreatic β cells and increased insulin biosynthetic capacity (Table 7.1).[56] The insulin secretory response to glucose stimulation both in vitro and in vivo is increased in the fetuses of mildly diabetic rats.[57] In adulthood, the offspring of mildly diabetic mothers display normal mass of endocrine tissue with a normal distribution of the four different cell types.[58] Plasma glucose and insulin levels are normal under basal conditions but when stimulated with glucose both the in vitro and in vivo insulin secretory response are decreased. In this model and in other models of perinatal hyperinsulinemia, adult glucose tolerance is impaired.[59–62]

Under conditions of a severe diabetic pregnancy the fetus encounters very high glucose concentrations, which induce β cell hyperactivity and hypertrophy (Table 7.1). Initially the fetuses demonstrate hyperinsulinemia but this adaptation is short lived as β cells become depleted of insulin and appear degranulated.[56] β cell exhaustion results in reduced fetal insulin levels.[57] The combined presence of hypoinsulinemia and reduced number of insulin receptors in target tissues result in reduced fetal glucose uptake.[62,63] Fetal protein synthesis is consistently lower in the progeny of a severely diabetic pregnancy.[64]

The growth of the pups born to a severely diabetic female is retarded and these rats remain small in size in adulthood compared to controls.[56] In adulthood the islet mass in the pancreas of these animals is greater than that of control animals and this increase is primarily due to an increase in the number of small-sized islets.[58] Insulin secretory capacity of these islets is enhanced when subject to stimulation both under in vitro and in vivo conditions.[56] Additionally, these rats demonstrate insulin resistance during a euglycemic hyperinsulinemic clamp and this resistance to the action of insulin is evident in liver as well as in extrahepatic tissues.[65,66]

The transmission of the diabetogenic tendency to the progeny (generational effect) by female offspring of mildly diabetic mothers has been demonstrated. Female offspring from a mildly diabetic pregnancy have increased plasma glucose concentrations when they are pregnant and the fetuses of such females are macrosomic, hyperinsulinemic and display islet hypertrophy.[56,60] In adult life, these rats have glucose intolerance.[56,60]

Concluding remarks on fetal programming

Forty-three cycles of cell division occur between fertilization and birth but only 5 cycles of cell division occur after birth in the rat, which indicates the crucial role of fetal life and the importance of an optimal intrauterine environment for proper fetal development.[11] The consequences of fetal programming, due to an adverse intrauterine environment, are mostly observed at periods in life when increased stimulation is present such as at puberty and pregnancy, or in adulthood when compensation for early alterations that occurred in fetal life is no longer sufficient due to a reduction in the vitality of the organism. The fetal plasma milieu derived from the maternal in utero environment can directly or indirectly regulate the development of various organs in the fetus. For example, although high glucose concentrations present in a diabetic pregnancy promote β cell replication, the β cell hyperplasia observed in fetal pancreas of a diabetic pregnancy occurs only in the presence of a functioning hypothalamo-hypophyseal system implicating a role for derived hormones for this process.[67] Under conditions of fetal hypoinsulinemia the impetus for the development of the insulin receptor system in the various organs is impeded and the alterations in the degree of this defect in specific tissues may have implications for pathological situations later in life. These studies indicate that the influence of the intrauterine metabolic environment of the mother on the development and functional capacities of specific organs of the fetus is complex, involving a network of interactions between direct and indirect effects of the deficiency or excess of specific components on target tissues. These early effects complemented by other factors associated with aging result in adult-onset diseases.[11]

Animal models for nutritional modification in the immediate postnatal period (suckling period). Over- or undernutrition by adjusting litter size

Studies on the long-term consequences of an altered nutrition during the suckling period in rodents are not many due to experimental difficulties in the successful rearing of rat pups away from the dam. Litter size manipulation was mainly used to achieve under- or overnutrition during the suckling period and the long-term consequences of these manipulations were evaluated. McCance was the first to demonstrate that an altered nutrition in the immediate postnatal life has permanent effects on body size and composition in adulthood.[68] Widdowson and McCance[69] showed that rat pups undernourished during the suckling period by being raised in large litters maintain a diminished growth pattern throughout life. Rats raised in small litters show increase in body weight gain during the suckling period, which is maintained in adulthood and is accompanied by hyperphagia, hyperinsulinemia and hyperleptinemia.[70–72] It has been proposed that raising rats in small litters causes an altered programming of the hypothalamic neuronal activity responsible for energy homeostasis resulting in adulthood obesity.[73]

In the context of glucose metabolism, it has been shown that although rats raised in different litter sizes have similar plasma glucose levels, their plasma insulin levels are altered depending on litter size.[74,75] Fasting serum insulin levels in adult mice raised in small litters were two-fold higher and 50% lower in mice raised in large litters compared with age-matched normal-sized litter mice.[76] A heightened insulin secretory response to a glucose load is observed in adult mice raised in small litters while in those mice raised in large litters the response is blunted.[76] More recently, Waterland and Garza demonstrated that under- or overnourishment (by adjusting litter size) in rats during the suckling period permanently modifies pancreatic islet function at the level of insulin secretion and gene expression (Table 7.2).[77]

Overfeeding during the suckling period by reduction of litter size in the rat also results in the malprogram-

ming of the hypothalamic neurons. For example, it has been shown that in overweight small litter rats the normal bimodal effect of melanin concentrating hormone to excite or inhibit hypothalamic neurons becomes unidirectional reflecting the plasticity of the hypothalamic neuronal system to adapt to different environmental conditions in early life (Table 7.2).[73] The authors have also demonstrated increased inhibition of ventromedial hypothalamic neurons by agouti-related peptide in rats overfed due to small litter size during the suckling period.[78]

Caloric redistribution in the suckling period: the HC rat ("Pup in a cup") model

Adjustment of litter size results only in the modification of availability of total calories during the suckling period. This method does not permit alterations in the quality of nutrition without affecting total caloric intake during this period. This difficulty was overcome by the development of the artificial rearing technique by Hall, which allows one to raise rat pups immediately after birth on any desired milk formula.[79] Artificial rearing of 4-day-old rat pups via intragastric feeding (pups have no further access to their dams) on a high carbohydrate (HC) milk formula (caloric distribution in HC milk formula: carbohydrate 56%, protein 24% and fat 20%; and in rat milk: carbohydrate 8%, protein 24% and fat 68%) results in the immediate onset (within the first 24 h) of hyperinsulinemia that persists into adulthood despite withdrawal of the nutritional stimulus on postnatal day 24.[2,80] Although the plasma insulin concentration is about 6-fold higher in 12-day-old HC rats compared with age-matched mother-fed (MF) rats (Figure 7.2), their plasma glucose levels and body weights are not significantly different from those of age-matched MF rats.[81] Hyperinsulinemia persists in adulthood and is accompanied by an increase in growth rate from day 55 onwards and full blown obesity by approximately postnatal day 100 (Figure 7.2).[82,83] Additionally the progeny of females raised on the HC formula spontaneously acquire the characteristics of chronic hyperinsulinemia and adult-onset obesity without the requirement for any dietary treatment.[84] As indicated in Figure 7.3, second generation HC rats demonstrate hyperinsulinemia from postnatal day 28 onwards and increased growth rate from postnatal day 55 onwards and full blown obesity by approximately postnatal day 100.

The results from the HC rat model will be discussed under three headings: during the period of dietary treatment, in adulthood and in the next generation.

Table 7.2. Summary of the consequences of an altered nutritional experience in the immediate postnatal period

Nutritional experience	References
Undernourishment in the immediate postnatal period (large-sized litters)	
Lower growth trajectories for life	67,68
Reduced fasting plasma insulin levels	75
Blunted insulin secretory response to a glucose stimulus	75
Altered global gene expression patterns	76
Overnourishment in the immediate postnatal period (small-sized litters)	
Increased body weight gain from the start and persisting in adulthood accompanied by hyperphagia, hyperleptinemia and hyperinsulinemia	69,71
Higher fasting plasma insulin levels in adults	75
Increased insulin secretory response to a glucose stimulus	75
Altered global gene expression patterns in islets	76
Altered programming of the hypothalamus	72,77
Caloric redistribution (High carbohydrate (HC) dietary intervention) in suckling period	
Immediate effects	
Increased plasma insulin levels but normal plasma glucose levels	81
Leftward shift in the insulin secretory response to a glucose-stimulus	81
Modified response to incretins and neuroendocrine effectors	85
Ability to secrete moderate amounts of insulin in the absence of glucose and calcium	85
Increased gene expression of preproinsulin and related transcription factors	88
Increased number of small-sized islets and alterations in apoptosis and neogenesis in islets and duodenum	93
Persistent effects	
Increased plasma insulin levels	83,94
Abnormal glucose-tolerance test	82
Leftward shift in the insulin secretory response to a glucose stimulus	94
Increased gene expression of preproinsulin and related factors	94
Increase in weight gain from day 55 and significantly obese by day 100	83
Generational effect	
Pups born to HC females spontaneously acquire chronic hyperinsulinemia and adult-onset obesity	84,96

Adaptations during the period of HC dietary intervention

Table 7.2 and Figure 7.2 provide an overview of the adaptations due to the HC dietary intervention during the suckling period. The HC dietary treatment in neonatal rat pups induces several adaptations at the biochemical level in pancreatic islets of HC rats, which support the altered secretory capacity of these islets. Normal islets secrete increasing amounts of insulin in response to increasing glucose concentrations but do not secrete any measurable amount of insulin at very low glucose concentrations. In HC islets the insulin secretory response is significantly altered. Islets isolated from 12-day-old HC rats secrete significant amounts of insulin at sub-basal glucose concentrations in addition to secreting increased amounts of insulin at basal and above-basal glucose concentrations compared with age-matched controls.[81] Also, the observed increase in hexokinase may likely contribute to the lowering of the glucose threshold for insulin secretion by HC islets. Non-nutrient stimulants such as glucagons-like peptide-1 and acetylcholine augment insulin release to a larger extent in HC islets compared with age-matched MF islets even under stringent Ca^{2+}-depleted conditions.[85] In HC islets a ten-fold increase in norepinephrine concentration is required to inhibit insulin secretion compared to MF islets, indicating reduced sensitivity to adrenergic signals (negative modulators of insulin secretion).[85] Interestingly, the HC dietary intervention imparts the unique property to neonatal HC islets such that basal insulin secretion is partly independent of the requirements of glucose metabolism and increases in intracellular Ca^{2+} levels. The HC islets secrete significant amounts of insulin in the absence of glucose and under a simultaneously stringent Ca^{2+}-depleted condition.[85] Collectively, the above findings suggest that significant alterations at proximal and distal sites of the insulin secretory pathway in HC islets support the hyperinsulinemic condition of these rats (Figure 7.2).[86,87]

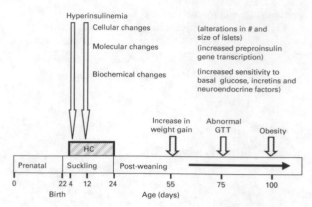

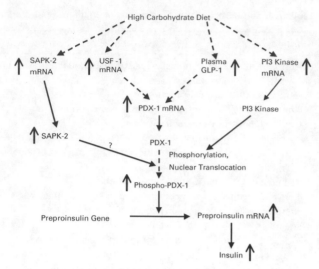

Figure 7.2. Summary of the immediate and persistent adaptations induced in the first generation HC rats in response to the HC dietary intervention during the suckling period. Rat pups were artificially reared on the HC formula from postnatal day 4 to 24 and weaned onto a standard lab chow ad libitum.

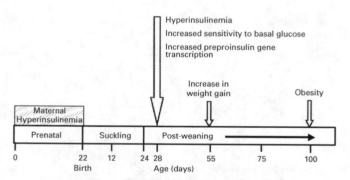

Figure 7.3. Summary of changes observed in the second generation HC rats due to the generational effect of the HC dietary modification in the immediate postnatal period of the dam. Pups born to HC females were reared naturally by normal foster nursing rats and the pups were weaned onto a standard lab chow ad libitum.

The altered dietary experience in the immediate postnatal life causes several molecular responses in islets, which may be essential for the persistence of the chronic hyperinsulinemic condition in this rat model. These include an increase in insulin biosynthesis and transcription of the preproinsulin gene in islets from neonatal HC rats and a significant increase in the gene expression of the components of the putative cascade of events such as PDX-1, USF-1, PI3 kinase, etc. implicated in the regulation of the transcription of the preproinsulin gene in neonatal HC islets.[88–91] Figure 7.4 illustrates the molecular adaptations induced in islets from 12-day-old HC rats and the possible interactions between them culminating in increased transcription of the preproinsulin gene via an increase in phospho-PDX-1. Additionally, global gene expression changes analyzed by

Figure 7.4. A postulated mechanism for the upregulation of the preproinsulin gene transcription in HC islets. Abbreviations are: SAPK-2: stress-activated protein kinase-2; USF-1: upstream stimulating factor-1; GLP-1: glucagon-like peptide-1; PDX-1: pancreatic duodenal homeobox transcription factor-1; PI3 kinase: phosphatidylinositol 3 kinase.

gene array analysis indicate that several clusters of genes involved in a wide array of cellular functions (e.g. cell cycle regulation, protein synthesis, ion channels and metabolic pathways) are upregulated in HC islets and may contribute to the onset of hyperinsulinemia in HC neonatal rats.[92]

The artificial rearing of neonatal rat pups on the HC milk formula also causes cellular alterations in the islets of these rats.[93] The significant cellular adaptations include (i) reduction in mean islet size in HC rats compared with age-matched MF controls and increase in the number of small-sized islets (Figure 7.5 A), (ii) increase in the number of islets per unit area (Figure 7.5 B), (iii) greater apoptotic rate in islets compared with ductal epithelium, a source of new islets by neogenesis and (iv) increase in islet cell replication, as indicated by the presence of proliferating cell nuclear antigen in 70–80% of the β cells.

In addition to the changes observed in the islets, the HC dietary modulation during the suckling period induces adaptations in other organs also. There is an increased deposition of glycogen in the liver of neonatal HC rats.[2] The lipogenic capacity of the liver is also increased in these rats.[82] Activities of glucokinase and malic enzyme are 77% and 96%, respectively, of adult levels in the liver of 10-day-old HC rats suggesting precocious induction of these enzymes by the HC dietary intervention (Figure 7.1).[2] Preliminary results suggest that the hypothalamus also responds to the HC nutritional experience and metabolic programming of the circuitry for energy

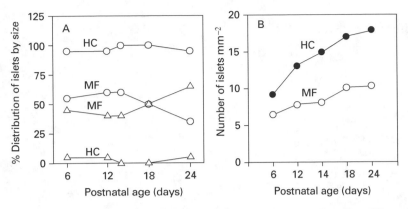

Figure 7.5. The alterations in the size (A) and number of islets (B) observed in 1-HC rats during the period of the dietary intervention. In (A) open triangle indicates large-sized islets (>10000 μm²) and open circle indicates small-sized islets (<10000 μm²). HC, high carbohydrate group; MF, mother-fed group.

homeostasis occurs in the neonatal HC rats (Shbeir, S and Patel, MS, unpublished observations).

Expression of programmed effects in adulthood

Artificially reared HC neonatal rats weaned onto lab chow on day 24 continue to be hyperinsulinemic into adulthood even after the withdrawal of the dietary modification that initiated hyperinsulinemia.[83] In addition, the growth rate of HC rats is higher than MF rats starting at day 55 and they are significantly obese by day 100.[84] Although normoglycemic, male HC rats display an aberrant response to a glucose tolerance test on day 75 compared with age-matched MF rats (Figure 7.2).[83]

Hyperinsulinemia in adulthood is supported by (i) a leftward shift (at a sub-basal level of glucose) in the insulin secretory response of islets from HC (100-day-old) v. age-matched MF rats, (ii) increased hexokinase activity and enhanced glucose- and Ca²⁺-independent insulin release,[94,95] (iii) increase in insulin-producing cell mass in HC pancreas,[82] (iv) increased preproinsulin gene transcription with concomitant increases in mRNA levels of PDX-1 and (v) significant increases in the expression of several clusters of genes as indicated by gene array analysis (Table 7.2).[92]

The onset of obesity is aided by the following observations. The epididymal adipose tissue weight is significantly higher in 100-day-old HC rats.[80] The lipogenic capacity of the liver and adipose tissue is significantly increased in HC rats as indicated by increases in the activity of fatty acid synthase and glucose-6-phosphate dehydrogenase (key enzymes in lipogenesis) as well as increased in vitro synthesis of lipids.[80] In addition there is a marked increase in the cell size in the epididymal and omental adipose tissues of 100-day-old male HC rats.[80]

Generational effects

A novel observation of the HC rat model is that HC females spontaneously transmit the HC phenotype (characteristics of chronic hyperinsulinemia and adult-onset obesity) to their progeny.[84] Figure 7.3 depicts the major adaptations in second generation HC (2-HC) rats due to fetal development in first generation HC (1-HC) female. 1-HC females are normoglycemic and hyperinsulinemic during pregnancy and lactation.[84] The plasma insulin levels of 2-HC rats are significantly increased (first observed on postnatal day 26).[96] Leftward shift in the insulin secretory response to a glucose stimulus, increase in hexokinase activity and increased preproinsulin gene transcription are observed in islets from 28-day-old 2-HC rats.[96] The body weight of 2-HC rats parallels that of age-matched MF rats up to postnatal day 55, but after then there is an increase in body weight of these rats with full-blown obesity being evident on approximately postnatal day 100 which correlates with a significant increase in the weight of the adipose tissues.[84] Concomitantly, there is an increase in the size of the adipocytes as well as an increase in the activities of the lipogenic enzymes (fatty acid synthase and glucose-6-phosphate dehydrogenase) in both liver and adipose tissue of 100-day-old 2-HC rats.[84] Liver and muscle glycogen content is reduced in 100-day-old 2-HC male rats and this is associated with a decrease in the activity of glycogen synthase.[97] The activities of the enzymes comprising the postulated upstream activators of glycogen synthase are also decreased in liver and muscle of 100-day-old 2-HC rats.[97] In contrast, in the epididymal adipose tissue of these rats glycogen synthase activity is increased with a concomitant increase in the activities of its postulated upstream activators.[98]

Potential mechanisms of metabolic programming

Adaptations in target tissues due to the overlap of an early nutritional stimulus or insult with the sensitive window of development of specific organs during early phases of life resulting in permanent alterations in the physiology and metabolism of target organs is termed metabolic programming. So far no specific mechanisms for metabolic programming are available. Potential mechanisms have been postulated and discussed by Lucas[3] and Waterland and Garza.[99] It has been suggested that structural alterations due to an altered dietary experience during the early developmental periods may be one of the mechanisms of metabolic programming.[22] For example it has been shown that occurrence of hyperinsulinemia during critical periods of brain development results in disorganization of the hypothalamus, which may be responsible for the later onset of pathological conditions.[100] Our results on the HC dietary intervention during the suckling period show that adaptations occur in pancreatic islets (hyperinsulinemia), gut (increased glucagon-like peptide-1 levels) and hypothalamus (alterations in the levels of neuropeptides) in 12-day-old HC rats in response to the HC milk formula. All of these organs are potentially important for maintaining glucose homeostasis. Figure 7.6 indicates the possible primary targets for the HC dietary intervention and the cross-talk between these organs that may be important for the establishment of the HC phenotype. It is proposed that in the HC rat model the increased availability of carbohydrate-derived calories in the HC milk formula induces responses in the gut, islets and hypothalamus all of which respond to the increased carbohydrate availability in the diet consumed. Glucagon-like peptide-1 via its effects on the islets could be augmenting the glucose effect on the islets. Additionally it has been shown that there are glucagon-like peptide-1 receptors in the brain and via this interaction specific responses could occur in the brain.[101] Insulin via interactions with its receptor in the hypothalamus could modulate hypothalamic programming. The HC dietary intervention results in increased availability of glucose to the brain. This could be a stimulus for altered programming of the energy circuitry in the brain. Neuroendocrine factors regulate insulin secretion and hyperinsulinemia in the HC rat could be a consequence of the altered neuroendocrine regulation of insulin secretion.[102] Such a hypothesis suggests a multifactorial mechanism for the onset and persistence of hyperinsulinemia in the HC rat. Hyperinsulinemia eventually results in insulin resistance leading to an altered glucose tolerance and obesity in adulthood.

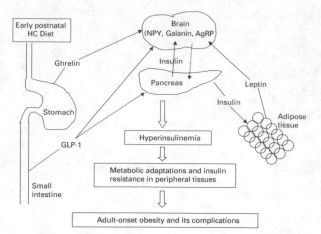

Figure 7.6. A diagrammatic representation of the probable sites of action of the high carbohydrate HC dietary modification and the interactions between these sites resulting in chronic hyperinsulinemia and adult-onset obesity and related complications.

An altered epigenetic programming has also been postulated as a possible mechanism for metabolic programming. Epigenetic mechanisms can be triggered by changes in the environment and can occur in both somatic and germ cell lineage during development.[103] Altered DNA methylation patterns have been reported to be caused by protein and folate deficiency.[104] Nutritional alterations early in life may induce altered cell-specific DNA methylation patterns causing changes in gene expression patterns in specific tissues. Such altered DNA methylation patterns can be transmitted to the daughter cells by replication facilitating perpetuation of the initial alterations.

Relevance to the high prevalence of the epidemic of obesity and the metabolic syndrome

Data from a plethora of human epidemiological studies resulted in the concept of "metabolic programming" which occurs as a consequence of the presence or often absence of a factor(s) during critical windows of development resulting in physiological effects in target organs that persist throughout life and cause adult-onset pathological conditions. Although the possible role of genetic and epigenetic factors in metabolic programming cannot be underestimated, epidemiological data strongly implicate an important role for environmental factors for this phenomenon. Amongst environmental factors, maternal/fetal malnutrition has been extensively investigated. Investigation of animal models such as the low protein diet, caloric restriction or hyperglycemia during fetal development have corroborated the observations from human epidemiological studies and underscored the importance of adequate nutrition during fetal development. Studies on over- or undernutrition and caloric redistribution without changes in total caloric intake (the HC rat model) in the immediate postnatal life also demonstrate the importance of proper nutrition during such periods for good health in adulthood. Collectively, the observations from different types of nutritional experiences in either the fetal or the immediate postnatal life as summarized above indicate that metabolic programming of target tissues such as pancreatic islets, hypothalamus, etc. during the period of exposure finally culminates in the appearance of the metabolic syndrome in adulthood with varying degrees of severity.

The precise mechanisms that prime an organism for adult-onset diseases due to an altered nutritional experience in early periods of life are not yet clearly understood. Such an understanding will aid in the design of treatments to overcome the epidemic situation of the metabolic syndrome. It is pertinent to decipher the initial hormonal and metabolic adaptations that occur in target tissues prior to the manifestation of the full-blown disease and which are essential for priming the individual for the eventual onset of these diseases. Such mechanistic approaches are a difficult proposition to investigate in human studies. For this purpose the various animal models described above are valuable tools to understand the mechanisms involved in metabolic programming of target organs by early life nutritional experiences, the interactions between them and interactions with adult life risk factors (sedentary life-style, over-eating, onset of puberty). The LP model is highly relevant to the biochemical mechanisms for high prevalence of type 2 diabetes, hypertension and cardiovascular diseases in impoverished populations especially in the developing countries. On the other hand, the HC rat model provides a unique opportunity to evaluate the underlying mechanisms involving adaptations in target organs and the crosstalk occurring between them beginning from the onset of hyperinsulinemia in the suckling period to the manifestation of abnormal growth rate (adult-onset obesity) and abnormal glucose tolerance much later in life. Results from such animal studies will also aid in the analysis of the consequences of altered dietary practices in human babies, which may provide a clue to the increase in the incidence of obesity, and other metabolic diseases specifically in the Western world. For example, in the light of the results obtained from the HC rat model, it is tempting to speculate that the changes in the weaning practice (formula feeding combined with early introduction of infant foods such as juices, fruits, cereals, etc.) for infants over

the past several decades, may have contributed in part to the observed epidemic of obesity in the United States. This, however, remains to be investigated.

Acknowledgments

We are grateful to Dr. Gail Willsky of this department and Dr. Satish Kalhan of Case Western Reserve University for their critical reading of the manuscript. Some of the studies reported in this chapter which were carried out in the author's laboratory were supported in part by National Institute of Child Health and Human Development Grant HD-11089 and National Institute of Diabetes and Digestive and Kidney Diseases Grants DK-51601 and DK-61518.

REFERENCES

1 Greengard, O. Enzymatic differentiation in mammalian tissues. *Essays Biochem.* 1971;**7**:159–205.

2 Haney, P. M., Raefsky-Estrin, C. R., Caliendo, A., Patel, M. S. Precocious induction of hepatic glucokinase and malic enzyme in artificially reared rat pups fed a high-carbohydrate diet. *Arch. Biochem. Biophys.* 1986;**244**:787–94.

3 Lucas, A. Programming by early nutrition in man. *CIBA Found. Symp.* 1991;**156**:38–55.

4 Kermack, W. O., McKendrick, A. G., McKinlay, P. L. Death-rates in Great Britain and Sweden. *Lancet* 1934;*i*:698–703.

5 Barker, D. J., Osmond, C. Infant mortality, childhood nutrition and ischaemic heart disease in England and Wales. *Lancet* 1986;*i*:1077–81.

6 Barker, D. J. P. Fetal origins of coronary heart disease. *Br. Med. J.* 1995;**311**:171–4.

7 Petry, C. J., Hales, C. N. Intrauterine development and its relationship with type 2 diabetes mellitus. In Hitman, G. A., ed. *Type 2 Diabetes: Prediction and Prevention.* New York, NY: John Wiley & Sons; 1999:153–68.

8 Hales, C. N., Barker, D. J. P. Type 2 (non-insulin-dependent) diabetes mellitus: the thrifty phenotype hypothesis. *Diabetologia* 1992;**35**:595–601.

9 Petry, C. J., Ozanne, S. E., Hales, C. N. Programming of intermediary metabolism. *Mol. Cell. Endocrinol.* 2001;**185**:81–91.

10 Holemans, A., Aerts, L., Van Assche, F. A. Lifetime consequences of abnormal fetal pancreatic development. *J. Physiol.* 2003;**547**:11–20.

11 Van Assche, F. A., Holemans, K., Aerts, L. Long-term consequences for offspring of diabetes during pregnancy. *Br. Med. Bull.* 2001;**60**:173–82.

12 Betram, C. E., Hanson, M. A. Animal models and programming of the metabolic syndrome. *Br. Med. Bull.* 2001;**60**:103–21.

13 Desai, M., Crowther, M. J., Lucas, A., Hales, C. N. Organ-selective growth in the offspring of protein-restricted mothers. *Br. J. Nutr.* 1996;**76**:591–603.

14 Kwong, W. Y., Wild, A. E., Roberts, P., Willis, A. C., Fleming, T. P. Maternal under nutrition during the pre-implantation period of rat development causes blastocyst abnormalities and programming of postnatal hypertension. *Development* 2000;**127**:4195–202.

15 Holeness, M. J. Impact of early growth retardation on glucoregulatory control and insulin action in mature rats. *Am. J. Physiol.* 1996;**270**:E946–54.

16 Snoeck, A., Remacle, C., Reucens, B., Hoet, J. J. Effect of a low protein diet during pregnancy on the fetal rat endocrine pancreas. *Biol. Neonate* 1990;**57**:107–18.

17 Dahri, S., Snoeck, A., Reucens-Billen, B., Remacle, C., Hoet, J. J. Islet function in offspring of mothers on low-protein diet during gestation. *Diabetes* 1991;**40**:115–20.

18 Cherif, H., Reucens, B., Dahri, S., Hoet, J. J., Remacle, C. Stimulatory effects of taurine on insulin secretion by fetal rat islets cultured *in vitro*. *J. Endocrinol.* 1996;**151**:501–6.

19 Berney, D. M., Desai, M., Palmer, D. J. *et al.* The effects of maternal protein deprivation on the fetal rat pancreas: major structural changes and their recuperation. *J. Pathol.* 1997;**183**:109–15.

20 Petrik, J., Reucens, B., Arany, E. *et al.* A low protein diet alters the balance of islet cell replication and apoptosis in the fetal and neonatal rat and is associated with a reduced pancreatic expression of insulin-like growth factor II. *Endocrinology* 1999;**140**:4861–73.

21 Arantes, V. C., Teixeira, V. P., Reis, M. A. *et al.* Expression of PDX-1 is reduced in pancreatic islets from pus of rat dams fed a low protein diet during gestation and lactation. *J. Nutr.* 2002;**132**:3030–5.

22 Bennis-Taleb, N., Remacle, C., Hoet, J. J., Reusens, B. A low-protein isocaloric diet during gestation affects brain development and alters permanently cerebral cortex blood vessels in rat offspring. *J. Nutr.* 1999;**129**:1613–9.

23 Plagemann, A., Harder, T., Rake, A. *et al.* Hypothalamic nuclei are malformed in weanling offspring of low protein malnourished rat dams. *J. Nutr.* 2000;**130**:2582–90.

24 Maloney, C. A., Gosby, A. K., Phuyal, J. L. *et al.* Site-specific changes in the expression of fat-partioning genes in weanling rats exposed to low-protein diet in utero. *Obes. Res.* 2003;**11**:461–8.

25 Shepherd, P. R., Crowther, N. J., Desai, M., Hales, C. N., Ozanne, S. E. Altered adipocyte properties in the offspring of protein malnourished rats. *Br. J. Nutr.* 1997;**78**:121–9.

26 Lucas, A., Baker, B. A., Desai, M., Hales, C. N. Nutrition in pregnant rats programs lipid metabolism in the offspring. *Br. J. Nutr.* 1996;**76**:605–12.

27 Ozanne, S. E., Wang, C. L., Petry, C. J., Smith, J. M., Hales, C. N. Ketosis resistance in the male offspring of protein-malnourished rat dams. *Metabolism* 1998;**47**:1450–4.

28 Petry, C. J., Dorling, M. W., Wang, C. L., Powlak, D. B., Ozanne, S. E. Catecholamine levels and receptor expression in low protein diet offspring. *Diabet. Med.* 2000;**17**:848–53.

29 Ozanne, S. E., Smith, G. D., Tikerpae, J., Hales, C. N. Altered regulation of hepatic glucose output in the male offspring of protein-malnourished rat dams. *Am. J. Physiol.* 1996;**270**:E559–64.

30 Desai, M., Byrne, C. D., Zhang, J., Petry, C. J. *et al.* Programming of hepatic insulin-sensitive enzymes in offspring of rat dams fed a protein-restricted diet. *Am. J. Physiol.* 1997;**272**:G1083–90.

31 Ozanne, S. E., Wang, C. L., Coleman, N., Smith, G. D. Altered muscle insulin sensitivity in the male offspring of protein malnourished rats. *Am. J. Physiol.* 1996;**271**:E1128–34.

32 Hales, C. N., Desai, M., Ozanne, S. E., Crowther, N. J. Fishing in the stream of diabetes: from measuring insulin to the control of fetal organogenesis. *Biochem. Soc. Trans.* 1996;**24**:341–50.

33 Ozanne, S. E., Nave, B. T., Wang, C. L. *et al.* Poor fetal nutrition causes long term changes in expression of insulin signaling components in adipocytes. *Am. J. Physiol.* 1997;**273**:E46–51.

34 Ozanne, S. E., Dorling, M. W., Wang, C. L., Petry, C. J. Depot-specific effects of early growth retardation on adipocyte insulin action. *Horm. Metab. Res.* 2000;**32**:71–5.

35 Ozanne, S. E., Wang, C. L., Dorling, M. W., Petry, C. J. Dissection of the metabolic actions of insulin in adipocytes from early growth-retarded male rats. *J. Endocrinol.* 1999;**162**:313–9.

36 Langley, S. C., Jackson, A. A. Increased systolic blood pressure in adult rats induced by fetal exposure to low protein diets. *Clin. Sci.* 1994;**86**:217–22.

37 Langley-Evans, S. C. Critical differences between two low protein diet protocols in the programming of hypertension in the rat. *Int. J. Food Sci. Nutr.* 2000;**51**:11–7.

38 Langley-Evans, S. C., Sherman, R. C., Welham, S. J. *et al.*. Intrauterine programming of hypertension: the role of rennin-angiotesin system. *Biochem. Soc. Trans.* 1999;**27**:88–93.

39 Woods, L. L. Fetal origins of adult hypertension: a renal mechanism? *Curr. Opin. Nephrol. Hypertens.* 2000;**9**:419–25.

40 Langley-Evans, S. C., Philips, G., Benediktsson, R. *et al.* Maternal dietary protein restriction, placental glucocorticoid metabolism and the programming of hypertension. *Placenta* 1996;**17**:169–72.

41 Iglesias-Barreira, V., Ahn, M. T., Reusens, B. *et al.* Pre- and postnatal low protein diet affect pancreatic islet blood flow and insulin release in adult rats. *Endocrinology* 1996;**137**:3797–801.

42 Petry, C. J., Ozanne, S. E., Wang, C. L., Hales, C. N. Effects of early protein restriction and adult obesity on rat pancreatic hormone content and glucose tolerance. *Horm. Metab. Res.* 2000;**32**:233–9.

43 Petry, C. J., Ozanne, S. E., Wang, C. L., Hales, C. N. Early protein restriction and obesity independently induce hypertension in 1-year-old rats. *Clin. Sci.* 1997;**93**:147–52.

44 Petry, C. J., Dorling, M. W., Powlak, D. B., Ozanne, S. E., Hales, C. N. Diabetes in old male offspring of rat dams fed a reduced protein diet. *Int. J. Expt. Diabetes Res.* 2001;**2**:139–43.

45 Holemans, K., Verhaeghe, J., Dequeker, J., Van Assche, F. A. Insulin sensitivity in adult female offspring of rats subjected

to malnutrition during the perinatal period. *J. Soc. Gyn. Invest.* 1996;**3**:71–7.

46 Holemans, K., Van Bree, R., Verhaeghe, J., Van Assche, F. A. Maternal under nutrition and streptozotocin-diabetes in the rat have different effects on *in vivo* glucose uptake by peripheral tissues in their female adult offspring. *J. Nutr.* 1997;**127**:1371–6.

47 Holemans, K., Gerber, R. T., Meurrens, K. *et al.* Maternal food restriction in the second half of pregnancy affects vascular function but not blood pressure of rat female offspring. *Br. J. Nutr.* 1999;**81**:73–9.

48 Bertin, E., Gangnerau, M. N., Bailbe, D., Portha, B. Glucose metabolism and beta-cell mass in adult offspring of rats protein or energy restricted during the last week of pregnancy. *Am. J. Physiol.* 1999;**277**:E11–7.

49 Garofano, A., Czernichow, P., Breant, B. Beta-cell mass and proliferation following late fetal and early postnatal malnutrition in the rat. *Diabetologia* 1998;**41**:1114–20.

50 Garofano, A., Czernichow, P., Breant, B. Effect of ageing on beta-cell mass and function in rats malnourished during the perinatal period. *Diabetologia* 1990;**42**:711–8.

51 Woodall, S. M., Johnston, B. M., Breier, B. H., Gluckman, P. D. Chronic maternal under nutrition in the rat leads to delayed postnatal growth and elevated blood pressure of offspring. *Pediatr. Res.* 1996;**40**:438–43.

52 Vickers, B. H., Breier, H., Cutfield, W. S., Hofman, P. L., Gluckman, P. D. Fetal origins of hyperphagia, obesity and hypertension and postnatal amplification by hyper caloric nutrition. *Am. J. Physiol.* 2000;**279**:E83–7.

53 Freinkel, N. Banting lecture. Of pregnancy and progeny. *Diabetes* 1980;**29**:1023–35.

54 Pederson, J. *The Pregnant Diabetic and her New Born. Problems and Management.* 2nd edn. Baltimore, MD: Williams and Wilkins;1977.

55 Van Assche, F. A., Holemans, K., Aerts, L. Fetal growth and consequences for later life. *J. Perinat. Med.* 1998;**26**:337–46.

56 Aerts, L., Holemans, K., Van Assche, F. A. Impaired insulin response and action in offspring of severely diabetes rats. In Shafrir, E., ed. *Frontiers in Diabetes Research. Lessons from Animal Diabetes III.* London: Smith-Gordon;1990:561–6.

57 Kervran, A., Guillaume, M., Jost, A. The endocrine pancreas of the fetus from diabetic pregnant rat. *Diabetologia* 1978;**15**:387–93.

58 Aerts, L., Vercruysse, L., Van Assche, F. A. The endocrine pancreas in virgin and pregnant offspring of diabetic pregnant rats. *Diabetes Res. Clin. Prac.* 1997;**38**:9–19.

59 Van Assche, F. A. Birthweight as risk factor for breast cancer. *Lancet* 1997;349:502.

60 Ktorza, A., Gauguier, D., Bihoreau, M. T., Berthault, M. F., Picon, L. Adult offspring from mildly hyperglycemic rats show impairment of glucose regulation and insulin secretion which is transmissible to the next generation. In Shafrir, E., ed. *Frontiers in Diabetes Research. Lessons from Animal Diabetes III.* London: Smith-Gordon; 1990:555–60.

61 Oh, W., Gelardi, N. L., Cha, C. J. Maternal hyperglycemia in pregnant rats: its effect on growth and carbohydrate metabolism in the offspring. *Metabolism* 1988;**37**:1146–51.

62 Philipps, A. F., Rosenkrantz, T. S., Grunner, M. L. *et al.* Effects of fetal insulin secretory deficiency on metabolism in fetal lamb. *Diabetes* 1986;**35**:964–72.

63 Plagemann, A., Heidrich, I., Rohde, W., Gotz, F., Dorner, G. Hyperinsulinism during differentiation of the hypothalamus is a diabetogenic and obesity risk factor in rats. *Neuroendocrinol. Lett.* 1992;**5**:373–8.

64 Canavan, J. P., Goldspink, D. F. Maternal diabetes in rats II. Effects on fetal growth and protein turnover. *Diabetes* 1988;**37**:1671–7.

65 Holemans, K., Aerts, L., Van Assche, F. A. Evidence for an insulin resistance in the adult offspring of streptozotocin-diabetic pregnant rats. *Diabetologia* 1991;**34**:81–5.

66 Holemans, K., Van Bree, R., Verhaeghe, J., Aerts, L., Van Assche, F. A. *In vivo* glucose utilization by individual tissues in virgin and pregnant offspring of severely diabetic rats. *Diabetes* 1993;**42**:530–6.

67 Van Assche, F. A. The fetal endocrine pancreas: a quantitative morphological approach. PhD thesis, University of Leuven; 1970.

68 McCance, R. A. Food, growth and time. *Lancet* 1962;**2**:271–2.

69 Widdowson, E. M., McCance, R. A. The effect of finite periods of under nutrition at different ages on the composition and subsequent development of the rat. *Proc. R. Soc. Lond. B. Biol. Sci.* 1963;**158**:329–42.

70 Faust, I. M., Johnson, P. R., Hirsh, J. Long-term effects of early nutritional experience on the development of obesity in rats. *J. Nutr.* 1980;**110**:2027–34.

71 Plagemann, A., Heidrich, I., Gotz, F., Rohde, W., Dorner, G. Obesity and enhanced diabetes and cardiovascular risk in adult rats due to early postnatal overfeeding. *Exp. Clin. Endocrinol.* 1992;**99**:154–8.

72 Plagemann, A., Harder, T., Rake, A., Voits, M., Fink, H., Rohde, W. Perinatal elevation of hypothalamic insulin, acquired malformation of hypothalamic galaninergic neurons, and syndrome X-like alterations in adulthood of neonatally overfed rats. *Brain Res.* 1999;**836**:146–55.

73 Davidowa, H., Li, Y., Plagemann, A. Hypothalamic ventromedial and arcuate neurons of normal and postnatally overnourished rats differ in their responses to melanin-concentrating hormone. *Reg. Peptides* 2002;**108**:103–11.

74 Cryer, A., Jones, H. M. The development of white adipose tissue. Effect of litter size on the lipoprotein lipase activity of four adipose-tissue depots, serum immunoreactive insulin and tissue cellularity during the first year of life in male and female rats. *Biochem. J.* 1980;**186**:805–15.

75 Hahn, P. Effect of litter size on plasma cholesterol and insulin and some liver and adipose tissue enzymes in adult rodents. *J. Nutr.* 1984;**114**:1231–4.

76 Aubert, R., Suquet, J. P., Lemonnier, D. Long-term morphological and metabolic effects of early under- and over-nutrition in mice. *J. Nutr.* 1980;**110**:649–61.

77 Waterland, R. A., Garza, C. Early postnatal nutrition determines adult pancreatic glucose-responsive insulin secretion and islet gene expression in rats. *J. Nutr.* 2002;**132**:357–64.

78 Li, Y., Plagemann, A., Davidowa, H. Increased inhibition by agouti-related peptide of ventromedial hypothalamic neurons in rats overweight due to early postnatal overfeeding. *Neurosci. Lett.* 2002;**330**:33–6.

79 Hall, W. G. Weaning and growth of artificially reared rats. *Science* 1975;**190**:1313–5.

80 Hiremagular, B. K., Vadlamudi, S., Johanning, G. L., Patel, M. S. Long-term effects of feeding of high carbohydrate diet in preweaning by gastrosomy: a new rat model for obesity. *Int. J. Obes.* 1993;**17**:495–502.

81 Aalinkeel, R., Srinivasan, M., Kalhan, S., Laychock, S. G., Patel, M. S. A dietary intervention (high carbohydrate) during the neonatal period causes islet dysfunction in rats. *Am. J. Physiol.* 1999;**277**:E1061–9.

82 Hiremagalur, B. K., Vadlamudi, S., Johanning, G. L., Patel, M. S. Alterations in hepatic lipogenic capacity in rat pups artificially reared on a milk-substitute formula high in carbohydrate or medium-chain triglycerides. *J. Nutr. Biochem.* 1992;**3**:474–80.

83 Vadlamudi, S., Hiremagalur, B. K., Tao, S., *et al.* Long-term effects on pancreatic functions of feeding a HC formula to rats during the preweaning period. *Am. J. Physiol. Endocrinol. Metab.* 1993;**265**:E565–71.

84 Vadlamudi, S., Kalhan, S. C., Patel, M. S. Persistence of metabolic consequences in the progeny of rats fed a HC formula in their early postnatal life. *Am. J. Physiol. Endocrinol. Metab.* 1995;**269**:E731–8.

85 Srinivasan, M., Aalinkeel, R., Song, F. *et al.* Adaptive changes in insulin secretion by islets from neonatal rats raised on a high-carbohydrate formula. *Am. J. Physiol. Endocr. Metab.* 2000;**279**:E1347–57.

86 Patel, M. S., Srinivasan, M. Metabolic programming: causes and consequences. *J. Biol. Chem.* 2002;**277**:1629–32.

87 Srinivasan, M., Laychock, S. G., Hill, D. J., Patel, M. S. Neonatal nutrition: metabolic programming of pancreatic islets and obesity. *Exp. Biol. Med.* 2003;**228**:15–23.

88 Srinivasan, M., Song, F., Aalinkeel, R., Patel, M. S. Molecular adaptations in islets from neonatal rats reared artificially on a high carbohydrate milk formula. *J. Nutr. Biochem.* 2001;**12**:575–84.

89 Marshak, S., Totary H., Cerasi, E., Melloul, D. Purification of the beta cell glucose-sensitive factor that transactivates the insulin gene differentially in normal and transformed islets cells. *Proc. Natl. Acad. Sci. USA.* 1996;**93**:15057–62.

90 MacFarlane, W. M., Mckinnon, C. M., Felton-Edkins, A. *et al.* Glucose stimulates translocation of the homeodomain transcription factor PDX-1 from the cytoplasm to the nucleus in pancreatic beta-cells. *J. Biol. Chem.* 1999;**274**:1011–6.

91 Qian, J., Kaytor, E. N., Towle, H. C., Olson, L. K. Upstream stimulatory factor regulates PDx-1 gene expression in differentiated pancreatic beta cells. *Biochem. J.* 1999;**341**:315–22.

92 Song, F., Srinivasan, M., Aalinkeel, R., Patel, M. S. Use of a cDNA array for the identification of genes induced in islets of suckling rats by a high-carbohydrate nutritional intervention. *Diabetes* 2001;**50**:2053–60.

93 Petrik, J., Srinivasan, M., Aalinkeel, R., *et al.* A long-term high-carbohydrate diet causes an altered ontogeny of pancreatic islets of Langerhans in the neonatal rat. *Pediatr. Res.* 2001;**49**:84–92.

94 Aalinkeel, R., Srinivasan, M., Song, F., Patel, M. S. Programming into adulthood of islet adaptations induced by early nutritional intervention in the rat. *Am. J. Physiol. Endocrinol. Metab.* 2001;**281**:E640–8.

95 Laychock, S. G., Vadlamudi, S., Patel, M. S. Neonatal rat dietary carbohydrate affects pancreatic islet insulin secretion in adults and progeny. *Am. J. Physiol.* 1995;**269**:E739–44.

96 Srinivasan, M., Aalinkeel, R., Song, F., Patel, M. S. Programming of islet functions in the progeny of hyperinsulinemic/obese rats. *Diabetes* 2003;**52**:984–90.

97 Srinivasan, M., Vadlamudi, S., Patel, M. S. Glycogen synthase regulation in hyperinsulinemic/obese progeny of rats fed a high carbohydrate formula in their infancy. *Int. J. Obesity.* 1996;**20**:981–9.

98 Srinivasan, M., Patel, M. S. Glycogen synthase activation in the epididymal adipose tissue from chronic hyperinsulinemic/obese rats. *Nutr. Biochem.* 1998;**9**:81–7.

99 Waterland, R. A., Garza, C. Potential mechanisms of metabolic imprinting that lead to chronic disease. *Am. J. Clin. Nutr.* 1999;**69**:179–97.

100 Harder, T., Plagemann, A., Rohde, W., Dorner, G. Syndrome X-like alterations in adult female rats due to neonatal insulin treatment. *Metabolism* 1998;**47**:855–62.

101 Kieffer, T. J., Habener, J. F. The glucagon-like peptides. *Endocrine Rev.* 1999;**20**:876–913.

102 Ahren, B. Autonomic regulation of islet hormone secretion–implications for health and disease. *Diabetologia* 2000;**43**:393–410.

103 Monk, M. Epigenetic programming of differential gene expression in development and evolution. *Dev. Genet.* 1995;**17**:188–97.

104 Jacob, R. A. Folate, DNA methylation and gene expression: factors of nature and nurture. *Am. J. Clin. Nutr.* 2000;**72**:903–4.

8

Nutrient regulation in brain development: glucose and alternate fuels

Camille Fung and Sherin U. Devaskar

Department of Pediatrics, David Geffen School of Medicine at UCLA, Los Angeles, CA

To maintain normal cerebral function and development, a sufficient amount of metabolizable substrate must be supplied to the brain at all times. Glucose is the primary energy substrate for the growing fetus, newborn and adult brain under physiologic conditions.[1,2] As much as 90% of all the energy consumed by the fetus is estimated to be derived from glucose.[3] Plasma glucose concentration of the fetus changes with that of the mother, i.e. a linear relationship exists between the glucose concentrations of the mother and the fetus.[4] At birth with umbilical cord clamping, the maternal supply of oxygen and nutrients ceases abruptly, which sets into motion the initiation of neonatal glucose production triggered by a surge in various circulating hormones. Most normal term and preterm infants are able to mobilize glycogen, initiate gluconeogenesis, and thereby produce glucose at 4–6 mg kg^{-1} min^{-1} in the immediate postnatal period.[5] When glucose deficiency occurs, other organic non-glucose substrates are utilized to sustain the normal energy balance of supply and demand. This chapter will address normal cerebral glucose metabolism focusing on the delivery of glucose by a family of facilitative glucose transporters, the role of alternate substrates when glucose availability is limited, cerebral adaptive responses to hypoglycemia, and finally hypoglycemia-induced brain cellular apoptosis and/or necrosis.

Difficulties in defining hypoglycemia

Abnormalities in glucose homeostasis continue to pose problems in the term and preterm newborn infant. The reported incidence of hypoglycemia varies depending on the definition of hypoglycemia and the test employed to measure glucose concentrations. It is becoming apparent that while statistical definitions of hypoglycemia have been traditionally used at the bedside, a neurophysiological definition that can predict an adverse developmental outcome is warranted. Sexson et al.[6] reported that 8.1% of the 232 newborn infants studied had glucose values < 30 mg dL^{-1} (1.6 mM) and 20.6% had glucose values < 40 mg dL^{-1} (2.2 mM). Glucose is the predominant metabolic fuel for the brain, thus a persistent lack of adequate circulating glucose results in significant neurological consequences.[7,8] Confusion regarding when to intervene in the case of neonatal hypoglycemia exists. This stems from the entity of "asymptomatic hypoglycemia" which may be due to hormonal depletion causing an inadequate counter-regulatory response or more realistically the nonspecific nature of symptoms that are less likely to be detected with the existent clinical acumen. What continues to be vague is the lack of precision pertaining to the level of hypoglycemia, the duration of hypoglycemia, and the contributory factors, that can injure the brain. Based on many reports,[9–11] transient hypoglycemia (25–45 mg dL^{-1} [1.4 to 2.5 mM]) in healthy infants is not associated directly with an abnormal neurodevelopmental outcome. However, measurement of auditory and sensory evoked potentials indicates that demonstrable neural dysfunction occurs with a blood glucose concentration of less than 2.6 mM, irrespective of whether any clinical signs are displayed.[12] While the accuracy of the blood glucose concentration relies on the site of sampling, the handling of the blood sample and the type of bedside testing employed, neural dysfunction relies more on the actual glucose

Neonatal Nutrition and Metabolism. Second Edition, ed. P. Thureen and W. Hay. Published by Cambridge University Press.

delivery and brain glucose extraction rather than on the blood glucose concentration which forms only the tip of an iceberg.

Normal cerebral glucose metabolism

The human brain is a highly metabolically active organ in the body. Despite making up only 2% of the total adult body weight, the brain represents up to 50% of the body's resting glucose consumption.[13] The main energy-consuming processes of the central nervous system include the biosynthesis and transport of ions and neurotransmitters (glutamate, acetylcholine and gamma-aminobutyric acid) required for neurotransmission. Of importance is the energy required for clearing glutamate from the brain extracellular compartment. Absence of energy leads to excessive glutamate accumulation that culminates in neuronal excitotoxicity causing cell injury and death.[14]

The mechanism by which glucose is transported from the blood into the brain was elucidated in the last 20 years. Studies in adult rats showed that the rate of unidirectional influx of glucose into the brain is about twice the rate of glucose utilization.[15] This excess of influx over utilization maintains brain glucose concentration at about 20% of the plasma value, so under normal circumstances, the concentration of brain glucose is far from limiting glycolysis. In fact, the rate-limiting step in glucose utilization appears to be the intracellular phosphorylation of glucose to glucose-6-phosphate by the mitochondrially bound hexokinase I and the glycolytic enzyme phosphofructokinase. The activity of these two key enzymes is increased by a lowering of the cellular adenosine triphosphate (ATP) content. Since processing of ATP is the basis of cellular energy extraction, the ATP content of neurons drives the uptake of glucose. It follows then that an increase in the rate of glycolysis and/or hypoglycemia with lowered ATP content could bring the rate of glucose influx close to matching the rate of cellular metabolism. In such situations, glucose transport becomes rate-limiting to neuronal energy extraction.[14]

Glucose transport

Glucose transport from blood across the endothelial cells of the blood–brain barrier and across the plasma membranes of neurons and glia is carried out by a family of structurally related membrane-spanning glycoproteins called the facilitative glucose transporters. The process of facilitative glucose transport is saturable and stereospecific, but is not concentrative, energy-dependent, or influenced by sodium.[16] To date, 13 GLUT isoforms have been identified and designated as GLUT 1–13 for the order in which they were cloned.[16] The two predominant isoforms detected in the brain are GLUT1 and GLUT3. GLUT1 ($Km = 1$–2 mM) in whole brain preparations can be resolved on sodium dodecyl sulfate (SDS)-polyacrylamide gel electrophoresis as two molecular mass isoforms of 45 and 55 kDa, the difference accounted for by the degree of glycosylation.[17–19] The 55 kDa isoform is expressed highly in the microvascular endothelium of the blood–brain barrier,[19–21] while the 45 kDa isoform has been detected in vascular-free brain membranes,[19,22] in synaptosome preparations[23] and in cultured glia.[24–26] GLUT3 ($Km = 0.03$ to 0.08 mM), on the other hand, is expressed primarily by neurons, particularly in the processes that form synapses.[25–27]

Many investigators, using the rodent model, have outlined changes in levels of expression of GLUT1 and GLUT3 during brain development.[17–19] This developmental change in expression must be viewed in the context of anatomical, biochemical, and functional changes that are occurring in the brain as it reflects the rate of regional cerebral glucose utilization. We know that the first barrier to the passage of glucose into the brain is the endothelial cells of the blood–brain barrier. Even though previous thinking has suggested that this barrier is poorly developed and "leaky" in the immature brain, it is now fairly well accepted that the rat brain endothelial cells begin barrier formation by day 16 of gestation,[28] and that fenestrations completely disappear by the end of gestation.[29] By having a system for glucose transport, namely with GLUT1 in the microvessels of the blood–brain barrier, the brain is able to continuously receive glucose. It has been shown that there is no significant regional variation in the expression of GLUT1 in the rat brain.[19] Similar investigations exist in the human brain as well demonstrating that GLUT1 is indeed the transporter of the blood–brain barrier.[30] Further GLUT 1 is asymmetrically distributed with a 3- to 4-fold higher abundance in the abluminal (facing the brain) relative to the luminal (facing the blood) surface of the endothelial cells. This distribution pattern provides a glucose gradient congenial for transport from blood into the extracellular compartment of the brain.[31,32] A substantial portion from this compartment is transported into glial cells that have processes (end feet) that surround the capillaries. The importance of the glial contribution is demonstrated by the facts that glial cells make up about half of the brain cells and possess a higher rate of basal glucose utilization (20 nmol mg^{-1} min^{-1}) than do neurons (8 nmol mg^{-1} min^{-1}). Once glucose is taken up by astrocytes, it can be stored as glycogen that can be converted into glucose upon stimulation of the beta-adrenergic receptors and transported back into the extracellular compartment to be available to fuel neuronal synapses. Thus, astrocytes have a small glycogen store with a high turnover rate and serve as the intermediate local storehouse that mediates the indirect glucose transfer from across the blood–brain barrier via the glial cells to the neurons.[14] In addition, GLUT3 mediates glucose transfer from the extracellular compartment directly into neurons.[26,27]

In terms of the developmental profile for GLUT3 in the rat and mouse, before the formation of barrier properties in the embryonic cerebral vasculature, only GLUT1 and not GLUT3 is expressed in the germinal neuro-epithelium which consists of proliferating progenitor cells.[33] Following the formation of the blood–brain barrier towards the end of gestation, GLUT3 expression begins and is found at low levels only in neurons. The regional variability of GLUT3 levels parallel the local glucose utilization rate with the subcortical structures of thalamus and hypothalamus demonstrating higher levels during early maturational stages and the cerebral cortex and hippocampus demonstrating an increase in GLUT3 later in development, corresponding to the period of neuronal maturation and synaptogenesis.[17,27,34] In addition, investigations targeted at deciphering the molecular mechanisms that mediate this developmental GLUT3 increase in the murine brain have revealed a role for both transcriptional and post-transcriptional mechanisms.[35–37] Particularly, stimulatory protein–3 (Sp3), cyclic AMP binding protein (CREB) and the mouse Y box protein 1 (MSY-1) transcriptionally regulate GLUT3 expression in neurons, thereby assigning an active role for this protein during neuronal cell differentiation and neurotransmission.[36,37] Of note is the developmental profile in which both GLUT1 and GLUT3 postnatally increase substantially towards the adult values at the time of weaning when there is an increasing proportion of carbohydrate intake with a concomitant decrease in alternate fuels such as ketones and when the cerebral energy demands increase dramatically.[17,35] A similar profile has been described in the human brain.[38]

In addition to GLUT1 and GLUT3, other isoforms have also been detected in brain. GLUT2 with a high Km is expressed in the hypothalamic region of the brain and GLUT4, the insulin-responsive isoform is observed in cortical neuronal processes. More recently one of the novel isoforms, namely GLUT8 has been detected in neuronal cell bodies with higher concentrations during the postnatal suckling phase when compared with the adult.[39,40] Further, GLUT8 demonstrates a predominantly intracellular distribution in neurons and its functional importance during development remains to be determined.[41] This is particularly evident when brain 2-deoxy-glucose uptake measurements predict the developmental changes in brain GLUT3 concentrations but not that of GLUT8.[17,35,40] Duffy et al.[42] noted the regional cerebral glucose utilization (rCGU)[43] in newborn dogs to be high in the brainstem grey matter structures which declined rostrally in the cerebral cortex. Employing ^{18}F-2-deoxy-glucose and PET scanning, Chugani et al.[44] demonstrated in newborn infants that the CGU was highest in the sensorimotor cortex, thalamus, midbrain-brainstem and cerebellar vermis at 5 weeks of age. At 3 months, maximal glucose utilization had shifted to the parietal, temporal and occipital cortices and in the basal ganglia. Further increases in frontal and association cortices occurred by 8 months of age, with little change in rCGU between 8 to 18 months, values being similar to that of the adult.[44] To date, a clinical GLUT1 deficiency syndrome has been described in which a genetic defect consisting of haplo-insufficiency (detected by FISH) results in hypoglycorrhachia with low cerebrospinal fluid lactate levels in the face of normoglycemia, developmental delays, incoordination and spasticity causing an abnormal gait, deceleration in head growth leading to acquired microcephaly, and seizures. These clinical manifestations occur during infancy and a ketogenic diet ameliorates the epileptic symptoms with no benefit to the behavioral complications.[45,46] Genomic DNA analysis in patients who have a negative FISH has revealed heterozygous mutations which include missense and nonsense mutations, insertions, microdeletions and splice-site mutations.[46] In addition to this genetic disorder, perturbations in circulating glucose concentrations are known to alter fetal ovine brain GLUT1 and GLUT3 concentrations,[47,48] thereby providing a compensatory response towards preserving the glucose supply.

Alternate substrates to glucose

Despite the predominant use of glucose in cerebral oxidative metabolism, situations do arise under physiologic conditions in which the supply of glucose may be limited. These situations include the immediate post-delivery period, suckling phase and fasting. Under such conditions, the neonatal brain utilizes alternate substrates, most notably the ketone bodies, β-hydroxybutyrate (β-OHB) and acetoacetate and lactic acid.

Much research concerning alternate brain fuels during postnatal development has focused upon the aforementioned ketone bodies and their relationship to glucose utilization. The generally accepted concepts arising from such research include the following: (1) although glucose may not always be the primary fuel, its uninterrupted supply is obligatory for normal growth and function, (2) at maximum, ketone bodies can only meet 50–60% of the brain's metabolic needs and (3) when taken together, glucose and ketones supply better than 88% of the brain's energy requirements.[49] As the brain is exposed to these changing levels of circulating substrates, it must adjust its metabolism in order to utilize the mix of fuels which is made available. As will be discussed later, this task is accomplished by a unique profile of monocarboxylate transporters and metabolic enzymes during development.

Although ketone bodies seem to play an important role in normal energy metabolism, it seems unlikely however that they do so under pathophysiological circumstances of glucose deprivation, since multiple studies have demonstrated the limited ability for hepatic ketone synthesis in the neonate[50,51] as well as the natural decline in blood–brain ketone transport seen in weaned animals.[1,52,53] During hypoglycemia, lactic acid then becomes an important source of energy. Hernandez et al.[54] showed in newborn dogs that during insulin-induced hypoglycemia along with a concomitant reduction in CGU, lactate was able to support 58% of cerebral oxidative metabolism. Other investigators have also demonstrated a preferential utilization of lactate over glucose or ketones in newborn animals, resulting in a sparing effect on glucose utilization during hypoglycemia.[49,55]

Monocarboxylate transporters

The energy substrates of ketone bodies and lactate are crucial substitutes but since they do not easily cross the blood–brain barrier, a transport system is required for them to reach the brain parenchyma. The monocarboxylate transporters (MCTs) serve the role of transport, with all these substrates competing for the same carrier. The first MCT cloned was named MCT1;[56] similar transporters from human, rat and mouse have now been cloned and sequenced. To date, nine isoforms of MCTs (MCT1– MCT9) have been identified in animal tissues with their levels of expression varying in the different tissues.[57,58] MCT1 and MCT2 are expressed in the central nervous system. Each MCT isoform is likely to have a unique pattern of expression and several isoforms are expressed in a single tissue reflecting their different specificities to allow for the import or export of particular monocarboxylates.[58] The developmental expression of MCTs in rodents[1,53,59] is opposite of that seen with the GLUTs. In the neonatal period soon after birth, the rat develops profound hypoglycemia with the interruption of the transplacental glucose supply (combined with low hepatic glycogenolysis and negligible

gluconeogenesis), thereafter spontaneously returning to normoglycemia by 3–4 hours. A similar phenomenon is seen in the human infant as well. Blood glucose falls progressively to hypoglycemic levels by 16 hours if suckling is withheld in the rat. The concentration of blood ketone bodies at birth is around 0.2–0.4 mM and increases ∼ 4-fold within 24 hours.[1] The ratio of β-hydroxybutyrate (OHB) to aceto-acetate remains constant until 4 hours at a value around 4.5 mM and then decreases to reach a value of ∼ 2 mM at 16 hours.[1] As a result of the high fat and low carbohydrate content of maternal milk, the newborn rat essentially develops a relative ketosis starting at birth and lasting through the suckling phase. β-OHB and aceto-acetate that rise sharply over the first 48 hours of postnatal life and stay high during suckling are actively utilized by the immature rat brain in proportion to their circulating concentrations. For this reason, the efficiency of the MCT system is very high in suckling rats and progressively decreases with weaning.

In the immature brain of the rat, ketone bodies not only serve as energy substrates but as precursors in the biosynthesis of both amino acids and lipids. They allow for sparing of glucose which is not available in high amounts during the suckling period and save it for preferential use by the pentose phosphate pathway, providing hydrogen equivalents which are necessary cofactors for the synthesis of myelin lipids, a process that is particularly active in neonatal rat brain. Ketone bodies along with glucose also act in synergy to support membrane protein and lipid formation in the brain. By about 15 days postnatally, the biosynthetic pathways of glycolysis and gluconeogenesis begin to develop and progressively reach their full capacities at the time of weaning. On the other hand, the activities of the enzymes involved in ketone metabolism are highest during suckling, and decrease after weaning to lower adult levels.

The age-pattern of lactate (and pyruvate) transport is similar to that of ketones, but is even more pronounced in the immature brain. Lactate is mostly consumed by the brain through the tricarboxylic acid (TCA) cycle during the first 2 hours after birth when this substrate is actively cleared from the blood. Although the immature rat brain is able to use ketones actively, the rat at birth is lacking white adipose tissue and thus active ketogenesis cannot occur as long as exogenous non-esterified fatty acids from maternal milk are not ingested.[1] Moreover, a transient inhibition of ketogenesis caused by the lack of ketogenic precursors or cofactors contributes to a low concentration of ketone bodies during the pre-suckling period. Lactate therefore has to serve as the immediate substrate before the onset of suckling. Indeed, lactate has been shown to accumulate in fetal rat blood during late gestation, reaching concentrations higher than 8 mM during the initial minutes of extra-uterine life.[1] However, most of the accumulated lactate during late gestation is used within the first 2 hours and the later evolution of lactate oxidation by the suckling brain is less clear. Experimental evidence in vitro however supports neuronal use of lactate via the monocarboxylate carrier, regardless of whether lactate arises from the periphery (bloodstream) or from neighboring astrocytes.[60]

Correlating with the fluxes of these various alternate substrates in brain, the 17-day-old suckling rat pups were noted to have 25 times more MCT1 labeling in the membranes of capillary endothelial cells than the adults.[59] This isoform was also shown to be equally distributed in luminal and abluminal surfaces of the endothelial cells with little MCT1 in the cytoplasm. This suggests that MCT1 up-regulation would most likely involve mechanisms such as enhanced transcription and/or translation rather than recruitment from cytoplasm stores as proposed for GLUT1.[31] Of interest is that the suckling rats had 19 times higher MCT1 concentrations in membranes associated with astrocytic end feet adjacent to the microvessels, the significance of which will be addressed later in this chapter. Similar developmental observations were established in the neonatal and adult murine brain,[53] but in addition, a detailed characterization of the regional expression of both MCT1 and MCT2 demonstrated that MCTs are particularly abundant in the cerebral cortex, hippocampus and cerebellum. Additionally, cellular expression patterns differ with MCT1 observed in astrocytes and MCT2 in neurons.[61]

Metabolic coupling

The concept of metabolic coupling between neurons and glia, particularly astrocytes, is aimed at maintaining cerebral metabolic homeostasis (Figure 8.1). This concept emerged when it was first noticed that the specialized astrocytic processes, the end-feet, are interposed between virtually all brain capillaries and neuronal processes. In this configuration, astrocytes are ideally positioned to provide coupling between neuronal activity and glucose uptake. The sequence of events occurs as follows: (1) at glutamatergic synapses, glutamate release depolarizes postsynaptic neurons by acting on its receptors; (2) the action of glutamate is subsequently terminated by an efficient glutamate-uptake system located primarily in astrocytes; (3) glutamate uptake causes Na^+ co-transport into astrocytes, causing an activation of the Na^+/K^+ ATPase; (4) activation of this ATPase stimulates glycolysis with the production of lactate as the end-product; (5) lactate, once released by astrocytes into extracellular space, is taken up by presynaptic or postsynaptic neurons and serves as an energy

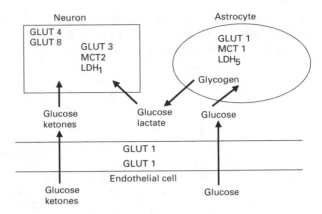

Figure 8.1. Metabolic coupling concept.

substrate.[62,63] Further evidence supporting this metabolic coupling comes from the notion that cell-specific distribution of lactate dehydrogenase (LDH) isoforms exists. LDH_5, which is present in cells/tissues that produce lactate glycolytically, is localized predominantly to astrocytes, whereas LDH_1, which is enriched in cells/tissues that use lactate as a substrate, is distributed mainly in neurons.[62] These observations taken together provide a cellular and molecular basis for the functional brain imaging results that show increased lactate signal after physiologic stimulation.[64,65]

Metabolic enzymes

The ultimate utilization of all substrates for energy lies in the development of competent enzyme systems of glycolysis and ketone body metabolism. In the case of aerobic glycolysis, the activities of most of these enzymes rise rapidly during the suckling period in the rat and reach adult activities shortly after weaning at 21–22 days postnatal age.[52] Included in this adaptation is the induction of the development of adult brain isoforms of both lactate dehydrogenase (M → H isoform) and pyruvate kinase (H → M isoform) enzymes. By contrast, the ketone body metabolic enzymes rise to a maximum during the suckling period and then decline to less than half of their maximal activity in the post-weaning period, reflective of the change to a high carbohydrate diet. Fatty acid oxidative enzymes, although relatively low in activity at the beginning, show an increase in activity with a profile similar to that of the aerobic glycolytic enzymes.[52] A key enzyme that marks the advent of neurological competence associated with the capability for complete dependence on and oxidation of glucose is the pyruvate dehydrogenase complex (PDHC), which acts as a major link between glycolysis and the TCA cycle. Marked increases of PDHC activity occur postnatally during the suckling period in the rat with the regulation modulated at the translational or post-translational level.

One other important function of astrocytes that was mentioned previously is their capacity for glycogen storage and mobilization. In comparison to liver or muscle brain contains only low concentrations of glycogen. The ratio of glycogen content in liver, muscle and brain is estimated to be 100 :10 : 1.[66] If the supply of glucose to the brain is interrupted, glycogen can support the activity of the brain only for 3 minutes.[67] Nonetheless, glycogen (and the main glycogenolytic enzyme, glycogen phosphorylase) found predominantly in astrocytes is the largest energy reserve available in the central nervous system.[68] Glycogen recycling is known to be highly regulated by neurohormones such that some promote glycogen breakdown while others enhance glycogen accumulation. Studies primarily in cell culture models[68,69] have characterized the role of glycogen in astrocytes during glucose deprivation and noted that glycogen is mobilized in the form of extracellular lactate during glucose deficiency to support the function of neighboring cells (i.e. neurons).[68] Astroglial cells express hexokinase (HK) and glucose-6-phosphatase with dramatically different K_m values for glucose of 40 μM and 9 mM respectively. Therefore, a glucose molecule generated by hydrolysis of glucose-6-phosphate (G-6-P) undergoes an almost inevitable rapid phosphorylation by HK, rendering it difficult to leave the astrocyte. In addition, the accumulation of glycogen in astrocytes augmented by insulin and methionine sulfoximine reduces neuronal damage following several hours of exposure to medium lacking glucose.[69] The protective effect in part may be explained by glycogen's ability to fuel astrocyte's reuptake of glutamate and aspartate released during glucose deprivation as well as to preserve astrocyte membrane pumps to help keep local K^+ concentration down, thereby reducing neuronal excitability.

In summary, brain energy homeostasis depends on three main variables: (1) substrate availability to the brain by the circulatory serum concentrations; (2) substrate availability to the brain via the transport systems across the blood–brain barrier and into the brain parenchymal cells; and (3) the activation of enzyme systems responsible for the metabolism of these energy substrates.

Physiological and biochemical responses to hypoglycemia

Before delving into the scientific data regarding the physiological and biochemical responses to hypoglycemia in the brain, it is pertinent to discuss the whole body's mechanisms of glucose counter-regulation first in the face of hypoglycemia since many gluco-regulatory mechanisms are in place to prevent the development of neuroglycopenia. The principles of glucose homeostasis include: (1) the prevention of hypoglycemia as a result of both insulin dissipation and counter-regulatory hormonal activation; (2) insulin is the dominant glucose-lowering agent, whereas numerous counter-regulators exist; and (3) a hierarchy of counter-regulatory mechanisms is evident.

The current understanding of glucose regulation in humans was first defined in a model of short-term hypoglycemia produced by rapid intravenous injection of insulin.[70,71] At first injection, insulin suppresses hepatic glucose production and stimulates glucose utilization by insulin-sensitive tissues. As a result, plasma glucose levels decrease. Soon, glucose utilization rate falls to baseline, and glucose production is seen to rise sharply above basal rate and above the glucose utilization rate. Thus, recovery from acute hypoglycemia is a direct result of a regulated increase in glucose production itself. During prolonged hypoglycemia, however, glucose utilization actually falls below that of baseline while glucose production continues. Hepatic glycogenolysis accounts for ~ 85% of glucose production over the first 3–4 hours. After ~ 2 hours, gluconeogenesis begins to participate as well and accounts for ~ 85% of hepatic glucose production later during hypoglycemia. Under normal physiological conditions in the adult, the threshold for the suppression of insulin secretion takes place at 83 ± 3 mg dL^{-1} (4.6 ± 0.2 mM).[72]. The glycemic thresholds for glucagon and epinephrine release are actually similar to the plasma glucose level at which brain glucose and oxygen uptake are first measurably decreased as hypoglycemia occurs (~ 3.7 mM). For symptoms to occur, Mitrakou *et al.*[73] determined the threshold to be 58 ± 2 mg dL^{-1} (3.2 ± 0.1 mM) for autonomic/neurogenic symptoms and 51 ± 3 mg dL^{-1} (2.8 ± 0.2 mM) for neuroglycopenic symptoms. Cognitive function is affected at 49 ± 2 mg dL^{-1} (2.7 ± 0.1 mM). Hence, the normal sequence of events in response to declining glucose concentrations in humans is (1) decreased insulin secretion; (2) increased glucagon and epinephrine (and to a lesser degree, growth hormone and cortisol) release; (3) symptoms; and (4) cognitive dysfunction. A further decrease in plasma glucose concentration will result in seizures, coma and ultimately death. These thresholds have been defined for the adult; whether similar thresholds exist for the newborn is less clear, although it appears that such thresholds would be lower in the immature animal when compared with the adult due to efficient alternate substrate utilization. It is also known that there are distinct differences between the newborn and adult with respect to the effect of insulin on hepatic glucose production and the role of counter-regulation.

The close-knit relationship of the brain and body in maintaining normal energy homeostasis (by balancing energy intake, expenditure and storage) must rely upon specialized metabolic sensor neurons to integrate afferent neural and metabolic signals. Two types of glucosensing neurons exist: glucose excited (GE) neurons increase their firing rate as brain glucose levels rise and glucose inhibited (GI) neurons decrease their firing rate as glucose levels rise.[74] Populations of GE and GI neurons are located in a variety of brain regions. The two best-studied areas include the hypothalamus and caudal brainstem, which receive a multitude of convergent signals from internal and external environments. Glucosensing neurons are primarily located in the hypothalamic ventromedial, arcuate (ARC), paraventricular, and suprachiasmatic nuclei and the lateral hypothalamus.[75] ARC neuropeptide Y (NPY) and pro-opiomelanocortin (POMC) neurons are prototypes of neurons which respond to both glucose and a variety of other metabolic signals from the central and peripheral nervous systems.[76] The mechanism of action for GE neurons relies upon an intact ATP-sensitive K^+ (K_{ATP}) channel. The K_{ATP} channel responds to the intracellular ATP/ADP ratio and is inactivated by direct binding to ATP (i.e. when glucose concentration is sufficient to maintain ATP production), which leads to K^+ accumulation and depolarization, followed by Ca^{2+} influx through a voltage-depending Ca^{2+} channel, thus leading to increased firing of cell bodies and increased neurotransmitter release at the nerve terminals.[77–79] Little is known however about the glucose sensing mechanism of GI neurons.

The physiological compensation associated with hypoglycemia has been elucidated in the newborn dog,[54,80,81] an animal model in which the neurological development is similar to that of the human infant at birth and is of a size adequate not only for monitoring systemic physiological function but also for preserving optimally labile metabolites in brain prior to and during hypoglycemia. The mean glucose in the normoglycemic group was 9.79 ± 2.58 mM, while that of the hypoglycemic group was 0.70 ± 0.03 mM, and the severe hypoglycemic group was 0.32 ± 0.10 mM. The results noted significant decreases in both arterial pH and pCO_2 in the hypoglycemic groups, the decline in pH was associated with elevations in mean arterial lactate concentration by 250% above the normoglycemic control, while the decrease in pCO_2 was attributed to the change in ventilatory support to correct for the metabolic acidosis. A 49% rise in cerebral lactate concentration was observed in the severe hypoglycemic group when compared to the normoglycemic group. The degrees of hypoglycemia obtained in this study demonstrated significant hypotensive effects, with the mean arterial blood pressure decreasing to 52% of the controls in the severe hypoglycemic group. Interestingly, cerebral blood flow (CBF) and CMR_{O2} did not change significantly with hypoglycemia despite the hypotension. In adult animals and in man, major neurological and cerebral metabolic disturbances would have occurred at the blood glucose concentrations achieved here, but in immature animals, cerebral autoregulation remained intact to support its metabolism. It is noteworthy to point out that the cerebral utilization of lactate did increase 10–12-fold in the experimental groups, but the utilization of μ-OHB did not change, reinforcing our prior discussion that the newborn brain shows tremendous versatility in the use of lactate which may contribute to the tolerance of the immature nervous system to the known deleterious effects of comparable degrees of hypoglycemia in adults.[54]

A separate investigation[81] extended the above observations by measuring regional CBF and regional CGU in newborn dogs during normoglycemia and insulin-induced hypoglycemia approximating 1 mM concentration. Blood flows to 16 brain structures were determined. In control animals, a hierarchy of CBF values was evident, with the pons and medulla exhibiting the highest flows, cerebral and cerebellar gray matter structures showing intermediate flows, and subcortical white matter having the lowest flow. Significant increases in all brain regions with hypoglycemia were measured, with the brainstem and diencephalon having the greatest flow, followed by cerebellum, cerebral cortex and hippocampus, and lastly subcortical white matter. Regional CGU showed a variable pattern, the rate was higher in hindbrain structures (brainstem and cerebellum) than forebrain structures (cerebral gray matter, subcortical white matter and diencephalon) in controls. In hypoglycemic animals, CGU was relatively unchanged in 11 of 16 structures. Only in occipital white matter and cerebellum was glucose utilization lower than corresponding controls. CGU was increased on the other hand in the pons and medulla. Thus, according to this study, hypoglycemia of 1 mM is noted with essentially a global increase in perinatal CBF, a concept that is established in mature animals including humans in which major metabolic stresses (such as hypoxia, hypercapnic acidosis and seizures) produce vasodilatation and a subsequent increase in CBF. In stark contrast to in-vivo investigations, in-vitro studies using cultured isolated neuronal cells demonstrate that glucose deficiency activates A1 adenosine receptors leading to neuronal adenosine release with changes in intracellular calcium concentrations which in turn induce pro-apoptotic enzymes leading to neuronal injury.[82] Thus mechanism(s) beyond the neurons appear to play a role in adapting and protecting these cells against hypoglycemic injury.

Another experimental study using the insulin-induced hypoglycemic newborn dog model examined the cerebral metabolic responses to hypoglycemia by the direct analysis of glycolytic intermediates and high-energy phosphate reserves in brain and blood.[80] Results showed that the decline in blood glucose from the mildly hypoglycemic group (1.0–1.5 mM) to the severe hypoglycemic group (< 0.5 mM) was associated with a greater decrease in brain glucose content such that brain/blood glucose ratios fell to very low levels. Further, glycolytic intermediates were not adversely affected by hypoglycemia when blood glucose concentrations remained above 1.0 mM, but partial depletion of all measured metabolites of glycolysis from G-6-P to lactate were seen below 1.0 mM. The reduction in G-6-P was proportionately greater than any of the other intermediates. With regard to cerebral high-energy phosphate compounds, these were relatively well preserved at all degrees of hypoglycemia. Taken together, these observations suggest reduced cerebral glucose consumption via the glycolytic pathway in the face of critical hypoglycemia, and given the lower energy requirements of the immature brain and its enhanced ability to use alternate substrates such as lactate for oxidative fuel, the energy status of the brain is sustained.

Switching focus from these acute hypoglycemic experiments, it seems pertinent to examine briefly the effects of repeated hypoglycemia on brain function. What is known with repeated hypoglycemia is that the glucose threshold at which the brain detects hypoglycemia and triggers neurohumoral responses is shifted downward in nondiabetic and diabetic individuals.[83,84] The glucose-sensing neurons are believed to adapt to repeated hypoglycemia, by a process of "synaptic adaptation." A series of in vitro studies to analyze synaptic function during repeated hypoglycemia in guinea pig hippocampal slices were carried out by Sakurai et al.[85] Using 14–28-day-old guinea pig hippocampal slices, metabolic substrates that fuel synaptic function and synaptic activity using electrophysiological techniques were estimated in response to repeated glucose deprivation (1.0 and 0.5 mM). In addition, the effect of lactate and pyruvate in the presence of glucose deficiency were tested. The extracellular recordings of the field postsynaptic population spike (PS) in the granule cell layer of the hippocampal dentate gyrus with 2 mM sodium chloride glass electrodes were assessed. Decreasing glucose concentrations produced slowly developing decreases in synaptic response (76.6 ± 4.2% and 50.3 ± 5.0% of control for 1.0 mM and 0.5 mM of glucose respectively). Upon complete removal of glucose, a complete elimination of the PS was achieved

within 30 minutes. When the standard medium (10 mM) was re-supplemented after 30 minutes of hypoglycemia, the recovery of the PS amplitude rose to 129.0 ± 5.9% of the control. Once glucose depletion recurred after stabilization, the PS amplitude was inhibited over a period of 80–90 minutes. In addition, exogenous lactate and pyruvate (10 mM) under control conditions did not sustain synaptic transmission but in hippocampal sections recovered from transient hypoglycemia, led to maintenance of synaptic activity. Thus monocarboxylates are able to sustain synaptic function during repeated hypoglycemia, reinforcing the concept of metabolic coupling between astrocytes and neurons. Despite studies such as this one[86,87] which explore the neural basis of synaptic adaptation, the relationship between the possible contribution of the hypoglycemic "synaptic adaptation" and the molecular mechanisms underlying the activation of the astrocyte-neuron monocarboxylate shuttle (metabolic coupling) in response to recurrent hypoglycemia remains to be elucidated. Further, these studies should not be misinterpreted to suggest that hypoglycemia, acute or chronic, will not impair brain function in the immature animal/human. Instead hypoglycemia causes multiple adaptations geared towards preservation of neuronal function. These adaptations protect within reason but are overcome easily by the severity of glucose deprivation, the length and repetition of episodes and the concomitant lack of adequate alternate substrates.

Neuronal apoptosis and/or necrosis when adaptive mechanisms fail

The body employs multiple mechanisms to compensate for nutrient deficiencies. Given that glucose plays such a critical role in cerebral metabolism, any sustained fall in blood glucose concentration will inevitably lead to a fall in brain metabolism and function, eventually becoming clinically evident as cognitive dysfunction, coma or even permanent brain injury and death. Current research has brought new insight into the intracellular cascade of events leading to brain injury associated with hypoglycemia. Depending on the conditions, the same triggering factors culminating in glucose deficiency can lead to either neuronal apoptosis and/or necrosis. The important concept emerging from all these studies is that the intensity and duration of the insult determines the ultimate fate of brain cells. Mild insults seem to yield apoptosis and severe ones necrosis, but significant overlap occurs in this continuum of cell death.

Apoptosis is an active, energy-dependent, programmed pathway, which accounts for the majority of physiological cell death. In contrast, necrosis typically involves an acute insult to the cell and does not require energy for its occurrence.[88] Morphologically, necrotic cells and their organelles are characteristically swollen. Early membrane damage occurs with eventual loss of plasma membrane integrity and leakage of cytosol into the extracellular space. Despite early clumping, the nuclear chromatin undergoes karyolysis. Because large groups of cells are involved and cellular content lost early into the extracellular space, necrotic tissues evoke vigorous inflammatory responses. On the other hand, apoptotic cells are shrunken and develop blebs containing dense cytoplasm. Membrane integrity is not lost until late, after cell death. Nuclear chromatin undergoes striking condensation and fragmentation leading to the formation of the 180 bp DNA ladder. The cytoplasm becomes divided to form apoptotic bodies containing organelles and/or nuclear debris. Terminally, apoptotic cells and fragments are engulfed by phagocytes, leading to little or no inflammation.[88] Despite this distinct morphological classification of apoptosis and necrosis, a blend of these processes is often seen in dying cells due to the variable expression of overlapping apoptotic and necrotic cells and the superimposition of secondary necrosis upon apoptosis.

A key component of apoptosis is the activation of a family of proteases named the caspases. These are cysteine proteases that bear a specificity to cleave after aspartic acid residues of their substrates.[88] Caspases share similar homology and generally are synthesized as inactive zymogens. Activation of caspases involves proteolytic cleavage between domains resulting in the removal of a pro-domain and a linker region, and the assembly of large and small subunits into active tetrameric complexes. A hierarchy of caspases exists with upstream initiator caspases capable of processing themselves as well as other downstream effector caspases to generate active enzymes. In cells undergoing apoptosis, caspases target two important groups of protein substrates: (1) regulatory proteins and (2) structural and "housekeeping" proteins. Cleavage of regulatory proteins reinforces apoptotic activation, whereas breakdown of structural proteins results in cellular disintegration. Examples of target regulatory proteins include DNA fragmentation factor (DFF-45), Bcl-2 and several important protein kinases. The latter group includes cytoskeletal proteins of actin and keratins, and nuclear proteins such as poly(ADP)-ribosylating protein (PARP), topoisomerases I and II, and U1-70 kDa subunit of small nuclear ribonucleoprotein.[88]

It has been shown in different cell types that the transport and metabolism of glucose are able to modify the apoptotic pathway. Three cell death paradigms linking a decrease in glucose transport to apoptosis

have recently been reviewed.[89] These paradigms include: (1) glucose deprivation-induced ATP depletion and stimulation of the mitochondrial death pathway cascade; (2) glucose deprivation-induced oxidative stress and triggering of Bax-associated events including c-jun N-terminal kinase/mitogen activated protein kinases (JNK/MAPK) signaling; and (3) hypoglycemia-regulated expression of hypoxia-inducible factor-1α (HIF-1α), causing a stabilization of p53 leading to an increase in p53-associated apoptosis. In brief, the first paradigm shows that decreased glucose uptake by cells can result in ATP depletion, which in turn triggers the mitochondrial death cascade involving the translocation of the pro-apoptotic protein, Bax, from the cytosol to the outer membrane of the mitochondria. This results in a loss of the mitochondrial membrane potential, followed by a release of cytochrome c (cyt c) into the cytoplasm, and subsequent activation of caspases which mediate PARP cleavage, DNA laddering and fragmentation.

The second paradigm relates to damage due to the endogenous production of reactive oxygen species (ROS) by the mitochondria causing an oxidative stress to the cell. Under normal conditions, a cell has developed systems for detecting and scavenging ROS. In glucose-deprived environments, an accumulation of pro-oxidants (superoxide and hydrogen peroxide) is seen as a result of the metabolic shift to oxidative phosphorylation. For example, during neurogenesis, multiple neurons generated by cell division from neuroblasts die while the rest of the neurons make functional connections with their targets. Neuronal survival is dependent upon trophic factors, nerve growth factor (NGF) being the preferred candidate. Using primary cultures from sympathetic superior cervical ganglion neurons, Deckwerth et al.[90] found that ROS increase within the first 6 hours of NGF withdrawal, coinciding with a concomitant decrease in 2-DG transport. This metabolic event took place 24 hours before a decline in cell viability, evidence of soma degeneration, or DNA fragmentation was evident. This experiment suggests that an altered redox state became the trigger for the downstream apoptotic cascade. Other cell systems used for this investigation extended the findings further by showing that oxidative stress triggered the activation of Lyn kinase (Lyn; a member of the *src* family of tyrosine kinases), JNK/MAPK signal transduction pathway, and eventually leading to the transcription of AP-1 dependent target genes.[91, 92] Increased Bax expression led to the completion of the apoptotic cascade including *c-fos* induction, caspase activation and PARP cleavage.

The last paradigm of apoptosis stemmed from the observation that hypoxia and/or hypoglycemia activated the expression of HIF-1α in affected cells in order to restore homeostasis by inducing glycolysis, erythropoiesis and angiogenesis. HIF-1α is found to associate directly with and stabilize p53, causing the upregulation of Bax transcription and subsequent apoptosis.

Our discussion up to this point has proposed that under hypoglycemia and other stresses (such as hypoxia-ischemia), cell death occurs by either apoptosis and/or necrosis. A study by Ouyang *et al.*[93] in rats undergoing hypoglycemic coma by insulin injection was carried out to address this particular question. They knew that hypoglycemia coma induced a characteristic distribution of the neuronal damage. It yields necrotic damage to neocortex layers 2–3, to hippocampal areas of the subiculum section of CA1, the tip of the dentate gyrus, and to the dorsolateral crescent of the caudoputamen.[94] The first question addressed was whether cyt c was released and caspase-3 was activated in the described regions in hypoglycemic rats. If these phenomena were true, the expressions of Bcl-xL (anti-apoptotic) and Bax (pro-apoptotic) would also be altered. The results demonstrated that although hypoglycemic coma led to cell death with morphological characteristics of necrosis, an apoptotic pathway seemed to be triggered as well. The time course of early expression of Bax (within 30 minutes of coma), release of cyt c (at 3 hours of recovery) and activation of caspase-3 (at 6 hours of recovery) in hypoglycemic rat brain suggests that translocation of Bax to the mitochondria triggered the release of cyt c, activating caspases and resulting in apoptotic cell death.

Conclusions

This review of cerebral metabolism in brain development is by no means exhaustive given the ongoing experiments in various laboratories. However, the importance of glucose as an obligate substrate for the developing brain is clear. When this crucial substrate is low in supply, physiological and biochemical pathways must respond to compensate. Organic substrates other than glucose are capable of at least partially supporting cerebral metabolism during periods of starvation, suckling and hypoglycemia. It must be emphasized however that all cerebral energy fuels, except glucose, require oxygen for their consumption to produce energy equivalents. Only glucose is able to sustain energy homeostasis under conditions of a total oxygen debt, owing to its capacity for consumption via anaerobic glycolysis with the production of lactic acid and ATP. It follows then if hypoglycemia was superimposed with hypoxia-ischemia, the end-result could certainly be even more devastating. The combined effects of this situation are beyond the scope of this chapter but one must be aware that hypoglycemia and hypoxia resulting from asphyxia are often intertwined in the clinical setting.

Acknowledgments

Some of the work described here was supported by grants from the National Institutes of Health HD 33997 (SUD), HD 25024 (SUD) and HD 41230 (SUD). Camille Fung was supported by a postdoctoral training grant from the National Institutes of Child Health and Human Development – HD 07549.

REFERENCES

1 Nehlig, A., Pereira de Vasconcelos, A. Glucose and ketone body utilization by the brain of neonatal rats. *Prog. Neurobiol.* 1993;**40**:163–221.

2 Nehlig, A. Respective roles of glucose and ketone bodies as substrates for cerebral energy metabolism in the suckling rat. *Dev. Neurosci.* 1996;**18**:426–33.

3 Kalhan, S. C., Raghavan, C. V. Metabolism of glucose in the fetus and newborn. In Polin, R. A., Fox, W. W., eds. *Fetal and Neonatal Physiology.* 2nd edn. Philadelphia, PA: W. B. Saunders & Co.; 1998:543–58.

4 Rosenblatt, J., Wolfe, R. R. Calculation of substrate flux using stable isotopes. *Am. J. Physiol.* 1988;**254**:E526–31.

5 Kalhan, S., Peter-Wohl, S. Hypoglycemia: what is it for the neonate? *Am. J. Perinatol.* 2000;**17**:11–18.

6 Sexson, W. R. Incidence of neonatal hypoglycemia: a matter of definition. *J. Pediatr.* 1984;**105**:149–50.

7 Anderson, J. M., Milner, R. D. G., Strich, S. J. Pathological changes in the nervous system in severe neonatal hypoglycemia. *Lancet* 1966;**13**:372–5.

8 Lucas, A., Morley, R., Cole, T. J. Adverse neurodevelopmental outcome of moderate neonatal hypoglycemia. *Br. Med. J.* 1988;**297**:1304–8.

9 Duvanel, C. B., Fawer, C.-L., Cotting, J. *et al.* Long-term effects of neonatal hypoglycemia on brain growth and psychomotor development in small-for-gestational age preterm infants. *J. Pediatr.* 1999;**134**:492–8.

10 Singh, M., Singhal, P. K., Paul, V. K. *et al.* Neurodevelopmental outcome of asymptomatic and symptomatic babies with neonatal hypoglycemia. *Indian J. Med. Res.* 1991;**94**:6–10.

11 Koivisto, M., Blanco-Sequeiros, M., Krause, U. Neonatal symptomatic and asymptomatic hypoglycaemia: a follow-up study in 151 children. *Dev. Med. Child Neurol.* 1972;**14**:603–14.

12 Koh, T. T. H. G., Aynsley-Green, A., Tarbit, M., Eyr, J. A. Neural dysfunction during hypoglycaemia. *Arch. Dis. Child.* 1988;**63**:1353–8.

13 Evans, M. L., Sherwin, R. S. Brain glucose metabolism and hypoglycaemia. *Diabetes Nutrition Metab.* 2002;**15**:294–6.

14 Messier, C. Glucose improvement of memory: a review. *Eur. J. Pharmacol.* 2004;**490**:33–57.

15 Cremer, J. E. Substrate utilization and brain development. *J. Cereb. Blood Flow Metab.* 1982;**2**:394–407.

16 Wood, S., Trayhurn, P. Glucose transporters (GLUT and SGLT): expanded families of sugar transport proteins. *Br. J. Nutr.* 2003;**89**:3–9.

17 Vannucci, S. J. Developmental expression of GLUT1 and GLUT3 glucose transporters in rat brain. *J. Neurochem.* 1994;**62**:240–6.

18 Sivitz, W. S., DeSautel, P. S., Pessin, J. E. Regulation of the glucose transporter in developing rat brain. *Endocrinology* 1989;**124**:1875–80.

19 Devaskar, S. U., Zahm, D. S., Holtzclaw, L., Chundu, K., Wadzinski, B. E. Developmental regulation of the distribution of rat brain insulin-insensitive (Glut 1) glucose transporter. *Endocrinology* 1991;**129**:1530–40.

20 Dick, A. P., Harik, S. I., Klip, A., Walker, D. M. Identification and characterization of the glucose transporter of the blood-brain barrier by cytochalasin B binding and immunological reactivity. *Proc. Natl Acad. Sci. USA* 1984;**81**:7233–7.

21 Pardridge, W. M., Boado, R. J., Farrell, C. R. Brain-type glucose transporter (Glut-1) is selectively localized to the blood-brain barrier. *J. Biol. Chem* 1990;**265**:18035–40.

22 Maher, F., Vannucci, S. J., Simpson, I. A. Glucose transporter isoforms in brain: absence of GLUT3 from the blood-brain barrier. *J. Cereb. Blood Flow Metab.* 1993;**13**:342–5.

23 Bhattacharyya, M. V., Brodsky, J. L. Characterization of the glucose transporter from rat brain synaptosomes. *Biochem. Biophys. Res. Commun.* 1988;**155**:685–91.

24 Sadiq, F., Holtzclaw, L., Chundu, K., Muzzafer, A., Devaskar, S. The ontogeny of the brain glucose transporter. *Endocrinology* 1990;**126**:2417–24.

25 Walker, P. S., Donovan, J. A., Van Ness, B. G. *et al.* Glucose dependent regulation of glucose transport activity, protein and mRNA in primary cultures of rat brain glial cells. *J. Biol. Chem.* 1988;**263**:15594–601.

26 Maher, F., Davies-Hill, T. M., Simpson, I. A. Expression of glucose transporters, GLUT 1 and GLUT 3, in cultured cerebellar neurons: evidence for neuron-specific expression of GLUT 3. *Mol. Cell Neurosci.* 1991;**2**:351–60.

27 Fields, H. M., Rinaman, L., Devaskar, S. U. Distribution of glucose transporter isoform-3 and hexokinase I in the postnatal murine brain. *Brain Res.* 1999;**846**:260–4.

28 Robertson, P. L., Dubois, M., Bowman, P. D. *et al.* Angiogenesis in developing rat brain: an in vivo and in vitro study. *Brain Res. Dev. Brain Res.* 1985;**23**:219–23.

29 Yoshida, Y., Yamada, M., Wakabayashi, K. *et al.* Endothelial fenestrae in the rat fetal cerebrum. *Brain Res. Dev. Brain Res.* 1988;**44**:211–19.

30 Mantych, G., Sotelo-Avila, C., Devaskar, S. The blood-brain barrier glucose transport system is conserved in the very low birth weight, preterm, and term newborn infants. *J. Clin. Endocrinol. Metab.* 1993;**77**:46–9.

31 Farrell, C. L., Pardridge, W. M. Blood-brain barrier glucose transporter is asymmetrically distributed in brain capillary endothelial luminal and abluminal membranes: an electron microscopic immunogold study. *Proc. Natl Acad. Sci. USA* 1991;**88**:5779–83.

32 Vorbrodt, A. W., Dobrogowska, D. H., Meeker, H. C., Carp, R. L. Immunogold study of regional differences in the distribution of glucose transporter (GLUT 1) in mouse brain associated with physiological and accelerated aging and scrapie infection. *J. Neurocytol.* 1999;**28**:711–19.

33 Bondy, C. A., Lee, W., Zhou, J. Ontogeny and cellular distribution of brain glucose transporter gene expression. *Mol. Cell Neurosci.* 1992;**3**:305–14.

34 Devaskar, S. U., Rajakumar, P. A., Mink, R. B. *et al.* Effect of development and hypoxic-ischemia upon rabbit brain glucose transporter expression. *Brain Res.* 1999;**823**:113–28.

35 Khan, J. Y., Rajakumar, R. A., McKnight, R. A., Devaskar, U. P., Devaskar, S. U. Developmental regulation of genes mediating brain glucose uptake. *Am. J. Physiol.* 1999;**45**:892–900.

36 Rajakumar, R. A., Thamotharan, S., Menon, R. K., Devaskar, S. U. Sp1 and Sp3 regulate transcriptional activity of facilitative glucose transporter isoform-3 gene in mammalian neuroblasts and trophoblasts. *J. Biol. Chem* 1998;**273**:27474–83.

37 Rajakumar, R. A., Thamotharan, S., Menon, R. K., Devaskar, S. U. Trans-activators regulating neuronal glucose transporter isoform-3 gene expression in mammalian neurons. *J. Biol. Chem.* 2004;**279**:26768–79.

38 Mantych, G., James, D. E., Chung, H. D., Devaskar, S. U. Cellular localization and characterization of Glut 3 glucose transporter isoform in human brain. *Endocrinology* 1992;**131**:1270–8.

39 Caryannopoulos, M., Chi, M. M.-Y., Cui, Y. *et al.* GLUT 8 is a glucose transporter responsible for insulin-stimulated glucose uptake in the blastocyst. *PNAS, USA.* 2000;**97**:7313–18.

40 Sankar, R., Thamotharan, S., Shin, D., Moley, K. H., Devaskar, S. Insulin-responsive glucose transporters – GLUT 8 and GLUT 4 are expressed in the developing mammalian brain. *Mol. Brain Res.* 2002;**107**:157–65.

41 Shin, B., McKnight, R. A., Devaskar, S. U. Glucose transporter – GLUT 8 translocation in neurons is not insulin responsive. *Neurosci. Res.* 2004;**75**:835–44.

42 Duffy, T. E., Cavazutti, M., Cruz, L. F. *et al.* Local cerebral glucose metabolism in newborn dogs: effects of hypoxia and halothane anesthesia. *Ann. Neurol.* 1982;**11**:233–46.

43 Sokoloff, L., Reivich, M., Kennedy, C. *et al.* The [^{14}C]deoxyglucose method for the measurement of local cerebral glucose utilization: theory, procedure, and normal values in the conscious and anesthetized albino rat. *J. Neurochem.* 1977;**28**:897–916.

44 Chugani, H. T., Phelps, M. E. Maturational changes in cerebral function in infants determined by [18]FDG positron emission tomography. *Science* 1986;**231**:840–3.

45 De Vivo, D. C., Trifiletti, R. R., Jacobson, R. I. *et al.* Defective glucose transport across the blood-brain barrier as a cause of persistent hypoglycorrhachia, seizures, and developmental delay. *N. Engl. J. Med.* 1991;**325**:703–9.

46 Pascual, J. M., Wang, D., Lecumberri, B. *et al.* GLUT 1 deficiency and other glucose transporter diseases. *Eur. J. Endocrinol.* 2004;**150**:627–33.

47 Das, U. G., Schroeder, R. E., Hay, W. W. Jr. Devaskar, S. U. Time-dependent and tissue-specific effects of circulating glucose on fetal ovine glucose transporters. *Am. J. Physiol.* 1999;**276**:R809–17.

48 Anderson, M. S., Flowers-Ziegler, J., Das, U. G., Hay, W. W. Jr, Devaskar, S. U. Glucose transporter protein responses to selective hyperglycemia or hyperinsulinemia in fetal sheep. *Am. J. Physiol.* 2001;**281**:R1545–52.

49 Dombrowski, G. J., Swiatek, K. R., Chao, K. L. Lactate, 3-Hydroxybutyrate, and glucose as substrates for the early postnatal rat brain. *Neurochem. Res* 1989;**14**:667–75.

50 Anday, E. K., Stanley, C. A., Baker, L. *et al.* Plasma ketones in newborn infants: absence of suckling ketosis. *J. Pediatr.* 1981;**98**:628–30.

51 Stanley, C. A., Anday, E. K., Baker, L. *et al.* Metabolic fuel and hormone responses to fasting in newborn infants. *Pediatrics* 1979;**64**:613–19.

52 Clark, J. B., Bates, T. E., Cullingford, T. *et al.* Development of enzymes of energy metabolism in the neonatal mammalian brain. *Dev. Neurosci.* 1993;**15**:174–80.

53 Pellerin, L., Pellegri, G., Martin, J. L. *et al.* Expression of mono-carboxylate transporter mRNAs in mouse brain: support for a distinct role of lactate as an every substrate for the neonatal vs. adult brain. *Proc. Natl Acad. Sci. USA* 1998;**95**:3990–5.

54 Hernandez, M. J., Vannucci, R. C., Salcedo, A. *et al.* Cerebral blood flow and metabolism during hypoglycemia in newborn dogs. *J. Neurochem.* 1980;**35**:622–8.

55 Maran, A., Cranston, I., Lomas, J. *et al.* Protection by lactate of cerebral function during hypoglycemia. *Lancet* 1994;**343**:16–20.

56 Kim, C. M., Goldstein, J. L., Brown, M. S. cDNA cloning of MEV, a mutant protein that facilitates cellular uptake of mevalonate, and identification of the point mutation responsible for its gain of function. *J. Biol. Chem.* 1992;**267**:23113–21.

57 Halestrap, A. P., Price, N. T. The proton-linked MCT family: structure, function and regulation. *Biochem. J.* 1999;**343**:281–99.

58 Price, N. T., Jackson, V. N., Halestrap, A. P. Cloning and sequencing of four new mammalian monocarboxylate transporter (MCT) homologues confirms the existence of a transporter family with an ancient past. *Biochem. J.* 1998;**329**:321–8.

59 Leino, R. L., Gerhart, D. Z., Drewes, L. R. Monocarboxylate transporter (MCT1) abundance in brains of suckling and adult rats: a quantitative electron microscopic immunogold study. *Dev. Brain Res.* 1999;**113**:47–54.

60 Dringen, R., Wiesinger, H., Hamprecht, B.. Uptake of L-lactate by cultured rat brain neurons. *Neurosci. Lett.* 1993;**163**:5–7.

61 Broer, S., Rahman, B., Pellegri, G. *et al.* Comparison of lactate transport in astroglial cells and monocarboxylate transporter 1 (MCT 1) expressing *Xenopus laevis* oocytes. Expression of two different monocarboxylate transporters in astroglial cells and neurons. *J. Biol. Chem.* 1997;**272**:30096–102.

62 Tsacopoulos, M., Magistretti, P. J. Metabolic coupling between glia and neurons. *J. Neurosci.* 1996;**16**:877–85.

63 Pellerin, L., Magistretti, P. J. Glutamate uptake into astrocytes stimulates aerobic glycolysis: a mechanism coupling neuronal activity to glucose utilization. *Proc. Natl Acad. Sci. USA* 1994;**91**:10625–9.

64 Prichard, J., Rothman, D., Novotny, E. *et al.* Lactate rise detected by ^{1}H NMR in human visual cortex during physiologic stimulation. *Proc. Natl Acad. Sci. USA* 1991;**88**:5829–31.

65 Fellows, L. K., Boutelle, M. G., Fillenz, M. Physiological stimulation increases nonoxidative glucose metabolism in the brain of the freely moving rat. *J. Neurochem.* 1993;**60**:1258–63.

66 Nelson, S. R., Schulz, D. W., Passonneau, J. V. *et al.* Control of glycogen levels in brain. *J. Neurochem.* 1968;**15**:1271–9.

67 Siesjo, B. K. *Brain Energy Metabolism.* New York, NY: John Wiley & Sons; 1978:162–4.

68 Dringen, R., Gebhardt, R., Hamprecht, B. Glycogen in astrocytes: possible function as lactate supply for neighboring cells. *Brain Res.* 1993;**623**:208–14.

69 Swanson, R. A., Choi, D. W. Glial glycogen stores affect neuronal survival during glucose deprivation in vitro. *J. Cereb. Blood Flow Metab.* 1993;**13**:162–9.

70 Clarke, W. L., Santiago, J. V., Thomas, L. *et al.* Adrenergic mechanisms in recovery from hypoglycemia in man: adrenergic blockade. *Am. J. Physiol.* 1979;**236**:E147–52.

71 Garber, A. J., Cryer, P. E., Santiago, J. V. *et al.* The role of adrenergic mechanisms in the substrate and hormonal response to insulin-induced hypoglycemia in man. *J. Clin. Invest.* 1976;**58**:7–15.

72 Schwartz, N. S., Clutter, W. E., Shah, S. D. *et al.* Glycemic thresholds for activation of glucose counterregulatory systems are higher than the threshold for symptoms. *J. Clin. Invest.* 1987;**79**:777–81.

73 Mitrakou, A., Ryan, C., Veneman, T. *et al.* Hierarchy of glycemic thresholds for counterregulatory hormone secretion, symptoms and cerebral dysfunction. *Am. J. Physiol.* 1991;**260**: E67–74.

74 Oomura, Y., Kimura, K., Ooyama, H. *et al.* Reciprocal activities of the ventromedial and lateral hypothalamic area of cats. *Science* 1964;**143**:484–5.

75 Levin, B. E. Glucosensing neurons: the metabolic sensors of the brain? *Diabetes Nutrition Metab.* 2002;**15**:274–81.

76 Devaskar, S. U. Neurohumoral regulation of body weight gain. *Pediatr. Diabetes* 2001;**2**:131–44.

77 Trapp, S., Ashcroft, F. M. A metabolic sensor in action: news from the ATP-sensitive K$^+$-channel. *News Physiol. Sci.* 1997;**12**:255–63.

78 Routh, V. H., McArdle, J. J., Levin, B. E. Phosphorylation modulates the activity of ATP-sensitive K$^+$-channel in the ventromedial hypothalamic nucleus. *Brain Res.* 1997;**778**:107–19.

79 Amoroso, S., Schmid-Antomarchi, H., Fosset, M. *et al.* Glucose, sulfonylureas, and neurotransmitter release: role of ATP-sensitive K$^+$-channels. *Science* 1990;**247**:852–4.

80 Vannucci, R. C., Nardis, E. E., Vannucci, S. J. *et al.* Cerebral carbohydrate and energy metabolism during hypoglycemia in newborn dogs. *Am. J. Physiol.* 1981;**240**:R192–9.

81 Mujsce, D. J., Christensen, M. A., Vannucci, R. C. Regional cerebral blood flow and glucose utilization during hypoglycemia in newborn dogs. *Am. J. Physiol.* 1989;**256**:H1659–66.

82 Turner, C. P., Blackburn, M. R. and Rivkees, S. A. A1 adenosine receptors mediate hypoglycemia-induced neuronal injury. *J. Mol. Endocrinol.* 2004;**32**:129–44.

83 Hvidberg, A., Fanelli, C. G., Hershey, T. *et al.* Impact of recent antecedent hypoglycemia on hypoglycemic cognitive dysfunction in nondiabetic humans. *Diabetes* 1996;**45**:1030–6.

84 Fanelli, C. G., Paramore, D. S., Hershey, T. *et al.* Impact of nocturnal hypoglycemia on hypoglycemic cognitive dysfunction in type I diabetes. *Diabetes.* 1998;**47**:1920–7.

85 Sakurai, T., Yang, B., Takata, T. *et al.* Synaptic adaptation to repeated hypoglycemia depends on the utilization of monocarboxylates in guinea pig hippocampal slices. *Diabetes* 2002;**51**:430–8.

86 Amiel, S. A. Hypoglycemia in diabetes mellitus: protecting the brain. *Diabetologia* 1997;**40** (Suppl. 2);S62–8.

87 Jacob, R. J., Dziura, J., Blumberg, M. *et al.* Effects of recurrent hypoglycemia on brain stem function in diabetic BB rats. *Diabetes* 1999;**48**:141–5.

88 Saikumar, P., Dong, Z., Mikhailov, V. *et al.* Apoptosis: definition, mechanisms, and relevance to disease. *Am. J. Med.* 1999;**107**:489–506.

89 Moley, K. H., Mueckler, M. M. Glucose transport and apoptosis. *Apoptosis* 2000;**5**:99–105.

90 Deckwerth, T. L., Johnson, E. M. Temporal analysis of events associated with programmed cell death (apoptosis) of sympathetic neurons deprived of nerve growth factor. *J. Cell. Biol.* 1993;**123**:1207–22.

91 Blackburn, R. V., Spitz, D. R., Liu, X. *et al.* Metabolic oxidative stress activates signal transduction and gene expression during glucose deprivation in human tumor cells. *Free Radic. Biol. Med.* 1999;**26**:419–30.

92 Lee, Y. J., Galoforo, S. S., Berns, C. M. *et al.* Glucose deprivation-induced cytotoxicity in drug resistant human breast carcinoma MCF-7/ADR cells: role of c-myc and bcl-2 in apoptotic cell death. *J. Cell Sci.* 1997;**110**:681–6.

93 Ouyang, Y. B., He, Q. P., Li, P. A. *et al.* Is neuronal injury caused by hypoglycemic coma of the necrotic or apoptotic type? *Neurochem. Res.* 2000;**25**:661–7.

94 Auer, R. N., Siesjo, B. K. Biological differences between ischemia, hypoglycemia, and epilepsy. *Ann. Neurol.* 1988;**24**:699–707.

9

Water and electrolyte balance in newborn infants

Shanthy Sridhar and Stephen Baumgart

Department of Pediatrics, State University of New York at Stony Brook, Stony Brook, NY

Water spaces – life processes

Up to 80% of body weight is water in neonates near term,[1] and even more may be water in premature babies (90%). Cell membranes separate intracellular water (ICW) and extracellular water (ECW) spaces. The ECW is separated further into plasma water and interstitial water across vascular endothelium. The ECW maintains ICW solute concentrations and cell nutrition. The ECW content is regulated physiologically by the heart and the kidneys, and is controlled by several hormone systems.

As shown in Figure 9.1,[2] water coming into the ECW carries mineral solutes, carbohydrates, fats and proteins.[3–6] Cellular wastes exiting the ECW with water and solutes constitute carbon dioxide (respiratory), urea and fixed acids (renal) and heat dissipation (integument). Also, some water is lost in stool, and a small amount is gained from substrate oxidation. Growth in the newborn also requires water, substrates and solutes for cell proliferation and differentiation. In this chapter, regulation of the cell's ICW, and the interfacing role of the ECW compartment in neonatal water metabolism will be discussed.

Inside the cell membrane – osmotic pressure

Water moves from higher to lower solute concentrations across the cell's membrane. In physiologic solutions, solute concentration is expressed in milliosmoles (mOsm) per kg of water. The movement of water across semipermeable membranes in response to small gradient changes regulates cell volume. Vant Hoff measured physiological osmotic pressure in living cells – determining one milliosmole per liter of water exerts 19.3 mmHg pressure.[7] Normal osmolality of the ECW and ICW pools is 270–300 mOsm; therefore, the osmotic pressure in each compartment is 5500 mmHg. If a cell were suddenly injected into pure water, a force equal to 5500 mmHg would drive water into the cell resulting in immediate cell lysis. So, preservation of physiologic osmolality is essential to water metabolism and life processes described in Figure 9.1.

Regulation of cell volume

The solutes found in the ICW comprise anionic proteins and organic phosphates, and balancing cations (predominantly calcium and potassium).[8] The cell membrane is impermeable to organic phosphates and the proteins, producing osmotic and electrochemical forces moving water into the cell. However, a membrane Na^+/K^+ ATPase pump maintains constant cell volume by balancing these forces, resulting in the distribution of potassium within the cell, and sodium outside the cell in the ECW. Energy stored across concentration differences for sodium and potassium between the ICW and the ECW also drives cellular work.

The volume of ICW is also regulated by production/degradation of intracellular organic osmolytes (polyols – sorbitol and myoinositol; amino acids – taurine, alanine and proline; and methyl amines – betaine, glyceryle and phosphoryl choline). Body solute distribution is different in fetal life, and water and solute redistribution occurs during transition to extrauterine existence.[1,9,10]

Neonatal Nutrition and Metabolism. Second Edition, ed. P. Thureen and W. Hay. Published by Cambridge University Press.
© Cambridge University Press 2006.

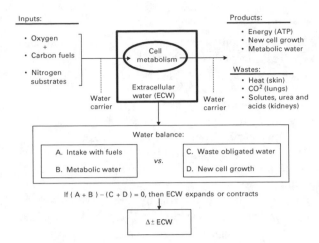

Inputs:
- Oxygen
- +
- Carbon fuels
- Nitrogen substrates

Cell metabolism

Extracellular water (ECW)

Water carrier

Water carrier

Products:
- Energy (ATP)
- New cell growth
- Metabolic water

Wastes:
- Heat (skin)
- CO_2 (lungs)
- Solutes, urea and acids (kidneys)

Water balance:

A. Intake with fuels

B. Metabolic water

vs.

C. Waste obligated water

D. New cell growth

If (A + B) − (C + D) = 0, then ECW expands or contracts

$\Delta \pm$ ECW

Figure 9.1. Summary of water metabolism. Adapted with permission.[2]

Outside the cell – the interstitial and plasma compartments of the ECW

The movement of water with nutrients, from the plasma compartment into the interstitial fluid is governed by the capillary endothelium. Two forces that drive fluids across this ECW exchange are hydrostatic pressure generated by the myocardium, and oncotic pressure resulting from proteins in the plasma.[11]

Oncotic pressure

Osmolality of body fluids is affected profoundly by large plasma proteins (colloids, e.g. fibrinogen and albumin) that do not cross semipermeable membranes. These proteins nevertheless exert an osmotic force and an electrical (anionic) force across the endothelial membrane. These osmotic and electrical forces cause an unequal distribution of smaller diffusible ions (crystalloids) between body compartments (e.g. Na^+, K^+, Cl^-). Governing this distribution is the Gibbs–Donnan Equilibrium.[13] Crystalloid cations (along with plasma protein anions) augment osmotic pressure in the plasma compartment. The total increase in pressure is called oncotic pressure. Plasma oncotic pressure in term neonates is only about 15–17 mmHg, compared with 25–28 mm Hg in adults due to lower plasma protein concentrations.[14,15]

Starling's equilibrium – hydrostatic and oncotic balance

Water movement across the capillary endothelium was first articulated by Starling[16] with the following equation: $J_V = K_F [(P_C - P_T) - \delta(\pi_P - \pi_T)]$, where J_V is the net flow across

the capillary endothelium, K_F is a water permeability co-efficient characteristic of each capillary membrane bed, P_C and P_T represent capillary and tissue (interstitial) hydrostatic pressures, δ is Stavermann's oncotic coefficient, and π_P and π_T represent plasma and tissue oncotic pressures.

Fluid movement from the plasma depends on capillary water permeability (K_F), and the difference between hydrostatic and oncotic pressures into or out of the capillary.[11,17] Water and solute leave the plasma at the arterial side of the capillary, and re-enter the plasma at the venous end as hydrostatic pressure falls across the capillary bed's resistance. Remaining interstitial fluid returns to the circulation via lymphatic flow driven by high lymphatic oncotic pressure. Capillaries impermeable to oncotic proteins (δ near 1) enhance oncotic pressure and thus maintain a more constant tissue volume (e.g. brain), while capillaries "leaking" oncotic proteins, e.g. liver sinusoids (low δ),[18,19] tend to change volume as changes in hydrostatic force move water from the interstitium. Edema formation in injured tissues is favored by capillary-interstitial and protein leak.[20] Lymphatic flow also influences edema formation, hence swelling occurs with immobility and lymphatic obstruction in tissue injury.

Regulation of ECW in the extrauterine environment

Regulation of ECW in the extrauterine environment requires basic cardiac and renal controls to maintain both the circulation (determined by cardiac output), and to keep ECW osmolality at ~ 280 mOsm kg^{-1} (in particular, serum sodium concentration).[21] The heart, the kidneys and the gastrointestinal tract (water intake stimulated by thirst and spontaneous feeding) accomplish these goals. In critically ill premature neonates, thirst and feeding are not regulated spontaneously, and intake is determined solely by the clinician. Therefore, a decrease in ECW volume (e.g. with dehydration), relative to a low fluid intake, results in lower circulating blood volume, that in turn results in reduced cardiac output. The kidney sees reduced perfusion pressure, and (glomerular filtration rate – GFR) urine volume diminishes to conserve ECW volume.

If the fluid loss is hypotonic (e.g. with increased transcutaneous water evaporation), then free water should be preferentially conserved by the kidney, and excess sodium preferentially excreted. Therefore, these cardiac and primarily the renal responses must be modified additionally by sympathetic catecholamines, the renin-angiotensin-aldosterone system (RAAS), arginine vasopressin (AVP), atrial natriuretic peptide (ANP), prostaglandins and numerous kinens. Conversely, if ECW volume is increased (e.g. with clinician-determined intake), then these cardiac and renal mechanisms (modulated appropriately) should compensate with increases in cardiac output and urine formation.[21–24]

Cardiac delivery of blood flow to the neonatal kidney improves with fetal and postnatal development, and adjusts acutely with the circulatory transition from intra- to extrauterine life (resulting in a physiologic diuresis during the first 2–3 days of life normally). Blood pressure in the fetus increases gradually as gestation progresses, and continues to increase after birth during the first several weeks. Renal blood flow parallels blood pressure as renal vascular resistance drops.[25, 26] Recent estimates suggest that neonatal kidneys receive 2% of cardiac output at term, 8.8% by 5 months and 9.6% by a year.[27] Although not as robust as with older children (the adult fraction is estimated at approximately 15%), within a narrow range of relatively high fluid intakes necessary for nutrition and growth, the neonate's cardiac output and renal response regulates ECW volume and osmolality well.

Nevertheless, term and preterm infants may exhibit blunted cardiac and renal responses to acute, severe volume loading or dehydration of the ECW space when compared with older children and adults.[28] Moreover, cardiorespiratory failure frequently attendant in critically ill, premature neonates causes further disruption of ECW volume control outside of normal regulatory capacity.

The neonatal kidney

Development of glomerular filtration

The nephrons in the fetal kidney proliferate from the juxtamedullary parenchyma until ~ 34–36 weeks' gestation approaching the adult number.[29] As a result, renal blood flow is diminished much before 34 weeks.[27] Immature glomeruli are small with less surface area for filtration.[30] Therefore, renal vascular resistance is high, also restricting renal blood flow, contributing to a lower glomerular filtration rate.

At birth, blood pressure increases in the first hours and days of life, and renal vascular resistance falls.[25, 26] Glomerular filtration rate rises through the first week of life with birth after 34 weeks.[31–34] Thereafter, the glomerulus matures further, generating a larger cortical nephron population. In premature infants < 34 weeks, however, glomerular function remains restricted with fewer and smaller juxtamedullary nephrons.[29, 31, 32] The result is a relative intolerance to water and salt loads from the ECW due to diminished glomerular filtration in prematures.

Proximal tubular development

Most ion transport mechanisms in the developing kidney are regulated through Na^+/K^+ ATP-ase activity in the proximal tubular cell wall.[27,35] Natriuresis and free water diuresis are controlled by Na^+/K^+ ATP-ase reclamation in the proximal tubule of $\geq 80\%$ of the filtered sodium load. Humoral factors may affect proximal tubular sodium balance. Tubular regulatory function increases with production of Na^+/K^+ ATP-ase activity.[36] Glucocorticoids enhance Na^+/K^+ ATP-ase activity in the lung and kidney both around the time of parturition in animal models, enhancing conservation of sodium.[37] Indomethacin inhibits sodium and water excretion, resulting in oliguria and diminished amniotic fluid, suggesting prostaglandins and glucocorticoids in part mediate the development of Na^+/K^+ ATP-ase activity in utero.[38,39]

Developing distal tubule and collecting system

Development of distal tubules occurs early in gestation.[29] With delivery of filtrate from the proximal tubule, the distal tubules and collecting system of premature infants readily produce a diluted urine. The limited capacity in premature neonates for excreting excess fluid loads is from limited glomerular filtration, rather than distal nephron dilution.[40]

In contrast, preterm infants concentrate urine poorly at < 600 mOsm/L.[25] This restriction results from low medullary urea concentration,[41, 42] shorter Loops of Henle [43] and blunted response to AVP.[41,43] Therefore, extremely premature neonates tolerate dehydration poorly, which may contribute toward hypertonicity in these babies.

Finally, the development of potassium secretion from the distal tubules requires Na^+/K^+ ATPase maturation, which increases potassium concentration within the distal tubular epithelium. Intracellular potassium promotes secretion into the tubular lumen.[27] Immaturity in distal tubular Na^+/K^+ ATPase activity is one cause suggested for poor potassium secretion in prematures, and therefore a tendency towards hyperkalemia developing commonly in the extremely low birthweight group.[44]

Sodium and water balance (ECW)

Before birth, urine production is restricted by low GFR and high renal vascular resistance.[30] Tubular re-absorption of filtered sodium increases through 20 weeks, with urine that is more dilute. Thereafter, AVP response develops, and urine volume decreases, as salt and water are conserved.[42, 45, 46] Facilitated water and active salt transports from the placenta increase ECW volume to match rapid cellular growth. By mid-gestation the fetus responds to ECW expansion by modulating proximal tubular solute and fluid resorption.[47] At term, human infants have positive sodium and water balances over a range of intakes,[45] that ensures growth. Despite this advantage, the kidney's bias for sodium and water retention may limit excretion with acute ECW loading that occurs sometimes in critically ill infants resuscitated from shock.[48]

Premature birth poses other problems in sodium and water balance. A preterm infant's sodium excretion is relatively high. Small increases in GFR produce natriuresis due to immature tubular resorption (aldosterone response), and to low aldosterone production.[49] The premature infant is therefore more susceptible to both sodium wasting (ECW dehydration) and ECW overload with a limited GFR.[45,48]

Potassium balance

The proximal tubule resorbs almost all filtered potassium through Na^+/K^+ ATP-ase. Potassium balance is therefore only in part dependent on glomerular filtration, and is more likely determined by chemical gradients and hormonal influences on distal tubular potassium secretion.[27,49] In extremely immature babies, the aldosterone effect on distal tubular transport is weak, reducing potassium secretion (with sodium wastage).[44,45] Contributing to poor potassium regulation, leakage from immature cells (immature Na^+/K^+ ATP-ase activity) may result in intrinsic hyperkalemia.[44,50–52]

Hormone regulation of water balance

Renin, angiotensin and aldosterone

Contracting ECW and plasma volume eventually lowers renal perfusion and filtration.[53] The juxtaglomerular apparatus responds to renin secretion. Renin cleaves angiotensinogen into angiotensin I, which is converted into angiotensin II by angiotensin converting enzyme (ACE). Angiotensin II increases systemic blood pressure with vasoconstriction, and shifts intra-renal blood flow favoring proximal tubular re-absorption. Angiotensin II also acts on the tubules to increase Na/K ATP-ase, further stimulating resorption.[36] Finally, angiotensin II stimulates aldosterone secretion, increasing distal reabsorption of salt and water. The sum effect of these actions replenishes circulating plasma volume.

In the developing newborn, plasma renin activity forms early in gestation, and high values occur after birth.[54,55] Premature infants have high renin activity, probably the result of immature feedback on renin production, and poor renal

tubular response.[56] Nevertheless, renin secretion is functional in neonates: hypoxia increases renin production, and volume combined with furosemide decreases renin.[57,58] ACE development parallels renin, decreasing with gestation, and high ACE levels occur in premature infants with RDS.[59] Aldosterone and angiotensin also parallel this pattern of development.[54,57,59]

Arginine vasopressin

Osmolality is the main stimulus for release of arginine vasopressin (AVP) from the neurohypophysis in the posterior pituitary. An increase in osmolality causes AVP release in mature subjects. Hypotension also stimulates AVP, increasing blood volume through affecting water concentration in the ECW, acting on the distal tubules and collecting system to increase water resorption from tubular filtrate, and concentrating the urine. During development, AVP production begins after 15 weeks' gestation and matures by the mid-trimester.[60] High AVP occurs at birth in both term and preterm deliveries, and urinary excretion does not vary with gestation.[61] After a sharp increase, levels drop in 24 hours and remain low after the first week.

AVP increases with pulmonary disease in preterm babies (respiratory distress syndrome (RDS), pneumonia, positive pressure ventilation), and in term infants (asphyxia, meconium aspiration, pneumothorax). Intraventricular hemorrhage and pain also increases AVP,[62,63] and the syndrome of inappropriate antidiuretic hormone (SIADH) contributes to hyponatremia sometimes seen with these conditions. Although hyponatremia may result from AVP release, immature distal tubular function in very preterm infants diminishes the effect of AVP release on blood pressure since urinary concentrating ability is limited, especially in the preterm baby. Inability to concentrate urine with AVP is probably the result of limited solute concentration in the renal medulla (primarily urea).[64–67]

Atrial natriuretic peptide

Stretch receptors in the left and right atria release ANP propeptide that is cleaved into active ANP in the plasma, and lowers blood pressure by stimulating natriuresis and diminishing renin production (and aldosterone secretion). ANP directly increases glomerular filtration, and reduces aldosterone's effect on the distal tubule, with urinary excretion of water and sodium.[68] At birth, such a volume surfeit results from acute expansion in ECW volume. Intracellular water shifts into the interstitium,[10] alveolar fluid is forced from the lung into pulmonary lymphatics, and a transfer of plasma occurs via the umbilical vein. After an initially low urine flow, urinary diuresis occurs after 24–48 hours, resulting in 10–15% body weight loss in the first week (more in extremely low birth weight premature infants).[69]

Although measurements of ANP shortly after birth demonstrate increased hormone levels, the natriuretic response to ANP is less certain.[70] ANP has been observed to initiate diuresis of excess edema in critically ill premature infants.[71] Ronconni *et al.* reported urinary AVP levels consistently higher in preterm neonates with RDS on mechanical ventilators, enhancing diuresis by day 5 of life.[72] In contrast, however, Rozicki *et al.* showed high ANP levels in premature babies with RDS, but no natriuretic effect.[73] Premature tubular response may be diminished in infants under 30 weeks' gestation.[70]

Prostaglandins

Prostaglandin-E_2 (vasodilator) is produced in renal tubules increasing renal blood flow and promoting natriuresis.[27] Neonatal urinary prostaglandin-E_2 is higher following premature birth.[74] Indomethacin is a prostaglandin synthesis inhibitor used to promote closure of the ductus arteriosus, and is advocated by some for prevention of intracranial hemorrhage. However, vasoconstriction with indomethacin occurs also in splanchnic and renal vascular beds, resulting in reduced intestinal blood flow, and even oliguria. Feeding intolerance (necrotizing enterocolitis), and electrolyte disturbances (hyponatremia and hypokalemia) may also occur with its use.

Kallikrein and bradykinins

Renal production of kallikrein increases salt and water resorption by the kidney through vascular effects.[27,75] Kallikrein hydrolyzes kininogens to bradykinins, which vasodilate and increase intrarenal blood flow causing natriuresis. In neonates, urine excretion of kallikrein is low, and lower in prematures. Plasma renin activity may be less with increased urine kallikrein, although functional changes in renal physiology may not be observed in the newborn.

Abnormalities in water balance with prematurity and disease

Respiratory distress syndrome and bronchopulmonary dysplasia

Premature infants with RDS have surfactant deficiency with poor mechanical lung compliance, increased pulmonary vascular resistance, reduced lung lymphatic drainage (with low albumin). The resulting elevation in transpulmonary hydrostatic pressure and low oncotic pressure favors movement of water into the pulmonary interstitium.[76,77] This disturbance results in interstitial fluid and protein leak (pulmonary edema formation with disruption of Starling's forces) and initiates a cascade of inflammation, further compromising lung function, and contributing to the development of bronchopulmonary dysplasia (BPD) as early as the second week of life.[14,15,60,76] High energy and protein needs, and impaired nutrition further contribute to hypoalbuminemia and capillary leak.

Although mechanical ventilation and oxygen toxicity contribute to alveolar and small airways injury, recent reports suggest also a role for excessive parenteral fluid administration in promoting pulmonary edema. In 1991, Palta *et al.* described an association between high fluid intake before 96 hours of life and oxygen dependence at 30 days.[78] Van Marter *et al.* also reported that volumes of crystalloid and colloid fluids administered early on during treatment for RDS was associated with subsequent development of BPD.[79] Oxygen toxicity or barotrauma were not significantly associated with chronic lung disease in their study. For many years, the association of high parenteral fluid volume administration and the development of a clinically significant patent ductus arteriosus has been known to be associated with pulmonary edema formation.[80]

Also implying a role for fluid imbalance in the pathogenesis of RDS, Langman *et al.* and Costarino *et al.* observed that a brief period of high volume urinary diuresis usually precedes a complete pulmonary recovery from RDS without BPD.[69,81] This significant volume diuresis was probably the result of a modest increase in GFR and sodium clearance in the Costarino study, with a much larger increase in free water clearance and contraction of the extracellular space, and a rise in serum sodium.[69] Finally, BPD has been found to occur most often in infants with delayed or late onset of diuresis past the fourth day of life, with water accumulation in the first 2 weeks being a major contributing factor to the pathogenesis of chronic lung changes in very premature infants.[82]

Attempts to force a diuresis to improve interstitial lung edema and pulmonary function using furosemide have only proved transiently effective.[83] Huet *et al.* suggest that theophylline may be used to augment diuresis with lung improvement.[84] If diuretics are used, mineral wasting of sodium, potassium, calcium and chloride should be anticipated, and aggressive nutritional support with parenteral nutrition and high protein/calorie formulas are advocated.[85,86] Use of antenatal steroids and postnatal surfactant has demonstrated altered fluid and electrolyte balance seen in infants recovering from

RDS.[87,88] Prenatal steroid administration promotes lung maturation and surfactant production, and may enhance lung sodium/potassium-ATPase activity with facilitated clearance of fetal lung fluid and expansion of the ECW space.[88,89]

In light of these findings, we and others have adopted a modified (and controversial) approach to parenteral fluid and electrolyte administration to premature babies with RDS in the first few days of life. We do not recommend routinely replacing all predicted/measured fluid losses (insensible, urine, stool) in order to maintain body weight within a narrow range of birth weight. Total body weight is permitted to contract (with an anticipated weight loss as high as 15–20%, and perhaps even more at lower gestation births) until the interstitial fluid compartment stabilizes at a new, "dry" equilibrium between the pulmonary capillary and the interstitium. Increasingly, evidence suggests that fluid restriction during the acute phase of RDS prevents later development of pulmonary edema, patent ductus arteriosus with congestive heart failure and bronchopulmonary dysplasia.[81,90–93]

Extremely low birth weight infants and the hyperosmolar state

Extremely low birth weight (ELBW) infants are described here as weighing < 700–800 grams at ≤ 25–26 weeks gestation, where water physiology is quite distinct from VLBW infants (>1000 grams comparatively). These ELBW babies have gelatinous and nonkeratinized epidermis at birth when they are immediately exposed to dry room or incubator air instead of the aqueous intrauterine environment. Therefore, ELBW babies' insensible (unregulated) water evaporation occurs transepidermally at a disproportionately high rate relative to VLBW infants who have more mature skin with keratin barrier function (Figure 9.2).[94,95] Contributing to disproportionate evaporation, an ELBW infant's body surface area to body mass ratio is six times greater than the adult's (Figure 9.3). Finally, the ELBW baby's body mass has a much larger interstitial water (and sodium rich) pool that evaporates transcutaneously. Recently, treatment with prenatal steroids has been shown to enhance the ELBW infant's integument maturation and to improve skin barrier function, thus abetting some of this immense transepidermal water loss during the first few days of life. Thereafter, stimulated by birth and air exposure, keratin production matures after 7–14 days. As a result of all these conditions, intravenous fluid management becomes quite hectic during the first week of life – no one prescription serves all patients.

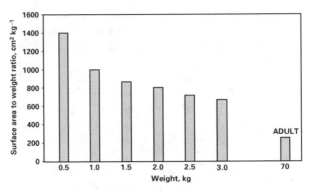

After Haycock: BSA, m² = W, kg.5378 x L, cm.3964 x .024265

Figure 9.2. Geometric increase in body surface area with diminishing body mass. Calculated from formula.[96]

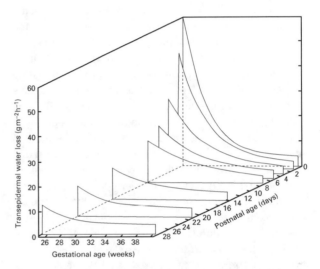

Figure 9.3. Transepidermal water loss measured for gestational age at birth, and postnatal age. Adapted with permission.[95]

Since free water evaporation from the interstitium may remain high for at least 48–72 hours (depending largely on incubator environment), interstitial sodium content is left behind promoting development of a hypernatremic, hyperosmolar state. Hyperglycemia often contributes to high osmolality since these babies are also often insulin insensitive. Worse yet, Gruskey *et al.* described high urinary fractional excretion of sodium associated with non-oliguric hyperkalemia developing by 1–2 days in ELBW infants, which they ascribed to aldosterone insensitivity in the distal tubule, thus restricting potassium secretion by the kidneys.[44] Others have suggested that significantly higher serum creatinine and lower calculated glomerular filtration results in both sodium and potassium retention by the ELBW baby's kidneys.[97] Finally, Stefano *et al.* have shown lower erythrocyte Na/K-ATPase activity in ELBW infants developing hyperkalemia when compared with a slightly more mature population who did not, suggesting an intra-to-extracellular potassium leak in their most immature subjects.[50] Compounding this latter effect, hypernatremia per se contributes to cellular potassium leak.

The intracellular compartment ultimately shares excessive water loss with a rise in osmotic pressure within this compartment (formed also in part by compensatory organic osmolyte up-regulation to maintain equilibrium). Thus, rapid lowering of sodium in the extracellular space with hypotonic fluid administration often puts these infants at high risk for developing cerebral edema and periventricular leukomalacia (PVL).[94] Serum sodium concentration reduction should probably not exceed 10 mEq L^{-1} 24 h^{-1}.

In managing therapy for this cascade of dramatic metabolic derangements in ELBW babies, we advocate first environmental and evaporative barrier manipulations to reduce the excessive skin water loss that (along with immature adaptation) is probably the primary source initiating this sequence of problems. Several artificial barriers have been used to minimize water loss, thereby avoiding the need to compensate with water loading. A variety of plastic shields have sometimes been effective in this regard,[98] a thin polyurethane membrane used as an artificial skin[99] has also been investigated, and petroleum-based emollients have been advocated as barriers for preventing water loss and infections; however, the latter technique has raised some recent concerns of altered bacterial flora and infection rates in anecdotal reports. The use of well-controlled humidified incubation has also gained acceptance more recently for preventing transepidermal water loss early in the first week of life; however, scrupulous care should be taken to avoid observable condensation within the ELBW baby's fragile environment, as water-borne bacterial contamination may occur.[100] We've seen an unfortunately common practice of increasing humidification in an incubator or under a plastic barrier shield on a radiant warmer bed until condensation appears (called "swamping" or "rainout") which should be avoided. Modern incubators are equipped to maintain set humidity near 70–80% in most nurseries without rainout. However, ambient dew points are unique to each location and temperature condition, so no one environmental recommendation replaces careful observation.

Our approach to fluid administration to ELBW infants is to accept a slow rise in serum sodium concentration during 48–72 hours of life into a high–normal range (145–149 mEq L^{-1}), while adjusting fluid volume intake every 6–8 hours while following serial serum electrolyte concentrations. No supplemental sodium or potassium is provided during this period as the hyperosmolar state is considered imminent. We hope to avoid hypotonic fluid overload and large intravenous volume replacements by these strategies, thereby minimizing the risks for developing patent ductus arteriosus, pulmonary edema and intraventricular hemorrhage with PVL.

Hyponatremia in VLBW (late onset) and ELBW (early onset) infants

Hyponatremia in growing VLBW premature infants was extensively researched by Sulyok et al.[101–103] Late-onset hyponatremia occurred during rapid growth phases about 4–6 weeks after birth while recovering from preterm birth at 1200–1500 grams. Mineral depletion from failure to complete gestation, and from chronic fluid and mineral restrictions during critical illness, along with diuretic use was felt to contribute to this syndrome. Unsupplemented breast milk and formula feedings resulted in further sodium deprivation, as did developing physiological anemia and hypoalbuminemia. Despite low sodium stores, these infants continued to lose urinary sodium due to renal tubular immaturity. Severe salt wasting retards bone mineralization which obligates sodium deposition as well. Serum sodium concentrations in Sulyok et al.'s infants were characteristically observed between 124–130 mEq L^{-1}, and have been associated by some authors with subsequent neurodevelopmental delays, although causative evidence is sketchy. Sulyok et al. felt routine sodium intake at 2–4 mEq kg^{-1} day^{-1} was insufficient to main a positive sodium balance and to compensate for these deficits. This author recommended sodium supplementation up to twice these intake values to promote normonatremia and growth.

In ELBW babies <1000 grams at birth (at between 23–26 weeks gestation), hyponatremia may not be of the late-onset type attributed to chronic sodium intake deprivation. These infants are more frequently sodium restricted during the first week of life due to their large extracellular sodium pool and high evaporative water losses tending towards the hypernatremic/hyperosmolar state described above. However, these babies are almost certainly not sodium depleted. Rather, as their epidermal barrier keratinizes after the first week of life (between weeks 2 and 3), free water replenishment from parenteral fluid volume replacement engenders a dilutional effect not well compensated by these infants' characteristically low GFR and poor tubular function (which results in some sodium loss with a characteristically negative salt balance).[104,105] Again, preliminary reports have suggested that developmental delays may

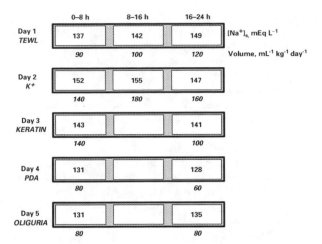

Figure 9.4. Conceptualized fluid volume intake management for extremely low birth weight infants during the first five days of life. Prescribed volume intake is adjusted every 8 hours according to measured serum sodium concentrations. Likely physiologic events that should be anticipated (in sequence) are shown at the left margin. Numerical values for actual day of life, serum sodium concentrations, and fluid volumes prescribed are likely to vary for individual patients from those shown here.

result from inappropriate management of this common electrolyte imbalance.[106]

A strategy brief to avoid electrolyte disturbances

To avoid the hypernatremia/hyponatremia sequence in VLBW and ELBW infants, we have proposed a therapeutic approach theoretically laid out in Figure 9.4. Initially, sodium-free water intake is judiciously applied as serially determined serum sodium concentrations rise into a high-normal range. Every effort is made to reduce environmental evaporative water loss and avoid hypernatremia/hyperosmolality during the first week of life (incubator humidification, saran plastic blankets or other semipermeable artificial skin barriers), while parenteral volume administered is minimized to avoid complications of fluid overload (PDA, pulmonary edema). Thereafter, sodium maintenance is provided (monitoring urinary sodium excretion and fractional excretion) while free water intake is aggressively restricted to avoid hyponatremia. The pathogenesis of these imbalances is not well enough characterized at the present time, however, to predict an individual infant's response to these fluid and environmental manipulations; hence, only close monitoring and response can perhaps avoid these disorders and their potential consequences.

REFERENCES

1 Friis-Hansen, B. Body water compartments in children. *Pediatrics* 1961;**28**:169–81.

2 Costarino, A. T., Baumgart, S. Neonatal water and electrolyte metabolism. In Cowett, R. M., ed. *Principles of Perinatal-Neonatal Metabolism.* 2nd edn. New York: Springer; 1998.

3 Dahlstrom, H. Basal metabolism and extracellular fluid. *Acta Physio. Scand.* 1950;**21**:7–80.

4 Wedgewood, R. J., Bass, D. E., Klincis, J. A., Kleeman, C. R., Quinn, M. Relationship of body composition to basal metabolic rate in normal man. *J. Appl. Physiol.* 1953;**6**:317–34.

5 Astrup, J. Energy-requiring cell functions in the ischemic brain. *J. Neuro. Surg.* 1982;**56**:282–97.

6 Valtin, H. *Renal Function: Mechanisms Preserving Fluid and Solute Balance in Health.* Boston: Little Brown; 1973.

7 Guyton, A. C. *Textbook of Medical Physiology* 6th edn. Philadelphia, PA: W. B. Saunders; 1981:339.

8 MacKnight, A. D. C., Leaf, A. Regulation of cellular volume. *Physiol. Rev.* 1977;**57**:510–73.

9 Strauss, J. Fluid and electrolyte composition of the fetus and newborn. *Pediatr. Clin. N. Am.* 1966;**13**:1077–102.

10 MacLaurin, J. C. Changes in body water distribution during the first two weeks of life. *Arch. Dis. Child.* 1966;**41**:286–91.

11 Landis, E. M., Pappenheimer, J. R. Exchange of substances through capillary walls. In *Handbook of Physiology. Circulation Section 2, Vol. 2.* Washington, DC: American Physiologic Society; 1963:961–1034.

12 Wiel, M. H., Henning, R. J., Puri, V. K. Colloid oncotic pressure: clinical significance. *Crit. Care Med.* 1979;**3**:113–16.

13 Webster, H. L. Colloid osmotic pressure: theoretical aspects and background. *Clin. Perinatol.* 1982;**9**:505–21.

14 Bhat, R., Javed, S., Malalis, L., Vidyasagar, D. Colloid osmotic pressure in healthy and sick neonates. *Crit. Care Med.* 1981;**9**:563–7.

15 Sola, A., Gregory, G. A. Colloid osmotic pressure of normal newborns and premature infants. *Crit. Care Med.* 1981;**9**:568–72.

16 Starling, E. H. On the absorption of fluid from the connective tissue spaces. *J. Physiol (Lond.)* 1896;**19**:312–26.

17 Civetta, J. M. A new look at the Starling equation. *Crit. Care Med.* 1979;**7**:84–91.

18 Taylor, A. E. Capillary fluid filtration. *Circ. Res.* 1981;**49**:557–75.

19 Granger, D. N., Miller, T., Allen, R. *et al.* Permselectivity of cat liver blood-lymph barrier to endogenous macromolecules. *Gastroenterology* 1979;**77**:103–9.

20 Nicoll, P. A., Taylor, A. E. Lymph formation and flow. *Annu. Rev. Physiol.* 1977;**39**:73–95.

21 Robertson, G. L., Berl, T. Water metabolism. In Brenner, B. M., Rector, F. C., eds. *The Kidney.* Philadelphia, PA: W. B. Saunders; 1986:385–431.

22 Hall, J. E., Guyton, A. C., Colemean, T. G., Mizelle, H. L., Woods, L. L. Regulation of arterial pressure: role of pressure natriuresis and diuresis. *Fed. Proc.* 1986;**45**:2897–903.

23 Mann, J. F. E., Johnson, A. K., Gantten, D., Eberhard, R. Thirst and the renin-angiotensin system. *Kidney Int.* 1987;**32**:S27–34.

24 Robertson, G. L., Shelton, R. L., Athar, S. The osmoregulation of vasopressin. *Kidney Int.* 1976;**10**:25–37.

25 Spitzer, A. Renal physiology and function development. In Edelman, C. M., Jr. ed. *The Kidney and Urinary Tract, Vol. 1.* 1978:25–128.

26 Cleary, G. M., Higgins, S. T., Merton, D. A., *et al.* Developmental changes in renal artery blood flow velocity during the first three weeks of life in preterm neonates. *J. Pediatr.* 1996;**129**:251–7.

27 Bailie, M. D. Development of the endocrine function of the kidney. *Clin. Perinat.* 1992;**19**:59–68.

28 Baylen, B. G., Ogata, H., Ikeganim, M. *et al.* Left ventricular performance and contractility before and after volume infusion: a comparative study in preterm and full-term newborns. *Circulation* 1986;**73**:1042–9.

29 Robillard, J. E., Matson, J. R., Sessions, C. *et al.* Maturational changes in the fetal glomerular filtration rate. *Am. J. Obstet. Gynecol.* 1975;**122**:601–6.

30 Chung, E. E., Moore, E. S., Cevallos, E. E. *et al.* The effect of gestational age and arterial pressure on renal function in utero. *Pediatr. Res.* 1976;**10**:437.

31 Leake, R. D., Trygstad, C. W. Glomerular filtration rate during the period of adaptation to extrauterine life. *Pediatr. Res.* 1977;**11**:959–62.

32 Aperia, A., Broberger, O., Elinder, G. *et al.* Postnatal development of renal function in pre-term and full-term infants. *Acta Pediatri. Scand.* 1981;**70**:183–7.

33 Guignard, J. P., Torrado, A., Mazouni, S. M., Gautier, E. Renal function in respiratory distress syndrome. *J. Pediatr.* 1976;**88**:845–50.

34 Seitel, H., Scopes, J. Rates of creatinine clearance in babies less than one week of age. *Arch. Dis. Child.* 1973;**48**:717–20.

35 Gaycock, G. B., Aperia, A. Salt and the newborn kidney. *Pediatr. Nephrol.* 1991;**5**:65–70.

36 Aperia, A., Holtback, U., Syren, M. L. *et al.* Activation/deactivation of renal Na$^+$, K$^+$ ATPase: a final common pathway for regulation of natriuresis. *FASEB J.* 1994;**8**:436–9.

37 Celsi, G., Wang, Z. M., Akusjarvi, G., Aperia, A. Sensitive periods for glucocorticoids' regulation of Na$^+$, K$^+$ ATPase mRNA in the developing lung and kidney. *Pediatr. Res.* 1993;**33**:5–9.

38 Norton, M. E., Merrill, J., Cooper, B. A. B. *et al.* Neonatal complications after the administration of indomethacin for preterm labor. *N. Engl. J. Med.* 1993;**329**:1602–7.

39 Van den Anker, J. N., Hop, W. C. J., de Groot, R. *et al.* Effects of prenatal exposure to betamethasone and indomethacin on the glomerular filtration rate in the preterm infant. *Pediatr. Res.* 1994;**36**:578–81.

40 Leake, R. D., Zakanddin, S., Trygstad, C. W. *et al.* The effects of large-volume intravenous fluid infusion on neonatal renal function. *J. Pediatr.* 1976;**89**:968–72.

41 Imbert-Teboul, M., Chabardes, D., Clique, A. *et al.* Ontogenesis of hormone-dependent adenylate cyclase in isolated rat nephron segments. *Am. J. Physiol.* 1984;**247**:F316–25.

42 Aperia, A., Broberger, O., Thodenius, K. *et al.* Development of renal control of salt and fluid homeostasis during the first year of life. *Acta Pediatr. Scand.* 1975;**64**:393–98.

43 Edelman, C. M., Barnett, H. L. Role of kidney in water metabolism in young infants. *J. Pediatr.* 1960;**56**:154–79.

44 Gruskay, J. A., Costarino, A. T., Polin, R. A., Baumgart, S. Non-oliguric hyperkalemia in the premature infant less than 1000 grams. *J. Pediatr.* 1988;**113**:381–6.

45 Spitzer, A. The role of the kidney in sodium homeostasis during maturation. *Kidney Int.* 1982;**21**:539–45.

46 Aperia, A., Elinder, G. Distal tubular sodium reabsorption in the developing rat kidney. *Am. J. Physiol.* 1981;**29**:F487–91.

47 Robillard, J. E., Sessions, C., Kennedy, R. L. *et al.* Interrelationships between glomerular filtration rate and renal transport of sodium and chloride during fetal life. *Am. J. Obstet. Gynecol.* 1977;**128**:727–33.

48 Aperia, A., Zetterstrom, R. Renal control of fluid homeostasis in the newborn infant. *Clin. Perinatol.* 1982;**9**:523–33.

49 DeFronzo, R. A., Bia, M., Smith, D. Clinical disorders of hyperkalemia. *Annu. Rev. Med.* 1982;**33**:521–54.

50 Stefano, J. L., Norman, M. E., Morales, M. C. *et al.* Decreased erythrocyte Na$^+$, K$^+$ ATPase activity associated with cellular potassium loss in extremely low birth weight infants with nonoliguric hyperkalemia. *J. Pediatr.* 1993;**122**:276–84.

51 Stefano, J. L., Norman, M. E. Nitrogen balance in extremely low birth weight infants with nonoliguric hyperkalemia. *J. Pediatr.* 1993;**123**:632–5.

52 Brion, L. P., Fleischman, A. R., Schwartz, G. J. Hyperkalemia in very low birthweight infants with non-oliguric renal failure. *Pediatr. Res.* 1985;**19**:336A.

53 Laragh, J. H. Atrial natriuretic hormone, the renin aldosterone axis and blood pressure – electrolyte homeostasis. *N. Engl. J. Med.* 1985;**313**:1330–40.

54 Kotchen, T. A., Strickland, A. L., Rice, M. S., Walters, D. R. A study of the renin-angiotensin system in newborn infants. *J. Peds.* 1972;**80**:938–46.

55 Richer, C., Hornych, H., Amiel-Tison, C. Plasma renin activity and its postnatal development in preterm infants. *Biol. Neonate* 1977;**31**:301–4.

56 Csaba, I., Ertyl, T., Nemeth, M. *et al.* Postnatal development of renin-angiotensin-aldosterone system, Raas, in relation to electrolyte balance in premature infants. *Ped. Res.* 1979;**13**:817–20.

57 Pipkin, F. B., Phil, D., Smales, O. R. C. A study of factors affecting blood pressure and angiotensin II in newborn infants. *J. Peds.* 1977;**91**:113–19.

58 Godard, C., Geering, J. M., Geering, K., Vallotton, M. B. Plasma renin activity related to sodium balance, renal function and urinary vasopressin in the newborn infant. *Pediat. Res.* 1979;**13**:742–5.

59 Bender, J. W., Davitt, M. K., Jose, P. Angiotensin-I converting enzyme activity in term and premature infants. *Biol. Neonate.* 1978;**34**:19–23.

60 Schubert, F., George, J. M., Rao, M. B. Vasopressin and oxytocin content of human fetal brain at different stages of gestation. *Brain Res.* 1981;**213**:111–17.

61 Wiriyathian, S., Rosenfeld, C. R., Arant, B. S. *et al.* Urinary arginine vasopressin: Pattern of excretion in the neonatal period. *Pediatr. Res.* 1986;**20**:103–8.

62 Stern, P., LaRochelle, F. T., Little, G. A. Vasopressin and pneumothorax in the neonate. *Pediatrics* 1981;**68**:499–503.

63 Leslie, G. I., Philips, J. B., Work, J., Ram, S., Cassady, G. The effect of assisted ventilation on creatinine clearance and hormonal control of electrolyte balance in very low birth weight infants. *Pediatr. Res.* 1986;**20**:447–52.

64 Kovacs, L., Sulyok, E., Lichardus, B., Mihajlovskij, N., Bircak, J. Renal response to arginine vasopressin in premature infants with late hyponatraemia. *Arch. Dis. Child.* 1986;**61**:1030–2.

65 Svenningsen, N. W., Aronson, A. S. Postnatal development of renal concentration capacity as estimated by DDAVP-test in normal and asphyxiated neonates. *Biol. Neonate* 1974;**25**:230–41.

66 Edelman, C. M., Barnett, H. L., Stark, H. Effect of urea on concentration of urinary nonurea solute in premature infants. *J. Appl. Physiol.* 1966;**21**:1021–5.

67 Sulyok, E., Kovacs, L., Lichardus, B. *et al.* Late hyponatremia in premature infants: role of aldosterone and arginine vasopressin. *J. Pediatr.* 1985;**106**:990–4.

68 Richards, A. M., Ikram, H., Yanckle, T. G. *et al.* Renal, hemodynamic, and hormonal effects of human alpha atrial natriuretic peptide in healthy volunteers. *Lancet.* 1985;**1**:545–8.

69 Costarino, A. T., Baumgart, S., Norman, M. E., Polin, R. A. Renal adaptation to extrauterine life in patients with respiratory distress syndrome. *Am. J. Dis. Child.* 1985;**139**:1060–3.

70 Ekblad, H., Kero, P., Vuolteenaho, O. *et al.* Atrial natriuretic peptide in the preterm infant: lack of correlation with natriuresis and diuresis. 1992;**81**:978–82.

71 Kojuma, T., Hirata Y., Fukuda, Y., Iwase, S., Kobayashi, Y. Plasma atrial natriuretic peptide and spontaneous diuresis in sick neonates. *Arch. Dis. Child.* 1987;**62**:667–70.

72 Ronconi, M., Fortunato, A., Soffiati, G. *et al.* Vasopressin, atrial natriuretic factor and renal water homeostasis in premature newborn infants with respiratory distress syndrome. *J. Perinat. Med.* 1995;**23d**:307–14.

73 Rozycki, H. J., Baumgart, S. Atrial natriuretic factor and renal function during diuresis in preterm infants. *Clin. Res.* 1987;**35**:556A.

74 Arant, B. S., Jr. Functional immaturity of the newborn kidney: paradox or prostaglandin? In Strauss, J., ed. *Homeostasis, Nephrotoxicity and Renal Anomalies in the Newborn.* Boston: Nihjoff; 1984:271.

75 el-Dhar, S. S. Development biology of the renal kallikrein-kinin system. *Pediatr. Nephrol.* 1994;**8**:624–31.

76 Jefferies, A. L., Coates, G., O'Brodovich, H. Pulmonary epithelial permeability in hyaline membrane disease. *N. Engl. J. Med.* 1984;**31**:1075–80.

77 Abman, S. H., Groothus, J. R. *et al.* Pathophysiology and treatment of BPD, current issues. *Pediatr. Clin. N. Am.* 1994;**41**:277.

78 Palta, M., Babbert, D., Weinstein, M. R., Peters, M. E. Multivariate assessment of traditional risk factors for chronic lung disease in very low birth weight neonates. *J. Pediatr.* 1991;**119**:285–92.

79 Van Marter, L. J., Pagano, M., Allred, E. N., Leviton, A., Kuban, K. C. K. Rate of bronchopulmonary dysplasia as a function of neonatal intensive care practices. *J. Pediatr.* 1992;**120**:938–46.

80 Bell, E. F., Warburton, D., Stonestreet, B. S., Oh, W. Effect of fluid administration on the development of symptomatic patent ductus arteriosus and congestive heart failure in premature infants. *N. Engl. J. Med.* 1980;**302**:598–604.

81 Langman, C. B., Engle, W. D., Baumgart, S., Fox, W. W., Polin, R. A. The diuretic phase of respiratory distress syndrome and its relationship to oxygenation. *J. Pediatr.* 1981;**98**:462–6.

82 Spitzer, A. R., Fox, W. W., Delivoria-Papadopoulos, M. *et al.* Maximum diuresis. A factor predicting recovery for RDS and development of BPD. *J. Pediatr.* 1981;**98**:476–9.

83 Heaf, D. P., Belik, J., Spitzer, A. R., Gewitz, M. H., Fox, W. W. Changes in pulmonary function during the diuretic phase of respiratory distress syndrome. *J. Pediatr.* 1982;**101**:103–7.

84 Huet, F., Semama, D., Grimaldi, M. *et al.* Effects of theophylline on renal insufficiency in neonates with respiratory distress syndrome. *Int. Care Med.* 1995;**21**:511–14.

85 Kurzner, S. I., Garg, M., Bautista, B. *et al.* Growth failure in bronchopulmonary dysplasia: elevated metabolic rates and pulmonary mechanics. *J. Pediatr.* 1988;**112**:73–80.

86 Periera, G. R., Baumgart, S., Bennett, M. J. *et al.* Use of high fat formula for premature infants with bronchopulmonary dysplasia, metabolic, pulmonary and nutritional studies. *J. Pediatr.* 1994;**124**:605–11.

87 Ballard, P. L., Ballard, R. A. Scientific basis and therapeutic regimens for use of antenatal glucocorticoids. *Am. J. Obstet. Gynecol.* 1995;**173**:254–62.

88 Padbury, J. F., Ervin, G., Polk, D. H. Extra pulmonary effects of antenatal administered steroids. *J. Pediatr.* 1996;**128**:167–72.

89 Omar, S. A., Decristofaro, J. D., Agarwal, B. I. *et al.* Effects of prenatal steroids on water and sodium homeostasis in extremely low birth weight neonates. *Pediatrics* 1999;**104**:482–8.

90 Tammela, O. K. T. Appropriate fluid regimen to prevent broncho pulmonary dysplasia. *Eur. J. Pediatr.* 1995;**154**:515.

91 Cornblath, M., Forbes, A. E., Pildes, R. S. *et al.* A controlled study of early fluid administration on survival of low birth-weight infants. *Pediatrics* 1966;**38**:547–54.

92 Spahr, R. C., Klein, A. M., Brown, D. R. *et al.* Fluid administration and bronchopulmonary dysplasia. *Am. J. Dis. Child.* 1980;**134**:958–60.

93 Gersony, W. M., Peckham, G. J., Ellison, R. C., Miettinen, O. S., Nadas, A. S. Effects of indomethacin in premature infants with patent ductus arteriosus: results of a national collaborative study. *J. Pediatr.* 1983;**102**:895–906.

94 Costarino, A. T., Baumgart, S. Modern fluid and electrolyte management of the critically ill premature infant. *Ped. Clin. N. Am.* 1986;**33**:153–78.

95 Hammarlund, K., Sedin, G. Transepidermal water loss in newborn infants: VIII. Relation to gestational age and post-natal age in appropriate and small for gestational age infants. *Acta Paediatr. Scand.* 1983;**72**:721–8.

96 Haycock, G. B., Schwartz, G. J., Wisotsky, D. H. Geometric method for measuring body surface areas: a height-weight

formula validated in infants, children and adults. *J. Pediatr.* 1978;**93**:62–6.

97 Shaffer, S. G., Kilbride, H. W., Hayen, L. K. *et al.* Hyperkalemia in very low birth weight infants. *J. Pediatr.* 1992;**121**:275–9.

98 Baumgart, S., Fox, W. W., Polin, R. A. Physiologic implications of two different heat shields for infants under radiant warmers. *J. Pediatr.* 1982;**100**:787–90.

99 Knauth, A., Gordin, M. S., McNelis, W., Baumgart, S. Semipermeable polyurethane membrane as an artificial skin for the premature neonate. *Pediatrics* 1989;**83**:945–50.

100 Harpin, A., Rutter, N. Humidification of incubators. *Arch. Dis. Child.* 1985;**60**:219–24.

101 Sulyok, E. The relationship between electrolyte and acid base balance in premature infants during early postnatal life. *Biol. Neonate* 1971;**95**:227–37.

102 Sulyok, E., Nemeth, M., Teny, I. F. *et al.* Relationship between maturity, electrolyte balance, and the function of renin-angiotensin-aldosterone system in newborn infants. *Biol. Neonate* 1979;**35**:60–5.

103 Sulyok, E., Rascher, W., Baranyai, Z. *et al.* Influence of NaCl supplementation on vasopressin secretion and water excretion in premature infants. *Biol. Neonate* 1993;**64**:201–8.

104 Lorenz, J. M., Kleinman, L. I., Ahmed, G., Markarian, K. Phases of fluid and electrolyte homeostasis in the extremely low birth weight infant. *Pediatrics* 1995;**96**:484–9.

105 Costarino, A. T., Gruskay, J. A., Corcoran, L., Polin, R. A., Baumgart, S. Sodium restriction versus daily maintenance replacement in very low birth weight premature neonates: a randomized, blind therapeutic trial. *J. Pediatr.* 1992;**120**:99–106.

106 Bhatty, S. B., Tsirka, A., Quinn, P. B., LaGamma, E. F., DeCristofaro, J. D. Rapid correction of hyponatremia in extremely low birth weight (ELBW) premature neonates is associated with long term developmental delay. *Pediatr. Res.* 1997;**41**: 140A.

10

Amino acid metabolism and protein accretion

Johannes B. van Goudoever

Department of Pediatrics, Erasmus MC/ Sophia Children's Hospital, Rotterdam, the Netherlands

Very-low-birth-weight (VLBW) infants face many diseases during the neonatal period that may affect their growth. The weight gain in utero between 24 and 36 weeks of gestation is higher than at any other time during life. In this period the average weight gain rates equal 15–17 g kg^{-1} day^{-1} with a more than 3-fold increase of weight over this period. Adequate nutrition in the neonatal period is therefore extremely important for growth.

As protein depletion is one of the factors limiting survival, accretion of body protein is the most important factor for growth if there is an excess of nutrients.[1] Quantifying the magnitude of protein deposition or loss is, therefore, vital if one wants to understand how the various diseases the very premature neonate faces directly after birth affect survival. The purpose of this chapter is to describe the available methods to follow dynamic changes in protein metabolism in the newborn and to interpret the results obtained from these methods. Noteworthily, as proteins or amino acids differ from glucose or fat only in the presence of nitrogen, studies on changes in body protein mass should focus on the nitrogen atom of amino acids.

The conventional method to follow changes in body protein status is the nitrogen (N) balance method. This routine method has been the golden standard for defining minimum levels of dietary protein and essential amino acid intake in humans of all ages, including infants.[2–6] In the studies in infants, neonates were fed mixtures of free amino acids based on the pattern of mother's milk proteins. Each of the amino acids, e.g. methionine, was eliminated for a while and reintroduced. The amount of methionine needed to reach a similar nitrogen retention as with the complete mixture was considered to be the minimal requirement.[7] A major limitation of the N balance method lies in the fact that it only defines the difference between N entering and N leaving the body. This is done by carefully recording all food consumed and collecting all material excreted: urine, feces, sputum and so on. The N from aliquots of each food, urine and fecal collection is tediously converted to ammonia by boiling the specimens in concentrated acid. The ammonia concentration is determined, after which N intake and excretion are calculated. This technique, however, is fraught with technical difficulties: N losses are routinely *underestimated* because in many cases not all urine and feces are collected and insensible losses through skin, sweat, intestinal urea hydrolysis and so on may occur; likewise, N intake is routinely *overestimated* because not all food may be consumed, and so on.[8,9] In addition to N balance studies, weight gain rates can be used to determine levels and quality of protein in the infant's diet. This may require days to weeks to be effective. Weight gain, however, is not only determined by protein intake but also by energy intake and the child's well-being. An additional drawback of this method is that it gives no information on the dynamics of amino acid metabolism.

The next best method to gain insight into body protein turnover is the quantification of 3-methylhistidine (3-MH) excretion in urine. This can be used to estimate muscle protein breakdown as 3-MH is a constituent of actin and the heavy chain of myosin.

The obvious limitation of this method is the fact that muscle protein is not the only source of 3-MH. The gastrointestinal tract can also contribute to the urinary excretion and meat in the diet might also serve as a major source of 3-MH. However, as infant formula feeding does not contain any 3-MH, this method is well suited to estimate myofibrillar protein degradation in infants. Ballard *et al.*[10]

Neonatal Nutrition and Metabolism. Second Edition, ed. P. Thureen and W. Hay. Published by Cambridge University Press.

measured 3-MH excretion in 36 premature infants, and also determined with the N balance, energy intake and weight gain rates. Autopsy data of 3-MH content of muscle protein revealed increased muscle protein degradation whenever infants were losing weight. Muscle protein degradation was found to be reduced, though not to be abolished during periods of weight gain. In addition, no effect of caloric intake on muscle protein degradation was observed. Similar findings were reported by others.[11–14]

A different approach to the study of amino acid and protein kinetics is to assume a single, free pool of amino acid–N with *two inflows* – amino acid from dietary protein and amino acid released from protein breakdown – and *two outflows* – amino acid oxidation to end products (carbon dioxide (CO_2), urea and ammonia) and amino acid uptake for protein synthesis. The model can be attributed to Schoenheimer and associates, who described it in the 1930s, and to Picou and Taylor-Roberts who later made adaptations.[15–17] This approach basically involves the administration of a single labeled amino acid (e.g. 15N-glycine) and next studying its fate. It is based on the fact that all protein in the body (structural, enzymes and so on) is constantly being made and being broken down. Most of the protein in the body, e.g. muscle protein, turns over slowly and can be considered to be a large amorphous donor of amino acids via protein breakdown as well as a large amorphous receiver of amino acids from the fast-turnover free amino acid–N pool. Lumping all body protein into a single entity is nevertheless a gross oversimplification. The body contains many different tissues, each with a wide range of proteins, which each has a different turnover rate. Following the individual fates of hundreds of proteins is an impossible task. However, because most of the important stores of N in the body turn over at similarly slow rates, it is possible to simplify the system into a conceptual model that can be dealt with.

Apart from nonessential amino acids specific representative essential amino acids can be used. Measuring the kinetics of such an essential amino acid is nowadays the commonest method to quantify amino acid metabolism. It is important, though, to note that different tracers yield different results when extrapolated to whole-body protein turnover.[18,19] While this underscores the differential contribution of various body proteins – represented by various amino acid tracers – to whole body protein turnover, it provides a strong argument to express amino kinetics for each specific amino acid. Numerous modifications of the technique using amino acids labeled with stable isotopes have been made, but a discussion of these is beyond the scope of this chapter.

Table 10.1. Leucine kinetics in amino acid deprived preterm infants, term infants and adults

	Leucine flux μmol kg⁻¹ h⁻¹	Leucine oxidation μmol kg⁻¹ h⁻¹	Change in protein mass
Preterm infants[27]*	201 ± 20	41 ± 13	-1.7 ± 0.5
Term infants[20]	164 ± 28	34 ± 11	-1.4 ± 0.4
Adults[20]	87 ± 15	15 ± 3	-0.6

Values are mean ± SD.
*Indicates study reference.

Effect of age and feeding

Due to the immaturity of the various enzyme systems, many metabolic processes are still underdeveloped in the first few weeks following premature birth. However, the birth itself and the effects of birth-associated stress cause a more rapid development of enzyme activity than would have occurred should the fetus have remained within the uterus. Thus, both gestational age and postnatal age have to be considered for their effects on amino acid metabolism and protein accretion. Another confounding factor is the intake of amino acids or proteins. Most studies on amino acid metabolism in adults are performed in the postabsorptive state. However, it is ethically unacceptable to starve newborn infants, especially preterm infants, for a prolonged period of time. For this reason there are hardly any data on amino acid metabolism in preterm infants during fasting; the available studies were done in infants receiving glucose intravenously. Yet a clear trend in amino acid metabolism emerges. Denne *et al.* studied healthy, term newborns during the first 3 days following birth using [1–13C]leucine tracer.[20] Table 10.1 compares the main findings from this study with findings from other studies using the same tracer in healthy adults and in premature "healthy" infants on the first day of life. It shows that the turnover rate of leucine, quantified by the dilution of the tracer in plasma, decreases with age. In term infants and adults, the contribution of leucine oxidation to energy generation was lower than that in preterm infants. Preterm infants had the highest rate of leucine oxidation, despite the fact that they were given small amounts of glucose, which also might serve as a fuel source. Indeed, glucose oxidation measured in a similar group of preterm infants under the same conditions accounted for approximately 40% of the energy expenditure although one would expect a certain protein-sparing effect of the additional glucose.[21] Glucose administration to

Table 10.2. The effect of amino acid administration on protein accretion in the first few days following birth

Study reference	Amino acid intake (g protein kg^{-1} day^{-1})	Number of infants studied	Postnatal age (days)	Non-protein energy intake (kcal kg^{-1} day^{-1})	Protein accretion[1]	Relative effect[2] (accretion/Δ intake) %
26	0	9	3	36 ± 11.1	−0.60 ± 0.20	
	2.3 ± 0.2	9	3	45 ± 9.6	1.40 ± 0.20	87
27	0	9	1	24.2 ± 5.2	−0.69 ± 0.28	
	1.15 ± 0.06	9	1	26.1 ± 6.3	0.06 ± 0.79	65
26	0	9	3	36 ± 11.1	−0.60 ± 0.20	
	2.3 ± 0.2	9	3	45 ± 9.6	1.40 ± 0.20	87
28	0.13 ± 0.04	11	3	36 ± 0.96	−0.83 ± 0.14	
	1.8 ± 0.09	10	3	45 ± 3.1	0.75 ± 0.04	95
29	0	8	3	38 ± 10	n.d.	
	1.5	11	3	48 ± 17	plasma AA ↑	
30	0	12	3	35 ± 12	−0.84 ± 0.28	
	1.6 ± 0.05	11	3	54 ± 11	0.55 ± 0.34	87
31	0.85 ± 0.08	13	2	41.5 ± 3.7	−0.26 ± 0.11	
	2.65 ± 0.13	15	2	49.1 ± 4.3	1.16 ± 0.15	79

[1] A negative number indicates a negative protein balance i.e. protein loss.

[2] The relative effect of amino acid administration is calculated by dividing the net protein gain (protein accretion at the high amino acid intake − protein accretion at the low or zero protein intake) by the difference in protein intake.

term healthy or premature infants did not reduce proteolysis either.[22,23] Extrapolating these data by assuming a fixed amount of 590 µmol leucine per gram body protein, the loss of protein mass brought about by cessation of amino acids is the most prominent in the youngest human. This has an even greater impact if the total mass of body proteins is taken into account. A preterm infant of 26 weeks has an average body protein store of only 80 grams, and thus loses 1–2% of its total protein store on every day of protein starvation. A term infant has a protein mass of approximately 400 grams and thus loses only 0.3%, whereas an adult loses only 0.01% of its protein mass daily. So from these studies a clear picture emerges: protein turnover and catabolism rates are the highest in the youngest with a major impact on body protein stores.

Considering the huge impact of starvation on protein mass, especially in preterm infants, investigators have begun introducing amino acids early after birth. The initial reluctance to start amino acid supplementation immediately following birth had sprung from reports on hyperammonemia, metabolic acidosis and uremia three decades ago.[24,25] These side effects appeared to be associated with the use of protein hydrolysates, which now have been replaced by crystalline solutions. These seem to be well tolerated by preterm infants and several studies have shown that amino acids can be safely administered early after

birth.[26–31] The effects of different amino acid intake and energy intake are summarized in Table 10.2. It shows that preterm infants apparently not only metabolize these amino acids without metabolic disturbances, but also use the administered amino acids for protein accretion. Some studies used stable isotope techniques to discriminate the positive effect on protein balance into either an increase in protein synthesis or a decrease in proteolysis. Although not clear in all studies, the predominant impression is one of increased protein synthesis with no significant effect on proteolysis.[26,31] These studies also show that amino acid supplementation does improve protein accretion despite a very low energy intake. Thus, it is indeed feasible to administer amino acids parenterally from birth onwards, with a positive effect on protein accretion.

Following a short period of parenteral feeding, preterm infants are fed enterally. The effect of enteral feeding on amino acid metabolism and protein accretion has been widely investigated. Term neonates respond by an increase in leucine turnover and synthesis, whereas leucine oxidation is not changed when newborns are fed.[32] This is in contrast to adults, whose first response to nutrient administration is suppression of protein breakdown. The response on protein metabolism of enteral feeding versus parenteral feeding has also been investigated by several groups.[33,34] Although Denne *et al.* found no differences in leucine turnover rates, it is obvious from a number of animal and human studies that the intestine absorbs a substantial amount of dietary amino acids (see below). In order to determine the appropriate quantity and quality of the dietary amino acid intake it is crucial to know to which extent dietary proteins are metabolized within the splanchnic tissues. However, before discussing the impact of intestinal metabolism on whole-body amino acid metabolism and protein accretion, it should be mentioned that many studies have attempted to determine the adequate amount of protein intake for optimal growth. Catzeflis et al.[35] described a linear relationship between nitrogen intake and nitrogen balance in 1– to 2-month-old preterm infants. Zello et al.[36] concluded that at least 0.73 g kg^{-1} day^{-1} should be administered to achieve a zero balance.

However, it is not only the protein and energy intake that are important;[37] the carbohydrate/fat ratio also significantly influences protein accretion and growth. In enterally fed preterm infants carbohydrate seems to be more effective in enhancing protein accretion than fat.[38,39]

Amino acid accretion of specific tissues

So far, amino acid metabolism accretion has been discussed at whole body level. However, different tissues obviously have different rates of protein turnover. Figure 10.1 shows different fractional synthetic rates for different tissues. These turnover rates also change with varying circumstances. Sepsis, for example, might increase the synthesis of hepatic protein for the purpose of acute phase protein production, and increase proteolysis in peripheral muscle.

The intestine as a whole, and the small intestinal mucosa in particular, has a high rate of protein synthesis and energy expenditure. Thus, although the portal-drained viscera constitute 3–6% of body weight, they account for 20–35% of cardiac output, whole body protein turnover and energy expenditure.[40–44] The intestinal mucosa is also a highly secretory and proliferative tissue, whose continual cell turnover and secretion has at least one major consequence. As not all intestinal secretions, such as cell fragments, mucins, glutathione, defensins, are recycled to the body, the intestine is essentially in a permanent state of net protein production. Thus, secretory protein synthesis, especially that of mucins, probably has a substantial impact on the requirements for some specific amino acids, and as such influences protein retention on a whole body level.

The core proteins of the major intestinal secretory mucins (MUC2 and MUC3) contain high quantities of cysteine, threonine, proline and serine.[45,46] It follows that

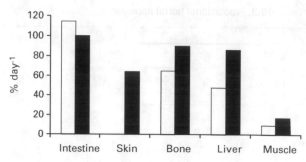

Figure 10.1. Fractional synthetic rate of different tissues in the body. Composed from references McNurlan et al.,[41] Preedy et al.,[56] Burrin et al.,[57] Seve et al.[58]. Open bars represent data obtained from pigs, closed bars from rats.

mucin secretion should have a measurable influence on the requirements for cysteine and threonine. Studies in newborn animals have provided evidence compatible with this proposition, i.e. the portal appearance of dietary threonine, when expressed as a proportion of intake, is uniformly lower that that of other essential amino acids (Table 10.3). Threonine requirement of piglets maintained by parenteral nutrition (a treatment that lowers intestinal mass and probably also mucin secretion) was less than 40% of that of piglets receiving enteral feedings.[47] On ethical grounds it is not feasible to measure portal availability of amino acids in neonates. The next best method to estimate intestinal and hepatic uptake of dietary nutrients is the dual tracer approach in which tracers are administered intravenously and enterally at the same time. The magnitude of the higher dilution of the enteral tracer is related to the proportion of tracer uptake in intestine and liver. This method was applied in a study in enterally fed preterm infants with mean gestational age 29 weeks and a birth weight of approximately 1000 grams who received threonine and lysine tracers. In first pass almost 20% of the administered lysine was utilized, versus 70% of the enterally administered threonine.[48,49] A lower enteral intake resulted in an increase in fractional first pass uptake of both lysine and threonine. Previous studies had already shown that 40–50% of the ingested leucine was absorbed in the splanchnic bed.[50,51] It is hard to believe that such high amounts of dietary amino acids are taken up for protein accretion, notwithstanding the fact that intestinal tissues grow very rapidly, especially during the first few weeks of life (Figure 10.2). Stoll et al. found that only 10–20% of the utilized amino acids were incorporated into the intestinal tissue, which indicates that most synthesized glyco-proteins are secretory and thus are not used for protein accretion.[52] This would imply a major loss of essential amino acids, however many of the secreted proteins are recycled.[53]

Table 10.3. Proportional portal appearance of dietary essential amino acids in the portal blood of piglets

	Portal balance of amino acid (per cent of intake)			
	Van der Schoor *et al.*[51]*	Van Goudoever *et al.*[43]	Reeds *et al.*[54] Stoll *et al.*[44]	Deutz *et al.*[55]
Body weight (kg)	9	7	8	21
Threonine	33	16	47	39
Lysine	64	54	53	61
Leucine	66	47	59	52
Phenylalanine	49	37	55	51
Valine	51	41	63	54
Methionine	75	ND	54	61
Isoleucine	30	28	62	56

*Indicates study reference.

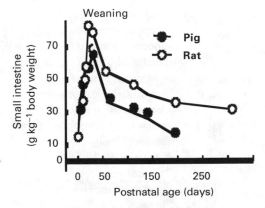

Figure 10.2. Weight gain rate of small intestine expressed per kilogram body weight in the postnatal period.

Summary

Over the last three decades different methods have been used to gain insight in the dynamic aspects of protein and amino acid metabolism in term and preterm neonates. Currently, tracer studies with stable isotopes are considered the best method to study these aspects. Studies using this method demonstrated that preterm infants have higher rates of protein turnover and breakdown than term infants, and that infants benefit from amino acid administration even directly from birth onwards. The different tissues in the body show different rates of protein turnover, with the intestinal tissues consuming up to 50% of dietary intake. Consequently, intestinal metabolism has a substantial impact on the systemic availability of dietary amino acids, which subsequently affects growth.

REFERENCES

1 Bier, D. M., Young, V. R. Assessment of whole-body protein kinetics in the human infant. In Fomon, S. J., Heird, W. C., eds. *Energy and Protein Needs During Infancy.* San Diego, CA: Academic Press, 1986:107–25.

2 Snyderman, S. E., Bayer, A., Norton, P. M., Roitman, E., Holt, L. E. The essential amino acid requirement of infants. X. Methionine. *Am. J. Clin. Nutr.* 1964;**15**:322–30.

3 Fomon, S. J., Ziegler, E. E., Nelson, S. E., Edwards, B. B. Requirement for sulfur containing amino acids in infancy. *J. Nutr.* 1986;**116**:1405–22.

4 Harper, A. E.. Origin of recommended dietary allowances: an historic overview. *Am. J. Clin. Nutr.* 1985;**41**:140–8.

5 Ziegler, E. E., Fomon, S. J. Methods in infant nutrition research: balance and growth studies. *Acta Paediatr Scand.* 1982;**299**:90–6.

6 Food and Nutrition Board. *National Research Council (US): Recommended Dietary Allowances.* 10th edn. Washington, DC: National Academy Press;1989:52–77.

7 Jurgens, P. Zum aminosuerebedarf Fruh und Neugeborener sowie junger Sauglinge bei enterale und parenterale Ernahung. In Bassler, K. H., Grunert, A., Kleinberger, G., eds. *Contributions to Infusion Therapy and Clinical Nutrition.* Basel: Karger; 1986;**16**:14–53.

8 Kopple, J. D. Uses and limitations of the balance technique. *J. Parenter. Enteral Nutr.* 1987;**11**:790–050.

9 Tomé, D., Bos, C. Dietary protein and nitrogen utilization. *J. Nutr.* 2000;**130**:1868S–73S.

10 Ballard, F. J., Thomas, F. M., Pope, L. M. *et al.* Muscle protein degradation in premature human infants. *Clin Sci.* 1979;**57**:535–44.

11 Pencharz, P. B., Masson, M., Desgranges, F., Papageorgiou, A. The effects of post-natal age on the whole body protein metabolism and the urinary 3-methyl-histidine excretion of premature infants. *Nutr. Res.* 1984;9–16.

12 Burgoyne, J. L., Ballard, F. J., Tomas, F. M. *et al.* Measurements of myofibrillar protein breakdown in newborn human infants. *Clin. Sci.* 1982;**63**:421–7.

13 Hulsemann, J., Kordass, U., Sander, G., Schmidt, E., Schoch, G. 3-Methylhistidine/creatinine ratio in urine from low-birth-weight infants. Clinical approach. *Ann. Nutr. Metab.* 1988;**32**:44–51.

14 Seashore, J. H., Huszar, G., Davis, E. M. Urinary 3-methylhistidine/creatinine ratio as a clinical tool: correlation between 3-methylhistidine excretion and metabolic and clinical states in healthy and stressed premature infants. *Metabolism* 1981;**30**:959–69.

15 Schoenheimer, R., Rastner, S., Rittenberg, D. Studies in protein metabolism; metabolic activity of body proteins investigated with 1-leucine containing 2 isotopes. *J. Biol. Chem.* 1939;**130**:730–2.

16 Schoenheimer, R., Rastner, S., Rittenberg, D. Protein metabolism (II): Synthesis of amino acids containing isotopic N. *J. Biol. Chem.* 1939;**130**:703.

17 Picou, D., Taylor-Roberts, T. The measurement of total protein synthesis and catabolism and nitrogen turnover in infants in different nutritional states and receiving different amounts of dietary protein. *Clin. Sci.* 1969;**36**:283–96.

18 Van Goudoever, J. B., Sulkers, E. J., Halliday, D. *et al.* Whole-body protein turnover in preterm appropriate for gestational age and small for gestational age infants: comparison of [15N]glycine and [1-(13)C]leucine administered simultaneously. *Pediatr. Res.* 1995;**37**:381–7.

19 Van Toledo-Eppinga, L., Kalhan, S. C., Kulik, W., Jakobs, C., Lafeber, H. N. Relative kinetics of phenylalanine and leucine in low birth weight infants during nutrient administration. *Pediatr. Res.* 1996;**40**:41–6.

20 Denne, S. C., Kalhan, S. C. Leucine metabolism in human newborns. *Am. J. Physiol.* 1987;**253**:E608–15.

21 van Goudoever, J. B., Sulkers, E. J., Chapman, T. E. *et al.* Glucose kinetics and glucoregulatory hormone levels in ventilated preterm infants on the first day of life. *Pediatr. Res.* 1993;**33**:583–9.

22 Denne, S. C., Karn, C. A., Wang, J., Liechty, E. A. Effect of intravenous glucose and lipid on proteolysis and glucose production in normal newborns. *Am. J. Physiol.* 1995;**269**:E361–7.

23 Hertz, D. E., Karn, C. A., Liu, Y. M., Liechty, E. A., Denne, S. C. Intravenous glucose suppresses glucose production but not proteolysis in extremely premature newborns. *J. Clin. Invest.* 1993;**92**:1752–8.

24 Heird, W. C., Dell, R. B., Driscoll, J. M., Grebin, B., Winters, R. W. Metabolic acidosis resulting from intravenous alimentation mixtures containing synthetic amino acids. *N. Engl. J. Med.* 1972;**287**:943–8.

25 Johnson, J. D., Albritton, W. L., Sunshine, P. Hyperammonaemia accompanying parenteral nutrition in newborn infants. *J. Pediatr.* 1972;**81**:154–61.

26 Van Lingen, R. A., van Goudoever, J. B., Luijendijk, I. H., Wattimena, J. L., Sauer, P. J. Effects of early amino acid administration during total parenteral nutrition on protein metabolism in preterm infants. *Clin. Sci.* 1992;**82**:199–203.

27 Van Goudoever, J. B., Colen, T., Wattimena, J. L. *et al.* Immediate commencement of amino acid supplementation in preterm infants: effect on serum amino acid concentrations and protein kinetics on the first day of life. *J. Pediatr.* 1995;**127**:458–65.

28 Saini, J., MacMahon, P., Morgan, J. B., Kovar, I. Z. Early parenteral feeding of amino acids. *Arch. Dis. Child.* 1989;**64**:1362–6.

29 Rivera, A. Jr, Bell, E. F., Stegink, L. D., Ziegler, E. E. Plasma amino acid profiles during the first three days of life in infants with respiratory distress syndrome: effect of parenteral amino acid supplementation. *J. Pediatr.* 1989;**115**:465–8.

30 Rivera, A. Jr, Bell, E. F., Bier, D. M. Effect of intravenous amino acids on protein metabolism of preterm infants during the first three days of life. *Pediatr. Res.* 1993;**33**:106–11.

31 Thureen, P. J., Melara, D., Fennessey, P. V., Hay, W. W. Jr. Effect of low versus high intravenous amino acid intake on very low birth weight infants in the early neonatal period. *Pediatr. Res.* 2003;**53**:24–32.

32 Denne, S. C., Rossi, E. M., Kalhan, S. C. Leucine kinetics during feeding in normal newborns. *Pediatr. Res.* 1991;**30**:23–7.

33 Denne, S. C., Karn, C. A., Liu, Y. M., Leitch, C. A., Liechty, E. A. Effect of enteral versus parenteral feeding on leucine kinetics and fuel utilization in premature newborns. *Pediatr. Res.* 1994;**36**:429–35.

34 Wykes, L. J., Ball, R. O., Menendez, C. E., Ginther, D. M., Pencharz, P. B. Glycine, leucine, and phenylalanine flux in low-birth-weight infants during parenteral and enteral feeding. *Am. J. Clin. Nutr.* 1992;**55**:971–5.

35 Catzeflis, C., Schutz, Y., Micheli, J. L. *et al.* Whole body protein synthesis and energy expenditure in very low birth weight infants. *Pediatr. Res.* 1985;**19**:679–87.

36 Zello, G. A., Menendez, C. E., Rafii, M. *et al.* Minimum protein intake for the preterm neonate determined by protein and amino acid kinetics. *Pediatr. Res.* 2003;**53**:338–44.

37 Kashyap, S., Schulze, K. F., Ramakrishnan, R., Dell, R. B., Heird, W. C. Evaluation of a mathematical model for predicting the relationship between protein and energy intakes of low-birth-weight infants and the rate and composition of weight gain. *Pediatr. Res.* 1994;**35**:704–12.

38 Kashyap, S., Ohira-Kist, K., Abildskov, K. *et al.* Effects of quality of energy intake on growth and metabolic response of enterally fed low-birth-weight infants. *Pediatr. Res.* 2001;**50**:390–7.

39 Kashyap, S., Towers, H. M., Sahni, R. *et al.* Effects of quality of energy on substrate oxidation in enterally fed, low-birth-weight infants. *Am. J. Clin. Nutr.* 2001;**74**:374–80.

40 Burrin, D. G., Ferrell, C. L., Britton, R. A., Bauer, M. Level of nutrition and visceral organ size and metabolic activity in sheep. *Br. J. Nutr.* 1990;**64**:439–48.

41 McNurlan, M. A., Garlick, P. J. Contribution of rat liver and gastrointestinal tract to whole-body protein synthesis in the rat. *Biochem. J.* 1980;**186**:381–3.

42 Lobley, G. E., Milne, V., Lovie, J. M., Reeds, P. J., Pennie, K. Whole body and tissue protein synthesis in cattle. *Br. J. Nutr.* 1980;**43**:491–502.

43 van Goudoever, J. B., Stoll, B., Henry, J. F., Burrin, D. G., Reeds, P. J. Adaptive regulation of intestinal lysine metabolism. *Proc. Natl Acad. Sci. USA.* 2000;**97**:11620–5.

44 Stoll, B., Burrin, D. G., Henry, J., Jahoor, F., Reeds, P. J. Phenylalanine utilization by the gut and liver measured with intravenous and intragastric tracers in pigs. *Am. J. Physiol.* 1997;**273**:G1208–7.

45 Chang, S. K., Dohrman, A. F., Basbaum, C. B. *et al.* Localization of mucin (MUC2 and MUC3) messenger RNA and peptide expression in human normal intestine and colon cancer. *Gastroenterology* 1994;**107**:28–36.

46 Van Klinken, B. J., Dekker, J., Buller, H. A., de Bolos, C., Einerhand, A. W. Biosynthesis of mucins (MUC2–6) along the longitudinal axis of the human gastrointestinal tract. *Am. J. Physiol.* 1997;**273**:G296–302.

47 Bertolo, R. F., Chen, C. Z., Law, G., Pencharz, P. B., Ball, R. O. Threonine requirement of neonatal piglets receiving total parenteral nutrition is considerably lower than that of piglets receiving an identical diet intragastrically. *J. Nutr.* 1998;**128**:1752–9.

48 Van der Schoor, S. R. D., Reeds P. J., Stellard F. *et al.* Lysine kinetics in preterm infants; the importance of enteral feeding. *Gut.* **53**:38–43.

49 Van der Schoor, S. R. D., Wattimena, D. L., Reeds, P. J. *et al.* Threonine kinetics in preterm infants: the gut takes nearly all (in press).

50 Beaufrere, B., Fournier, V., Salle, B., Putet, G. Leucine kinetics in fed low-birth-weight infants: importance of splanchnic tissues. *Am. J. Physiol.* 1992;**263**:E214–20.

51 Darmaun, D., Roig, J. C., Auestad, N., Sager, B. K., Neu, J. Glutamine metabolism in very low birth weight infants. *Pediatr. Res.* 1997;**41**:391–6.

52 Stoll, B., Henry, J., Reeds, P. J. *et al.* Catabolism dominates the first-pass intestinal metabolism of dietary essential amino acids in milk protein-fed piglets. *J. Nutr.* 1998;**128**:606–14.

53 Van Der Schoor, S. R., Reeds, P. J., Stoll, B. The high metabolic cost of a functional gut. *Gastroenterology* 2002;**123**:1931–40.

54 Reeds, P. J., Burrin, D. G., Jahoor, F. *et al.* Enteral glutamate is almost completely metabolized in first pass by the gastrointestinal tract of infant pigs. *Am. J. Physiol.* 1996;**270**:E413–18.

55 Deutz, N. E., Bruins, M. J., Soeters, P. B. Infusion of soy and casein protein meals affects interorgan amino acid metabolism and urea kinetics differently in pigs. *J. Nutr.* 1998;**128**:2435–45.

56 Preedy, V. R., McNurlan, M. A., Garlick, P. J. Protein synthesis in skin and bone of the young rat. *Br. J. Nutr.* 1983;**49**:517–23.

57 Burrin, D. G., Wester, T. J., Davis, T. A., Fiorotto, M. L., Chang, X. Dexamethasone inhibits small intestinal growth via increased protein catabolism in neonatal pigs. *Am. J. Physiol.* 1999;**276**:E269–77.

58 Seve, B., Reeds, P. J., Fuller, M. F., Cadenhead, A., Hay, S. M. Protein synthesis and retention in some tissues of the young pig as influenced by dietary protein intake after early-weaning. Possible connection to the energy metabolism. *Reprod. Nutr. Dev.* 1986;**26**:849–61.

11

Carbohydrate metabolism and glycogen accretion

Rebecca A. Simmons

Department of Pediatrics, University of Pennsylvania, Philadelphia, PA

Metabolism of glucose in the fetus

Glucose is a vital substrate for the growing and developing fetus. It is required by most cells for oxidative and nonoxidative ATP production and serves as a precursor for other carbon-containing compounds. It is the primary fuel used for several specialized cells and is the major fuel used by the brain. Its storage in the liver as glycogen provides a means by which glucose homeostasis can be maintained, particularly during the neonatal period. The fetal requirement for glucose is met almost, if not entirely, by transplacental transport from the mother to the fetus.[1,2] At birth, there is an abrupt loss of the maternal supply of substrates and nutrients and the newborn has to mobilize glucose and other substrates to meet its energy needs.

A number of studies in a variety of species, including humans, have shown that fetal plasma glucose concentrations are significantly lower than that of the mother.[3–5] Furthermore, there is a direct relationship between maternal and fetal plasma glucose concentrations and the supply of glucose to the fetus is highly dependent upon maternal glycemia.[6–12] Thus, the supply of glucose to the fetus is likely to be diminished in the case of maternal hypoglycemia and to be increased in the case of maternal hyperglycemia. However, the placenta has a large capacity for glucose storage in the form of glycogen which blunts glucose transfer to the fetus when significant maternal hyperglycemia occurs.

There are a limited number of studies examining the effect of altered uterine blood flow upon fetal glucose concentrations and glucose utilization. When umbilical blood flow is decreased acutely in the fetal lamb (at 116–120 days' gestation), blood glucose and lactate concentrations rise, and there is a trend toward increased glucose delivery and uptake by the fetal hind limb.[13,14] Similar results have been obtained in the fetal rat subjected to an abrupt decrease in blood flow.[15] However, during more severe glucose deprivation, placental transfer and fetal uptake of glucose are constrained in proportion with maternal supply.

Placental glucose transport

Transfer of glucose from maternal to fetal blood occurs along a concentration gradient by facilitated, carrier-mediated diffusion via the placental villi and is most likely mediated by the glucose transporter, GLUT1. GLUT1 is abundantly expressed in the plasma membranes of both the basal and apical sides of the syncytiotrophoblast. GLUT1 may facilitate the entry of glucose into the cytoplasm of the syncytiotrophoblast from maternal blood, while GLUT1 at the basal plasma membrane may aid in the exit of glucose from the cytoplasm of the syncytiotrophoblast to the pericapillary space of the fetus. GLUT1 on the endothelial cell of the capillary then transfers glucose into the fetal circulation.[16–19] Protein and mRNA levels of GLUT1 increase in the placenta as the fetus matures underscoring the importance of this transporter in fetal development.[17,19] GLUT3 is distributed throughout placental villous tissue and decreases during gestation.[17,19] While GLUT3 mRNA is abundantly expressed in villous tissue, GLUT3 protein is primarily localized to the vascular endothelium. The low Km of GLUT3 may facilitate its role in transporting glucose from mother to fetus following trans-syncytial transport.

The asymmetrical distribution of membrane transporters between the maternal and fetal facing surface of the

Neonatal Nutrition and Metabolism. Second Edition, ed. P. Thureen and W. Hay. Published by Cambridge University Press.
© Cambridge University Press 2006.

syncytiotrophoblast is a basic feature of the transplacental transport system.[20] There is a higher expression of GLUT1 protein in the microvillous as compared with the basal membrane of the syncytiotrophoblast.[16,17] In addition to the increased density of GLUT1, a 6-fold larger surface area of the microvillous covering [21] leads to a several times higher total transport capacity across the syncytial compared with the basal membrane.[17] The high overall capacity of uptake across the apical membrane of the syncytium assures an intracellular glucose concentration which is maintained close to the maternal plasma level in spite of a high rate of glucose consumption by the syncytium. This mechanism seems to be of central importance for a continuous flux of glucose from the mother to the fetus.[22]

Carrier-mediated transport favoring the flux of glucose from the mother to the fetus and restricting movement in the opposite direction plays an important role in maintaining a stable glucose environment for fetal tissues, especially in situations of maternal hypoglycemia. Transport across the basal membrane is thought to be the rate-limiting step in the transplacental flux of glucose.[17] Therefore, alterations in GLUT1 density in the basal membrane could theoretically determine the rate of flux across the placenta from the mother to the fetus. GLUT1 levels in the microvillous membrane do not change during pregnancy whereas basal membrane GLUT1 levels double as pregnancy progresses, which has been linked to the overall rise of placental glucose transport in late pregnancy.[17]

As gestation advances, there is a lowering of glucose concentration in the fetus and the transplacental gradient is increased since the maternal glucose values do not change during pregnancy.[4,23] This physiological decrease in fetal glucose concentrations is an important contributing factor to meet the increased need of glucose by the rapidly growing fetus.

There are obviously many factors in addition to the asymmetry of surface area and density of GLUT1 in the microvillous and the basal membrane of the syncytiotrophoblast that contribute to the polarity of glucose transport across the human placenta. Tissue components of the barrier separating maternal from fetal blood like the basement membrane and the endothelial layer of the villous capillaries may influence flux, although a number of investigators have shown that these layers do not contribute significantly to the flux of small hydrophilic molecules.[24-26] Glucose moves across the capillary wall into the fetal circulation via paracellular clefts in the endothelial layer.[27] The overall surface area of this microvasculature plays an important role in transplacental diffusion of solutes and diseases such as diabetes and pre-eclampsia influence the extent of vascularization and capillary diameter.[28-32]

Glucose supply to the fetus

A number of studies in the sheep fetus have shown that under basal conditions, during maternal euglycemia, maternal glucose is the only source of fetal glucose and that fetal glucose production under these circumstances either does not occur or is negligible[33,34] until the last few days of gestation.[10,35,36] Using tracer methodology, endogenous glucose production was measured in chronically catheterized sheep fetuses during normal fed conditions at different gestational ages. In normal fed conditions, the rate of fetal glucose production was negligible until 143–145 days (term 145 days) when it increased significantly to account for close to 50% of the glucose used by the fetus.[36]

Data are limited with respect to sources of glucose for the human fetus. One study using glucose labeled with ^{13}C infused to pregnant women undergoing elective cesarean section at term showed that the fetal glucose pool was in equilibrium with the maternal glucose pool and that maternal glucose was the only source of glucose for the human fetus at term gestation.[37]

In many species, the activities of key gluconeogenic enzymes, such as glucose-6-phosphatase and phosphoenolpyruvate carboxykinase (PEPCK), increase towards term in the fetal liver and kidney.[38-41] In fetal sheep, the ontogenic increments in tissue G6P and PEPCK activities are known to be dependent on the prepartum cortisol surge.[41] The increases in hepatic and renal G6P and PEPCK seen close to term are prevented by fetal adrenalectomy, and are stimulated prematurely by an exogenous infusion of cortisol earlier in gestation.[41]

Glycogen metabolism in the fetus

In the fetus, as in the adult, the major storage form of glucose is glycogen. Glycogen is stored in liver, skeletal and cardiac muscle, kidney, intestine, brain, lung and placenta. Glycogen is present in very low quantities in the human fetus in early gestation and slowly increases until approximately 36 weeks.[42,43] Peak values in lung, heart, kidney and placenta are attained at this gestational age. In liver and skeletal muscle, glycogen reaches maximum concentration at term.[44,45]

The accumulation of glycogen stores parallels the increase in activity of the rate-limiting enzyme for glycogen synthesis, glycogen synthase.[43] Recent studies have further elucidated the steps in the glycogenetic cascade. Two recently identified proteins have been demonstrated to be involved in glycogenesis in the adult: the glucosyltransferase glycogenin [46] and the stable glycogen-precursor proglycogen.[47] Based on these findings, the following sequence of glycogen metabolism is proposed: glycogenin transfers glucose from UDPglucose to the hydroxyl of its Tyr-194 and then adds further residues to form protein-bound maltosaccharides. This fully glycosylated glycogenin serves as the primer for the synthesis of proglycogen by a putative proglycogen synthase (distinct from the well-recognized glycogen synthase) and branching enzyme with UDPglucose as substrate. Subsequently, the classical glycogen synthase and branching enzyme take proglycogen to glycogen.[48] It remains to be determined whether this pathway exists in the fetus and newborn.

In the adult, a significant proportion of glycogen is derived from the gluconeogenic precursors, lactate, pyruvate and alanine.[49,50] Since the fetal liver has little capacity for gluconeogenesis, other substrates including glucose and serine may contribute to the synthesis of glycogen.[51-53] Glucose has been shown to be incorporated in glycogen in fetal rat liver and in isolated fetal rat hepatocytes [51] and incorporation of ^{14}C-glucose into glycogen is much greater in fetal hepatocytes compared with adult hepatocytes. [54] Serine and glycine are cycled between fetal liver and placenta, providing another substrate for glycogen accretion.[55] The role of lactate as a glycogenic precursor has been examined in ovine fetuses using [^{14}C]lactate and D-[3[3]H]glucose infusions. These investigators concluded that glycogenesis from glucose is partly through the indirect gluconeogenic route and that lactate may be an important glycogenic precursor in the ovine fetus.[56]

Glycogen accretion in the fetal liver is dependent upon substrate supply and hormonal regulation. Insulin and cortisol are two of the more important hormones regulating glycogen synthesis in adults. However, the effect of insulin in the fetus may differ from that in the adult. While insulin has been shown to stimulate glycogen synthesis in isolated fetal hepatocytes,[57,58] the presence of cortisol is required. Adult hepatocytes can synthesize glycogen in response to insulin in the absence of cortisol.[57] Furthermore, fetal rats can maintain glycogen synthesis despite chronic hypoinsulinemia.[59] Other hormones such as epidermal growth factor and insulin-like-growth factor I (IGF-I) have been shown to stimulate fetal hepatic glycogen synthesis in the rat.[60-62] Studies using IGF-II knockout mice suggest that IGF-II also plays an important role in regulating glycogen deposition in the fetus.[63] IGF-II knockout mice have very low levels of hepatic glycogen at birth which is paralleled by low enzymatic activities of glycogen synthase.[63] It is not known whether IGF-II is mediating its effects via the IGF-I or the insulin receptor in the fetal liver.

Mobilization of hepatic glycogen stores in the perinatal period is crucial in order to maintain glucose homeostasis. Release of glucose from degradation of liver glycogen requires the activities of the two enzymes phosphorylase and glucose-6-phosphatase. The initial step in glycogen degradation is catalyzed by glycogen phosphorylase, which exists as three genetically distinct isozymes referred to as muscle, liver and brain isoforms. The brain and liver isoforms of glycogen phosphorylase may be involved in mobilization of type II cell glycogen during late fetal lung development.[64] In fetal liver and kidney, glycogen breakdown with subsequent release of glucose into the fetal circulation can be induced by catecholamines or glucagon or by stimuli such as cold stress or hypoxia. Whether such glucose release occurs physiologically and the precise conditions that lead to such release in vivo remain to be determined. In other organs such as the placenta, lung and heart, phosphorylase, but not glucose-6-phosphatase, is present, and glycogen is available only for intracellular consumption. This is particularly important in organs that have high energy demands such as the heart and placenta, and the lung where glycogen is used for surfactant synthesis by type II pneumocytes.[65]

Glucose metabolism in the newborn

Development of carbohydrate homeostasis in the newborn infant results from a balance between hormonal, enzymatic, neural regulation and substrate availability. The newborn infant must supply its own substrate to meet the energy requirements for maintenance of body temperature, respiration, muscular activity and regulation of blood glucose. The concentration of glucose in the umbilical venous blood approximates 70–80% of that in the mother and is higher than in the umbilical arterial blood. During the first 4–6 hours of postnatal life, glucose values fall, stabilizing between 50–60 mg dL^{-1}.[66] This decrease in glucose is even greater in preterm or small-for-gestational-age infants. By 2–3 days of age, plasma glucose values average 70–80 mg dL^{-1}.

Blood glucose concentration is normally maintained at a relatively constant level by a fine balance between hepatic glucose output and peripheral glucose uptake. Hepatic glucose output depends on adequate glycogen stores, sufficient supplies of endogenous gluconeogenic precursors, a normally functioning hepatic gluconeogenic and glycogenolytic system, and a normal endocrine system for modulating these processes.

At birth the neonate has glycogen stores that are greater than those in the adult. However, because of a two-fold greater basal glucose utilization, these stores are rapidly depleted and begin to decline within 2–3 hours after birth, remain low for several days, and then gradually rise to adult levels. Both serum glucagon and catecholamines increase 3-fold to 5-fold in response to umbilical cord cutting. Circulating insulin levels usually decrease in the immediate newborn period and remain low for several days. The depressed serum insulin and elevated glucagon and epinephrine levels along with elevated serum growth hormone levels at birth favor glycogenolysis, lipolysis and gluconeogenesis. Changes in various hormone receptors also modulate these processes. Hepatic glucagon receptors increase in number and become functionally linked with cyclic 3′ 5′ adenosine monophosphate protein kinase (cAMP) responses. Neonatal glucose homeostasis also requires appropriate enzyme maturation and response in the newborn. After birth, glycogen phosphorylase activity is increased whereas glycogen synthetase activity is decreased, thus allowing for the rapid depletion of hepatic glycogen. Phosphoenolpyruvate carboxykinase activity, the rate-limiting enzyme for gluconeogenesis, also increases during the immediate postnatal period. Thus, hormonal and enzymatic activities in the fetus provide for anabolism and substrate accretion, whereas those in the newborn period provide for the maintenance of glucose homeostasis in response to the abrupt interruption of maternal glucose supply.

Mobilization of liver glycogen stores

Prior to birth the fetus accumulates large quantities of hepatic glycogen, with these stores mobilized as glucose in the early postnatal period to sustain the newborn until the onset of suckling and gluconeogenesis. The liver acts to mobilize glycogen in the early neonatal period and gradually adjusts to the alternating supply of nutrients that results from the onset of a feeding cycle. At birth, degradation of hepatic glycogen occurs rapidly, with almost complete depletion within 12 hours in the human newborn.[67] Hepatic glycogen is converted to glucose via glucose-6-phosphatase, which is in abundant supply in the liver just prior to birth. Because of the rapid depletion of glycogen, liver glycogenolysis can only support glucose homeostasis for a short period of time and maintenance of the newborn's blood glucose levels requires active liver gluconeogenesis.

Mobilization of glycogen stores in skeletal muscle is a much longer process and due to the lack of glucose-6-phosphatase, glycogen stores can only be used by muscle itself.[68] However, lactate, formed by glycolysis, can leave muscle and be converted into glucose in the liver or oxidized by other tissues.

A number of factors initiate liver glycogenolysis at birth, however the precise mechanisms have not been completely elucidated. Glycogenolysis occurs when glycogen synthase (GS) is inactivated and glycogen phosphorylase (GP) is inactivated. The ratio of active forms of these enzymes is determined by their phosphorylation state which is mediated by cAMP. Levels of smooth endoplasmic reticulum (SER)-associated synthase phosphatase and phosphorylase phosphatase activities are diminished from high prenatal levels, contributing to these changes in activation of GS and GP.[69]

Studies using a rat strain with a deficiency of a phosphorylase b kinase have been used to assess the importance of liver glycogen in glucose homeostasis of the newborn. In normal rats the mean blood glucose concentration of the fetus measured at various times up to 24 h after natural birth ranged between 3.7 and 5.4 mM. In contrast, fetuses of the affected rats were hypoglycemic before birth (2.02 ± 0.15 mM), and by 1 h after birth the blood glucose had decreased to 0.74 ± 0.14 mM. Concentrations increased by 4 h to 1.48 ± 0.17 mM and by 24 h reached values not significantly different from the normal newborn rats. Changes in plasma insulin over the perinatal period were similar in both groups although concentrations were always significantly lower in the affected rats. The findings demonstrate the crucial role of the fetal liver glycogen store in the maintenance of normoglycemia in the newborn. Rats with the glycogen storage disorder experienced severe hypoglycemia without any apparent effects, which raises questions concerning alternative fuels available to and utilized by the newborn.[70]

At birth, the concomitant rise in glucagon and fall in plasma insulin coincide with activation of glycogen phosphorylase activity.[71–73] Injection of glucagon to the rat fetus induces a marked decrease in fetal liver glycogen content[74] and exogenous glucagon stimulates glycogenolysis in isolated fetal hepatocytes.[75] In vivo administration of insulin partially inhibits hepatic glycogenolysis, and insulin antiserum accelerates glycogen breakdown.[74]

The rapid changes in insulin and glucagon plasma concentrations that occur at birth are likely due to the considerable increase in circulating levels of catecholamines.[76–78] Since there appears to be significant glucagon resistance in the newborn, increased plasma catecholamine levels have been suggested to be the primary mediators of the sudden increase in hepatic glucose output.[78] This effect is believed to be mediated by the beta-adrenergic-cAMP signal transduction system. Removal of the adrenal glands in the fetal sheep results in low blood glucose values in the newborn, which fail to rise.[79] However, newborn rats adrenalectomized at birth show normal hepatic glycogenolysis.[74] These conflicting results may be due to species differences or differences in experimental design.

The autonomic nervous system is involved in the regulation of hepatic glucose metabolism in the adult and may also contribute to glucose homeostasis in the newborn. It has been demonstrated that electrical stimulation of the vagus nerves induces activation of the liver enzyme glycogen synthase, which in turn increases glycogen synthesis and reduces glucose output.[80] Conversely, electrical stimulation of the splanchnic nerve induces activation of the liver enzyme glycogen phosphorylase, which in turn increases glycogenolysis and glucose output.[81] Vagal blockade acutely modulates hepatic glucose production by inhibiting glycogenolysis in awake fasted dogs.[82] Taken together, these data have been interpreted to suggest that activation of the parasympathetic nervous system promotes glucose uptake and hepatic glycogen deposition while activation of the sympathetic nervous system promotes glycogenolysis and glucose output.

Development and regulation of gluconeogenesis

After birth, with the loss of the continuous umbilical glucose supply, the newborn must eventually rely on gluconeogenesis (GNG) to maintain glucose homeostasis. Of the four gluconeogenic enzymes present in liver (pyruvate carboxylase, phosphoenolpyruvate carboxykinase, fructose-1, 6-bisphosphatase and glucose-6-phosphatase), pyruvate carboxylase and phosphoenolpyruvate carboxykinase are present in the liver at negligible levels before birth but appear rapidly after birth, consistent with the onset of gluconeogenesis.[83–85]

The pathway of gluconeogenesis is shown in Figure 11.1. The formation of glucose from pyruvate involves the entry of pyruvate into the mitochondria, where it is converted by pyruvate carboxylase into oxaloacetate. The latter is a common intermediate for GNG and oxidation in the tricarboxylic cycle. The oxaloacetate exits the mitochondria via malate and is converted to phosphoenolpyruvate (PEP) by phosphoenolpyruvate carboxykinase (PEPCK). PEP is then converted via a number of steps into fructose 1, 6-biphosphate, which is the precursor for fructose-6-phosphate, a reaction catalyzed by fructose 1, 6-biphosphatase. Glucose-6-phosphatase catalyzes the conversion of glucose-6-phosphate into glucose. The above four enzymatic reactions are irreversible and absence or mutations in these enzymes (pyruvate carboxylase, PEPCK, fructose 1, 6-biphosphatase, glucose-6-phosphatase) results in the inhibition of GNG with the subsequent development of hypoglycemia.

Pyruvate carboxylase

There are two tissue-specific promoters responsible for the production of multiple transcripts with 5′-end heterogeneity for rat pyruvate carboxylase.[86] The abundance of PC mRNAs is low in fetal rat, sheep and guinea pig liver but increases by 2–4-fold within 7 days after birth, concomitant with an 8-fold increase in the amount of immunoreactive PC and its activity and then decreases to adult levels during the weaning period.[39,41,87–89] The mechanisms that control the production of PC during postnatal development are unknown but are potentially complicated, involving switching of two promoters.[87] The transcript generated from the proximal promoter is the major form that is increased during the suckling period, concomitant with an increased amount of PC and its activity. During this period gluconeogenesis occurs at the highest rate. This suggests that the proximal promoter of the PC gene is activated to supply the demand of cells producing PC to fully participate in gluconeogenesis during such a period. However, during the weaning period and in adults, when the gluconeogenic rate has decreased, the proximal promoter activity decreases.[87] Increase in glucagon and catecholamine and fall in insulin levels at birth increased PC expression whereas increased insulin levels during weaning represses PC transcription.[90] Insulin selectively inhibits the expression of the proximal promoter of rat PC.[86]

Phosphoenol pyruvate carboxykinase

PEPCK is the last gluconeogenic enzyme to be expressed in liver development and is rate limiting in the liver's capacity for gluconeogenesis at this time. The hormonal factors that coordinate the complex pattern of development of these processes are only partly understood. In fetal sheep, the ontogenic increments in hepatic PEPCK activity are dependent on the prepartum cortisol surge.[41] The increases in PEPCK seen close to term are prevented by fetal adrenalectomy, and are stimulated prematurely by an exogenous infusion of cortisol earlier in gestation.[41] PEPCK can be activated in rat fetuses by increasing the glucagon/insulin ratio to a state that is similar to that which prevails at birth,[74] injecting fetuses with either cAMP[91] or agents that reduce insulin, such as streptozotocin or anti-insulin serum.[92,93] Furthermore, the chromatin conformation of the PEPCK gene in the liver undergoes a gradual transition from a "compact" conformation on day 19 of gestation to an "open" conformation just prior to the initiation of its transcription at birth.[94] Injecting 19-day fetal rats with Bt2cAMP induces both this process and the expression of the gene for PEPCK in the fetal liver.[94]

The regulator sites for control of PEPCK gene expression are localized within a region between −500 and +73

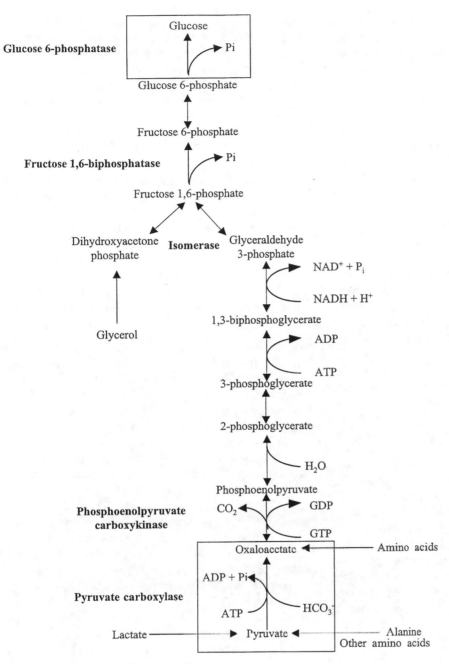

Figure 11.1. Reactions of gluconeogenesis.

base pairs of the PEPCK promoter. The activation of PEPCK gene transcription at birth correlates with the late appearing transcription factors from the C/EBP family.[94–97] However, in addition to activation, other data imply that the hepatic gene transcription might be repressed prior to birth.[98,99] Recent studies suggest that two mechanisms regulate the correct onset of hepatic PEPCK gene expression after birth: (a) activation of the gene expression by distinct liver-enriched transcription factors which, in turn, appear relatively late in development; (b) prevention of a premature onset of expression, via specific regulatory sequences and their cognate transcription factors.[100]

Glucose-6-phosphatase

Hepatic glucose-6-phosphatase (G6P) system catalyzes the last step of both gluconeogenesis and glycogenolysis and plays a pivotal role in the maintenance and regulation of blood glucose levels. G6Pase is tightly associated with the endoplasmic reticulum and the nuclear membranes of both liver and kidney.[101] Since the G6Pase active site faces the ER lumen glucose-6-phosphate must be transported from the cytoplasm across the ER membranes before hydrolysis can occur.[102,103] A recent study indicates that the orientation of the catalytic subunit is different in the fetal liver in comparison with the adult form. It appears that the components of the glucose-6-phosphatase system are already present, although to a lower extent, in fetal liver, but they are functionally uncoupled by the extravesicular orientation of the catalytic subunit.[104]

Studies in 250 human fetal liver biopsy samples have determined that G6P enzyme activity develops at 11 weeks' gestation and slowly increases to approximately 10% of adult activity at term. In the first week after birth, activity rises to adult values. Increases in enzyme activity coincide with increasing concentrations of the G6P enzyme protein. The phosphate/pyrophosphate transport protein of the human hepatic G6P complex develops at a different rate from that of the enzyme.[105]

Several factors can contribute to the fetal-to-neonatal transition of the glucose-6-phosphatase system. The postnatal drop in plasma glucose levels and the consequently high glucagon/insulin ratio may have a primary role.[106] It has also been reported that dibutyryl cyclic AMP stimulates the transcription of the glucose-6-phosphatase gene in cultured fetal hepatocytes.[106] In this same study, long chain fatty acids contributed to the induction of G6Pase by the stabilization of the transcript.[106] However, the rise in the amount of mRNA and enzyme protein is lower than the dramatic elevation of the activity,[107] indicating that other, post-transcriptional factors can also affect the protein(s) of the glucose-6-phosphatase system around the birth. Intraperitoneal administration of thyroid hormones to the rat fetus accelerates the normal maturational increase in hepatic G6P activity.[108] A recent study suggests that T3 may be primarily responsible for the cortisol-induced rise in G6P enzyme activity in fetal sheep liver.[109] It remains to be determined as to whether similar factors induce G6Pase activity and expression in the human.

Gluconeogenic substrates

The contribution of exogenous glucose supplied via the milk to neonatal glucose requirements can be measured with stable or radioactive tracers. Methodology and application of these techniques in the newborn have been thoroughly reviewed by Kalhan and Parimi.[110] Glucose obtained from hydrolysis of lactose provides approxi-

mately 6.1 g kg^{-1} day^{-1} of glucose, which is approximately 20–50% of the estimated glucose requirements of the newborn.[111,112] Of the remaining gluconeogenic substrates, galactose provides the largest amount, with smaller amounts available from lactate, amino acids and glycerol.[113] Galactose is actively transported by the enterocyte by the sodium-coupled glucose transporter SGLUT1 [114] and delivered to the liver where it is mainly converted to glucose by glucose-6-phosphatase.[115] Uptake is independent of insulin concentration, and clearance is very rapid compared with that of glucose: 6.9% disappearance per minute compared with 1.4% per minute.[116]

Human newborns can metabolize galactose rapidly which is accompanied by a rise in blood glucose, consistent with conversion of galactose to glucose.[117] Incubation of fetal and neonatal liver slices with galactose leads to rapid incorporation of glycogen in rats and sheep.[118] Galactose also affects glycogen metabolism in fetal and neonatal rats and monkeys by activating glycogen synthase.[119,120]

Glycerol

The initial step of glycerol metabolism is phosphorylation to glycerol-3-phosphate catalyzed by glycerol kinase. The development of glycerol kinase before and after birth has been investigated in liver and kidney of rat and hamster. In rat liver, enzyme activity increases very slowly before birth and rapidly thereafter, reaching adult values at day 6 of postnatal life. In hamster liver, glycerol kinase was considerably elevated already in utero, increased dramatically within day 1 of postnatal life and reached adult values at the end of the first week.[121] These studies also indicate that the first step of gluconeogenesis from glycerol in liver and kidney is not influenced by glucagon, insulin and glucocorticoids, which are generally believed to regulate the rate of gluconeogenesis from non-glycerol precursors, but probably by the change in blood glycerol concentration.[121]

Tracer studies performed in normal newborn infants have estimated that glycerol accounts for approximately 10–20% of systemic glucose production.[122–126] Glycerol may also be used as a substrate for gluconeogenesis in preterm infants, although in this particular study, the infants were receiving intravenous glucose.[126]

Lactate and pyruvate

Until recently GNG has only been estimated indirectly in the human newborn by quantifying the glucose carbon recycling. However, methods have now been developed to measure GNG directly in the newborn using the method of deuterium labeling of body water.[127,128] The deuterium incorporation in the hydrogens of C-6 of glucose quantifies the contribution of pyruvate to glucose and does not include the contribution of glycerol.[127,128] Kalhan *et al.* [129] quantified the rate of glucose turnover (Ra) and gluconeogenesis via pyruvate 4 by use of [^{13}C6]glucose and ^{2}H$_2$O in full-term healthy babies between 24 and 48 h after birth and in low-birth-weight infants on days 3 and 5. The contribution of GNG to glucose production was measured by the appearance of ^{2}H on C-6 of glucose. Glucose Ra in full-term babies was 30 ± 1.7 (SD) μmol kg^{-1} min^{-1}. Gluconeogenesis via pyruvate contributed $\sim 31\%$ to glucose Ra. These estimates are of a similar magnitude to those seen in normal healthy adults after an overnight fast.[130,131] In an additional group of infants, lactate turnover and its incorporation into glucose were measured within 4–24 h of birth by use of [^{13}C3]lactate tracer. The rate of lactate turnover was 38 μmol kg^{-1} min^{-1}, and lactate C, not corrected for loss of tracer in the tricarboxylic acid cycle, contributed $\sim 18\%$ to glucose C. There was a large contribution of GNG to glucose production in preterm babies as well, even when the endogenous rate of glucose production was low, e.g. infants infused with glucose plus amino acids with or without lipids. It is of interest that, in these babies also, GNG via pyruvate contributed 20–40% to endogenous production of glucose.[129]

GNG from lactate is apparent soon after birth in the healthy newborn infant and it contributes $\sim 30\%$ of the total glucose produced.[129] The Ra of lactate turnover was almost 2-fold the Ra of glucose turnover. This is in contrast to the data in adults,[132–134] in which lactate turnover has been reported to be much lower than the rate of glucose turnover (in lactate equivalents). The investigators suggest that the high turnover in lactate indicates either a rapid rate of equilibrium of the tracer between various compartments of lactate (plus pyruvate plus alanine) in babies or an influx of carbon into the lactate pool from non-glucose sources, e.g. amino acids.

Alanine

Only one study has measured the contribution of alanine to glucose production in the human newborn.[135] Frazer *et al.* estimated the rate of alanine turnover and its contribution to gluconeogenesis from [2, 3-^{13}C2]alanine in the human neonate by determination of ^{13}C2 enrichment in blood glucose during the constant infusion of tracer [2, 3-^{13}C2]alanine between 4 and 8 h of postnatal age. Alanine flux, calculated from the steady-state blood [2, 3-^{13}C2]alanine enrichment, was 16.6 +/−

1.3 (SE) μmol kg^{-1} min^{-1}. At 8 h of age, 9.3 +/− 2.3% of blood glucose was derived from alanine.

REFERENCES

1 Hay, W. W. Jr, Sparks, J. W., Quissell, B. J., Battaglia, F. C., Meschia, G.. Simultaneous measurements of umbilical uptake, fetal utilization rate, and fetal turnover rate of glucose. *Am. J. Physiol.* 1981;**240**:E662–8.

2 Hay, W. W. Jr, Myers, S. A., Sparks, J. W. *et al.* Glucose and lactate oxidation rates in the fetal lamb. *Proc. Soc. Exp. Biol. Med.* 1983;**173**:553–63.

3 Aynsley-Green, A., Soltesz, G., Jenkins, P. A., Mackenzie, I. Z. The metabolic and endocrine milieu of the human fetus at 18–21 weeks of gestation. II. Blood glucose, lactate, pyruvate and ketone body concentrations. *Biol. Neonate* 1985;**47**:19–25.

4 Bozzetti, P., Ferrari, M. M., Marconi, A. M. *et al.* The relationship of maternal and fetal glucose concentrations in the human from midgestation until term. *Metabolism* 1988;**37**:358–63.

5 James, E. J., Raye, J. R., Gresham, E. L. *et al.* Fetal oxygen consumption, carbon dioxide production, and glucose uptake in a chronic sheep preparation. *Pediatrics* 1972;**50**:361–71.

6 Goodner, C. J., Conway, M. J., Werrbach, J. H. Relation between plasma glucose levels of mother and fetus during maternal hyperglycemia, hypoglycemia, and fasting in the rat. *Pediatr. Res.* 1969;**3**:121–7.

7 Bossi, E., Greenberg, R. E. Sources of blood glucose in the rat fetus. *Pediatr. Res.* 1972;**6**:765–72.

8 Kalhan, S. C., D'Angelo, L. J., Savin, S. M., Adam, P. A. Glucose production in pregnant women at term gestation. Sources of glucose for the human fetus. *J. Clin. Invest.* 1979;**63**:388–94.

9 Anand, R. S., Ganguli, S., Sperling, M. A. Effect of insulin induced maternal hypoglycemia on glucose turnover in maternal and fetal sheep. *Am. J. Physiol.* 1980;**238**:E524–32.

10 Hay, W. W. Jr, Sparks, J. W., Wilkening, R. B., Battaglia, F. C., Meschia, G. Fetal glucose uptake and utilization as functions of maternal glucose concentration. *Am. J. Physiol.* 1984;**246**:E237–42.

11 Battaglia, F. C., Meschia, G. Foetal and placental metabolisms: their interrelationship and impact upon maternal metabolism. *Proc. Nutr. Soc.* 1981;**40**:99–113.

12 Hauguel, S., Desmaizieres, V., Challier, J. C. Glucose uptake, utilization, and transfer by the human placenta as functions of maternal glucose concentration. *Pediatr. Res.* 1986;**20**:269–73.

13 Boyle, D. W., Lecklitner, S., Liechty, E. A. Effect of prolonged uterine blood flow reduction on fetal growth in sheep. *Am. J. Physiol.* 1996;**270**:R246–53.

14 Gardner, D. S., Giussani, D. A. Enhanced umbilical blood flow during acute hypoxemia after chronic umbilical cord compression: a role for nitric oxide. *Circulation* 2003;Epub: Jun 30.

15 Lueder, F. L., Ogata, E. S. Uterine artery ligation in the maternal rat alters fetal tissue glucose utilization. *Pediatr. Res.* 1990;**28**:464–8.

16 Takata, K.. Localization of erythrocyte/HepG2-type glucose transporter (GLUT-1) in human placental villi. *Cell Tissue Res.* 1992;**267**:407–12.

17 Jansson, T., Wennergren, M., Illsley, N. P. Glucose transporter protein expression in human placenta throughout gestation and in intrauterine growth retardation. *J. Clin. Endocrinol. Metab.* 1993;**77**:1554–62.

18 Jansson, T., Ekstrand, Y., Wennergren, M., Powell, T. L. Placental glucose transport in gestational diabetes mellitus. *Am. J. Obstet. Gynecol.* 2001;**184**:111–16.

19 Arnott, G., Coghill, G., McArdle, H. J., Hundal, H. S. Immunolocalization of GLUT1 and GLUT3 glucose transporters in human placenta. *Biochem. Soc. Trans.* 1994;**22**:272S.

20 Illsley, N. P. Glucose transporters in the human placenta. *Placenta* 2000;**21**:14–22.

21 Teasdale, F., Jean-Jacques, G. Intrauterine growth retardation: morphometry of the microvillous membrane of the human placenta. *Placenta* 1988;**9**:47–55.

22 Schneider, H., Reiber, W., Sager, R., Malek, A. Asymmetrical transport of glucose across the in vitro perfused human placenta. *Placenta* 2003;**24**:27–33.

23 Molina, R. D., Meschia, G., Battaglia, F. C., Hay, W. W. Jr. Gestational maturation of placental glucose transfer capacity in sheep. *Am. J. Physiol.* 1991;**261**:R697–704.

24 Takata, K., Hirano, H. Mechanism of glucose transfer across the human and rat placental barrier: a review. *Micros. Res. Tech.* 1997;**38**:145–52.

25 Leach, L., Firth, J. A. Advances in understanding permeability in fetal capillaries of the human placenta: a review of organization of the endothelial paracellular clefts and their junctional complexes. *Reprod. Fert. Dev.* 1995;**7**:1451–6.

26 Eaton, B. M., Leach, L., Firth, J. A. Permeability of the fetal villous microvasculature in the isolated perfused term human placenta. *J. Physiol.* 1993;**463**: 141–55.

27 Leach, L., Firth, J. A. Structure and permeability of human placental microvasculature. *Micros. Res. Tech.* 1997;**38**:137–44.

28 Burton, G. J., Palmer, M. E., Dalton, K. J. Morphometric differences between the placental vasculature of non-smokers, smokers and ex-smokers. *Br. J. Obstet. Gynaecol.* 1989;**96**: 907–15.

29 Mayhew, T. M., Jackson, M. R., Haas, J. D. Microscopical morphology of the human placenta and its effects on oxygen diffusion: a morphometric model. *Placenta* 1986;**7**:121–31.

30 Mayhew, T. M., Sorensen, F. B., Klebe, J. G., Jackson, M. R. Growth and maturation of villi in placentae from well-controlled diabetic women. *Placenta* 1994;**15**:57–65.

31 Teasdale, F. Histomorphometry of the human placenta in maternal preeclampsia. *Am. J. Obstet. Gynecol.* 1985;**152**: 25–31.

32 Teasdale, F. Histomorphometry of the human placenta in preeclampsia associated with severe intrauterine growth retardation. *Placenta* 1987;**8**:119–28.

33 Anand, R. S., Sperling, M. A., Ganguli, S., Nathanielsz, P. W. Bidirectional placental transfer of glucose and its turnover in fetal and maternal sheep. *Pediatr. Res.* 1979;**13**:783–87.

34 Hay, W. W. Jr. Regulation of placental metabolism by glucose supply. *Reprod. Fertil. Dev.* 1995;**7**:365–75.

35 Owens, J. A., Falconer, J., Robinson, J. S. Glucose metabolism in pregnant sheep when placental growth is restricted. *Am. J. Physiol.* 1989;**257**:R350–7.

36 Fowden, A. L., Mundy, L., Silver, M. Developmental regulation of glucogenesis in the sheep fetus during late gestation. *J. Physiol.* 1998;**508**:937–47.

37 Kalhan, S. C., D'Angelo, L. J., Savin, S. M., Adam, P. A. Glucose production in pregnant women at term gestation. Sources of glucose for human fetus. *J. Clin. Invest.* 1979;**63**:388–94.

38 Mersmann, H. J. Glycolytic and gluconeogenic enzyme levels in pre- and postnatal pigs. *Am. J. Physiol.* 1971;**220**: 1297–302.

39 Jones, C. T., Ashton, I. K. The appearance, properties, and functions of gluconeogenic enzymes in the liver and kidney of the guinea pig during fetal and early neonatal development. *Arch. Biochem. Biophys.* 1976;**174**:506–22.

40 Fowden, A. L., Mijovic, J., Ousey, J. C., McGladdery, A., Silver, M. The development of gluconeogenic enzymes in the liver and kidney of fetal and newborn foals. *J. Dev. Physiol.* 1992;**18**: 137–42.

41 Fowden, A. L., Mijovic, J., Silver, M. The effects of cortisol on hepatic and renal gluconeogenic enzyme activities in the sheep fetus during late gestation. *J. Endocrinol.* 1993;**137**:213–22.

42 Capkova, A., Jirasek, J. E. Glycogen reserves in organs of human fetuses in the first half of pregnancy. *Biol. Neonat.* 1968;**13**:129–42.

43 Devi, B. G., Habeebullah, C. M., Gupta, P. D. Glycogen metabolism during human liver development. *Biochem. Int.* 1992;**28**:229–37.

44 Shelley, H. J. Blood sugars and tissue carbohydrate in fetal and infant lambs and rhesus monkeys. *J. Physiol.* 1960;**153**:527.

45 Shelley, H. J. Glycogen reserves and their changes at birth and in anoxia. *Br. Med. Bull.* 1961;**17**:137.

46 Whelan, W. J. The initiation of glycogen synthesis. *Bioessays* 1986;**5**:136–40.

47 Lomako, J., Lomako, W. M., Whelan, W. J. Proglycogen: a low-molecular-weight form of muscle glycogen. *FEBS Lett.* 1991;**279**:223–8.

48 Hahn, D., Blaschitz, A., Korgun, E. T. *et al.* From maternal glucose to fetal glycogen: expression of key regulators in the human placenta. *Mole. Hum. Reprod.* 2001;**12**:1173–8.

49 Katz, J., McGarry, J. D. The glucose paradox. Is glucose a substrate for liver metabolism? *J. Clin. Invest.* 1984;**74**:1901–9.

50 Magnusson, I., Chandramouli, V., Schumann, W. C. *et al.* Quantitation of the pathways of hepatic glycogen formation on ingesting a glucose load. *J. Clin. Invest.* 1987;**80**:1748–54.

51 Bourbon, J., Gilbert, M. Role of fetal insulin in glycogen metabolism in the liver of the rat fetus. *Biol. Neonate* 1981;**40**:38–45.

52 Plas, C., Forest, N., Pringault, E., Menuelle, P. Contribution of glucose and gluconeogenic substrates to insulin-stimulated glycogen synthesis in cultured fetal hepatocytes. *J. Cell Physiol.* 1982;**113**:475–80.

53 Bismut, H., Plas, C. Role of serine biosynthesis and its utilization in the alternative pathway from glucose to glycogen during the response to insulin in cultured foetal-rat hepatocytes. *Biochem. J.* 1991;**276**:577–82.

54 Zheng, Q., Levitsky, L. L., Fan, J., Ciletti, N., Mink, K. Glycogenesis in the cultured fetal and adult rat hepatocyte is differently regulated by medium glucose. *Pediatr. Res.* 1992;**32**:714–18.

55 Cetin, I., Fennessey, P. V., Sparks, J. W., Meschia, G., Battaglia, F. C. Fetal serine fluxes across fetal liver, hindlimb, and placenta in late gestation. *Am. J. Physiol.* 1992;**263**:E786–93.

56 Levitsky, L. L., Paton, J. B., Fisher, D. E. Precursors to glycogen in ovine fetuses. *Am. J. Physiol.* 1988;**255**:E743–7.

57 Plas, C., Nunez, J. Role of cortisol on the glycogenolytic effect of glucagon and on the glycogenic response to insulin in fetal hepatocyte culture. *J. Biol. Chem.* 1976;**251**:1431–7.

58 Gruppuso, P. A., Brautigan, D. L. Induction of hepatic glycogenesis in the fetal rat. *Am. J. Physiol.* 1989;**256**:E49–54.

59 Girard, J. R., Ferre, P., Gilbert, M. *et al.* Fetal metabolic response to maternal fasting in the rat. *Am. J. Physiol.* 1977;**232**:E456–63.

60 Freemark, M. Epidermal growth factor stimulates glycogen synthesis in fetal rat hepatocytes: comparison with the glycogenic effects of insulin-like growth factor I and insulin. *Endocrinology* 1986;**119**:522–6.

61 Plas, C., Duval, D. Dexamethasone binding sites and steroid-dependent stimulation of glycogenesis by insulin in cultured fetal hepatocytes. *Endocrinology* 1986;**118**:587–94.

62 Menuelle, P., Binoux, M., Plas, C. Regulation by insulin-like growth factor (IGF) binding proteins of IGF-II-stimulated glycogenesis in cultured fetal rat hepatocytes. *Endocrinology* 1995;**136**:5305–10.

63 Lopez, M. F., Dikkes, P., Zurakowski, D., Villa-Komaroff, L., Majzoub, J. A. Regulation of hepatic glycogen in the insulin-like growth factor II-deficient mouse. *Endocrinology* 1999;**140**:1442–8.

64 Rannels, S. R., Liu, L., Weaver, T. E. Expression of glycogen phosphorylase isozymes in developing rat lung. *Am. J. Physiol.* 1997;**273**:L389–94.

65 Maniscalco, W. M., Wilson, C. M., Gross, I. *et al.* Development of glycogen and phospholipid metabolism in fetal and newborn rat lung. *Biochim. Biophys. Acta* 1978;**530**:333–46.

66 Srinivasan, G., Pildes, R. S., Cattamanchi, G., Voora, S, Lilien, L. D. Plasma glucose values in normal neonates: a new look. *J. Pediatr.* 1986;**109**:114–17.

67 Shelley, H. J., Neligan, G. A. Neonatal hypoglycaemia. *Br. Med. Bull.* 1966;**22**:34–9.

68 Shelley, H. J. Carbohydrate metabolism in the foetus and the newly born. *Proc. Nutr. Soc.* 1969;**28**:42–9.

69 Margolis, R. N., Tanner, K. Glycogen metabolism in neonatal liver of the rat. *Arch. Biochem. Biophys.* 1986;**249**:605–10.

70 Gain, K. R., Malthus, R., Watts, C. Glucose homeostasis during the perinatal period in normal rats and rats with a glycogen storage disorder. *J. Clin. Invest.* 1981;**67**:1569–73.

71 Biondi, R., Viola-Magni, M.P. Regulatory mechanisms of hepatic phosphorylase in fetal and neonatal livers of rats. *Am. J. Physiol.* 1977;**232**:E370–4.

72 Kawai, Y., Arinze, I. J. Activation of glycogenolysis in neonatal liver. *J. Biol. Chem.* 1981;**256**:853–8.

73 Margolis, R. N. Hepatic glycogen synthase phosphatase and phosphorylase phosphatase activities are increased in obese (fa/fa) hyperinsulinemic Zucker rats: effects of glyburide administration. *Life Sci.* 1987;**41**:2615–22.

74 Girard, J. R., Caquet, D., Bal, D., Guillet, I. Control of rat liver phosphorylase, glucose-6-phosphatase and phosphoenolpyruvate carboxykinase activities by insulin and glucagon during the perinatal period. *Enzyme* 1973;**15**:272–85.

75 Plas, C., Nunez, J. Glycogenolytic response to glucagon of cultured fetal hepatocytes. Refractoriness following prior exposure to glucagon. *J. Biol. Chem.* 1975;**250**:5304–11.

76 Ktorza, A., Bihoreau, M. T., Nurjhan, N., Picon, L., Girard, J. Insulin and glucagon during the perinatal period: secretion and metabolic effects on the liver. *Biol. Neonate* 1985;**48**:204–20.

77 Padbury, J. F., Diakomanolis, E. S., Hobel, C. J., Perelman, A., Fisher, D. A. Neonatal adaptation: sympatho-adrenal response to umbilical cord cutting. *Pediatr. Res.* 1981;**15**:1483–87.

78 Padbury, J. F., Polk, D. H., Newnham, J. P., Lam, R. W. Neonatal adaptation: greater sympathoadrenal response in preterm than full-term fetal sheep at birth. *Am. J. Physiol.* 1985;**248**:E443–9.

79 Padbury, J. F., Ludlow, J. K., Ervin, M. G., Jacobs, H. C., Humme, J. A. Thresholds for physiological effects of plasma catecholamines in fetal sheep. *Am. J. Physiol.* 1987;**252**:E530–7.

80 Shimizu, T. Regulation of glycogen metabolism in the liver by autonomic nervous system. Activation of glycogen synthetase by vagal stimulation. *Biochim. Biophys. Acta* 1971;**252**:28–38.

81 Shimizu, T., Fukuda, A. Increased activities of glycogenolytic enzymes in liver after splanchnic-nerve stimulation. *Science* 1965;**150**:1607–8.

82 Cardin, S., Walmsley, K., Neal, D. W., Williams, P. E., Cherrington, A. D. Involvement of the vagus nerves in the regulation of basal hepatic glucose production in conscious dogs. *Am. J. Physiol. Endocrinol. Metab.* 2002;**283**:E958–64.

83 Stevenson, R. E., Morriss, F. H. Jr, Adcock, E. W. 3rd, Howell, R. R. Development of gluconeogenic enzymes in fetal sheep liver and kidney. *Dev. Biol.* 1976;**52**:167–72.

84 Marsac, C., Augereau, C., Boue, J., Vidailhet, M. Antenatal diagnosis of pyruvate-carboxylase deficiency. *Lancet* 1981;**1**:675.

85 Greengard, O. Enzymic differentiation of human liver: comparison with the rat model. *Pediatr. Res.* 1977;**11**:669–76.

86 Jitrapakdee, S., Booker, G. W., Cassady, A. I., Wallace, J. C. The rat pyruvate carboxylase gene structure. Alternate promoters

generate multiple transcripts with the 5′-end heterogeneity. *J. Biol. Chem.* 1997;**272**:20522–30.

87 Jitrapakdee, S., Gong, Q., MacDonald, M. J., Wallace, J. C. Regulation of rat pyruvate carboxylase gene expression by alternate promoters during development, in genetically obese rats and in insulin-secreting cells. Multiple transcripts with 5′-end heterogeneity modulate translation. *J. Biol. Chem.* 1998;**273**:34422–8.

88 Rolph, T. P., Jones, C. T. Delayed development of gluconeogenic capacity and the appearance of hypoglycaemia in the newborn guinea-pig after intra-uterine growth restriction. *J. Dev. Physiol.* 1982;**4**:1–21.

89 Chang, L. O. The development of pyruvate carboxylase in rat liver mitochondria. *Pediatr. Res.* 1977;**11**:6–8.

90 Lynch, C. J., McCall, K. M., Billingsley, M. L. *et al.* Pyruvate carboxylase in genetic obesity. *Am. J. Physiol.* 1992;**262**:E608–18.

91 Hanson, R. W., Reshef, L., Ballard, J. Hormonal regulation of hepatic P-enolpyruvate carboxykinase (GTP) during development. *Fed. Proc.* 1975;**34**:166–71.

92 Mencher, D., Shouval, D., Reshef, L. Premature appearance of hepatic phosphoenolpyruvate carboxykinase in fetal rats, not mediated by adenosine 3′:5′-monophosphate. *Eur. J. Biochem.* 1979;**102**:489–95.

93 Mencher, D., Cohen, H., Benvenisty, N., Meyuhas, O., Reshef, L. Primary activation of cytosolic phosphoenolpyruvate carboxykinase gene in fetal rat liver and the biogenesis of its mRNA. *Eur. J. Biochem.* 1984;**141**:199–203.

94 Benvenisty, N., Reshef, L. Developmental acquisition of DNase I sensitivity of the phosphoenolpyruvate carboxykinase (GTP) gene in rat liver. *Proc. Natl. Acad. Sci. USA* 1987;**84**:1132–6.

95 Birkenmeier, E. H., Gwinn, B., Howard, S. *et al.* Tissue-specific expression, developmental regulation, and genetic mapping of the gene encoding CCAAT/enhancer binding protein. *Genes Dev.* 1989;**3**;1146–56.

96 Descombes, P., Schibler, U. A liver-enriched transcriptional activator protein, LAP, and a transcriptional inhibitory protein, LIP, are translated from the same mRNA. *Cell* 1991;**67**:569–79.

97 Croniger, C., Trus, M., Lysek-Stupp, C. *et al.* Role of the iso-forms of CCAAT/enhancer-binding protein in the initiation of phosphoenolpyruvate carboxykinase (GTP) gene transcription at birth. *J. Biol. Chem.* 1997;**272**:26306–12.

98 Friedman, A. D., Landschultz, W. H., McKnight, S. L. CCAAT/enhancer binding protein activates the promoter of the serum albumin gene in cultured hepatoma cells. *Genes Dev.* 1989;**3**:767–76.

99 Yanuka-Kashles, O., Cohen, H., Trus, M. *et al.* Transcriptional regulation of the phosphoenolpyruvate carboxykinase gene by cooperation between hepatic nuclear factors. *Mol. Cell Biol.* 1994;**14**:7124–33.

100 Cassuto, H., Aran, A., Cohen, H., Eisenberger, C. L., Reshef, L. Repression and activation of transcription of phosphoenolpyruvate carboxykinase gene during liver development. *FEBS Lett.* 1999;**457**:441–4.

101 Nordlie, R. C., Stepanik, P. A., Traxinger, R. R. Comparative reactivity of carbamyl phosphate and glucose 6-phosphate with the glucose-6-phosphatase of intact microsomes. *Biochim. Biophys. Acta* 1986;**881**:300–4.

102 Nilsson, O. S., Arion, W. J., Depierre, J. W., Dallner, G., Ernster, L. Evidence for the involvement of a glucose-6-phosphate carrier in microsomal glucose-6-phosphatase activity. *Eur. J. Biochem.* 1978;**82**:627–34.

103 Pan, C. J., Lei, K. J., Annabi, B., Hemrika, W., Chou, J. Y. Transmembrane topology of glucose-6-phosphatase. *J. Biol. Chem.* 1998;**273**:6144–8.

104 Puskas, F., Marcolongo, P., Watkins, S. L. *et al.* Conformational change of the catalytic subunit of glucose-6-phosphatase in rat liver during the fetal-to-neonatal transition. *J. Biol. Chem.* 1999;**274**:117–22.

105 Burchell, A., Gibb, L., Waddell, I. D., Giles, M., Hume, R. The ontogeny of human hepatic microsomal glucose-6-phosphatase proteins. *Clin. Chem.* 1990;**36**:1633–7.

106 Girard, J., Pegorier, J. P. An overview of early post-partum nutrition and metabolism. *Biochem. Soc. Trans.* 1998;**26**:69–74.

107 Chatelain, F., Pegorier, J. P., Minassian, C. Development and regulation of glucose-6-phosphatase gene expression in rat liver, intestine, and kidney: in vivo and in vitro studies in cultured fetal hepatocytes. *Diabetes* 1998;**47**:882–9.

108 Greengard, O. Enzymic differentiation in mammalian liver injection of fetal rats with hormones causes the premature formation of liver enzymes. *Science* 1969;**163**:891–5.

109 Forhead, A. J., Poore, K. R., Mapstone, J., Fowden, A. L. Developmental regulation of hepatic and renal gluconeogenic enzymes by thyroid hormones in fetal sheep during late gestation. *J. Physiol.* 2003;**548**:941–7.

110 Kalhan, S., Parimi, P. Gluconeogenesis in the fetus and newborn. *Semin. Perinatol.* 2000;**24**:94–106.

111 Sparks, J. W. Augmentation of the glucose supply in the fetus and newborn. *Semin. Perinatol.* 1979;**3**:141–55.

112 Hay, W. J. Fetal and neonatal glucose homeostasis and their relation to the small for gestational age infant. *Semin. Perinatol.* 1984;**8**:101–16.

113 Cohn, R. M., Segal, S. Galactose metabolism and its regulation. *Metabolism* 1973;**22**:627–42.

114 Wright, E. M., Turk, E., Martin, M. G. Molecular basis for glucose-galactose malabsorption. *Cell Biochem. Biophys.* 2002;**36**:115–21.

115 Kliegman, R. M., Sparks, J. W. Perinatal galactose metabolism. *J. Pediatr.* 1985;**107**:831–41.

116 Battaglia, F. C., Sparks, J. W. Perinatal nutrition and metabolism. In Boyd, R. D. H., Battaglia, F. C., eds. *Pediatrics 2: Perinatal Medicine*. London: Butterworths; 1983: 145–71.

117 Mulligan, P. B., Schwartz, R. Hepatic carbohydrate metabolism in the genesis of neonatal hypoglycemia. *Pediatrics* 1961;**30**:125–35.

118 Ballard, F. J., Oliver, I. T. Carbohydrate metabolism in liver from fetal and neonatal sheep. *Biochem. J.* 1965;**95**:191–200.

119 Sparks, J. W., Lynch, A., Chez, R. A., Glinsmann, W. H. Glycogen regulation in isolated perfused near term monkey liver. *Pediatr. Res.* 1976;**10**:51–6.

120 Sparks, J. W., Lynch, A., Glinsmann, W. H. Regulation of rat liver glycogen synthesis and activities of glycogen cycle enzymes by glucose and galactose. *Metabolism* 1976;**25**:47–55.

121 Seitz, H. J., Porsche, E., Tarnowski, W. Glycerolkinase – a regulatory enzyme of gluconeogenesis? *Acta Biol. Med. Ger.* 1976;**35**:141–54.

122 Patel, D., Kalhan, S. Glycerol metabolism and triglyceride-fatty acid cycling in the human newborn: effect of maternal diabetes and intrauterine growth retardation. *Pediatr. Res.* 1992;**31**:52–8.

123 Bougneres, P. F., Karl, I. E., Hillman, L. S., Bier, D. M. Lipid transport in the human newborn. Palmitate and glycerol turnover and the contribution of glycerol to neonatal hepatic glucose output. *J. Clin. Invest.* 1982;**70**:262–70.

124 Sunehag, A., Ewald, U., Larsson, A., Gustafsson, J. Attenuated hepatic glucose production but unimpaired lipolysis in newborn infants of mothers with diabetes. *Pediatr. Res.* 1997;**42**:492–7.

125 Sunehag, A., Gustafsson, J., Ewald, U. Glycerol carbon contributes to hepatic glucose production during the first eight hours in healthy term infants. *Acta Paediatr.* 1996;**85**:1339–43.

126 Sunehag, A., Ewald, U., Gustafsson, J. Extremely preterm infants (<28 weeks) are capable of gluconeogenesis from glycerol on their first day of life. *Pediatr. Res.* 1996;**40**:553–7.

127 Chandramouli, V., Ekberg, K., Schumann, W. C. *et al.* Quantifying gluconeogenesis during fasting. *Am. J. Physiol. Endocrinol. Metab.* 1997;**273**: E1209–15.

128 Landau, B. R., Wahren, J., Chandramouli, V. *et al.* Use of $2H^2O$ for estimating rates of gluconeogenesis. Application to the fasted state. *J. Clin. Invest.* 1995;**95**:172–8.

129 Kalhan, S. C., Parimi, P., Van Beek, R. *et al.* Estimation of gluconeogenesis in newborn infants. *Am. J. Physiol. Endocrinol. Metab.* 2001;**281**:E991–7.

130 Haymond, M. W., Sunehag, A. L. The reciprocal pool model for the measurement of gluconeogenesis by use of [U-^{13}C]glucose. *Am. J. Physiol. Endocrinol. Metab.* 2000;**278**:E140–5.

131 Tayek, J. A., Katz, J. Glucose production, recycling, and gluconeogenesis in normals and diabetics: a mass isotopomer [U-^{13}C]glucose study. *Am. J. Physiol. Endocrinol. Metab.* 1996;**270**:E709–17.

132 Consoli, A., Kennedy, F., Miles, J., Gerich, J. Determination of Krebs cycle metabolic carbon exchange in vivo and its use to estimate the individual contributions of gluconeogenesis and glycogenolysis to overall glucose output in man. *J. Clin. Invest.* 1987;**80**:1303–10.

133 Diraison, F., Large, V., Brunengraber, H., Beylot, M. Noninvasive tracing of liver intermediary metabolism in normal subjects and in moderately hyperglycaemic NIDDM subjects. Evidence against increased gluconeogenesis and hepatic fatty acid oxidation in NIDDM. *Diabetologia* 1998;**41**:212–20.

134 Lecavalier, L., Bolli, G., Gerich, J. Glucagon-cortisol interactions on glucose turnover and lactate gluconeogenesis in normal humans. *Am. J. Physiol. Endocrinol. Metab.* 1990;**258**:E569–75.

135 Frazer, T. E., Karl, I. E., Hillman, L. S., Bier, D. M. Direct measurement of gluconeogenesis from [2,3]^{13}C2]alanine in the human neonate. *Am. J. Physiol.* 1981;**240**:E615–21.

12

Energy requirements and protein-energy metabolism and balance in preterm and term infants

Sudha Kashyap and Karl F. Schulze

Department of Pediatrics, College of Physicians and Surgeons, Columbia University, New York, NY

Energy is required for all vital functions of the body at the cellular and organ level and this need is met by the dietary intake of energy substrates. Energy produced during oxidation of nutrients is generally converted to ATP (adenosine-5-triphosphate) that, in turn, provides the energy for necessary activities when it is hydrolyzed to ADP (adenosine-5-diphosphate). In this chapter some general aspects of energy metabolism are summarized briefly. This review is followed by discussions on energy needs of term and preterm infants. Finally, protein-energy metabolism and balance with specific attention to protein-energy interaction are discussed.

The energy requirement for an individual has been defined as: the amount of energy intake from food that will balance energy expenditure and exogenous energy losses when the individual's body size and composition and physical activity profile is consistent with long-term good health. In children and pregnant or lactating women, the energy requirements also include the energy needs associated with deposition of tissues or secretion of milk consistent with good health.[1] Requirements for energy during the neonatal period when referenced to body weight are higher than any time later in life, primarily because of high rates of growth.

Energy requirements can be best understood by examining the energy balance equation: Gross Energy intake = Energy excreted + Energy expended + Energy stored. The gross energy intake is the energy provided by the diet. The energy provided by milk as determined by combustion in a bomb calorimeter is 5.65 kcal g^{-1} of protein, 3.95 kcal g^{-1} of carbohydrate and 9.25 kcal g^{-1} of fat.[2] Energy excreted is the energy lost in stool and urine. Fat accounts for most of the energy excreted in stool with small contributions from

carbohydrate and protein. The term *digestible energy* refers to gross energy intake minus the energy lost in stool. Most of the energy lost in urine is from urea. The term *metabolizable energy* refers to gross energy intake minus energy lost in stool and urine. The energy expended includes energy expenditure for basal or resting metabolism, thermoregulation, physical activity and diet-induced thermogenesis which includes a prominent contribution from the energy expended in synthesis of new tissue. Energy stored is energy stored in new tissue, mainly as fat and protein. The various components of the energy balance equation are shown in Figure 12.1.

Methods of measuring energy expenditure

Direct calorimetry estimates energy expenditure from the heat produced by the combustion of energy substrates which, in turn, is transferred directly to the environment as heat energy. The infant is placed in a thermally isolated closed system and the sum of the heat lost by radiation, convection, conduction and evaporation is then determined. Although this method has been used by some investigators,[3–5] it is impractical as it allows limited access to the infants and requires sophisticated equipment and frequent calibration.

Indirect calorimetry, the method most often used to estimate energy expenditure, determines indirectly the heat produced during oxidative metabolism by the measurement of oxygen consumption (VO$_2$) and carbon dioxide production (VCO$_2$), usually combined with estimates of protein catabolism made from urinary nitrogen excretion. VO$_2$ and VCO$_2$ are measured using open-circuit indirect

Neonatal Nutrition and Metabolism. Second Edition, ed. P. Thureen and W. Hay. Published by Cambridge University Press.

Table 12.1. Energy produced on oxidation of energy substrates and respiratory quotient.[a]

Energy substrate	Energy produced per liter of oxygen (kcal)	Respiratory quotient
Glucose[b]	5.02	1.0
Palmitate[b]	4.66	0.7
Amino acids[b]	4.17	0.81

[a]Adapted from Ferrannini.[6]

[b] Caloric value may vary according to the type of carbohydrate, fat and protein.

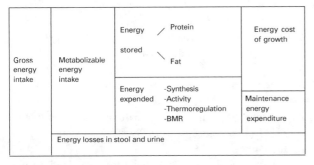

Figure 12.1. Schematic representation of the energy balance equation. BMR, basal metabolic rate.

calorimetry. The removal of oxygen from and the addition of carbon dioxide to a bias flow of gas is estimated using the Fick principle. The difference in concentration of O_2 and CO_2 when multiplied by the total flow of gas through the respiratory chamber (with some small corrections) will, assuming complete capture of exhaled gases, estimate the rate of flux of these gases into or out of the subject. In addition to estimates of total energy expenditure, it is often useful to use these measurements to calculate the rate of oxidation of the macronutrients: carbohydrate, fat and protein in the diet, as the amount of energy produced per liter of oxygen consumed differs with each macronutrient (Table 12.1). The macronutrient mix being combusted can be determined by measuring the nonprotein respiratory quotient (RQ) which is the ratio VCO_2/VO_2. The RQ for carbohydrate is 1.0, for fat 0.7 and for protein 0.8. Knowing the rate of VO_2 and VCO_2 and subtracting the amount of each due to the catabolism of protein allows one to determine the rate of energy expenditure as well as the relative proportions of fat and carbohydrate being oxidized. Measurements of energy expenditure by indirect calorimetry and by direct calorimetry have been shown to be equivalent.[7, 8]

Since this method is noninvasive and has open circuitry it allows adequate access to the infants for routine care and can be used to measure energy expenditure over long periods. Studies have suggested that 6-hour determinations of energy expenditure by indirect calorimetry can be used with acceptable accuracy to compute 24–48 hour energy balance.[9–11] This method of determining energy expenditure has limitations that have been extensively reviewed.[12,13] At desirable rates of gas flow, the measured changes in the concentration of O_2 and CO_2 are small, thus requiring highly accurate measurements of the concentrations in the inspired and expired gases. For accurate measurements of VO_2, the concentration of O_2 in the inspired gas needs to be constant. This is particularly critical for infants receiving supplemental O_2 or when making measurements in an ICU setting where oxygen is used for the treatment of nearby patients.

Doubly labeled water technique determines total energy expenditure averaged over several days. This method involves administration of a dose of two stable nontoxic, nonradioactive tracers (^2H and ^{18}O) and tracking the washout kinetics of the tracers in daily body fluid samples (urine in infants) using isotope ratio mass spectrometry. The principle is that ^2H is a tracer for water flux whereas ^{18}O is a tracer for flux of water and CO_2 combined.[14] The difference between the flux rates of the two isotopes gives an estimate of CO_2 production rate. Using the CO_2 production rate and an assumed RQ, the energy expenditure can be calculated. This method rests on several assumptions that have been critically reviewed.[15–17] Though this technique of measuring CO_2 production rate has been validated by comparison with similar measurements made by indirect calorimetry in animals,[18] human adults[19] and preterm infants,[20] the individual variability in the estimation of energy expenditure by both methods was large.[21] Concerns also have been raised in the use of this technique in extremely low birth weight (ELBW) infants in the immediate neonatal period since the method requires relatively stable total body water. Before using this technique it is recommended that all assumptions on which it is based be reviewed with special attention being paid to the peculiarities of the population under study. One should not rely on validating data from stable subjects when investigating distressed and unstable infants. The propagation of errors involved in estimating energy balance and the relatively small differences in energy storage that can, over time, be clinically important call for high standards of accuracy in all measurements.

Infrared thermographic calorimetry uses infrared scans to measure mean body surface temperature and, in conjunction with heat loss theory, estimates directly heat lost by radiation, conduction and convection and thereby determines energy expenditure. This method has recently been validated against indirect calorimetry in healthy preterm infants.[22] This method has the theoretical advantage of measuring heat loss directly.

Factors influencing energy expenditure

Age

Expressing energy expenditure per kg body weight does not take into consideration the changes in body composition that occur with age. Considerably higher rates of energy expenditure are reported in neonates than in adults (50 kcal kg^{-1} day^{-1} versus 25 kcal kg^{-1} day^{-1}). It is unclear whether the changes with age are related to age alone or are influenced by other factors that change with age like rate of growth, body composition, surface area to body mass ratio, and dietary intake. Various attempts to define the reference standard for energy expenditure have utilized many parameters of body mass and surface area, but the ease of simple measurements of weight has led to their dominant use in clinical studies.

Although it is thought that resting energy expenditure of term and preterm infants increases during the first several months of life, there are no longitudinal studies to support this. Based on cross-sectional data it has been suggested that resting energy expenditure of infants increases from birth, peaking at 2–6 months of age, and then declines.[23,24] This suggestion is supported by data from term infants studied at 3 days of age and again at 3 months of age.[25] In preterm infants also, increase in energy expenditure from the first few days of life to 5–6 weeks of age has been reported.[5,26–29] However, there is a strong suggestion from the studies in preterm infants that the increase in energy expenditure observed with age during the first few weeks of life is due to the increase in energy intake.[5,27–29]

Dietary intake

The energy expended for digestion, absorption, transportation, utilization and storage of nutrients in the diet has been referred to as the thermic effect of food, diet-induced thermogenesis (DIT), or specific dynamic action (SDA). This is generally estimated in the neonate by determining the baseline (fasting) rate of energy expenditure and then estimating the area under the curve during the postprandial rise and fall in energy expenditure. DIT is assumed to end when energy expenditure returns to baseline or when the next feed is administered. As it is not feasible to achieve a true fasting state in the infant, determina-

tions of DIT are certain to be underestimated. Diet-induced thermogenesis generally peaks 50–80 minutes after a feed in the neonate[23,30] and is estimated to increase resting energy expenditure by 10–15%.[30–33]

The magnitude of diet-induced thermogenesis has been reported to be significantly correlated with weight gain[30,33,34] and energy intake of the diet.[35–37] It is important to consider all possible energy requiring processes that comprise DIT in any given subject. For example, biochemical processes necessary for growth require oxygen as well as protein and energy. Transport of oxygen to growing or dividing cells is associated with increases in both cardiac output and minute ventilation, that are achieved primarily by increases in heart rate and respiratory rate respectively (these measurements track the metabolic rate very closely). Since these additional heart beats and breaths would not otherwise occur, the energy expended in the associated myocardial and respiratory work will be included in estimates of diet-induced thermogenesis, comprising a cardiorespiratory cost of growth. It is difficult to separate the effects of all such subtle contributions to diet-induced thermogenesis.

Since metabolic rate of adults continues to fall during days and weeks of fasting[38] it is necessarily arbitrary as to how to label this change in metabolic rate. Is this continuing withdrawal of DIT or an alteration in basal metabolic rate? The energy content of the diet has also been shown to have an effect on overall energy expenditure in addition to the immediate response seen after a feed. Higher rates of energy expenditure have been reported with higher energy intakes.[27–29,39–41] It is unclear to what extent the effect of growth, age and diet-induced thermogenesis can explain this relationship. In some of the studies, the gestational and postnatal ages were relatively well controlled,[39–41] however, infants receiving the higher energy intake had greater rates of weight gain. It is clear, however, that any comparison of rates of energy expenditure among or within subjects must take the energy and protein intake and growth rate of the infant into account.

Physical activity

In term infants it has been estimated that physical activity contributes approximately 20–25% to the total energy expenditure.[42,43] As infants grow, activity expenditure increases.[44] Since preterm infants sleep 80–90% of the time, physical activity is a smaller component of their energy expenditure. The primary effects of physical activity in these infants are those related to the sleep cycle, i.e. the rhythmic change between active (rapid eye movement: REM) and quiet (non-rapid eye movement: NREM) sleep.

Lower rates of energy expenditure during quiet sleep have been reported when compared with those of active sleep in adults,[45] term infants[46] and in preterm infants.[47] It has been estimated that physical activity contributes approximately 10% to the energy expenditure of the low birth weight infant.[5,48,49] Crying or extreme restlessness is associated with increase in energy expenditure of approximately 50–70%.[50]

Environmental temperature

Increases in energy expenditure in the neonate have been associated with environments that are too cool or too warm.[51] The changes in the energy expenditure associated with changes in environment temperature have been reported to occur promptly and may occur without any changes in core temperature.[52]

Neutral thermal environment is defined as thermal conditions under which oxygen consumption (metabolic rate) is minimal while core temperature is maintained within the normal range. Here again, there are problems in separating various contributions to overall metabolic rate. Recent evidence indicates that preterm,[53] term and young infants[54] are warmer when laying in the prone body position, yet their expenditure of energy is reduced. Does this mean that they are not thermoneutral in the supine position or is this due to a change in physical activity (quiet sleep is increased in the prone position). Maintenance of thermoneutral conditions while providing care to preterm infants will decrease their energy needs for thermoregulation, however, it is difficult to maintain a thermoneutral environment continually as infants require frequent nursing care, procedures and handling. Dietary energy intakes of 5–10 kcal kg^{-1} day^{-1} have been recommended to meet the daily cost of thermoregulation.

Size for gestational age

Though higher rates of energy expenditure have been observed by some investigators in small-for-gestational-age (SGA) infants when compared with appropriate-for-gestational-age (AGA) infants,[55,56] others have reported either no differences between the two groups of infants[57,58] or an insignificant trend toward higher energy expenditure in SGA infants.[59] There are two opposing influences impacting the metabolic rate of small-for-dates infants. First, depending on their age and diet, SGA infants will be growing at different rates than AGA infants, and the energy expended in tissue synthesis (DIT) will be correspondingly different. For example, by definition, at birth the SGA will be growing more slowly than the AGA infant and, hence, would be expected to expend less energy in tissue synthesis. This component of energy expenditure may well change during catch-up growth. Second, the question of a proper reference standard is particularly important in comparing these infants. Body weight alone is likely to be misleading as a denominator and probably should be replaced by a higher level model, including some estimate of cranial volume or body composition.

Clinical status

Increases in energy expenditure by 20–90% for up to 3 weeks have been reported in septic adults compared with controls.[60–62] Although data from infants are limited, increases in energy expenditure for the first few days in term infants with sepsis, have also been observed.[63] Though a positive correlation between VO_2 and degree of illness in neonates (gestational age 34–41 weeks) was observed by Mrozek et al., no difference was seen between the infants who were septic compared with those who were not.[64] The increase in energy expenditure in septic adults is believed to be secondary to the systemic inflammatory response.[62] The increase in heart and respiratory rates observed in septic subjects may also contribute to the increase in energy expenditure.

Although increases in energy expenditure with the increase in intensity of respiratory support[65] have been reported, decreases in energy expenditure with continous positive airway pressure (CPAP) were observed in preterm infants compared with spontaneously breathing infants of similar age.[28] No differences in respiratory rates were observed, however, the spontaneously breathing infants spent a greater amount of time in active REM sleep than infants on CPAP. In ventilated preterm infants, 25% of the VO_2 observed has been attributed to increased VO_2 of the injured lung.[66] Increased energy expenditure has also been associated with chronic lung disease.[67,68] Use of methylxanthines for apnea of prematurity has also been observed to be associated with increases in energy expenditure by some investigators[28,69,70] and not by others.[71]

In the ill preterm infants, especially those requiring various degrees of respiratory support, energy expenditure measurements are extremely difficult studies to perform using any existing measurement technique. In evaluating all clinical studies, the reader should determine to his/her satisfaction that the experimental design and methods are sound and all covariables, particularly macronutrient intake, have been identified and controlled.

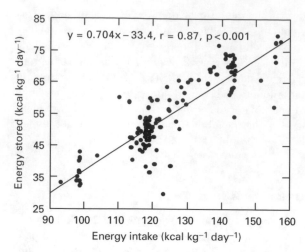

Figure 12.2. Relationship between gross energy intake and energy stored of low birth weight infants enrolled in enteral feeding studies.[41,91,92,104]

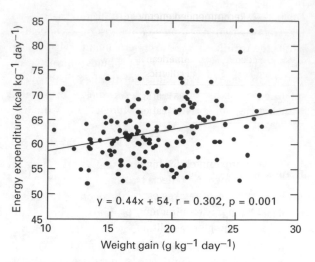

Figure 12.3. Relationship between weight gain and energy expenditure of low birth weight infants enrolled in enteral feeding studies.[41,91,92,104] The slope of the line represents the estimate of the energy required for tissue deposition or synthesis.

Energy cost of growth

The energy cost of growth comprises two components: the energy equivalent of new tissue stores added during growth and the energy expended in the process of depositing these new growth tissues. The energy equivalent of deposited tissue i.e. energy stored (ES), can be calculated as the difference between the metabolizable energy intake and energy expended. In growing low birth weight (LBW) infants, energy stored is a linear function of gross energy intake as shown in Figure 12.2. The composition of the tissue deposited as protein and fat (ignoring the small changes in carbohydrate storage) can be estimated from the nitrogen balance and ES.

Protein stored (g kg^{-1} day^{-1}) = 6.25 × Nitrogen balance (g/kg^{-1} day^{-1}). Fat stored (g kg^{-1} day^{-1}) = ES − (5.65 × protein stored)/ 9.25; where 5.65 and 9.25 are energy equivalents of a gram of protein and fat.

The energy cost of tissue deposition or synthesis cannot be determined directly. Estimates from studies of weight gain, macronutrient storage and energy expenditure in LBW infants have been derived.[5,29,36,49,72–75] As shown in Figure 12.3, the energy expenditure of a large group of growing LBW infants is strongly related to their rate of weight gain, and the slope of the line represents the estimate of the energy required for tissue deposition or synthesis. The energy cost of tissue deposition or synthesis per gram of weight gain as estimated from the regression relationship has been reported to be 0.23 to 0.68 kcal g^{-1}.[73–75]

Roberts and Young estimated energy expenditure required for deposition of protein and fat in preterm infants using pooled data from several studies to relate

metabolizable energy intake and energy expenditure to estimates of protein and fat stored. They concluded that the energy expended for protein and fat synthesis was approximately 7.75 and 1.55 kcal g^{-1} respectively.[72] Using a regression model where independent measures of all independent variables were used, Towers *et al.* reported energy expended in protein and fat synthesis to be 5.5 ± 1.1 kcal g^{-1} and 1.6 ± 0.3 kcal g^{-1}.[75] The estimates of energy cost of synthesis obtained by the above methods are several times greater than theoretical estimates made using the Atkinson's metabolic pricing system; this is especially true for protein synthesis. Many have attributed this difference to the fact that protein accretion is a dynamic, bidirectional process. Tracer studies suggest that net protein synthesis requires 5-fold turnover of tissue protein, i.e. for every gram of protein accreted, 5 g of protein is synthesized and catabolized.[76]

The energy cost of growth can be estimated from the sum of energy stored and the energy cost of tissue deposition or synthesis. In growing LBW infants, energy cost of growth can be substantial and mean values as high as 74 kcal kg^{-1} day^{-1} are reported.[75] Approximately 73% of this was stored energy as protein and fat and 27% was expended in protein and fat deposition.

Energy requirements of term infants

The energy requirements of term infants have been based on the intakes of healthy thriving infants.[77] Recommendations made by the Food and Agriculture Organization and

Table 12.2. Recommended energy intakes for preterm infants.

Recommended energy intake	American Academy of Pediatrics[83]	Canadian Pediatric Society[84]	European Society for Gastroenterology and Nutrition[87]	Life Science Research Office[86]
Minimum	105 kcal kg^{-1} day^{-1}	105 kcal kg^{-1} day^{-1}	98 kcal kg^{-1} day^{-1}	110 kcal kg^{-1} day^{-1}
Maximum	130 kcal kg^{-1} day^{-1}	135 kcal kg^{-1} day^{-1}	128 kcal kg^{-1} day^{-1}	135 kcal kg^{-1} day^{-1}

WHO are approximately 5% higher than the actual reported intakes.[1] This increase reflects the correction for assumed underestimation of intakes especially those of breast-fed infants. The energy requirements of the infants, when estimated from energy expenditure measurements made by doubly labeled water and energy stored calculated from the reference values of body composition,[78] or derived from total body fat and fat free mass gain determined by total body electrical conductivity and TOBEC,[79] have been reported to be lower than the recommended intakes. For infants 0–3 months' age, energy intakes ranging from 100–116 kcal kg^{-1} day^{-1} have been recommended.[1,80–82]

Energy requirements of preterm infants

Recommendations for energy and other nutrient intakes for preterm infants are based on the assumption that postnatal growth of these infants should be at intrauterine growth rates.[83–85] In the event it is not possible to provide these intakes initially, as may happen in the first few weeks after birth, it may be necessary to provide greater intakes to allow for catch-up growth.

Based on energy balance and growth data in the literature the Expert Panel for the American Society for Nutritional Sciences, Life Sciences Research Office recently recommended energy intakes for preterm infants in the range of 110–135 kcal kg^{-1}.[86] Similar recommendations have been made by the American Academy of Pediatrics Committee on Nutrition[83] and committees such as the Canadian Pediatric Society[84] and the European Society for Gastroenterology and Nutrition[87] and are shown in Table 12.2.

Protein–energy metabolism and balance

Protein requirements cannot be determined without considering concurrent energy intake and energy requirements cannot be determined without consideration of simultaneous protein intake. The interaction between protein and energy has been addressed in the human adult, by studying the effects of varying energy intake on nitrogen balance, effects of varying protein intake on nitrogen balance, and the effects of other nutrients on the protein–energy interaction. It has been shown that at adequate energy intakes, increasing protein intake increases nitrogen retention and at adequate protein intakes increasing energy intake also increases nitrogen retention. However, if either of the intakes are inadequate, increasing energy without increasing protein or increasing protein without increasing energy will be without benefit; i.e. for any specific nitrogen intake, there is a concomitant energy intake beyond which further increases will not further improve nitrogen retention.

Effect of varying energy and protein intake on nitrogen balance

The effect of energy intake on protein utilization has been studied extensively in animals and, to some extent, in human adults.[88–90] However, few data from human infants are available. The reported studies of the effect of concomitant energy intake on protein utilization of LBW infants suggest that the principles outlined above apply, however, they fall short of defining the quantitative aspects of this interaction.

Kashyap et al., in a series of controlled enteral feeding studies examined the effects of independent and systematic variations in the absolute amount and relative proportion of protein and energy intake on the rate and composition of weight gain and metabolic response. The importance of these studies derives from their use of specially prepared formulas with widely varying absolute amounts of protein, energy and protein-energy ratios. Taken together, the data from these prospective, randomized, double-blind studies, which typically spanned the period from full enteral intake until weight reached 2200 g, allow for reliable analysis of the separate effects of the amount and relative proportions of these macronutrients on weight gain and nitrogen retention over a wide range of intakes. The number of infants in each study cell typically numbered 9–15.

Initial studies, employing enteral protein intakes of 3.5–3.6 g kg^{-1} day^{-1} with a concomitant energy intake of either 120 or 150 kcal kg^{-1} day^{-1} demonstrated no statistically significant difference in nitrogen retention.[91] However, the blood urea nitrogen concentration and the plasma concentration of several amino acids were somewhat lower in the group that received the higher energy intake, suggesting that the higher energy intake was at least minimally beneficial in enhancing nitrogen utilization. Subsequent studies of infants at higher protein intakes of either 3.8 or 3.9 g kg^{-1} day^{-1} revealed that nitrogen retention of infants who received a concomitant energy intake of 142 kcal kg^{-1} day^{-1} was significantly higher than that of infants who received the same protein intakes with an energy intake of 120 kcal kg^{-1} day^{-1}.[41] However, at still higher protein intakes of 4.2–4.3 g kg^{-1} day^{-1}, despite the fact that urinary nitrogen excretion was lower at high energy intakes (141 kcal kg^{-1} day^{-1}), nitrogen retention of the infants was not different from those receiving the same protein intake with concomitant energy intake of 117 kcal kg^{-1} day^{-1}.[92] This raises the possibility that protein intakes greater than 4 g kg^{-1} day^{-1} may exceed the capacity of LBW infants for protein utilization regardless of accompanying energy intake or that even higher energy intake is required for significantly better utilization of such protein intakes.

The data from the same series of studies also demonstrated that the rate and composition of the weight gained by these infants was predictable from the composition of their diets. The rate of weight gain was dependent on the absolute intakes of protein and energy.[92] The multiple regression equation summarizing this relationship is:

$$\Delta Wt = 0.095 \, Ein + 3.6 \, Pin - 0.00468 \, BW + 1.699;$$

$$(r^2 = 0.62; \text{ residual error} = 3.34 \text{ g/kg}^1 \text{ day}^1)$$

where Ein is the energy intake (kcal kg^{-1} day^{-1}), Pin is protein intake (g kg^{-1} day^{-1}) and BW is the birth weight. The relative composition of the weight gained as protein stored and fat stored was dependent on the protein–energy ratio of the diet as shown in Figure 12.4.

Also, as shown in Figure 12.5, urinary nitrogen excretion and hence nitrogen retention of these LBW infants is a continuous function of the protein to energy ratio of the intake, supporting the notion that, for any given protein intake, increasing energy intake will decrease nitrogen excretion and thus improve nitrogen retention. However, since the protein–fat ratio of newly synthesized tissue parallels the protein–energy ratio of the intake, increasing energy intake will also result in greater fat deposition. Urinary nitrogen excretion is also influenced by the quality of the non-protein energy of the diet. LBW infants fed high carbohydrate diets, in a study similar to those described above, were noted to have lower urinary nitrogen excretion

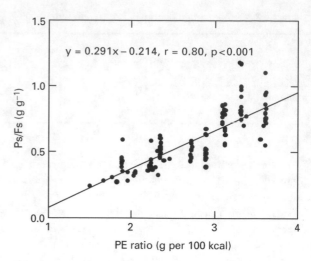

Figure 12.4. Relationship between protein energy (PE) ratio of the dietary intake and protein stored and fat stored ratio (Ps/Fs) of LBW infants enrolled in enteral feeding studies.[41,91,92,104]

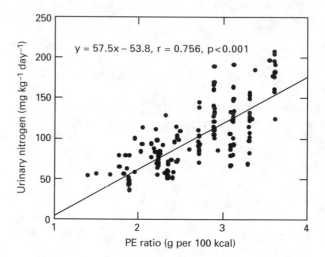

Figure 12.5. Relationship between protein energy (PE) ratio of the dietary intake and urinary nitrogen excretion of LBW infants enrolled in enteral feeding studies.[41,91,92,104]

(hence greater nitrogen retention) than infants fed high fat diets at the same protein–energy ratio.[93]

In LBW infants receiving total parenteral nutrition, Zlotkin *et al.* observed higher nitrogen retention with an amino acid intake of 3.1 g kg^{-1} day^{-1} at energy intakes of 50–60 kcal kg^{-1} day^{-1} than those reported by Anderson *et al.* in infants receiving amino acid intake of 2.5 g kg^{-1} day^{-1} at the same energy intake.[94,95] Further increasing the amino acid intake to 4g kg^{-1} day^{-1} at the same energy intake resulted in no further increase in nitrogen retention.[94] However, the utilization of both intakes of

3 and 4 g kg^{-1} day^{-1} in parenterally fed infants was greater when energy intake was 80 versus 50–60 kcal kg^{-1} day^{-1}.[94] Other investigators have also reported improved utilization of parenterally delivered amino acid intakes of 2.5–2.9 g kg^{-1} day^{-1} with concomitant energy intakes of 80–90 kcal kg^{-1} day^{-1} compared with 60–70 kcal kg^{-1} day^{-1}.[96,97]

Based on these data from LBW infants, it is not possible to precisely predict the energy intake required to assure maximal utilization of a specific protein or amino acid intake. However, it appears that energy intake of 120 kcal kg^{-1} day^{-1} is sufficient to assure near-maximal utilization of an enteral protein intake of 3.6 g kg^{-1} day^{-1}. Also, an energy intake of 80 kcal kg^{-1} day^{-1} is sufficient to assure near-maximal utilization of a parenteral amino acid intake of 2.7 g kg^{-1} day^{-1} and an energy intake of 60 kcal kg^{-1} day^{-1} is sufficient to assure reasonable utilization. From these data, it seems safe to conclude that utilization of the protein content of an enterally administered regimen will be quite efficient if the energy-protein ratio of the regimen is at least 30 kcal g^{-1} and that utilization of the amino acid content of a parenterally administered regimen will be quite efficient, although perhaps not maximally efficient, if the energy–amino acid ratio of the regimen is at least 20–25 kcal g^{-1}. These energy–protein ratios, however, may not be optimal for maximal utilization of protein and amino acid intakes outside the range of intakes from which they were calculated. Also, the ratio may be different if the distribution of energy intake between carbohydrate and fat is different from the distribution of these nutrients in the regimens for which the ratios were calculated. In this regard, there is considerable evidence that carbohydrate is more effective than fat in promoting nitrogen retention.[89,93,98] There is no apparent benefit of an energy intake much in excess of that necessary to assure utilization of the concomitant protein intake. Such intakes result simply in excessive fat deposition relative to protein deposition[40,41,73,88,99,100] or worse, at marginal protein intakes, may be associated with low albumin concentrations.[101]

Balance studies in enterally fed LBW infants have been used to estimate protein and energy requirements of these infants. A number of studies have provided considerable insight into the growth and nutrient accretion rates incident to a variety of protein intakes as well as the effects of various protein intakes on other indices of protein adequacy or excess. Thus, it is possible to define the protein intake required to achieve a variety of goals.

The American Academy of Pediatrics Committee on Nutrition,[83] the Canadian Pediatric Society[84] and the European Society of Pediatric Gastroenterology and Nutrition[85] have recommended protein intakes for preterm infants to be sufficient to support the intrauterine rate of nitrogen accretion as a goal. The protein intakes of preterm infants fed 180 ml kg^{-1} day^{-1} of either term or preterm human milk providing $\sim$ 2 g kg^{-1} day^{-1} and $\sim$2.5 g kg^{-1} day^{-1} respectively are insufficient to support the intrauterine rate of nitrogen accretion.[102–104]

Increasing nitrogen retention has been reported with increasing protein intake both in parenterally and enterally fed LBW infants.[94,105,106] In healthy enterally fed preterm infants the efficiency of protein utilization at adequate energy intakes has been estimated to be approximately 70%.[99,107,108] An enteral protein intake of approximately 2.8 g kg^{-1} day^{-1} is close to the minimal intake needed to insure intrauterine rates of weight gain and nitrogen retention. This intake has also been shown to maintain acceptable plasma albumin and transthyretin concentrations.[41,91] The blood urea nitrogen concentration and the plasma concentration of most amino acids in infants receiving this intake are only minimally different from concentrations observed in infants fed preterm human milk.[104]

A protein intake of 3.5–4 g kg^{-1} day^{-1} results in rates of both weight gain and nitrogen accretion well in excess of intrauterine rates and also maintains acceptable plasma albumin and transthyretin concentrations.[41,91] Although the blood urea nitrogen and plasma amino acid concentrations of infants fed these intakes are higher than those of infants fed lower intakes, blood urea nitrogen concentrations are within the acceptable range (8.1 $\pm$ 2.3 mgDL^{-1}), and the plasma concentrations of only a few amino acids exceed the concentrations of cord plasma[109] or plasma obtained at fetoscopy.[110] As a general guide to the adequacy of enteral protein intake, clinicians should pay close attention to the blood urea nitrogen concentrations. If a stable infant is on marginal intakes and the blood urea nitrogen concentration is low, the total volume of formula should be increased. If the volume of intake is deemed to be adequate and the blood urea nitrogen concentration is low, supplementation with protein should be considered.

Today, most LBW infants in the USA are fed either preterm human milk fortified with protein and other nutrients, one of several formulas designed specifically for LBW infants, or a combination of human milk and one of the preterm formulas. When volumes sufficient to provide an energy intake of 120 kcal kg^{-1} day^{-1} are fed, the LBW infant formulas currently available in the USA provide protein intakes ranging from 3.25–3.6 g kg^{-1} day^{-1}. Infants fed these formulas gain weight and retain nitrogen at rates equal to, or slightly in excess of, intrauterine rates without appreciable "metabolic stress".[111–113] However, recent data indicate that most conventionally managed infants who weigh less than 1500 g at birth, although appropriate size for gestational age at birth, weigh less than the 10th percentile of intrauterine standards at hospital discharge.[114] This suggests that they fail to compensate for the lack of growth or actual weight loss of most such infants during the first 2–4 weeks of life.

The Life Sciences Research Office (LSRO) Expert Panel on Assessment of Nutrient Requirements for Preterm Infant Formulas[115] recommended minimum and maximum protein contents of 2.5 and 3.6 g 100 kcal^{-1}, respectively. At an energy intake of 120 kcal kg^{-1} day^{-1} these recommendations equate to protein intakes of 3–4.3 g kg^{-1} day^{-1}.

Effect of other nutrient intakes on nitrogen balance

Inadequate intake of any nutrient required for new tissue synthesis will also limit the extent to which protein can be deposited as new tissue. This has been best demonstrated in the study of Rudman et al.[116] in adults receiving exclusively parenteral nutrition. In this study, withdrawal of sodium, potassium or phosphorus from an otherwise complete parenteral nutrition regimen resulted in lower nitrogen retention and a lower rate of weight gain. Though no such data are available for term or preterm infants, significant correlations between nitrogen retention and electrolytes and minerals have been reported,[117] suggesting that an inadequate intake of any nutrient required for production of new tissue is likely to interfere with the LBW infant's utilization of protein and/or amino acid intake.

Kashyap et al.[91] suggested this possibility to explain apparent differences between the results of their studies on effects of protein intake on growth and metabolic response of LBW infants when compared with those reported by Räihä and colleagues.[118] Kashyap and associates observed marked difference in rates of weight gain as well as in nitrogen retention between infants fed protein intakes of 2.25 g kg^{-1} day^{-1} versus 3.6 g kg^{-1} day^{-1}, with an energy intake of 120 kcal kg^{-1} day^{-1}. However, Räihä et al. found no difference in rates of weight gain of LBW infants fed protein intakes of 2.25 vs. 4.5 g kg^{-1} day^{-1} with an energy intake of 120 kcal kg^{-1} day^{-1}. The only apparent difference between the two studies was the electrolyte and mineral contents of the formulas fed to the infants. The sodium and phosphorus intakes of infants studied by Räihä and co-workers were considerably lower and were similar to those provided by human milk. Based on the intrauterine relationships between sodium and phosphorus accretion and the accretion of nitrogen,[119] the sodium and phosphorus intakes of the infants studied by Räihä et al., even if 100% absorbed, were insufficient to permit utilization of the higher protein intake. In contrast, the sodium and phosphorus intakes of the infants studied by Kashyap and associates were higher and retention of sodium and phosphorus relative to the

retention of nitrogen was roughly the same as the intrauterine relationships.

Although few data concerning this potentially important relationship are available, it seems reasonable to conclude that inadequate intake of any nutrient required for synthesis and/or deposition of new tissue is likely to inhibit utilization of protein for production of lean body mass.

Though protein energy balance studies in preterm infants have provided information to enable recommendations of protein and energy intakes for specific short-term goals, effects of these intakes on long-term outcomes on growth, body composition, neurodevelopment and clinical susceptibility to adult onset diseases are lacking.

REFERENCES

1 FAO/WHO/UNU Expert Consultation. Energy and Protein Requirements. WHO Technical Bulletin #724. Geneva, Switzerland: World Health Organization;1985.

2 Food and Agricultural Organization of the United Nations, Ad Hoc Committee, Energy and protein requirements. FAO Food Nutr. 1973;7:1024.

3 Rao, M., Blass, E. M., Brignol, M. M. et al. Reduced heat loss following sucrose ingestion in premature and normal human newborns. Early Hum. Dev. 1997;48:109–16.

4 Rao, M., Koenig, E., Li, S. et al. Direct calorimetry for the measurement of heat release in preterm infants: methods and applications. J. Perinatol. 1995;15:375–81.

5 Sauer, P. J., Dane, H. J., Visser, H. K. Longitudinal studies on metabolic rate, heat loss, and energy cost of growth in low birth weight infants. Pediatr. Res.1984;18:254–9.

6 Ferrannini, E. The theoretical bases of indirect calorimetry: a review. Metabolism 1988;37:287–301.

7 Webb, P., Annis, J. F., Troutman, S. J. Jr. Energy balance in man measured by direct and indirect calorimetry. Am. J. Clin. Nutr. 1980;33:1287–98.

8 Seale, J. L., Rumpler, W. V., Conway, J. M. et al. Comparison of doubly labeled water, intake-balance, and direct- and indirect-calorimetry methods for measuring energy expenditure in adult men. Am. J. Clin. Nutr. 1990;52:66–71.

9 Schulze, K., Stefanski, M., Masterson, J. et al. An analysis of the variability in estimates of bioenergetic variables in preterm infants. Pediatr. Res. 1986;20:422–7.

10 Bell, E. F., Rios, G. R., Wilmoth, P. K. Estimation of 24-hour energy expenditure from shorter measurement periods in premature infants. Pediatr. Res. 1986;20:646–9.

11 Perring, J., Henderson, M., Cooke, R. J. Factors affecting the measurement of energy expenditure during energy balance studies in preterm infants. Pediatr. Res. 2000;48:518–23.

12 Sinclair, J. C. Energy needs during infancy. In Fomon, S. J., Heird, W. C., eds. Energy and Protein needs during Infancy. Bristol-Myers Nutrition Symposia: Academic Press;1986: 41–51.

13 Swyer, P. R. Assumptions used in measurements of energy metabolism. *J. Nutr.* 1991;**121**:1891–6.

14 Lifson, N., Gordon, G. B., McClintock, R. Measurement of total carbon dioxide production by means of D2O18. *J. Appl. Physiol.* 1955;**7**:704–10.

15 Schoeller, D. A. Measurement of energy expenditure in free-living humans by using doubly labeled water. *J. Nutr.* 1988;**118**:1278–89.

16 Wells, J. C. K. Energy metabolism in infants and children. *Nutrition* 1998;**14**:817–20.

17 Speakman, J. R. Principles, problems and a paradox with the measurement of energy expenditure of free-living subjects using doubly-labeled water. *Stat. Med.* 1990;**9**:1365–80.

18 Speakman, J. R., Perez-Camargo, G. *et al.* Validation of the doubly-labeled water technique in the domestic dog (*Canis familiaris*). *Br. J. Nutr.* 2001;**85**:75–87.

19 Klein, P. D., James, W. P., Wong, W. W. *et al.* Calorimetric validation of the doubly-labeled water method for determination of energy expenditure in man. *Hum. Nutr. Clin. Nutr.* 1984;**38**:95–106.

20 Roberts, S. B., Coward, W. A., Schlingenspeisen, K. H. *et al.* Comparison of the doubly labeled water (2H$_2$(18)O) method with indirect calorimetry and a nutrient-balance study for simultaneous determination of energy expenditure, water intake, and metabolizable energy intake in preterm infants. *Am. J. Clin. Nutr.* 1986;**44**:315–22.

21 Jensen, C. L., Butte, N. F., Wong, W. W. *et al.* Determining energy expenditure in preterm infants: comparison of 2H$_2$(18)O method and indirect calorimetry. *Am. J. Physiol.* 1992;**263**:R685–92.

22 Adams, A. K., Nelson, R. A., Bell, E. F. *et al.* Use of infrared thermographic calorimetry to determine energy expenditure in preterm infants. *Am. J. Clin. Nutr.* 2000;**71**:969–77.

23 Schulze, K. A model of variability in metabolic rate of neonates. In Fomon, S. J., Heird, W. C., eds. *Energy and Protein Needs during Infancy.* Bristol-Myers Nutrition Symposia: Academic Press;1986:19–40.

24 Schofield, W. N. Predicting basal metabolic rate, new standards and review of previous work. *Hum. Nutr. Clin. Nutr.* 1985;**39**:S5–41.

25 Roberts, S. B., Savage, J., Coward, W. A., Chew, B., Lucas, A. Energy expenditure and intake in infants born to lean and overweight mothers. *N. Engl. J. Med.* 1988;**318**:461–6.

26 DeMarie, M. P., Hoffenberg, A., Biggerstaff, S. L. *et al.* Determinants of energy expenditure in ventilated preterm infants. *J. Perinat. Med.* 1999;**27**:465–72.

27 Bauer, J., Maier, K., Hellstern, G., Linderkamp, O. Longitudinal evaluation of energy expenditure in preterm infants with birth weight less than 1000 g. *Br. J. Nutr.* 2003;**89**:533–7.

28 Bauer, K., Laurenz, M., Ketteler, L., Versmold, H. Longitudinal study of energy expenditure in preterm neonates < 30 weeks' gestation during the first three postnatal weeks. *J. Pediatr.* 2003;**142**:390–6.

29 Chessex, P., Reichman, B. L., Verellen, G. J. *et al.* Influence of postnatal age, energy intake, and weight gain on energy metabolism in the very low-birth-weight infant. *J. Pediatr.* 1981;**99**:761–6.

30 Rubecz, I., Mestyan, J. Postprandial thermogenesis in human milk-fed very low birth weight infants. *Biol. Neonate* 1986;**49**:301–6.

31 Danforth, E. Jr. Diet and obesity. *Am. J. Clin. Nutr.* 1985;**41**:S1132–45.

32 Stothers, J. K., Warner, R. M. Effect of feeding on neonatal oxygen consumption. *Arch. Dis. Child* 1979;**54**:415–20.

33 Brooke, O. G., Alvear, J. Postprandial metabolism in infants of low birth weight. *Hum. Nutr. Clin. Nutr.* 1982;**36**:167–75.

34 Brooke, O. G., Ashworth, A. The influence of malnutrition on the postprandial metabolic rate and respiratory quotient. *Br. J. Nutr.* 1972;**27**:407–15.

35 Mestyan, J., Jarai, I., Fekete, M. The total energy expenditure and its components in premature infants maintained under different nursing and environmental conditions. *Pediatr. Res.* 1968;**2**:161–71.

36 Brooke, O. G. Energy balance and metabolic rate in preterm infants fed with standard and high-energy formulas. *Br. J. Nutr.* 1980;**44**:13–23.

37 Kinabo, J. L., Durnin, J. V. Thermic effect of food in man: effect of meal composition, and energy content. *Br. J. Nutr.* 1990;**64**:37–44.

38 Flatt, J. P. Assessment of energy metabolism in health and disease. In Kinny, J. M., ed. *Report of the First Ross Conference on Medical Research.* Columbus, OH: Ross Laboratories;1980:79.

39 Roberts, S. B., Lucas, A. Energetic efficiency and nutrient accretion in preterm infants fed extremes of dietary intake. *Hum. Nutr. Clin. Nutr.* 1987;**41**:105–13.

40 Schulze, K. F., Stefanski, M., Masterson, J. *et al.* Energy expenditure, energy balance and composition of weight gain in low birth weight infants fed diets of different protein and energy content. *J. Pediatr.* 1987;**110**:753–9.

41 Kashyap, S., Schulze, K. F., Forsyth, M. *et al.* Growth, nutrient retention and metabolic response in low birth weight infants fed varying intakes of protein and energy. *J. Pediatr.* 1988;**113**:713–21.

42 Wells, J. C., Davies, P. S. Energy cost of physical activity in twelve week old infants. *Am. J. Hum. Biol.* 1995;**7**:85–92.

43 Butte, N. F., Wong, W. W., Ferlic, L. *et al.* Energy expenditure and deposition of breast-fed and formula-fed infants during early infancy. *Pediatr. Res.* 1990;**28**:631–40.

44 Waterlow, J. C. Basic concepts in the determination of nutritional requirements of normal infants. In Tsang, R. C., Nichols, B. L., eds. *Nutrition during Infancy.* Philadelphia, PA: Hanley & Belfus:1988:1–19.

45 Brebbia, D. R., Altshuler, K. Z. Oxygen consumption rate and electroencephalographic stage of sleep. *Science* 1965;**150**:1621–3.

46 Stothers, J. K., Warner, R. M. Oxygen consumption and neonatal sleep states. *J. Physiol.* 1978;**278**:435–40.

47 Schulze, K., Kairam, R., Stefanski, M. *et al.* Spontaneous variability in minute ventilation oxygen consumption and heart rate of low birth weight infants. *Pediatr. Res.* 1981;**15**:1111–6.

48 Brooke, O. G., Alvear, J., Arnold, M. Energy retention, energy expenditure, and growth in healthy immature infants. *Pediatr. Res.* 1979;**13**:215–20.

49 Reichman, B. L., Chessex, P., Putet, G. *et al.* Partition of energy metabolism and energy cost of growth in the very low-birth-weight infant. *Pediatrics* 1982;**69**:446–51.

50 Murlin, J. R., Conklin, R. E., Marsh, M. E. Energy metabolism of normal newborn babies, with special reference to the influence of food and of crying. *Am. J. Dis. Child.* 1925;**29**:1–28.

51 Day, R. Respiratory metabolism in infancy and childhood. Regulation of body temperature of premature infants. *Am. J. Dis. Child.* 1943;**65**:376.

52 Bruck, K. Temperature regulation in the newborn infant. *Biol. Neonate* 1961;**3**:65.

53 Masterson, J., Zucker, C., Schulze, K. Prone and supine positioning effects on energy expenditure and behavior of low birth weight neonates. *Pediatrics* 1987;**80**:689–92.

54 Chong, A., Murphy, N., Matthews, T. Effect of prone sleeping on circulatory control in infants. *Arch. Dis. Child.* 2000;**82**:253–6.

55 Sinclair, J. C., Silverman, W. A. Relative hypermetabolism in undergrown human neonates. *Lancet* 1964;**41**:49.

56 Chessex, P., Reichman, B., Verellen, G. *et al.* Metabolic consequences of intrauterine growth retardation in very low birth-weight infants. *Pediatr. Res.* 1984;**18**:709–13.

57 Picaud, J. C., Putet, G., Rigo, J., Salle, B. L., Senterre, J. Metabolic and energy balance in small- and appropriate-for-gestational-age, very low-birth-weight infants. *Acta. Paediatr. Suppl.* 1994;**405**:54–9.

58 Lafeber, H. N., Sulkers, E. J., Chapman, T. E., Sauer, P. J. Glucose production and oxidation in preterm infants during total parenteral nutrition. *Pediatr. Res.* 1990;**28**:153–7.

59 Bohler, T., Kramer, T., Janecke, A. R., Hoffmann, G. F., Linderkamp, O. Increased energy expenditure and fecal fat excretion do not impair weight gain in small-for-gestational-age preterm infants. *Early Hum. Dev.* 1999;**54**:223–34.

60 Kreymann, G., Grosser, S., Buggischn, P. *et al.* Oxygen consumption and resting metabolic rate in sepsis, sepsis syndrome, and septic shock. *Crit. Care Med.* 1993;**21**:1012–19.

61 Plank, L. D., Connolly, A. B., Hill, G. L. Sequential changes in the metabolic response in severely septic patients during the first 23 days after the onset of peritonitis. *Ann. Surg.* 1998;**228**:146–58.

62 Moriyama, S., Okamoto, K., Tabira, Y. *et al.* Evaluation of oxygen consumption and resting energy expenditure in critically ill patients with systemic inflammatory response syndrome. *Crit. Care Med.* 1999;**27**:2133–6.

63 Bauer, J., Hentschel, R., Linderkamp, O. Effect of sepsis syndrome on neonatal oxygen consumption and energy expenditure. *Pediatrics* 2002;**110**:e69.

64 Mrozek, J. D., Georgieff, M. K., Blazar, B. R., Mammel, M. C., Schwarzenberg, S. J. Effect of sepsis syndrome on neonatal protein and energy metabolism. *J. Perinatol.* 2000;**20**:96–100.

65 Wahlig, T. M., Gatto, C. W., Boros, S. J. *et al.* Metabolic response of preterm infants to variable degrees of respiratory illness. *J. Pediatr.* 1994;**124**:283–8.

66 Schulze, A., Abubakar, K., Gill, G., Way, R. C., Sinclair, J. C. Pulmonary oxygen consumption: a hypothesis to explain the increase in oxygen consumption of low birth weight infants with lung disease. *Intens. Care Med.* 2001;**27**:1636–42.

67 Kurzner, S. I., Garg, M., Bautista, D. B. *et al.* Growth failure in infants with bronchopulmonary dysplasia: nutrition and elevated resting metabolic expenditure. *Pediatrics* 1988;**81**:379–84.

68 Yeh, T. F., McClenan, D. A., Ajayi, O. A., Pildes, R. S. Metabolic rate and energy balance in infants with bronchopulmonary dysplasia. *J. Pediatr.* 1989;**114**:448–51.

69 Carnielli, V. P., Verlato, G., Benini, F. *et al.* Metabolic and respiratory effects of theophylline in the preterm infant. *Arch. Dis. Child Fetal Neonatal Edn.* 2000;**83**:F39–43.

70 Bauer, J., Maier, K., Linderkamp, O., Hentschel, R. Effect of caffeine on oxygen consumption and metabolic rate in very low birth weight infants with idiopathic apnea. *Pediatrics* 2001;**107**:660–3.

71 Fjeld, C. R., Cole, F. S., Bier, D. M. Energy expenditure, lipolysis, and glucose production in preterm infants treated with theophylline. *Pediatr. Res.* 1992;**32**:693–8.

72 Roberts, S. B., Young, V. R. Energy costs of fat and protein deposition in the human infant. *Am. J. Clin. Nutr.* 1988;**48**:951–5.

73 Reichman, B., Chessex, P., Putet, G. *et al.* Diet, fat accretion and growth in premature infants. *N. Engl. J. Med.* 1981;**305**:1495–500.

74 Gudinchet, F., Schutz, Y., Micheli, J. L., Stettler, E., Jequier, E. Metabolic cost of growth in very low-birth-weight infants. *Pediatr. Res.* 1982;**16**:1025–30.

75 Towers, H. M., Schulze, K. F., Ramakrishnan, R., Kashyap, S. Energy expended by low birth weight infants in the deposition of protein and fat. *Pediatr. Res.* 1997;**41**:584–9.

76 Young, V. R., Steffee, W. P., Pencharz, P. B., Winterer, J. C., Scrimshaw, N. S. Total human body protein synthesis in relation to protein requirements at various ages. *Nature* 1975;**253**:192–4.

77 Whitehead, R. G., Paul, A. A., Cole, T. J. A critical analysis of measured food energy intakes during infancy and early childhood in comparison with current international recommendations. *J. Hum. Nutr.* 1981;**35**:339–48.

78 Prentice, A. M., Lucas, A., Vasquez-Velasquez, L., Davies, P. S., Whitehead, R. G. Are current dietary guidelines for young children a prescription for overfeeding? *Lancet* 1988;**2**:1066–9.

79 de Bruin, N. C., Degenhart, H. J., Gal, S. *et al.* Energy utilization and growth in breast-fed and formula-fed infants measured prospectively during the first year of life. *Am. J. Clin. Nutr.* 1998;**67**:885–96.

80 Food and Nutrition Board. *Commission on Life Sciences, National Research Council. Recommended Dietary Allowances, 10th Edition.* Washington, DC: National Academy Press; 1989.

81 Committee on Medical Aspects of Food Policy. *Dietary Reference Values for Food Energy and Nutrients for United Kingdom.* London: HMSO;1991.

82 Health and Welfare Canada. *Nutrition Recommendations. The Report of the Scientific Review Committee.* Ottawa, ONT; 1990: Supply and Services.

83 American Academy of Pediatrics Committee on Nutrition. Nutritional needs of preterm infants. In Kleinman, R. E., ed. *Pediatric Nutrition Handbook American Academy of Pediatrics.* Elk Grove Village, IL; 1998:55–87.

84 Canadian Pediatric Society Nutrition Committee. Nutrition needs and feeding of premature infants. *Can. Med. Assoc. J.* 1995;**152**:1765.

85 European Society for Gastroenterology and Nutrition, Committee on Nutrition of the Preterm Infant. Nutrition and feeding of preterm infants. *Acta. Paediatr. Scand.* 1987;**336**:1.

86 The Life Sciences Research Office (LSRO) Expert Panel on Assessment of Nutrient Requirements for Preterm Infant Formulas. *J. Nutr.* 2002;**132**:1413S.

87 European Society for Gastroenterology and Nutrition. Comment on the content and composition of lipids in infant formulas. *Acta. Paediat. Scand.* 1991;**80**:887–96.

88 Millward, D. J., Bates, P. C., Coyer, P. *et al.* The effect of dietary energy and protein on growth as studied in animal models. In Fomon, S. J., Heird, W. C., eds. *Energy and Protein Needs During Infancy.* New York, NY: Academic Press; 1986: 127–56.

89 Munro, H. N. General aspects of the regulation of protein metabolism by diet and by hormones. III. Influence of dietary carbohydrate and fat on protein metabolism. In Munro, H. N., ed. *Mammalian Protein Metabolism.* New York, NY: Academic Press;1964:412–47.

90 Calloway, D. H., Spector, H. Nitrogen balance as related to calorie and protein intake in active young men. *Am. J. Clin. Nutr.* 1954;**2**:405–12.

91 Kashyap, S., Forsyth, M., Zucker, C. *et al.* Effects of varying protein and energy intakes on growth and metabolic response in low birth weight infants. *J. Pediatr.* 1986;**108**:955–63.

92 Kashyap, S., Schulze, K. F., Ramakrishnan, R., Dell, R. B., Heird, W. C. Evaluation of a mathematical model for predicting the relationship between protein and energy intakes of low birth weight infants and the rate and composition of weight gain. *Pediatr. Res.* 1994;**35**:704–12.

93 Kashyap, S., Ohira-Kist, K., Abildskov, K. *et al.* Effects of quality of energy on growth and metabolic response in enterally fed low birth weight infants. *Pediatr. Res.* 2001; **50**:390–7.

94 Zlotkin, S. H., Bryan, M. H., Anderson, G. H. Intravenous nitrogen and energy intakes required to duplicate in utero nitrogen accretion in prematurely born human infants. *J. Pediatr.* 1981;**99**:115–20.

95 Anderson, T. L., Muttart, C. R., Bieber, M. A., Nicholson, J. F., Heird, W. C. A controlled trial of glucose versus glucose and amino acids in premature infants. *J. Pediatr.* 1979;**94**:947–51.

96 Duffy, B., Gunn, T., Collinge, J., Pencharz, P. The effect of varying protein quality and energy intake on the nitrogen metabolism of parenterally fed very low birth weight (less than 1600 g) infants. *Pediatr. Res.* 1981;**15**:1040–4.

97 Pineault, M., Chessex, P., Bisaillon, S., Brisson, G. Total parenteral nutrition in the newborn: impact of the quality of infused energy on nitrogen metabolism. *Am. J. Clin. Nutr.* 1988;**47**:298–304.

98 Long, J. M. 3rd, Wilmore, D. W., Mason, A. D. Jr, Pruitt, B. A. Jr. Effect of carbohydrate and fat intake on nitrogen excretion during total intravenous feeding. *Ann. Surg.* 1977;**185**:417–22.

99 Reichman, B., Chessex, P., Verellen, G. *et al.* Dietary composition and macronutrient storage in preterm infants. *Pediatrics* 1983;**72**:322–8.

100 Whyte, R. K., Haslam, R., Vlainic, C. *et al.* Energy balance and nitrogen balance in growing low birth weight infants fed human milk or formula. *Pediatr. Res.* 1983;**17**:891–8.

101 Lunn, P. G., Austin, S. Dietary manipulation of plasma albumin concentration. *J. Nutr.* 1983;**113**:1791–802.

102 Roberts, S. B., Lucas, A. The effects of two extremes of dietary intake on protein accretion in preterm infants. *Early Hum. Dev.* 1985;**12**:301–7.

103 Atkinson, S. A., Bryan, M. H., Anderson, G. H. Human milk feeding in premature infants: protein, fat, and carbohydrate balances in the first two weeks of life. *J. Pediatr.* 1981;**99**:617–24.

104 Kashyap, S., Schulze, K. F., Forsyth, M. *et al.* Growth, nutrient retention and metabolic response of low-birth-weight infants fed supplemented and unsupplemented preterm human milk. *Am. J. Clin. Nutr.* 1990;**52**:254–62.

105 Kashyap, S., Heird, W. C. Protein requirements of low birthweight, very low birthweight, and small for gestational age infants. In Räihä, N. C. R., ed. *Protein Metabolism During Infancy, Nestlé Nutrition Workshop Series, Vol 33.* New York, NY: Nestec Ltd, Vevey/Raven Press, Ltd; 1994:133.

106 Zello, G. A., Menendez, C. E., Rafii, M. *et al.* Minimum protein intake for the preterm neonate determined by protein and amino acid kinetics. *Pediatr. Res.* 2003;**53**:338–44.

107 Catzeflis, C., Schutz, Y., Micheli, J. L. *et al.* Whole body protein synthesis and energy expenditure in very low birth weight infants. *Pediatr. Res.* 1985;**19**:679–87.

108 Heird, W. C., Kashyap, S., Schulze, K. F. *et al.* Nutrient utilization and growth in LBW infants. In Goldman, A. *et al.*, eds. *Human Lactation 3: The Effects of Human Milk on the Recipient Infant.* New York, NY: Plenum Press; 1987:9–21.

109 Pittard, W. B. 3rd, Geddes, K. M., Picone, T. A. Cord blood amino acid concentrations from neonates of 23–41 weeks gestational age. *JPEN.* 1988;**12**:167–9.

110 McIntosh, N., Rodeck, C. H., Heath, R. Plasma amino acids of the mid-trimester human fetus. *Biol. Neonate* 1984;**45**:218–24.

111 Schanler, R. J., Oh, W. Nitrogen and mineral balance in preterm infants fed human milks or formula. *J. Pediatr. Gastroenterol Nutr.* 1985;**4**:214–19.

112 Shenai, J. P., Reynolds, J. W., Babson, S. G. Nutritional balance studies in very low birth weight infants: enhanced nutrient retention rates by an experimental formula. *Pediatrics* 1980;**66**:233–8.

113 Tyson, J. E., Lasky, R. E., Mize, C. E. *et al.* Growth, metabolic response and development in very low birth weight infants fed banked human milk or enriched formula. I. Neonatal findings. *J. Pediatr.* 1983;**103**:95–104.

114 Ehrenkranz, R. A., Younes, N., Lemons, J. A. *et al.* Longitudinal growth of hospitalized very low birth weight infants. *Pediatrics* 1999;**104**:280–9.

115 The Life Sciences Research Office (LSRO) Expert Panel on Assessment of Nutrient Requirements for Preterm Infant Formulas. *J. Nutr.* 2002;**132**:1423S–4S.

116 Rudman, D., Millikan, W. J., Richardson, T. J. *et al.* Elemental balances during intravenous hyperalimentation of underweight adult subjects. *J. Clin. Invest.* 1975;**55**:94–104.

117 Kashyap, S., Forsyth, M., Zucker, C. *et al.* Relationship between nitrogen retention and retention of electrolytes and minerals in low birth weight infants. *Pediatr. Res.*, 1986; **20**:413A.

118 Räihä, N. C., Heinonen, K., Rassin, D. K., Gaull, G. E. Milk protein quality in low-birthweight infants. I. Metabolic responses and effects on growth. *Pediatrics* 1976;**57**:659–84.

119 Widdowson, E. M. Changes in body proportion and composition during growth. In Davis, J., Dobbing, J., eds. *Scientific Foundations of Pediatrics*. Philadelphia, PA: W.B. Saunders Co; 1974:153–63.

13

The role of essential fatty acids in development

William C. Heird

Department of Pediatrics, Children's Nutrition Research Center and Baylor College of Medicine, Houston, TX

Fatty acids are aliphatic monocarboxylic acids. They are classified as saturated, monounsaturated or polyunsaturated fatty acids depending upon the number of double bonds in the carbon chain. Saturated fatty acids have no double bonds, monounsaturated fatty acids have 1 double bond and polyunsaturated fatty acids have 2 or more, but usually no more than 6, double bonds. Most fatty acids can be synthesized endogenously but the major source is from dietary fat which accounts for approximately half the energy content of breast milk and infant formulas. Triglycerides, which have three, usually different, fatty acid molecules esterified to a molecule of glycerol, are the major components of dietary fat; the remainder includes phospholipids, monoglycerides, diglycerides and sterols. These are hydrolyzed in the intestinal lumen, the released fatty acids are reassembled within the enterocyte and the reassembled triglycerides, phospholipids, monoglycerides and sterol esters are absorbed primarily into the thoracic duct from which they eventually reach the bloodstream where they circulate as components of the various lipoproteins. Some free fatty acids also are absorbed and circulate bound to albumen.

All fatty acids have common names but, by general convention, they are identified by a "shorthand" system indicating their number of carbon atoms, their number of double bonds and the site of the first double bond from the terminal methyl group of the molecule. For example, palmitic acid, a 16-carbon saturated fatty acid is designated 16:0 and oleic acid, an 18-carbon monounsaturated fatty acid with its single double bond located between the ninth and tenth carbon from the methyl terminal, is designated $18:1\omega9$. Linoleic acid (LA) and α-linolenic acid (ALA) are designated $18:2\omega6$ and $18:3\omega3$, respectively. Both are 18-carbon polyunsaturated fatty acids. Linoleic acid has 2 double bonds, the first between the sixth and seventh carbon from the methyl terminal, and ALA has 3 double bonds, the first between the third and fourth carbon from the methyl terminal. The common names as well as the shorthand designations of several dietary fatty acids are shown in Table 13.1.

Essential fatty acids

Fatty acids with double bonds at the $\omega6$ and $\omega3$ positions cannot be synthesized endogenously by the human species.[1] Therefore, specific $\omega6$ and $\omega3$ fatty acids or their precursors with double bonds at these positions, i.e. LA ($18:2\omega6$) and ALA ($18:3\omega3$), must be provided in the diet. Both LA and ALA are metabolized by the same series of desaturases and elongases to longer chain, more unsaturated fatty acids[2] but $\omega6$ fatty acids cannot be converted to $\omega3$ fatty acids and vice versa. This pathway is outlined in Figure 13.1. As indicated, two desaturation – elongation steps result in formation of $22:4\omega6$ and $22:5\omega3$. However, instead of being desaturated exclusively by Δ^4-desaturase to $22:5\omega6$ and $22:6\omega3$, as formerly believed, $22:4\omega6$ and $22:5\omega3$ are, first, elongated to $24:4\omega6$ and $24:5\omega3$ which are desaturated by Δ^6-desaturase to $24:5\omega6$ and $24:6\omega3$. $22:5\omega6$ and $22:6\omega3$ are then formed from $24:5\omega6$ and $24:6\omega3$ by partial β-oxidation. This alternate pathway was described in the early 1990s by Voss *et al.*[3] and its involvement in formation of $22:5\omega6$ and $22:6\omega3$ from labeled $18:2\omega6$ and $18:3\omega3$, respectively, was confirmed in infants by Sauerwald *et al*[4]

Collectively, the longer chain, more unsaturated fatty acids synthesized from LA and ALA are referred to as

Neonatal Nutrition and Metabolism. Second Edition, ed. P. Thureen and W. Hay. Published by Cambridge University Press.

Table 13.1. Common names and numerical nomenclature of selected fatty acids

Common name	Numerical nomenclature
Caprylic acid	8:0
Capric acid	10:0
Lauric acid	12:0
Myristic acid	14:0
Palmitic acid	16:0
Stearic acid	18:0
Oleic acid	18:1ω9*
Linoleic acid	18:2ω6*
γ-linolenic acid	18:3ω6
Dihomogamma-linolenic acid	20:3ω6
Arachidonic acid	20:4ω6
α-linolenic acid	18:3ω3*
Eicosapentaenoic acid	20:5ω3
Docosahexaenoic acid	22:6ω3

*ω9, ω6, and ω3 are used interchangeably with n-9, n-6, and n-3.

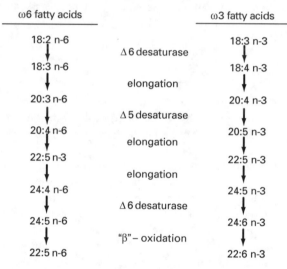

Figure 13.1. Metabolic pathways of 6 and 3 fatty acids.

long chain (i.e. more than 18 carbons), polyunsaturated fatty acids (LC-PUFA). Important metabolites of LA include γ-linolenic acid (GLA; 18:3ω6), dihomogamma linolenic acid (DHLA; 20:3ω6) and arachidonic acid (ARA; 20:4ω6). Eicosapentaenoic acid (EPA; 26:5ω3) and docosahexaenoic acid (DHA; 22:6ω3) are the most important metabolites of 18:3ω3. In vivo, LA and ALA are found in storage lipids, cell membrane phospholipids, intracellular cholesterol esters and plasma lipids. In contrast, LC-PUFA synthesized from these precursors are found primarily in specific cell membrane phospholipids. In addition, DHLA, ARA and EPA are immediate precursors of eicosanoids,[1,5] each being con-verted to a different series with different biological activities and/or functions.

Linoleic acid has been recognized as an essential nutrient for the human species for almost 75 years.[6,7] The primary symptoms of deficiency are poor growth and scaly skin lesions. Although the essentiality of ALA has been suspected for some time, it was not recognized as an essential nutrient until approximately 20 years ago. In animals, deficiency of this fatty acid results in visual and neurological abnormalities.[8-11] Neurological abnormalities also were observed in a human infant who had been maintained for several weeks on a parenteral nutrition regimen containing LA but lacking ALA[12] and in elderly nursing home residents who were receiving intragastric feedings of an elemental formula with no ALA.[13] These symptoms were reversed by administration of ALA.

Although symptoms related to deficiency of the two series of essential fatty acids seem to differ, many studies of ω6 fatty acid deficiency employed a fat-free or very low fat diet rather than a diet deficient in only LA. Thus, there may be some overlap in symptoms of LA and ALA deficiency. The clinical symptoms of ω6 fatty acid deficiency can be corrected by LA, GLA, DHLA or ARA; those related specifically to ALA deficiency can be corrected by ALA, EPA or DHA. Whether LA and ALA have specific functions that cannot be met by their metabolites is not clear.

The same series of enzymes that catalyze desaturation and elongation of ω6 and ω3 fatty acids also catalyze desaturation and elongation of ω9 fatty acids. Since the substrate preference of these enzymes is ω3, followed by ω6 and, finally, ω9,[2] competition between the ω9 fatty acids and either the ω6 or ω3 fatty acids is rarely an issue. However, if the concentrations of LA and ALA are low, oleic acid (18:1ω9) is readily desaturated and elongated to eicosatrienoic acid (20:3ω9). The plasma ratio of this fatty acid to ARA, i.e. the triene/tetraene ratio, is a diagnostic index of ω6 fatty acid deficiency. A ratio of > 0.4 is definitely indicative of deficiency,[14] but since this ratio usually is < 0.1, a ratio of > 0.2 is thought to be a more reasonable indicator of deficiency. In the few documented cases of isolated ALA deficiency in which it was measured, the triene/tetraene ratio was not elevated.

The minimum requirement for LA is thought to be from 2–4% of total energy intake or, for most infant diets, from 4–8% of total fatty acids.[15] The minimum requirement for ALA is less well defined but is thought to be about 1% of total energy intake, or about 2% of the total fatty acids of most infant diets.[16] LA comprises about 15–20% of the total fatty acids of infant formulas available in the USA. Although little emphasis was placed on the ALA content of infant formulas until recently and many with virtually no ALA were

Table 13.2. Fatty acid composition of common vegetable oils*

Fatty acid	Canola	Corn	Coconut	Palm olein	Safflower[†]	Soy	High oleic sunflower
6:0–12:0	–	0.1	62.1	0.2	–	–	–
14:0	–	0.1	18.1	1.0	0.1	0.1	–
16:0	4.0	12.1	8.9	39.8	6.8	11.2	3.7
18:0	2.0	2.4	2.7	4.4	2.4	0.4	5.4
18:1	55.0	32.1	6.4	42.5	12.5	22.0	81.3
18:2	26.0	50.9	1.6	11.2	76.8	53.8	9.0
18:3	10.0	0.9	–	0.2	0.1	7.5	–
Other	2.0	1.0	–	<1.6	<1.0	<1.0	<1.0

* Per cent of total fatty acids (g 100 g^{-1}).
† High oleic safflower oil contains ~77% 18:1 and 12.5% 18:2.

available as recently as a decade ago, ALA now comprises 1.5–2% of the total fatty acid content of most formulas. The LA and ALA contents of human milk are more variable than the contents in formulas. On average, LA comprises ~ 16% of the total fatty acid content of the milk of USA women and ALA comprises about 1%.[17] Human milk also contains small amounts of a number of longer-chain, more unsaturated metabolites of both LA and ALA including ARA and DHA.

Maternal diet has a marked impact on the concentration of all fatty acids in human milk, particularly that of DHA. The concentration of DHA in the milk of women consuming a typical North American diet is generally in the range of 0.1–0.3% of total fatty acids and the concentration of ARA ranges from 0.4–0.6%.[17] The milk of vegetarian women contains less DHA[18] and that of women whose dietary fish consumption is high, or who take ω3 fatty acid supplements, is higher.[19–21] The ARA content of human milk is less variable and appears to be less dependent on maternal ARA intake, perhaps reflecting the relatively high LA intake of most populations.

Corn, coconut, safflower, palm olein and soy oils as well as high oleic safflower and sunflower oils are commonly used in the manufacture of infant formulas available in the USA (Table 13.2). All except coconut oil provide adequate amounts of LA but only soybean oil contains an appreciable amount of both LA and ALA (~ 50% and ~ 7% of total fatty acids, respectively). Canola oil, a component of many formulas available outside the USA, contains somewhat less LA and more ALA.

Recent recommendations for the minimal content of LA in infant formulas range from 2.7–8% of total fatty acids and those for the maximum content range from 21–35% of total fatty acids.[22,23] The recommendations for the minimum and maximum contents of ALA in infant formulas are 1.75% and 4% of total fatty acids, respectively.[23] To maintain

a reasonable balance between the two fatty acids, it is recommended that the LA/ALA ratio be between 5–6 and 15–16.[22,23] As mentioned above, the term and preterm infant formulas currently available in the USA contain 15%–20% of total fatty acids as LA and 1.5%–2% as ALA; hence, their LA/ALA ratios are ~10. Formulas containing the long chain polyunsaturated fatty acids, DHA and ARA, also are available for both term and preterm infants.

LC-PUFA

Interest in the role of LC-PUFA in infant nutrition intensified about 15 years ago when a number of investigators reported that plasma and erythrocyte lipid contents of DHA and ARA were lower in formula-fed than in breast-fed infants.[24–27] Since these fatty acids are present in human milk but not formulas, the lower plasma and erythrocyte lipid contents of these fatty acids in formula-fed infants were interpreted as indicating that infants cannot synthesize DHA and ARA or cannot synthesize enough to meet ongoing needs. Concurrent and earlier observations of better cognitive function of breast-fed v. formula-fed infants[28–31] focused attention on the possibility that the lower cognitive function of formula-fed infants also might be related to inadequate intake of LC-PUFA.

This possibility is supported by the facts that DHA and ARA are the major ω3 and ω6 fatty acids, respectively, of neural tissues[32–34] and DHA is the major fatty acid of retinal photoreceptor membranes.[34] Further, postmortem studies of infants who died suddenly during the first year of life[35–37] indicate that the cerebral content of DHA, but not ARA, is lower in formula-fed v. breast-fed term infants. However, the DHA content of the retina of breast-fed and formula-fed term infants does not appear to differ,[37] perhaps because the content of DHA in retina reaches adult levels at approximately term whereas the adult level in cerebrum is not reached until much later.[34] In one of the postmortem studies, the cerebral DHA content of infants fed a formula with a relatively high ALA content was greater than that of infants fed a formula with less ALA.[36] This is consistent with data from studies in piglets showing that an ALA intake greater than 1.75% of total fatty acids maintains normal brain levels of DHA[38] and studies in infants showing a positive relationship between ALA intake and the appearance of labeled DHA in plasma following administration of labeled ALA.[39]

A major supply of LC-PUFA to the fetus during gestation is actively transported from maternal plasma.[40,41] Thus, the preterm infant who is born early in the third trimester of pregnancy and, hence, receives less LC-PUFA prior to birth than the infant who is born at term, is thought to have a higher LC-PUFA requirement than the term infant. However, the daily rates of accumulation of these fatty acids in the developing central nervous system change minimally between mid-gestation and 18–24 months of age[34] suggesting that the total daily needs of preterm and term infants are likely to be similar. On the other hand, since preterm infants are smaller, their daily needs per kilogram, or per 100 kcal, are undoubtedly greater, particularly during early life.

Both term and preterm infants can convert LA to ARA and ALA to DHA.[4,39,42–45] This was established by studies in which the precursor fatty acids labeled with stable isotopes of either carbon (^{13}C) or hydrogen (^{2}H) were administered to infants and blood levels of the labeled precursors as well as labeled metabolites of each were measured by gas chromatography/mass spectrometry (Figure 13.1). The studies of Sauerwald *et al.*[4,39] and Uauy *et al.*,[45] which included both term and preterm infants, suggest that the overall ability of preterm infants to convert LA and ALA to LC-PUFA is at least equal to that of term infants. However, since the amount of LC-PUFA synthesized is a function of both the rate of synthesis and the pool size of the precursor, the preterm infant's greater apparent rate of conversion of LA and ALA to ARA and DHA, respectively, may not be sufficiently great to compensate for its smaller pool of precursor. Moreover, there is considerable variability in conversion among both preterm and term infants fed the same formula. Further, since measurement of the enrichment of DHA and ARA following administration of labeled precursors is limited to plasma, which represents only a small fraction of the body pool of both the precursor and product fatty acids and may not be representative of the fatty acid pools of other tissues, the amounts of LC-PUFA that either preterm or term infants can synthesize are not known.

The higher DHA and ARA content of the plasma lipids of breast-fed infants and infants fed formulas supplemented with LC-PUFA v. infants fed unsupplemented formulas suggests that the amounts of LC-PUFA formed endogenously are less than the amounts provided by human milk or supplemented formulas. However, the extent to which the concentration of individual LC-PUFA in plasma reflects the content of these fatty acids in tissues, particularly the brain, is not known. In piglets, the brain content of LC-PUFA is not correlated as highly with the content in plasma as is the content in erythrocytes, skeletal muscle and liver.[46,47] In contrast, one of the postmortem studies of human infants showed a weak, but statistically significant, correlation between brain and erythrocyte contents of DHA.[37] The correlation between the erythrocyte content of this fatty acid and its content in other tissues was not reported.

Studies in isolated cell systems suggest that precursors of DHA (e.g. 20:5ω3; 22:5ω3) are transferred from plasma to astrocytes where they are converted to DHA which, in turn, is transferred to neurons.[48,49] Whether direct synthesis of DHA within the central nervous system occurs in humans is not known but limited findings of in vivo studies in animals are compatible with this possibility.[50]

Although far from definitive, the findings discussed above support the possibility that failure to provide preformed LC-PUFA during early infancy, perhaps longer, may compromise development. Thus, for the past several years, studies have focused on differences in visual acuity and neurodevelopmental indices between breast-fed and formula-fed infants as well as between infants fed LC-PUFA-supplemented and unsupplemented formulas. Human milk, of course, contains a number of factors other than LC-PUFA that might affect visual acuity or neurodevelopmental indices; thus, studies comparing outcomes of breast-fed v. formula-fed infants cannot help resolve the role of LC-PUFA in infant development. On the other hand, studies taking advantage of the natural variability in milk contents of LC-PUFA or enhanced variability secondary to maternal supplementation and, hence, differences in LC-PUFA intake of the recipient infants[51–55] appear to be helpful. The following discussion is limited to findings from these types of studies and findings from studies in which LC-PUFA-supplemented v. unsupplemented formulas were compared.

LC-PUFA intake and visual function

Early studies in rodents established the importance of ω3 fatty acids for normal retinal function[8,9] and subsequent studies confirmed this in primates.[10,11] More recently, studies have focused on the effect of ω3 fatty acids on retinal function and/or overall visual function of human infants. However, whereas the abnormal retinal/visual function of ω3 fatty acid-deficient animals clearly resulted from an inadequate intake of ALA and were reversed by ALA, the more recent studies in human infants have focused primarily on the effects of DHA intake on retinal and/or visual function. Studies have been conducted in both term and preterm infants and have utilized both behaviorally based and electrophysiologically based methods for assessing visual function.

Preferential looking tests of visual acuity are the most commonly utilized behaviorally based methods. These tests take advantage of the innate tendency to look toward a discernible pattern rather than a blank field.[56–58] The Teller Acuity Card procedure, a rapid measure of resolution acuity that combines forced-choice preferential looking and operant preferential looking procedures, is usually used. The test is performed by showing the subject a series of cards with stripes (gratings) of different widths on one side and a blank field on the other while observing his/her looking behavior through a peephole in the center of the card. Cards with wider stripes are shown initially followed by cards with progressively decreasing stripe widths. Scoring or evaluation of visual acuity is based on the finest grating toward which the infant clearly looks preferentially. This is assumed to be the finest grating that the subject can resolve.

The electrophysiologically based tests utilize visual evoked potentials (VEP). These measure the activation of the visual cortex in response to visual information processed by the retina and transmitted along the geniculostriate pathway to the visual cortex.[59] The presence of a reliable evoked response indicates that the stimulus information was resolved up to the point in the visual pathway (i.e. the visual cortex) where the response is processed. Use of VEPs to assess visual acuity requires measuring the electrical potentials of the visual cortex in response to patterns of contrast reversal with vertical square wave gratings or checkerboards. During the presentations, the frequency of the gratings or checkerboards is decreased from low to high (large to small) and the visual acuity threshold is estimated by linear regression of the VEP amplitudes versus the frequency, or size, of the grating or checkerboard stimulus.[60] Data are recorded as the $\log_{10}$ of the minimum angle of resolution (logMAR) with smaller logMAR values indicative of better visual acuity. A rapid VEP method (sweep VEP) has been developed for use in infant populations.[59,61] The standard VEP also allows assessment of latency, or the time between presentation of the stimulus and the peak of the electrical potential. This reflects the rate of transmission of the stimulus and, hence, should be useful for assessing the effects of LC-PUFA (or other intervention).

However, it has been used for this purpose by only a few investigators.[55,62–65]

Unlike the Teller Acuity Card and VEP procedures, which measure the response of the entire visual system to a stimulus, electroretinography measures only the activity of the retina. The primary components of the electroretinogram generated in response to a flash of light are the a-wave, which is produced by hyperpolarization of the photoreceptor, and the b-wave, which reflects the subsequent activation of retinal neurons. Performance is quantified by a number of parameters, some measured directly and some calculated.[66,67] Among these are the threshold (the minimal intensity of light necessary to elicit a small amplitude), the implicit time or peak latency (the time from the presentation of a brief flash of light to the response peak), the maximal amplitude, and the sensitivity (the intensity of light that elicits a response of half the maximal amplitude). This methodology is somewhat more invasive and time consuming than the other methods and has been used to assess effects of LC-PUFA in only a few studies.[63,68,69]

Meta-analyses of data from studies in both term and preterm infants using both behavioral and electrophysiological methods of assessment have been reported.[70,71] The meta-analysis of behaviorally based tests of visual acuity obtained in randomized studies of term infants showed a statistically significant advantage of DHA-supplemented v. unsupplemented formula at 2 months of age but not at other ages. Meta-analysis of data from term infant studies utilizing electrophysiologically based tests showed no statistically significant advantage of supplementation at any age. A recently reported multicenter study,[72] which was not included in the meta-analysis, showed no advantages of DHA (0.14% of total fatty acids) plus ARA (0.46% of total fatty acids) supplementation on visual function as assessed by the Teller Acuity Card procedure at 2, 4, 6 or 12 months of age. This study did not include electrophysiologically based tests of visual function. Whether inclusion of these additional data in a future meta-analysis will change the conclusions is not clear.

Another recent study[52] showed an apparent relationship between DHA intake and visual acuity. In this study of term infants who were breast-fed exclusively for at least 3 months following birth and, then, weaned to a standard formula, there was a statistically significant positive correlation between visual acuity assessed by the Teller Acuity Card procedure at 2 and 12 months of age and the DHA content of erythrocyte phosphatidylethanolamine at 2 months of age. There was no correlation at either 4 or 6 months of age. In addition, infants with an erythrocyte phosphatidylethanolamine DHA concentration >10.78 g $\cdot$ 100 g^{-1} at 2 months of age (i.e. the upper tertile) had significantly better acuity at 2 and 12 but not at 4 and 6 months of age than those with an erythrocyte phosphatidylethanolamine DHA content < 8.53 g 100 g^{-1} at 2 months of age (i.e. the lowest tertile).

Birch et al.[73] recently reported results of a randomized controlled trial of supplemented (0.36% of total fatty acids as DHA and 0.72% as ARA) v. unsupplemented formula following near-exclusive breastfeeding (1 feeding per day of formula allowed) for the first 6 weeks of life. Visual acuity of the 2 groups as measured by sweep VEP was similar at enrollment but that of the supplemented group was better at 17, 26 and 52 weeks of age. Random dot stereoacuity of the supplemented group also was better at 17 weeks of age but not at 26 and 52 weeks of age. Random dot stereopsis, which reflects processing in the visual cortex, is not present before 3 months of age and matures rapidly between 3 and 5 months of age. It is thought to be particularly sensitive to differences in maturation of the visual cortex between 3 and 5 months of age.

In a similar study, Hoffman et al.[74] assigned infants to the same formulas after 4–6 months of near-exclusive breastfeeding. Visual acuity of the supplemented group as assessed by sweep VEP was better at 12 months of age. As expected, there was no difference in random dot stereoacuity between the two groups, presumably because the period of rapid development of the visual cortex ended prior to enrollment. The findings of this study and that of Birch et al.,[73] indicate a possible need for DHA beyond 4–6 months of age, the maximum duration of supplementation in many previous studies.

In another recent study of 435 children who were born at term, stereoacuity at 3.5 years of age was greater in children who had been breast-fed for at least 4 months than in those who had not been breast-fed.[75] Among infants who had been breast-fed, stereoacuity at 3.5 years of age was greater in those whose mothers ate oily fish during pregnancy than in those whose mothers did not eat oily fish. The content of DHA in maternal erythrocyte phospholipid prior to birth also was related to maternal intake of fatty fish during pregnancy.

The meta-analysis of data from randomized studies in preterm infants showed an advantage of DHA-supplemented v. unsupplemented formulas on both behaviorally based and electrophysiologically based measurements of visual acuity.[71] Advantages with behaviorally based tests were apparent at 2 and 4 months corrected age but not at other ages. Electrophysiologically based measurements showed an advantage of DHA supplementation at 4 months corrected age but not at other ages. A recent randomized, controlled trial in preterm infants[76] showed no advantage of ARA and DHA supplementation (0.26%

and 0.42% of total fatty acids, respectively, from birth to term and, then, 0.16% and 0.42%, respectively, through the first year of life) on visual acuity at 2, 4 or 6 months of age as assessed by the Teller Acuity Card procedure. However, in a subset of infants, there was an advantage of supplementation on acuity as assessed by sweep VEP at 6 but not at 4 months post-term. Another recent multicenter study in which supplemented (0.36% of total fatty acids as DHA and 0.72% as ARA) v. unsupplemented formulas were fed to preterm infants for an average of ~ 28 days during hospitalization showed no effect on visual acuity as assessed by the Teller Acuity Card procedure at either 48 or 57 weeks postmenstrual age.[77] Electrophysiological assessments were not performed.

In apparent contrast to some of the findings discussed above, recent Cochrane reviews of much, but not all, of the same data concluded that there were no consistent effects of LC-PUFA on visual acuity of either term[78] or preterm infants.[79] Gibson et al.[80] in reviewing most reported randomized controlled trials of supplemented v. unsupplemented formulas concluded that the evidence for a beneficial effect of LC-PUFA supplementation on visual function of preterm infants was "reasonably compelling" whereas the evidence of a beneficial effect on visual function of term infants was less so. This conclusion seems to be a valid interpretation of the available data.

LC-PUFA and cognitive/behavioral development

Most studies addressing the cognitive/behavioral development of infants fed LC-PUFA-supplemented v. unsupplemented formulas have utilized the Bayley Scales of Infant Development and/or the Fagan Test of Infant Intelligence (FTII). The Bayley Scales provide standardized indices of both mental (MDI) and psychomotor development (PDI). They have been used for years and are considered the "gold standard" for assessing global abilities of infants from birth to approximately 3 years of age. However, the relationship between cognitive and/or psychomotor function as assessed by the Bayley Scales early in life and later function is poor, particularly for "normal" infants.[81]

The Fagan Test of Infant Intelligence assesses novelty preference.[82] The infant is shown a single stimulus (usually a face) for a standardized, age-based period and, then, is shown this stimulus along with a "novel" one. If the infant has "learned" the original stimulus prior to the novelty test, the typical response is to look selectively toward the "novel" v. the "familiar" image. Scores on this test during infancy are somewhat more predictive of later cognitive function than the Bayley MDI; however, the internal consistency (reproducibility) of the test is relatively poor.[83] Look duration during the familiarization and the paired comparison phases of the test also is a modest predictor of both concurrent performance on other tests during infancy and later tests of intelligence;[83] shorter look durations during the familiarization phase predict better concurrent as well as later cognitive performance.

One, sometimes both, of these tests has been utilized in most studies of LC-PUFA supplementation in both term and preterm infants. Some of these studies showed advantages of supplementation with both tests, some with one but not the other and still others with neither. Available studies in term infants were reviewed in 1998 by an Expert Panel appointed by the Life Sciences Research Organization (LSRO) to assess the nutrient requirements for term infant formulas.[23] As a group, the studies available at that time were criticized for including too few infants, failing to control adequately for confounding factors, failing to assess function at more than one age, failing to examine individual differences in development, and failing to follow the infants for a sufficiently long period (e.g. none of the studies cited in the report included data beyond 1 year of age). Based on this review, the Panel did not recommend addition of LC-PUFA to term infant formulas but suggested that the issue be re-evaluated in about 5 years.

The four randomized trials in term infants published since 1998[72,84–86] have not resolved many of these difficulties. The largest of these[84] compared developmental outcomes of infants assigned randomly to be fed a formula supplemented with both ARA and DHA (0.3 and 0.32% of total fatty acids, respectively, from purified egg phospholipid and triglyceride fractions) or an unsupplemented formula for the first 6 months of life. At 18 months of age, the mean Bailey MDIs of the supplemented group ($n = 125$), the control group ($n = 125$) and a breast-fed reference group ($n = 104$) were 95.5 ± 1.2 (SE), 94.5 ± 1.2 and 96.0 ± 1.0, respectively. Mean Bayley PDIs of the three groups, respectively, were 96.4 ± 0.9, 95 ± 0.8 and 94.4 ± 1.20. These small differences among groups obviously are not statistically significant and, probably, are not biologically significant.

A smaller trial[85] included a breast-fed reference group ($n = 46$) and groups assigned to a control formula (no LC-PUFA, $n = 21$), a formula supplemented with only DHA (0.35% of total fatty acids as tuna oil; $n = 23$) or a formula supplemented with both DHA and ARA (0.34% of total fatty acids as each from egg yolk phospholipid; $n = 24$). The formulas were fed through 12 months of age at which time neither the MDI nor the PDI differed among groups. Scores of the three formula groups also did not differ at 24 months of age but the scores of all were lower than scores of the breast-fed reference group.

Another small trial[86] included three formula-fed groups but no breast-fed reference group: a control group (no LC-PUFA; $n = 20$); a group fed a DHA-supplemented formula (0.35% of total fatty acids as an algal-derived triglyceride; $n = 17$); a group fed a formula supplemented with both DHA and ARA (0.36% and 0.72% of total fatty acids, respectively, as a mixture of algal- and fungal-derived triglycerides; $n = 19$). All were fed the assigned formula through 4 months of age. The mean Bayley MDI of the group fed the formula supplemented with both DHA and ARA was 7.3 points higher than that of the control group at 18 months of age (105.6 ± 11.8 (SD) v. 98.3 ± 8.2; $P < 0.05$) and 3.2 points higher than that of the DHA-supplemented group (102.4 ± 7.5; NS). Bayley PDIs of the three groups did not differ.

The most recently reported trial in term infants[72] included a reference group of breast-fed infants ($n = 165$) and groups of infants fed a control formula ($n = 77$) or one of two formulas with the same contents of DHA and ARA (0.14% and 0.46% of total fatty acids, respectively) from either a combination of fish oil and egg triglyceride ($n = 80$) or a combination of fish and fungal oil ($n = 82$). The formulas were fed for the first year of life during which time there were no differences among groups in visual acuity (see above), information processing (Fagan Test of Infant Intelligence) or temperament (Infant Behavior Questionnaire). General development assessed by Bayley Scales of Infant Development at 12 months of age and language development assessed by MacArthur Communicative Development Inventories at 14 months of age also did not differ among groups.

Reasons for the discrepant results among these recent studies (and other older studies) are not clear. The trials differed with respect to the source of LC-PUFA supplementation, the duration of supplement and the amounts of DHA and ARA supplementation as well as the ratio of ARA/DHA. There also were some differences in the LA and ALA contents of the control and experimental formulas. The variance in Bayley MDI and PDI scores also varied among studies. Interestingly, the variance was quite small in the study showing that infants who received a formula supplemented with DHA + ARA for the first 4 months of life had a higher Bayley MDI score at 18 months of age than infants who received an unsupplemented formula.[86]

Even fewer studies are available in preterm infants fed LC-PUFA supplemented v. unsupplemented formulas and these are subject to many of the same criticisms levied against studies in term infants. However, the available data, including those from recently reported, large, multicenter studies,[76,87] suggest that preterm infants are more likely to benefit from supplementation than term infants.

One of the recently reported trials[76] included infants who weighed between 750–1800 g at birth and were assigned randomly, before initiation of enteral feeding, to be fed one of three formulas until 12 months of age: a control formula ($n = 144$); a formula with 0.26% of total fatty acids as DHA and 0.46% as ARA as a combination of fish and fungal oils until term and, then, 0.16% and 0.46% of total fatty acids as DHA and ARA, respectively, from the same sources ($n = 140$); a formula with the same DHA and ARA contents as a combination of fish oil and egg triglyceride ($n = 143$). Infants fed human milk exclusively through term served as a reference group ($n = 43$). The effects of the supplemented formulas on visual acuity are described above. The group supplemented with a combination of fish oil and egg triglyceride had a higher mean Fagan Test of Novelty Preference score at 6 months corrected age than either the control group or the group supplemented with fish and fungal oils; but there was no difference in mean scores among groups at 9 months corrected age. There also was no difference in mean Bayley MDI among groups at 12 months corrected age. However, among infants who weighed <1250 g at birth, the mean Bayley PDI of those assigned to the fish and fungal oil supplement was higher than that of the control group at 12 months corrected age. The mean Bayley PDI of the subgroup who weighed <1250 g at birth and were assigned to the fish oil and egg triglyceride supplement (and, interestingly, had a higher Fagan Test of Novelty Preference score at 6 months corrected age), however, was not different from either the control or the other supplemented group at 12 months corrected age. If twins and infants from Spanish speaking families were excluded, both supplemented groups had better vocabulary comprehension at 14 months corrected age than the control group; however, without these exclusions, there was no difference in vocabulary comprehension among groups.

The second recent trial in LBW infants, so far reported only as an abstract,[87] included infants with birthweights <1500 g who were assigned shortly after birth to a control formula ($n = 83$), a formula with DHA (0.34% of total fatty acids) and ARA (0.68% of total fatty acids), both from single cell oils ($n = 72$), or a formula with the same amounts of DHA and ARA from a combination of fish and single cell oils ($n = 90$). A group of breast-fed term infants ($n = 105$) also was followed. The assigned formulas, either preterm, post-discharge or term, depending upon the wishes of the infants' physicians or parents, were fed through 92 weeks postmenstrual age (PMA). They were fed as sole diets until 57 weeks PMA, after which addition of biekost was permitted. Bayley MDI and PDI of both supplemented groups at 118 weeks PMA, although lower than those of the term breast-fed infants studied concurrently, were higher than

those of the control group. There were no differences in Bayley MDI or PDI between the two supplemented groups.

A few methods other than the Bayley Scales of Infant Development and the Fagan Test of Infant Intelligence have been used to assess the effects of LC-PUFA on development. For example, Willats et al.[88] found that term infants assigned to a formula supplemented with both DHA and ARA v. an unsupplemented formula had better visual habituation scores at 4 months of age and performed better on a means-end problem-solving test at 10 months of age. The supplemented group not only had more intentional solutions to items of this test but also scored higher than those assigned to the control formula, findings that have been related to higher intelligence quotient scores later in childhood.

Innis et al.,[52] studying breast-fed term infants with a range of DHA and ARA as well as LA and ALA intakes and, hence, a range of plasma and erythrocyte lipid DHA and ARA contents, found no statistically significant relationships between infant DHA or ARA status at 2 months, when all infants were exclusively breast-fed, and scores on an object-search test at either 6 or 12 months of age. There also was no statistically significant relationship at either 6 or 12 months of age between infant DHA or ARA status at 2 months of age and novelty preference, Bayley MDI or Bayley PDI scores. However, there was a relationship between ability to discriminate non-native retroflex and phonetic contrasts at 9 months of age and the DHA content of both plasma phospholipid and erythrocyte phosphatidylethanolamine at 2 months of age. This finding is thought to indicate more rapid language development in those with higher plasma and erythrocyte lipid levels of DHA at 2 weeks of age.

Two other studies of the effect of maternal DHA supplementation and, hence, intake of DHA by the breastfeeding infant are relevant. Gibson et al.[51] supplemented breastfeeding mothers with varying amounts of DHA, achieving breast milk DHA concentrations ranging from 0.1–1.7% of total fatty acids and, hence, a wide range in DHA content of infant plasma lipids. However, there was no relationship between DHA content of milk or infant plasma lipids and VEP acuity at either 12 or 16 weeks of age. On the other hand, Bayley MDI at 12 months of age, but not at 24 months of age, was weakly correlated with milk DHA content.

In a somewhat similar study, Jensen et al.[53] assigned breastfeeding mothers to receive DHA (~ 250 mg day^{-1} as an algal-derived triglyceride) or a placebo for the first 4 months postpartum. At 4 months of age, plasma phospholipid DHA content of infants whose mothers had received DHA was approximately 50% higher than that of infants whose mothers received the placebo. However, there was no difference in visual acuity between the 2 groups at either 4 or 8 months of age, whether assessed by sweep VEP or the Teller Acuity Card procedure. There also was no difference between groups in scores on a variety of neurodevelopmental tests at 12 and 18 months of age but at 30 months of age, the mean Bayley PDI of the group whose mothers received DHA was 8 points higher than that of the group whose mothers received placebo ($P < 0.01$). There was no statistically significant difference in mean Bayley MDI between the two groups at 30 months of age and there was no statistically significant relationship between PDI scores at 30 months of age and plasma phospholipid content of DHA at 4 months of age.

Helland et al.,[54] examining the effect of supplementing women with either cod liver oil ($\sim$1.2 g day^{-1} of DHA and 0.8 mg day^{-1} of EPA) or corn oil from week 18 of pregnancy until 3 months after delivery, found that children whose mothers received cod liver oil scored higher at 4 years of age on the Mental Processing Composite of Kaufman Assessment Battery for Children (106.4 ± 7.4; $n = 48$) than children whose mothers received corn oil (102.3 ± 11.3; $n = 36$). In a multiple regression model, maternal intake of DHA during pregnancy was the only variable related significantly to the mental processing scores of the children at 4 years of age.

In a somewhat similar study, Malcolm et al.[55] assigned pregnant women to fish oil ($n = 50$) or placebo capsules ($n = 50$) from week 15 of pregnancy through term. The fish oil capsules provided about 200 mg DHA per day. Although the DHA content of maternal erythrocytes at birth was $\sim$50% higher in the DHA group, umbilical cord erythrocyte DHA content of the two groups did not differ between groups at either 50 or 66 weeks postconceptional age. However, maturity of the pattern-reversal VEP at 50 and 66 weeks postconceptional age was related to the DHA status of the infants at birth. Specifically, infants with higher erythrocyte DHA content at birth had shorter P 100 peak latencies than those with lower erythrocyte DHA content at birth.

The effects of LC-PUFA supplementation of infant formulas on other aspects of brain development also have been examined. Three studies of the effects on brain auditory evoked potentials of preterm infants showed no effects of supplementation.[63,64,89] In one of these,[64] supplemented infants had slower peripheral nerve conduction than infants fed human milk but not slower than those fed the control formula. A very recent study[90] investigated the effect of supplemented (0.3% of total fatty acids (by weight) as DHA and 0.45% as ARA from a mixture of egg yolk, tuna oil and a fungal oil) v. unsupplemented formula during the first 2 months of life on the quality of the infants' general movements at 3 months of age as assessed from videotapes made at that time. The unsupplemented group had mildly abnormal general movements significantly more often than the supplemented group or a breast-fed group that was studied concurrently (31%, 19% and 20%, respectively). The frequency of "normal optimal" movements did not differ between supplemented and unsupplemented groups (18% and 21%, respectively) but was less in both than observed in the breast-fed group (34%). Although not familiar to those not versed in infant and child development, the quality of general movements has been shown to be useful for evaluating the quality of brain function in young infants.

Only one study has examined the effect of LC-PUFA supplementation on structural brain development.[65] In this study, preterm infants were assigned randomly to receive either a standard formula ($n = 20$) or a formula supplemented with 0.34% and 0.70% of total fatty acids as DHA and ARA, respectively ($n = 22$), both from single cell oils, until a corrected age of 6 months (preterm formula until weight reached 3000 g and a term formula thereafter). Brain structural development, assessed by MRI at 3 and 12 months corrected age, did not differ between groups at either age. This method essentially assesses the degree of myelination, and in this study neither global myelination nor myelination of the cerebral visual system differed between groups. This may not be surprising since the LC-PUFA content of myelin is low. However, myelin deposition is dependent on close interaction among neurons, their axons and oligodendrocytes which are rich in LC-PUFA. Thus, myelination is thought to reflect the functional maturity of all these components. Visual acuity and neurodevelopment was also assessed by the Teller Acuity Card procedure and the Dutch version of the Bayley Scales of Infant Development, respectively; neither differed between groups at 3, 6, 12 or 24 months of age. VEP latency and amplitude, assessed at 3 and 12 months of age also did not differ.

Adverse effects of long-chain polyunsaturated fatty acids

The observation by Carlson et al. in the early 1990s that preterm infants assigned to a formula supplemented with fish oil (0.3% of total fatty acids as EPA and 0.2% as DHA) v. an unsupplemented formula weighed less and had a lower weight-for-length at various times during the first year of life than infants assigned to an unsupplemented formula[91] has generated considerable concern. In this study, weight at 12 months corrected age correlated with plasma phospholipid ARA content at various times during the first year of life.[92] Interestingly, a smaller study conducted at about the same time did not show differences in growth between supplemented and unsupplemented preterm infants although the supplemented group received even more of a similar fish oil.[93] However, the duration of this study may not have been sufficient to permit detection of weight differences. A less marked effect on growth also was observed by Carlson et al.[94] in preterm infants fed a formula supplemented with low-EPA fish oil v. an unsupplemented formula. In this study, there was no correlation between ARA status and growth but there was a correlation between weight at some ages and the plasma phospholipid ratio of ARA/DHA. Ryan et al.[95] observed lower rates of growth in preterm male, but not female, infants fed a formula supplemented with the same low-EPA fish oil (0.2% of total fatty acids as DHA) v. a control formula from shortly before hospital discharge until 59 weeks postmenstrual age (PMA). In this study, plasma phospholipid ARA content of the supplemented group was lower through 59 weeks PMA but there was no statistically significant correlation between plasma phospholipid ARA content and any aspect of growth. Rather, rates of increase in both weight and length of male infants were inversely correlated with plasma phospholipid DHA content. A lower weight at 4 months of age also was observed in term infants fed formulas with a LA:ALA ratio of ~4 v. ~40 and, in this study, weight at 4 months of age was correlated with plasma phospholipid ARA content.[62]

More recently, Innis et al.,[52] studying infants who were breast-fed exclusively for the first 3 months of life, reported a statistically significant inverse correlation between erythrocyte phosphatidyl choline and phosphatidyl ethanalamine contents of DHA and weight at 6 but not 12 months of age. There was no statistically significant relationship between DHA or ARA contents of plasma lipids and size at any age.

In contrast to these observations of an apparent adverse effect of $\omega 3$ fatty acids on growth, Innis et al.[77] observed more rapid growth of preterm infants fed formula supplemented with both DHA (0.33% of fat as an algal oil) and ARA (0.6% of fat as a fungal oil) v. a DHA-supplemented (0.34% of fat as an algal oil) or a control formula for at least 28 days prior to hospital discharge and followed until 57 weeks PMA. Another recent study also showed a positive growth effect of formulas supplemented with both DHA and ARA, either as single cell oils or a mixture of fish and fungal oils.[87] In this study, weight of the group supplemented with single cell oils was greater than that of the control group from 66 through 118 weeks substitute and equal to that of breast-fed term infants at 118 weeks PMA. Length of this group also was greater than that of either the control group or the group supplemented with fish and fungal oil at 79 and 92 weeks PMA and equal to that of the breast-fed term infants by 79 weeks PMA.

Possible reason(s) for an inhibitory effect of $\omega 3$ fatty acids or, perhaps, a stimulatory effect of $\omega 6$ fatty acids on growth are not clear. Those that have been suggested include inhibition of desaturation and elongation of LA to ARA by the $\omega 3$ fatty acids, inhibition of eicosanoid synthesis from ARA by the intake of preformed EPA or endogenous synthesis of EPA from a moderately high intake of ALA, and effects of $\omega 3$ and $\omega 6$ fatty acids on transcription of genes controlling lipolysis and lipogenesis.[96]

In addition to concerns about adverse effects of $\omega 3$ fatty acids on growth, a number of theoretical concerns, all related to the known biological effects of $\omega 6$ and $\omega 3$ LC-PUFA, have been raised.[97] Among these is the possibility that supplementation with highly unsaturated fatty acids and their subsequent incorporation into cell membranes will increase the likelihood of oxidant damage. This is because peroxidation occurs at the site of double bonds making membranes with more unsaturated fatty acids likely to be more vulnerable to oxidant damage. If so, LC-PUFA supplementation might increase the incidence of conditions thought to be related to oxidant damage (e.g. necrotizing enterocolitis; bronchopulmonary dysplasia; retrolental fibroplasia). There also is concern that unbalanced supplementation with $\omega 3$ and $\omega 6$ LC-PUFA will result in altered eicosanoid metabolism with potential effects on a variety of physiological mechanisms (e.g. blood clotting; infection). In addition to these potential effects, a higher content of polyunsaturated fatty acids in muscle cell membranes has been related to enhanced insulin sensitivity[98,99] and specific LC-PUFA have been shown to inhibit transcription of some genes and enhance transcription of others.[100] Unfortunately, there are few data to either support or allay these theoretical concerns with respect to the small amounts of LC-PUFA likely to be added to infant formulas.

Recently reported, multicenter randomized, controlled, double-blind trials in preterm infants[76,77,87,101–103] have shown no difference in the incidence of bronchopulmonary dysplasia, necrotizing enterocolitis or other common neonatal morbidities between infants assigned to formulas supplemented with either DHA or both DHA and ARA from a variety of sources (single cell oils; low-EPA fish oil; egg yolk phospholipid; egg yolk triglyceride) and infants receiving unsupplemented formula. Further, as discussed above, these studies showed no adverse effects on growth although the apparent stimulation of growth observed in two of the studies perhaps should be as disturbing as the minimal adverse effects on growth. Together, these studies included more than 1000 infants assigned to supplemented or unsupplemented formulas. Thus, despite the relative absence of definitive data concerning the validity of theoretical safety concerns related to the known biological effects of LC-PUFA, the fact that supplemented formulas in the studies of preterm infants cited above did not result in a greater incidence of conditions thought to be related etiologically to the theoretical concerns suggests that the amounts of the sources of LC-PUFA used in these studies are safe, at least over the short term.

Conclusions

It is clear that supplementation of infant formulas with DHA and ARA from a variety of sources results in DHA and ARA contents of plasma and erythrocyte lipids that are similar to those observed in breast-fed infants. Although less clear, there is some evidence that supplementation may also maintain tissue contents of these fatty acids, including contents in the central nervous system. However, whether maintaining plasma and, perhaps, tissue contents of these fatty acids equal to those of breast-fed infants confers functional benefits is not at all clear. Some studies have shown benefits and some have not. Moreover, those that demonstrated benefits often did so with one functional test but not with another intended to assess the same functional domain. Further, some studies have shown benefits at one age but not at another. Although some of these apparent discrepancies can be explained by the nature of the assessment method and/or the complex nature of infant development, no study reported to date is without problems.

Nonetheless, formulas supplemented with DHA and ARA are now available worldwide. These differ with respect to amounts of added DHA and ARA as well as the sources of the added DHA and ARA. Although the efficacy of such formulas in improving visual and/or cognitive development of term or preterm infants remains uncertain, they appear to be safe, at least for the short-term. Further, the large coefficients of variation reported in all studies suggest that the apparent rates of conversion of ALA and LA to DHA and ARA, respectively, are quite variable. The maternal LC-PUFA status and, hence, the amounts transferred to the developing fetus also are quite variable. Thus, it is likely that some infants cannot form sufficient LC-PUFA endogenously and will benefit from supplementation whereas others can form sufficient LC-PUFA and will not benefit. Unfortunately, those likely to benefit cannot be identified easily by current methodologies. This possibility that some infants may benefit from LC-PUFA supplementation is probably the best argument for availability of LC-PUFA supplemented infant formulas. On the other hand,

several recent studies suggest that LC-PUFA supplementation in early infancy as well as during gestation may have effects that are not detectable until well beyond the period of supplementation. Nonetheless, those who expect supplemented formulas to be as efficacious as breastfeeding are likely to be disappointed.

REFERENCES

1 Innis, S. M. Essential fatty acids in growth and development. *Prog. Lipid Res.* 1991;**30**:39–103.

2 Holman, R. T. Nutritional and biochemical evidences of acyl interaction with respect to essential polyunsaturated fatty acids. *Prog. Lipid Res.* 1986;**25**:29–39.

3 Voss, A., Reinhart, M., Sankarappa, S., Sprecher, H. The metabolism of 7, 10, 13, 16, 19-docosahexaenoic acid to 4, 7, 10, 13, 16, 19-docosahexaenoic acid in rat liver is independent of a 4-desaturase. *J. Biol. Chem.* 1991;**266**:19995–20000.

4 Sauerwald, T. U., Hachey, D. L., Jensen, C. L. *et al.* Intermediates in endogenous synthesis of C22:6ω3 and C20:4ω6 by term and preterm infants. *Pediatr. Res.* 1997;**41**:183–7.

5 Oliw, E., Gramström, E., Änggärd, E. The prostaglandins and essential fatty acids. In Pace-Asciak, C., Gramström, E., eds. *Prostaglandins and Related Substances.* Amsterdam: Elsevier; 1983:1–19.

6 Burr, G. O., Burr, M. M. A new deficiency disease produced by the rigid exclusion of fat from the diet. *J. Biol. Chem.* 1929;**82**:345–67.

7 Hansen, A. E., Steward, R. A., Hughes, G. *et al.* The relation of linoleic acid to infant feeding, a review. *Acta Paediatr.* 1962;**51**:1–41.

8 Benolken, R. M., Anderson, R. E., Wheeler, T. G. Membrane fatty acids associated with the electrical response in visual excitation. *Science* 1973;**182**:1253–4.

9 Wheeler, T. G., Benolken, R. M. Visual membranes: specificity of fatty acid precursors for the electrical response to illumination. *Science* 1975;**188**:1312–14.

10 Neuringer, M., Connor, W. E., Van Petten, C. *et al.* Dietary omega-3 fatty acid deficiency and visual loss in infant Rhesus monkeys. *J. Clin. Invest.* 1984;**73**:272–6.

11 Neuringer, M., Connor, W. E., Lin, D. S. *et al.* Biochemical and functional effects of prenatal and postnatal ω3 fatty acid deficiency on retina and brain in Rhesus monkeys. *Proc. Natl Acad. Sci. USA* 1986;**83**:4021–5.

12 Holman, R. T., Johnson, S. B., Hatch, R. F. A case of human linolenic acid deficiency involving neurological abnormalities. *Am. J. Clin. Nutr.* 1982;**35**:617–23.

13 Bjerve, K. S., Fischer, S., Alme, K. Alpha-linolenic acid deficiency in man: effect of ethyl linolenate on plasma and erythrocyte fatty acid composition and biosynthesis of prostanoids. *Am. J. Clin. Nutr.* 1987;**46**:570–6.

14 Holman, R. T. The ratio of trienoic: tetraenoic acids in tissue lipids as a measure of essential fatty acid requirement. *J. Nutr.* 1960;**70**:405–10.

15 Holman, R. T., Caster, W. O., Wiese, H. F. The essential fatty acid requirement of infants and the assessment of their dietary intake of linolenate by serum fatty acid analysis. *Am. J. Clin. Nutr.* 1964;**14**:70–5.

16 Innis, S. M. Fat. In Tsang, R. C., Lucas, A., Uauy, R., Zlotkin, S., eds. *Nutritional Needs of the Preterm Infant.* Baltimore: Williams and Wilkins; 1993:65–86.

17 Jensen, R. G. Lipids in human milk. *Lipids* 1999;**34**:1243–71.

18 Sanders, T. A. B., Reddy, S. The influence of a vegetarian diet on the fatty acid composition of human milk and the essential fatty acid status of the infant. *J. Pediatr.* 1992;**120**:S71–7.

19 Henderson, R. A., Jensen, R. G., Lammi-Keefe, C. J. *et al.* Effect of fish oil on the fatty acid composition of human milk and maternal and infant erythrocytes. *Lipids* 1992;**27**:863–9.

20 Makrides, M., Neumann, M. A., Gibson, R. A. Effect of maternal docosahexaenoic acid (DHA) supplementation on breast milk composition. *Eur. J. Clin. Nutr.* 1996;**50**:352–7.

21 Jensen, C. L., Maude, M., Anderson, R. E., Heird, W. C. Effect of docosahexaenoic acid supplementation of lactating women on milk total lipid, and maternal and infant plasma phospholipid fatty acids. *Am. J. Clin. Nutr.* 2000;**71**:292S–9S.

22 ESPGAN Committee on Nutrition. Comment on the content and composition of lipids in infant formulas. *Acta Paediatr. Scand.* 1991;**80**:887–96.

23 Raiten, D. J., Talbot, J. M., Waters, J. H. LSRO Report: assessment of nutrient requirements for infant formulas. *J. Nutr.* 1998;**128**:2059S–2093S.

24 Carlson, S. E., Rhodes, P. G., Ferguson, M. G. Docosahexaenoic acid status of preterm infants at birth and following feeding with human milk or formula. *Am. J. Clin. Nutr.* 1986;**44**:798–804.

25 Innis, S. M., Akrabawi, S. S., Diersen-Schade, D. A. *et al.* Visual acuity and blood lipids in term infants fed human milk or formulae. *Lipids* 1997;**32**:63–72.

26 Jrgensen, M. H., Hernell, O., Lund, P. *et al.* Visual acuity and erythrocyte docosahexaenoic acid status in breast-fed and formula-fed term infants during the first four months of life. *Lipids* 1996;**31**:99–105.

27 Ponder, D. L., Innis, S. M., Benson, J. D. *et al.* Docosahexaenoic acid status of term infants fed breast milk or infant formula containing soy oil or corn oil. *Pediatr. Res.* 1992;**32**:683–8.

28 Lucas, A., Morley, R., Cole, T. J. *et al.* Early diet in preterm babies and developmental status at 18 months. *Lancet* 1990;**335**:1477–81.

29 Lucas, A., Morley, R., Cole, T. J. Randomised trial of early diet in preterm babies and later intelligence quotient. *Br. Med. J.* 1998;**317**:1481–7.

30 Morrow-Tlucak, M., Haude, R. H., Ernhart, C. B. Breastfeeding and cognitive development in the first 2 years of life. *Soc. Sci. Med.* 1988;**26**:635–9.

31 Rogan, W. J., Gladen, B. C. Breast-feeding and cognitive development. *Early Hum Dev.* 1993;**31**:181–93.

32 Clandinin, M. T., Chappell, J. E., Leong, S. *et al.* Intrauterine fatty acid accretion rates in human brain: implications for fatty acid requirements. *Early Hum. Dev.* 1980;**4**:121–9.

33 Clandinin, M. T., Chappell, J. E., Leong, S. *et al.* Extrauterine fatty acid accretion in infant brain: implications for fatty acid requirements. *Early Hum. Dev.* 1980;**4**:131–8.

34 Martinez, M. Tissue levels of polyunsaturated fatty acids during early human development. *J. Pediatr.* 1992;**120**: S129–38.

35 Farquharson, J., Cockburn, F., Patrick, W. A. *et al.* Infant cerebral cortex phospholipid fatty-acid composition and diet. *Lancet* 1992;**340**:810–13.

36 Jamieson, E. C., Abbasi, K. A., Cockburn, F. *et al.* Effect of diet on term infant cerebral cortex fatty acid composition. *World Rev. Nutr. Diet.* 1994;**75**:139–41.

37 Makrides, M., Neumann, M. A., Byard, R. W. *et al.* Fatty acid composition of brain, retina, and erythrocytes in breast- and formula-fed infants. *Am. J. Clin. Nutr.* 1994;**60**:189–94.

38 Arbuckle, L. D., MacKinnon, M. J., Innis, S. M. Formula 18:2 (n-6) and 18:3 (n-3) content and ratio influence long-chain polyunsaturated fatty acids in the developing piglet liver and central nervous system. *J. Nutr.* 1994;**124**:289–98.

39 Sauerwald, T., Hachey, D. L., Jensen, C. L. *et al.* Effect of dietary α-linolenic acid intake on incorporation of docosahexaenoic and arachidonic acids into plasma phospholipids of term infants. *Lipids* 1996;**31**:S131–5.

40 Berghaus, T. M., Demmelmair, H., Koletzko, B. Fatty acid composition of lipid classes in maternal and cord plasma at birth. *Eur. J. Pediatr.* 1998;**157**:763–8.

41 Dutta-Roy, A. K. Transport mechanisms for long-chain polyunsaturated fatty acids in the human placenta. *Am. J. Clin. Nutr.* 2000;**71**:315S–22S.

42 Carnielli, V. P., Wattimena, D. J., Luijendijk, I. H. *et al.* The very low birth weight premature infant is capable of synthesizing arachidonic and docosahexaenoic acids from linoleic and linolenic acids. *Pediatr. Res.* 1996;**40**:169–74.

43 Demmelmair, H., von Schenck, U., Behrendt, E. *et al.* Estimation of arachidonic acid synthesis in full term neonates using natural variation of ^{13}C content. *J. Pediatr. Gastroenterol. Nutr.* 1995;**21**:31–6.

44 Salem, N., Jr, Wegher, B., Mena, P. *et al.* Arachidonic and docosahexaenoic acids are biosynthesized from their 18-carbon precursors in human infants. *Proc. Natl Acad. Sci. USA* 1996;**93**:49–54.

45 Uauy, R., Mena, P., Wegher, B. *et al.* Long chain polyunsaturated fatty acid formation in neonates: effect of gestational age and intrauterine growth. *Pediatr. Res.* 2000;**47**:127–35.

46 Rioux, F. M., Innis, S. M., Dyer, R. *et al.* Diet-induced changes in liver and bile but not brain fatty acids can be predicted from differences in plasma phospholipid fatty acids in formula and milk fed piglets. *J. Nutr.* 1997;**127**:370–7.

47 Blank, C., Neumann, M. A., Makrides, M., Gibson, R. A. Optimizing DHA levels in piglets by lowering the linoleic acid to α-linolenic acid ratio. *J. Lipid Res.* 2002;**43**:1537–43.

48 Moore, S. A., Yoder, E., Murphy, S. *et al.* Astrocytes, not neurons, produce docosahexaenoic acid ($22:6\omega3$) and arachidonic acid ($20:4\omega6$). *J. Neurochem.* 1991;**56**:518–24.

49 Moore, S. A. Cerebral endothelium and astrocytes cooperate in supplying docosahexaenoic acid to neurons. *Adv. Exp. Med. Biol.* 1993;**331**:229–33.

50 Pawlosky, R. J., Denkins, Y., Ward, G., Salem, N. Jr. Retinal and brain accretion of long-chain polyunsaturated fatty acids in developing felines: the effects of corn oil-based maternal diets. *Am. J. Clin. Nutr.* 1997;**65**:465–72.

51 Gibson, R., Neumann, M., Makrides, M. Effect of increasing breast milk docosahexaenoic acid on plasma and erythrocyte phospholipid fatty acids and neural indices of exclusively breast-fed infants. *Eur. J. Clin. Nutr.* 1997;**51**:578–84.

52 Innis, S. M., Gilley, J., Werker, J. Are human milk long-chain polyunsaturated fatty acids related to visual and neural development in breast-fed term infants? *J. Pediatr.* 2001;**139**: 532–8.

53 Jensen, C. L., Voigt, R. G., Prager, T. C. *et al.* Effects of maternal docosahexaenoic acid (DHA) supplementation on visual function and neurodevelopment of breast-fed infants. *Pediatr. Res.* 2001;**49**:448A.

54 Helland, I. B., Smith, L., Saarem, K., Saugstad, O. D., Drevon, C. A. Maternal supplementation with very-long-chain n-3 fatty acids during pregnancy and lactation augments children's IQ at 4 years of age. *Pediatrics* 2003;**111**: e39–44.

55 Malcolm, C. A., McCulloch, D. L., Montgomery, C., Shepherd, A., Weaver, L. T. Maternal docosahexaenoic acid supplementation during pregnancy and visual evoked potential development in term infants: a double blind, prospective, randomised trial. *Arch. Dis. Child Fetal Neonatal Ed.* 2003;**88**:F383–90.

56 Dobson, V. Clinical applications of preferential looking measures of visual acuity. *Behav. Brain. Res.* 1983;**10**:25–38.

57 Dobson, V., Teller, D. Y. Visual acuity in human infants: a review and comparison of behavioral and electrophysiological studies. *Vision Res.* 1978;**18**:1469–83.

58 McDonald, M. A., Dobson, V., Sebris, S. L. *et al.* The acuity card procedure: a rapid test of infant acuity. *Invest. Ophthalmol. Vis. Sci.* 1985;**26**:1158–62.

59 Norcia, A. M., Tyler, C. W. Spatial frequency sweep VEP: visual acuity during the first year of life. *Vision Res.* 1985;**25**:1399–408.

60 Uauy, R., Birch, E., Birch, D., Peirano, P. Visual and brain function measurements in studies of n-3 fatty acid requirements of infants. *J. Pediatr.* 1992;**120**:S168–80.

61 Sokol, S., Hansen, V. C., Moskowitz, A. *et al.* Evoked potential and preferential looking estimates of visual acuity in pediatric patients. *Ophthalmology* 1983;**90**:552–62.

62 Jensen, C. L., Prager, T. C., Fraley, J. K. *et al.* Effect of dietary linoleic/alpha-linolenic acid ratio on growth and visual function of term infants. *J. Pediatr.* 1997;**131**:200–9.

63 Faldella, G., Govoni, M., Alessandroni, R. *et al.* Visual evoked potentials and dietary long chain polyunsaturated fatty acids in preterm infants. *Arch. Dis. Child.* 1996;**75**:F108–12.

64 Bougle, D., Denis, P., Vimard, F. *et al.* Early neurological and neuropsychological development of the preterm infant and polyunsaturated fatty acids supply. *Clin. Neurophysiol.* 1999;**110**:1363–1370.

65 Van Wezel-Meijler, G., van der Knapp, M. S., Huisman, J. *et al.* Dietary supplementation of long-chain polyunsaturated fatty acids in preterm infants: effects on cerebral maturation. *Acta Paediatr.* 2002;**91**:942–50.

66 Hood, D. C., Birch, D. G. The a-wave of the human electroretinogram and rod receptor function. *Invest. Ophthalmol. Vis. Sci.* 1990;**31**:2070–81.

67 Naka, K. I., Rushton, W. A. H. S-potentials from colour units in the retina of fish (cyprindae). *J. Physiol.* 1966;**185**:536–55.

68 Birch, D. G., Birch, E. E., Hoffman, D. R., Uauy, R. D. Retinal development in very-low-birth-weight infants fed diets differing in omega-3 fatty acids. *Invest. Ophthalmol. Vis. Sci.* 1992;**33**:2365–76.

69 Hoffman, D. R., Birch, E. E., Birch, D. G. *et al.* Impact of early dietary intake and blood lipid composition of long-chain polyunsaturated fatty acids on later visual development. *J. Pediatr. Gastroenterol. Nutr.* 2000;**31**:540–53.

70 SanGiovanni, J. P., Berkey, C. S., Dwyer, J. T., Colditz, G. A. Dietary essential fatty acids, long-chain polyunsaturated fatty acids, and visual resolution acuity in healthy fullterm infants: a systematic review. *Early Hum. Dev.* 2000;**57**:165–88.

71 SanGiovanni, J. P., Parra-Cabrera, S., Colditz, G. A. *et al.* Meta-analysis of dietary essential fatty acids and long-chain polyunsaturated fatty acids as they relate to visual resolution acuity in healthy preterm infants. *Pediatrics* 2000;**105**: 1292–8.

72 Auestad, N., Halter, R., Halla, R. T. *et al.* Growth and development in term infants fed long-chain polyunsaturated fatty acids: a double-masked, randomized, parallel, prospective, multivariate study. *Pediatrics* 2001;**108**:372–81.

73 Birch, E. E., Hoffman, D. R., Castañeda, Y. S. *et al.* A randomized controlled trial of long-chain polyunsaturated fatty acid supplementation of formula in term infants after weaning at 6 wk of age. *Am. J. Clin. Nutr.* 2002;**75**:570–80.

74 Hoffman, D. R., Birch, E. E., Castañeda, Y. S. *et al.* Visual function in breast-fed term infants weaned to formula with or without long-chain polyunsaturates at 4 to 6 months: a randomized clinical trial. *J. Pediatr.* 2003;**142**:669–77.

75 Williams, C., Birch, E. E., Emmett, P. M., Northstone, K., (ALSPAC) Study Team. Stereoacuity at age 3.5 y in children born full-term is associated with prenatal and postnatal dietary factors: a report from a population-based cohort study. *Am. J. Clin. Nutr.* 2001;**73**:316–22.

76 O'Connor, D. L., Hall, R., Adamkin, D. *et al.* Growth and development in preterm infants fed long-chain polyunsaturated fatty acids: a prospective, randomized controlled trial. *Pediatrics* 2001;**108**:359–71.

77 Innis, S. M., Adamkin, D. H., Hall, R. T. *et al.* Docosahexaenoic acid and arachidonic acid enhance growth with no adverse effects in preterm infants fed formula. *J. Pediatr.* 2002;**140**: 547–54.

78 Simmer, K., Cochrane Neonatal Group. Long-chain polyunsaturated fatty acid supplementation in infants born at term. *Cochrane Database of Systematic Reviews.* 2001; Issue 3.

79 Simmer, K., Cochrane Neonatal Group. Long-chain polyunsaturated fatty acid supplementation in preterm infants. *Cochrane Database of Systematic Reviews*. 2001; Issue 2.

80 Gibson, R. A., Chen, W., Makrides, M. Randomized trials with polyunsaturated fatty acid interventions in preterm and term infants: functional and clinical outcomes. *Lipids* 2001;**36**: 873–83.

81 McCall, R. B., Mash, C. W. Long-chain polyunsaturated fatty acids and the measurement and prediction of intelligence (IQ). In Dobbing, J., ed. *Developing Brain and Behaviour*. London: Academic Press;1997:295–338.

82 Fagan, J. F. III, Singer, L. T. Infant recognition memory as a measure of intelligence. *Adv. Infancy Res*. 1983;**2**:31–78.

83 Colombo, J. Individual differences in infant cognition: methods, measures, and models. In Dobbing, J., ed. *Developing Brain and Behaviour*. London: Academic Press;1997:339–85.

84 Lucas, A., Morley, R. Efficacy and safety of long-chain polyunsaturated fatty acid supplementation of infant-formula milk: a randomised trial. *Lancet* 1999;**354**:1948–54.

85 Makrides, M., Neumann, M. A., Simmer, K. *et al.* A critical appraisal of the role of dietary long-chain polyunsaturated fatty acids on neural indices of term infants: a randomized, controlled trial. *Pediatrics* 2000;**105**:32–8.

86 Birch, E. E., Garfield, S., Hoffman, D. R. *et al.* A randomized controlled trial of early dietary supply of long-chain polyunsaturated fatty acids and mental development in term infants. *Devel. Med. Child Neurol*. 2000;**42**:174–81.

87 Clandinin, M., Van Aerde, J., Antonson, D. *et al.* Formulas with docosahexaenoic acid (DHA) and arachidonic acid (ARA) promote better growth and development scores in very-low-birth-weight infants (VLBW). *Pediatr. Res*. 2002;**51**: 187A–8A.

88 Willats, P., Forwyth, J. S., DiModugno, M. K., Varma, S., Colvin, M. Effect of long-chain polyunsaturated fatty acids in infant formula on problem solving at 10 months of age. *Lancet* 1998;**352**:688–91.

89 Uauy, R., Hoffman, D. R., Peirano, P., Birch, D. G., Birch, E. E. Essential fatty acids in visual and brain development. *Lipids* 2001;**36**:885–95.

90 Bouwstra, H., Dijck-Brouwer, D. A. J., Wildeman, J. A. L. *et al.* Long-chain polyunsaturated fatty acids have a positive effect on the quality of general movements of healthy term infants. *Am. J. Clin. Nutr*. 2003;**78**:313–18.

91 Carlson, S. E., Cooke, R. J., Werkman, S. H. *et al.* First year growth of preterm infants fed standard compared to marine oil n-3 supplemented formula. *Lipids* 1992;**27**:901–7.

92 Carlson, S. E., Werkman, S. H., Peeples, J. M. *et al.* Arachidonic acid status correlates with first year growth in preterm infants. *Proc. Natl Acad. Sci. USA*. 1993;**90**:1073–7.

93 Uauy, R. D., Hoffman, D. R., Birch, E. E. *et al.* Safety and efficacy of omega-3 fatty acids in the nutrition of very-low-birth-weight infants: soy oil and marine oil supplementation of formula. *J. Pediatr*. 1994;**124**:612–20.

94 Carlson, S. E., Werkman, S. H., Tolley, E. A. Effect of long-chain n-3 fatty acid supplementation on visual acuity and growth of preterm infants with and without bronchopulmonary dysplasia. *Am. J. Clin. Nutr*. 1996;**63**:687–9.

95 Ryan, A. S., Montalto, M. B., Groh-Wargo, S. *et al.* Effect of DHA-containing formula on growth of preterm infants to 59 weeks postmenstrual age. *Am. J. Hum. Biol*. 1999;**11**:457–87.

96 Lapillonne, A., Clarke, S. D., Heird, W. C. Plausible mechanisms for effects of long-chain polyunsaturated fatty acids on growth. *J. Pediatr*. 2003;**143** (4 Suppl.): S9–16.

97 Heird, W. C., Biological effects and safety issues related to long-chain polyunsaturated fatty acids in infants. *Lipids* 1999;**34**:207–14.

98 Borkman, M., Storlien, L. H., Pan, D. A. *et al.* The relationship between insulin sensitivity and the fatty-acid composition of skeletal muscle phospholipids. *New Engl. J. Med*. 1993;**328**:238–44.

99 Pan, D. A., Hylbert, A. J., Storlien, L. H. Dietary fats, membrane phospholipids and obesity. *J. Nutr*. 1994;**124**:1555–65.

100 Clarke, S. D., Jump, D. B. Polyunsaturated fatty acid regulation of hepatic gene transcription. *J. Nutr*. 1996;**126**:1105–9.

101 Vanderhoof, J., Gross, S., Hegyi, T. Evaluation of a long-chain polyunsaturated fatty acid supplemented formula on growth tolerance, and plasma lipids in preterm infants up to 48 weeks postconceptional age. *J. Pediatr. Gastroenterol. Nutr*. 1999;**29**:318–26.

102 Vanderhoof, J., Gross, S., Hegyi, T., for the Multicenter Study Group. A multicenter long-term safety and efficacy trial of preterm formula supplemented with long-chain polyunsaturated fatty acids. *J. Pediatr. Gastroenterol. Nutr*. 2000;**31**:121–7.

103 Lim, M., Antonson, D., Clandinin, M. *et al.* Formulas with docosahexaenoic acid (DHA) and arachidonic acid (ARA) for low-birth-weight infants (LBW) are safe. *Pediatr. Res*. 2002;**51**:319A.

14

Vitamins

Frank R. Greer

University of Wisconsin, Madison, WI

Vitamins are organic compounds required in trace amounts in the diet for the maintenance of normal growth and development. They are divided into fat-soluble and water-soluble groups. For term infants, the daily requirement is based on the content of human milk with the exceptions of vitamins D and K for which human milk is clearly deficient.

Newborn deficiencies of the fat-soluble vitamins A, D, E and K are well described. The fat-soluble vitamins require the presence of pancreatic enzymes and bile acids in the gut for their absorption. They are stored in the body and thus clinical deficiency may require some time to develop unless stores are inadequate at birth as in the preterm infant. On the other hand, excessive intakes accumulate in the body and have the potential for toxicity. All of the fat-soluble vitamins have been used in pharmacologic quantities in the newborn for treatment or prevention of disease processes, though clear indications for their use in this fashion remain areas of neonatal nutritional controversy. Vitamin D, unique to this family of compounds, functions more like a prohormone in that it can be synthesized in the skin and carried to other organs where the metabolic effects occur.

As for the water-soluble vitamins and vitamin-like cofactors, the same statements cannot be made. Requirements for term infants are based on the concentrations in human milk. Deficiency or toxicity is very rare in developed countries. As for the premature infant, there continues to be very little information on which to make intake recommendations regardless of feeding method, and deficiency states have generally not been described in this population.

Fat-soluble vitamins A, E, and K

Vitamin A

The term vitamin A refers to a number of compounds that include both the naturally occurring and synthetically derived retinoids. Its biologic activity is diverse. It is essential for vision, growth, healing, reproduction, cell differentiation, and immunocompetency. This multiplicity of effects is due to its mechanism of action through gene regulation. Vitamin A's action is similar to that of steroid hormones in that a specific retinoic-acid-receptor protein complex becomes bound to nuclear DNA, resulting in regulation of specific genes.[1] Dietary intake is quantitated in terms of retinal equivalents (RE), one RE equaling 1 µg of all trans-retinol.[2] One International Unit (IU) is equivalent to 0.3 µg of preformed retinol, or 0.3 RE. Retinol is the naturally occurring alcohol formed in vivo from its precursor ß-carotene, found in plants. Vitamin A is transported in plasma as retinol, bound to retinol-binding protein (RBP), a specific carrier protein synthesized in the liver. For ß-carotene there is little specific information on its uptake or its metabolism to vitamin A during the perinatal period. However, it has been known for years that ß-carotene can meet the fetal and newborn growth requirements for vitamin A.

The mechanism and regulation of retinol transport from the maternal circulation to the fetus through the human placenta is not well described. In humans, significant correlations between maternal and cord blood RBP concentrations have not been reported consistently.[3,4] Cord blood concentrations of vitamin A are generally lower in preterm

Neonatal Nutrition and Metabolism. Second Edition, ed. P. Thureen and W. Hay. Published by Cambridge University Press.
© Cambridge University Press 2006.

than term infants.[5] The ratio of maternal to fetal concentrations of plasma vitamin A in healthy pregnancies is approximately 2:1.[6-10] Fetal plasma vitamin A concentrations appear to be maintained within a normal range despite variations in the maternal vitamin A status and intake.[6,11]

Ingested carotene and dietary retinyl esters are converted to free retinol in the proximal small intestine after the action of hydrolases from the pancreas and intestinal brush border. These enzymes may have low activity in the premature infant in the early days of life. After solubilization with bile salts into mixed micelles, retinol is absorbed into the intestinal cells, re-esterified, and incorporated into chylomicrons that are transported via lymph (thoracic duct) into the circulation, as with all fat-soluble vitamins. Intraluminal bile acids, important for this process, are decreased in premature infants and may lead to inadequate micelle formation and affect retinol absorption.[12]

After absorption, chylomicrons, containing lipoprotein-bound retinyl esters, are taken up by the liver, the main storage organ for retinol (90% of body stores).[2] The normal liver vitamin A concentration in healthy human adults ranges from 100–300 $\mu g\,g^{-1}$.[13] Premature infants are potentially born with low or marginal liver vitamin A stores.[14,15] In one study of 25 preterm infants who died within the first 24 hours of life, 37% had liver concentrations less than 20 $\mu g\,g^{-1}$.[14] Thus, the ability of many preterm infants to offset an inadequate intake of vitamin A from liver stores would be limited.

Following retinol hydrolysis in the liver, the subsequent transport of retinol to other tissues for metabolism is dependent on liver RBP synthesis and secretion.[16] After secretion of the RBP-retinol complex, RBP binds with plasma transthyretin, reducing the chance for glomerular filtration and renal catabolism of RBP. The circulating retinol-RBP-transthyretin complex is delivered to target tissues. At the time of birth, plasma RBP concentration was lower in a group of 39 preterm infants (gestational age 24–36 weeks) compared with a group of 32 term infants (2.8 ± 1.2 $\mu g\,dL^{-1}$ v. 3.6 ± 1.1 $\mu g\,dL^{-1}$, mean ± SD, p < 0.001).[17] In this same study, mean plasma vitamin A was also lower in preterm compared with full term infants (16.0 ± 6.2 μg dL^{-1} v. 23.9 ± 10.2 $\mu g\,dL^{-1}$, mean ± SD, p < 0.001).

The vitamin A content of human milk varies somewhat, depending on postpartum age and the volume of fat content of milk. Ninety per cent or more of the vitamin A in human milk is in the form of retinyl esters contained in milk fat globules.[18] Vitamin A is higher in colostrum than in mature human milk (1200–1800 $\mu g\,L^{-1}$ v. 180–600 $\mu g\,L^{-1}$) (Table 14.1).[19] The vitamin A content of preterm human milk reported is quite variable, but generally is compar-

Table 14.1. Vitamin content of human milk per liter[170]

	<28 days (Early milk)	>28 days (Mature milk)
Fat-soluble vitamins		
Vitamin A (retinol) $\mu g\,L^{-1}$	1200–1800	300–600
Vitamin E $mg\,L^{-1}$	8–12	2–4
Vitamin K $\mu g\,L^{-1}$		
Vitamin D $\mu g\,L^{-1}$		0.33
Water-soluble vitamins		
Thiamine (B1) $\mu g\,L^{-1}$	20	220
Riboflavin (B2) $\mu g\,L^{-1}$		400–600
Pyridoxine (B6) $\mu g\,L^{-1}$		90–310
Cobalamin (B12) $\mu g\,L^{-1}$		0.5–1.0
Folate $\mu g\,L^{-1}$		80–140
Niacin $mg\,L^{-1}$	0.5	1.8–6.0
Biotin $\mu g\,L^{-1}$		5–9
Pantothenic acid $mg\,L^{-1}$		2.0–2.5
Vitamin C $mg\,L^{-1}$		100

able with that of mature milk, particularly after the first few weeks of lactation.

Neonatal requirements

As noted, even term infants are relatively deficient in vitamin A at the time of birth compared with older children. Based on the vitamin A content of human milk, recommended intake for term infants is 400–500 $\mu g\,day^{-1}$ (Table 14.5). This intake is easily met by term infant formulas that contain approximately 600 $\mu g\,L^{-1}$.

Recommended supplements for the VLBWI are in the 200–450 $\mu g\,kg^{-1}$ day^{-1} range, whether enteral or parenteral, with 450 $\mu g\,kg^{-1}$ day^{-1} being preferable (Tables 14.5 and 14.6). Most infant formulas for the VLBWI will easily supply this amount of intake as they contain about 3000 $\mu g\,L^{-1}$ (Table 14.2). Even formulas for preterm infants after discharge contain 1020 $\mu g\,L^{-1}$. All of the commercially available human milk fortifiers contain vitamin A (Table 14.3).

The vitamin A content of a typical multivitamin oral supplement used for preterm infants is 450 $\mu g\,ml^{-1}$. Thus, the recommended intake for the orally fed preterm infant can be met with preterm infant formula, fortified human milk or multivitamin preparations.

Using either of two standard multivitamin preparations for total parenteral nutrition (TPN) solutions provides 690 μg of vitamin A for term infants (Table 14.4). However, administration of vitamin A by this method is very inefficient because of loss of vitamin A by photodegradation and binding to intravenous tubing.[21,22] Net losses by an in

Table 14.2. Vitamins provided by selected formulas per liter

	Similac Special Care 24 Liquid (Ross, Columbus, OH)	Enfamil Premature 24 Liquid (Mead Johnson, Evansville, IN)	Neosure 22 cal Liquid (Ross, Columbus, OH)	Enfacare 22 cal Liquid (Mead Johnson, Evansville, IN)	Enfamil®/Enfamil® with Iron (Mead Johnson, Evansville, IN)	Good Start (Nestle, Glendale, CA)	Similac® Low Iron/with Iron* (Ross, Columbus, OH)
Fat soluble							
A IU	10,150	10,150	3422	3330	2000	2027	2027
D IU	1218	2200	521	590	410	405	405
E IU	32	51	27	30	13.5	8	10.1
K µg	100	65	82	59	54	55	54
Water soluble							
Thiamine (B_1) µg	2030	1620	1488	1480	540	405	676
Riboflavin (B_2) µg	5030	2400	1116	1480	950	912	1014
Pyridoxine µg	2030	1220	744	740	410	507	405
B_{12} µg	4.5	2	3.0	2.2	2.0	1.5	1.7
Niacin mg	40.6	32	14.5	14.8	6.8	5.1	7.1
Folic acid µg	300	280	186	192	108	61	101
Pantothenic acid mg	15.4	9.7	5.9	6.3	3.4	3.0	3.04
Biotin µg	300	32	67	44	20	14.9	29.7
C (ascorbic acid) mg	300	162	111	118	81	54.1	61

Table 14.3. Vitamins in human milk fortifiers for premature infant fed human milk – nutrients provided when added to 100 ml of human milk

	Enfamil Human Milk Fortifier (4 pkt per 100 ml)	Similac Human Milk Fortifier (4 pkt per 100 ml)	Similac Natural Care Fortifier (Liquid, 100 ml)*
Fat soluble			
Vitamin A µg	285	186	165
Vitamin D µg	3.75	3.0	3.0
Vitamin E mg	4.6	3.2	3.2
Vitamin K µg	4.4	8.3	10
Water soluble			
Vitamin C (ascorbate) mg	12	25	30
Thiamin µg	150	233	203
Riboflavin µg	220	417	503
Pyridoxine µg	115	211	203
Niacin mg	3	3.57	4
Pantothenate mg	0.73	1.5	1.5
Biotin µg	2.7	2.6	3.0
Folate µg	25	23	30
Vitamin B_{12} µg	0.18	0.64	0.45

* Similac Natural Care is to be diluted 1:1 with human milk which will decrease concentrations by 50% in the feedings.

Table 14.4. TPN vitamin solutions

	MVI Pediatric		Infuvite	
			Vial #1	
Vitamin	Amount provided per 5 ml	Amount provided per 2 ml	Amount provided per 4 ml	Amount provided per 2 ml
Vitamin A (retinal)	690 µg	276 µg	690 µg	345 µg
Vitamin D	10 µg	4 µg	10 µg	5 µg
Vitamin E	7.0 mg	2.8 mg	7.0 mg	3.5 mg
Vitamin K_1	200 µg	80 µg	200 µg	100 µg
Thiamine (vitamin B_1)	1200 µg	480 µg	1200 µg	600 µg
Riboflavin (vitamin B_2)	1400 µg	560 µg	1400 µg	700 µg
Pyridoxine (vitamin B_6)	1000 µg	400 µg	1000 µg	500 µg
Niacinamide	17.0 mg	6.8 mg	17 mg	8.5 mg
Dexpanthenol	5 mg	2.0 mg	5 mg	2.5 mg
Ascorbic acid (vitamin C)	80 mg	32 mg	80 mg	40 mg
			Vial #2	
			Amount provided per 1 ml	Amount provided per 0.5 ml
Folic acid	140 µg	56 µg	140 µg	70 µg
Biotin	20 µg	8 µg	20 µg	10 µg
Vitamin B_{12}	1.0 µg	0.4 µg	1 µg	0.5 µg

vitro study in this system estimated vitamin A losses between 62% and 89%.[23,24] M.V.I. Pediatric or Infuvit supply 275–345 μg to preterm infants on TPN. This will be decreased to 200 μg if typical photodegradation occurs (Tables 14.4 and 14.6).

For premature infants with significant lung disease, recommendations for a larger intake of vitamin A can be justified at this time from the available clinical trials.[25] Thus, a parenteral or enteral dose of 600–900 μg kg^{-1} day^{-1} has been recommended, with 900 μg being preferred. However, it should be noted that there is no satisfactory preparation for administering this dose enterally at this time, and an intramuscular injection is required.

High dose vitamin A supplementation for the preterm infant

Experimental supplementation of premature infants with 450 μg kg^{-1} day^{-1} results in "normalization" of serum retinol and RBP.[26,27] One of the more controversial neonatal issues is whether or not this level of supplementation or an even higher one may ameliorate bronchopulmonary dysplasia.[26–30] It is clear that intramuscular vitamin A is more effective than the enteral route in premature infants for delivering these large doses.[31,32] Pertinent to the use of vitamin A for the amelioration of bronchopulmonary dysplasia in addition to its tissue healing effects, is that retinol, retinyl palmitate, and retinoic acid are all potential antioxidants.

Randomized trials using large doses of parenteral vitamin A ($\geq$ 450 μg kg^{-1} day^{-1}) to prevent chronic lung disease, have recently been reviewed.[25] To date, six randomized trials have been published,[26,28,33–36] though one of these[35] has a sample size four times larger than all the others combined and enrolled the smallest and most premature infants (birthweights 401–1000 g). Also, a total of 554 infants treated with vitamin A have been compared with 543 control infants in a recent meta-analysis.[25]

Overall, the results of these studies are mixed. No study has found a significant effect on mortality, differences in days of assisted ventilation, or length of hospital stay.[26,28,33–36] The pooled data for all six studies showed a trend towards reduction in oxygen use at one month in survivors that does not reach statistical significance (RR 0.93 [0.86, 1.01]).[25] The study with largest number of infants reported no significant difference in the combined outcomes of death and oxygen use at 36 weeks (RR 0.89 [0.79, 1.0]).[35] However, there was a significant reduction of oxygen use in the vitamin A group at 36 weeks (RR 0.85 [0.73, 0.98]). The need for supplemental oxygen at 36 weeks postmenstrual age declined from 62% in the unsupplemented controls to 55% in the supplemented infants. Using these data, it would require treatment of 14.5 infants with supplemental vitamin A to benefit one patient.[35] Concern has also been expressed for the invasiveness of repeated intramuscular injections of vitamin A in return for this very modest benefit, though no side effects from the high dose vitamin A supplements were reported from any of these studies. These included clinical monitoring of anterior fontanel pressure and biochemical evidence of vitamin A toxicity.

Vitamin A deficiency/toxicity

Vitamin A deficiency is not common in infants in developed countries in the absence of malabsorption, though it is not uncommon in other parts of the world. It may be part of generalized malnutrition. The first signs of deficiency in an infant are xerosis of the cornea and conjunctivitis, followed by keratomalacia, ulceration and ultimate destruction of the eye.

The "adequate" concentration of serum vitamin A in VLBWI is not known. Serum concentrations below 20.0 μg dL^{-1} (0.70 μmol L^{-1}) have been considered as deficient in premature infants and concentrations below 10.0 μg dL^{-1} (0.35 μmol L^{-1}) as indicating severe deficiency with depleted liver stores. Unfortunately, a single plasma retinol value does not correlate well with liver stores until they become very low [< 10.0 μg dL^{-1} (< 0.35 μmol L^{-1})] [15,37,38] or extremely low [< 5 μg dL^{-1} (< 0.17 μmol L^{-1})].[39] Many authors have noted this problem, but the use of a single plasma retinol concentration continues in the evaluation of premature infants.

In one study, a high percentage of preterm infants, up to 77%, had plasma RBP below 3.0 μg dL^{-1}, which may be indicative of vitamin A deficiency.[17] Both the plasma RBP response[27] and the relative rise in serum retinol concentration[40] following intramuscular vitamin A administration have been described as useful tests to assess functional vitamin A status. This is a better method of confirming actual low vitamin A storage than random plasma concentrations.[40]

In the very large study by Tyson, 25% of infants receiving supplemental vitamin A (1500 μg three times per week) and 54% of controls (approximately 300 μg day^{-1}) had vitamin A concentrations below 20.0 μg dL^{-1} on day 28.[35] Similar percentages, 22% of those receiving supplemental vitamin A and 45% of controls, had a relative dose response of > 10% following an intramuscular dose of 600 μg. From these data it was suggested than an even higher dose of vitamin A may be required to achieve vitamin A sufficiency in very premature infants (birth weights < 1000 g).

The studies reviewed above, with high dose vitamin A supplements did not report any vitamin A toxicity as noted.[26,28,33–36] Dosages used in these studies were roughly twice the recommended RDA for premature infants. Another report states that one oral dose of 15 000 µg given to newborns was associated only with an asymptomatic bulging anterior fontanel in 4–5% of the infants.[41] However, clinical assessment of toxicity in preterm infants has not been really studied, so guidelines in this area must be made carefully.

It has been known for years that excess maternal vitamin A may cause congenital anomalies in animal fetuses,[42,43,44] and retinoic acid seems especially teratogenic.[17] Women who take more than 3000 µg of vitamin A per day as a supplement have an increased frequency of birth defects. The highest frequency of defects was related to high consumption before the 7th week of gestation.[45] The defects (mostly craniofacial, cardiac, and thymic) resulted in a high mortality rate.[46–48]

Laboratory assessment of vitamin A status

A number of methods can be used to measure plasma vitamin A, the usual method for assessing vitamin A status. Generally, plasma levels only decline after liver reserves have been depleted. Levels less than 20 µg dL^{-1} are considered deficient and 10 µg dL^{-1} are associated with signs of deficiency. A method of confirming actual low vitamin A stores in the liver is the determination of the relative dose response (RDR) following either oral or intramuscular administration of vitamin A (change in serum retinol concentration divided by the pre-injections concentration).[38]

Vitamin E

The term vitamin E refers to eight naturally occurring compounds. Though the biological activities of vitamin E isomers vary considerably, they all show antioxidant capability with the ability to protect cellular and subcellular membranes from oxidative destruction initiated at the molecular level by lipid peroxidation.[49] To be effective, tocopherol must be localized in membrane sites exposed to free radicals. The most abundant and active isomer is alpha-tocopherol. On the basis of in vivo bioassays, the approximate relative potencies of the other vitamin E isomers compared with dl-α-tocopherol are β 40–50%, γ 10–30%, δ about 1%. The original international standard of vitamin E, synthesized from natural phytol and initially designated dl-α-tocopherol acetate, is defined as having 1 IU mg^{-1}. The corresponding value for naturally occurring α-tocopherol is 1.49 IU mg^{-1}.

A relatively low concentration of vitamin E is found in fetal tissues until body fat increases in late gestation. Total body content of tocopherol in the human fetus increases from about 1 mg at 5 months gestation to approximately 20 mg at term.[50] Although pregnancy is associated with a high maternal concentration of circulating vitamin E proportional to rising plasma lipids, transplacental delivery of tocopherols to the fetus is limited. Administering large doses of vitamin E to women in the last weeks of pregnancy has little effect on cord vitamin E levels.[51,52] The ratio of maternal to fetal tocopherol concentration in blood is approximately 4:1, with the former concentration averaging 1.5 mg dl^{-1} and the latter 0.38 mg dl^{-1} in five studies.[53] Similarly, neonatal tissues show a relative paucity of vitamin E isomers. In premature neonates the low proportion of adipose tissue further limits the total body vitamin E content.

The absorption of tocopherols is variable depending on total lipid absorption as with the other fat-soluble vitamins.[54] Bile salts and pancreatic enzymes are essential to the absorption process.[55,56] In general the efficiency of absorption decreases as larger amounts of tocopherol are consumed.[57] Decreased absorption of fat, as seen in the premature neonate, results in a parallel loss of tocopherols.[54] Factors important in the absorption of vitamin E by the neonate include gestational age, the fat component of the diet, and the preparation of vitamin E given. Little is known about passage of vitamin E through the absorptive cells of the mucosa as no intestinal transfer proteins have been identified for tocopherol. After micelle formation with bile salts, vitamin E is absorbed, incorporated into chylomicrons and transported with fat along with the other fat-soluble vitamins via lymphatic vessels into the venous system. The concentration of tocopherol in plasma varies depending on the amount of associated lipoproteins.

Liver, adipose tissue, and skeletal muscle are the major storage organs for the vitamin. At the cellular level, it must be integrated into lipid droplets, cellular membranes, and organelles to be effective. It is concentrated wherever there is abundant fatty acid, especially in phospholipid membrane-containing structures (e.g., mitochondrial, microsomal, and plasma membranes). Fat accumulates α-tocopherol and can sequester it.[58] When the intake of vitamin E is high, the liver is a major repository, but the tocopherol pool in adipose tissue is much larger. Although adipose tissue is sometimes considered a "store" of vitamin E, the tocopherol present in adipocytes is not readily available to other tissues.[59]

In the liver, newly absorbed lipids are incorporated into very low-density lipoproteins (VLDL), and VLDL particles secreted by the liver are preferentially enriched with α-tocopherol. The liver is responsible for the control and release of α-tocopherol into human plasma[60,61] via the hepatic cytosolic α-tocopherol transfer protein (TTP).[62] The gene for this protein has been localized to the

8q13.1–13.3 region of chromosome 8.[63,64] Human deficiencies of this protein have now been reported.[65–68]

There is a large inter-individual variation in the human milk content of vitamin E (Table 14.1). Colostrum contains relatively high concentrations of tocopherol isomers averaging 8–12 mg L^{-1}.[69] After two weeks of lactation, the vitamin E concentration of human milk declines. Mature human milk contains all the expected isomers of tocopherol, but the isomers other than α-tocopherol account for only about 2% of the vitamin E activity.[70] Generally, mature human milk contains 2–4 mg L^{-1} of α-tocopherol (Table 14.1).[69] The amount of vitamin E ingested daily (approximately 2 mg of α-tocopherol equivalents in 750 ml of mature milk) appears to be adequate to prevent antioxidant deficiency in the term neonate. For the preterm infant, however, with lower initial stores and reduced intestinal absorption, human milk may not provide sufficient vitamin E.

Neonatal requirements

Because the neonate, especially the premature neonate, is born with low stores of α-tocopherol in addition to a decreased blood concentration, early provision of vitamin E is necessary to correct the depleted state and prevent adverse consequences attributable to insufficient antioxidants. In the term neonate with normal intestinal absorption, it has been calculated from data obtained in studies of milk-fed neonates that 2 mg day^{-1} is sufficient to raise blood and tissue levels. The amount is higher per kilogram than the 10–15 mg recommended for older children and adults.[71] It is clear that normal blood and tissue concentrations of tocopherol can be achieved promptly in term neonates fed the usual volume of either breast milk or commercial formula. Commercial formulas for term infants contain 1.3–2.5 mg L^{-1} (Table 14.2).

The situation is different for premature neonates. The decreased intestinal absorption that has been demonstrated makes it necessary to give larger amounts (i.e., 6–12 mg kg^{-1} day^{-1}) when vitamin E supplements are provided enterally.[72] In studies of enteral nutrition, it has been shown that a daily dose of 10–25 mg of water-miscible α-tocopherol acetate given to 0.6- to 1.5-kg neonates may be required to produce and maintain normal vitamin E status.[73–76] Even some premature neonates on this regimen (10–25 mg day^{-1}) may not maintain a plasma tocopherol concentration above 0.5 mg dl^{-1}, especially if they receive iron-fortified formula. Data from studies of enterally fed neonates are generally more difficult to interpret in relation to the dose and time required to correct a low blood vitamin E concentration. Special formulas for preterm infants for use in the hospital contain 32 to 51 mg L^{-1} (Table 14.2).

Those for use after hospital discharge contain 27–30 mg L^{-1}. The commercially available human milk fortifiers all contain vitamin E (Table 14.3).

In intravenously nourished neonates, 1 mg kg^{-1} day^{-1} eventually corrects the vitamin E deficiency state, but up to 7–10 days may be required.[77–79] Parenteral α-tocopherol acetate at 3 mg kg^{-1} day^{-1} rapidly corrects low vitamin E levels and abnormal peroxide hemolysis tests within 24 hours.[80,81] Once a normal blood concentration of vitamin E is achieved, 1–2 mg kg^{-1} day^{-1} can be given to maintain vitamin E sufficiency, but without continued provision of tocopherol in the parenterally fed infant, insufficiency quickly develops.[81] Current multivitamin solutions for pediatric TPN solutions provide 7 mg day^{-1} to term infants when used as recommended (Table 14.6).

From studies of parenterally and enterally nourished premature neonates, it is reasonable to conclude that the immediate requirement of such neonates for "deliverable or absorbable" vitamin E is 2–3 mg kg^{-1} day^{-1} and that 1 mg kg^{-1} day^{-1} suffices once the initial deficiency state is corrected and tissue stores are established. Using one of two multivitamin solutions available for pediatric TPN solutions, 2.8–3.5 mg of vitamin E (α-tocopherol) are provided when used as recommended (Tables 14.4 and 14.6).

It is recommended that premature infants receive 2.8–3.5 mg kg^{-1} day^{-1} vitamin E parenterally and 6–12 mg kg^{-1} day^{-1} enterally (Tables 14.5 and 14.6).[82] These intakes are approximated with the present formulas and multivitamin

Table 14.5. Dietary reference intakes for fat-soluble and water-soluble vitamins

	Term infant per day[71,172]	Preterm infant per 100 kcal[83]
Fat-soluble vitamins		
Vitamin A (retinol)	400–500 µg	200–450 µg
Vitamin E	4–5 mg	6–12 mg
Vitamin K	2.0–2.5 µg	7–9 µg
Vitamin D	5 µg	5–10 µg
Water-soluble vitamins		
Thiamine (B1)	200–300 µg	150–200 µg
Riboflavin (B2)	300–400 µg	200–300 µg
Pyridoxine (B6)	100–300 µg	125–175 µg
Cobalamin (B12)	0.4–0.5 µg	0.25 µg
Folate	65–80 µg	21–42 µg
Niacin	2–4 mg	3–4 mg
Biotin	5–6 µg	3–5 µg
Pantothenic acid	1.7–1.8 mg	1.0–1.5 mg
Vitamin C (Ascorbic acid)	40–50 mg	15–20 mg

Table 14.6. Vitamin intakes for infants receiving total parenteral nutrition*

	Term infant per day*	Preterm infant per day
Fat-soluble vitamins		
Vitamin A (retinol)	690 µg	275–345 µg
Vitamin E	7 mg	2.8–3.5 mg
Vitamin K	200 µg	100 µg
Vitamin D	10 µg	4–5 µg
Water-soluble vitamins		
Thiamine (B1)	1200 µg	480–600 µg
Riboflavin (B2)	1400 µg	560–700 µg
Pyridoxine (B6)	1000 µg	400–500 µg
Cobalamin (B12)	1 µg	0.4–0.5 µg
Folate	140 µg	56–70 µg
Niacin	17 mg	6.8–8.5 mg
Biotin	20 µg	8–10 µg
Pantothenic acid	5 mg	2–2.5 mg
Vitamin C (Ascorbic acid)	80 mg	32–40 mg

* Intake based on the currently available TPN vitamin solutions (see Table 14.4). For term infants, 5 ml of MVI pediatric is recommended. For preterm infants, 2 ml of MVI is recommended. For Infuvite, 4 ml of Vial #1 and 1 ml Vital #2 is recommended for term infants. For preterm infants receiving Infuvite, 2 ml of Vial #1 and 0.5 ml of Vial #2 is recommended.

preparations. The American Academy of Pediatrics Committee on Nutrition has recommended that formulas provide a minimum of 1 mg of vitamin E per gram of linoleic acid and 0.7 mg per 100 kcal, though the special formulas with iron for premature infants contain 4–6 mg per 100 kcal, because of the higher requirement for vitamin E with these formulas.[83]

Vitamin E deficiency in the neonate

Several adverse consequences potentially attributable to vitamin E deficiency have been described in the medical literature in infants and children.[84–96] Unfortunately, controversy has surrounded almost all of the conditions attributed to human vitamin E deficiency, though a deficiency state in premature infants is the most convincing. Recent studies have demonstrated that vitamin E deficiency is common among premature neonates receiving intensive care.[72,73,80,97,98] Some of these investigations have defined methods of correcting or preventing vitamin E deficiency in the critically ill, low birth weight neonate,[74–76,81,99–101] but they have also identified toxicity associated with excess doses of tocopherol preparations.[102]

The absorption of vitamin E in premature neonates has been studied primarily by the technique of administering large single dosages and measuring the blood concentration sequentially. From these results, it appears that neonates less than 32 weeks gestation have significant malabsorption of tocopherol compared with term neonates and older children.[103] Prematurely delivered neonates may show evidence of vitamin E deficiency owing to several factors, including limited tissue storage at birth, intestinal malabsorption, and rapid growth rates that increase nutritional requirements in general. Many premature neonates may not be given enteral or even parenteral vitamin E for several days because of severe respiratory disorders requiring ventilatory assistance. Even when they are given tocopherol supplements, premature neonates with respiratory distress syndrome may have a low blood tocopherol concentration.[72,80,97,103,104]

Oski and Barness have incriminated tocopherol deficiency as a responsible factor in hemolytic anemia of prematurity.[84] As described in detail elsewhere, the conclusions from hematological studies of vitamin E supplementation in premature neonates differ depending on other variables that influence vitamin E status and requirements.[98,105] Nevertheless, the careful investigations of Gross and Melhorn indicated the following: (1) an abnormal degree of hemolysis occurs in association with vitamin E deficiency; (2) supplementation of premature neonates with 25 mg of α-tocopherol acetate per day decreases the hemolysis and leads to a modest but significant increase in blood hemoglobin content; and (3) the hemolytic anemia associated with vitamin E deficiency is aggravated by ingestion of iron in iron-fortified formulas.[106] It has been established that vitamin E deficiency under certain nutritional dietary conditions contributes to accelerated hemolysis and caused prolonged anemia in premature neonates.

High dose vitamin E therapy in preterm infants/toxicity

A potential role of vitamin E supplementation in preventing or ameliorating retinopathy of prematurity was proposed in 1949 by Owens and Owens and has remained controversial.[107] In its severe form, retinopathy of prematurity causes retinal scarring, detachment and blindness. Tocopherols are concentrated in the retinal tissue, where lipid concentrations are high and clearly can interrupt oxidation reactions that conceivably initiate the injury process. A recent meta-analysis[108] of six randomized controlled trials with a total sample of 704 VLBW infants treated with vitamin E and 714 VLBW controls,[87,88,95,109–111] found no difference in the overall incidence of ROP between the two groups. However, there was a significant difference in the incidence of Grade III ROP between the two groups, 2.4% in the vitamin E v. 5.5% in the controls (pooled odds ratio 0.44, 95% CI 0.21–0.81, p < 0.02). However, the total number of infants with severe ROP was very small and the authors recommended that further studies be done on the smallest infants (birth weight below 1000 g). It must be concluded that at present there is no clear benefit of giving large doses of vitamin E for the intended purpose of preventing severe retinal disease.

Bronchopulmonary dysplasia is another condition of premature neonates that was reported to be preventable by vitamin E therapy.[86] Further investigation of the role of vitamin E in bronchopulmonary dysplasia did not lead to confirmation of the original data, by either the same investigators[94] or others.[112,113] The rationale for this proposed effect is again logical, as tocopherols prevent oxidation-related injury of pulmonary membrane systems. However, it cannot be claimed that vitamin E in large doses prevents bronchopulmonary dysplasia in preterm infants.

There are also data supporting the suggestion that vitamin E supplementation, if given in the first 12 hours of life, can reduce the incidence of intraventricular hemorrhage.[92,93,114,115] The hypothesis is that the effect is related to the vitamin's ability to scavenge free radicals, which then protects brain matrix capillary endothelial cells from hypoxic-ischemic injury. However, vitamin E in large doses cannot be recommended to prevent intraventricular hemorrhage at this time. Further study is required.[77]

Serious toxicity has been associated with megavitamin E supplements in premature neonates.[102] As reviewed elsewhere,[98] the adverse effects may be attributable to the vehicle used for megavitamin E supplementation rather than the tocopherol preparation per se. Doses of vitamin E exceeding 3.5 mg kg^{-1} day^{-1} by the parenteral route or 25 mg kg^{-1} day^{-1} by the enteral route should be regarded as experimental and having potentially more risk than benefit for premature neonates at this time. It must be emphasized there is no compelling evidence to treat the premature infant with pharmacologic doses of vitamin E to prevent any condition.

Laboratory assessment

Ninety per cent or more of the circulating vitamin E is normally α-tocopherol, and serum or plasma samples can be measured. A concentration of at least 0.5 mg dL^{-1} indicates adequate nutritional status.[105] Most would agree that vitamin E concentration in tissue is the most appropriate parameter to measure to assess vitamin E status, though this is not usually available in infants.

Adequate vitamin E concentration is dependent on the concentration of plasma lipids. Tocopherol data have been expressed as a function of lipid concentration in many studies.[116–118] These investigations have demonstrated that, although children have significantly lower levels of plasma vitamin E than adults, a tocopherol/total lipid ratio of 0.6–0.8 mg g^{-1} indicates adequate nutritional status.[116,117] This ratio would be important to measure in the very premature infant in whom marked changes in lipid levels occur, ranging from very low at birth to high during intravenous feedings of fatty acids. However, this ratio requires measurement of cholesterol, triglycerides and phospholipids, and requires considerable amounts of blood for a very small premature infant. Part of the explanation for low circulating tocopherol in premature infants relates to decreased plasma lipids compared with the lipid concentration in adults.

To characterize the apparent vitamin E deficiency of premature neonates, the hydrogen peroxide hemolysis test has been recommended.[97] However, a very recent study in premature infants (mean 33 weeks gestation) compared plasma and erythrocyte vitamin E levels, vitamin E to lipid ratios, and two variations of the hydrogen peroxide hemolysis test. The investigators concluded that there was no satisfactory method for the clinical assessment of vitamin E deficiency in the premature infant.[119] It is important to differentiate between tocopherol-sufficient and tocopherol-deficient premature neonates, particularly as parenteral vitamin E is being advocated in high doses for prophylaxis against neonatal disorders associated with oxygen toxicity.

Vitamin K

Compared with the other fat-soluble vitamins, there is little specific information regarding the infant requirements for vitamin K. It is also the only vitamin routinely administered in large quantities at the time of birth. Its concentration in cord blood is not reliably detectable by present assay techniques at any gestational age. The vitamin K concentration of human milk is very low, and for the newborn breastfeeding infant, a deficiency state has been described. Thus, there is not a "gold standard" for assessing the nutritional needs of this vitamin in infants. It is only recently that even longitudinal serum levels have been determined in term and preterm infants.

Vitamin K exists in two forms: (1) Vitamin K_1 or phylloquinone which is the plant form of the vitamin, and (2) vitamin K_2, a series of compounds with unsaturated side chains of varying length, synthesized by bacteria and collectively referred to as menaquinones. The vitamin functions postribosomally as a cofactor in the metabolic conversion of intracellular precursors of vitamin K-dependent proteins to active forms. The coagulation factors II (prothrombin), VII, IX and X were the first of these proteins to be described. Other vitamin K-dependent proteins in plasma include proteins C, S, and Z. Vitamin K-dependent proteins have been identified in nearly all tissues of the body. These include osteocalcin or bone gla protein as well as matrix gla protein of the skeleton, and kidney gla protein.[120]

All of the known vitamin K-dependent proteins have in common gamma-carboxyglutamic acid (Gla), the unique amino acid formed by the postribosomal action of vitamin K-dependent carboxylase. These Gla residues are located in the homologous amino-terminal domain with a high degree of amino acid sequence identity seen in all vitamin K-dependent proteins.[121] They are required for the calcium mediated interaction of these proteins and are the location of specific calcium binding sites. An overview of the current knowledge of vitamin K metabolism can be found in more detail elsewhere.[120,122]

There is very little information on menaquinones in the perinatal period. Most of the bacteria comprising the normal intestinal flora of human milk fed infants do not produce menaquinones, including *Bifidobacterium*, *Lactobacillus*, and *Clostridium* species. Bacteria which produce menaquinones include *Bacteroides fragilis* and *Escherichia coli* which are more common in formula fed infants. Both phylloquinone and menaquinone are actually more prevalent in the stools of formula-fed infants (all formulas in the US are fortified with phylloquinone) compared with breast-fed infants.[123,124] In the newborn liver, unlike adults, phylloquinone predominates over menaquinones (81 ± 73 v. 9 ± 2 pmol per g of liver).[125] Menaquinones are not readily available from the hepatic pool,[126] compared with phylloquinone. Little is known about their absorption from the intestinal tract, plasma transport, or clearance from circulation. Most of the gut bacterial pool of menaquinones, located within bacterial membranes, is probably not available for absorption.

Vitamin K_1 has been reported to be present in low (<2 µg ml^{-1}) to undetectable concentrations in cord blood.[124,127-129] Recent data have shown that out of 156 cord bloods in term infants, none had measurable vitamin K.[130] Thus, there is no correlation between maternal and cord blood levels. From all of the available evidence it appears that only very small quantities of vitamin K cross the placenta from mother to fetus. Indeed, even maternal pharmacological doses of vitamin K have unpredictable effects on cord blood concentration.[124,127-129]

Vitamin K is absorbed from the intestine into the lymphatic system, requiring the presence of both bile salts and pancreatic secretions.[131] The lymphatic system is the major route of intestinal transport of absorbed phylloquinone in association with chylomicrons. Little is known of the existence of carrier proteins. In the neonate, 29% of an oral dose of vitamin K_1 is reportedly absorbed from the intestine.[132] The importance of the enterohepatic circulation of vitamin K in the human is unknown. Compared with other fat-soluble vitamins, relatively small amounts of vitamin K have been reported in the liver of the neonate. However, vitamin K is found in relatively high concentrations in liver, heart, and bone compared with other tissues.[133,134] In adult humans it has been demonstrated with labeled vitamin K_1 that the total body pool of vitamin K is replaced approximately every 2.5 hours.[135] There is no information in the infant.

Vitamin K is found in the milk fat globules. Human milk generally contains less than 10 µg L^{-1}, and there is no significant difference between mature milk and colostrum (Table 14.1).[19] However, human milk concentration is affected by maternal supplements. A recent report found a concentration 3.0 ± 2.3 µg L^{-1} (SD) in six mothers delivering between 26 and 30 weeks gestation.[136] By supplementing these mothers with 2.5 mg phylloquinone a day orally for two weeks the vitamin K concentration of the milk was increased to 64.2 ± 31.4 µg L^{-1} (SD).[136] In term infants, supplements of vitamin K to mothers will increase vitamin K in both breast milk and infant serum.[137]

Neonatal requirements

Though the official DRI for infants is 2–2.5 µg day^{-1}, it seems prudent to continue 1 mg of phylloquinone intramuscularly at birth to all infants including the premature infant greater than 1000 g birth weight.[20] For preterm infants with birth weights <1000 g, 0.3 mg kg^{-1} intramuscularly would be sufficient. This amount of vitamin K should sustain the infant at least through the first 2 weeks of life.

Though human milk does not supply the DRI for vitamin K of 2–2.5 µg day^{-1} for exclusively breast fed infants, these infants generally do not show any signs of deficiency during the first 3 months of life if they received prophylactic vitamin K at birth.[130] Formulas for term infants with added vitamin K supply 7–9 µg kg^{-1} day^{-1} exceeding the RDA.

As all infant formulas for low birth weight infants contain large amounts of vitamin K (65–100 µg L^{-1}, Table 14.2), 150 ml kg^{-1} day^{-1} would supply 9.6–15.0 µg kg^{-1} day^{-1}. For the VLBWI on vitamin K supplemented formula, no additional vitamin K is needed. The available human milk fortifiers for the VLBWIs in the USA all contain vitamin K (Table 14.3). Premature infants on formula or fortified human milk by 40 weeks post-conceptional age, have plasma vitamin K concentrations and intakes comparable with those of term infants on fortified formula.[138]

For term infants on TPN solutions, M.V.I. Pediatrics or Infuvite will supply 200 μg day^{-1} (Tables 14.4 and 14.6). There would appear to be little justification for term infants on TPN to receive these large amounts of vitamin K. Preterm infants receiving 2 ml of M.V.I. Pediatric or Infuvite receive 80–100 μg day^{-1} in addition to the 10 μg kg^{-1} day^{-1} from 3 g kg^{-1} day^{-1} of Intralipid (20%) (Table 14.6). Intralipid contains about 70 μg dL^{-1}. Again these large doses do not seem justified. A recent report found very high plasma levels (124.4 ± 101.1 ng ml^{-1}, adult normal <1 ng ml^{-1}) in preterm infants receiving TPN at 2 weeks of age.[138] Presently, no available oral, liquid vitamin preparation containing vitamin K is available for infants.

High dose vitamin K for infants/toxicity

A number of studies have tried to associate periventricular-intraventricular hemorrhage PIVH in the VLBWI with vitamin K deficiency.[139–144] Maternal supplements of vitamin K have been given as a result.[145–147] However, given the very low transfer rate of vitamin K across the placenta even when given in large doses to the mother, and the mixed results of these studies, one cannot conclude that PIVH in the premature infant is secondary to vitamin K deficiency at birth. In fact, it is clear that many cases of PIVH occur in infants 3 or more days after receiving the customary prophylactic dose of phylloquinone at birth, implying that vitamin K does not prevent PIVH. To date, toxicity from vitamin K has not been reported in the premature infant with the presently available formulations.

Pharmacologic doses of the vitamin are used in the newborn period for prevention of hemorrhagic disease. Historically, hyperbilirubinemia and kernicterus were reported in premature infants in the 1960s prophylactically treated with large quantities of a highly protein-bound form of the vitamin (menadione), no longer in clinical use.[148] In term infants given 1 mg intramuscularly for newborn prophylaxis, there was an association reported with the onset of childhood leukemia, but this initial report has not been confirmed.[149]

Vitamin K deficiency

Vitamin K deficiency with hemorrhage in the newborn is a worldwide problem, though it is not a major problem in the USA where nearly all infants receive prophylactic vitamin K at the time of birth. As formulas are all fortified with vitamin K, it is largely a disease of breast-fed infants who often have another disorder associated with malabsorption such as biliary atresia or alpha-1-antitrypsin deficiency. In the classic form of the disease, hemorrhage occurs between days 2 and 10 of life, and intracranial hemorrhage is uncommon. It is hallmarked by generalized ecchymosis or gastrointestinal bleeding. Bleeding from a circumcision site or umbilical cord stump is also common. A second form of the disease, late hemorrhagic disease, is less benign. Again, this form occurs mostly in breast-feeding infants between 6 weeks and 6 months of life and is associated with intracranial hemorrhage with devastating sequelae.[150]

Laboratory assessment of vitamin K status

In the neonate the concentrations of the vitamin K-dependent clotting factors (factors II, VII, IX, and X) are generally 25%–70% of normal adult concentrations, and there is little difference at the time of birth between 30 and 40 weeks gestational age infants.[151,152] Normal adult concentrations of these factors are not achieved until 6 months of age, and if anything, premature infants show an accelerated postnatal maturation towards adult levels compared with term infants. The prothrombin time shows a wider range and variability in the newborn at birth (11–16 seconds) compared with the adult (11–14 seconds), and this persists through the first 6 months of life. The activated partial thromboplastin time shows a similar pattern compared with adults through the first 6 months of life.[151,152] Interestingly enough, in the neonate injections of vitamin K$_1$ do not significantly alter these tests or the measurements of the individual clotting factors.[129,153] Thus, the differences in coagulation between adults and newborns cannot totally be ascribed to vitamin K "deficiency". The coagulation differences may be limited by the availability of precursor proteins for the synthesis of vitamin K-dependent carboxylase enzyme of the vitamin K cycle, rather than the availability of vitamin K$_1$.

Human vitamin K deficiency results in the secretion of partially carboxylated prothrombin into the plasma, referred to as abnormal prothrombin, or PIVKA-II (protein induced by vitamin K absence or antagonism).[154] PIVKA-II is a heterogeneous molecule. It consists of a pool of partially carboxylated prothrombin, as well as some completely acarboxylated prothrombin.[155] Detection rates of PIVKA-II in cord blood have ranged from 10% to 30%.[156–159] PIVKA-II values in a large series of full-term newborn infants in the USA at the time of birth have recently been reported. Of 148 cord bloods, 49/148 (33%) were positive for PIVKA-II (≥0.2 AU ml^{-1}).[130] Similarly, in another study of 13 premature infants (27–36 weeks gestation) and 46 term infants (37–41 weeks), there was no correlation between gestation age and PIVKA-II values in cord blood.[160] Thirty-one infants (52%) had elevated PIVKA-II in cord blood. Finally, in a recent report in premature infants (24–36 weeks gestation),

PIVKA-II levels were elevated in cord blood in 19/69 samples (27.5%).[138]

The usefulness of this measurement for showing a subclinical vitamin K deficiency is a point of controversy. A number of studies have shown that prophylactic vitamin K administered to the newborn results in near elimination of the positive PIVKA-II values that were present in cord blood.[161–164] Similarly, in preterm infants PIVK-II is not detected at 2 and 6 weeks after birth with high intakes of vitamin K.[138] In a recent study of exclusively breast feeding infants who received vitamin K prophylaxis at birth (either orally or intramuscularly), there was no significant correlation between measurable PIVKA-II levels and low plasma vitamin K levels during the first 3 months of life.[130]

Water-soluble vitamins

Water soluble vitamins include vitamin C or ascorbic acid and the B complex vitamins. As a group, these vitamins function physiologically as prosthetic groups for enzymes involved in a broad variety of metabolic functions, including amino acid metabolism, energy production, and nucleic acid synthesis. With the exceptions of folic acid and vitamin B_{12} which are stored in the liver, these vitamins are not stored to any great extent. Thus, they must be supplied at frequent intervals. Excesses are largely excreted in the bile and urine. They are all inactivated by heat and ionizing radiation. Unfortunately, determination of appropriate enteral and parenteral vitamin intake based on scientific data especially for preterm infants is lacking. Even the amounts supplied in TPN solutions are dictated not necessarily by the actual requirement, but by the concentrations available in multivitamin preparations (M.V.I. Pediatrics and Infuvite) (Table 14.4). The full implications of parenterally administered vitamins, particularly in large quantities, are unknown. For term infants, the vitamin content of human milk is the intake standard. Maternal diet may affect vitamin sufficiency in the fetus and breast-fed infant. The gastrointestinal tract and liver modify the orally ingested water-soluble vitamins.

Thiamine (vitamin B$_1$)

Thiamine is absorbed in the proximal small intestine by both active and passive mechanisms, the carrier mediated process occurring in low concentrations (less than 2 μM) and the passive process at higher concentrations.[165,166] After absorption thiamine is converted in the liver to its primary active cofactor, thiamine pyrophosphate (TPP), necessary for three enzyme complexes essential for carbohydrate metabolism. These are pyruvate dehydrogenase

and alpha-ketoglutarate in the Krebs cycle, and transketolase which is involved in the production of ribose for the synthesis of RNA and also provides NADPH required for fatty acid synthesis. Further phosphorylation of TPP occurs in the CNS to form thiamine triphosphate (TTP), thought to facilitate nerve conduction by its influence on membrane sodium ion conductance.[165,167,168] Thiamine appears to readily cross the placenta, in that fetal concentrations are approximately 7 times those of maternal plasma concentration.[169] Human milk concentration of thiamine increases from 20 μg L^{-1} in colostrum to 220 μg L^{-1} in mature milk (Table 14.1). In well-nourished women, the thiamine concentration in human milk is not affected by diet.[170]

Neonatal requirements

The need for thiamine is directly related to the amount of carbohydrate consumed. Thiamine deficiency in breast-fed neonates of well-nourished mothers has not been reported. The daily recommended intake (DRI) for term infants is 200–300 μg day^{-1} (Table 14.5) which is based on the amount in human milk (220 μg L^{-1}) (Table 14.1).[171,172] As standard infant formulas contain 75–100 μg per 100 kcal, formula-fed infants will easily meet the DRI (Table 14.2).

For the premature infant, the recommended thiamine intake is 150–200 μg per 100 kcal (Table 14.5).[82,83,172] Preterm infant formula contains 200–250 μg per 100 kcal so will meet even the highest of these recommendations and this appears to be an adequate amount (Table 14.2).[174] Commercially available human milk fortifiers provide an equivalent amount of thiamine when used to fortify human milk to 24 per cal per oz (Table 14.3). Human milk on the other hand (220 μg L^{-1}) may not meet the needs of the premature infant especially where milk banking and/or heat treatment is required. Preterm infants have increased metabolic needs compared with the term infant.

The recommendations for thiamine intake for newborn infants on parenteral nutrition are much less precise and there are very little data on which to base these recommendations.[82] Five ml of M.V.I. Pediatric or 4 ml of Infuvite supplies 1200 μg day^{-1} which would seem to be more than adequate for a term infant (Tables 14.4 and 14.6). When given in the recommended amounts for preterm infants, 2 ml provides 480–600 μg day^{-1} of thiamine to a premature infant, again an intake which seems very adequate.[174]

Deficiency/toxicity

Deficiency or toxicity of thiamine in the western world is almost unheard of in the newborn infant. Deficiency has been reported in those parts of the world where the diet consists of un-enriched white rice or flour, but even in these countries, it is extremely rare in the newborn. An infantile form of beriberi may occur in the first 4 months of life in breast-fed infants whose mothers have a deficient thiamine intake.[175] Symptoms include weak swallowing, nuchal rigidity, apnea, spasticity, ophthalmoplegia, hypothermia, and coma. In adults, toxicity rarely has included an anaphylactic reaction and large parenteral doses have been associated with respiratory depression.

Laboratory assessment

The most reliable index of thiamine status is whole blood thiamine level. The classic test for thiamine deficiency is the erythrocyte transketolase assay, in which transketolase is measured before and after addition of thiamine pyrophosphate.[176] However, this method does not detect marginal or elevated concentrations of the vitamin which may be a concern when assessing parenteral needs.

Riboflavin (vitamin B₂)

Riboflavin and its coenzymes flavin mononucleotide (FMN) and flavin adenine dinucleotide (FAD) function as electron donors and acceptors in oxidation-reduction systems. They are important for energy metabolism, glycogen synthesis, erythrocyte production, and conversion of folate to its active coenzyme. Absorption of riboflavin mostly occurs in the proximal small intestine and is under very tight control. Uptake occurs largely via a high-affinity, low-capacity carrier which allows for efficient absorption at low gut concentrations while preventing excessive absorption. In the intestinal mucosa riboflavin is phosphorylated to FMN. Further phosphorylation produces FAD. Riboflavin is transported via serum albumin and stored primarily in the liver and kidney in small quantities. It is eliminated primarily by the kidneys.[177] Riboflavin, FMN, and FAD appear to cross the placenta from mother to infant against a concentration gradient but no detailed information is known about this transport process.[178]

The concentration in human milk is 400–600 μg L⁻¹ (Table 14.1). It remains nearly constant throughout lactation.[170] It is subject to photodegradation. Standard term formulas contain 150 μg per 100 kcal, while preterm formulas contain 300–620 μg per 100 kcal (Table 14.2). Commercially available human milk fortifiers provide 250–500 μg per 100 kcal when used to fortify human milk to 24 cal per oz (Table 14.3)

Neonatal requirements

The DRI for enteral riboflavin in neonates is 300–400 μg day⁻¹ (Table 14.5) an amount not likely to be achieved by breast-feeding infants if the human milk concentration of riboflavin is 400–600 μg L⁻¹.[172] However, breast-feeding infants do not show signs of riboflavin deficiency. Preterm infants have higher intake requirements due to the need for phototherapy and the exposure of stored milk to light. The recommended enteral intake for preterm infants varies from 200–300 μg per 100 kcal (Table 14.5).[83,173]

The recommended intake for parenteral nutrition for term neonates is 1400 μg (Table 14.6), the amount supplied by 5 ml of M.V.I. Pediatric or 4 ml of Infuvite (Table 14.4).[82] Two ml of these vitamin solutions provide 560–700 μg to the preterm infant (Table 14.6). A dose of 150 μg day⁻¹ has been suggested as appropriate,[82] but this cannot be provided with presently available multivitamin solutions. High blood levels of riboflavin have been reported in preterm infants whether receiving formula or TPN, which quickly normalize when riboflavin is removed from the diet.[179]

Deficiency/toxicity

Isolated riboflavin deficiency does not usually occur. Principal manifestations are dermatologic and ophthalmologic, including angular stomatitis, cheilosis, glossitis, seborrhea, photophobia, and increased corneal vascularity. Overt signs of deficiency are very rare in the developed countries. Though there are no known toxic effects of this vitamin, plasma levels in preterm infants receiving multivitamins had serum levels 100 times the cord blood levels, and in theory could cause urinary precipitation of riboflavin and obstructive tubular damage.[173] Some biochemical deficiency (decreased erythrocyte glutathione reductase activation coefficient) has been reported in preterm infants receiving unsupplemented human milk but this is of unknown clinical significance.[180]

Laboratory assessment

A classic screen for riboflavin deficiency can be obtained by measuring erythrocyte glutathione reductase activity both in the presence and absence of excess added active cofactor FAD. An increase in activity of more than 20% indicates riboflavin deficiency.[181] A better measure of riboflavin status (both deficiency and excess), is measuring riboflavin and its cofactors FMN and FAD in plasma and red blood cells, along with urinary riboflavin concentrations. However, even "normal" blood levels in infants have not been established.[174]

Vitamin B₆ (Pyridoxine)

Vitamin B₆ refers to three naturally occurring pyridines – pryridoxine (PN), pyridoxal (PL), and pyridoxamine (PM) and their phosphorylated derivatives.[182] The dephosphorylated forms are all absorbed passively in the proximal jejunum, and transported to the liver where conversion to the active forms occurs. Vitamin B₆ serves as a cofactor in a large number of reactions involved in the synthesis, inter-conversion, and metabolism of amino acids. It is also necessary for the synthesis of niacin, various neurotransmitters, heme, and prostaglandins. It is stored in small amounts and very sensitive to heat and photodegradation.

Vitamin B_6 readily crosses the placenta from mother to infant, though details of this transport are not known. There is accumulation of vitamin B_6 in the fetus with increasing gestation and this is important for the breast-fed infant.[183] Daily supplementation of the mother during pregnancy with >2 mg of pyridoxine is associated with normal vitamin status in infants through 4 months of age.[183] In general, because of the extra protein allowance for pregnancy, a supplement of 0.6 mg per day is recommended during pregnancy as well as lactation (DRI).[172]

The human milk concentration of vitamin B_6 can be related to maternal intake. In mothers not taking supplements, the concentration is 70–150 μg L^{-1} (Table 14.1).[170] Formulas for term infants contain 60 μg per 100 kcal and formulas for preterm infants contain up to 2030 μg L^{-1} (Table 14.2). Commercial human milk fortifiers add 1280 μg L^{-1} to human milk (Table 14.3).

Requirements

Requirements are directly proportional to protein intake (Table 14.5). For term infants, the DRI for vitamin B_6 should be between 100–300 μg day^{-1}.[172] If the vitamin intake of the mother is adequate during pregnancy and lactation, then the breast-fed term infant needs no additional vitamin B_6. Preterm infants, however, need more vitamin B_6 than would normally be supplied by human milk. Though there are little data on which to base the recommendations, recommended enteral intakes in preterm infants range from 125–175 μg per 100 kcal.[83] Formula-fed infants, whether preterm or term, receive adequate intakes via the appropriate formula, though some have suggested that the levels in preterm formulas may be too high.[174,184]

Parenteral requirements for term infants on TPN are estimated to be 1000 μg day^{-1} (Table 14.6). For preterm infants, parenteral recommendations of 400–500 μg day^{-1} are easily met with presently available solutions (Tables 14.4 and 14.6). A dose of 300 μg kg^{-1} day^{-1} provides very high blood levels of this vitamin, and some have raised concerns about this level of intake.[82,174]

Deficiency and toxicity

Due to the availability of this vitamin, deficiency is quite uncommon in infants. Symptoms of deficiency include hypochromic microcytic anemia, vomiting, diarrhea, failure to thrive, irritability, and seizures. Several conditions associated with abnormalities of vitamin B_6 metabolism

that require pharmacologic doses (200–600 mg day^{-1}) of the vitamin have been described in infants.[185–187] These include pyridoxine-dependent seizures, pyridoxine-responsive hypochromic microcytic anemia, xanthurenic aciduria, cysthathioninuria, and homocystinuria. Toxicity even with these megadoses of the vitamin, has not been reported in infants.

Laboratory assessment

High-performance liquid chromatography methods to quantify all the vitamins in plasma and erythrocytes provide the most accurate and reliable measure of vitamin B_6 status.[188] Measurement of pyridoxal phosphate (most abundant blood isomer) has been proposed to assess the vitamin B_6 status in preterm infants.[189] Because of the requirement for the vitamin in the normal metabolism of tryptophan, a measurement of certain urinary metabolites has been used as a functional test for vitamin deficiency.[82]

Vitamin B_{12} (Cobalamin)

Vitamin B_{12} is unique in a number of ways compared with the other water-soluble vitamins. It is produced in nature by bacteria and not contained in plants, leading to deficiency in vegans, including those who are lactating. It occurs in two forms: methylcobalamin and adenosylcobalamin.[177] Methylcobalamin is the form found in body fluids including breast milk. It is a cytoplasmic cofactor which transfers a methyl group from tetrahydrofolate to homocysteine for the synthesis of methionine. Vitamin B_{12} is necessary for the regeneration of tetrahydrofolate such that in the deficiency state folate is trapped in its demethylated form and is unavailable for pyrimidine synthesis. Thus, a deficiency of Vit B_{12} is responsible for the cellular folate deficiency.[177] Adenosylcobalamin is present in the mitochondria of solid tissues and is involved in the formation of myelin sheaths in neural tissue.[190] It participates in the reduction of purine and pyrimidine ribonucleotides to their corresponding deoxyribonucleotides necessary for DNA synthesis.

The absorption and storage of vitamin B_{12} is also unique.[177] Upon ingestion the vitamin is released from food at gastric pH and complexed with the salivary R binder. Under the alkaline conditions of the jejunum, pancreatic enzymes digest the R binder.[191] Vitamin B_{12} is then bound to intrinsic factor, which facilitates its calcium dependent absorption across the ileal mucosa. Once absorption occurs, the vitamin circulates bound to a specific family of binding proteins, the transcobalamins. It is also the only water-soluble vitamin that is stored to any significant degree in the body, and a very effective enterohepatic circulation accounts for its very long half life. Little is known about its transfer from the mother to the fetus across the placenta, but this obviously occurs.

Reported values for human milk range from 0.16–0.97 μg L^{-1}.[170] An average value from the literature would be 0.7 μg L^{-1} (Table 14.1). The vitamin B$_{12}$ content of human milk decreases with increasing time of lactation and maternal supplementation in a repleted state does not have much effect on milk concentration. Standard formulas for term infants have about 0.25 μg per 100 kcal and formulas for preterm infants contain 2.0–4.5 μg L^{-1} (Table 14.2). Fortification of human milk with human milk fortifiers (24 cal per oz) for preterm infants will supply at least 2.5 μg L^{-1} (Table 14.3).

Requirements

Human milk and formula provide adequate vitamin B$_{12}$ for the term infant. Exceptions would be human milk from vegan mothers with inadequate intake of the vitamin. The DRI of 0.4–0.5 μg day^{-1} provides a substantial margin of sufficiency (Table 14.5).[172] There is no information available on what to base the recommendations for the preterm infant. Hence, they are about the same as for a term infant for enteral feeding. The parenteral requirements for term neonates are 0.75–1.0 μg day^{-1} (0.1 μg per 100 kcal) (Table 14.6).[82] Preterm infants receiving 0.65 μg kg^{-1} day^{-1} (0.85 μg per 100 kcal) have elevated plasma levels.[192,193] Though 0.3 μg kg^{-1} day^{-1} has been estimated to be adequate for the preterm infant, standard TPN multivitamin solutions will deliver 0.4–0.5 μg to a 1000 g infant (Tables 14.4 and 14.6).

Deficiency/toxicity

Deficiency is almost unheard of in infants except in those situations where breast-feeding mothers are strict vegans who take no vitamin supplements or have pernicious anemia.[194] The deficiency state results in ineffective DNA synthesis which results in hypersegmented neutrophils and megaloblastic anemia. Infants present with failure to thrive and neurologic symptoms which include regression of milestones and hypotonia.[194] Toxicity has never been described.

Laboratory assessment

Plasma vitamin B$_{12}$ can be measured as a good indicator of overall vitamin B$_{12}$ status. The Schilling test, in which radio-labeled vitamin B$_{12}$ is given orally is also helpful in evaluating deficiency.[190]

Folate

Folate refers to a family of compounds synthesized by bacteria and plants, consisting of a pteroic acid moiety conjugated to a variable number of 11 glutamic acid residues.[177] Folic acid refers to pteroylglutamic acid, the monoglutamate, though most naturally occurring folates exist as polyglutamates. It participates in the biosynthesis of purines and pyrimidines, in the metabolism of some amino acids and in the catabolism of histidine.[195]

The vitamin is primarily absorbed from the jejunum by an active process. Homeostasis is regulated in part by a very efficient enterohepatic circulation. It is not stored to any significant degree. It accumulates in the fetus during the third trimester of pregnancy, so that term infants have higher levels and are at lower risk for the development of deficiency than the preterm infant.[196,197]

The folate content of human milk is tightly regulated and remains relatively constant even in mothers with marginal status. Its concentration in human milk increases during the first 3 months of lactation. The reported folate concentration in human milk ranges from 80–140 μg L^{-1} (Table 14.1).[170] Term infant formulas contain 15 μg per 100 kcal and preterm formulas contain 300 μg L^{-1} (Table 14.2). Commercially available human milk fortifiers (24 cal per oz) add 300 μg L^{-1} of folate (Table 14.3).

Requirements

The DRI for term infants is 65–80 μg day^{-1} (9 μg kg^{-1} day^{-1}) (Table 14.5).[172] Four μg per 100 kcal results in normal red blood cell morphology in full term infants.[198] The folate requirements of preterm infants remain undetermined, though 21 42 μg per 100 kcal is recommended by the AAP.[171] At least two studies of high (65 μg day^{-1} –100 μg day^{-1}) v. low (3.5 μg day^{-1}–15 μg day^{-1}) failed to show any advantage of the higher intake in preterm infants.[199,200] Preterm infants fed human milk probably need a supplement which can be provided by the human milk fortifier (300 μg L^{-1}) (Table 14.3).

Parenteral requirement for TPN therapy in term infants is 140 μg day^{-1}, the amount contained in 5 ml of M.V.I. Pediatric (Table 14.6).[82] There is little on which to base a recommendation for preterm infants, but the standard doses of TPN multivitamins will deliver 56–70 μg day^{-1}.

Deficiency/toxicity

Folate deficiency is one of the most common vitamin deficiencies reported during the perinatal period and supplementation of pregnant women is known to reduce the incidence of neural tube defects in the fetus.[195,201] Though the deficiency is uncommon in infants from developed countries, the deficiency state produces growth retardation, megaloblastic anemia, alterations in neurologic status, and small intestinal morphology. Toxicity has not been described, though hypersensitivity reactions have been described in adults.

Laboratory assessment
Folate status is best assessed by measuring concentrations of the vitamin in sera and erythrocytes.[190]

Niacin

Niacin is a term used to describe two equivalent compounds, nicotinic acid and nicotinamide.[177,190] Niacin is converted in the liver to the active cofactors nicotinamide adenine dinucleotide (NAD) and nictotinamide adenine dinucleotide phosphate (NADP). These coenzymes are essential in two-electron transfers and are involved in fat synthesis, intracellular respiratory metabolism, and glycolysis. Technically, niacin is not a vitamin as it is synthesized in the body from excess dietary tryptophan. This process is catalyzed by riboflavin and vitamin B_6. Transport to tissues occurs largely in red blood cells.[190] There is no known storage form of the vitamin.

Human milk contains 1.8–6.0 mg L^{-1} or 0.17–0.27 mg per 100 kcal of niacin (Table 14.1).[170] Perhaps more importantly, the breast milk concentration of tryptophan is 220 mg L^{-1} or about 3.8 niacin equivalents per liter (1 niacin equivalent equals 60 mg tryptophan). Formulas for term infants contain 1.1 mg per 100 kcal (Table 14.2). Those for preterm infants contain 32–40 mg L^{-1}, and breast milk fortifiers (24 cal per oz) add 32 mg L^{-1} (Table 14.3).

Requirements

Requirements are dependent on the dietary intake of tryptophan as well as riboflavin and vitamin B_6 status. There are not good guidelines for precise dietary requirements in infants. The DRI for term infants is 2–4 mg day^{-1} (Table 14.5).[172] The recommended intake for preterm infants is 3–4 mg per 100 kcal.[171] Breast milk and formulas obviously meet the dietary requirements (Tables 14.1 and 14.2).

The parenteral requirement of niacin in term infants is met by the 17 mg in 5 ml of M.V.I. Pediatric (Tables 14.4 and 14.6).[82] For a 1000 g preterm infant receiving 2 ml of M.V.I. Pediatric or Infuvite, 6.8–8.5 mg is provided (Table 14.6). The quantities of tryptophan in TPN solutions do not influence niacin requirements.

Deficiency/toxicity

Niacin deficiency, or pellagra, does not occur in neonates in the developed world. There are also no described cases of toxicity in the neonate.

Laboratory assessment

Niacin is converted to multiple metabolites in the liver. The most commonly employed method of determining niacin deficiency is the measurement of the liver metabolite N^1-methyl nicotinamide in the urine.[202]

Biotin

Biotin is important for mammalian enzymes involved in carboxylation and carbon dioxide transfer reactions. It plays an important role in the synthesis of amino acids and fatty acids as well as being a cofactor in gluconeogenesis. Though little is known about its intestinal absorption in humans, it is thought to be passively absorbed from the small intestine. It is transported bound to plasma proteins. When biotin-containing enzymes are degraded, the biotin can be recovered by the liver and plasma biotinidase. This method of conservation makes deficiency very uncommon.[177,203]

The biotin content of human milk is reported to be 5–9 μg L^{-1} (Table 14.1).[170] Formulas for term infants contain 2.2–4.5 μg per 100 kcal (Table 14.2). Formulas for preterm infants contain a wide range, 32–300 μg L^{-1}, while breast milk fortifiers (24 cal per oz) for preterm infants add 26 μg L^{-1} to human milk (Table 14.3).

Requirements

There are very little data on which to base the DRI for neonates. The current DRI for term infants is 5–6 μg day^{-1} (Table 14.5).[172] Human milk and formula provide adequate amounts of biotin. Parenteral administration of 20–90 μg day^{-1} to term infants maintains normal plasma levels for 90 days.[82] Premature infants receiving 12 μg kg^{-1} day^{-1} have elevated plasma biotin levels. Five ml of M.V.I. Pediatric supplies 20 μg (Table 14.6);[192] 2 ml of M.V.I. Pediatric would supply 8 μg to the 1000 g preterm infant; and 0.5 ml of Infuvite supplies 10 μg (Table 14.6).

Deficiency/toxicity

Biotin deficiency has not been reported in breast-fed or formula-fed infants, though several inborn errors of metabolism affect the biotin-dependent enzymes which can be treated with large doses of biotin.[204] Biotin deficiency has been reported in parenterally fed infants receiving biotin deficient TPN solutions.[205] These symptoms include alopecia, exfoliative dermatitis, and conjunctivitis. Toxicity has not been reported.

Laboratory assessment

Plasma levels can be measured by a number of methods to assess biotin status.[190]

Pantothenic acid

Pantothenic acid, widely distributed in plant and animal tissues, is an integral part of coenzyme A, which functions in acyl group transfers in the synthesis of fatty acids, pyruvate, and alpha-ketoglutarate, and other acetylation reactions.[190,206] It is typically ingested in the coenzyme A form, undergoing intestinal hydrolysis prior to absorption. It is transported in blood as pantothenic acid and then re-synthesized to coenzyme A in target tissues. The plasma concentration in neonatal cord blood is several-fold higher than maternal blood, inferring active transport across the placenta from mother to fetus.[207]

The concentration of pantothenic acid in human milk is 2.0–2.5 mg L^{-1} (Table 14.1). Supplementation affects milk concentration only in malnourished mothers. Formulas for term infants supply 0.4–0.5 mg per 100 kcal, while formulas for preterm infants generally supply 10–15 mg L^{-1} (Table 14.2). Human milk fortifiers (24 cal per oz) add 11.3 mg L^{-1} (Table 14.3).

Requirements

The DRI for term infants is 1.7–1.8 mg day^{-1} (Table 14.5).[172] Recommended enteral intake for preterm infants is 1–1.5 mg per 100 kcal (Table 14.5). Parenteral requirements for infants on TPN are met with 5 mg day^{-1} for term infants and 2.0–2.5 mg day^{-1} for preterm infants, the amounts contained in the recommended amounts of pediatric multivitamins for TPN solutions (Table 14.6).[82]

Deficiency/toxicity

Neither isolated deficiency nor toxicity of pantothenic acid have been reported in infants. Inborn errors of metabolism have not been reported.

Laboratory assessment

Plasma levels using a number of techniques can be measured to assess status.[82]

Vitamin C (ascorbic acid)

L-ascorbic acid is the biologically active form of vitamin C. It is an antioxidant and accelerates hydroxylation reactions in many biosynthetic pathways.[208] At the tissue level, a major function is synthesis of collagen, proteoglycans, and other organic constituents of the intercellular matrix in such diverse tissues as tooth, bone, and capillary endothelium. It is readily absorbed from the small intestine by an energy-dependent process that is saturable and dose-dependent. It is ubiquitously distributed throughout tissues.[209] Fetal blood levels are higher than maternal levels which implies an active placental transport process as well.[210] As glucose competes with ascorbic acid for transport, maternal hyperglycemia may decrease the supply of ascorbic acid to the developing fetus.

Human milk concentrations exceed plasma concentrations. The vitamin C content of milk depends somewhat on maternal intakes. It averages 100 mg L^{-1}, depending on maternal intake (Table 14.1).[170] The vitamin C content of formulas for term infants is 8–9 mg per 100 kcal (Table 14.2). Formulas for preterm infants contain more: 160–300 mg L^{-1} (Table 14.2). Human milk fortifiers (24 cal per oz) will supply 166 mg L^{-1} of ascorbic acid (Table 14.3). Some have suggested that for preterm infants, even greater amounts of vitamin C should be added to preterm formulas or human milk fortifiers based on serum concentrates of vitamin C, which are low in some infants on these intakes.[174]

Requirements

The RDA for vitamin C for healthy term newborn infants is 340–350 mg day^{-1} which is based on the vitamin C content of human milk (Table 14.5).[172] To achieve this intake, breast-fed infants would have to ingest about 500 ml of milk per day. Between 15–20 mg per 100 kcal is also appropriate for the preterm infant unless they are receiving a high protein diet (see below) (Table 14.5). For full-term infants on TPN, 80 mg day^{-1} will maintain normal plasma levels.[82] This is the amount supplied by 5 ml of M.V.I. Pediatric or 4 ml of Infuvite (Table 14.4). Two ml of M.V.I. Pediatric or 0.5 ml of Infuvite will supply 32–40 mg to the 1000 g infant which appears to be sufficient for the smaller preterm infant (Table 14.6).

Deficiency/toxicity

Vitamin C deficiency results in scurvy. Historically this was seen in both term and preterm infants fed pasteurized formula or human milk without the addition of vitamin C, as ascorbic acid is very sensitive to heat treatment.[177,210]

Infantile scurvy is characterized by irritability and tenderness, swelling, and pseudoparalysis of the lower extremities. A scaly dermatitis, anorexia and failure to thrive have also been reported. Hypertyrosinemia has been reported in formula-fed premature infants resulting from a low vitamin C intake relative to a high protein (5–6 g kg^{-1} day^{-1}) intake in the past.[211] This was corrected with the addition of larger amounts of vitamin C to formulas for preterm infants as well as lowering protein intakes.[212] No toxic effects of the doses given to newborn infants have ever been reported.

Laboratory assessment

Both plasma and leukocyte concentrations can be assayed to determine vitamin C status.[208,210] Serum concentrations less than 6 mg per 100 ml are indicative of deficiency, though concentrations less than this are not uncommon in preterm infants receiving recommended intakes.[174]

REFERENCES

1 Mangelsdorf, D. J., Umesono, K., Evans, R. M. The retinoid receptors. In Sporn, M. B., Roberts, A. B., Goodman, D. S., eds. *The Retinoids.* 2nd edn. Orlando, FL: Academic Press; 1994:319–50.

2 Blomhoff, R. Transport and metabolism of vitamin A. *Nutr. Rev.* 1994;**52**:513–23.

3 Dostalova, L. Correlation of the vitamin status between mother and newborn at delivery. *Dev. Pharmacol. Ther.* 1982;**4**:45–7.

4 Hustead, V. A., Gutcher, G. R., Anderson, S. A. *et al.* Relationship of vitamin A (retinol) status to lung disease in the preterm infant. *J. Pediatr.* 1984;**105**:610–15.

5 Tammela, O., Aitola, M., Ikonen, S. Cord blood concentrations of vitamin A in preterm infants. *Early Hum. Dev.* 1999;**56**:39–47.

6 Lund, C. J., Kimble, M. S. Plasma vitamin A and carotene of the newborn infant with consideration of fetal-maternal relationships. *Am. J. Obstet. Gynecol.* 1943;**46**:207–21.

7 Baker, H., Thompson, F. O., Langer, A. D. *et al.* Vitamin profile of 174 mothers and newborns at parturition. *Am. J. Clin. Nutr.* 1975;**28**:59–65.

8 Baker, H., Thind, I. S., Frank, O. *et al.* Vitamin levels in low birth-weight newborn infants and their mothers. *J. Obstet. Gynecol.* 1977;**129**:521–4.

9 Vahlquist A., Rask L., Peterson, P. A., Berg, T. The concentrations of retinol-binding protein, prealbumin, and transferrin in sera of newly delivered mothers and children of various ages. *Scand. J. Clin. Lab. Invest.* 1975;**35**:569–75.

10 Jansson L., Nilsson, B. Serum retinol and retinol-binding protein in mothers and infants at delivery. *Biol. Neonate.* 1983;**43**:269–71.

11 Barnes, A. C. The placental metabolism of vitamin A. *Am. J. Obstet. Gynecol.* 1951;**61**:368–372.

12 Ong, D. E. Absorption of vitamin A. In Blomhoff, R., ed. *Vitamin A in Health and Disease.* New York, NY: Marcel Dekker, Inc.; 1994:37–72.

13 Hugue, T. A survey of human liver reserves of retinol in London. *Br. J. Nutr.* 1982;**47**:165–172.

14 Shenai, J. P., Chytil, F., Stahlman, M. T. Liver vitamin A reserves of very low birth weight neonates. *Pediatr. Res.* 1985;**19**:892–3.

15 Olson, J. A., Gunning, D. B., Tilton, R. A. Liver concentrations of vitamin A and carotenoids, as a function of age and other parameters of American children who died of various causes. *Am. J. Clin. Nutr.* 1984;**39**:903–10.

16 Soprano, D. R., Blaner, W. S. Plasma retinol-binding proteins. In Sporn, M. B., Roberts, A. B., Goodman, D. S., eds. The Retinoids. 2nd edn. Orlando, FL: Academic Press; 1994:257–82.

17 Shenai, J. P., Chytil, F., Jhaveri, A. *et al.* Plasma vitamin A and retinol binding protein in premature and term neonates. *J. Pediatr.* 1981;**99**:302–5.

18 Thompson, S. Y., Kon, S. K., Mawson, E. H. The application of chromatography to the study of carotenoids of human and cow's milk. *Biochem. J.* 1942;**36**:17–18.

19 Canfield, L. M., Giuliano, A. R., Graver, E. J. Carotenoids, retinoids, and vitamin K in human milk. In Jensen, R. G., ed. *Handbook of Milk Composition.* San Diego, CA: Academic Press; 1995:693–705.

20 Food and Nutrition Board, Institute of Medicine. *Dietary Reference Intakes for Vitamin A, Vitamin K, Arsenic, Boron, Chromium, Copper, Iodine, Manganese, Molybdenum, Silicon, Vanadium and Zinc.* Washington, DC: National Academic Press; 2002.

21 Howard, L., Chu, R., Feman, S. *et al.* Vitamin A deficiency from long-term parenteral nutrition. *Ann. Intern. Med.* 1980;**93**:576–7.

22 Silvers, K. M., Sluis, K. B., Darlow, B. A. *et al.* Limiting light-induced lipid peroxidation and vitamin loss in infant parenteral nutrition by adding multivitamin preparations to intralipid. *Acta Paediatr.* 2001;**90**:242–9.

23 Shenai, J. P., Stahlman, M. T., Chytil, F. Vitamin A delivery from parenteral alimentation solution. *J. Pediatr.* 1981;**99**:661–3.

24 Gillis, J., Jones, G., Pencharz, P. Delivery of vitamins A, D, and E in total parenteral nutrition solutions. *J. Parenter. Enteral Nutr.* 1983;**7**:11–14.

25 Darlow, B. A., Graham, P. J. Vitamin A supplementation for preventing morbidity and mortality in very low birthweight infants (Cochrane Review). *The Cochrane Library.* Issue 2. Oxford, UK: Update Software; 2001.

26 Shenai, J. P., Kennedy, K. A., Chytil, F. *et al.* Clinical trial of vitamin A supplementation in infants susceptible to bronchopulmonary dysplasia. *J. Pediatr.* 1987;**111**:269–77.

27 Shenai, J. P., Rush, M. G., Stahlman, M. T. *et al.* Plasma retinol binding protein response to vitamin A administration in infants susceptible to bronchopulmonary dysplasia. *J. Pediatr.* 1990;**116**:607–14.

28 Pearson, E., Bose, C., Snidow, T. *et al.* Trial of vitamin A supplementation in very low birth weight infants at risk for bronchopulmonary dysplasia. *J. Pediatr.* 1992;**121**:420–7.

29 Shenai, J. P., Rush, M. G., Stahlman, M. T., Chytil, F. Vitamin A supplementation and bronchopulmonary dysplasia – revisited. *J. Pediatr.* 1992;**121**:399–401.

30 Robbins, S. T., Fletcher, A. B. Early vs. delayed vitamin A supplementation in very-low-birth-weight infants. *J. Parenter. Enteral Nutr.* 1993;**17**:220–5.

31 Rush, M. G., Shenai, J. P., Parker, R. A. *et al.* Intramuscular versus enteral vitamin A supplementation in very low birth weight neonates. *J. Pediatr.* 1994;**125**:458–62.

32 Schwartz, K. B., Cox, J. M., Clement, L. *et al.* Possible antioxidant effect of vitamin A supplementation in premature infants. *J. Pediatr. Gastroenterol. Nutr.* 1997;**25**:408–14.

33 Bental, R. Y., Cooper, P. A., Cummins, R. R. *et al.* Vitamin A therapy-effects on the incidence of bronchopulmonary dysplasia. *S. Afr. J. Food Sci. Nutr.* 1994;**6**:141–5.

34 Paragaroufalis, C., Cairis, M., Pantazatou, E. *et al.* A trial of vitamin A supplementation in infants susceptible to bronchopulmonary dysplasia. *Pediatr. Res.* 1988;**23**:518A.

35 Tyson, J. E., Wright, L. L., Oh, W. *et al.* Vitamin A supplementation for extremely-low-birth-weight infants. *N. Engl. J. Med.* 1999;**340**:1962–8.

36 Wardle, S. P., Hughes, A., Chen, S. *et al.* Randomized controlled trial of oral vitamin A supplementation in preterm infants to prevent chronic lung disease. *Arch. Dis. Child. Fetal Neonatal Ed.* 2001;**84**:F9-13.

37 Olson, J. A. Serum levels of vitamin A and carotenoids as reflectors of nutritional status. *J. Natl. Cancer. Inst.* 1984;**73**: 1439–44.

38 Meyer, K. A., Popper, H., Steigmann, F. *et al.* Comparison of vitamin A of liver biopsy specimens with plasma vitamin A in man. *Proc. Soc. Exp. Biol. Med.* 1942;**49**;589–91.

39 Montreewasuwat, N., Olson, J. A. Serum and liver concentrations of vitamin A in Thai fetuses as a function of gestational age. *Am. J. Clin. Nutr.* 1979;**32**:601–6.

40 Zachman, R. D., Samuels, D. P., Brand, J. M. *et al.* Use of the intramuscular relative dose response test to predict bronchopulmonary dysplasia in premature infants. *Am. J. Clin. Nutr.* 1996;**63**:123–9.

41 Agaoestina, T., Humphrey, J. H., Taylor, G. A. *et al.* Safety of one 52-μmol (50,000 IU) oral dose of vitamin A administered to neonates. *Bull. World Health Org.* 1994;**72**:859–68.

42 Robens, J. R. Teratogenic effects of hypervitaminosis A in the hamster and guinea pig. *Toxicol. Appl. Pharmacol.* 1970;**16**;88–94.

43 Geelan, J. C. A. Hypervitaminosis A-induced teratogenesis. *CRC Crit. Rev. Toxicol.* 1979;**6**:351–75.

44 Shenefelt, R. E. Morphogenesis of malformations in hamsters caused by retinoic acid: relation to dose and stage at treatment. *Teratology* 1972;**5**:103–18.

45 Rothman, K. J., Moore, L. L., Singer, M. R. *et al.* Teratogenicity of high vitamin A intake. *N. Engl. J. Med.* 1995;**333**: 1369–73.

46 Lammer, E. J., Chen, D. T., Hoar, R. M. *et al.* Retinoic acid embryopathy. *N. Engl. J. Med.* 1985;**313**:837–41.

47 Benke, P. J. The isotretinoin teratogen syndrome. *J. Am. Med. Assoc.* 1984;**251**:3267–9.

48 Lott, I. T., Bocian, M., Pribram, H. W. *et al.* Fetal hydrocephalus and ear anomalies associated with maternal use of isotretinoin. *J. Pediatr.* 1984;**105**:597–602.

49 Burton, G. W., Traber, G. W. Vitamin E: antioxidant activity, biokinetics and bioavailability. *Annu. Rev. Nutr.* 1990;**10**:357–82.

50 Dju, M. Y., Mason, K. I., Filer, L. I. Vitamin E (tocopherol) in human fetuses and placentae. *Etudes Neonatales* 1952;**1**:46–62.

51 Cruz, C. S., Wimberley, P. D., Johansen, K., Friis-Hansen, B. The effect of vitamin E on erythrocyte hemolysis and lipid peroxidation in newborn premature infants. *Acta Paediatr. Scand.* 1983;**72**:823–6.

52 Mino, M., Nishimo, H. Fetal and maternal relationship in serum vitamin E level. *J. Nutr. Sci. Vitaminol.* 1973;**19**:475–82.

53 Farrell, P. M. Vitamin E. In Shils, M., Young, V., ed. *Modern Nutrition in Health and Disease.* Philadelphia, PA: Lea & Febiger; 1988;340–54.

54 Farrell, P. M., Zachman, R. D., Gutcher, G. R. Fat soluble vitamins A, E, and K in the premature infant. In Tsang, R. C., ed. *Vitamin and Mineral Requirements in Preterm Infants.* New York, NY: Marcel Dekker; 1985;63–98.

55 Bieri, J. G., Farrell, P. M. Vitamin E. *Vitam. Horm.* 1976;**34**:31–75.

56 Farrell, P. M., Bieri, J. G., Fratantoni, J. F. *et al.* The occurrence and effects of human vitamin E deficiency: a study in patients with cystic fibrosis. *J. Clin. Invest.* 1977;**60**:233–41.

57 Losowky, M. S., Kelleher, J., Walker, B. E. Intake and absorption of tocopherol. *Ann. NY Acad. Sci.* 1972;**203**:212–22.

58 Bieri, J. G., Evarts, R. P. Effect of plasma lipid levels and obesity on tissue stores of α-tocopherol. *Proc. Soc. Exp. Biol. Med.* 1975;**149**:500–2.

59 Bieri, J. G. Kinetics of tissue α-tocopherol depletion and repletion. *Ann. NY Acad. Sci.* 1972;**203**:181–91.

60 Traber, M. G., Burton, G. W., Hughes, L. *et al.* Discrimination between forms of vitamin E by humans with and without genetic abnormalities of lipoprotein metabolism. *J. Lipid. Res.* 1992;**33**:1171–82.

61 Traber, M. G., Sokol, R. J., Kohlschutter, A. *et al.* Impaired discrimination between stereoisomers of α-tocopherol in patients with familial isolated vitamin E deficiency. *J. Lipid. Res.* 1993;**34**:201–10.

62 Traber, M. G. Determinants of plasma vitamin E concentrations. *Free Rad. Biol. Med.* 1994;**16**:229–39.

63 Arita, M., Sato, Y., Miyata, A. *et al.* Human alpha-tocopherol transfer protein: cDNA cloning, expression and chromosomal localization. *Biochem. J.* 1995;**306**:437–43.

64 Doerflinger, N., Linder, C., Puahchi, K. *et al.* Ataxia with vitamin E deficiency: refinement of genetic localization and analysis of linkage disequilibrium by using new markers in 14 families. *Am. J. Hum. Genet.* 1995;**56**:1116–24.

65 Sokol, R. J., Kayden, H. J., Bettis, D. B. *et al.* Isolated vitamin E deficiency in the absence of fat malabsorption – familial and sporadic cases: characterization and investigation of causes. *J. Lab. Clin. Med.* 1988;**111**:548–59.

66 Ben Hamida, C., Doerflilnger, N., Belal, S. *et al.* Localization of Friedreich ataxia phenotype with selective vitamin E deficiency to chromosome 8q by homozygosity mapping. *Nature Genet.* 1993;**5**:195–200.

67 Ben Hamida, M., Belal, S., Sirugo, G. *et al.* Friedreich's ataxia phenotype not linked to chromosome 9 and associated with selective autosomal recessive vitamin E deficiency in two inbred Tunisian families. *Neurology* 1993;**43**:2179–83.

68 Ouahchi, K., Arita, M., Kayden, H. *et al.* Ataxia with isolated vitamin E deficiency is caused by mutations in the α-tocopherol transfer protein. *Nature Genet.* 1995;**9**:141–5.

69 Lammi-Keefe, C. J. Vitamin D and E in human milk. In Jensen, R. G., ed. *Handbook of Milk Composition.* San Diego, CA: Academic Press; 1995:706–17.

70 Kobayaski, H., Kanno, C., Yamauchi, K. *et al.* Identification of alpha-, beta-, gamma-, and delta-tocopherols and their contents in human milk. *Biochim. Biophys. Acta.* 1975;**380**: 282–90.

71 Food and Nutrition Board, Institute of Medicine. *Dietary Reference Intakes for Vitamin C, Vitamin E, Selenium, and Carotinoids.* Washington, DC: National Academy Press; 2000:186–283.

72 Huijbers, W. A. R., Schrijver, J., Speek, A. J. *et al.* Persistent low plasma vitamin E levels in premature infants surviving respiratory distress syndrome. *Eur. J. Pediatr.* 1986;**145**: 170–1.

73 Gross, S. J., Gabriel, E. Vitamin E status in preterm infants fed human milk or infant formula. *J. Pediatr.* 1985;**106**:634–40.

74 Hittner, H. M., Speer, M. E., Rudolph, A. J. *et al.* Retrolental fibroplasia and vitamin E in the preterm infant – comparison of oral versus intramuscular administration. *Pediatrics* 1984;**73**:238–49.

75 Ronnholm, K. A. R., Dostalova, L., Simes, M. A. Vitamin E supplementation in very-low-birth-weight infants: Long-term follow-up at two different levels of vitamin E supplementation. *Am. J. Clin. Nutr.* 1989;**49**:121–6.

76 Friedman, C. A., Wender, D. F., Temple, D. M. *et al.* Serum alpha-tocopherol concentrations in preterm infants receiving less than 25 mg kg^{-1} day^{-1} alpha-tocopherol acetate supplements. *Dev. Pharmacol. Ther.* 1988;**11**:273–80.

77 Laro, M. R., Wojewardine, K., Wald, N. J. Is routine vitamin E administration justified in very low-birthweight infants? *Dev. Med. Child. Neurol.* 1990;**32**:442–50.

78 Farrell, P. M. Vitamin E deficiency in premature infants. *J. Pediatr.* 1979;**95**:869–72.

79 Banagale, R. C., Bray, J. J., Erenberg, A. P. Serum free tocopherol levels in premature infants (PI) receiving total parenteral nutrition (TPN). *Pediatr. Res.* 1981;**15**:492A.

80 Phillips, B., Franck, L. S., Greene, H. L. Vitamin E levels in premature infants during and after intravenous multivitamin supplementation. *Pediatrics* 1987;**80**:680–3.

81 Gutcher, G. R., Farrell, P. J. M. Early intravenous correction of vitamin E deficiency in premature infants. *J. Pediatr. Gastroenterol. Nutr.* 1985;**4**:604–9.

82 Greene, H. L., Hambridge, K. M., Schanler, R., Tsang, R. C. Guidelines for the use of vitamins, trace elements, calcium, magnesium, and phosphorus in infants and children receiving total parenteral nutrition: report of the Subcommittee on Pediatric Parenteral Nutrient Requirements from the Committee on Clinical Practice Issues of The American Society for Clinical Nutrition. *Am. J. Clin. Nutr.* 1988;**48**:1324–42.

83 American Academy of Pediatrics, Committee on Nutrition. *Nutritional Needs of Preterm Infant. Pediatric Nutrition Handbook.* 5th edn. AAP; 2003.

84 Oski, F. A., Barness, L. A. Vitamin E deficiency: a previously unrecognized cause of hemolytic anemia in the premature infant. *J. Pediatr.* 1967;**70**:211–20.

85 Horwitt, M. K., Bailey, P. Cerebellar pathology in an infant resembling chick nutritional encephalomalacia. *Arch. Neural Psychiatr.* 1959;**95**:869–72.

86 Ehrenkranz, R. A., Bonta, B. W., Ablow, R. C. *et al.* Amelioration of bronchopulmonary dysplasia after vitamin E administration: a preliminary report. *N. Engl. J. Med.* 1978;**229**: 564–9.

87 Johnson, L., Schaffer, D., Quinn, G. *et al.* Vitamin E supplementation and the retinopathy of prematurity. *Ann. NY Acad. Sci.* 1982;**393**:473–84.

88 Hittner, H. M., Godio, L. B., Rudolph, A. J. *et al.* Retrolental fibroplasia: efficacy of vitamin E in a double-blind clinical study of preterm infants. *N. Engl. J. Med.* 1981;**305**:1365–71.

89 Hittner, H. M., Godio, L. B., Speer, M. I. *et al.* Retrolental fibroplasia: Further clinical evidence and ultrastructural support for efficacy of vitamin E in the preterm infant. *Pediatrics* 1983;**71**:423–32.

90 Kretzer, F. L., Hittner, J. M., Johnson, A. T. *et al.* Vitamin E and retrolental fibroplasia: ultrastructural support of clinical efficacy. *Ann. NY Acad. Sci.* 1982;**393**:145–64.

91 Sokol, R. J. Vitamin E deficiency and neurologic disease. *Am. Rev. Nutr.* 1988;**8**:351–73.

92 Chiswick, M. L., Johnson, M., Woodhall, C. *et al.* Protective effect of vitamin E (dl-alpha-tocopherol) against intraventricular hemorrhage in premature babies. *Br. Med. J.* 1983;**287**: 81–4.

93 Speer, M. E., Blifeld, C., Rudolph, A. J. *et al.* Intraventricular hemorrhage and vitamin E in the very low-birth-weight infant: evidence of efficacy of early intramuscular vitamin E administration. *Pediatrics* 1984;**74**:1107–12.

94 Ehrenkranz, R. A., Ablow, R. C., Warshaw, J. B. Effect of vitamin E on the development of oxygen-induced lung injury in neonates. *Ann. NY Acad. Sci.* 1982;**393**:452–65.

95 Phelps, D. L., Rosenbaum, A. L., Isenberg, S. J. *et al.* Tocopherol efficacy and safety for preventing retinopathy of prematurity: a randomized, controlled, double-masked trial. *Pediatrics* 1987;**79**:489–500.

96 Bell, E. F. Prevention of bronchopulmonary dysplasia: vitamin E and other antioxidants. In Farrell, P. M., Tausing, L. M., ed.

Bronchopulmonary Dysplasia and Related Chronic Respiratory Disorders. Report of the Ninetieth Ross Conference on Pediatric Research. Columbus, OH: Ross Laboratories; 1986;77–82.

97 Gutcher, G. R., Raynor, W. J., Farrell, P. M. An evaluation of vitamin E status in premature infants. *Am. J. Clin. Nutr.* 1984;**40**:1078–89.

98 Slagle, T. A., Gross, S. J. Vitamin E. In Tsang, R. C., Nichols, B. L., ed. *Nutrition during Infancy*. Philadelphia, PA: Hanley & Belfus; 1988:277–88.

99 Greene, H. L., Moore, M. E. C., Phillips, B. *et al*. Evaluation of a pediatric multiple vitamin preparation for total parenteral nutrition. II. Blood levels of vitamins A, D, and E. *Pediatrics* 1986;**77**:539–47.

100 Bougle, D., Boutroy, M. J., Heng, J. *et al*. Plasma kinetics of parenteral tocopherol in premature infants. *Dev. Pharmacol. Ther.* 1986;**9**:310–16.

101 Knight, M. E., Roberts, R. J. Disposition of intravenously administered pharmacologic doses of vitamin E in newborn rabbits. *J. Pediatr.* 1986;**108**:145–50.

102 Balistreri, W. F., Farrell, M. K., Bove, K. E. Lessons from the E-ferol tragedy. *Pediatrics* 1986;**78**:503–6.

103 Melhorn, D. K., Gross, S. Vitamin E-dependent anemia in the premature infant. II. Relationships between gestational age and absorption of vitamin E. *Pediatrics* 1971;**79**:581–8.

104 Gutcher, G. R., Lax, A. M., Farrell, P. M. Tocopherol isomers in intravenous lipid emulsions and resultant plasma concentrations. *J. Parenter. Enteral Nutr.* 1984;**8**:269–73.

105 Farrell, P. M. Vitamin E. A comprehensive treatise. In Machlin, L. J., ed. *Human Health and Disease*. New York, NY: Marcel Dekker; 1980:519–620.

106 Gross, S., Melhorn, D. K. Vitamin E, red cell lipids and red cell stability in prematurity. *Ann. NY Acad. Sci.* 1972;**203**:141–62.

107 Owens, W. C., Owens, E. U. Retrolental fibroplasia in premature infants. *Am. J. Ophthalmol.* 1949;**32**:1631–7.

108 Taju, T. N. K., Langenberg, P., Bhutani, V., Quinn, G. E. Vitamin E prophylaxis to reduce retinopathy of prematurity: a reappraisal of published trials. *J. Pediatr.* 1997;**131**:844–50.

109 Milner, R. A., Watts, J. L., Paes, B., Zipursky, A. RLF in < 1500 gram neonates. Part of a randomized clinical trial of the effectiveness of vitamin E. In *Retinopathy of Prematurity Conference*. Columbus, OH: Ross Laboratories; 1981:703–16.

110 Finer, N. N., Schindler, R. F., Grant, G., Hill, G. B., Peters, K. L. Effect of intramuscular vitamin E on frequency and severity of retrolental fibroplasia. A controlled trial. *Lancet* 1982;**1**:1087–91.

111 Puklin, J. E., Simon, R. M., Ehrenkranz, R. A. Influence on retrolental fibroplasia of intramuscular vitamin E administration during respiratory distress syndrome. *Ophthalmology* 1982;**89**:96–103.

112 Saldanha, R. L., Cepeda, E. E., Poland, R. L. The effect of vitamin E prophylaxis on the incidence and severity of bronchopulmonary dysplasia. *J. Pediatr.* 1982;**101**:89–93.

113 Watts, J. L., Milner, R., Zipursky, A. *et al*. Failure of supplementation with vitamin E to prevent bronchopulmonary dysplasia in infants <1500 g birthweight. *Eur. Respir. J.* 1991;**4**:188–90.

114 Chiswick, M., Gladman, G., Sinba, S. *et al*. Vitamin E supplementation and periventricular hemorrhage in the newborn. *Am. J. Clin. Nutr.* 1991;**53**:370S–2S.

115 Fish, W. H., Cohen, M., Franzek, E. *et al*. Effect of intramuscular vitamin E on mortality and intracranial hemorrhage in neonates of 1,000 grams or less. *Pediatrics* 1990;**85**;578–84.

116 Farrell, P. M., Levine, S. L., Murphy, M. D. *et al*. Plasma tocopherol levels and tocopherol-lipid relationships in a normal population of children as compared with healthy adults. *Am. J. Clin. Nutr.* 1978;**31**:1720–6.

117 Horwitt, M. K., Harvey, C. C., Dahm, C. H. Jr *et al*. Relationship between tocopherol and serum lipid levels for determination of nutritional adequacy. *Ann. NY Acad. Sci.* 1972;**203**:223–6.

118 Sokol, R. J., Heubi, J. E., Iannacone, S. T. *et al*. Vitamin E deficiency with normal serum vitamin E concentrations in children with chronic cholestasis. *N. Engl. J. Med.* 1984;**310**:1209–12.

119 Van Zoeren-Grobben, D., Jacobs, N. J. M., Houdkamp, E. *et al*. Vitamin E status in preterm infants: assessment by plasma and erythrocyte vitamin E-lipid ratios and hemolysis tests. *J. Pediatr. Gastro. Nutr.* 1998;**26**:73–9.

120 Greer, F. R., Zachman, R. D. Neonatal vitamin metabolism. Fat soluble. In Cowett, R. M., ed. *Principles of Perinatal-Neonatal Metabolism*. New York, NY: Springer; 1998:943–75.

121 Suttie, J. W. Synthesis of vitamin K-dependent proteins. *FASEB J.* 1993;**7**:445–52.

122 Dowd, P., Ham, S. W., Naganathan, S., Hershline, R. The mechanism of action of vitamin K. *Ann. Rev. Nutr.* 1995;**15**:419–40.

123 Fujita, K., Kakuya, F., Ito, S. Vitamin K_1 and K_2 status and fecal flora in breast-fed and formula fed 1-month-old infants. *Eur. J. Pediatr.* 1993;**152**:852–5.

124 Greer, F. R., Mummah-Schendel, L. L., Marshall, S., Suttie, J. W. Vitamin K_1 (phylloquinone) and vitamin K_2 (menaquinone) status in newborn during the first week of life. *Pediatrics* 1988;**81**:137–40.

125 Kayata, S., Kindberg, C., Greer, F. R. *et al*. Vitamin K_1 and K_2 in infant human liver. *J. Pediatr. Gastroenterol. Nutr.* 1989;**8**:304–7.

126 Suttie, J. W. The importance of menaquinones in human nutrition. *Annu. Rev. Nutr.* 1995;**15**:399–417.

127 Pietersma-deBruyn, A. L. J. M., Van Haard, P. M. M. Vitamin K_1 in the newborn. *Clin. Chim. Acta.* 1985;**150**:95–101.

128 Shearer, M. J., Barkhan, P., Rahim, S. *et al*. Plasma vitamin K_1 in mothers and their newborn babies. *Lancet* 1982;**2**:460–3.

129 Mandelbrot, L., Guillaumont, M., Leclercq, M. *et al*. Placental transfer of vitamin K1 and its implication in fetal hemostasis. *Thromb. Haemost.* 1988;**60**:39–43.

130 Greer, F. R., Marshall, S. P., Severson, R. R. *et al*. A new mixed-micellar preparation for oral vitamin K prophylaxis. Comparisons with an intramuscular formulation in breast-fed infants. *Arch. Dis. Child.* 1998;**79**:300–5.

131 Blomstrand, R., Forsgren, L. Vitamin K_1 ^{3}H in man: its intestinal absorption and transport in the thoracic duct lymph. *Int. Z. Vitam. Forschung.* 1968;**38**:45–64.

132 Sann, L., Leclercq, M., Guillaumont, M. *et al.* Serum vitamin K_1 concentrations after oral administration of vitamin K_1 in low birth weight infants. *J. Pediatr.* 1985;**107**:608–11.

133 Thijssen, J. W., Drittij-Reijnders, M. J., Fischer, M. A. J. G. Phylloquinone and menaquinone-4 distribution in rats: synthesis rather than uptake determines menaquinone-4 organ concentrations. *J. Nutr.* 1996;**126**:537–43.

134 Hodges, S. J., Bejui, J., Leclercq, M. *et al.* Detection and measurement of vitamins K_1 and K_2 in human cortical and trabecular bone. *J. Bone Miner. Res.* 1993;**8**:1005–8.

135 Bjornsson, T. D., Meffin, P. G., Swezey, S. E. *et al.* Disposition and turnover of vitamin K_1 in man. In Suttie, J. W., ed. *Vitamin K Metabolism and Vitamin K-Dependent Proteins.* Baltimore, MD: University Park Press; 1980:328–32.

136 Bolisetty, S., Gupta, G. G., Salonikas, C., Naidoo, D. Vitamin K in preterm breastmilk with maternal supplementation. *Acta Paediatr.* 1998; **87**:960–2.

137 Greer, F. R., Marshall, S., Suttie, J. W. Improving the vitamin K status of breast-feeding infants with maternal vitamin K supplements. *Pediatrics* 1997;**99**:88–92.

138 Kumar, D., Greer, F. R., Super, D. M., Suttie, J. W., Moore, J. J. Vitamin K status of premature infants. Implications for current recommendations. *Pediatrics* 2001;**108**:1117–22.

139 Gray, O. P., Ackerman, A. Fraser, A. J. Intracranial hemorrhage and clotting defects in low-birth-weight infants. *Lancet* 1968;**1**:545–8.

140 Cole, V. A., Durbin, M., Olaffson, A. *et al.* Pathogenesis of intraventricular haemorrhage in newborn infants. *Arch. Dis. Child.* 1974;**49**:722–8.

141 Setzer, E. S., Webb, I. B., Wassenaar, J. W. *et al.* Platelet dysfunction and coagulopathy in intraventricular hemorrhage in the premature infant. *J. Pediatr.* 1982;**100**:599–605.

142 MacDonald, M. M., Johnson, M. L., Rumack, C. M. *et al.* Role of coagulopathy in newborn intracranial hemorrhage. *Pediatrics* 1984;**74**:26–32.

143 Beverly, D. W., Chance, G. W., Inwood, M. J., Shaus, M., O' Keefe, B. Intraventricular haemorrhage and haemostasis defects. *Arch. Dis. Child.* 1984;**59**:444–8.

144 Van de Bor, M., Van Bel, F., Lineman, R., Ruys, J. H. Perinatal factors and periventricular haemorrhage in preterm infants. *Am. J. Dis. Child.* 1986;**140**:1125–30.

145 Pomerance, J. J., Teal, J. G., Gogolok, J. F., Brown, S., Stewart, M. E. Maternally administered antenatal vitamin K_1: effect on neonatal prothrombin activity, partial thromboplastin time, and intraventricular hemorrhage. *Obstet. Gynecol.* 1987;**70**:235–41.

146 Morales, W. J., Angel, J. L., O' Brien, W. F., Knuppel, R. A., Marsalis, F. The use of antenatal vitamin K in the prevention of early neonatal intraventricular hemorrhage. *Am. J. Obstet. Gynecol.* 1988;**159**:774–9.

147 Kazzi, N. J., Ilagan, N. B., Liang, K. C. *et al.* Maternal administration of vitamin K does not improve coagulation profile of preterm infants. *Pediatrics* 1989;**84**:1045–50.

148 Committee on Nutrition American Academy of Pediatrics. Vitamin K compounds and their water-soluble analogues:

Use in therapy and prophylaxis in pediatrics. *Pediatrics* 1961;**28**:501–7.

149 Klebanoff, M. A., Read, J. S., Mills, J. L. *et al.* The risk of childhood cancer after neonatal exposure to vitamin K. *N. Engl. J. Med.* 1989;**329**:905–8.

150 Greer, F. R. Vitamin K deficiency and hemorrhage in infancy. *Clin. Perinatol.* 1995;**22**:759–78.

151 Andrew, M., Paes, B., Milner, R. *et al.* Development of the human coagulation system in the full-term infant. *Blood* 1987;**70**:165–72.

152 Andrew, M., Paes, B., Milner, R. *et al.* Development of the human coagulation system in the healthy premature infant. *Blood* 1988;**72**:1651–7.

153 Göbel, U., Sonnenschein-Kosenow, S., Petrich, C. *et al.* Vitamin K deficiency in the newborn. *Lancet* 1977;**2**:187–8.

154 Von Kries, R., Greer, F. P., Suttie, J. W. Assessment of vitamin K status of the newborn infant. *J. Pediatr. Gastroenterol. Nutr.* 1993;**16**:231–8.

155 Liska, D. J., Suttie, J. W. Location of gamma-carboxyglutamyl residues in partially carboxylated prothrombin preparations. *Biochemistry* 1988;**27**:8636–41.

156 Von Kries, R., Shearer, M. J., Widdershoven, J. *et al.* Desgamma-carboxyprothrombin (PIVKA-II) and plasma vitamin K_1 in newborns and their mothers. *Thromb. Haemost.* 1992;**68**:383–7.

157 Bovill, E. G., Soll, R. F., Lynch, M. *et al.* Vitamin K_1 metabolism and the production of descarboxyprothrombin and protein C in the term and premature neonate. *Blood* 1993;**81**: 77–83.

158 Motahara, K., Endo, F., Matsuda, I. Effect of vitamin K administration on carboxyprothrombin (PIVKA-II) levels in newborns. *Lancet* 1985;**2**:242–4.

159 Motohara, K., Takayi, S., Endo, F. *et al.* Oral supplementation of vitamin K for pregnant women and effects on levels of plasma vitamin K and PIVKA-II in the neonate. *J. Pediatr. Gastroenterol. Nutr.* 1990;**11**:32–6.

160 Greer, F. R., Costakos, D. T., Suttie, J. W. Determination of desgamma-carboxy-prothrombin (PIVKA II) in cord blood of various gestational ages with the STAGO antibody – a marker of vitamin K deficiency? *Pediatr. Res.* 1999;**45**:283A.

161 Widdershoven, J., Lambert, W., Motohara, K. *et al.* Plasma concentrations of vitamin K1 and PIVKA-II in bottle-fed and breast-fed infants with and without vitamin K prophylaxis at birth. *Eur. J. Pediatr.* 1988;**148**:139–42.

162 Cornelissen, E., Kollée, L., DeAbreu, R. *et al.* Effects of oral and intramuscular vitamin K prophylaxis on vitamin K_1, PIVKA-II and clotting factors in breast-fed infants. *Arch. Dis. Child.* 1992;**67**:1250–4.

163 Cornelissen, E., Kollée L., DeAbreu, R. *et al.* Prevention of vitamin K deficiency in infancy by weekly administration of vitamin K. *Acta Pediatr.* 1983;**82**:656–9.

164 Cornelissen, E., Kollée, L., van Lith, T. *et al.* Evaluation of a daily dose of 25 mg vitamin K_1 to prevent vitamin K deficiency in breast-fed infants. *J. Pediatr. Gastroenterol. Nutr.* 1993;**16**: 301–5.

165 Moran, J. R., Greene, H. L. The B vitamins and vitamin C in human nutrition I. General considerations and "obligatory" B vitamins. *Am. J. Dis. Child.* 1979;**133**:192–9.

166 Rindi, G., Ventura, U. Thiamine intestinal transport. *Physiol. Rev.* 1972;**52**:821–7.

167 Gubler, C. J. Thiamine. In Machlin, L. J., ed. *Handbook of Vitamins*. New York City, NY: Marcel Dekker; 1991:233–82.

168 Davis, R. E., Icke, G. C. Clinical chemistry of thiamine. *Adv. Clin. Chem.* 1983;**23**:93–140.

169 Link, G., Zempleni, J., Bitsch, I. The intrauterine turnover of thiamin in preterm and full-term infants. *Int. J. Vit. Nutr. Res.* 1998;**68**:242–8.

170 Picciano, M. F. Breastfeeding 2001, Part I. Representative values for constituents of human milk. *Pediatr. Clin. N. Am.* 2001;**48**:263–4.

171 American Academy of Pediatrics. Vitamins. *Pediatric Nutrition Handbook*. 5th Edn. AAP; 2003.

172 Food and Nutrition Board, Institute of Medicine. Dietary reference intakes for thiamin, riboflavin, niacin, vitamin B6, folate, vitamin B12, pantothenic acid, biotin, and choline. Washington, DC: National Academy Press; 2000.

173 Greene, H. L., Porcelli, P., Adcock, E., Swift, L. Vitamins for newborn infant formulas: a review of recommendations with emphasis on data from low-birth-weight infants. *Eur. J. Clin. Nutr.* 1992;**46**:S1–8.

174 Friel, J. K., Bessie, J. C., Belkhode, S. L. *et al*. Thiamine, riboflavin, pyridoxine, and vitamin C status in premature infants receiving parenteral and enteral nutrition. *J. Parenter. Gastroenterol. Nutr.* 2001;**33**:64–9.

175 Rascoff, H. Beriberi heart in a 4 month old infant. *J. Am. Med. Assoc.* 1942;**120**:1292–3.

176 Sauberlich, H. E. Biochemical alterations in thiamine deficiency: their interpretation. *Am. J. Clin. Nutr.* 1967;**20**:528–46.

177 Moran, J. R., Greene, H. L. Nutritional biochemistry of water-soluble vitamins. In Grand, R. J., Sutphen, J. L., Dietz, W. H. Jr, eds. *Pediatric Nutrition, Theory and Practice*. Boston, MA: Butterworths; 1987:51–67.

178 Zempleni, J., Link, G., Bitsch, I. Intrauterine vitamin B$_2$ uptake of preterm and full-term infants. *Pediatr. Res.* 1995;**38**:585–91.

179 Porcelli, P. J., Rosser, M. L., DelPaggio, D. *et al*. Plasma and urine riboflavin during riboflavin-free nutrition in very-low-birth-weight infants. *J. Parenter. Gastroenterol. Nutr.* 2001;**31**:142–8.

180 Lucas, A., Bates, C. J. Occurrence and significance of riboflavin deficiency in preterm infants. *Biol. Neonate*. 1987;**52**:113–18.

181 Ramos, J. L. A., Barretto, O. C., Nonoyama, K. Vitamin dependent erythrocyte enzymes in newborns in relation to gestational age and birth weight. *J. Perinat. Med.* 1996;**24**:221–5.

182 Wilson, R. G., Davis, R. E. Clinical chemistry of vitamin B6. *Adv. Clin. Chem.* 1983;**23**:1–68.

183 Contractor, S. F., Shane, B. Blood and urine levels of vitamin B$_6$ in the mother and fetus before and after loading of the mother with vitamin B$_6$. *Am. J. Obstet. Gynecol.* 1970;**107**:635–40.

184 Porcelli, P. J., Adcock, E. W., DelPaggio, D. *et al*. Plasma and urine riboflavin and pyridoxine concentrations in enterally fed very-low-birth-weight-neonates. *J. Parenter. Gastroenterol. Nutr.* 1996;**23**:141–6.

185 Bessey, O. A., Adam, D. J. D., Hansen, A. E. Intake of vitamin B$_6$ and infantile convulsions: a first approximation of requirements of pyridoxine in infants. *Pediatrics* 1957;**20**:33–44.

186 Molony, C. J., Parmelee, A. H. Convulsions in young infants as a result of pyridoxine (vitamin B$_6$) deficiency. *J. Am. Med. Assoc.* 1954;**154**:405–6.

187 Bartlett, K. Vitamin-responsive inborn errors of metabolism. *Adv. Clin. Chem.* 1986;**23**:141–98.

188 Ubbink, J. B., Schnell, A. M. Assay of erythrocyte enzyme activity levels involved in vitamin B6 metabolism by high-performance liquid chromatography. *J. Chromatogr.* 1988;**431**:406–12.

189 Raiten, D. J., Reynolds, R. D., Andon, M. B. *et al*. Vitamin B-6 metabolism in premature infants. *Am. J. Clin. Nutr.* 1991;**53**:78–83.

190 Brewster, M. A. Vitamins. In Kaplan, L., Pesce, A., eds. *Clinical Chemistry*. St Louis, MO: C. V. Mosby Co; 1984:656–8.

191 Herbert, V. The 1986 Herman Award Lecture. Nutrition science as a continually unfolding story: The folate and vitamin B-12 paradigm. *Am. J. Clin. Nutr.* 1987;**46**:387–402.

192 Moore, M. C., Greene, H. L., Phillips, B. *et al*. Evaluation of a pediatric multiple vitamin preparation for total parenteral nutrition in infants and children: I. Blood level of water-soluble vitamins. *Pediatrics* 1986;**77**:530–8.

193 Monagle, P. T., Tauro, G. P. Infantile megaloblastosis secondary to maternal vitamin B$_{12}$ deficiency. *Clin. Lab. Haem.* 1997;**19**:23–5.

194 Graham, S. M., Arvela, O. M., Wise, G. A. Long-term neurologic consequences of nutritional vitamin B$_{12}$ deficiency in infants. *J. Pediatr.* 1992;**121**:710–4.

195 Davis, R. E. Clinical chemistry of folic acid. *Adv. Clin. Chem.* 1986;**25**:233–94.

196 Ek, J. Plasma and red cell folate values in newborn infants and their mothers in relation to gestational age. *J. Pediatr.* 1980;**97**:288–92.

197 Hoffbrand, A. V. Folate deficiency in premature infants. *Arch. Dis. Child.* 1970;**45**:441–4.

198 Ek, J. Folic acid and vitamin B$_{12}$ requirements in premature infants. In Tsang, R. C., ed. *Vitamin and Mineral Requirements in Preterm Infants*. New York, NY: Marcel Dekker; 1985:23–38.

199 Stevens, D., Burman, D., Strelling, K., Morris, A. Folic acid supplementation in low birth weight infants. *Pediatrics* 1979;**64**:333–5.

200 Ek, J., Behneke, L., Halvorsen, K. S., Magnus, E. Plasma and red cell folate values and folate requirements in formula-fed premature infants. *Eur. J. Pediatr.* 1984;**142**:78–82.

201 Mulinare, J., Cordero, J. F., Erickson, J. D., Berry, R. J. Periconceptional use of multivitamins and the occurrence of neural tube defects. *J. Am. Med. Assoc.* 1988;**260**:3141–5.

202 Sauberlich, H. E., Skala, J. H., Dowdy, R. P. *Laboratory Tests for the Assessment of Nutritional Status*. Cleveland, OH: CRC Press; 1974.

203 Roth, K. S. Biotin in clinical medicine – a review. *Am. J. Clin. Nutr.* 1981;**34**:1967–74.

204 Wolf, B., Heard, G. S., Weissbecker, K. A. *et al*. Biotinidase deficiency: initial clinical features and rapid diagnosis. *Ann. Neurol.* 1985;**18**:614–17.

205 Mock, D. M., DeLorimer, A. A., Liebman, W. M. *et al*. Biotin deficiency: an unusual complication of parenteral alimentation. *N. Engl. J. Med.* 1981;**304**;820–3.

206 Fox, H. M. Pantothenic acid. In Machlin, L. J., ed. *Handbook of Vitamins*. New York, NY: Marcel Dekker; 1984:437–58.

207 Gross, S. J. Choline, pantothenic acid, and biotin. In Tsang, R. C., ed. *Vitamin and Mineral Requirements in Preterm Infants*. New York, NY: Marcel Dekker; 1985:191–201.

208 Olson, J. A., Hodges, R. E. Recommended dietary intakes (RDI) of vitamin C in humans. *Am. J. Clin. Nutr.* 1987;**45**:693–703.

209 Kallner, A., Hartmann, D., Hornig, D. On the absorption of ascorbic acid in man. *Int. J. Vitam. Nutr. Res.* 1977;**47**:383–8.

210 Ingalls, T. H. Ascorbic acid requirements in early infancy. *N. Engl. J. Med.* 1938;**218**:872–5.

211 Irwin, M. I., Hutchins, B. K. A conspectus of research on vitamin C requirements of man (2). *J. Nutr.* 1976;**106**:823–79.

212 Light, I. J., Berry, H. K., Sutherland, J. M. Aminoacidemia of prematurity. *Am. J. Dis. Child.* 1966;**112**:229–36.

15

Normal bone and mineral physiology and metabolism

Oussama Itani[1] and Reginald Tsang[2]

[1] Michigan State University and Kalamazoo Center for Medical Studies, and Borgess Medical Center, Kalamazoo, MI
[2] Department of Pediatrics, Children's Hospital Medical Center, Cincinnati, OH

Introduction

Perinatal calcium (Ca), phosphorus (P), and magnesium (Mg) metabolism involves an intricate and complex biological system of interrelated hormones and growth factors that regulate the concentrations of these minerals in the tissues of the mother, fetus, and neonate. Mineral metabolism depends on the availability of mineral substrates and interactions with hormones and growth factors including parathyroid hormone (PTH), calcitonin (CT), 1,25 dihydroxyvitamin D (1,25(OH)2D), insulin-like growth factors (IGFs) and possibly leptins. Understanding of the perinatal physiology of these minerals is important in the prevention and management of mineral disorders in the neonate.[1-6]

In this chapter we review the perinatal physiology of Ca, P, and Mg metabolism in the fetus and neonate and offer a practical approach to the pathophysiology and management of Ca, P, and Mg disorders. We also review the current nutritional requirements of these minerals for enteral as well as parenteral nutrition. Finally, we review normal bone physiology, and discuss the pathophysiology, prevention, and management of metabolic bone disease or rickets/ osteopenia of prematurity.

Mineral, vitamin D and bone physiology

Body mineral content

Calcium is the fifth most abundant inorganic element in the human body. The adult human body contains about 1200 g of calcium (19 g of Ca per kg body weight). The total body Ca content in a full-term newborn is approximately 28 g, almost all of which (99%) resides in bone (8 g of Ca per kg body weight) where it serves structural and metabolic functions. The remainder resides in body fluids and serves a crucial role in a multitude of physiologic processes involving muscular contraction, neurotransmission, membrane transport, enzyme reactions, hormone secretion, and blood coagulation.[1,3-5,7-9]

Total body phosphorus (P) in the term newborn infant is 16 g (4.5 g of P per kg body weight), 80% of which is concentrated in the hydroxyapatite microcrystalline lattice of bone, 9% in the skeletal muscle and the remainder in the viscera and extracellular fluid. Normally, calcium and phosphorus are deposited in bone in a Ca/P ratio of 2:1.[7,8] Most of the body's Ca and P (80%) are acquired during the last trimester of pregnancy at a rate of 150 mg Ca per kg fetal weight day^{-1} (Figure 15.1) and 75 mg P per kg of fetal weight day^{-1} (Figure 15.2).

Magnesium is the fourth most abundant cation and the second most abundant intracellular cation (next to potassium) within the body. Total body Mg content in the newborn amounts to 0.8 g (0.22 g of Mg/kg body weight), most of which (50 to 60%) is concentrated in bone tissue, not as an integral component, but on the surface of the hydroxyapatite lattice, 30 to 40% in the intracellular space and 1% in the extracellular fluid compartment. About 80% of Mg is acquired during the last trimester of pregnancy at a rate of 3 mg/kg of fetal weight/day (Figure 15.3).[8] About 20% of total body Mg is concentrated in muscle and another 20% is in the intracellular compartment of blood cells and other body tissues. Changes in total body Mg content are largely reflected in changes in skeletal Mg and to a lesser extent in serum Mg concentrations. Magnesium has a significant regulatory role in a multitude of biologic processes

Neonatal Nutrition and Metabolism. Second Edition, ed. P. Thureen and W. Hay. Published by Cambridge University Press.
© Cambridge University Press 2006.

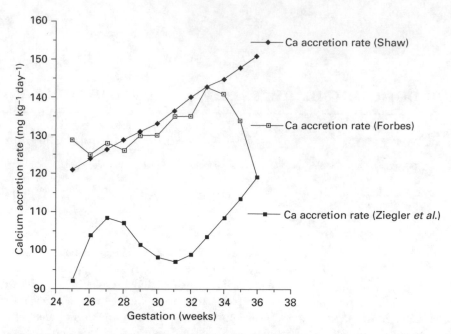

Figure 15.1. Calcium accretion in the human fetus during the latter half of gestation. In general, the rate of calcium accretion in the fetus increases with gestation, most remarkably in the third trimester. Data adapted.[9–11]

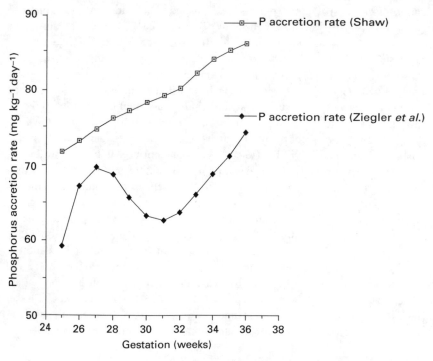

Figure 15.2. Phosphorus accretion in the human fetus during the latter half of gestation. In general, the rate of phosphorus accretion in the fetus increases with gestation, most remarkably in the third trimester. Data adapted.[10,11]

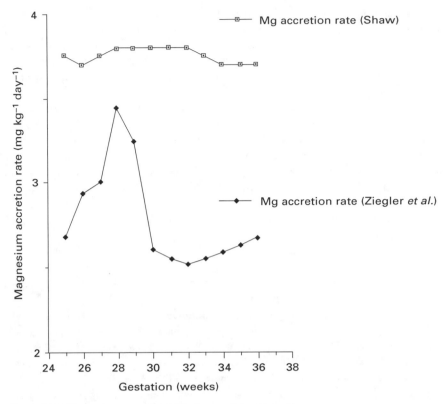

Figure 15.3. Magnesium accretion in the human fetus during the latter half of gestation. Data adapted.[10,11]

involved in storage, transfer, and production of energy. Further, Mg plays a significant role in calcium and bone homeostasis. Mg cations may contribute to the control of the onset of bone matrix and osteoid matrix vesicle-induced mineralization.[13,14]

Serum mineral concentrations

Less than 1% of the total body content of each of calcium, phosphorus, and magnesium is in the circulation. In the circulation, calcium exists in three forms: 50% of total serum calcium is the biologically active ionized calcium, 40% is protein-bound mainly to albumin, and 10% is complexed to anions (phosphate, lactate, citrate).[4] Total serum calcium concentration is accurately assayed by atomic absorption spectrophotometry. However, determination of serum ionized calcium (iCa) concentration is more desirable because it is a better physiologic indicator of Ca homeostasis. Serum ionized calcium concentrations in term 1-day-old infants range from 4.3 – 5.4 mg dL^{-1}.[15] In the term newborn, cord blood total Ca concentration is 10.2 mg^{-1}dL^{-1} and iCa concentration is 5.8 mg dL^{-1}. By 24–36 hours serum Ca decreases

to a nadir of 9 mg dL^{-1}, and serum iCa drops to a nadir of 4.9 mg dL^{-1}. Thereafter, a gradual rise in serum Ca and iCa concentrations occurs and by one week of life reach relatively stable values throughout life.[16] In the preterm newborn, mean cord serum iCa ranges from 5.74–5.86 mg dL^{-1}. After a drop during the first 24 36 hours of life, serum iCa rises to stable values by the end of the first week of life. Summer-born infants have lower serum total calcium than winter-born infants.[17] This may be due to a complex interaction of calciotropic hormones early in fetal life.

Serum phosphorus concentration is higher in children than in adults. It is relatively low at birth; then it rises shortly after birth to reach older newborn and infant values (8 mg dL^{-1}) by 1 week of age. Then it decreases from infancy (8 mg dL^{-1}) to childhood and adulthood (3.0–4.5 mg dL^{-1}).[18] Serum inorganic phosphorus exists in three forms: 55% is ionized (free phosphate ions), 10% is protein-bound, and 35% is complexed to sodium (Na), Ca, and Mg.

Total serum Mg concentration in infancy and early childhood is 1.5–2.8 mg dL^{-1}.[19] In the cord blood of term newborns, serum Mg concentration is 1.45–1.83 mg dL^{-1}.[20] Magnesium in the plasma exists in three forms: 55% is ionized (free Mg ions), 30% is protein-bound, and 15%

is complexed to anions (phosphate, oxalate).[21] Ionized Mg is the fraction that is important for biochemical processes. Because Mg is predominantly an intracellular cation, serum Mg concentrations as determined by atomic absorption spectrophotometry may not reflect total body Mg content. Mononuclear blood cell Mg might be a better predictor of intracellular Mg and total body Mg status than the concentration of Mg in plasma or erythrocytes.[22] Normally, Mg exchange occurs between the extracellular fluid compartment and bone in response to changes in serum Mg concentration.[23] About one third of bone Mg content is on the surface of hydroxyapatite crystals and may be freely available for exchange. Magnesium homeostasis is only partly understood. It does not appear to be primarily controlled through hormonal mechanisms, and plasma concentrations seem to be predominantly under renal control.[24]

Bone physiology

Bone structure

The skeletal system is a dynamic organ that serves two interdependent roles: provision of support and maintenance of mineral homeostasis.[4,25] Both functions are successfully achieved by continuous bone remodeling. Any disturbances in the balance and nature of bone formation and resorption produce a variety of bone diseases. Dense cortical bone provides strength needed for structural support, and the spicules of trabecular bone provide a large surface area for bone synthesis and resorption and provide a reservoir of minerals for the maintenance of mineral homeostasis.

Bone contains three major types of mature cells, osteoblasts, osteocytes, and osteoclasts.[25,26] Osteoblasts,[27,28] found along surfaces of both cortical and trabecular bone, synthesize bone matrix. The plasma membrane of the osteoblast is very rich in alkaline phosphatase, the activity of which is an index of bone formation. Osteoblasts have receptors for PTH, $1,25(OH)^2D$ and estrogen but not for calcitonin. Stimulation by PTH, $1,25(OH)^2D$, growth hormone, and estrogen cause osteoblasts to produce insulin-like growth factor I (IGF-I), which has a significant role in local bone regulation and modeling. IGF is an essential autocrine factor that increases the rate of cell division and plays a critical role in normal postnatal skeletal growth. Mutations in the growth hormone receptor results in Laron dwarfism, which is characterized by very low serum IGF-I concentrations.[29,30]

As osteoblasts become embedded in bone matrix, they differentiate into mature osteocytes. Osteocytes synthesize small amounts of matrix continuously to maintain bone integrity, and they are able to resorb bone (osteocytic osteolysis) in exceptional circumstances when normal mineral homeostasis is altered. Regulation of osteoblast differentiation is mediated and orchestrated by local factors such as bone morphogenetic proteins (BMPs) and hedgehogs and the transcription factor, core-binding factor alpha-1 (Cbfa1).[31] BMPs are the most potent regulators of osteoblast differentiation among the local factors. BMPs induce the differentiation of mesenchymal cells toward cells of the osteoblastic lineage and enhance the differentiated function of the osteoblast. The activity of BMPs is tempered by intracellular and extracellular antagonists.[28] BMPs are important to up-regulate Cbfa1 expression. They also interact with Sonic and Indian hedgehogs. Cbfa1, a member of the runt domain gene family, plays a major role in the processes of determination of osteoblast cell lineage and maturation of osteoblasts, and is an essential transcription factor for osteoblast differentiation and bone formation.

Osteoclasts[32,33] contain enzymes that demineralize and digest bone matrix. Osteoclastic bone resorption occurs at a special part of the osteoclast cell membrane, "the ruffled border," which comprises a sealed lysosomal compartment. Because of their acidic pH, lysosomes dissolve bone crystals, and their proteolytic enzymes digest bone matrix. Although bone resorption is primarily affected by the osteoclast, other cells influenced by bone-resorbing hormones can direct the osteoclasts. Both osteoblasts and osteoclasts have receptors for bone-resorbing hormones and appear to play a significant role in bone resorption.

Only a small portion of bone is cellular; calcified matrix predominates. This matrix is primarily composed of collagen fibers (mostly type I), a glycosaminoglycans-containing ground substance, and noncollagenous proteins. Type I collagen is the major collagen produced by osteoblasts and represents more than 90% by weight of the nonmineral component of bone. Osteocalcin is the major component of bone's noncollagen proteins (see below). Although most bone proteins are synthesized by osteoblasts, some proteins, such as $alpha_2$-HS- glycoprotein, are produced by the liver and absorbed by bone matrix. Spindle-shaped hydroxyapatite, $Ca_{10}(PO_4)_6(OH)_2$, crystals are present in the ground substance and aligned on and within collagen fibers. Glycosaminoglycans are highly anionic complexes that may play a major role in the calcification process and the fixation of hydroxyapatite crystals to collagen fibers. Approximately one-fourth of the amino acids present in collagen are either proline or hydroxyproline, neither of which is present to any great extent in other tissues. When collagen is metabolized, hydroxyproline-containing oligopeptides are excreted in the urine, and the amount present correlates with the amount of bone turnover. The mineral elements of bone consist mostly of crystals of calcium and phosphate arranged either amorphously or as hydroxyapatite. A wide range of other elements may be present, including sodium, magnesium, copper, zinc, lead, and fluoride.

The growth plate is the final target organ for longitudinal growth and results from chondrocyte proliferation and differentiation. During the first year of life, longitudinal growth rates are high, followed by a decade of modest longitudinal growth. The age at onset of puberty and the growth rate during the pubertal growth spurt (which occurs under the influence of estrogens and GH) contribute to sex difference in final height between boys and girls. At the end of puberty, growth plates fuse, thereby ceasing longitudinal growth. Receptors for many hormones such as estrogen, GH, and glucocorticoids are present in or on growth plate chondrocytes, suggesting that these hormones may influence processes in the growth plate directly. Growth factors and cytokines such as IGF-I, Indian hedgehog, PTH related peptide (PTHrP), fibroblast growth factors, bone morphogenetic proteins, and vascular endothelial growth factor, may have crucial regulatory roles of chondrocyte proliferation and differentiation.[34]

Both osteoblasts and osteoclasts have receptors for estrogen which is the key hormone for maintaining bone mass.[35] Both sex steroids, estrogen and testosterone, are important for developing peak bone mass, but estrogen deficiency is the major determinant of age-related bone loss in both sexes. Together with GH and IGF-I, sex steroids initiate a 3- to 4-year pubertal growth spurt that doubles skeletal mass. Although estrogen is required for the attainment of maximal peak bone mass in both sexes, the additional action of testosterone on stimulating periosteal apposition accounts for the larger size and thicker cortices of the adult male skeleton.

Biomechanics and bone

Frost[36] proposed the mechanostat/mechanical loading model of postnatal bone formation, which states that the primary factor in the development of bone strength is the load (force) placed on the bone. The load causes a strain on the bone, which is transmitted to the mechanostat as an input signal. The mechanostat is a sensor within bone that can evaluate the input of strain from a given load placed on bone and then direct an appropriate output to the effector cells, osteoblasts, and osteoclasts. Strain is the proportional change in length caused by a load and can be from compression, tension, or shearing loads.

The mechanostat functions as a feedback or regulatory system to keep bone strength commensurate with the loads placed on bone. The mechanostat processes the strain input and compares it with preset, threshold levels of strain for increasing bone strength or decreasing bone strength. The mechanostat generates appropriate output signals to effector cells to bring about the needed change in bone strength to align the strain within given limits. Effector cells are osteoblasts that produce bone and osteoclasts that resorb bone. Excessive loads that exceed the threshold for increasing bone strength trigger the mechanostat to signal the effector cells to increase bone strength. If significantly decreased loads that exceed the threshold for decreasing bone strength are placed on a bone, then the mechanostat signals the effector cells to decrease bone strength. If the strain does not exceed either of these thresholds, then the effector cells operate at a status quo, or baseline, level of activity. Osteoblast and osteoclast activity can change bone strength through either altering bone density or altering bone architecture through two distinctly different processes of bone physiology: bone modeling and bone remodeling. Both modeling and remodeling are processes that respond to bone loading through the mechanostat.[36–38]

Modeling is the process by which bone is sculpted to the most advantageous geometry, both for bone strength and for appropriate attachment of muscles and tendons. As bone grows, some bone must be added to certain surfaces and some bone must be removed from other surfaces. The bone achieves this result through formation drifts and resorption drifts. Formation drifts influence osteoblasts to build up some bone surfaces, whereas resorption drifts influence osteoclasts to remove bone from some bone surfaces. Modeling results in changes of bone size or shape or both and thus is a prominent process in bone development during fetal life and in childhood. In bone modeling, osteoblasts and osteoclasts function independent of each other, and each cell type responds to a certain preset modeling threshold within the mechanostat. Modeling almost always increases bone strength either by increasing bone mass or by favorably altering bone architecture. Remodeling is the process whereby fatigued bone is efficiently removed and then replaced by new, intact bone by the sequential activity of osteoclasts to resorb the fatigued bone followed by osteoblasts to produce new bone. In bone remodeling, osteoblasts and osteoclasts act cooperatively in a coupled manner in a unit called a basic multicellular unit. This coordinated activity is also realized when a certain preset threshold of strain is sensed by the mechanostat.

There are two types of bone loading. The first is associated with the direct contact or impact of bone against another object, such as the increased load that the leg bones realize during running, or from the resistance that a bone might experience such as the extremities realize in swimming. The second is associated with the active and passive load that the bone senses from the muscles attached to it. The muscles that attach to a bone exert a small but continuing load on the bone even when the muscle is not actively moving the bone. The loading of the skeletal system from attached muscles is critical in maintaining bone density. Weightlifters have greater bone density than nonweightlifters.[39] Children with chronic, neuromuscular diseases associated with muscle paralysis and muscle weakness, have osteopenia and an increased risk for fracture.[40]

Frost's model of bone development the "Utah paradigm," includes nutritional, hormonal, cellular, biochemical, and biomechanical factors.[37] Through the mechanostat regulatory activity, bone strives to have optimal density. Rauch[41,42] proposed a functional model of bone development in which the genome only provides positional information for the basic outline of the skeleton as a cartilaginous template. Thereafter, bone cell action is coordinated by the mechanical requirements of the bone. When mechanical challenges exceed an acceptable level (the mechanostat set point), bone tissue is added at the location where it is mechanically necessary. The main mechanical challenges during growth result from increases in bone length and in muscle force. Hormones, nutrition, and environmental factors exert an effect on bone either directly by modifying the mechanostat system or indirectly by influencing longitudinal bone growth or muscle force. Predictions based on this model are in accordance with observations on prenatal, early postnatal, and pubertal bone development.

Bones are formed in two distinct steps.[37] The first step is the embryogenesis of the skeletal system. Between 5 and 12 weeks of gestation, multiple, specific genes direct condensations of mesenchyme to specific anatomic locations that are destined to become the precursor tissues of bone that will eventually chondrify and ossify.[43] In a similar period during the first trimester, other specific genes direct ventral and dorsal condensations of somitic mesoderm to become precursor tissues of skeletal muscle, and these will eventually attach to their appropriate bones. By 16 weeks of gestation, the anatomy, anatomical relationships, and biologic machinery for adaptation of bones are in place. This state of bone is called the baseline condition.

The second step of bone formation, beginning during the midportion of the second trimester, is the state of responsiveness of the skeletal system to genetically defined bone proteins and humoral mediators, nutrient considerations, and mechanical factors. Long bones grow both in length and in diameter. Linear bone growth of the long

bones is determined primarily by specific genes through enchondral ossification. However, long bones assume their final, normal geometry, through the process of modeling, which uses osteoblasts to form bone and osteoclasts to remove bone. Diametrical bone growth of long bones occurs through modeling in which osteoclasts remove bone from the endosteum and osteoblasts form bone along the periosteum. Flat bones, such as the scapula, pelvis, and skull, grow through intramembranous bone formation. Modeling that is responsive to bone loading occurs in enchondral and intramembranous bone formation in both the prenatal and postnatal periods. During the second and third trimesters, bone modeling also responds to increasing muscle forces. As the skeletal system ages, the adaptations for any given bone, which include growth, modeling, and remodeling, are added to the baseline conditions of the bone.

At the same time that bone modeling begins, fetal movement commences at approximately week 16 of gestation. Bone modeling is strongly influenced by bone loading, which in turn is determined primarily by fetal movement. Bone strength, density, and architecture are directly related to fetal movement. Diminished fetal movement results in decreased bone strength of the fetus and newborn through changes in bone density and bone architecture. This paradigm is supported by the following observations: (1) Infants with congenital neuromuscular disease in which there is both decreased fetal movement and decreased fetal muscle mass and function have osteopenia and decreased cortical bone thickness of long bones, suggesting diminished subperiosteal bone formation in infants with prenatal-onset neuromuscular disease.[44,45] (2) In an experimental rat model, fetuses paralyzed during the last trimester were found to have short umbilical cords and osteopenia at birth.[46] (3) Diminished fetal movement and intrauterine confinement have been put forth as the underlying basis of temporary brittle bone disease.[38,47,48] This observation has led to the suggestion that prenatal bone loading in the form of fetal movement can influence postnatal bone strength during the first year of life and that infants who had significantly decreased fetal movement may be at risk for incurring fractures with physical forces that might not ordinarily cause a fracture, especially in the first 4 months of life.

The fetus has a functioning musculoskeletal system by 16 weeks of gestation. Genetic, hormonal, nutritional, and biomechanical factors influence bone physiology after 16 weeks of gestation and into postnatal existence. Miller[38] suggests that biomechanical factors have a critical role in determining ultimate bone strength. The extent of in utero bone loading will determine the ultimate skeletal strength of the fetus, especially during the last trimester, when there is rapid bone growth and bone mineralization. Fetal movement in the third trimester is the critical event that endows the newborn infant with normal bone loading and, thus, normal skeletal strength. The term infant who has an intact neuromuscular system realizes the full influence of this fetal movement on bone formation. The intrauterine loading of the fetal musculoskeletal system through fetal movement activates the mechanostat to increase bone strength through the process of modeling. Fetal movement also promotes muscle growth, which contributes to bone loading and thus also influences bone modeling. Extreme prematurity deprives the infant of much of this musculoskeletal bone loading in utero. After birth, the markedly preterm infant is often hypotonic and has decreased movements compared with the term infant.[49] Decreased bone loading in the VLBW, preterm infant theoretically will lead to a lower input strain to the mechanostat. Postnatal modulation of the mechanostat occurs to increase resorption and decrease bone formation. The markedly preterm, VLBW infant is, therefore, at a distinct biomechanical disadvantage in bone formation by losing weeks of meaningful intrauterine movement that promotes bone formation and replacing this period with that of an earlier-than-expected encounter with the extrauterine environment, which is probably less favorable for bone formation.

The pathophysiology of rib fractures associated with preterm birth is probably the same as that for long bone fractures. Bone loading of ribs probably can occur from the following: (1) fetal movement and kicking that likely is transmitted along the skeleton to the ribs; (2) active or passive breathing, which would provide some bone loading through the ribs expanding in inspiration and contracting in expiration; and (3) the muscles attached to the ribs, which indirectly would get stronger with active breathing but probably would not get stronger if breathing were assisted by mechanical ventilation. Rodriguez et al.[44] found that the periosteal diameter of the fifth rib in infants with prenatal-onset neuromuscular disease was significantly lower than that of control infants, which supports the concept that prenatal bone loading does influence rib strength.

Factors affecting fetal and neonatal bone mineral content

Changes in maternal bone during pregnancy may affect fetal bone mineralization. The biphasic changes in maternal bone histology (temporary loss of cancellous bone in early pregnancy restored by term gestation) are consistent with corresponding blood biochemistry changes; increased bone resorption markers in the first trimester, while bone formation markers are increased in the last

trimester. Postpartum bone mineral density (BMD) by dual-energy x-ray absorptiometry (DEXA) is increased at cortical bone and decreased at trabecular bone sites compared with prepregnancy values. The mean reduction of spine BMD is 3.5% from prepregnancy to immediate postpartum. Neonatal bone mineral content (BMC) is different by season of birth, low weight relative to gestation, and having a diabetic mother. Lower total body BMC and high bone resorption marker in winter v. summer-born newborns was related to low vitamin D, indicating alterations of fetal bone metabolism by maternal D deficiency. Maternal vitamin D deficiency may affect fetal bone mineralization. Korean winter-born newborn infants have lower serum 25-hydroxyvitamin D (25-OHD), increased bone resorption as indicated by high serum C-propeptide of Type 1 collagen (ICTP) and lower total body BMC than summer-born newborn infants.[50,51] Infant total body BMC was positively correlated with cord serum 25-OHD and inversely correlated with ICTP, which was also negatively correlated with vitamin D status. This is in contrast to studies of North American neonates, which showed lower BMC in summer newborn infants compared with winter newborn infants. The reason for conflicting BMC results might be the markedly different maternal vitamin D status of the North American and Korean women. Seasonal differences in bone markers have also been reported in adult women by Douglas.[52] Serum osteocalcin concentrations were lower in autumn than in spring while serum bone specific alkaline phosphatase concentration was higher in autumn than in spring.

There is evidence of decreased bone mineralization in small-for-gestational age (SGA) infants manifested by reduced BMC, cord serum osteocalcin and 1,25 (OH)2D, but no alterations in indices of fetal bone collagen metabolism. In theory, reduced utero-placental blood flow in SGA infants may result in reduced transplacental mineral supply and reduced fetal bone formation.[17] Bone mineral content is consistently increased with increasing body weight and length in infants. Race and gender differences in BMC appear in early life, but not at birth. Ethanol consumption and smoking by the mother during pregnancy affect fetal skeletal development.[50,51]

Regulation of postnatal longitudinal bone growth

Longitudinal bone growth is achieved by endochondral ossification, a complex, multi-step process whereby the cartilaginous template of the axial and appendicular skeleton is replaced by bone.[53] This process is initiated when chondrocytes at the epiphyseal growth plate are stimulated to proliferate and then proceed through stages of maturation and hypertrophy. In the region of cellular hypertrophy, the surrounding matrix and vascular tissue undergo calcification. The hypertrophic chondrocytes degenerate and give way to invading osteoblasts, and bone and bone marrow subsequently replace the calcified cartilage at the metaphysis.

This growth plate activity is subject to complex and intricate regulation by a number of factors, including genetic, endocrine, paracrine, or autocrine origin. These stimuli include various hormones such as growth hormone,[54] thyroid hormones (T3),[55] and parathyroid hormone/parathyroid hormone related peptide (PTH/ PTHrP),[56,57] as well as several growth factors and cytokines, such as IGF-I, basic fibroblast like growth factor, transforming growth factor Beta, and Indian hedgehog (Ihh). The two main stimulatory peptides contributing to longitudinal bone growth are growth hormone and IGF-I. Growth hormone directly promotes differentiation of chondrocyte progenitor cells, and indirectly increases the responsiveness of proliferative cells to the stimulatory effects of IGF-I. Ihh is a regulatory protein secreted by chondrocytes and has a key role in embryonic patterning. It promotes chondrocyte proliferation and activates a negative feedback loop mediated by PTHRrP.[57] Ihh and PTHrP target PTH/PTHrP receptor (PTHR/PTHrPR) expressing growth plate chondrocytes in a negative feedback loop to regulate the coordinated progression of chondrocyte maturation and hypertrophy.[58] Thyroxine plays a role in chondrocyte maturation by inducing the synthesis of Type-X collagen, an effect that is probably mediated by bone morphogenetic protein-2.[29] Mutations involving the genes encoding fibroblast growth factor receptors may be responsible for craniosynostosis syndromes.[58]

Bone mass

About 45% of the adult skeleton is built and enlarged during adolescence.[4,59] The concept of peak bone mass has become crucial in understanding osteoporosis, especially postmenopausal osteoporosis.[60] Peak bone mass is determined by several factors including genetics, nutrition, mechanics, and environment.[61] The genetic effect on adult bone mass may be mediated largely through effects on bone formation rather than through effects on resorption. There is a strong positive relationship between current and past calcium intake and the peak bone mass achieved.[62–65] Higher calcium intake during adolescence theoretically may optimize, within genetic limits, peak bone mass. Physical activity,[61] use of estrogenic oral contraceptives and dietary calcium intake exert a positive effect on bone gain in children and young adult women. Androgens and estrogen are important determinants of peak bone density in young women. The optimal dietary calcium intake for bone growth is a debatable issue. Calcium retention require-

ments for growth are as follows: an average of 100 mg day^{-1} must be retained during childhood, 220 mg day^{-1} during adolescence, and probably 20 to 30 mg day^{-1} during early adulthood from 20 to 30 years of age.[62]

Inherent to bone physiology is the process of "coupling" of the processes of bone formation and resorption.[25] Bone is a dynamic organ, which is constantly remodeling. "Remodeling" continues throughout life and requires a balance between bone formation and resorption. At any time approximately 10% of bone mass participates in bone remodeling. The processes of bone formation and resorption continue throughout life, but are more rapid during periods of skeletal growth. Childhood and adolescence are characterized by highly active bone remodeling. Infancy is the period of life with the highest linear growth velocity. It is associated with extensive bone remodeling. Growth is associated with predominance of bone formation over bone resorption, resulting in increased bone mass and bone deposition. In young adults, the processes of bone resorption and formation are equal. With aging, bone resorption exceeds bone formation thereby predisposing to net bone loss and osteoporosis. "Remodeling" determines the size and shape of a particular bone, and involves simultaneous widening of long bone and development of the medullary cavity by bone formation at the periosteal surface and resorption at the endosteal surface, respectively.

Determinants of bone health

Growth in bone size and strength occurs during childhood, but bone accumulation is not completed until the third decade of life, after the cessation of linear growth. The bone mass attained early in life is perhaps the most important determinant of life-long skeletal health.[4] Individuals with the highest peak bone mass after adolescence have the greatest protective advantage when the declines in bone density associated with increasing age, illness, and diminished sex-steroid production take their toll. Bone mass may be related not only to osteoporosis and fragility later in life but also to fractures in childhood and adolescence. Genetic factors exert a strong influence on peak bone mass, but physiological, environmental, and lifestyle factors[66] can also play a significant role. Among these are adequate nutrition and body weight, exposure to sex hormones at puberty, and physical activity. Thus, maximizing bone mass early in life presents a critical opportunity to reduce the impact of bone loss related to aging. Childhood is also a critical time for the development of lifestyle habits conducive to maintaining good bone health throughout life.

Cigarette smoking, which usually starts in adolescence, may have a deleterious effect on achieving bone mass as well as on the growing fetus.[67,68] Good nutrition is essential for normal bone growth and health. Supplementation of calcium and vitamin D may be necessary. Calcium is most important for attaining peak bone mass and for preventing and treating osteoporosis.[69] Although the Institute of Medicine recommends calcium intakes of 800 mg day^{-1} for children ages 3 to 8 and 1300 mg day^{-1} for children and adolescents ages 9 to 17, only about 25% of boys and 10% of girls ages 9 to 17 are estimated to meet these recommendations. Factors contributing to low calcium intakes are restriction of dairy products, insufficient fruit and vegetable consumption, and a high intake of low calcium beverages such as sodas. Wyshak[70,71] reported a positive relationship between cola beverage intake and bone fracture, and a protective effect of high calcium intake against bone fracture in adolescent boys and girls. For older adults, calcium intake should be maintained at 1000 to 1500 mg day^{-1}; yet only about 50%–60% of this population meets this recommendation.

Vitamin D is required for optimal calcium absorption and bone health. Most infants and young children in the US have adequate vitamin D intake because of supplementation and fortification of milk. During adolescence, when consumption of dairy products decreases, vitamin D intake is less likely to be adequate, and this may adversely affect calcium absorption. Vitamin D intake of 400–600 IU day^{-1} has been recommended for adults.

High dietary protein, caffeine, phosphorus, and sodium can adversely affect calcium balance, but their effects appear not to be important in individuals with adequate calcium intakes. Exercise and physical activity early in life contributes to higher peak bone mass.[61] Evidence indicates that resistance and high impact exercise are most beneficial in promoting bone formation.[72 74] There are few studies on the effects of exercise during the middle years of life on BMD. Exercise during the later years, in the presence of adequate calcium and vitamin D intake, probably has a modest effect on slowing the decline in BMD.

Gonadal steroids secreted during puberty increase BMD and peak bone mass.[75] Osteoblasts have receptors for estrogen.[76] Gonadal steroids influence skeletal health throughout life in both women and men.[77] In adolescents and young women, sustained production of estrogens is essential for the maintenance of bone mass. Reduction in estrogen production with menopause is the major cause of loss of BMD during later life. Timing of menarche, absent or infrequent menstrual cycles, and the timing of menopause influence both the attainment of peak bone mass and the preservation of BMD. Testosterone production in adolescent boys and men is similarly important in achieving and maintaining maximal bone mass. Estrogens have also been implicated in the growth and maturation of the male skeleton. Delayed onset of puberty is a risk factor for diminished bone mass in men, and hypogonadism in adult men results in osteoporosis. From recent clinical as well as molecular evidence there appears to be a synergistic anabolic effect of calcitriol and estriol on osteoblasts.[78] Combined treatment with estrogen and 1,25-dihydroxyvitamin D3 increases femoral neck bone mass density more than treatment with estrogen alone in postmenopausal osteoporotic women. The increase in cell viability of cultured human osteoblast-like cells caused by treatment with estriol was significantly augmented by combined treatment with calcitriol. Estriol may up-regulate the cell viability of osteoblast cells, and concomitant treatment of estriol and calcitriol further augments the cell viability associated with an estriol-induced increase in calcitriol receptor mRNA expression in those cells.[78]

Growth hormone and IGF-I, which are maximally secreted during puberty, play a role in acquisition and maintenance of bone mass and determination of body composition into adulthood.[54] Growth hormone deficiency is associated with a decrease in BMD. Children and youth with low body mass index (BMI) are likely to attain lower-than-average peak bone mass. Although there is a direct association between BMI and bone mass throughout the adult years, it is not known whether the association between body composition and bone mass is due to hormones, nutritional factors, higher impact during weight-bearing activities, or other factors. Observational studies of fractures in older persons show an inverse relationship between fracture rates and BMI. Metabolic acidosis increases urine calcium excretion without increase in calcium absorption, resulting in net loss of bone mineral density. The mechanism of bone demineralization is increased production of prostaglandins.[79]

Assessment of bone mineral content and bone density

Several groups of children and adolescents may be at risk for compromised bone health. Premature and low birth weight infants have lower-than-expected bone mass in the first few months of life, but long-term implications are unknown. Bone growth is related to protein and energy supply necessary for osteoid matrix synthesis. Growth in bone area may reflect a difference in body weight gain. In contrast, bone mineral content is considered as a measure of hydroxyapatite content, and gain in bone mineral content is a reflection of mineral accretion. In Pieltain's validation study, calcium to bone mineral content ratio was 46.5%. Whole body calcium content was accurately measured by DEXA with an error of estimation of only 4.4%. Using the same type of conversion equation, the whole body calcium content estimated in preterm and term infants at birth was similar to the intrauterine reference values.[80]

Earlier studies of bone mineralization used x-rays with the main purpose to identify infants with rickets. However, with x-ray examination the BMC cannot be measured and size correction is not possible. By use of single-photon absorptiometry (SPA), it became possible to measure BMC, but only in a small part of the skeleton. With the development of dual energy X- ray absorptiometry (DEXA), it has become possible to measure whole-body BMC with high precision and minimal radiation dose.[81–83] DEXA is currently the "gold standard" for determining BMC because of its high precision and accuracy.

There are methodological differences between SPA and DEXA. SPA measures cortical bone, thus excluding metaphyseal areas, whereas DEXA measures cortical and trabecular bones. The measurements with SPA are localized to a small part of the skeleton, which represents less than 2% of the total bone mass, and it has been shown in neonates that data obtained from a small site of the skeleton do not necessarily correlate well with those obtained for the whole body.[84] Thus, results observed at a very small site of the body should be considered with caution when compared with results of whole body DEXA scan.

Total BMC values in healthy mature infants range from 60–70 g or 18–20 g kg^{-1}.[85,86] Bone mineralization in a premature infant after birth is different than that of intrauterine life. Calcium retention from enteral feeding of unfortified formula is limited to approximately 70–80 mg kg^{-1} day^{-1},[87] while intrauterine calcium retention in the last trimester is approximately 140 mg kg^{-1} day^{-1} as calculated from carcass analysis.[10] Bone strength is determined by bone density and bone quality. Bone density is expressed as grams of mineral per area or volume and in any given adult is determined by peak bone mass and amount of bone loss. Bone quality refers to architecture, turnover, damage accumulation (e.g., microfractures) and mineralization. A fracture occurs when a failure-inducing force (e.g., trauma) is applied to bone. Osteopenia is a significant risk factor for skeletal fracture. Bone loss in adults commonly occurs with aging. An individual who does not reach an optimal peak bone mass during childhood and adolescence may develop osteoporosis without occurrence of accelerated bone loss. Hence suboptimal bone growth in childhood and adolescence is as important as bone loss to the development of osteoporosis in adults.

Currently there is no accurate measure of overall bone strength. Bone mineral density (BMD) accounts for approximately 70% of bone strength. The World Health Organization (WHO) operationally defines osteoporosis as bone density 2.5 standard deviations below the mean for young white adult women. It is not clear how to apply this diagnostic criterion to men, children, and across ethnic groups. There is also difficulty in accurate measurement and standardization between instruments and sites.

Postnatal development of bone mineral status during infancy has been studied by Koo[88] using DEXA scan. In a cross-section observational study of total body bone mineral content (TB BMC) and density (TB BMD), Koo and coworkers demonstrated that during infancy (up to 1 year of life), average TB BMC increased by 389% and TB BMD increased by 157%. In this study the best determinant of bone mineral status is body weight, which accounted for 97% of TB BMC, 98% of TB area, and 86% of TB BMD variation. Postnatal age and body length jointly added only 1%, <1% and 2.5%, respectively, to the explained variation of these DEXA measurements; race, gender, and season all failed to reach statistical significance.

Principles of bone densitometry

Measurement of body composition including bone density has reached fundamental importance in the nutritional management of preterm infants. Several techniques have evolved for this purpose.[89–93] Metabolic balance studies and indirect calorimetry allowed the composition of weight gain in preterm infants to be defined.[94,95] However, these techniques are complex and laborious. DEXA has emerged as an accurate, precise, and reproducible technique for measuring whole body composition in vivo in humans. This valuable tool has made feasible the determination of lean body mass, fat mass, bone area, and bone mineral content.[85,96–99] Reference values of body composition in preterm and term infants at birth have been reported.[97,100]

DEXA is a safe and noninvasive method for measuring bone mineral content and density. Using DEXA, Salle and coworkers[101] assessed BMC and BMD of the lumbar spine (5 vertebrae) in newborns and infants (1–24 months of age). A modified high-resolution program allows assessment of BMC and BMD with a precision higher than 2.4% and 1.5%, respectively. In newborns, BMC and BMD correlated positively with birth weight, body area, length, and gestational age. In infants, both BMC and BMD correlated highly with weight, age, length, and body area over 2 years.

DEXA scans are analyzed using infant whole body software. Whole body composition data analysis provides measurements of bone mineral density (g), bone area (cm^2), fat mass (g), and lean body mass (g), whereas the software calculates body weight and BMC. Bone mineral density, calculated as bone mineral content per unit area of bone, is highly dependent on anthropometric variables. Molgaard and coworkers use BMC adjusted for bone area[80,102] or BMDI [bone mineral content (mg)/(bone area $(cm^2))^{1.7}$], which enables them to obtain a density index independent of anthropometric variables. These measurements have been made in preterm and term infants at birth.[100,103]

Most studies that use total body DEXA in children rely on areal bone mineral density (BMD = bone mineral content [BMC]/bone area [BA]) and compare the output with age- and sex-specific normative data. However, this approach is prone to size-related misinterpretation. Hogler et al. studied the interrelations among BMC, body size (height), and lean tissue mass (LTM). [104] LTM/height tended to be greater in males than in females. Gender effect was still evident as BMC/LTM ratio was greater in females than in males, even after adjustment for age and height. Therefore these researchers recommend that total body DEXA in children should be interpreted in four steps: (1) BMD or BMC/age, (2) height/age, (3) LTM/height, and (4) BMC/LTM ratio for height.

Bone densitometry is based on the principle that if the body is exposed to radiation, different tissues will absorb the radiation to different extents. If the amount of radiation the body (or part of the body is exposed to) is known and the amount of radiation that has not been absorbed is also known, then it should be possible to calculate the amount of energy that has been absorbed by the body. As bone and soft tissue absorb radiation to different degrees, it is possible to calculate the amount of soft tissue and bone tissue by exposing the body to two different levels of radiation. When a DEXA is performed, the body is exposed to two different energy levels (dual energy), the energy used is derived from the conversion of ordinary electricity to a soft x-ray energy (x-ray), and the amount of radiation absorbed is calculated (absorption). The energy beamed at the part of the body scanned can be either in the form of a very narrow beam of energy (pencil-beam) which systematically scans the part of the body, or in the form of a burst of energy which reaches the part to be scanned at one point in time (fan-beam). The pencil beam technique is more time consuming because the entire part of the body is scanned one small section at a time, whereas in the fan-beam technique the exposure is only during a very brief period, similar to that in ordinary x-rays. The dual energy can either be obtained by alternating the strength of the energy at two different levels, or by using alternating filters which block only one level of energy at a time. Z scores are determined as $(X - M)/S$, where X = individual anthropometric and DEXA values, M = mean value of the reference according to gestational age[105] and body weight,[100] and S = SD of the reference. Koo[106] has recently validated the use of pencil beam DEXA and its ability to determine relative changes in bone mass

and body composition measurements over a much greater range of body weight than previous reports, although its use as a direct indicator of nutrient requirement may be limited.

Newer measures of bone strength, such as ultrasound, have been introduced for the diagnosis and monitoring of osteoporosis[107] and successfully adapted to assess bone strength in premature infants.[108–110] Bone strength is determined using quantitative ultrasound measurement of bone speed of sound (SOS) at the middle left tibial shaft. The instrument measures the speed of propagation of ultrasound waves (SOS, meters (second^{-1})) along a fixed longitudinal distance of the cortical layer at the bone shaft. Tibial SOS is a precise method of assessing bone status without exposing the patient to sources of radiation. In contrast to SPA and DEXA, which measure mainly quantitative aspects of bone such as mineral density, this method additionally measures other qualitative bone properties, such as cortical thickness, elasticity, and microarchitecture, thus providing a more complete picture of bone strength.[111–114] Tibial SOS significantly correlated with age, time since menopause in women, height, and weight, as well as with BMD at the radius, spine, and femur.

In VLBW infants tibial SOS correlates positively with gestational age but inversely with postnatal age.[116] They have significant postnatal decrease in bone strength concomitant with biochemical evidence for new bone formation (increase in bone-specific alkaline phosphatase (BSAP) and a decrease in ICTP) during the first 8 postnatal weeks.[115] However, changes in the biochemical bone markers could not predict the changes in bone strength as there was no correlation between levels of bone markers and bone SOS. The postnatal decrease in bone SOS was attenuated by a 4-week exercise program consisting of early range-of-motion intervention (extension and flexion range of motion against passive resistance of the upper and lower extremities).[109] The same exercise program was also associated with further increase in bone formation postnatally as indicated by a further rise in bone formation markers (BSAP and C-terminal propeptide type 1 procollagen – PICP) and decrease in bone resorption markers (ICTP).[116] Using quantitative ultrasound techniques at the humerus, Rubinacci[110] demonstrated that SOS correlated positively with gestational age, length, and weight but negatively with postconceptional age. The authors of this study suggested that the latter part of pregnancy is characterized with increasing fetal bone mineralization that is halted by premature delivery.

In general, clinical trials of pharmacologic therapies have utilized DEXA, rather than QUS, for entry criterion for studies, and there is uncertainty regarding whether the results of these trials can be generalized to patients identified by QUS to have high risk of fracture. Several professional organizations have been working on establishing a standard of comparability of different devices and sites for assessing fracture risk. With this approach, measurements derived from any device or site could be standardized to predict hip fracture risk. However, the values obtained from different instruments cannot be used to predict comparable levels in bone mass. Limitations in precision and low correlation among different techniques will require appropriate validation before this approach can be applied to different skeletal sites and to different age groups.

Risk factors for bone disease in infants and children

The most important risk factor for suboptimal bone growth and mineralization is deficient dietary mineral intake. Hereditary and genetic causes of osteopenia and rickets (such as osteogenesis imperfecta, osteopetrosis hypophosphatasia) are discussed elsewhere.[4,117,118] A partial list of diseases that may predispose to bone disease in children and adults include hyperparathyroidism, rheumatologic and connective tissue disorders, hypogonadism, paretic and paralytic conditions, thyroid dysfunction, osteomalacia, diabetes mellitus, neoplastic disorders, malabsorption, and malnutrition (Table 15.1).

Glucocorticoids[119] are commonly used in the neonatal intensive care unit (NICU) to improve pulmonary mechanics in infants with chronic lung disease and in older children for the treatment of childhood inflammatory diseases. The bone effects of this treatment need to be considered when steroid use is required chronically. The long-term effects on bone health of intermittent courses of systemic steroids or the chronic use of inhaled steroids, as are often used in asthma, are not well described. Cystic fibrosis, celiac disease, and inflammatory bowel disease (IBD) are associated with malabsorption and resultant osteopenia.[120] The osteoporosis of cystic fibrosis is also related to the frequent need for corticosteroids as well as to other undefined factors. Reduced bone mass and the increased risk of fracture in gastrointestinal diseases have a multifactorial pathogenesis. Undoubtedly, genetics play an important role, but other factors such as systemic inflammation, malnutrition, hypogonadism, glucocorticoid therapy in IBD and other lifestyle factors, such as smoking or being sedentary, may contribute to reduced bone mass. At a molecular level the proinflammatory cytokines that contribute to the intestinal immune response in IBD and probably also in coeliac disease are also known to enhance bone resorption. The discovery of the role of the interaction of the Receptor to Activated NFkappaB (RANK) with

Table 15.1. Risk factors for bone disease in infants

Dietary
  Deficient mineral or Vitamin D intake
  Malnutrition
Gastrointestinal
  Malabsorption
  Liver disease, cholestasis
  Prolonged hyperalimentation
Genetic
  Hereditary bone disease
    Osteogenesis imperfecta
    Skeletal dysplasia (e.g. achondroplasia)
    Hypophosphatasia
    Osteopetrosis
Endocrine
  Parathyroid gland disorders
  Thyroid gland dysfunction
  Diabetes mellitus
    Hypogonadism
    Turner syndrome
  Anorexia nervosa in older children
  Adrenal gland dysfunction
  Vitamin D-dependent rickets (Type I and II)
  Growth hormone deficiency
Renal
  Tubular disorders
    Fanconi syndrome
    Hypophosphatemic rickets
  Chronic renal failure
    Renal osteodystrophy and secondary hyperparathyroidism
Rheumatologic
  Connective tissue disease
Drugs
  Glucocorticoids
  Anticonvulsants
  Diuretics
  Aluminum
  Chemotherapy
  Prostaglandins
  Vitamin A and D toxicity
Mechanical
  Immobilization and decreased mechanical load on bone
  Neuromuscular disorders, hypotonia
  Cerebral palsy

its ligand RANKL, in orchestrating the balance between bone resorption and formation may link mucosal and systemic inflammation with bone remodeling, since RANK-RANKL is also involved in lymphopoiesis and T-cell apoptosis. Low circulating leptin in response to weight loss in any gastrointestinal disease may be an important factor in reducing bone mass.[120] Although hypogonadism is an important feature of anorexia nervosa[121] predisposing to decreased bone density, profound undernutrition and nutrition-related factors also play a critical role. This latter point is evidenced, in part, by the failure of estrogen replacement to correct the bone loss.

Several medications affect bone metabolism.[4] Corticosteroids are used to variable degrees in preterm infants with chronic lung disease. Daily exogenous glucocorticoids are capable of slowing growth in children, an effect that is variably counterbalanced by growth hormone treatment.[122] The cause of this growth suppressing effect is multifactorial,[123] including a direct suppressive effect on matrix production and synthesis of local growth factors, and antagonism of growth hormone action by downregulation of growth hormone receptor mRNA expression and binding capacity with reduction in local production of IGF-I.[124] Dexamethasone decreased BMC in animals[125] and human infants. Ward[119] demonstrated lower bone mineral content measured by DEXA at term-corrected age in dexamethasone-treated infants with chronic lung disease compared with preterm and term reference infants. Dexamethasone treatment markedly suppresses collagen turnover (decreases PICP and ICTP) in preterm infants with chronic lung disease.[126, 127]

Other mechanisms by which steroids impair bone growth and mineralization include: (1) Direct inhibition of the osteoblasts and their precursors, leading to a reduction of the rate of bone formation and decreased serum osteocalcin concentrations.[128] (2) Reduced intestinal absorption of calcium probably by interfering with the active transcellular transport of calcium. (3) Reduced renal tubular reabsorption of calcium resulting in hypercalciuria and increased risk of nephrocalcinosis.[129] (4) Reduced production of estrogen and testosterone by inhibiting the pituitary secretion of follicle-stimulating hormone and luteinizing hormone and by direct inhibition of the granulosa cells in the ovaries and testicles. (5) Reducing the production of androstenedione and dehydroepiandrosterone by the adrenal glands. (6) Inhibition of the actions of vitamin D by altering the vitamin D receptors. (7) Possibly the inhibition of prostaglandins, interleukin-1, interleukin-6, growth hormone, and insulin-like growth factor.

Furosemide and other loop diuretics increase renal calcium loss and therefore induce a negative calcium balance. This is the opposite of thiazide diuretics, which increase the renal retention of calcium and induce a positive calcium balance. Prolonged administration of heparin has been associated with decreased bone density. The rate of bone resorption is increased, while that of bone formation is reduced. The incidence of heparin-induced osteopenia is unknown. The mechanisms by which heparin causes osteopenia include decreasing osteoblastic activity resulting in defective ossification, abnormal vitamin D metabolism, and secondary hyperparathyroidism (PTH-dependent increased bone resorption). Heparin directly affects osteoclast development and activity. Heparin may have a direct effect on stimulation of osteoblastic collagenase synthesis linked to increased bone resorption. Excessive thyroid supplementation increases the rate of bone resorption. This is a consideration in infants treated for congenital hypothyroidism or hypothyroxinemia of prematurity.

Prolonged use of anticonvulsant therapy has been associated with rachitic bone disease and proximal myopathy in children.[130, 131] It is estimated that up to 30% of epileptic children receiving phenobarbital and/or phenytoin may develop rickets. Biochemically, these patients may have low serum and urine calcium concentrations, low serum P, and low serum 25-OHD concentrations. Serum alkaline phosphatase, osteocalcin, and PTH concentrations are elevated. Radiologically these patients may have rachitic bone changes. Mechanistically, anticonvulsants increase hepatic metabolism of vitamin D by increasing hydroxylation, glucuronidation, and excretion of the metabolites of vitamin D and 25-OHD, therefore resulting in lower serum concentrations of vitamin D and 25-OHD. They inhibit calcitriol-dependent active intestinal calcium transport, possibly by blunting the response of target organ receptors to calcitriol. High serum calcitriol concentrations may be encountered in these patients, and are explained partly by target organ resistance to calcitriol and a compensatory increased renal synthesis of calcitriol. Effective therapy of this disease is achievable by administration of supraphysiologic doses of vitamin D compounds (Vitamin D, 25-OHD or calcitriol).

Excessive aluminum intake from parenteral hyperalimentation inhibits the rate of bone turnover (see below). Lithium stimulates the production of parathyroid hormone and increases the rate of bone resorption. Cytotoxic medications inhibit bone turnover and predispose to bone resorption,[132] probably through a direct effect on the response of chondrocytes to changes in the growth hormone–IGF-I axis. Methotrexate is a commonly used antineoplastic agent particularly in childhood leukemias. It decreases osteoblastic activity in animals, and increases bone resorption in humans. Consequently prolonged use of this agent may induce osteopenia. An excessive amount of vitamin D increases the rate of bone resorption.

Biochemical measurements of bone turnover

Biochemical measurements of bone turnover (Table 15.2) are helpful in the study of the pathophysiology of skeletal

Table 15.2. Biochemical markers of bone turnover

Bone formation markers
  Serum osteocalcin
  Serum alkaline phosphatase (ALP), Bone specific ALP
  Serum procollagen I extension peptides
Bone resorption markers
  Urine hydroxyproline
  Urine deoxypyridinoline
  Urine pyridinoline
  Type I collagen telopeptides (peptides containing crosslinks)
    N-terminal telopeptide to helix in urine (NTX-I)
    C-terminal telopeptide-1 to helix in serum (ICTP)
    C-terminal telopeptide-2 in urine and serum (CTX)
  Serum tartrate-resistant acid phosphatase
  Hydroxylysine and its glycosides

metabolism and growth.[4,133–138] However, interpretation of their results is difficult because they depend on age, pubertal stage, growth velocity, mineral accrual, hormonal regulation, nutritional status, circadian variation, day-to-day variation, method of expression of results of urinary markers, specificity for bone tissue, and sensitivity and specificity of assays. The accuracy of these markers for diagnosis and monitoring of bone disorders is inferior to bone mineral density measurements. Therefore accuracy concerns have hampered their widespread use. Furthermore, there are no well-established neonatal or pediatric reference ranges for many of the markers. Measurement of these markers in conjunction with clinical evaluation and radiological findings may aid in the initial investigation of bone disorders and possibly assist in monitoring therapy. Due to their multiple limitations, bone metabolism markers should not be relied on exclusively to make important clinical decisions. Measurement of several indices at once, as well as serial measurements, may help to overcome some of these limitations. Table 15.2 summarizes several laboratory assays for bone metabolism markers.

Markers of bone formation include osteocalcin, alkaline phosphatase and its skeletal isoenzyme, and procollagen I extension peptides. Bone resorption markers include hydroxyproline, deoxypyridinoline, and pyridinoline; peptides containing these cross links such as N-telopeptide to helix in urine (NTX), C-terminal telopeptide-1 to helix in serum (ICTP) and C-terminal telopeptide-2 in urine and serum (CTX); tartrate-resistant acid phosphatase; hydroxylysine and its glycosides.

Alkaline phosphatase (ALP) is synthesized and released by intestinal, hepatic, osteoblast, placental, and splenic cells. It is the most commonly used serum marker of osteoblastic activity, and bone formation. However, it lacks sensitivity and specificity, particularly in patients with osteoporosis, where serum ALP is commonly normal. The most common sources of elevated serum alkaline phosphatase concentration are the liver, the skeletal system, and the placenta. Often total activity in the serum is measured, which does not determine the source of the enzyme. Isoenzyme separation by heat denaturation or electrophoresis can distinguish between bone and hepatic isoenzymes, but this is a tedious process and may be associated with analytic difficulties. Serum ALP concentrations are affected by age, sex, and hormonal factors. It is elevated in diseases characterized by increased osteoblastic activity including Paget's disease, osteitis fibrosa cystica, and osteomalacia.

Osteocalcin is the major noncollagenous bone protein. It is a noncollagenous 49-amino acid protein synthesized by osteoblasts and is a marker of bone formation. It contains gammacarboxyglutamic acid, which is a vitamin K-dependent calcium-binding amino acid. Most of synthesized osteocalcin is incorporated in bone where it constitutes 1% of the organic matrix of bone. Minute amounts, however, circulate in blood and can be measured by radioimmunoassay or immunoradiometric assay.[139] Osteocalcin in the circulation is derived from new protein synthesis rather than from resorption of bone matrix. Serum osteocalcin concentration is determined by the amount of newly synthesized protein not incorporated in bone, and released into the circulation. The role of osteocalcin in the skeletal system is not well understood. However, its presence in embryonic bone at a time of rapid bone mineralization, its association with the hydroxyapatite crystal lattice and its chemoattractant property for osteoclasts suggest that osteocalcin may have a role in bone turnover.[140] The synthesis of osteocalcin is stimulated by 1,25(OH)2D. Circulating osteocalcin concentration correlates with osteoblastic activity. Serum osteocalcin concentration parallels the growth velocity curve during childhood and adolescence.[141]

Clinically, serum osteocalcin concentration is elevated in bone diseases characterized by increased osteoblastic activity including Paget's disease, osteomalacia, osteitis fibrosa, renal osteodystrophy, and it correlates with other markers of bone formation (i.e., serum alkaline phosphatase, bone histomorphometry, calcium kinetic studies, x-ray, densitometry). Decreased serum concentrations of PTH, thyroid hormone or growth hormone are associated with decrease in serum osteocalcin concentration, while the reverse is true: thyrotoxicosis, acromegaly, and hyperparathyroidism are associated with elevated serum osteocalcin concentrations. Puberty is associated with a rise in serum osteocalcin concentration, consistent with the increase in osteoblastic activity that accompanies the pubertal growth spurt and gonadal hormone surges. Circadian variation in serum osteocalcin concentration (peak levels at 4 am and nadir at 5 pm) as well as in serum markers of bone formation and resorption have been reported but the etiology and physiological implications of these observations are unknown.[142] Physiologically, serum osteocalcin is increased in children, particularly during the first year of life and during puberty, and is related to physical growth velocity. Serum osteocalcin levels parallel the height velocity curve, with higher values in childhood and during adolescence. Osteocalcin is a highly specific, reliable and useful marker for evaluation of the growth spurt and is not influenced by nonosseous disorders.[143]

Procollagen I extension peptides:[144, 145] procollagen, a precursor of collagen, undergoes cleavage to collagen and extension proteins before collagen becomes incorporated into bone matrix. These proteins serve as indicators of osteoblastic activity. For instance, serum concentration of Type I procollagen is elevated in Paget's disease. However, assay of procollagen propeptides as an indicator of bone formation is less sensitive and specific than serum osteocalcin and bone isoenzyme of alkaline phosphatase.

Urine hydroxyproline is mainly used as an index of greatly increased rate of bone resorption. However, it is not a specific test because sources of hydroxyproline include bone, diet, connective tissues, serum proteins, and degradation of propeptides from collagen biosynthesis. This test correlates poorly with bone resorption as assessed by bone histomorphometric and calcium kinetic studies. Urine hydroxylysine glycosides are released to a great extent from bone and their concentration increases greatly during osteoporosis. However, this test has the same problem of nonspecificity as urine hydroxyproline.

Serum tartrate-resistant acid phosphatase (TRAP)[146] is the portion of serum acid phosphatase derived from osteoclasts. The isoform TRAP 5b is a good and specific marker for osteoclastic bone resorption. Tissues other than bone produce acid phosphatase (prostate, pancreas, and blood cells). Bone acid phosphatase is differentiated from that of other tissues by determining its mobility on acrylamide gel and the resistance of its activity to tartrate. Elevated serum concentrations of tartrate-resistant acid phosphatase occur with high bone turnover diseases such as primary hyperparathyroidism and osteopetrosis. This assay is not widely available and normative data are lacking.

Urine collagen pyridinoline cross-linking amino acids[147–149] are among the best available specific biomarkers of bone resorption. These compounds, which include hydroxylysylpyridinoline and lysylpyridinoline, are released upon degradation of mature collagen from skeletal tissues. The hydroxypyridinium collagen cross-links, pyridinoline and deoxypyridinoline are released upon degradation of mature collagen. In urine these compounds are either free (nonpeptide bound) (40%) or peptide-bound (60%). Assays are available to measure type I collagen telopeptides (with carboxy or amine terminals) in urine and serum.

Urinary N-telopeptides[150] are the peptide fragments of the protein that link the collagen bundles in bones. These fragments are liberated into the circulation as a result of the breakdown of collagen in the bones, and they are excreted unchanged in the urine. Urine levels of N-telopeptides therefore reflect the degree of bone resorption. Because there are diurnal variations in the degree of bone resorption, with the highest levels occurring during the night, the N-telopeptides are best measured either in a 24-hour urine sample or in the early morning sample. Pyridinium cross-links and collagen telopeptides involving the cross-linking site are the best indices of bone resorption. Demarini[151] reported higher telopeptide of type I collagen (ICTP), normal cord blood propeptide of type I procollagen (PICP), and lower bone mineral content in infants of diabetic mothers (IDMs) at birth indicating increased bone resorption/modeling. Pratico[152] measured serum (ICTP) concentration from 1 (cord blood) to 90 days of life. During this period serum ICTP concentration was about tenfold higher than in adulthood. During the first 3 months of life serum ICTP concentration shows a progressive increase from 0 to 7 days, remains unchanged until day 30, then decreases until day 45, and maintains similar values from days 45–90 of life. The trend of serum ICTP in the first week of life may reflect increased bone resorption, probably to maintain normocalcemia following delivery, then a gradual decrease and reach of baseline equilibrium as bone formation increases.

Bone Sialoprotein (BSP) accounts for 5–10% of noncollagenous bone matrix. It may play a role in cell-matrix adhesion processes and organization of the extracellular matrix of mineralized tissues. In adults and children serum BSP drops following bisphosphonate therapy, possibly reflecting decreasing bone resorption activity. The usefulness of this marker is still not well studied. BSP might be a useful marker of noncollagenous organic bone matrix in laboratory assessment of bone turnover, being inversely related to BMD and showing significant correlations to established markers of bone turnover like B-ALP and OC.

Changes of bone turnover during growth have been described during infancy, prepubertal period, puberty, and the postpubertal period. Pubertal changes of bone markers are described with special attention to gender differences and hormonal mechanisms of the growth spurt, which determine differences related to the pubertal stage. From available data, biochemical markers of bone remodeling may be useful in the clinical investigation of bone turnover in children in health and disease. However, their use in everyday clinical practice is not advised at present.[133] Although these markers have found significant utility in the evaluation of adults with metabolic bone diseases, their application in children has been limited due to great variability in normal ranges that reflect the changes in skeletal metabolism induced by age, growth rate, gender, and pubertal state.[134]

Single measurements of bone markers cannot predict bone density. Recently, van der Sluis[153] provided reference data of biochemical markers of bone turnover and vitamin D metabolites for children and young adults, taking into consideration the effects of gender and age: serum calcium and vitamin D levels were independent of age. The peak concentrations for collagen type I cross-linked N-telopeptide, cross-linked telopeptide of type I collagen, carboxy-terminal propeptide of type I procollagen, N-terminal propeptide of type I procollagen, alkaline phosphatase, and osteocalcin were found during puberty, in girls approximately 2.5 years earlier than in boys. Strong correlations were found between the markers of bone turnover, while no correlation was found among the markers of bone turnover and bone mineral density measured by DEXA.

Koo[154] studied molar ratios of peptide-bound and free hydroxyproline : creatinine (OHPr : Cr) in urine over the first year of life in VLBW infants, with or without radiographically confirmed fractures and (or) rickets (F/R). The urinary peptide-bound OHPr : Cr ratio varied widely and was greatest at 3 months. The ratio decreased with increasing postnatal age and was not statistically different between infants with or without F/R. The urinary free OHPr : Cr ratio also was greatest at age 3 months, rapidly decreasing afterwards, and was not statistically different between infants with or without F/R. The authors of this study suggest that, in VLBW infants, bone turnover as indicated by the urinary peptide-bound OHPr : Cr ratio is highest during early infancy; however, it appears from the wide range of values for this ratio that its use alone is not sufficient for detection of F/R in VLBW infants. The rapid decrease in free OHPr : Cr ratio is presumably related to the maturation of renal tubular function.

In a longitudinal study, Pittard[155] measured BMC via photon absorptiometry and serum osteocalcin and skeletal alkaline phosphatase (BALP) concentrations from birth to 16 weeks in very low birth weight infants. All serum values were measured in mothers at delivery. The results of this study showed that (1) cord blood osteocalcin concentrations were significantly greater than corresponding maternal concentrations, and by 1 week had significantly increased from birth values; (2) the increase in serum osteocalcin concentration, from birth to 1 week, was significantly correlated with simultaneous increase in (OH) 2D concentrations; (3) there was no correlation between the change in BMC, over the first 4 mo of life and serum concentrations of OC and BALP; and (4) a significant negative correlation between serum osteocalcin and BALP concentrations at week 4; and, although not significant, a negative correlation from 1–16 weeks of age.

There is an inverse correlation between gestational age and markers of bone turnover in cord blood or amniotic fluid.[156–162] Ogueh[157] measured umbilical cord concentrations of PICP and ICTP at the time of delivery from healthy women at different gestations. They found a significant inverse correlation between cord blood PICP or ICTP concentration and gestational age; and between ICTP and birth weight. Birth weight effect is a function of gestational age. These findings suggest that both bone formation and resorption decrease with gestational age. Such changes may be due to the shift from growth to maintenance of bone during the last trimester.

Ogueh[163] studied the effect of gestational diabetes on maternal and fetal bone metabolism. Plasma PICP and ICTP were obtained from mothers with or without gestational diabetes and umbilical cord blood at the time of delivery. Although there was a significant correlation between 1 hour postprandial blood glucose and maternal ICTP concentration, there was no significant difference in maternal or fetal PICP and ICTP concentrations between study and control groups. There was a significant correlation between maternal and fetal ICTP, but not between maternal and fetal PICP concentrations. From this study, although maternal ICTP concentration was related to the 1 hour postprandial blood glucose level, gestational diabetes did not affect maternal or umbilical cord serum concentrations of markers of bone metabolism.

Harrast[162] investigated the effects of gestational age on markers of fetal bone turnover (PICP, ICTP) in the amniotic fluid, and the relationship of bone mass at birth in small-for-gestational-age (SGA) infants and infants of diabetic mothers (IDMs). Biochemical markers of decreased bone formation or increased bone resorption were examined. Both PICP and ICTP concentrations in amniotic fluid were inversely associated with gestational age. Amniotic fluid concentrations of PICP increased exponentially in relation to infant birthweight. SGA infants had lower amniotic fluid PICP concentrations than controls. The presence of diabetes in the mother was not associated with alterations in amniotic fluid PICP or ICTP concentrations. Although maturational effects on clearance of bone markers from amniotic fluid cannot be excluded, these data are consistent with a high turnover of bone matrix early in fetal life, and a reduction in bone formation when fetal growth is compromised.

Namgung[164] measured markers of bone collagen type I biosynthesis and degradation, PICP and ICTP, in SGA infants. SGA infants have lower bone mineral content (BMC), lower serum IGF-I and lower serum osteocalcin compared with appropriate-for-gestational-age (AGA) infants. There were no differences between SGA and AGA infants in serum PICP or ICTP concentrations. Serum ICTP was correlated with osteocalcin and with PICP in SGA infants but not in AGA infants. Thus, serum biochemical indices of bone collagen type I biosynthesis and degradation in term SGA infants are similar to those in term AGA infants. From these findings the authors suggest that the reduced bone mineral content in SGA infants is predominantly related to a lower supply of minerals rather than defective regulation of bone collagen type I metabolism.

Yamaga[165] reported an increase in bone resorption during pregnancy and lactation by measuring pyridinoline (Pyr) and deoxypyridinoline (D-Pyr), urinary excretions of C-telopeptide (CTX) and cross-linked N-telopeptide (NTX) of type I collagen. These markers significantly increased in the third trimester of pregnancy and remained high during the puerperium. The same researchers investigated the relationship between maternal and neonatal bone turnover markers,[166] including bone formation markers (intact osteocalcin, bone-specific alkaline phosphatase) and bone resorption markers (C-telopeptide of type I collagen; CTX) in maternal and umbilical cord venous blood. The concentrations of all markers of bone turnover, including CTX, in cord serum were significantly higher than those in maternal serum. There was no significant correlation between maternal and cord serum levels for any marker. These results indicate that fetal bone turnover is markedly enhanced compared with maternal bone turnover and is independent of maternal bone metabolism in late pregnancy.

Yasumizu[167] measured PICP, ICTP and osteocalcin in mother-infant pairs and age-matched nonpregnant women. Serum PICP and ICTP of term women at delivery were significantly higher and serum osteocalcin was significantly lower than in nonpregnant women. The ratio of PICP to ICTP was essentially the same for term and nonpregnant women. Serum PICP, ICTP, and osteocalcin were virtually the same in the umbilical arteries and vein. PICP, ICTP, and osteocalcin were much higher in fetal than maternal circulation, and fetal bone marker concentrations did not correlate with maternal concentrations, or with birth weight. Thus, during pregnancy, either osteoclastic or osteoblastic

activity would appear to increase slightly, but the balance between bone formation and resorption is maintained. During fetal life, bone turnover may be greatly accelerated and bone metabolism may occur independently of maternal bone metabolism.

Mora[159] studied bone markers to monitor bone turnover rate during the perinatal period. They evaluated bone turnover rate, assessed by the measurement of urinary N-terminal telopeptide of type I collagen (NTX) concentrations, at different gestational ages, and documented bone turnover rate in the first days after birth in term and preterm newborns and infants of diabetic mothers (IDMs). There is a strong association between gestational age and NTX concentrations at birth. NTX concentrations progressively decrease after birth, reaching a nadir between weeks 38 and 42 of gestation. Preterm infants had NTX excretion values at birth significantly higher than full term infants, whereas NTX excretion rates of IDMs were not different. The authors of this study suggest that gestational age seems to be the major determinant of bone turnover in neonates; NTX excretion rate is higher before term, slows in proximity of delivery, and increases significantly during the first 48 hours of life. Preterm infants have higher bone turnover rate than full term infants. NTX excretion rate of IDMs was comparable to those of the control subjects.

In a longitudinal study, Crofton investigated the relationship of bone and collagen markers (bone-specific alkaline phosphatase-ALP, C-terminal propeptide of type I collagen – PICP, N-terminal propeptide of type III procollagen – PNP, C-terminal telopeptide of type I collagen, urinary pyridinoline – Pyd, and deoxypyridinoline – Dpd) to growth and bone mineral content in preterm infants over the first 10 weeks of life.[168] Concentrations of all collagen markers were 10-fold higher than in older children. Each marker showed a distinctive pattern of postnatal change, with early increases in PICP and PNP and decreases in ICTP reflecting postnatal growth. Once markers reached a plateau during weeks 4–10, type III procollagen (PNP) was positively correlated, whereas urinary pyridinoline (Pyd) and deoxypyridinoline (Dpd) were negatively correlated with the rate of weight gain. Type III procollagen was also positively correlated with overall linear growth. PICP was strongly correlated with mean BMC and with total BMC attained by 10 weeks of age. Bone ALP was positively correlated with the rate of bone mineral accretion. From this study it appears that PNP, a marker of soft-tissue collagen formation, is a good marker for overall ponderal and linear growth in preterm infants, whereas the markers of collagen breakdown, Pyd and Dpd, have inverse relationships with weight gain. PICP and bone ALP seem to be good surrogate markers for bone mineralization in preterm infants. These markers may provide information on whole-body turnover of bone and collagen that is complementary to traditional physical measures of growth and bone mineralization.

In osteogenesis imperfecta,[169] markers of bone formation (PICP, osteocalcin and alkaline phosphatase) and bone resorption [ICTP and hydroxypyridinium cross-links, pyridinoline (Pyr) and deoxypyridinoline (Dpyr)] correlate with the severity of the disease: bone resorption becomes excessive in severe disease coupled with decreased bone formation. Shiff[170] measured circulating bone turnover markers (osteocalcin, BSAP, PICP, and ICTP) in preterm infants during the first 10 weeks of life. Markers of osteoblastic activity increased markedly during the first 3 weeks of life, and then continued to increase gradually until week 10 of life, indicating increased bone formation in premature infants in the first 3 months of life. Circulating ICTP levels increased in the first week of life and then decreased gradually over the following 9 weeks. Serum concentrations of osteocalcin (in weeks 2–5 of life), PICP (weeks 3–5), and ICTP (weeks 2–3) were significantly higher in VLBW (1000–1250 g) than ELBW (<1000 g) preterm infants. Increased bone turnover in VLBW compared with ELBW preterm infants may be due to higher morbidity in ELBW preterm infants in the first few weeks of life.

Lapillonne[171] and coworkers evaluated bone resorption in infants by measuring urinary collagen type 1 cross-linked N-telopeptide (NTX) excretion normalized to creatinine (NTX/Cr) in a spot urine sample as a reflection of daily NTX production in infants, and computed normative values for NTX excretion from birth to 1 year of age. Spot urine NTX/Cr values significantly and linearly correlated with daily NTX excretion. In healthy infants, NTX excretion is low at birth, increases dramatically and significantly during the first 10 days of life, remains significantly elevated for approximately 3 months, and then decreases progressively to return to values similar to that observed at birth by 1 year of age. The normative data demonstrate significant age-related variations in this marker, which probably reflect adaptation to extrauterine life and accelerated bone turnover in infancy, and which should be considered for interpretation of this noninvasive bone resorption marker in the clinical setting.

Leptin may play a role in fetal bone metabolism as part of its effect on fetal growth and development.[172] Hassink[173] showed a positive correlation between umbilical cord blood leptin concentration and newborn weight and body mass index. Matsuda[174] demonstrated that leptin concentrations in preterm newborns were lower than those in term newborns and tended to increase according to gestational age and birth weight, especially from the late stage of gestation. Leptin concentrations in pregnant women increased from the first trimester and then remained higher than those in non-pregnant women throughout the remainder of pregnancy even after controlling for body mass index. The leptin concentrations of newborns declined rapidly and were extremely low by the day 6 of life.

Ogueh and coworkers[175] investigated the relationship between leptin and fetal bone metabolism. They measured fetal blood levels of leptin, PICP and ICTP from 18–35 weeks' gestation. There was a positive correlation between leptin concentration and gestational age and a negative correlation between both PICP and ICTP and gestational age. Also, there was a negative correlation between the concentrations of leptin and both PICP and ICTP. The increase in leptin concentration with gestational age is consistent with adipose tissue development and the subsequent accumulation of fat mass. The negative correlation between fetal leptin and ICTP suggests that leptin may decrease bone resorption with the overall effect of increasing bone mass.

Furmaga-Jablonski[176] investigated the correlation between serum concentrations of leptin, markers of bone formation (osteocalcin and PICP) and selected anthropometric traits in AGA newborns between 27 to 42 weeks' gestation. These investigators found significant correlations between leptin, osteocalcin, PICP and overall physical growth in AGA newborns but no correlations between serum leptin concentration and markers of bone formation.

Maternal smoking during pregnancy and maternal obesity may have a negative impact on fetal bone formation. Hogler[67] investigated the effect of maternal smoking and weight gain on fetal bone turnover. The authors evaluated the relationship of bone marker concentrations to maternal and fetal variables as well as maternal smoking and assessed the short-term change in bone markers during the first days of life. Serum markers of bone formation (osteocalcin and BSAP) and bone resorption (C-terminal telopeptide of type I collagen) were measured in cord blood and at discharge (median of day 3 of life) in healthy term neonates. Concentrations of BSAP were significantly lower in neonates of smokers compared with nonsmokers, both at birth and at discharge. Both cord blood osteocalcin and BSAP were negatively related to maternal weight and maternal body mass index. Maternal smoking and pregnancy weight gain were significant predictors of cord BSAP. C-terminal telopeptide of type I collagen and osteocalcin increased significantly from birth to discharge, whereas BSAP levels remained the same. The significant increase of osteocalcin and C-terminal telopeptide of type I collagen may result either from an increase in bone turnover or altered renal clearance.

Colak has also demonstrated negative effect of maternal smoking on fetal bone metabolism.[68] They measured osteocalcin (OC), bone isoenzyme of alkaline phosphatase (BALP), and procollagen type 1 C-terminal propeptide (PICP) in maternal serum and umbilical cord blood. Infants of smoker women have significantly lower umbilical cord blood OC and BALP concentrations than infants of non-smoking women. All bone markers except total ALP were significantly higher in umbilical cord blood than maternal blood. Smoking-induced altered fetal bone metabolism may be due to chronic hypoxia resulting in the suppression of bone matrix synthesis or placental synthesis as reflected by low OC and BALP concentrations in umbilical cord blood of infants of women who smoke.

Fares and coworkers evaluated the impact of puberty, gender, and vitamin D status on biochemical markers of bone remodeling.[177] They measured serum osteocalcin (OC), bone alkaline phosphatase (BAP), C-terminal telopeptide of type I collagen crosslinks (S-CTX), and 25-OHD. Adolescent boys achieve a higher peak bone mass than girls and had higher concentrations of bone markers. In girls, all markers of bone turnover changed significantly with pubertal stage, were maximal at midpuberty, and decreased toward adult levels by Tanner stage V. Conversely in boys, these markers increased during early pubertal stages but had not normalized by Tanner stage V. Levels of all biochemical markers were significantly higher in boys compared with girls even after adjustment for age, body weight, and Tanner stage. Adolescent girls with vitamin D insufficiency had much higher serum levels of BAP and S-CTX. However, gender remains the only consistent correlate of all three markers of bone remodeling. Nutritional status and leptin concentrations are involved in the regulation of growth factors and biochemical markers of bone formation. Bini[178] investigated the relationship of leptin to growth factors and biochemical markers of bone turnover of prepubertal overweight children, specifically the relationships between circulating serum leptin concentration and insulin-like growth factor I (IGF-I), insulin growth factor binding protein-3 (IGFBP-3) and biochemical markers of bone turnover (OC, PICP and ICTP). Overweight children had higher concentrations of leptin, IGF-I and IGFBP-3, and lower OC concentrations. Weight reduction is associated with a significant reduction of serum leptin and IGFBP-3 concentrations and an increase in serum OC and PICP, but not of ICTP concentration. Leptin, corrected by BMI and sex, has a significant negative correlation with PICP, IGF-I and height velocity but not with OC, ICTP, and IGFBP-3.

Sorva[179] investigated the relationship of serum collagen markers and serum osteocalcin to pubertal growth in healthy boys. The soft tissue marker, serum amino-terminal propeptide of type III procollagen (PIIINP) increased when boys reached Tanner stage G3, which may predict a normal pubertal growth spurt. Markers of bone collagen matrix increased only at advanced pubertal stage indicating higher bone turnover. Bone formation markers, carboxy-terminal and amino-terminal propeptides of type I procollagen, and degradation marker, ICTP carboxy-terminal telopeptide of type I collagen were higher only at stage G4. Serum osteocalcin was higher only at Stage G4 associated with the pubertal growth spurt. There is evidence of increased bone turnover in pre-eclampsia as evidenced by increased concentrations of ICTP and PICP during the third trimester.[180] However these markers did not correlate with body mass index, blood pressure, serum uric acid levels, or platelet count.

Hormonal regulation of bone remodeling

Bone mass is constantly regulated by a dynamic balance between bone formation and resorption. These processes are under influence of systemic and local regulators. Systemic regulators (Table 15.3) of bone homeostasis include primarily the calciotropic hormones. Local regulation (Table 15.4) of bone homeostasis involves prostaglandins[181] and growth factors such as insulin-like growth factors I and II (IGF-I and II)[182] which act as autocrine or paracrine effectors of bone formation by increasing osteoblastic proliferation and bone matrix biosynthesis. IGF-I mediates the linear growth-promoting actions of GH. IGF binding proteins play significant and complex roles, primarily via modulation of IGF actions.[183]

Insulin is one of the most important systemic hormones modulating normal skeletal growth. It does not regulate bone resorption, but it causes a marked stimulation of bone

Table 15.3. Systemic regulation of bone remodeling*

	Bone resorption	Bone formation
PTH	Increase	Increase in low doses
		Decrease in high doses
1,25(OH)2D	Increase	Increase in low doses
		Decrease in high doses
Calcitonin	Decrease	Increase
Estrogen	Decrease	Increase
Growth hormone/IGF	Increase	Increase
Insulin/IGF	No effect	Increase
Thyroid hormone	Increase	Increase
Glucocorticoids	Increase	Decrease

*Adapted from data.[408]

Table 15.4. Local regulation of bone remodeling*

	Bone resorption	Bone formation
Growth factors		
IGF-I	–	Increase
TGF-Beta	–	Increase
Fibroblast Growth Factor (FGF)	–	Increase
Platelet derived growth factor (PDGF)	–	Increase
PTHrP	Increase	Increase
Cytokines that cause bone loss		
Interleukin-1	Increase	–
Interleukin-6	Increase	–
Interleukin-11	Increase	–
TNF alpha	Increase	–
Osteoclast Differentiation Factor (ODF)	Increase	–
Cytokines that decrease bone loss		
Interleukin-4	Decrease	–
Interleukin-13	Decrease	–
Interleukin-18	Decrease	–
Osteoprotegerin	Decrease	–
BMP	–	Increase
Prostaglandin E2	Increase	Increase
Vitamin A	Increase	–
Cathepsins	Increase	–

*Adapted from data.[408] IGF-I, insulin-like growth factors I; PTHrP, parathyroid related peptide.

matrix synthesis and cartilage formation.[184–186] Insulin also increases IGF-I production by the liver; it is well known that IGF-I enhances bone collagen and matrix synthesis and stimulates the replication of cells of the osteoblast lineage.[184]

Parathyroid hormone and 1,25(OH)2D play an important role in activating bone remodeling. The process requires activation of existing osteoclasts and generation of new osteoclasts from precursor cells. Osteoclast precursor cells have receptors for both PTH and 1,25(OH)2D. Activation of these receptors results in releasing hydrolytic enzymes and lowering bone pH, thus dissolving bone mineral. PTH stimulates the secretion of lysosomal enzymes, which dissolve the osteoid matrix. It also stimulates the release of collagenase from osteoblasts. However, PTH has a biphasic effect on bone homeostasis. On the one hand, intermittent administration of PTH stimulates bone formation possibly through production of IGF-I and IGF-II.[187] On the other hand continuous PTH administration has a catabolic effect on bone and favors bone resorption.

Prostaglandins, particularly of the E series, are potent local bone resorbing agents. TGF-beta appears to have an essential role in normal postnatal growth and development. It is secreted by chondrocytes and may have a regulatory role in chondrocyte differentiation.[29] Calcitriol 1,25(OH)2D also has a biphasic effect on bone: it increases bone formation through the effect of IGF-I, but it also increases the number and activity of osteoclasts, thus promoting bone resorption. Growth hormone[188] also has an anabolic effect on bone metabolism. It increases bone formation by increasing local concentrations of IGF-I.[189]

Estradiol and progesterone stimulate osteoblastic activity to increase bone formation,[190] and estrogen has been demonstrated to increase production of both IGF-I and IGF-II. Several cytokines have osteoclast-activating effect most likely mediated by osteoblasts. Cytokines which promote bone resorption include interleukin I, tumor necrosis factors alpha and beta, and differentiation-inducing factor. Osteoclasts carry receptors for calcitonin. Calcitonin directly inhibits bone resorption by binding specific receptors on osteoclasts to inhibit osteoclast formation, motility, and activity.[25, 191]

Thyroid hormones have a biphasic effect on bone homeostasis.[193] In vitro studies demonstrate an increase in bone mass because of an increase in osteoblastic activity with low doses of triiodothyronine (T3), and a decrease in bone mass because of increased osteoclastic activity.[192] Receptors for T3 have been identified on osteoblastic cell lines. T3 increases bone turnover. In physiologic doses, it increases osteoblastic activity reflected biochemically in a rise in serum alkaline phosphatase and osteocalcin concentrations, and histologically in an increase in osteoid formation and mineralization rate. However, excessive T3 as in thyrotoxicosis has an additional effect of increasing osteoclastic activity and bone resorption resulting in an overall decrease in bone mass.[194] Thyrotoxicosis is a significant risk factor for osteoporosis.

Vitamin A metabolites have a significant impact on bone homeostasis. Vitamin A deficiency results in increased bone mass; excessive vitamin A intake causes increased bone resorption and decreased bone mass.[195] The mechanism of vitamin A-induced bone resorption is by direct stimulation of osteoclasts by vitamin A metabolites, retinol, and retinoic acid, mediated by specific cytosolic receptors.

Recently cathepsins have been described to have a major role in osteoclastic bone resorption.[196] Cathepsin K is essential for normal bone resorption; humans lacking cathepsin K exhibit pycnodysostosis, which is characterized by short stature and osteosclerosis. Cathepsin K knockout mice develop osteopetrosis and display features characteristic of pycnodysostosis, and osteoclasts isolated from these mice exhibit impaired bone resorption in vitro. Bone resorption depends upon the synthesis of cathepsin K by osteoclasts and its secretion into the extracellular compartment at the attachment site between osteoclasts and the bone surface, wherein the organic matrix is subsequently degraded by cathepsin K. Factors that directly modulate osteoclastic bone resorption, including cytokines (RANK ligand, tumor necrosis factor-alpha and interferon gamma), hormones (retinoic acid and estrogen) and nuclear transcriptional factors (c-jun and Mitf), also regulate cathepsin K gene expression.

The osteoclast is a bone-degrading polykaryon that derives from a monocyte/macrophage precursor. Osteoclast formation requires permissive concentrations of macrophage-colony stimulating factor and is driven by contact with mesenchymal cells in bone that bear the TNF-family ligand RANKL.[33] Osteoclast precursors express RANK, and the interaction between RANKL and RANK is the major determinant of osteoclast formation. PTH/PTHrP, glucocorticoids and 1,25(OH)2D, and humoral factors, including TNF-alpha, interleukin-1, TGFs and prostaglandins, influence osteoclast formation by altering expression of these molecular factors. TNF-alpha, IL-6, and IL-11 promote osteoclast formation by RANKL-independent processes. RANKL-dependent/independent osteoclast formation is likely to play an important role in conditions where there is pathological bone resorption. Osteoclast functional defects cause sclerotic bone disorders, many of which have recently been identified as specific genetic defects. Osteoclasts express specialized proteins including a vacuolar-type H+-ATPase that drives HCl secretion for dissolution of bone mineral. One v-ATPase component, the 116 kD V0 subunit, has several isoforms. Only one isoform, TCIRG1, is upregulated in osteoclasts. Defects in TCIRG1 are common causes of osteopetrosis. HCl secretion is dependent on chloride channels; a chloride channel homologue, CLCN7, is another common defect in osteopetrosis. Humans who are deficient in carbonic anhydrase II or who have defects in phagocytosis also have variable defects in bone remodeling. Organic bone matrix is degraded by thiol proteinases, principally cathepsin K, and abnormalities in cathepsin K cause another sclerotic bone disorder, pycnodysostosis. Thus, bone turnover in normal subjects depends on relative expression of key cytokines, and defects in osteoclastic turnover usually reflect defects in specific ion transporters or enzymes that play essential roles in bone degradation.

Leptin is a hormone secreted by adipocytes that can regulate bone mass through a central, neuroendocrine signaling pathway.[197] Leptin is a powerful inhibitor of bone formation in vivo. This antiosteogenic function involves leptin binding to its receptors on ventromedial hypothalamic neurons, the autonomous nervous system and beta-adrenergic receptors on osteoblasts. However, the mechanisms whereby leptin controls the function of ventromedial hypothalamic antiosteogenic neurons remain unclear.[198] Chondrocytes possess leptin receptors, which mediate its effect in enhancing chondrocyte proliferation and subsequent cell differentiation.[199] Serum leptin concentration is elevated in obesity and decreased in malnutrition and malabsorption. Leptin may stimulate growth even in the presence of caloric restriction independently of peripheral IGF-I.[200]

The concept of peak bone mass has become crucial in understanding bone disorders. It is generally defined as the highest level of bone mass achieved in life as a result of normal growth. Using DEXA techniques, Van der Sluis et al.[153] as well as others[65] showed that peak bone mass was virtually achieved by the end of the second decade. Therefore, peak bone mass, which is attained in early adulthood, is an important determinant of postmenopausal osteoporosis later in life. It is determined by a number of factors including genetic, nutritional, mechanical, and environmental factors.[66] The relative contribution of each of these determinants to peak bone mass is difficult to assess. The genetic effect on adult bone mass may be mediated largely through effects on bone formation rather than through effects on resorption. About 45% of the adult skeleton is built and enlarged during adolescence. There is a strong positive relationship between calcium intake and peak bone mass achieved.[201] Better calcium intake during adolescence may optimize, within genetic limits, peak bone mass.[202] Physical activity, use of estrogenic oral contraceptives and dietary calcium intake exert a positive effect on bone gain in young adult women.[61] Androgens and estrogen are important determinants of peak bone density in young women.[203] Reduced dietary calcium intake results in a drop in serum ionized calcium concentration, which promptly stimulates PTH secretion to correct the perturbed homeostasis. PTH in turn increases renal synthesis of calcitriol to increase renal calcium reabsorption and intestinal calcium absorption, and also stimulates bone resorption to release bone calcium into the circulation and normalize serum ionized calcium. However, adaptation to suboptimal calcium intake is limited and if dietary calcium intake is not improved secondary hyperparathyroidism and bone disease result. The optimal dietary calcium intake for bone growth is a debatable issue. Calcium retention requirements for growth are as follows: an average of 100 mg day^{-1} must be retained during childhood, 220 mg day^{-1} during adolescence, and probably 20–30 mg day^{-1} during early adulthood from ages 20 to 30 years. Environmental determinants of bone mass include smoking, alcohol, and medications.[66] Important increments in bone mass may result from physical activity during childhood.[61]

Hormonal regulation of mineral metabolism

Parathyroid hormone

Parathyroid hormone (PTH) is an 84 amino acid polypeptide (molecular weight of 9500 daltons) synthesized in the parathyroid glands, which develop early in gestation from the third and fourth branchial pouches. Production of PTH, demonstrated histologically by the presence of electron-dense secretory granules, first appears at the 6–7 centimeter-long stage (6–10 g weight) of embryologic development,[204] and gradually increases during gestation. In rats, the parathyroid glands are well differentiated by day 17 of gestation.[205] Human fetal parathyroid glands elaborate PTH as early as 10 weeks of gestation; immunoreactive-PTH staining cells are demonstrated early in fetal development using antibodies specific to the carboxyl terminal PTH.[206]

The PTH gene is located on the short arm of chromosome 11. It codes for pre-pro-PTH, which undergoes two enzymatic cleavages before it yields PTH. Calcium-sensing receptors are membrane-bound G protein coupled receptors in parathyroid cells, C cells of the thyroid gland and kidney cells.[207–209] Serum ionized calcium (iCa) concentration is the main determinant of PTH secretion: a drop in serum iCa concentration is detected by calcium-sensing receptors,[210] which in turn stimulate PTH secretion. Conversely, a rise in serum iCa concentration is transduced by calcium-sensing receptors to suppress PTH secretion. However other ions and hormones influence PTH secretion by the parathyroid glands: for instance, a rise in serum 1,25(OH)2D decreases PTH secretion. An acute drop in serum Mg concentration stimulates PTH secretion but to a much smaller extent (10-fold less) compared with the effect of acute hypocalcemia.[211] Chronic hypomagnesemia impairs PTH secretion and causes blunting of PTH action at target organs.[212–216] Magnesium ions are essential for adenylate cyclase mediated secretion of secretory granules from the parathyroid chief cells. Therefore, magnesium deficiency may cause secondary hypocalcemia. Hypermagnesemia also suppresses PTH secretion.[217,218] Aluminum inhibits PTH secretion in vitro.[219]

Full biological activity resides in the amino-terminal 1–34 peptide; the middle and carboxy-terminal sequence (35–85 amino acids) are biologically inert although immunologically highly reactive. PTH regulates serum concentrations of Ca and P by modulating the activity of specific cells in bone and kidney, generating intracellular cyclic adenosine monophosphate. Known actions of PTH include: (1) stimulation of the release of calcium and phosphorus from bone into circulation. The most obvious histological action of PTH is an increase in osteoclast number and activity[220,221] thus increasing osteoclastic bone resorption. Although osteoclasts may carry receptors for PTH, it is likely that osteoclastic bone resorption is affected by a PTH–osteoblast–osteoclast interaction mechanism. PTH has a synergistic effect with 1,25(OH)2D in stimulating bone resorption. (2) Enhancement of fractional reabsorption of calcium from the glomerular filtrate. (3) Stimulation of renal 1-alpha hydroxylase activity to increase 1,25(OH)2D synthesis which leads to increased intestinal Ca and P absorption. (4) Action on renal tubules to decrease reabsorption of P resulting in significant phosphaturia and an overall decrease in serum phosphorus concentration, despite PTH-induced bone resorption and release of bone phosphorus into the circulation. Parathyroid hormone has dual effects on bone homeostasis: anabolic (increase bone formation) and catabolic (increase bone resorption). Both intermittent and continuous PTH administration increase bone formation independent of its resorption effects. However, increase in bone mass and calcium accretion rate was consistent with intermittent PTH administration (which mimics the physiologic pulsatile secretion of PTH) but not with continuous PTH administration.[222]

Parathyroid hormone-related peptide (PTHrP)

Parathyroid hormone-related peptide (PTHrP)[223] was first demonstrated with cytochemical bioassay and discovered to have a major role in the etiology of hypercalcemia of malignancy.[224–226] Parathyroid hormone and PTHrP genes are members of the same gene family; the amino terminal of PTHrP has a sequence homology of eight amino acids in the PTH amino terminal. It is also equipotent to that of PTH when assessed by cytochemical bioassay and in situ biochemistry.[227] PTHrP is produced by normal keratinocytes and has been demonstrated in in vivo histochemical studies of the skin and detected in the medium of keratinocytes cultured in vitro. Squamous cells, which originate in keratinocytes, are a common source of PTHrP and have a common association with hypercalcemia of malignancy. From several studies it appears that this peptide may have a significant physiological role. One of the major production sites of PTHrP is lactating breast tissue. PTHrP is present in large quantities in milk. The release of parathyroid hormone-like peptides has been detected in cultures of fetal rat long bones.[228]

In normal adults, plasma PTHrP concentrations by radioimmunoassay ranged from less than 2 to 5 pmol l^{-1}. Infusion of PTHrP causes an elevation in serum 1,25(OH)2D concentration and an increase in bone formation parameters. PTHrP activates the PTH receptor and mimics the biological effects of PTH on bone, kidney, and the gut.[221] It stimulates osteoclastic bone resorption and promotes renal tubular calcium reabsorption.

PTHrP has a critical role in local osteolysis[221] and in the regulation of chondrocyte proliferation and differentiation.[229,230] Genetic manipulations of the PTHrP, PTH, and the PTH/PTHrP receptor genes, respectively, have demonstrated the critical role of these proteins in regulating both the switch between proliferation and differentiation of chondrocytes, and their replacement by bone cells.[231] In cultures of fetal rat long bones, PTHrP causes a rise in cAMP concentration and bone resorption, which is qualitatively and quantitatively similar to that induced by PTH. It is possible that PTH and PTHrP act on the same receptor.[232] In vivo rat experiments also demonstrate PTHrP effects to be similar to PTH, namely increased bone resorption and formation (by histomorphometric techniques), and hypercalcemia and hypophosphatemia.[233] Inactivation of PTHrP gene in mice leads to severe chondrodysplasia and premature epiphyseal closure, supporting the role of PTHrP in bone and cartilage development. Karaplis[234] demonstrated lethal skeletal dysplasia from targeted disruption of the parathyroid hormone-related peptide gene. Mutations in the PTH/PTHrP receptor have been identified as the cause of Jansen metaphyseal chondrodysplasia and Blomstrand's lethal chondrodysplasia, dwarfing conditions associated with delays in growth plate mineralization and hypercalcemia.[231] There is decreased expression of PTHrP in achondroplasia and a potential salutary effect by addition of PTHrP or IGF-1.[235]

PTHrP is produced in the fetal parathyroid glands and placenta and may be responsible for stimulation of placental calcium transport. The midregion peptide of PTHrP is essential to maintain the calcium gradient across the placenta. PTHrP gene is expressed in the rat myometrium, with a major peak in PTHrP mRNA expression occurring in the 48 hours immediately preceding parturition.[236] PTHrP mRNA has been demonstrated in the myometrium by in situ hybridization histochemistry. The rise in myometrial PTHrP mRNA in late gestation was dependent on intrauterine occupancy; the myometrium of nongravid uterine horns had greatly reduced or absent PTHrP mRNA. It is possible that the expression of the PTHrP gene in the myometrium is dependent on local factors. PTHrP has been demonstrated in human fetal tissues, serum and amniotic fluid.[237,238]

PTHrP has a role in the development of mammary glands. It is expressed in lactating rat mammary glands after suckling, possibly as a result of rises in serum prolactin concentration rather than suckling per se.[239] Thiede and Rodan found PTHrP mRNA and PTH-like bioactivity in the breast tissue of lactating mice. Although several studies demonstrated significant amounts of PTHrP in breast milk,[240–242] the precise role of PTHrP in breast milk remains unclear. PTHrP may play a role in stimulating calcium transport into breast milk, and it may enhance intestinal calcium absorption in breastfeeding infants.[240] Lactation is associated with a rapid, but reversible, reduction in bone mass due to accelerated bone resorption.[243,244] Nursing women lose 6–8% of vertebral bone mass during the first 6 postpartum months. This bone loss during lactation is not dependent on either of the classical calciotropic hormones, vitamin D and PTH.[243–245] Regulation of bone loss in this setting has remained enigmatic. Sowers[246] reported a negative correlation between bone mass and PTHrP levels in lactating women. Several lines of evidence have suggested that PTHrP might be a mediator of increased bone resorption,[246–251] yet not all data support this hypothesis.[252,253]

Some authors suggest an endocrine role for PTHrP during lactation. Concurrent with increases in systemic PTHrP levels, hypoparathyroid patients have been shown to require reductions in doses of calcium and vitamin D during lactation.[254,255] During lactation, large amounts of calcium are transferred to milk by a poorly understood mechanism. This demand results in negative calcium balance in lactating mothers and is associated with rapid bone loss. VanHouten[256] demonstrated that PTHrP production and calcium transport in mammary epithelial cells are regulated by extracellular calcium acting through the calcium-sensing receptor (CaR). The CaR becomes expressed on mammary epithelial cells at the transition from pregnancy to lactation. Increasing concentrations of calcium suppress PTHrP secretion by mammary epithelial cells in vitro, whereas in vivo, systemic hypocalcemia increases PTHrP production. Hypocalcemia also reduces overall milk production and calcium content, presumably through other mechanisms. Thus the lactating mammary gland can sense calcium and adjusts its secretion of calcium and PTHrP in response to changes in extracellular calcium concentration. Some researchers suggest the presence of a homeostatic system that helps to match milk production to the availability of calcium.

The mechanisms of bone loss during lactation are only partly understood. Secretion of PTHrP by lactating mammary glands might regulate bone turnover during lactation. VanHouten[257] demonstrated in mice that removal of PTHrP from the lactating mammary glands resulted in reductions in levels of circulating PTHrP and 1,25 (OH) 2D and urinary cAMP. In addition, bone turnover was reduced and bone loss during lactation was attenuated. Thus it appears that during lactation mammary epithelial cells produce circulating PTHrP that promotes bone loss by increasing rates of bone resorption.

Calcitonin (CT)

Calcitonin is a 32-amino acid polypeptide with a molecular weight of 3500 daltons. It is secreted by the parafollicular C-cells of the thyroid gland which develop embryologically from a neural crest origin.[258] The calcitonin gene peptide superfamily consists of calcitonin (CT), calcitonin gene-related peptide (CGRP), and amylin. CT and CGRP derive from the CT/CGRP gene, which is encoded on chromosome 11. Alternative splicing of the primary RNA transcript leads to the translation of CGRP and CT peptides in a tissue-specific manner.

Secretion of CT is affected by several factors. Serum Ca concentration is the most important regulator of CT secretion. Plasma CT concentration increases when serum ionized Ca concentration rises, and declines when it falls. Secretion of CT is also induced by gastrin, cholecystokinin, and glucagon.[258–260] The physiologic role of these secretagogues in CT regulation is not clear. Vitamin D has a direct regulatory (inhibitory) effect on CT gene expression and CT secretion; receptors for 1,25(OH)2D have been demonstrated on parafollicular C-cells.[261] The CT receptor has been cloned and is structurally similar to the PTH/PTHrP and secretin receptors.[221]

The best recognized physiologic effect of CT is to counteract the action of PTH at several organ sites in the human body. At the bone level, receptors specific for CT have been demonstrated on bone osteoclasts.[262] CT antagonizes PTH-mediated bone resorption by suppressing osteoclastic activity.[263,264] Consequently, CT decreases the flux of Ca and P from bone into the circulation. CT is the most potent peptide inhibitor of osteoclast-mediated bone resorption. Therefore it may have a critical role in protecting the skeleton during periods of "calcium stress" such as growth, pregnancy, and lactation.[191] At the kidney level, CT may enhance Ca, Mg, and P excretion. CT also acts on vitamin D metabolism; it enhances 1,25(OH)2D production by proximal renal tubules.[265,266] The overall effects of CT are to decrease serum Ca and P concentrations.

Calcitonin gene-related peptide

Calcitonin gene-related peptide (CGRP) is another product of the translation of the calcitonin gene.[267] It is a 37 amino acid peptide, which has little amino acid sequence homology with calcitonin and is the most potent endogenous vasodilatory peptide discovered so far. CGRP receptors are widely distributed in the body. CGRP synthesis occurs in neural tissues, where it is likely to have a role in neurotransmission. CGRP causes redistribution of blood flow in humans. Using Doppler techniques, Jager[268] demonstrated that CGRP increases regional blood flow to the brain and the skin at the expense of the gastrointestinal tract. CGRP receptors have been identified in syncytiotrophoblast membranes of the human placenta,[269] but the role of CGRP in perinatal mineral homeostasis is not very well understood.

In rats, CGRP lowers plasma calcium concentration and inhibits bone resorption by isolated rat osteoclasts. Bevis[270] demonstrated that rat CGRP elevates plasma calcium concentration in the chick. In another study, they found that human CGRP (alpha) and PTH produce a concentration-dependent elevation of plasma calcium concentrations. However, the two peptides did not follow precisely the same time course. Whereas at 15 minutes CGRP produced hypocalcemia, at 30 minutes both CGRP and PTH produced hypercalcemia. Bevis and coworkers suggested that CGRP initially interacts with the calcitonin receptor to produce early hypocalcemia due to a calcitonin-like effect, followed by delayed hypercalcemia possibly because of a regulatory effect of CGRP on endogenous circulating calcitonin.

Vitamin D metabolism

The human body obtains vitamin D from two major sources: (a) endogenous from the skin where vitamin D synthesis occurs under the effect of ultraviolet light, and (b) exogenous from dietary vitamin D_2 (derived from plant sterols) and D_3 (from animal or synthetic origin). Vitamins D_2 and D_3 are virtually equipotent in humans and can be included under the general name vitamin D. When present in the diet, fat-soluble vitamin D is efficiently absorbed with neutral lipids in the small intestine and transferred to the lymphatic system in chylomicrons. When formed in the skin, cholecalciferol is transported in blood, bound by an alpha$_2$-globulin, to the liver to undergo further metabolism.[271–273] Normally, in adults at least 90% of vitamin D requirement is provided by endogenous photosynthesis in the skin,[274] which amounts to 2.5–10 ug day^{-1} (100–400 I.U. day^{-1}).[275]

The synthesis of vitamin D comprises a sequence of biochemical reactions in several organs that start with cholesterol and end up with the formation of 1,25(OH)2D, the most active vitamin D metabolite. Under the effect of small intestinal mucosal dehydrogenase, dietary cholesterol is converted into 7-dehydrocholesterol, which is then transported to the Malpighian layer of the skin.[276] Ultraviolet light (of wavelengths 290–320 nm) penetrates the skin to break the C9–C10 bond of 7-dehydrocholesterol (Provitamin D_3) to form pre-vitamin D_3. Pre-vitamin D_3 undergoes several reactions: it may be photoisomerized to lumisterol and tachysterol or converted by a temperature-dependent isomerization to cholecalciferol (vitamin D_3). Cholecalciferol is then released in the circulation where it is bound to vitamin D binding protein and transported to the liver. Less than 1% of vitamin D is free and the rest is bound. Vitamin D is cleared rapidly from the blood and lymphatics in the liver, where it undergoes a first hydroxylation at the carbon in position 25 to yield 25-hydroxyvitamin D, the main circulating form of vitamin D (25-OHD),[277] which is released into the circulation once again before reaching the kidney. Under normal circumstances, circulating concentrations of 25-OHD can be regarded as a good index of overall vitamin D status (sufficiency or insufficiency). In the mitochondria of the proximal nephrons, 25-OHD undergoes 1-alpha-hydroxylation (by a complex cytochrome P mitochondrial enzyme system) to produce 1,25(OH)2D, the most important and biologically active metabolite, that plays a major role in maintaining appropriate blood calcium and phosphorus concentrations,[278] or 24-hydroxylation to form 24,25-dihydroxyvitamin D [24,25(OH)2D]. The role of 24,25(OH)2D in mineral and vitamin D homeostasis is not very well known, but there is evidence that it may have an important role in normal intramembranous bone formation.[279] Reduced serum 24,25(OH)2D concentrations are correlated with histological evidence of bone loss in diabetic rats.[280] The activity of renal 1-alpha hydroxylase is stimulated by PTH,[281] IGF-I,[282] and hypophosphatemia, by periods of high calcium demand such as growth,[283,284] pregnancy, or low calcium intake,[281,284,285] and may be inhibited by calcitonin, 1,25(OH)2D, and other vitamin D metabolites.[286]

Decreased circulating concentrations of calcium increase serum parathyroid hormone (PTH) synthesis and secretion, which in turn stimulates the renal hydroxylation of 25-OHD to 1,25 (OH)2D. High concentrations of 1,25(OH)2D may inhibit the hydroxylation of 25-hydroxyvitamin D and the secretion of PTH. 1,25(OH)2D promotes the active intestinal absorption of calcium and phosphorus and enhances PTH effects on the nephron to promote renal tubular Ca reabsorption; the combined action of 1,25(OH)2D and PTH is to stimulate calcium mobilization from bones.[271–273] Chronic hypomagnesemia may suppress PTH secretion and induce end-organ resistance to the effect of PTH, in particular renal resistance with secondary drop in renal synthesis of 1,25(OH)2D.[287] Magnesium supplementation restores parathyroid and calcitriol responses to low calcium diet.[288]

Calcitriol [1,25(OH)2D] is the major active vitamin D metabolite. It acts on several organ systems where specific vitamin D receptors are located: gut, bone, kidney, parathyroid glands, and immune system.[289] It increases calcium and phosphorus absorption from the small intestine[290] and the kidney tubules, mobilizes Ca and P from bone, and induces a specific calcium-binding protein in the intestines, calbindin D. Calcitriol may have a synergistic effect with PTH in stimulating osteoclastic bone resorption. Calcitriol also has an anabolic effect on bone. It stimulates osteoblastic activity and bone formation, directly through its effects on osteoblasts, and possibly indirectly through its stimulation of prostaglandin E2 secretion.[291]

Calcitriol has a regulatory effect on PTH and CT gene transcription: it decreases PTH mRNA and CT mRNA concentrations in vitro and in vivo in rats. In humans with secondary hyperparathyroidism, intravenous 1,25(OH)2D administration leads to a marked reduction in serum PTH concentration.[292] Oral administration of calcitriol to children with hypophosphatemic rickets and secondary hyperparathyroidism also has an inhibitory effect on PTH secretion.[293] Calcitriol upregulates its own receptor in the parathyroid glands: in vivo and in vitro 1,25(OH)2D administration increases the concentration of vitamin D receptor mRNA in the parathyroid gland.[289]

Perinatal mineral and vitamin D homeostasis

Maternal physiology

Pregnancy is associated with a number of physiological adaptations that provide an optimal milieu for fetal growth and preservation of maternal homeostasis.[294,295] The extracellular fluid compartment expands, and renal blood flow and glomerular filtration rate increase. Serum total Ca concentration decreases gradually throughout pregnancy parallel to serum albumin concentration, reaching a nadir by the mid-third of gestation and rising slightly thereafter. In contrast, serum ionized Ca remains constant or drops slightly after 30 weeks gestation and postpartum. Martinez[296] demonstrated lower serum ionized Ca concentrations in the second and third trimesters of pregnancy, and at delivery. Serum P concentration also declines during pregnancy and parallels that of serum Ca.

Studies applying radioimmunoassays (targeting the amino terminal) demonstrated that serum PTH concentration may rise during pregnancy and a state of "physiological hyperparathyroidism" appears to set in,[297] possibly a response to compensate for the increasing transfer of Ca from the mother to the fetus across the placenta. However, such RIAs are insensitive and often detect inactive PTH fragments, so that the correlation between PTH immunoreactivity and bioactivity is poor. Newer studies using immunoradiometric assay (IRMA) of the intact PTH molecule reported a gestational drop,[298] no change,[299] or a rise in serum PTH concentration. In a longitudinal study from Denmark, serum PTH rose significantly from 13 to 36 weeks gestation and continued for 12 months postpartum. In other studies, serum PTH declined toward mid-pregnancy and increased thereafter.[300]

Gallacher[299] demonstrated that serum PTHrP and alkaline phosphatase concentrations rose during pregnancy. Serum osteocalcin and PTH concentrations remained unchanged during pregnancy but rose significantly postpartum. Martinez[300] investigated perinatal calciotropic hormones in normal as well as diabetic pregnancies. In normal pregnant women serum PTH concentrations increased during the third trimester and total calcitriol increased at delivery. Serum osteocalcin concentrations decreased in the second trimester but returned to normal values during the third trimester. In contrast, in diabetic women serum PTH concentration remained constant throughout pregnancy, serum calcitriol concentration increased to a smaller extent, serum osteocalcin concentrations in the second and third trimester were lower. Infants of diabetic mothers showed lower PTH and osteocalcin concentrations than infants of normal pregnant women, whereas their serum calcitriol concentrations were similar. From these data it appears that diabetes mellitus decreases bone turnover during pregnancy in the mother and during the neonatal period in their offspring.

Serum CT does not change significantly during pregnancy but serum CGRP concentration shows a significant increase during pregnancy and a fall to preconceptional values after delivery.[301] Halhali[302] demonstrated significantly lower circulating PTHrP and CGRP concentrations in women with preeclampsia, which may contribute to the development and maintenance of hypertension during pregnancy. Magnesium sulfate treatment resulted in a significant increase in maternal circulating CGRP but not PTHrP concentrations.

Maternal serum 25-OHD concentration is little affected during pregnancy. It is mainly influenced by ultraviolet light exposure and dietary vitamin D intake. Serum vitamin D binding protein concentration doubles during pregnancy.

Nevertheless, toward the end of human pregnancy, there is an increase in the amount of free 1,25(OH)2D. At term, concentrations of free 1,25(OH)2D in plasma of mother and fetus are correlated.[303] Serum concentration of calcitriol is high early in pregnancy and rises steadily with advancing gestation.[304–306] This is explained partly because of a rise in vitamin D binding-protein concentration and possibly from rises in serum PTH concentration, and is thought to increase the synthesis of intestinal calcium binding proteins and intestinal absorption of calcium and phosphorus, to meet the mineral requirements of the developing fetus. Further, placental tissues are capable of 1-alpha-hydroxylation of 25-OHD and may significantly contribute to the rise in serum 1,25(OH)2D concentration during pregnancy.[307–309] This mechanism is supported by the fact that patients with pseudohypoparathyroidism who previously required vitamin D therapy were able to maintain normal serum 1,25(OH)2D and Ca concentrations during pregnancy even without vitamin D therapy.

Although most studies have found that serum concentrations of calcitriol are not increased in lactating women[310–314] there appears to be a small trend of increasing calcitriol concentrations over the course of lactation.[315–317] In Kalkwarf's study,[316] serum calcitriol concentrations increased over the course of lactation, were 16% greater in lactating than in nonlactating postpartum women by 6 months postpartum, and did not correlate with bone density changes in lactating women.[318] Kalkwarf et al.[319] found that the increase in calcitriol after weaning was associated with increased intestinal calcium absorption. The first 3–6 mo of lactation are, or can be, associated with increased renal conservation of calcium, phosphorus, and magnesium but not with increased intestinal absorption of these minerals.[321]

Early in pregnancy serum osteocalcin concentration is low and declines further towards mid-pregnancy.[322,323] Then it increases in late pregnancy. Serum osteocalcin concentration declined from the first trimester until term and acutely increased in the puerperium.[324] Rodin[323] demonstrated a significant rise in serum bone alkaline phosphatase during the third trimester suggesting increased bone turnover. Osteocalcin values declined in the second trimester, but returned to nonpregnant levels late in the third trimester. Osteocalcin does not cross the placenta.[295] In Cole's study[322] no significant correlations were found between maternal osteocalcin concentrations and serum phosphorus, alkaline phosphatase, or iPTH, but significant negative correlations were found between osteocalcin and total calcium and total protein. Serum osteocalcin and ICTP concentrations are elevated in pregnant women with pre-eclampsia suggesting alterations in bone metabolism with pre-eclampsia.[325]

In a longitudinal study Naylor[326] evaluated changes in bone mineral density (BMD) and bone turnover during pregnancy and postpartum. They measured total-body BMD and biochemical markers of bone resorption (urinary pyridinium crosslinks and telopeptides of type I collagen) and bone formation (serum bone alkaline phosphatase, propeptides of type I procollagen (PINP) and osteocalcin), as well as maternal serum PTH, IGF-I, and human placental lactogen. Postpartum, BMD increased in the arms and legs but decreased in the pelvis and spine compared with prepregnancy values. All biochemical markers, with the exception of osteocalcin concentration, increased during pregnancy. The change in IGF-I at 36 weeks was related to the change in biochemical markers. These findings indicate that pregnancy is a high-bone-turnover state, that IGF-I levels may be an important determinant of bone turnover during pregnancy, and that elevated bone turnover may explain trabecular bone loss during pregnancy.

Maternal serum osteocalcin concentrations increased sharply after delivery,[295,322] yet serum iPTH concentrations remained normal. There was no correlation between serum osteocalcin and calcium or iPTH concentrations in lactating women. These changes are compatible with a sequence in which bone turnover is reduced during early pregnancy, rebounds in the third trimester, and increases in postpartum lactating women to meet calcium needs of the fetus during the third trimester and the nursing infant.[322] Salle[295] suggests that low osteocalcin concentrations during pregnancy may be due to placental trapping as there is evidence of high osteocalcin content measured in the placenta.

In another longitudinal study,[327] serum 1,25(OH)2D concentration was high early in pregnancy and increased with advancing gestation. Parathyroid hormone and osteocalcin levels were low in early pregnancy. They declined toward the middle of pregnancy, but increased in late pregnancy. In contrast to Cole's study, the serum osteocalcin level correlated with the parathyroid hormone level at the end of the pregnancy. Serum PTHrP concentration remains constant during pregnancy.[328]

More[329] evaluated bone turnover during pregnancy and 1 year postpartum. Bone turnover markers (PICP, OC, BSAP, urine deoxypyridinoline) increased during pregnancy and failed to reach baseline level even 12 months postpartum. There was a significant increase in PTH concentrations at 12 months postpartum although they remained within normal range. Urinary calcium/creatinine and serum calcium, phosphate and 25-OHD concentrations remained constant. From these findings the authors concluded that the calcium needed for infant growth during pregnancy and lactation may be drawn at least in part from the maternal skeleton.

The synthesis of osteocalcin by osteoblasts is stimulated by the action of 1,25(OH)2D, and serum osteocalcin levels are also related to the levels of parathyroid hormone. During early and mid pregnancy, the stimulatory effect of 1,25(OH)2D on the synthesis of osteocalcin may be overridden by the inhibitory effect of declining parathyroid hormone levels. The increase in osteocalcin level in late pregnancy may be a consequence of increasing levels of both parathyroid hormone and 1,25(OH)2D. PTH may influence the synthesis of osteocalcin indirectly by increasing osteoclast-mediated bone resorption. 1,25(OH)2D directly increases the synthesis of osteocalcin.

Pregnancy is stressful to maternal bone because it consumes a significant part of maternal mineral stores. Significant calcium transfer from mother to fetus or infant occurs during pregnancy and lactation. During pregnancy, intestinal calcium absorption increases to meet much of the fetal calcium needs. Maternal bone loss also may occur in the last months of pregnancy, a time when the fetal skeleton is rapidly mineralizing. As much as 10 g of net bone loss may occur during normal pregnancy. However, it is regained by the end of lactation.

Lactating women secrete approximately 250 mg of calcium in breast milk each day with some women having losses as much as 450 mg day^{-1}.[320] Maternal calcium need for breast milk production is met through increased renal calcium conservation and, to a greater extent, by mobilization of calcium from the maternal skeleton. Women experience a transient loss of approx 3%–9% of their bone density during lactation, which is regained after weaning 12–18 months postpartum. In contrast, non-lactating postpartum women have little change in their bone density during this same period.

The rate and extent of recovery are influenced by the duration of lactation and postpartum amenorrhea and differ by skeletal site studied. Additional calcium intake does not prevent bone loss during lactation or enhance the recovery after weaning. The recovery of bone is complete for most women and occurs even with shortly spaced pregnancies. Lactation-induced bone loss appears to be obligatory and under hormonal regulation, as it occurs even when calcium intake is high. Bone mineral is recovered after lactation ceases or menses resumes. Current data point to estrogen and PTHrP as regulating bone mobilization during lactation. The typical calcium regulatory hormones, parathyroid hormone, calcitriol, and calcitonin, do not appear to stimulate bone resorption during lactation. Restoration of ovarian hormone production and decreased production of PTHrP are likely to result in the recovery of bone mineral after lactation has ceased. Epidemiological studies have found that pregnancy and lactation are not associated with an increased risk of osteoporotic fractures.[318] In most recent studies serum PTH concentrations were moderately suppressed during lactation, especially early lactation, or unchanged;[253,313,315,330] and there was no correlation between serum PTH and bone changes during lactation.[246,316] Further, there is an increasing awareness of the clinical benefits of optimal calcium and magnesium homeostasis in the perinatal period. Calcium supplementation during pregnancy has been associated with lower incidence of prematurity and pregnancy-induced hypertension (PIH), possibly due to a relaxing effect of calcium on vascular smooth muscle fibers.[331] Trials of magnesium supplementation during pregnancy showed decreased incidence of PIH and prematurity.[332] Recently, Koo et al. demonstrated that maternal calcium supplementation of up to 2 g day^{-1} during the second and third trimesters can increase fetal bone mineralization in women with low dietary calcium intake. However, calcium supplementation in pregnant women with adequate dietary calcium intake is unlikely to result in major improvement in fetal bone mineralization.[333] Changes in bone turnover, and consequent bone loss and recovery during lactation and the postweaning period, are likely modulated by varying estrogen levels during these periods. Bone loss most likely occurs in the beginning of the postpartum period.

Holmberg-Marttila[334] measured serum biochemical markers of bone formation (bone-specific ALP, PICP, osteocalcin), of bone resorption (ICTP), and serum female sex hormones (estradiol, luteinizing hormone, and follicle-stimulating hormone) in healthy mothers postpartum and for 1 year after resumption of menses. During postpartum amenorrhea bone mineral density decreased significantly, but subsequently recovered. Bone turnover marker concentrations were elevated at parturition and still at the end of postpartum amenorrhea. Subsequent to parturition bone resorption marker concentration showed a decreasing trend while bone formation marker concentrations continued increasing over the first few months postpartum. Both lactation and hormonal status modulated bone turnover marker levels.

Fetal physiology

Fetal mineral homeostasis is closely linked to that of the mother. In the pregnant woman and the fetus there is an intimate and delicate relationship amongst the calciotropic hormones PTH, CT, calcitriol, and possibly PTHrP and the minerals Ca, P, and Mg. Any perturbation of maternal homeostatic mineral balance may affect that of the fetus

and may have metabolic sequelae on the fetus, manifesting in the neonatal period and infancy. The fetus relies on maternal resources to acquire minerals and vitamin D metabolites that are indispensable for optimal fetal mineral and bone homeostasis. In the rat, radiocalcium studies demonstrated that up to 92% of fetal calcium is acquired from maternal diet. In human pregnancy, stable calcium isotope studies demonstrated doubling of intestinal absorption from the end of the second trimester to term. Little transfer of minerals occurs during early gestation in rats and humans. Fetal acquisition of these minerals increases exponentially during gestation, and most remarkably during the third trimester. There is enough evidence showing that minerals, primarily Ca, P,[335,336] and Mg, are actively transported across the placenta from maternal to fetal circulation against a concentration gradient.

In humans cord blood Ca concentration at birth exceeds the corresponding maternal blood Ca concentration throughout the third trimester of pregnancy.[328,337,338] Serum total calcium concentration in the fetus as estimated by cord blood analysis is 5.5 mg dL^{-1} in the second trimester and approaches 11 mg dL^{-1} by the end of the third trimester.[294] It is possible that the rising fetal serum Ca concentration during pregnancy, in parallel with fetal Ca accretion, will facilitate deposition of Ca into rapidly growing and ossifying bone.[338] This is supported by finding higher serum osteocalcin and urine pyridinoline in the newborn than the mother.[338] The recent findings of higher serum calcium and osteocalcin but lower serum PTH concentrations in cord blood than in maternal circulation at delivery, and higher urine pyridinoline concentrations in the newborn than in the mother are consistent with increased fetal bone turnover in the last trimester. Atalas[337] also demonstrated higher osteocalcin concentration in cord blood than maternal blood at delivery.

Seki[328] demonstrated higher serum total and ionic calcium and PTHrP and lower PTH concentrations in cord blood compared with maternal blood. Higher PTHrP concentration in umbilical arterial blood than in umbilical venous blood is consistent with fetal production of PTHrP which stimulates placental calcium transfer from mother to fetus in animals and probably humans. Cord blood P[337] and Mg concentrations at birth are higher than corresponding maternal blood concentrations. In contrast to serum Ca concentration which increases with increasing gestational age, cord blood serum P concentration decreases from about 14 mg dL^{-1} in the second trimester to about 6 mg dL^{-1} at term.[294] Yet, total body P content increases directly with increasing gestational age.

The chemical analysis of dead fetuses at different gestational ages for Ca, Mg, and P[7] made possible a rough estimation of the fetal mineral accretion rate during pregnancy. The fetal accretion rate for these minerals increases exponentially during the last trimester of pregnancy (24–38 weeks). The peak mineral accretion rate is reached at 34–36 weeks' gestation and amounts to 117 mg of Ca, 74 mg of P, and 2.7 mg of Mg per kg fetal weight day^{-1}. In fact, more than two-thirds of fetal body calcium content is acquired during the third trimester of gestation at a rate of up to 150 mg kg^{-1} day^{-1}.[12]

In cord blood, the concentrations of Ca, Ca^{++}, P, Mg, CT and iPRL are all higher, and the concentrations of PTH lower than in the maternal blood. There is a significant positive correlation between cord Ca^{++} and maternal Ca or Ca^{++}, and a significant negative correlation between Ca^{++} and iPRL in cord blood, which may be consistent with an inhibitory effect of relative hypercalcemia on PRL secretion in the fetus.[339] The placenta plays a major role in regulating the active transfer of minerals from mother to fetus. Calcium transport across the placenta to the fetus may involve an ATPase-dependent active transport mechanism.[340,341] Receptors for calcitriol[342] and PTH[343] have been demonstrated on placental cells. Calcium binding proteins (CaBP) may play a significant role in perinatal mineral homeostasis. These proteins are primarily synthesized by calcium transporting tissues such as intestine, kidney, and placenta. They have been isolated from mouse and mammalian kidneys, mammalian placenta[344] and yolk sac, rat uterus and growth cartilage and osteoblasts, brain, pancreas, lung, and avian eggshell gland of the egg-laying hen. Major subclasses of calbindins are calbindin D9k in mammals and calbindin D28k in avian and other species. Synthesis of intestinal and renal calbindins is vitamin D dependent and calbindin concentrations rise in response to rising blood concentration of 1,25(OH)2D in pregnancy. The concentration of these peptides is tightly regulated by vitamin D status: vitamin D deficiency reduces their concentrations while vitamin D supplementation increases their concentrations. A high-calcium diet suppresses PTH and 1,25(OH)2D synthesis and intestinal CaBP concentrations and calcium absorption. In rat and mice, intestinal CaBP concentration increases progressively with advancing gestation, reaching a peak concentration in late gestation at a time when calcium transfer to the fetus and fetal bone mineralization are at their highest rate. Peak intestinal CaBP concentrations parallel those of maternal plasma 1,25(OH)2D concentrations and maternal intestinal calcium absorption.

Placental calcium binding protein (CaBP) is similar but not identical to intestinal calcium binding protein.[344] Placental CaBP concentration increases with gestation in parallel with the increasing transplacental calcium transfer to the fetus.[345] Theoretically, in analogy with intestinal CaBP, placental CaBP which is also 1,25(OH)2D-dependent[345–347] may play a role in the regulation of transplacental calcium transfer to the fetus, particularly because its concentration increases late in gestation in parallel with 1,25(OH)2D.

Fetal bone physiology is not completely understood. Most of the body minerals are stored in bone, which serves both as a mechanical support organ and as a metabolic reservoir for these minerals. Osteocalcin is a major component of the noncollagenous bone proteins and a sensitive indicator of osteoblastic activity. Immunocytochemical localization of osteocalcin in human fetal bones has been demonstrated as early as 12 weeks of development.[348] These studies demonstrate that osteocalcin is most actively synthesized by osteoblasts early in fetal life, and then is deposited on collagen fibers of the osteoid and bone matrix by 17 weeks of gestation. Localization of calbindins in bone and cartilage may potentially mean they have a significant role in bone formation and ossification. Calbindins have been immunocytochemically localized to chondrocytes of the growth plate in rats and chick, and rat and human osteoblasts. Calbindin D9k has been localized in the cytoplasm of maturing rat chondrocytes, and in the extracellular lateral edges of longitudinal septa, where mineralization of cartilage is initiated and where matrix vesicles are preferentially located. From these studies it is suggested that calbindins may be involved in cartilage ossification. From several immunocytochemical studies it appears that calbindins play a role in the movement of intracellular calcium in the chondrocyte and in the movement of calcium toward extracellular sites of calcification in the growth plate.

Perinatal placental physiology

The placenta transfers calcium ions from mother to fetus against a concentration gradient resulting in relative fetal hypercalcemia, and higher cord blood calcium concentration than in maternal blood.[349,350] In the rat, calcium fluxes are bi-directional and passive transfer accounts for the majority of placental calcium movement; however, an additional active component results in a net calcium movement favoring calcium deposition in the fetus. It is unclear whether bi-directional fluxes of calcium across the placenta exist in the human, or whether transport is entirely unidirectional from mother to fetus. Evidence supports an active energy-dependent process of transplacental Ca transfer to the fetus.[351,352] An intrinsic placental calcium binding protein (CaBP, calbindin) has been demonstrated in animals.[353,354] Calbindin synthesis is vitamin D-dependent: these proteins are present only in the presence of specific receptors for 1,25(OH)2D, which have been demonstrated in human placenta[355] and human fetal gut.[356] Calcium-dependent adenosine triphosphatase systems have been demonstrated in animal as well as in human placental tissue[357–359] and calcium ions have been localized in placental plasma membrane vesicles and mitochondria within the fetal capillary endothelium. It is likely that calbindin may play a significant role in the active transplacental transport of calcium to the fetus. Phosphorus and magnesium are also actively transported across the placenta to the fetus although the exact molecular mechanisms involved are unclear.[349,350,360]

The plasma Ca concentration of the fetus is maintained higher than maternal levels by active placental transport. Ca, Mg, and PO4 accumulation by the fetus is mainly associated with skeletal growth. The fetal parathyroid glands are essential for maintenance of elevated plasma Ca, which is necessary for the stimulation of fetal osteoblasts and mineralization of cartilage and osteoid. Theoretically, since PTH does not cross the placenta,[361–363] the relative fetal hypercalcemia should suppress the fetal parathyroid glands. Paradoxically, fetal PTH secretion is not suppressed. Cord blood PTH concentrations are lower than,[364–367] or similar to[368–370] maternal values in paired maternal samples. The inconsistency in PTH assay results stems from the use of different PTH antisera; assays may detect the amino- or carboxy-terminal or midmolecule of the PTH molecule. A possible explanation for the nonsuppressible PTH secretion, despite relative fetal hypercalcemia, is that the negative feedback system regulating PTH secretion by calcium concentration operates with a higher "set-point" in the fetus in such a way that suppression of PTH secretion in the fetus requires higher serum calcium concentrations than after birth. Although serum PTH concentrations by radioimmunoassay are often lower in the fetus than in the mother, PTH-like bioactivity, measured by a sensitive cytochemical assay, is higher in the fetus than in the mother.[371]

It is possible that PTH or PTH-related peptide (PTHrP) may have a significant role in placental transport of calcium.[372,373] Receptors for PTH have been demonstrated in human placenta.[343] Transcription and splicing of the PTHrP gene give rise to three peptides consisting of 139, 141, and 173 amino acids respectively. The amino-terminal 13 amino acids of each of these peptides are 70% homologous with the corresponding region of PTH. Unlike PTH, of which synthesis in normal subjects is restricted to the parathyroid glands, PTHrP messenger RNA is widely distributed in normal tissues, including the skin, thyroid, bone marrow, hypothalamus, pituitary, parathyroid, adrenal cortex, adrenal medulla, and stomach.[374] In thyroparathyroidectomized (with thyroxine replacement) pregnant sheep, fetal parathyroidectomy results in acute drop in fetal serum calcium concentration and a reversal of the maternal fetal calcium gradient; the lambs are born rachitic.[375] Interestingly, parathyroid extracts but not immunoreactive PTH infusions normalize the maternal fetal calcium gradient. From these experiments it was suggested that PTHrP might have a putative role in maintaining the transplacental maternal fetal calcium gradient.[376] It is interesting to note that PTHrP (1–34) is ineffective in increasing calcium transport across the sheep placenta, whereas PTHrP (1–84), PTHrP (1–108), and PTHrP (1–141) are effective, suggesting that specific receptors for PTHrP bind to the protein at a site distal to amino acid 34.[377]

MacIsaac et al.[378] demonstrated that fetal thyroparathyroidectomy results in decreased placental Ca transfer. Extracts of fetal parathyroid glands and purified PTHrP, as well as recombinant PTHrP (1–84, 1–108 and 1–141), stimulate Ca and Mg but not P transport across the placenta of thyroparathyroidectomized fetuses. Parathyroid hormone (PTH) and the N-terminal region of PTHrP do not stimulate placental Ca and Mg transport. The authors of these studies concluded that a mid-molecule region of PTHrP may be required to stimulate placental Ca transfer and contribute to the regulation of fetal Ca homeostasis.

Both PTH and PTHrP may have a significant role in promoting normal fetal bone mineralization.[379,380] PTH-deficient fetal mice have diminished cartilage matrix mineralization and reduced metaphyseal osteoblasts and trabecular bone, whereas mice lacking PTHrP died at birth with dyschondroplasia. From fetal mice experiments[380,381] it appears that (1) both PTH and PTHrP have a significant role in fetal blood calcium homeostasis; (2) PTHrP may play a more dominant role than PTH in regulation of placental calcium transfer, and differentiation of the cartilaginous growth plate into endochondral bone; (3) PTH may play a more dominant role than PTHrP in regulating fetal blood calcium; (4) blood calcium and PTH levels are rate-limiting determinants of skeletal mineral accretion; and (5) PTH is essential for skeletal mineralization. Fetal mice deficient in both PTH and PTHrP have severe growth restriction, limb shortening, greater reduction of fetal blood calcium, and reduced mineralization.

In the human fetus, the thyroid C-cells appear to be well developed by 14 weeks of gestation.[382] However, the role of CT in fetal mineral and bone homeostasis is not very well understood. Maternal serum calcitonin concentration may be elevated or unchanged during pregnancy. Calcitonin does not cross the placenta,[383] and, as with PTH, fetal CT function may be autonomous from that of the mother. Fetal production of CT is indirectly inferred from the observations that cord blood CT concentrations are significantly higher than corresponding maternal values in all trimesters,[383–389] and that arterial cord blood CT is higher than venous cord blood concentration.[383] The human fetal thyroid contains a larger number of C-cells than the adult thyroid.[390] Immunocytochemical evidence for CT in the thyroid gland has been demonstrated and confirmed by direct radioimmunoassay in human[391] fetuses. Because cord blood CT concentrations are elevated at birth in term and preterm infants[392] and presumably during the last trimester of gestation, it is speculated that elevated fetal blood CT concentration may play a significant role in promoting fetal bone mineralization.[393] In rats, thyroidectomy of the pregnant rat results in lower bone density. Calcitonin possibly plays a role in protecting bone mineralization in the mother as well as in the fetus.

The role of vitamin D metabolites in fetal mineral homeostasis is not completely understood.[294,295] There is evidence that vitamin D metabolites are necessary for optimal fetal and maternal bone mineralization. The fetus is entirely dependent on the mother for its supply of 25(OH)2D, which is believed to cross the placenta.[295] Serum concentrations of 25(OH)2D are a rate-limiting factor in the synthesis of 1,25(OH)2D by the kidneys as well as by decidual cells of the placenta to permit increased calcium absorption during pregnancy. Vitamin D deficiency results in osteomalacia and rickets in the mother and the infant respectively and can be prevented by dietary vitamin D supplementation. The fetus is totally dependent on maternal supplies of vitamin D. In humans, a supplement of 400 IU of vitamin D per day results in normal serum vitamin D concentration in the pregnant woman.[394]

Normally, the human newborn has undetectable plasma vitamin D concentration. Placental transfer of radiolabelled vitamin D has been assessed in the rat and the sheep.[395,396] These studies demonstrated limited placental transfer of vitamin D from maternal to fetal circulation: less than 10% of vitamin D activity was present in rat fetus in the form of unchanged vitamin D (5% in the sheep). The major vitamin D metabolite that crosses the placenta is 25-OHD in all species studied.[395,397,398]

Maternal serum 25-OHD concentration is mainly influenced by dietary vitamin D intake and ultraviolet light exposure. Serum concentration of calcitriol rises steadily in pregnancy, and is thought to increase the synthesis of intestinal calcium binding proteins and intestinal absorption of calcium and phosphorus, to meet the mineral requirements of the developing fetus. Fetal or cord plasma 25-OHD concentrations are lower than, and correlate positively with corresponding maternal plasma concentration,[360,387,388,399] supporting the thesis that fetal and neonatal plasma 25-OHD concentrations are dependent on maternal 25-OHD status. Although pregnancy in animals (sheep, rats, rabbits) is associated with a drop in plasma

25-OHD concentrations, presumably because of increased utilization of 25-OHD for synthesis of 1,25(OH)2D, this effect is not apparent in human pregnancy.

In animals and humans, cord plasma 24,25(OH)2D concentrations are lower than corresponding maternal values.[387,388,400] It is not known whether the origin of fetal 24,25(OH)2D is from endogenous fetal synthesis, or from maternal origin. Fetoplacental tissues have the enzymatic system to synthesize 24,25(OH)2D in vitro,[395,398,401] and there is evidence that fetoplacental synthesis of this compound may occur in vivo, at least in rats. Salle found that placental vein 25-hydroxyvitamin D and 24,25-dihydroxyvitamin D concentrations correlate significantly with those found in the maternal circulation, implying that these two secosteroids diffuse easily across the placental barrier and that the vitamin D metabolite pool of the fetus depends entirely on that of the mother.[295] However, the role of this metabolite in human fetal mineral and bone homeostasis is not known.

The role of 1,25(OH)2D in the fetal handling of calcium and other minerals is at present controversial. Maternal serum calcitriol concentrations are elevated during pregnancy possibly to increase maternal intestinal absorption of calcium to meet the requirements during pregnancy for fetal bone mineralization. There is no general agreement regarding transplacental passage of maternal 1,25(OH)2D.[387,403] In a longitudinal study of perinatal vitamin D homeostasis[404] four common vitamin D metabolites – 25-OHD, 1,25(OH)2D, 24,25(OH)2D, and 25,26(OH)2D – were determined simultaneously in mothers and infants from delivery to several months postpartum. At delivery, total vitamin D metabolites in maternal and fetal plasma were closely correlated, maternal concentrations being higher. Free (nonprotein bound) vitamin D metabolite concentrations were higher in fetal than in maternal plasma, except for free 1,25(OH)2D concentrations which were equal. Therefore transplacental maternal fetal transfer of 25-OHD, 24,25(OH)2D, and 25,26(OH)2D may be effected by an active transport system and that of 1,25(OH)2D by a passive transport system. With pharmacologic administration of 1,25(OH)2D in the mother for treatment of hypoparathyroidism, transplacental transfer of 1,25(OH)2D may occur.[295]

Longitudinal study of calcium homeostasis and bone metabolism during pregnancy, lactation, and postweaning was done by Cross and coworkers.[405] Maternal fractional intestinal calcium absorption and concentrations of 1,25(OH)2D were higher in the second and third trimesters. Total urinary calcium was higher during pregnancy and lower postweaning. Parathyroid hormone (PTH) concentrations were higher only postweaning. Markers of bone turnover increased in the third trimester and during lactation for serum tartrate resistant acid phosphatase, bone specific alkaline phosphatase, and urinary deoxypyridinoline. Serum procollagen I carboxypeptides increased only in the third trimester. Bone mineral density by single-photon absorptiometry did not differ by period. Absorption and urinary excretion of calcium increased during pregnancy, whereas bone turnover increased during late pregnancy and lactation, and renal changes consistent with an increase in PTH were seen postweaning.

In a longitudinal study[406] of calcium homeostasis during pregnancy and lactation and after the resumption of menses, Ritchie *et al.* concluded that fetal calcium demand is met by increased maternal intestinal absorption during pregnancy, and calcium supply for lactation was provided by postpartum maternal renal calcium conservation and an increase in maternal bone turnover resulting in reduced bone density, that was recovered 5 months after lactation was discontinued. Similarly, O'Brien *et al.* demonstrated that intestinal calcium absorption in adolescents was significantly higher during the third trimester of pregnancy than in the early postpartum period, and higher calcium intakes during pregnancy appeared to be protective against loss of trabecular bone at the lumbar spine.[407]

REFERENCES

1 Itani, O., Tsang, R. Calcium, phosphorus and magnesium in the newborn: pathophysiology and management. In Hay, W., ed. *Neonatal Nutrition and Metabolism*. St. Louis: Mosby-Year Book; 1991:171–202.

2 Itani, O., Tsang, R. C. Calcium and mineral metabolism in the fetus. In Thorburn, G. D., Harding, R., eds. *Textbook of Fetal Physiology*. Oxford: Oxford University Press; 1994:368–87.

3 Itani, O., Mehta, K., Tsang, R. C. Calcium, phosphorus and magnesium in parenteral nutrition. In Baker, R., Baker, S., Davis, A., eds. *Pediatric Parenteral Nutrition*. New York: Chapman & Hall; 1997:149–74.

4 Itani, O., Tsang, R. C. Bone disease. In Kaplan, L. A., Pesce, A. J., eds. *Clinical Chemistry: Theory, Analysis and Correlation*. 4th edn. St. Louis: Mosby-Year Book; 2003:507–34.

5 Koo, W. K., Tsang, R. C. Building better bones: calcium, magnesium, phosphorus and vitamin D. In Tsang, R. C., Zlotkin, S. H., Nichols, B. L., Hansen, J. W., eds. *Nutrition During Infancy*. Cincinnati, OH: Digital Educational Publishing, Inc.; 1997:175–207.

6 Koo, W. K., Tsang, R. C. Calcium, magnesium, phosphorus and vitamin D. In Tsang, R., Lucas, A., Uauy, R., Zlotkin, S., eds. *Nutritional Needs of the Preterm Infant: Scientific Basis and Practical Guidelines*. Baltimore: Williams & Wilkins, Inc.; 1993:135–55.

7 Widdowson, E., Spray, C. Chemical development in utero. *Arch. Dis. Child.* 1951;**26**:205–14.

8 Widdowson, E. M., Southgate, D. A., Hey, E. Fetal growth and body composition. In Linblad, B. S., ed. *Perinatal Nutrition*. New York: Academic Press; 1988:3–14.

9 Forbes, G. B. Calcium accumulation by the human fetus. *Pediatrics* 1976;**57**:976–7.

10 Ziegler, E. E., O'Donnell, A. M., Nelson, S. E., Fomon, S. J. Body composition of the reference fetus. *Growth* 1976;**40**:329–41.

11 Shaw, J. Parenteral nutrition in the management of sick low birth-weight infants. *Pediatr. Clin. N. Am.* 1973;**20**:333–58.

12 Shaw, J. Evidence for defective skeletal mineralization in low birth weight infants; the absorption of calcium and fat. *Pediatrics* 1976;**57**:16–25.

13 Schwartz, R., Reddi, A. Influence of magnesium depletion on matrix-induced endochondral bone formation. *Calcif. Tissue. Int.* 1979;**29**:15–20.

14 Wuthier, R., Gore, S. Partition of inorganic ions and phospholipids in isolated cell, membrane and matrix vesicle fractions: evidence for Ca-Pi acidic phospholipid complexes. *Calcif Tissue Res.* 1977;**24**:163–71.

15 Loughead, J., Mimouni, F., Tsang, R. Serum ionized calcium concentrations in normal neonates. *Am. J. Dis. Child.* 1988;**142**:516–18.

16 Wandrup, J., Kroner, J., Pryds, O., Kastrup, K. W. Age-related reference values for ionized calcium in the first week of life in premature and full-term neonates. *Scand. J. Clin. Lab. Invest.* 1988;**48**:255–60.

17 Namgung, R., Tsang, R. C., Specker, B. L., Sierra, R. I., Ho, M. L. Low bone mineral content and high serum osteocalcin and 1,25-dihydroxyvitamin D in summer-versus winter-born newborn infants: an early fetal effect? *J. Pediatr. Gastroenterol. Nutr.* 1994;**19**:220–7.

18 Specker, B. L., Lichtenstein, P., Mimouni, F., Gormley, C., Tsang, R. C. Calcium-regulating hormones and minerals from birth to 18 months of age: a cross-sectional study. II. Effects of sex, race, age, season, and diet on serum minerals, parathyroid hormone, and calcitonin. *Pediatrics* 1986;**77**:891–6.

19 Tsang, R. C. Neonatal magnesium disturbances. *Am. J. Dis. Child.* 1972;**124**:282–93.

20 Anast, C. S. Serum magnesium levels in the newborn. *Pediatrics* 1964;**33**:969–74.

21 Aikawa, J. K. *Magnesium: its Biological Significance*. Boca Raton: CRC Press; 1981;43–56.

22 Yang, X., Hosseini, J., Ruddel, M., Elin, R. Comparison of magnesium in human lymphocytes and mononuclear blood cells. *Magnesium* 1989;**8**:100–5.

23 Quamme, G., Dirks, J. Magnesium metabolism. In Maxwell, M., Kleeman, C., Narins, R., eds. *Clinical Disorders of Fluid and Electrolyte Metabolism*. 4th edn. New York: McGraw-Hill; 1987:297.

24 Quamme, G. Renal handling of magnesium: drug and hormone interactions. *Magnesium* 1986;**5**:248–72.

25 Rodan, G. Introduction to bone biology. *Bone* 1992;**13**:3–6.

26 Martin, T., Wah, K. Bone cell physiology. *Endocrin. Metab. Clin. N. Am.* 1989;**18**:833–58.

27 Canalis, E. Growth factors and their potential clinical value. *J. Clin. Endocrinol. Metab.* 1992;**75**:1–4.

28 Canalis, E., Economides, A. N., Gazzerro, E. Bone morphogenetic proteins, their antagonists, and the skeleton. *Endocr. Rev.* 2003;**24**:218–35.

29 Ballock, T. R., O'Keefe R. J. The biology of the growth plate. *J. Bone Joint Surg. Am.* 2003;**85-A**:715–26.

30 Ballock, R. T., O'Keefe, R. J. Physiology and pathophysiology of the growth plate. *Birth Defects Res. Part C Embryo Today* 2003;**69**:123–43.

31 Yamaguchi, A., Komori, T., Suda, T. Regulation of osteoblast differentiation mediated by bone morphogenetic proteins, hedgehogs, and Cbfa1. *Endocr. Rev.* 2000;**21**:393–411.

32 Roodman, G. D. Advances in bone biology: the osteoclast. *Endocr. Rev.* 1996;**17**:308–32.

33 Blair, H. C., Athanasou, N. A. Recent advances in osteoclast biology and pathological bone resorption. *Histol. Histopathol.* 2004;**19**:189–99.

34 Van der Eerden, B. C., Karperien, M., Wit, J. M. Systemic and local regulation of the growth plate. *Endocr. Rev.* 2003;**24**:782–801.

35 Riggs, B. L., Khosla, S., Melton, L. J. 3rd. Sex steroids and the construction and conservation of the adult skeleton. *Endocr. Rev.* 2002;**23**:279–302.

36 Frost, H. M. Perspectives: a proposed general model of the "mechanostat" (suggestions from a new paradigm). *Anat. Rec.* 1996;**244**:139–47.

37 Frost, H. M. From Wolff's law to the Utah paradigm: insights about bone physiology and its clinical applications. *Anat. Rec.* 2001;**262**:398–419.

38 Miller, M. E. The bone disease of preterm birth: a biomechanical perspective. *Pediatr. Res.* 2003;**53**:10–15.

39 Conroy, B. P., Kraemer, W. J., Maresh, C. M. *et al.* Bone mineral density in elite junior Olympic weightlifters. *Med. Sci. Sports Exerc.* 1993;**25**:1103–9.

40 Larson, C. M., Henderson, R. C. Bone mineral density and fractures in boys with Duchenne muscular dystrophy. *J. Pediatr. Orthop.* 2000;**20**:71–4.

41 Rauch, F., Schoenau, E. The developing bone: slave or master of its cells and molecules? *Pediatr. Res.* 2001;**50**:309–14.

42 Rauch, F., Schoenau, E. Skeletal development in premature infants: a review of bone physiology beyond nutritional aspects. *Arch. Dis. Child. Fetal Neonat. Ed.* 2002;**86**:F82–5.

43 Larsen, W. J. *Essentials of Human Embryology.* New York: Churchill Livingstone; 1998:207–16.

44 Rodriguez, J. I., Garcia-Alix, A., Palacios, J. *et al.* Changes in the long bones due to fetal immobility caused by neuromuscular disease. A radiographic and histological study. *J. Bone. Joint. Surg. [Am].* 1988;**70**:1052–60.

45 Rodriguez, J. I., Palacios, J., Garcia-Alix, A. *et al.* Effects of immobilization on fetal bone development. A morphometric study in newborns with congenital neuromuscular diseases with intrauterine onset. *Calcif. Tissue. Int.* 1988;**43**:335–9.

46 Rodriguez, J. I., Palacios, J., Ruiz, A. *et al.* Morphological changes in long bone development in fetal akinesia deformation sequence: an experimental study in curarized rat fetuses. *Teratology* 1992;**45**:213–21.

47 Rodriguez, J. I., Palacios, J. Pathogenetic mechanisms of fetal akinesia deformation sequence and oligohydramnios sequence. *Am. J. Med. Genet.* 1991;**40**:284–9.

48 Miller, M. E., Hangartner, T. N. Temporary brittle bone disease: association with decreased fetal movement and osteopenia. *Calcif. Tissue Int.* 1999;**64**:137–43.

49 Kakebeeke, T. J., von Siebenthal, K., Largo, R. H. Differences in movement quality at term among preterm and term infants. *Biol. Neonate* 1997;**71**:367–78.

50 Namgung, R., Tsang, R. C. Factors affecting newborn bone mineral content: in utero effects on newborn bone mineralization. *Proc. Nutr. Soc.* 2000;**59**:55–63.

51 Namgung, R., Tsang, R. C. Bone in the pregnant mother and newborn at birth. *Clin. Chim. Acta.* 2003;**333**:1–11.

52 Douglas, A. S., Miller, M. H., Reid, D. M. *et al.* Seasonal differences in biochemical parameters of bone remodelling. *J. Clin. Pathol.* 1996;**49**:284–9.

53 Hunziker, E. B. Mechanism of longitudinal bone growth and its regulation by growth plate chondrocytes. *Microsc. Res. Tech.* 1994;**28**:505–19.

54 Ohlsson, C., Bengtsson, B. A., Isaksson, O. G., Andreassen, T. T., Slootweg, M. C. Growth hormone and bone. *Endocr. Rev.* 1998;**19**:55–79.

55 Williams, G. R., Robson, H., Shalet, S. M. Thyroid hormone actions on cartilage and bone: interactions with other hormones at the epiphyseal plate and effects on linear growth. *J. Endocrinol.* 1998;**157**:391–403.

56 Lanske, B., Karaplis, A. C., Lee, K. *et al.* PTH/PTHrP receptor in early development and Indian hedgehog-regulated bone growth. *Science* 1996;**273**:663–6.

57 Vortkamp, A., Lee, K., Lanske, B. *et al.* Regulation of rate of cartilage differentiation by Indian hedgehog and PTH-related protein. *Science* 1996;**273**:613–22.

58 Horton, W. A. Skeletal development: insights from targeting the mouse genome. *Lancet* 2003;**362**:560–9.

59 Chan, G. M. Calcium needs during childhood. *Ped. Annals.* 2001;**30**;666–70.

60 Steelman, J., Zeitler, P. Osteoporosis in pediatrics. *Pediatr. Rev.* 2001;**22**:56–65.

61 Slemenda, C., Miller, J., Hui, S., Reister, T., Johnston, C. Role of physical activity in the development of skeletal mass in children. *J. Bone. Min. Res.* 1991;**6**:1227–33.

62 Committee on Nutrition. Calcium requirements of infants, children, and adolescents. *Pediatrics* 1999;**104**:1152–57.

63 Matkovic, V., Fonatana, D., Tominac, C., Goel, P., Chestnut, C. I. Factors that influence peak bone mass formation: a study of calcium balance and the inheritance of bone mass in adolescent females. *Am. J. Clin. Nutr.* 1990;**52**:878–88.

64 Matkovic, V. Calcium intake and peak bone mass. *N. Engl. J. Med.* 1992;**327**:119–20.

65 Martin, A. D., Bailey, D. A., McKay, H. A. *et al.* Bone mineral and calcium accretion during puberty. *Am. J. Clin. Nutr.* 1997;**66**:611–15.

66 Krall, E., Dawson-Hughes, B. Heritable and life style determinants of bone mineral density. *J. Bone. Min. Res.* 1993;**8**:1–9.

67 Hogler, W., Schmid, A., Raber, G. *et al.* Perinatal bone turnover in term human neonates and the influence of maternal smoking. *Pediatr. Res.* 2003;**53**:817–22.

68 Colak, O., Alatas, O., Aydogdu, S., Uslu, S. The effect of smoking on bone metabolism: maternal and cord blood bone marker levels. *Clin. Biochem.* 2002;**35**:247–50.

69 Johnston, C., Miller, J., Slemenda, C. *et al.* Calcium supplementation and increases in bone mineral density in children. *N. Engl. J. Med.* 1992;**327**:82–7.

70 Wyshak, G., Frisch, R. E. Carbonated beverages, dietary calcium, the dietary calcium/phosphorus ratio, and bone fractures in girls and boys. *J. Adolesc. Health* 1994;**15**:210–15.

71 Wyshak, G. Teenaged girls, carbonated beverage consumption, and bone fractures. *Arch. Pediatr. Adolesc. Med.* 2000;**154**:610–13.

72 Simkin, A., Ayalon, J., Leichter, I. Increased bone density due to bone-loading exercises in postmenopausal osteoporotic women. *Calcif. Tissue Int.* 1987;**40**:59–63.

73 Burger, E., Klein-Nulend, J., Veldhuijzen, J. P. Mechanical stress and osteogenesis in vitro. *J. Bone. Min. Res.* 1992;**7**:S397–401.

74 Pead, M., Skerry, T., Lanyon, L. Direct transformation from quiescence to bone formation in the adult periosteum following a single brief period of bone loading. *J. Bone. Min. Res.* 1988;**3**:647–56.

75 Buchanan, J., Myers, C., Loyd, T., Leuenberger, P., Demers, L. Determinants of peak trabecular bone density in women: the role of androgens, estrogen, and exercise. *J. Bone. Min. Res.* 1988;**3**:673–80.

76 Eriksen, E., Colvard, D., Berg, N. *et al.* Evidence of estrogen receptors in normal human osteoblast-like cells. *Science* 1988;**241**:84–6.

77 Lindsay, R. The effect of estrogens in prevention and treatment of osteoporosis. In Munro, H., Schlierf, G., ed. *Nutrition of the Elderly. Nestlé Nutrition Workshop Series, V 29.* New York: Raven Press; 1992:161–7.

78 Yamanaka, Y., Matsuo, H., Mochizuki, S. *et al.* Effects of estriol on cell viability and 1,25-dihydroxyvitamin D_3 receptor mRNA expression in cultured human osteoblast-like cells. *Gynecol. Endocrinol.* 2003;**17**:455–61.

79 Krieger, N. S., Bushinsky, D. A., Frick, K. K. Cellular mechanisms of bone resorption induced by metabolic acidosis. *Semin. Dial.* 2003;**16**:463–6.

80 Pieltain, C., De Curtis M., Gérard, P., Rigo, J. Weight gain composition in preterm infants with dual energy x-ray absorptiometry. *Pediatr. Res.* 2001;**49**:120–4.

81 Koo, W. W. K., Walter, J., Bush, A. J. Technical considerations of dual-energy x-ray absorptiometry based on bone mineral measurements for pediatric studies. *J. Bone Miner. Res.* 1995;**10**:1998–2004.

82 Koo, W. W. K., Massom, L. R., Walters, J. Validation and accuracy and precision of dual energy x-ray absorptiometry for infants. *J. Bone Miner. Res.* 1995;**10**:1111–15.

83 Brunton, J. A., Weiler, H. A., Atkinson, S. A. Improvement in the accuracy of dual energy x-ray absorptiometry for whole body and regional analysis of body composition: validation using piglets and methodologic considerations in infants. *Pediatr. Res.* 1997;**41**:590–6.

84 Venkataraman, P. S., Ahluwalia, B. W. Total bone mineral content and body composition by x-ray densitometry in newborns. *Pediatrics* 1992;**90**:767–70.

85 Faerk, J., Petersen, S., Petersen, B., Michaelsen, K. F. Diet and bone mineral content at term in premature infants. *Pediatr. Res.* 2000;**47**:148–56.

86 Lapillonne, A., Braillon, P., Chatelain, P. G., Delams, P. D., Salle, B. L. Body composition in appropriate and in small for gestational age infants. *Acta Paediatr.* 1997;**86**:196–200.

87 Bronner, F., Salle, B. L., Putet, G., Rigo, J., Senterre, J. Net calcium absorption in premature infants: results of 103 metabolic balance studies. *Am. J. Clin. Nutr.* 1992;**56**:1037–44.

88 Koo, W. W., Bush, A. J., Walters, J., Carlson, S. E. Postnatal development of bone mineral status during infancy. *J. Am. Coll. Nutr.* 1998;**17**:65–70.

89 Spady, D. W., Filipow, L. J., Overton, T. R., Szymanski, W. A. Measurement of total body potassium in premature infants by means of a whole-body counter. *J. Pediatr. Gastroenterol. Nutr.* 1986;**5**:750–5.

90 Tang, W., Modi, N., Clark, P. Dilution kinetics of H_2 ^{18}O for the measurement of total body water in preterm babies in the first week after birth. *Arch. Dis. Child.* 1993;**69**:28–31.

91 Tang, W., Ridout, D., Modi, N. Assessment of total body water using bioelectrical impedance analysis in neonates receiving intensive care. *Arch. Dis. Child.* 1997;**77**:123–6.

92 De Bruin, N. C., van Velthoven, K. A. M., de Ridder, M. *et al.* Standards for total body fat and fat-free mass in infants. *Arch. Dis. Child.* 1996;**74**:386–99.

93 Fusch, C., Slotboom, J., Fuehrer, U. *et al.* Neonatal body composition: dual-energy x-ray absorptiometry, magnetic resonance imaging, and three-dimensional chemical shift imaging versus chemical analysis in piglets. *Pediatr. Res.* 1999;**46**:465–73.

94 Putet, G., Salle, L., Rigo, J., Senterre, J. Nutrient balance, energy utilization, and composition of weight gain in very-low-birth-weight infants fed pooled human milk or a preterm formula. *J. Pediatr.* 1984;**105**:79–85.

95 Putet, G., Salle, L., Rigo, J., Senterre, J. Supplementation of pooled human milk with casein hydrolysate: energy and nitrogen balance and weight gain composition in very-low-birth-weight infants. *Pediatr. Res.* 1987;**21**:458–61.

96 Picaud, J. C., Rigo, J., Nyamugabo, K., Milet, J., Senterre, J. Evaluation of dual energy x-ray absorptiometry (DEXA) for body composition assessment in piglets and term human neonates. *Am. J. Clin. Nutr.* 1996;**63**:157–63.

97 Koo, W. W. K., Walters, J., Bush, A. J., Chesney, R. W., Carlson, S. E. Dual-energy-x-ray absorptiometry studies of

bone mineral status in newborn infants. *J. Bone. Min. Res.* 1996;**11**:997–1002.

98 Rigo, J., Nyamugabo, K., Picaud, J. C. *et al.* Reference values of body composition obtained by dual energy x-ray absorptiometry in preterm and term neonates. *J. Pediatr. Gastroenterol. Nutr.* 1998;**27**:184–90.

99 Cooke, R. J., McCormick, K., Griffin, I. J. *et al.* Feeding preterm infants after hospital discharge: effect of diet on body composition. *Pediatr. Res.* 1999;**46**:461–4.

100 Rigo, J., De Curtis, M., Nyamugabo, K. *et al.* Premature bone. In Bonjour, J. P., Tsang, R. C., eds. *Nutrition and Bone. Nestlé Nutrition Workshop Series, V 41.* New York: Raven Press; 1998:83–98.

101 Salle, B. L., Braillon, P., Glorieux, F. H. *et al.* Lumbar bone mineral content measured by dual energy X-ray absorptiometry in newborns and infants. *Acta Paediatr.* 1992;**81**:953–8.

102 Molgaard, C., Thomsen, B. L., Prentice, A., Cole, T. J. Whole-body bone mineral content in healthy children and adolescents. *Arch. Dis. Child.* 1997;**76**:9–15.

103 Rigo, J., De Curtis, M., Pieltain, C. *et al.* Bone mineral metabolism in the micropremie. *Clin Perinatol.* 2000;**27**:147–70.

104 Hogler, W., Briody, J., Woodhead, H. J., Chan, A., Cowell, C. T. Importance of lean mass in the interpretation of total body densitometry in children and adolescents. *J. Pediatr.* 2003;**143**:81–8.

105 Usher, R., McLean, F. Intrauterine growth of liveborn Caucasian infants at sea level: standard obtained from measurements in 7 dimensions of infants born between 25 and 44 weeks of gestation. *J. Pediatr.* 1969;**74**:901–10.

106 Koo, W. W. K., Hammami, M., Hockman, E. M. Validation of bone mass and body composition measurements in small subjects with pencil beam dual energy x-ray absorptiometry. *J. Am. Coll. Nutr.* 2004;**23**:79–84.

107 Foldes, A. J., Rimon, A., Keinan, D. D., Popovtzer, M. M. Quantitative ultrasound of the tibia: a novel approach for assessment of bone status. *Bone* 1995;**17**:363–7.

108 Nemet, D., Dolfin, T., Wolach, B., Eliakim, A. Quantitative ultrasound measurements of bone speed of sound in premature infants. *Eur. J. Pediatr.* 2001;**160**:737–40.

109 Litmanovitz, I., Dolfin, T., Friedland, O. *et al.* Early physical activity intervention prevents decrease of bone strength in very low birth weight infants. *Pediatrics* 2003;**112**:15–19.

110 Rubinacci, A., Moro, G. E., Boehm, G. *et al.* Quantitative ultrasound for the assessment of osteopenia in preterm infants. *Eur. J. Endocrinol.* 2003;**14**:307–15.

111 Foldes, A. J., Rimon, A., Keinan, D. D., Popovtzer, M. M. Quantitative ultrasound of the tibia: a novel approach for assessment of bone status. *Bone* 1995;**17**:363–77.

112 Kang, C., Speller, R. Comparison of ultrasound and dual energy X-ray absorptiometry measurements in the calcaneus. *Br. J. Radiol.* 1998;**56**:861–7.

113 Prins, S. H., Jorgensen, H. L., Hassager, C. The role of quantitative ultrasound in the assessment of bone: a review. *Clin. Physiol.* 1998;**18**:3–17.

114 Pearce, S., Hurtig, M. B., Runciman, J., Dickey, J. Effect of age, anatomic site and soft tissue on quantitative ultrasound. *J. Bone Miner. Res.* 2000;**15**:S407.

115 Litmanovitz, I., Dolfin, T., Regev, R. *et al.* Bone turnover markers and bone strength during the first weeks of life in very low birth weight premature infants. *J. Perinat. Med.* 2004;**32**:58–61.

116 Nemet, D., Dolfin, T., Litmanowitz, I. *et al.* Evidence for exercise-induced bone formation in premature infants. *Int. J. Sports Med.* 2002;**23**:82–5.

117 Kornak, W., Mundlos, S. Genetic disorders of the skeleton: a developmental approach. *Am. J. Hum. Genet.* 2003;**73**:447–74.

118 Whyte, M. P. Hypophosphatasia and the role of alkaline phosphatase in skeletal mineralization. *Endocr. Rev.* 1994;**15**:439–61.

119 Ward, W. E., Atkinson, S. A., Donovan, S., Paes, B. Bone metabolism and circulating IGF-1 and IGFBPs in dexamethasone-treated preterm infants. *Early Hum. Dev.* 1999;**56**:127–41.

120 Bernstein, C. N., Leslie, W. D. The pathophysiology of bone disease in gastrointestinal disease. *Eur. J. Gastroenterol. Hepatol.* 2003;**15**:857–64.

121 Bachrach, L., Guido, D., Katzman, D., Litt, I., Marcus, R. Decreased bone density in adolescent girls with anorexia nervosa. *Pediatrics* 1990;**86**:440–7.

122 Allen, D. B. Growth suppression by glucocorticoid therapy. *Endocrinol. Metab. Clin. N. Am.* 1996;**25**:699–717.

123 Kruse, K., Busse, M., Kracht, U., Kruse, U., Wohlfart, K. Disorders of calcium and bone metabolism in glucocorticoid treatment. *Monatsschr Kinderheilkd.* 1988;**136**:237–42.

124 Jux, C., Leiber, K., Hugel, U. *et al.* Dexamethasone impairs growth hormone (GH)-stimulated growth by suppression of local insulin-like growth factor (IGF)-I production and expression of GH- and IGF-I-receptor in cultured rat chondrocytes. *Endocrinology* 1998;**139**:3296–305.

125 Weiler, H., Wang, Z., Atkinson, S. Dexamethasone treatment impairs calcium regulation and reduces bone mineralization in infant pigs. *Am. J. Clin. Nutr.* 1995;**61**:805–11.

126 Crofton, P. M., Shrivastava, A., Wade, J. C. *et al.* Effects of dexamethasone treatment on bone and collagen turnover in preterm infants with chronic lung disease. *Pediatr. Res.* 2000; **48**:155–62.

127 Saarela, T., Risteli, J., Koivisto, M. Effects of short-term dexamethasone treatment on collagen synthesis and degradation markers in preterm infants with developing lung disease. *Acta Paediatr.* 2003;**92**:588–94.

128 Ekenstam, E., Stalenheim, G., Hallgren, R. The acute effect of high dose corticosteroid treatment on serum osteocalcin. *Metabolism* 1988;**37**:141–4.

129 Cranefield, D. J., Odd, D. E., Harding, J. E., Teele, R. L. High incidence of nephrocalcinosis in extremely preterm infants treated with dexamethasone. *Pediatr. Radiol.* 2004;**34**:138–42.

130 Takeshita, N., Seino, Y., Ishida, H. *et al.* Increased circulating levels of gamma-carboxyglutamic acid-containing protein and decreased bone mass in children on anticonvulsant therapy. *Calcif. Tissue Int.* 1989;**44**:80–5.

131 Matsuda, I., Higashi, A., Inotsume, N. Physiologic and metabolic aspects of anticonvulsants. *Pediatr. Clin. N. Am.* 1989;**36**:1099–11.

132 Robson, H. Bone growth mechanisms and the effects of cytotoxic drugs. *Arch. Dis. Child.* 1999;**81**:360–4.

133 Szulc, P., Seeman, E., Delmas, P. D. Biochemical measurements of bone turnover in children and adolescents. *Osteoporos. Int.* 2000;**11**:281–94.

134 Levine, M. A. Biochemical markers of bone metabolism: application to understanding bone remodeling in children and adolescents. *J. Pediatr. Endocrinol. Metab.* 2003;**16**:661–72.

135 Kent, N. G. Markers of bone turnover. *J. Int. Fed. Clin. Chem.* 1997;**9**:31–5.

136 Watts, N. B. Clinical utility of biochemical markers of bone remodeling. *Clin. Chem.* 1999;**45**:1359–68.

137 Delmas, P. Biochemical markers of bone turnover for the clinical assessment of metabolic bone disease. *Endocrinol. Metab. Clin. N. Am.* 1990;**19**:1–18.

138 Deftos, L. Bone protein and peptide assays in the diagnosis and management of skeletal disease. *Clin. Chem.* 1991;**37**:1143–48.

139 Garnero, P., Grimaux, M., Demiaux, B. *et al.* Measurement of serum osteocalcin with a human-specific two-site immunoradiometric assay. *J. Bone. Min. Res.* 1992;**7**:1389–98.

140 Ritter, N., Farach-Carson, M., Butler, W. Evidence for the formation of a complex between osteopontin and osteocalcin. *J. Bone. Min. Res.* 1992;**7**:877–85.

141 Michaelsen, K., Johansen, J., Samuelson, G., Price, P., Christiansen, C. Serum bone gamma-carboxyglutamic acid protein in a longitudinal study of infants: lower values in formula-fed infants. *Pediatr. Res.* 1992;**31**:401–5.

142 Hassager, C., Risteli, J., Risteli, L., Jensen, S., Christiansen, C. Diurnal variation in serum markers of type I collagen synthesis and degradation in healthy premenopausal women. *J. Bone Min. Res.* 1992;**7**:1307–11.

143 Kanbur, N. O., Derman, O., Sen, T. A., Kinik, E. Osteocalcin. A biochemical marker of bone turnover during puberty. *Int. J. Adolesc. Med. Health.* 2002;**14**:235–44.

144 Ebeling, P., Peterson, J., Riggs, B. Utility of type I procollagen propeptide assays for assessing abnormalities in metabolic bone diseases. *J. Bone. Min. Res.* 1992;**7**:1243–50.

145 Hassager, C., Jensen, L., Johansen, J. *et al.* The carboxyterminal propeptide of type I procollagen in serum as a marker of bone formation: the effect of nandrolone decanoate and female sex hormones. *Metabolism* 1991;**40**:205–8.

146 Allen, S., Nuttleman, P., Ketcham, C., Roberts, R. Purification and characterization of human bone tartrate-resistant acid phosphatase. *J. Bone. Min. Res.* 1989;**4**:47–55.

147 Uebelhart, D., Gineyts, E., Chapuy, M., Delmas, P. Urinary excretion of pyridinium crosslinks: a new marker of bone resorption in metabolic bone disease. *Bone Miner.* 1990;**8**:87–96.

148 Body, J., Delmas, P. Urinary pyridinium cross-links as markers of bone resorption in tumor-associated hypercalcemia. *J. Clin. Endocrinol. Metab.* 1992;**74**:471–5.

149 Seibel, M., Robins, S., Bilezikian, J. Urinary pyridinium crosslinks of collagen. Specific markers of bone resorption in metabolic bone disease trends. *J. Clin. Endocrinol. Metab.* 1992;**3**:263–70.

150 Hanson, D., Weis, M., Bollen, A. *et al.* A specific immunoassay for monitoring human bone resorption: Quantitation of type I collagen cross-linked N-telopeptides in urine. *J. Bone. Min. Res.* 1992;**7**:1251–58.

151 Demarini, S., Specker, B. L., Sierra, R. I., Miodovnik, M., Tsang, R. C. Evidence of increased intrauterine bone resorption in term infants of mothers with insulin-dependent diabetes. *J. Pediatr.* 1995;**126**:796–8.

152 Pratico, G., Caltabiano, L., Palano, G. M., Zingale, A. Normal levels of collagen-type-I telopeptide in the first 90 days of life. *Pediatr. Med. Chir.* 1998;**20**:193–5.

153 Van der Sluis, I. M., de Ridder, M. A., Boot, A. M. *et al.* Reference data for bone density and body composition measured with dual energy x-ray absorptiometry in white children and young adults. *Arch. Dis. Child.* 2002;**87**:341–7.

154 Koo, W. W., Krug Wispe, S. K., Succop, P. *et al.* Urinary hydroxyproline in infants with and without fractures/rickets. *Clin. Chem.* 1990;**36**:642–4.

155 Pittard, W. B. 3rd, Geddes, K. M., Hulsey, T. C., Hollis, B. W. Osteocalcin, skeletal alkaline phosphatase, and bone mineral content in very low birth weight infants: a longitudinal assessment. *Pediatr. Res.* 1992;**31**:181–5.

156 Kajantie, E., Dunkel, L., Risteli, J., Pohjavuori, M., Andersson, S. Markers of type I and III collagen turnover as indicators of growth velocity in very low birth weight infants. *J. Clin. Endocrinol. Metab.* 2001;**86**:4299–306.

157 Ogueh, O., Khastgir, G., Studd, J. *et al.* The relationship of fetal serum markers of bone metabolism to gestational age. *Early Hum. Dev.* 1998;**51**:109–12.

158 Hytinantti, T., Rutanen, E. M., Turpeinen, M., Sorva, R., Andersson, S. Markers of collagen metabolism and insulin-like growth factor binding protein-1 in term infants. *Arch. Dis. Child. Fetal Neonat. Ed.* 2000;**83**:F17–20.

159 Mora, S., Prinster, C., Bellini, A. *et al.* Bone turnover in neonates: changes of urinary excretion rate of collagen type I cross-linked peptides during the first days of life and influence of gestational age. *Bone* 1997;**20**:563–6.

160 Tsukahara, H., Watanabe, Y., Hirano, S. *et al.* Assessment of bone turnover in term and preterm newborns at birth: measurement of urinary collagen crosslink excretion. *Early Hum. Dev.* 1999;**53**:185–91.

161 Seibold-Weiger, K., Wollmann, H. A., Ranke, M. B., Speer, C. P. Plasma concentrations of the carboxyterminal propeptide of type I procollagen (PICP) in preterm neonates from birth to term. *Pediatr. Res.* 2000;**48**:104–8.

162 Harrast, S. D., Kalkwarf, H. J. Effects of gestational age, maternal diabetes, and intrauterine growth retardation on markers of fetal bone turnover in amniotic fluid. *Calcif. Tissue. Int.* 1998;**62**:205–8.

163 Ogueh, O., Khastgir, G., Studd, J. *et al.* Maternal and fetal plasma levels of markers of bone metabolism in gestational diabetic pregnancies. *Early Hum. Dev.* 1998;**53**:155–61.

164 Namgung, R., Tsang, R. C., Sierra, R. I., Ho, M. L. Normal serum indices of bone collagen biosynthesis and degradation

in small for gestational age infants. *J. Pediatr. Gastroenterol. Nutr.* 1996;**23**:224–8.

165 Yamaga, A., Taga, M., Minaguchi, H. Changes in urinary excretions of C-telopeptide and cross-linked N-telopeptide of type I collagen during pregnancy and puerperium. *Endocr. J.* 1997;**44**:733–8.

166 Yamaga, A., Taga, M., Hashimoto, S., Ota, C. Comparison of bone metabolic markers between maternal and cord blood. *Horm. Res.* 1999;**51**:277–9.

167 Yasumizu, T., Kato, J. Concentrations of serum markers of type I collagen synthesis and degradation and serum osteocalcin in maternal and umbilical circulation. *Endocr. J.* 1996;**43**: 191–5.

168 Crofton, P. M., Shrivastava, A., Wade, J. C. *et al.* Bone and collagen markers in pretrem infants: relationship with growth and bone mineral content over the first 10 weeks of life. *Pediatr. Res.* 1999;**46**:581–7.

169 Lund, A. M., Hansen, M., Kollerup, G. *et al.* Collagen-derived markers of bone metabolism in osteogenesis imperfecta. *Acta Paediatr.* 1998;**87**:1131–37.

170 Shiff, Y., Eliakim, A., Shainkin-Kestenbaum, R. *et al.* Measurements of bone turnover markers in premature infants. *J. Pediatr. Endocrinol. Metab.* 2001;**14**:389–95.

171 Lapillonne, A., Travers, R., DiMaio, M., Salle, B. L., Glorieux, F. H. Urinary excretion of cross-linked N-telopeptides of type 1 collagen to assess bone resorption in infants from birth to 1 year of age. *Pediatrics* 2002;**110**:105–9.

172 Whipple, T., Sharkey, N., Demers, L., Williams, N. Leptin and the skeleton. *Clin. Endocrinol. (Oxf).* 2002;**57**:701–11.

173 Hassink, S. G., de Lancey, E., Sheslow, D. V. *et al.* Placental leptin: an important new growth factor in intrauterine and neonatal development? *Pediatrics* 1997;**100**:E1.

174 Matsuda, J., Yokota, I., Iida, M. *et al.* Dynamic changes in serum leptin concentrations during the fetal and neonatal periods. *Pediatr. Res.* 1999;**45**:71–5.

175 Ogueh, O., Sooranna, S., Nicolaides, K. H., Johnson, M. R. The relationship between leptin concentration and bone metabolism in the human fetus. *J. Clin. Endocrinol. Metab.* 2000;**85**:1997–9.

176 Furmaga-Jablonska, W., Kulik-Rechberger, B., Kozlowska, M. Association between leptin, markers of bone formation and physical growth of newborns. *Ann. Hum. Biol.* 2003;**30**:250–61.

177 Fares, J. E., Choucair, M., Nabulsi, M. *et al.* Effect of gender, puberty, and vitamin D status on biochemical markers of bone remodeling. *Bone* 2003;**33**:242–7.

178 Bini, V., Igli Baroncelli, G., Papi, F. *et al.* Relationships of serum leptin levels with biochemical markers of bone turnover and with growth factors in normal weight and overweight children. *Horm. Res.* 2004;**61**:170–5.

179 Sorva, R., Anttila, R., Siimes, M. A. *et al.* Serum markers of collagen metabolism and serum osteocalcin in relation to pubertal development in 57 boys at 14 years of age. *Pediatr. Res.* 1997;**42**:528–32.

180 Anim-Nyame, N., Sooranna, S. R., Jones, J. *et al.* Biochemical markers of maternal bone turnover are elevated in pre-eclampsia. *Br. J. Obstet. Gynaecol.* 2001;**108**:258–62.

181 Vrotsos, Y., Miller, S. C., Marks, S. C. Jr. Prostaglandin E – a powerful anabolic agent for generalized or site-specific bone formation. *Crit. Rev. Eukaryot. Gene Expr.* 2003;**13**:255–63.

182 Canalis, E., McCarthy, T., Centrella, M. The role of growth factors in skeletal remodeling. *Endocrinol. Metab. Clin. N. Am.* 1989;**18**:903–18.

183 Jones, J. I., Clemmons, D. R. Insulin-like growth factors and their binding proteins: biological actions. *Endocr. Rev.* 1995;**16**:3–34.

184 Canalis, E. Effect of insulin-like growth factor I on DNA and protein synthesis in cultured rat calvaria. *J. Clin. Invest.* 1980;**66**:709–19.

185 Canalis, E. Regulation of bone remodeling. In Favus, M. J., ed. *Primer on the metabolic bone diseases and disorders of mineral metabolism.* New York: Raven Press;1993:33–7.

186 Yano, H., Ohya, K., Amajasa, T. Effects of insulin on in vitro bone formation in fetal rat perinatal bone. *Endocr. J.* 1994;**41**:293–300.

187 Canalis, E., Centrella, M., Burch, W., McCarthy, T. Insulin-like growth factor I mediates selective anabolic effects of parathyroid hormone in bone cultures. *J. Clin. Invest.* 1989;**83**: 60–5.

188 Chenu, C., Valentin-Opran, A., Chavassieux, P. *et al.* Insulin growth factor I hormonal regulation by growth hormone and by 1,25-(OH)2D3 and activity on human osteoblast-like cells in short-term cultures. *Bone* 1990;**11**:81–6.

189 Wong, G., Kotliar, D., Schlaeger, D., Brandes, S. IGF-I production by mouse osteoblasts. *J. Bone. Min. Res.* 1990;**5**:133–40.

190 Scheven, B., Damen, C., Hamilton, N., Verhaar, H., Duursma, S. Stimulatory effects of estrogen and progesterone on proliferation and differentiation of normal human osteoblast-like cells in vitro. *Biochem. Biophys. Res. Commun.* 1992;**186**:54–60.

191 Zaidi, M., Moonga, B. S., Abe, E. Calcitonin and bone formation: a knockout full of surprises. *J. Clin. Invest.* 2002;**110**:1769–71.

192 Mosekilde, L., Eriksen, E., Charles, P. Effects of thyroid hormones on bone and mineral metabolism. *Endocrinol. Metab. Clin. N. Am.* 1990;**19**:35–63.

193 Soskolne, W., Schwartz, Z., Goldstein, M., Ornoy, A. The biphasic effect of triiodothyronine compared to bone resorbing effect of PTH on bone modelling of mouse long bone in vitro. *Bone* 1990;**11**:301–7.

194 Ongphiphadhanakul, B., Alex, S., Braverman, L., Baran, D. Excessive L-Thyroxine therapy decreases femoral bone mineral densities in the male rat: effect of hypogonadism and calcitonin. *J. Bone. Min. Res.* 1992;**7**:1227–31.

195 Oreffo, R., Teti, A., Francis, M., Carano, A., Zallone, A. Effect of vitamin A on bone resorption: evidence for direct stimulation of isolated chicken osteoclasts by retinol and retinoic acid. *J. Bone. Min. Res.* 1988;**3**:203–10.

196 Troen, B. R. The role of cathepsin K in normal bone resorption. *Drug News Perspect.* 2004; **17**:19–28.

197 Hamrick, M. W., Pennington, C., Newton, D., Xie, D., Isales, C. Leptin deficiency produces contrasting phenotypes in bones of the limb and spine. *Bone* 2004;**34**:376–83.

198 Elefteriou, F., Takeda, S., Ebihara, K. *et al.* Serum leptin level is a regulator of bone mass. *Proc. Natl. Acad. Sci. USA.* 2004;**101**:3258–63.

199 Nakajima, R., Inada, H., Koike, T., Yamano, T. Effects of leptin to cultured growth plate chondrocytes. *Horm. Res.* 2003;**60**:91–8.

200 Gat-Yablonski, G., Ben-Ari, T., Shtaif, B. *et al.* Leptin reverses the inhibitory effect of caloric restriction on longitudinal growth. *Endocrinology* 2004;**145**:343–50.

201 Matkovic, V. Calcium intake and peak bone mass. *N. Engl. J. Med.* 1992;**327**:119–20.

202 Sentipal, J., Wardlaw, G., Mahan, J., Matkovic, V. Influence of calcium intake and growth indexes on vertebral bone mineral density in young females. *Am. J. Clin. Nutr.* 1991;**54**:425–8.

203 Recker, R., Davies, K., Hinders, S. *et al.* Bone gain in young adult women. *J. Am. Med. Assoc.* 1992;**268**:2403–8.

204 Altenahr, E., Wohler, J. Ultrastrukturell untersuchungen zur funktionellen epithelkorperchen-differenzierung wahrend der embryanal-fetal- und neonatal-periode. *Verh. Dtsch. Ges. Pathol.* 1971;**55**:160–6.

205 Stoeckel, M., Porte, A. Observations ultrastructurales sur la parathyroide de mammifere et d'oiseau dans les conditions normales et experimentales. *Arch. Anat. Microsc. Morphol. Exp.* 1973;**62**:55–88.

206 Leroyer-Alizon, E., David, L., Anast, C., Dubois, P. Immuno-cytological evidence for parathyroid hormone in human parathyroid glands. *J. Clin. Endocrinol. Metab.* 1981;**52**:513–16.

207 Brown, E. M. Calcium receptor and regulation of parathyroid hormone secretion. *Rev. Endocr. Metab. Disord.* 2000;**1**:307–15.

208 Brown, E. M., MacLeod, R. J. Extracellular calcium sensing and extracellular calcium signaling. *Physiol. Rev.* 2001;**81**:239–97.

209 Brown, E. M., Gamba, G., Riccardi, D. *et al.* Cloning and characterization of an extracellular Ca^{2+}-sensing receptor from bovine parathyroid. *Nature* 1993;**366**:575–80.

210 Raisz, L. G. The hunting of the snark: the elusive calcium receptor(s). *J. Clin. Invest.* 2003;**111**:945–7.

211 Buckle, R., Care, A., Cooper, C. The influence of plasma magnesium concentration on parathyroid hormone secretion. *J. Endocrinol.* 1968;**42**:529–34.

212 Suh, S., Tashjian, Jr. A., Matsuo, N. *et al.* Pathogenesis of hypocalcemia in primary hypomagnesemia: Normal end-organ responsiveness to parathyroid hormone, impaired gland function. *J. Clin. Invest.* 1973;**52**:153–60.

213 MacManus, J., Heaton, F., Lucas, P. A decreased response to parathyroid hormone in magnesium deficiency. *J. Endocrinol.* 1971;**49**:253–8.

214 Freitag, J., Martin, K., Conrades, M. *et al.* Evidence for skeletal resistance to parathyroid hormone in magnesium deficiency. *J. Clin. Invest.* 1979;**64**:1238–44.

215 Anast, C., Mohs, J., Kaplan, S., Burns, T. Evidence for parathyroid failure in magnesium deficiency. *Science* 1972;**177**:606–8.

216 Anast, C., Winnacker, J., Forte, L., Burns, T. Impaired release of parathyroid hormone in magnesium deficiency. *J. Clin. Endocrinol. Metab.* 1976;**42**:707–17.

217 Massry, S. G., Coburn, J. W., Kleeman, C. R. Evidence for suppression of parathyroid gland activity by hypermagnesemia. *J. Clin. Invest.* 1970;**49**:1619–29.

218 Cholst, I., Steinberg, S., Tropper, P. *et al.* The influence of hypermagnesemia on serum calcium and parathyroid hormone levels. *N. Engl. J. Med.* 1984;**301**:1221–5.

219 Morrissey, J., Slatopolsky, E. Effect of aluminum on parathyroid hormone secretion. *Kidney Int.* 1986;**29**:41–4.

220 Mundy, G., Roodman, G. Osteoclast ontogeny and function. In Peck, W., ed. *Bone and Mineral Research.* Amsterdam: Elsevier; 1987:209–80.

221 Mundy, G. R., Guise, T. A. Hormonal control of calcium homeostasis. *Clin. Chem.* 1999;**45**:1347–52.

222 Hock, J. M., Gera, I. Effects of continuous and intermittent administration and inhibition of resorption on the anabolic response of bone to parathyroid hormone. *J. Bone. Min. Res.* 1992;**7**:65–72.

223 Strewler, G. J. The physiology of parathyroid hormone-related protein. *N. Engl. J. Med.* 2000; **342**:177–85.

224 Kukreja, S., Shevrin, D., Wimbidcus, S. *et al.* Antibodies to parathyroid hormone-related protein lower serum calcium in athymic mouse models of malignancy-associated hypercalcemia due to human tumors. *J. Clin. Invest.* 1988;**82**:1798–1802.

225 Broadus, A., Mangin, M., Ikeda, K. *et al.* Humoral hypercalcemia of cancer: identification of a novel parathyroid hormone-like peptide. *N. Engl. J. Med.* 1988;**319**:556–63.

226 Wysolmerski, J. J., Broadus, A. E. Hypercalcemia of malignancy: the central role of parathyroid hormone-related protein. *Annu. Rev. Med.* 1994:**45**:189–200.

227 Loveridge, N., Dean, V., Goltzman, D., Hendy, G. Bioactivity of parathyroid hormone and parathyroid hormone-like peptide: agonist and antagonist activities of amino-terminal fragments as assessed by the cytochemical bioassay and in situ biochemistry. *Endocrinology* 1991;**128**:1938–46.

228 Bergmann, P., Nijs De Wolf, N., Pepersack, T., Corvilain, J. Release of parathyroid hormone-like peptides by fetal rat long bones in culture. *J. Bone Miner. Res.* 1990;**5**:741–53.

229 Ballock, T. R., O'Keefe, R. J. The biology of the growth plate. *J. Bone. Joint. Surg. Am.* 2003;**85**:715–26.

230 Ballock, R. T., O'Keefe, R. J. Physiology and pathophysiology of the growth plate. *Birth Defects Res. Part C Embryo Today* 2003;**69**:123–43.

231 Schipani, E., Provot, S. PTHrP, PTH, and the PTH/PTHrP receptor in endochondral bone development. *Birth Defects Res. Part C Embryo Today* 2003;**69**:352–62.

232 Raisz, L., Simmons, H. A., Vargas, S. J., Kemp, B. E., Martin, T. J. Comparison of the effects of amino-terminal synthetic parathyroid hormone-related peptide (PTHrP) of malignancy and parathyroid hormone on resorption of cultured fetal rat long bones. *Calcif. Tissue. Int.* 1990;**46**:233–8.

233 Rosol, T., Capen, C., Horst, R. Effects of infusion of human parathyroid hormone-related protein-(1–40) in nude mice: histomorphometric and biochemical investigations. *J. Bone Min. Res.* 1988;**3**:699–706.

234 Karaplis, A. C., Luz, A., Glowacki, J. *et al.* Lethal skeletal dysplasia from targeted disruption of the parathyroid hormone-related peptide gene. *Genes Dev.* 1994;**8**:277–89.

235 Yamanaka, Y., Ueda, K., Seino, Y., Tanaka, H. Molecular basis for the treatment of achondroplasia. *Horm. Res.* 2003;**60**:60–4.

236 Thiede, M., Daifotis, A., Weir, E. *et al.* Intrauterine occupancy controls expression of the parathyroid hormone-related peptide gene in preterm rat myometrium. *Proc. Natl. Acad. Sci. USA.* 1990;**87**:6969–73.

237 Moniz, C., Burton, P., Malik, A. *et al.* Parathyroid hormone-related peptide in normal human fetal development. *J. Mol. Endocrinol.* 1990;**5**:259–66.

238 Moseley, J., Hayman, J., Danks, J. *et al.* Immunohistochemical detection of parathyroid hormone-related protein in human fetal epithelia. *J. Clin. Endocrinol. Metab.* 1991;**73**:478–84.

239 Thiede, M., Rodan, G. Expression of a calcium-mobilizing parathyroid hormone-like peptide in lactating mammary tissue. *Science* 1988;**242**:278–80.

240 Budayr, A., Halloran, B., King, J. *et al.* High levels of a parathyroid hormone-like protein in milk. *Proc. Natl. Acad. Sci. USA* 1989;**86**:7183–85.

241 Burtis, W., Brady, T., Orloff, J. *et al.* Immunochemical characterization of circulating parathyroid hormone-related protein in patients with humoral hypercalcemia of cancer. *N. Engl. J. Med.* 1990;**322**:1106–12.

242 Khosla, S., Johansen, K. L., Ory, S. J., O' Brien P. C., Kao, P. C. Parathyroid hormone-related peptide in lactation and umbilical cord. *Mayo Clin. Proc.* 1990;**65**:1408–14.

243 Prentice, A. Calcium in pregnancy and lactation. *Annu. Rev. Nutr.* 2000;**20**:249–72.

244 Kovacs, C. S., Kronenberg, H. M. Maternal-fetal calcium and bone metabolism during pregnancy, puerperium, and lactation. *Endocr. Rev.* 1997;**18**:832–72.

245 Sowers, M., Zhang, D., Hollis, B. W. *et al.* Role of calciotrophic hormones in calcium mobilization of lactation. *Am. J. Clin. Nutr.* 1998;**67**:284–91.

246 Sowers, M. F., Hollis, B. W., Shapiro, B. *et al.* Elevated parathyroid hormone-related peptide associated with lactation and bone density loss. *J. Am. Med. Assoc.* 1996;**276**:549–54.

247 Yamamoto, M., Duong, L. T., Fisher, J. E. *et al.* Suckling-mediated increases in urinary phosphate and 3′,5′-cyclic adenosine monophosphate excretion in lactating rats: possible systemic effects of parathyroid hormone-related protein. *Endocrinology* 1991;**129**:2614–22.

248 Ratcliffe, W. A., Thompson, G. E., Care, A. D., Peaker, M. Production of parathyroid hormone-related protein by the mammary gland of the goat. *J. Endocrinol.* 1992;**133**:87–93.

249 Lippuner, K., Zehnder, H. J., Casez, J. P., Takkinen, R., Jaeger, P. PTH-related protein is released into the mother's bloodstream during location. evidence for beneficial effects on maternal calcium-phosphate metabolism. *J. Bone. Min. Res.* 1996;**11**:1394–99.

250 Grill, V., Hillary, J., Ho, P. M. *et al.* Parathyroid hormone-related protein: a possible endocrine function in lactation. *Clin. Endocrinol. (Oxf).* 1992;**37**:405–10.

251 Bucht, E., Rong, H., Bremme, K. *et al.* (1995). Midmolecular parathyroid hormone-related peptide in serum during pregnancy, lactation and in umbilical cord blood. *Eur. J. Endocrinol.* 1995;**132**:438–43.

252 Caplan, R. H., Wickus, G. G., Sloane, K., Silva, P. D. Serum parathyroid hormone-related protein levels during lactation. *J. Reprod. Med.* 1995;**40**:216–18.

253 Dobnig, H., Kainer, F., Stepan, V. *et al.* Elevated parathyroid hormone-related peptide levels after human gestation: relationship to changes in bone and mineral metabolism. *J. Clin. Endocrinol. Metab.* 1995;**80**:3699–707.

254 Anai, T., Tomiyasu, T., Takai, N., Miyakawa, I. Remission of idiopathic hypoparathyroidism during lactation: a case report. *J. Obstet. Gynaecol. Res.* 1999;**25**:271–3.

255 Mather, K. J., Chik, C. L., Corenblum, B. Maintenance of serum calcium by parathyroid hormone-related peptide during lactation in a hypoparathyroid patient. *J. Clin. Endocrinol. Metab.* 1999;**84**:424–7.

256 VanHouten, J., Dann, P., McGeoch, G. *et al.* The calcium-sensing receptor regulates mammary gland parathyroid hormone-related protein production and calcium transport. *J. Clin. Invest.* 2004;**113**:598–608.

257 VanHouten, J. N., Dann, P., Stewart, A. F. *et al.* Mammary-specific deletion of parathyroid hormone-related protein preserves bone mass during lactation. *J. Clin. Invest.* 2003;**112**:1429–36.

258 Deftos, L. Calcitonin secretion in humans. In Cooper, C., ed. *Current Research on Calcium Regulating Hormones.* Austin TX: University of Texas Press; 1987:79–100.

259 Cooper, C., Schwesinger, W., Mahgoub, A., Ontjes, D. Thyrocalcitonin stimulation of secretion by pentagastrin. *Science* 1971;**172**:1238–40.

260 Roos, B., Deftos, L. Calcitonin secretion in vitro II. Regulating effects of enteric mammalian polypeptide hormones on tract C-cell cultures. *Endocrinology* 1976;**98**:1284–8.

261 Freake, H., MacIntyre, I. Specific binding of 1,25 dihydroxycholecalciferol in human medullary thyroid carcinoma. *Biochem. J.* 1982;**206**:181–4.

262 Nicholson, G., Moseley, J., Sexton, P., Mendelsohn, F., Martin, T. Abundant calcitonin receptors in isolated rat osteoclasts. Biochemical and autoradiographic characterization. *J. Clin. Invest.* 1986;**78**:355–9.

263 Raisz, L. Bone metabolism and its hormonal regulation. *Triangle* 1983;**22**:81–92.

264 Deftos, L., Glowacki, J. Mechanisms of bone metabolism. In Kem, D., Frohlich, E., eds. *Pathophysiology.* Philadelphia, PA: JB Lippincott Co.; 1984:445–68.

265 Kawashima, H., Torikai, S., Kurokawa, K. Calcitonin selectively stimulates 25-hydroxyvitamin D3-1-hydroxylase in proximal straight tubules of rat kidney. *Nature* 1981;**291**:327–9.

266 Galante, L., Colston, K., MacAuley, S., MacIntyre, I. Effect of calcitonin on vitamin D metabolism. *Nature* 1972;**238**:271–3.

267 Wimalawansa, S. J. Calcitonin gene-related peptide and its receptors: molecular genetics, physiology, pathophysiology, and therapeutic potentials. *Endocr. Rev.* 1996;**17**:533–85.

268 Jager, K., Muench, R., Seifert, H. *et al.* Calcitonin gene-related peptide (CGRP) causes redistribution of blood flow in humans. *Eur. J. Clin. Pharmacol.* 1990;**39**:491–4.

269 Lafond, J., St-Pierre, S., Masse, A., Savard, R., Simoneau, L. Calcitonin gene-related peptide receptor in human placental syncytiotrophoblast brush-border and basal plasma membranes. *Placenta* 1997;**18**:181–8.

270 Bevis, P. J., Zaidi, M., MacIntyre, I. A dual effect of calcitonin gene-related peptide on plasma calcium levels in the chick. *Biochem. Biophys. Res. Commun.* 1990;**169**:846–50.

271 Horst, R. L. Vitamin D metabolism. In Feldman, D., Glorieux, F. H., Wesley Pike, J., eds. *Vitamin D.* New York: Academic Press; 1997:13–31.

272 De Luca, H. F., Schnoes, H. K. Vitamin D: recent advances. *Annu. Rev. Biochem.* 1985;**52**:411–39.

273 Clemens, T. L., Holick, M. F. Recent advances in the hormonal regulation of calcium and phosphorus in adult animals and humans. In Holick, M. F., Anast, C. S., Gray, T. K., eds. *Perinatal Calcium and Phosphorus Metabolism.* Amsterdam: Elsevier; 1983:1–24.

274 Tojo, R., Pavon, P., Antelo, J. *et al.* Vitamin D and its metabolites. Advances in the diagnosis and treatment of rickets. *Acta Vitaminol. Enzymol.* 1982;**4**:1–11.

275 Coburn, J., Slatopolsky, E. Vitamin D, parathyroid hormone, and renal osteodystrophy. In Rector, B., ed. *The Kidney.* Philadelphia, PA: W. B. Saunders Co; 1986:1657–729.

276 Bachrach, S. Vitamin D deficiency rickets in American children. *Compr. Ther.* 1981;**7**:29–34.

277 Felsenfeld, A., Llach, F. Vitamin D and metabolic bone disease: a clinicopathologic overview. *Pathol. Annu.* 1982;**17**:383–410.

278 Akiba, T., Endou, H., Koseki, C. *et al.* Localization of 25-hydroxyvitamin D3-1ahydroxylase activity in the mammalian kidney. *Biochem. Biophys. Res. Commun.* 1980;**94**:313–18.

279 St-Arnaud, R., Arabian, A., Travers, R. *et al.* Deficient mineralization of intramembranous bone in vitamin D-24-hydroxylase-ablated mice is due to elevated 1,25-dihydroxyvitamin D and not to the absence of 24,25-dihydroxyvitamin D. *Endocrinology* 2000;**141**:2658–66.

280 Umeda, F., Inoue, K., Hirano, K. *et al.* Alterations in femoral bone histomorphometry and vitamin D metabolism in neonatal streptozotocin-induced diabetic rat. *Fukuoka Igaku Zasshi.* 1992;**83**:403–8.

281 Garabedian, M., Holick, M., DeLuca, H., Boyle, I. Control of 25-hydroxycholecalciferol metabolism by parathyroid glands. *Proc. Natl. Acad. Sci. USA* 1972;**69**:1673–6.

282 Nesbitt, T., Drezner, M. Insulin-like growth factor-I regulation of renal 25-hydroxyvitamin D-1-hydroxylase activity. *Endocrinology* 1993;**132**:133–8.

283 Chesney, R., Rosen, J., Hamstra, A., DeLuca, H. Serum 1,25-dihydroxyvitamin D levels in normal children and in vitamin D disorders. *Am. J. Dis. Child.* 1980;**134**:135–9.

284 Armbrecht, H., Forte, L., Halloran, B. Effect of age and dietary calcium on renal 25(OH)D metabolism, serum 1,25(OH)2D and PTH. *Am. J. Physiol.* 1984;**246**:E266–70.

285 Ribovich, M., DeLuca, H. The influence of dietary calcium and phosphorus on intestinal calcium transport in rats given vitamin D metabolites. *Arch. Biochem. Biophys.* 1975;**170**: 529–35.

286 Lovinger, R. Rickets. *Pediatrics* 1980;**66**:359–65.

287 Fatemi, S., Ryzen, E., Flores, J., Endres, D., Rude, R. Effect of experimental human magnesium depletion on parathyroid hormone secretion and 1,25-dihydroxyvitamin D metabolism. *J. Clin. Endocrinol. Metab.* 1991;**73**:1067–72.

288 Saggese, G., Federico, G., Bertelloni, S., Baroncelli, G., Calisti, L. Hypomagnesemia and the parathyroid hormone-vitamin D endocrine system in children with insulin-dependent diabetes mellitus: effects of magnesium administration. *J. Pediatr.* 1991;**118**:220–5.

289 Pike, J. The vitamin D receptor and its gene. In Feldman, D., Glorieux, F. H., Wesley Pike, J., eds. *Vitamin D.* New York: Academic Press;1997:105–25.

290 Walling, M. Intestinal calcium and phosphate transport: differential responses to vitamin D3 metabolites. *Am. J. Physiol.* 1977;**233**:E488–94.

291 Schwartz, Z., Dennis, R., Bonewald, L. *et al.* Differential regulation of prostaglandin E2 synthesis and phospholipase A2 activity by 1,25-(OH)2D3 in three osteoblast-like cell lines (MC-3T#-E1, ROS 17/2.8, and MG-63). *Bone* 1992;**13**:51–8.

292 Slatopolsky, E., Weerts, C., Thielan, J. *et al.* Marked suppression of secondary hyperparathyroidism by intravenous administration of 1,25-dihydroxy- cholecalciferol in uremic patients. *J. Clin. Invest.* 1984;**74**:2136–43.

293 Betinelli, A., Bianchi, M., Mazzuchi, E., Gandolini, G., Appiani, A. Acute effects of calcitriol and phosphate salts on mineral metabolism in children with hypophosphatemic rickets. *J. Pediatr.* 1991;**118**:372–6.

294 Pitkin, R. Calcium metabolism in pregnancy and the perinatal period: a review. *Am. J. Obstet. Gynecol.* 1985;**151**:99–109.

295 Salle, B. L., Delvin, E. E., Lapillonne, A., Bishop, N. J., Glorieux, F. H. Perinatal metabolism of vitamin D. *Am. J. Clin. Nutr.* 2000;**71**:1317S–24S.

296 Martinez, M. E., Sanchez, C., Salinas, M. *et al.* Ionic calcium levels during pregnancy, at delivery and in the first hours of life. *Scand. J. Clin. Lab. Invest.* 1986;**46**:27–30.

297 Allgrove, J., Adami, S., Manning, R., O' Riordan, J. Cytochemical bioassay of PTH in maternal and cord blood. *Arch. Dis. Child.* 1985;**60**:110–15.

298 Davis, O. K., Hawkins, D. S., Rubin, L. P. *et al.* Serum parathyroid hormone (PTH) in pregnant women determined by an immuno-radiometric assay for intact PRH. *J. Clin. Endocrinol. Metab.* 1988;**67**:850–2.

299 Gallacher, S. J., Fraser, W. D., Owens, O. J. *et al.* Changes in calciotrophic hormones and biochemical markers of bone turnover in normal human pregnancy. *Eur. J. Endocrinol.* 1994;**131**:369–74.

300 Martinez, M. E., Catalan, P., Lisbona, A. *et al.* Serum osteocalcin concentrations in diabetic pregnant women and their newborns. *Horm. Metab. Res.* 1994;**26**:338–42.

301 Saggese, G., Bertelloni, S., Baroncelli, G. I., Pelletti, A., Benedetti, U. Evaluation of a peptide family encoded by the

calcitonin gene in selected healthy pregnant women. A longitudinal study. *Horm. Res.* 1990;**34**:240–4.

302 Halhali, A., Wimalawansa, S. J., Berentsen, V. *et al.* Calcitonin gene- and parathyroid hormone-related peptides in preeclampsia: effects of magnesium sulfate. *Obstet. Gynecol.* 2001;**97**:893–7.

303 Bouillon, R., Van Assche, F. A., Van Baelen, H. V. *et al.* Influence of the vitamin D-binding protein on the serum concentration of 1,25-dihydroxyvitamin D$_3$: significance of the free 1,25-dihydroxyvitamin D$_3$ concentration. *J. Clin. Invest.* 1981;**67**:589–96.

304 Delvin, E. E., Glorieux, F. H., Salle, B. L. *et al.* Control of vitamin D metabolism in preterm infants: feto-maternal relationships. *Arch. Dis. Child.* 1982;**57**:754–7.

305 Fleischman, A. R., Rosen, J. F., Cole, J. *et al.* Maternal and fetal serum 1,25-dihydroxyvitamin D levels at term. *J. Pediatr.* 1980;**97**:640–2.

306 Care, A. D. Vitamin D in pregnancy, the fetoplacental unit, and lactation. In Feldman, D., Glorieux, F. H., Wesley Pike, J., eds. *Vitamin D.* New York:Academic Press;1997:437–43.

307 Weisman, Y., Harell, A., Edelstein, D. *et al.* 1,25-Dihydroxyvitamin D$_3$ and 24,25-dihydroxyvitamin D$_3$ in vitro synthesis by human decidua and placenta. *Nature* 1979;**281**:317–19.

308 Delvin, E. E., Arabian, A., Glorieux, F. H. *et al.* In vitro metabolism of 25-OH-hydroxycholecalciferol by isolated cells from human decidua. *J. Clin. Endocrinol. Metab.* 1985;**60**:880–5.

309 Delvin, E. E., Arabian, A. Kinetics and regulation of 25-hydroxycholecalciferol 1-hydroxylase from cells isolated from human term decidua. *Eur. J. Biochem.* 1987;**163**:659–62.

310 Ritchie, L. D., Fung, E. B., Halloran, B. P. *et al.* A longitudinal study of calcium homeostasis during human pregnancy and lactation and after resumption of menses. *Am. J. Clin. Nutr.* 1998;**67**:693–701.

311 Kent, G. N., Price, R. I., Gutteridge, D. H. *et al.* Human lactation: forearm trabecular bone loss, increased bone turnover, and renal conservation of calcium and inorganic phosphate with recovery of bone mass following weaning. *J. Bone Min. Res.* 1990;**5**:361–9.

312 Cross, N. A., Hillman, L. S., Allen, S. H., Krause, G. F., Vieira, N. E. Calcium homeostasis and bone metabolism during pregnancy, lactation, and postweaning: a longitudinal study. *Am. J. Clin. Nutr.* 1995;**61**:514–23.

313 Prentice, A., Jarjou, L. M. A., Stirling, D. M. S., Buffenstein, R., Fairweather-Tait, S. Biochemical markers of calcium and bone metabolism during 18 months of lactation in Gambian women accustomed to a low calcium intake and in those consuming a calcium supplement. *J. Clin. Endocrinol. Metab.* 1998;**83**:1059–66.

314 Specker, B., Tsang, R., Ho, M. Changes in calcium homeostasis over the first year postpartum: effect of lactation and weaning. *Obstet. Gynecol.* 1991;**78**:56–62.

315 Krebs, N. F., Reidinger, C. J., Robertson, A. D., Brenner, M. Bone mineral density changes during lactation: maternal, dietary, and biochemical correlates. *Am. J. Clin. Nutr.* 1997;**65**:1738–46.

316 Kalkwarf, H. J. Hormonal and dietary regulation of changes in bone density during lactation and after weaning in women. *J. Mammary Gland Biol. Neoplasia* 1999;**4**:319–29.

317 Greer, F. R., Tsang, R. C., Searcy, J. E., Levin, R. S., Steichen, J. J. Mineral homeostasis during lactation – relationship to serum 1,25-dihydroxyvitamin D, 25-hydroxyvitamin D, parathyroid hormone, and calcitonin. *Am. J. Clin. Nutr.* 1982;**36**:431–7.

318 Kalkwarf, H. J., Specker, B. L. Bone mineral changes during pregnancy and lactation. *Endocrine* 2002;**17**:49–53.

319 Kalkwarf, H. J., Specker, B. L., Heubi, J. E., Vieira, N. E., Yergey, A. L. Intestinal calcium absorption of women during lactation and after weaning. *Am. J. Clin. Nutr.* 1996;**63**:526–31.

320 Kalkwarf, H. J., Specker, B. L., Ho, M. Effects of calcium supplementation on calcium homeostasis and bone turnover in lactating women. *J. Clin. Endocrinol. Metab.* 1999;**84**:464–70.

321 Prentice, A. Micronutrients and the bone mineral content of the mother, fetus and newborn. *J. Nutr.* 2003;**133**:1693S–99S.

322 Cole, D. E., Gundberg, C. M., Stirk, L. J. *et al.* Changing osteocalcin concentrations during pregnancy and lactation: implications for maternal mineral metabolism. *J. Clin. Endocrinol. Metab.* 1987;**65**:290–4.

323 Rodin, A., Duncan, A., Quartero, H. W. P. *et al.* Serum concentrations of alkaline phosphatase isoenzymes and osteocalcin in normal pregnancy. *J. Clin. Endocrinol. Metab.* 1989;**68**:1123–27.

324 Fukuoka, H., Mukai, S., Kobayashi, Y., Jimbo, T. Dynamic changes in serum osteocalcin levels in the perinatal periods. *Nippon Naibunpi Gakkai Zasshi.* 1989;**65**:1116–22.

325 Gorzelak, M., Darmochwal-Kolarz, D., Jablonski, M. *et al.* The concentrations of osteocalcin and degradation products of type I collagen in pregnant women with pre-eclampsia. *Eur. J. Obstet. Gynecol. Reprod. Biol.* 2001;**98**:23–7.

326 Naylor, K. E., Iqbal, P., Fledelius, C., Fraser, R. B., Eastell, R. The effect of pregnancy on bone density and bone turnover. *J. Bone. Min. Res.* 2000;**15**:129–37.

327 Seki, K., Makimura, N., Mitsui, C., Hirata, J., Nagata, I. Calcium-regulating hormones and osteocalcin levels during pregnancy: a longitudinal study. *Am. J. Obstet. Gynecol.* 1991;**164**:1248–52.

328 Seki, K., Wada, S., Nagata, N., Nagata, I. Parathyroid hormone-related protein during pregnancy and the perinatal period. *Gynecol. Obstet. Invest.* 1994;**37**:83–6.

329 More, C., Bhattoa, H. P., Bettembuk, P., Balogh, A. The effects of pregnancy and lactation on hormonal status and biochemical markers of bone turnover. *Eur. J. Obstet. Gynecol. Reprod. Biol.* 2003;**106**:209–13.

330 Kovacs, C. S. Calcium and bone metabolism in pregnancy and lactation. *J. Clin. Endocrinol. Metab.* 2001;**86**:2344–8.

331 Villar, J., Repke, J. Calcium supplementation during pregnancy may reduce preterm delivery in high-risk populations. *Am. J. Obstet. Gynecol.* 1990;**163**:1124–31.

332 Repke, J. Calcium, magnesium, and zinc supplementation and perinatal outcome. *Clin. Obstet. Gynecol.* 1991;**34**:262–7.

333 Koo, W. W., Walters, J. C., Esterlitz, J. *et al.* Maternal calcium supplementation and fetal bone mineralization. *Obstet. Gynecol.* 1999;**94**:577–82.

334 Holmberg-Marttila, D., Leino, A., Sievanen, H. Bone turnover markers during lactation, postpartum amenorrhea and resumption of menses. *Osteoporos. Int.* 2003;**14**:103–9.

335 Economou-Mavrou, C., McCance, R. Calcium, magnesium and phosphorus in fetal tissues. *Biochem. J.* 1958;**68**: 573.

336 Garel, J., Gilbert, M. Dietary calcium and phosphorus manipulations in thyroparathyroidectomized pregnant rats and fetal liver glycogen stores. *Reprod. Nutr. Rev.* 1981;**21**:969–72.

337 Alatas, O., Colak, O., Alatas, E. *et al.* Osteocalcin metabolism in late fetal life: fetal and maternal osteocalcin levels. *Clin. Chim. Acta.* 1995;**239**:179–83.

338 de Toro Salas, A., Duenas Diez J., de Jaime Revuelta, E. Concentrations of calcium and bone remodeling biomarkers in umbilical cord blood and urine of newborn infants during delivery. *An. Esp. Pediatr.* 2000;**54**:290–6.

339 Nishiyama, S., Fujimoto, S., Kodama, M., Matsuda, I. The negative correlation between prolactin and ionic calcium in cord blood of full term infants. *Endocrinol. Jpn.* 1985;**32**: 9–15.

340 Whitsett, J., Tsang, R. Calcium uptake and binding by membrane fractions of the human placenta: ATP-dependent calcium accumulation. *Pediatr. Res.* 1980;**14**:769–75.

341 Fisher, G., Kelley, L., Smith, C. ATP-dependent calcium transport across basal plasma membranes of human placental trophoblast. *Am. J. Physiol.* 1987;**252**:C38–46.

342 Pike, J. W., Gooze, L. L., Haussler, M. R. Biochemical evidence for 1,25-dihydroxyvitamin D receptor macromolecules in parathyroid, pancreatic, pituitary, and placental tissues. *Life Sci.* 1980;**26**:407–14.

343 Lafond, J., Auger, D., Fortier, J., Brunette, M. Parathyroid hormone receptors in human placental syncytiotrophoblasts brush border and basal plasma membranes. *Endocrinology* 1988;**123**:2834–40.

344 Umeki, S., Nagao, S., Nozawa, Y. The purification and identification of calmodulin from human placenta. *Biochem. Biophys. Acta.* 1981;**674**:319–26.

345 Bruns, M., Fausto, S., Avioli, L. Placental calcium-binding proteins in rats. *J. Biol. Chem.* 1978;**253**:3186–90.

346 Bruns, M., Vollmer, S., Wallshein, V., Bruns, D. Vitamin D-dependent calcium-binding protein. *J. Biol. Chem.* 1981;**256**:4649–53.

347 Lester, G. Cholecalciferol and placental calcium transport. *Fed. Proc.* 1986;**45**:2524–7.

348 Ohta, T., Mori, M., Ogawa, K., Matsuyama, T., Ishii S. Immunocytochemical localization of BGP in human bones in various developmental stages and pathological conditions. *Virchows Arch. A. Pathol. Anat. Histopathol.* 1989;**415**:459–66.

349 Khattab, A., Forfar, J. Interrelationships of calcium, phosphorus and glucose levels in mother and newborn infant. *Biol. Neonate.* 1970;**15**:26–36.

350 Cockburn, F., Belton, N., Purvis, R. *et al.* Maternal vitamin D intake and mineral metabolism in mothers and their newborn infants. *Br. Med. J.* 1980;**281**:11–14.

351 Croley, T. The intracellular localization of calcium within the mature human placental barrier. *Am. J. Obstet. Gynecol.* 1973;**117**:926–32.

352 Shami, Y., Messer, H., Copp, D. Calcium uptake by placental plasma membrane vesicles. *Biochim. Biophys. Acta* 1975;**401**:256–64.

353 Bruns, M., Fausto, S., Avioli, L. Placental calcium-binding proteins in rats. *J. Biol. Chem.* 1978;**253**:3186–90.

354 Bruns, M., Vollmer, S., Wallshein, V., Bruns, D. Vitamin D-dependent calcium-binding protein. *J. Biol. Chem.* 1981;**256**:4649–53.

355 Norman, A., Roth, J., Orci, L. The vitamin D endocrine system: steroid metabolism, hormone receptors, and biological response (calcium binding proteins). *Endocr. Rev.* 1982;**3**:331–66.

356 Delvin, E., Richard, P., Pothier, P., Menard, D. Presence and binding characteristics of calcitriol receptors in human fetal gut. *FEBS* 1990;**262**:55–7.

357 Shami, Y., Radde, I. Calcium-stimulated ATPase of guinea pig placenta. *Biochim. Biophys. Acta.* 1971;**249**:345–52.

358 Whitsett, J., Tsang, R. Calcium uptake and binding by membrane fractions of the human placenta: ATP-dependent calcium accumulation. *Pediatr. Res.* 1980;**14**:769–75.

359 Miller, R., Berndt, W. Evidence for Mg2+-dependent, Na+ + K+-activated ATPase and Ca2+-ATPase in the human term placenta. *Proc. Soc. Exp. Biol. Med.* 1973;**143**: 118–22.

360 Gupta, M., Kuppuswamy, G., Subramanian, A. Transplacental transfer of 25-hydroxycholecalciferol. *Postgrad. Med. J.* 1982;**58**:408–10.

361 Krukowsky, M., Lehr, D. Parathyroid hormone and the placental barrier. *Arch. Int. Pharmacodyn. Ther.* 1963;**146**: 245–65.

362 Garel, J., Dumont, C. Distribution and inactivation of labeled parathyroid hormone in the rat fetus. *Horm. Metab. Res.* 1972;**4**:217–21.

363 Northrop, G., Misenheimer, H., Becker, F. Failure of parathyroid hormone to cross the non-human primate placenta. *Am. J. Obstet. Gynecol.* 1979;**129**:449–53.

364 Root, A., Gruskin, A., Reber, R. *et al.* Serum concentrations of parathyroid hormone in infants, children, and adolescents. *Pediatrics* 1974;**85**:329–36.

365 Hillman, L., Slatopolsky, E., Haddad, J. Perinatal vitamin D metabolism: IV. Maternal and cord serum 24,25-dihydroxy vitamin D concentrations. *J. Clin. Endocrinol. Metab.* 1977;**47**:1073–77.

366 Reitz, R., Daane, T., Woods, J. *et al.* Calcium, magnesium, phosphorus, and parathyroid hormone interrelationships in pregnancy and newborn infants. *Obstet. Gynecol.* 1977;**50**:701–5.

367 Samaan, N., Wigoda, C., Castillo, S. Human serum calcitonin and parathyroid hormone levels in the maternal, umbilical

cord blood and postpartum. *Proceedings of the Fourth International Symposium on Endocrinology.* London: William Heinemann; 1973:364–72.

368 Watney, P., Rudd, B. Calcium metabolism in pregnancy and in the newborn. *J. Obstet. Gynecol. Br. Commonw.* 1974;**81**:210–19.

369 Lequin, R., Hackeng, W., Schopman, W. A radioimmunoassay for parathyroid hormone in man. II. Measurement of parathyroid hormone concentrations in human plasma by means of a radioimmunoassay for bovine hormone. *Acta Endocrinol.* 1970;**63**:655–66.

370 Tsang, R., Chen, I., Friedman, M. *et al.* Neonatal parathyroid function: role of gestational age and postnatal age. *J. Pediatr.* 1973;**83**:728–38.

371 Allgrove, J., Adami, S., Manning, R., O'Riordan, J. Cytochemical bioassay of PTH in maternal and cord blood. *Arch. Dis. Child.* 1985;**60**:110–15.

372 Robinson, N., Sibley, C., Mughal, M., Boyd, R. Fetal control of calcium transport across the rat placenta. *Pediatr. Res.* 1989;**26**:109–15.

373 Rodda, C., Kubota, M., Heath, J. *et al.* Evidence for a novel parathyroid hormone-related protein in fetal lamb parathyroid glands and sheep placenta: comparisons with a similar protein implicated in humoral hypercalcemia of malignancy. *J. Endocrinol.* 1988;**117**:261–71.

374 Ikeda, K., Weir, E., Mangin, M. *et al.* Expression of messenger ribonucleic acids encoding a parathyroid hormone-like peptide in normal human and animal tissues with abnormal expression in human parathyroid adenomas. *Mol. Endocrinol.* 1988;**2**:1230–36.

375 Care, A., Caple, I., Abbas, S., Pickard, D. The effect of fetal thyroparathyroidectomy on the transport of calcium across the ovine placenta. *Placenta* 1986;**7**:417–24.

376 Martin, T. A novel parathyroid hormone-related protein: role in pathology and physiology. In Peterlik, M., Bronner, F., eds. *Molecular and Cellular Regulation of Calcium and Phosphate Metabolism: Proceedings of the Symposium on Molecular and Cellular Regulation of Calcium and Phosphate Metabolism, held in Vienna, November 17, 1988.* New York:Wiley-Liss;1990:1–37.

377 Abbas, S., Pickard, D., Rodda, C. *et al.* Stimulation of ovine placental calcium transport by purified natural and recombinant parathyroid hormone-related protein (PTHrP) preparations. *Q. J. Exp. Physiol.* 1989;**74**:549–52.

378 MacIsaac, R. J., Heath, J. A., Rodda, C. P. *et al.* Role of the fetal parathyroid glands and parathyroid hormone-related protein in the regulation of placental transport of calcium, magnesium and inorganic phosphate. *Reprod. Fertil. Dev.* 1991;**3**:447–57.

379 Miao, D., He, B., Karaplis, A. C., Goltzman, D. Parathyroid hormone is essential for normal fetal bone formation. *J. Clin. Invest.* 2002;**109**:1173–82.

380 Kovacs, C. S., Chafe, L. L., Fudge, N. J., Friel, J. K., Manley, N. R. PTH regulates fetal blood calcium and skeletal mineralization

independently of PTHrP. *Endocrinology* 2001;**142**:4983–93.

381 Kovacs, C. S., Manley, N. R., Moseley, J. M., Martin, T. J., Kronenberg, H. M. Fetal parathyroids are not required to maintain placental calcium transport. *J. Clin. Invest.* 2001;**107**:1007–15.

382 Chan, A., Conen, P. Ultrastructural observations on cytodifferentiation of parafollicular cells in the human fetal thyroid. *Lab. Invest.* 1971;**53**:249–59.

383 Samaan, N., Anderson, G., Adam-Mayne, M. Immunoreactive calcitonin in the mother, neonate, child, and adult. *Am. J. Obstet. Gynecol.* 1975;**121**:622–5.

384 Whitehead, M., Lane, G., Young, O. *et al.* Interrelations of calcium-regulating hormones during normal pregnancy. *Br. Med. J.* 1981;**283**:10–31.

385 Drake, T., Kaplan, R., Lewis, T. The physiologic hyperparathyroidism of pregnancy: is it primary or secondary? *Obstet. Gynecol.* 1979;**53**:746–9.

386 Stevenson, J., Hillyard, C., MacIntyre, I. *et al.* The physiological role for calcitonin: protection of the maternal skeleton. *Lancet* 1979;**2**:769–70.

387 Wieland, P., Fisher, J., Trechsel, U. *et al.* Perinatal parathyroid hormone, vitamin D metabolites and calcitonin in man. *Am. J. Physiol.* 1980;**239**:E385–90.

388 Seino, Y., Ishida, M., Yamaoka, K. *et al.* Serum calcium regulating hormones in the perinatal period. *Calcif. Tissue. Int.* 1982;**34**:131–5.

389 Hillman, L., Rojanasathit, S., Slatopolsky, E., Haddad, J. Serial measurements of serum calcium, magnesium, parathyroid hormone, calcitonin, and 25-hydroxyvitamin D in premature and term infants during the first week of life. *Pediatr. Res.* 1977;**11**:739–44.

390 Pearse, A. Calcitonin. In Taylor, S., Foster, G., eds. *Calcitonin, Proceedings of the Second International Symposium.* London: Heinemann Medical;1969:125.

391 Leroyer-Alizon, E., David, L., Dubois, P. Evidence for calcitonin in the thyroid gland of normal and anencephalic human fetuses: immunocytological localization, radioimmunoassay and gel filtration of thyroid extracts. *J. Clin. Endocrinol. Metab.* 1980;**50**:316–21.

392 Venkataraman, P., Tsang, R., Chen, I., Sperling, M. Pathogenesis of early neonatal hypocalcemia: Studies of serum calcitonin, gastrin and plasma glucagon. *J. Pediatr.* 1987;**110**:599–603.

393 Barlet, J. Calcitonin may modulate placental transfer in ewes. *J. Endocrinol.* 1985;**104**:17–21.

394 Hollis, B., Pittard, W. Evaluation of total fetomaternal vitamin D relationships at term. Evidence for racial differences. *J. Clin. Endocrinol. Metab.* 1984;**59**:652–7.

395 Ross, R., Care, A., Taylor, C., Pele, B., Sommerville, B. The transplacental movement of metabolites of vitamin D in the sheep. In Norman, A., Schaefer, K., Coburn, J., eds. *Vitamin D. Basic Research and its Clinical Application.* Berlin: DeGruyter;1979:341–4.

396 Clements, M., Fraser, D. Vitamin D supply to the rat fetus and neonate. *J. Clin. Invest.* 1988;**81**:1768–73.

397 Ron, M., Levitz, M., Chuba, J., Dancis, J. Transfer of 25-hydroxyvitamin D3 across the perfused human placenta. *Am. J. Obstet. Gynecol.* 1984;**148**:370–4.

398 Ross, R. Calcium regulating hormones. In Polin, R., Fox, W., eds. *Fetal and Neonatal Physiology, Vol.* 2. Philadelphia, PA: W. B. Saunders Co; 1992:1698–734.

399 Hillman, L., Haddad, J. Human perinatal vitamin D metabolism: I. 25-hydroxy-vitamin D in maternal and cord blood. *J. Pediatr.* 1974;**84**:742–9.

400 Weisman, Y., Occhipinti, M., Knox, G., Reiter, E., Root, A. Concentrations of 24,25-dihydroxyvitamin D and 25-hydroxyvitamin D in paired maternal-cord sera. *Am. J. Obstet. Gynecol.* 1978;**130**:704–7.

401 Ross, R. Dorsey, J. Postnatal changes in plasma 1,25-dihydroxyvitamin D3 in sheep: role of altered clearance. *Am. J. Physiol.* 1991;**261**:E635–41.

402 Weisman, Y., Sapir, R., Harell, A., Edelstein, S. Maternal-perinatal interrelationships of vitamin D in rats. *Biochem. Biophys. Acta.* 1976;**428**:388–95.

403 Gertner, J., Glassman, M., Coustan, D., Goodman, D. Fetomaternal, vitamin D relationships at term. *J. Pediatr.* 1980;**97**:637–40.

404 Hoogenboezem, T., Degenhart, H., De Muinck Keizer-Schrama, S. *et al.* Vitamin D metabolism in breast-fed infants and their mothers. *Pediatr. Res.* 1989;**25**:623–8.

405 Cross, N. A., Hillman, L. S., Allen, S. H., Krause, G. F., Vieira, N. E. Calcium homeostasis and bone metabolism during pregnancy, lactation, and postweaning: a longitudinal study. *Am. J. Clin. Nutr.* 1995;**61**:514–23.

406 Ritchie, L. D., Fung, E. B., Halloran, B. P. *et al.* A longitudinal study of calcium homeostasis during human pregnancy and lactation and after resumption of menses. *Am. J. Clin. Nutr.* 1998;**67**:693–701.

407 O'Brien, K. O., Nathanson, M. S., Mancini, J., Witter, F. R. Calcium absorption is significantly higher in adolescents during pregnancy than in the early postpartum period. *Am. J. Clin. Nutr.* 2003;**78**:1188–93.

408 Raisz, L. G. Physiology and pathophysiology of bone remodeling. *Clin. Chem.* 1999;**45**:1353–8.

16

Disorders of mineral, vitamin D and bone homeostasis

Oussama Itani[1] and Reginald C. Tsang[2]

[1] Michigan State University and Kalamazoo Center for Medical Studies, and Borgess Medical Center, Kalamazoo, MI
[2] Department of Pediatrics, Children's Hospital Medical Center, Cincinnati, OH

Disorders of mineral homeostasis

Fetal mineral homeostasis is closely linked to that of the mother. In the pregnant woman and the fetus there is an intimate and delicate relationship amongst the calciotropic hormones, growth factors, and the minerals Ca, P, and Mg. Any perturbation of maternal or placental homeostatic mineral balance may affect that of the fetus and may have metabolic sequelae in the fetus manifesting in the neonatal period and infancy.

Disorders of calcium homeostasis

A wide variety of factors can cause significant disturbances in calcium and bone homeostasis in the fetus and neonate.

Maternal hypocalcemia

Maternal hypocalcemia results in fetal hypocalcemia, which stimulates the fetal parathyroid glands to synthesize and secrete more parathyroid hormone (PTH to achieve normocalcemia. PTH does not appear to cross the placenta in either direction. Causes of maternal hypocalcemia are listed in Table 16.1. Impaired secretion of PTH because of hypoparathyroidism or magnesium depletion and resistance to PTH because of mutant receptors, as in pseudohypoparathyroidism, result in maternal hypocalcemia. Hypocalcemia may also be a manifesting feature of abnormal vitamin D deficiency; in particular, maternal vitamin D deficiency may be caused by insufficient sunlight exposure, inadequate dietary intake, or malabsorption. Maternal liver disease may be associated with defective 25-hydroxylase

activity resulting in low serum 25-hydroxyvitamin D (25-OHD) concentration, hypocalcemia, and rickets.

Defective 1 alpha-hydroxylase activity may be caused by renal or parathyroid gland diseases. Renal hypophosphatemic rickets is a familial disorder characterized by decreased reabsorption of phosphate in the proximal renal tubules resulting in hypophosphatemia and rickets. It often has an X-linked dominant mode of inheritance. Serum Ca concentration is either normal or low. Serum PTH concentration is either normal or elevated. Serum 1.25 dihydroxyvitamin D(1,25(OH)2D) concentration may be normal or low.

Chronic renal failure is associated with hyperphosphatemia, hypocalcemia, and depressed 1 alpha-hydroxylase activity with low serum 1,25(OH)2D which results in secondary hyperparathyroidism. Vitamin D-dependent rickets type I is a familial disorder with an autosomal recessive inheritance pattern. It is characterized by depressed renal 1 alpha-hydroxylase activity, hypocalcemia, low serum 1,25(OH)2D concentration, and elevated serum PTH concentration. Vitamin D-dependent rickets type II is a rare disease characterized by defective target organ response to 1,25(OH)2D which is attributed to a defect in the cellular and nuclear uptake of 1,25(OH)2D. Receptors for 1,25(OH)2D are either absent or defective and bind abnormally to DNA molecules because of the expression of a point mutation in the gene coding for these receptors. Patients with this disease have elevated serum 1,25(OH)2D concentration and associated alopecia which may occur early in the neonatal period and precede any biochemical abnormalities.[1] Maternal hypoparathyroidism is associated with defective renal 1 alpha-hydroxylase activity, hypocalcemia, and low

Neonatal Nutrition and Metabolism. Second Edition, ed. P. Thureen and W. Hay. Published by Cambridge University Press.
© Cambridge University Press 2006.

Table 16.1. Causes of maternal hypocalcemia

Abnormal parathyroid gland function
    Impaired secretion of PTH
        Absent glands
        Magnesium deficiency
    Resistance to PTH action
        Magnesium deficiency
        Pseudohypoparathyroidism
Abnormal vitamin D metabolism
    Vitamin D deficiency
        Inadequate sunshine exposure or vitamin D intake
        Intestinal malabsorption
    Reduced 25-hydroxylase activity
        Hepatic disease
    Reduced 1 alpha-hydroxylase activity
        Hyperphosphatemia
        Renal disease
          Chronic renal failure
          Hypophosphatemic rickets
          Vitamin D-dependent Rickets type I
        Parathyroid gland-related
          Hypoparathyroidism
          Pseudohypoparathyroidism
        Reduced response to 1,25 dihydroxyvitamin D
    Vitamin D-dependent rickets Type II
Miscellaneous
    Tumor-induced osteomalacia
    Anticonvulsant therapy
    Acute pancreatitis
    Phosphate therapy
    Chemotherapy and tumor lysis syndrome

Table 16.2. Causes of neonatal hypocalcemia.

Early neonatal hypocalcemia
    Prematurity
    Birth asphyxia
    Infant of diabetic mothers
    Hypoparathyroidism secondary to maternal
        hyperparathyroidism
    Phototherapy
    Gestational exposure to anticonvulsants
    Congenital rickets and abnormal maternal-fetal vitamin D
        metabolism
Late neonatal hypocalcemia
    Excessive phosphorus intake
        Cow milk formulas
        High P-containing cereals
        High P-containing enemas
        Phosphate therapy
Decreased dietary calcium intake
Excessive calcium losses
    Renal: diuretics
    Intestinal: malabsorption
Maternal factors
    Decreased vitamin D intake
    Decreased sunlight exposure
    Advanced age and parity
    Low socioeconomic status
Hypoparathyroidism
    Congenital/Primary
        Sporadic
        Hereditary
    Acquired/secondary
        Maternal hyperparathyroidism
        Maternal insulin-dependent diabetes mellitus
        Acute hypermagnesemia
        Chronic hypomagnesemia
Abnormal vitamin D metabolism
    Vitamin D deficiency
        Inadequate sunshine exposure or vitamin D intake
        Intestinal malabsorption
    Reduced 25-hydroxylase activity:
        Hepatic disease
    Reduced 1 alpha hydroxylase activity
        Hyperphosphatemia
        Renal disease
          Chronic renal failure
          Hypophosphatemic rickets
          Vitamin D-dependent rickets type I
        Parathyroid gland-related
          Hypoparathyroidism
          Pseudohypoparathyroidism
        Reduced response to 1,25 dihydroxyvitamin D
    Vitamin D-dependent rickets Type II
Miscellaneous
    Exchange transfusion with citrate-containing blood
    Tumor-induced osteomalacia
    Acute pancreatitis
    Tumor lysis syndrome
    Osteopetrosis

serum 1,25(OH)2D concentration but the impact on the fetus may be a transient hyperparathyroidism state with hypercalcemia.

Neonatal hypocalcemia

Neonatal hypocalcemia is defined by serum total calcium concentration below 7 mg dL^{-1} (1.75 mmol dL^{-1}) for preterm and below 8 mg dL^{-1} (2 mmol dL^{-1}) for term infants as determined by atomic absorptiometry or serum ionized Ca concentration below 3.0–4.4 mg dL^{-1} (0.75–1.1 mmol L^{-1}).[2] Serum ionized Ca concentration as determined by ion-selective electrodes is a better indicator of physiologic calcium activity than total serum calcium concentration measurement.

Causes of hypocalcemia are listed in Table 16.2. Neonatal hypocalcemia is classified as early and late, based on the time of its occurrence after birth. Neonates with hypocalcemia may be asymptomatic or may display signs of exaggerated neuromuscular excitability (muscular twitches, jitteriness, positive Chvostek's and Trousseau's signs) or even seizures in severe cases. Early neonatal hypocalcemia occurs in the first few days of life. Its cause is uncertain. It is considered as an exaggeration of the physiologic drop in serum Ca concentration that usually occurs after birth and reaches a nadir by 24–48 hours of life. Early reports provided data consistent with transient neonatal hypoparathyroidism but reports of bio-assayed PTH appear to indicate a significant rise of circulating PTH concentration in response to hypocalcemia in preterm infants.[3] Prematurity is the most common cause of early neonatal hypocalcemia,[4,5] which occurs in 30–90% of preterm neonates.[4,5] The incidence of early hypocalcemia is inversely related to gestational age and birth weight.[4,6]

Hypercalcitoninemia was suggested to have a significant role in the development of early neonatal hypocalcemia.[7–9] However, from later studies, there is no correlation between neonatal serum Ca or the postnatal fall in serum Ca concentration and serum CT concentration in normal term infants and in infants of diabetic mothers.[4,10] In a case-control study of hypocalcemia, Mimouni found that risk factors for neonatal hypocalcemia include a low gestational age, low 5-minutes Apgar score, and white race.[11] The reason for increased risk for hypocalcemia among white infants compared with black infants is only speculative: (a) black infants have lower serum phosphorus concentrations which could lead to a higher serum calcium concentration, to maintain constant Ca × P product and (b) black infants may have increased bone mass contributing to the calcium pool. Asphyxia neonatorum is a risk factor for early neonatal hypocalcemia, which occurs in 30% of neonates who had an Apgar score below 5 at 1 minute of age.[12]

Mothers with insulin-dependent diabetes mellitus have excessive urinary magnesium losses especially if euglycemia is not maintained. Consequently these mothers – and theoretically their fetuses – may be magnesium-depleted. Hypomagnesemia impairs PTH secretion[13] and may explain the transient neonatal hypoparathyroidism and hypocalcemia that may develop in about 50% of infants of diabetic mothers.[14–16] Hypocalcemia in infants of diabetic mothers appears during the very early hours of life and changes little after 24 hours of life. This hypocalcemia tends to be more severe than the early neonatal hypocalcemia observed in preterm infants and tends to persist longer.[17] Infants of diabetic mothers (IDM) have low bone mineral context (BMC) at birth,[18] which correlates inversely with poor control of diabetes in the mother, specifically first trimester maternal mean capillary blood glucose concentration, implying that factors early in pregnancy might

have an effect on fetal BMC. The low BMC in IDM may be related to the decreased transplacental mineral transfer. Cord serum C-propeptide of type 1 collagen (ICTP) concentrations were higher in IDM than in control subjects, implying increased intrauterine bone resorption.[19] In contrast to Mimouni's finding of decreased BMC in IDM measured by single photon absorptiometry (SPA),[18] Lapillonne demonstrated higher bone mass in infants of diabetic mothers at birth using dual-energy x-ray absorptiometry (DEXA) scans.[20] The difference in these findings could be due to methodological differences between SPA and DEXA, different patient populations and different management of maternal diabetes. Because infants of diabetic mothers are hyperinsulinemic, especially the large-for-gestational-age (LGA) infants, any increase in fetal mineralization might be explained by the anabolic effect of insulin and insulin-like growth factor I (IGF-I) on bone formation. One author suggested the increased bone mass of these infants might be responsible for their increased calcium needs and subsequently for the neonatal hypocalcemia.[21] Early neonatal hypocalcemia that occurs in babies with intrauterine growth retardation (IUGR) is caused by prematurity or asphyxia and not IUGR itself.[22,23] Using DEXA scans, Lapillonne[24] showed that the total body fat, the lean mass, and the BMC of small-for-gestational-age (SGA) infants were decreased significantly in comparison with those of appropriate-for-gestational-age (AGA) infants with the same gestational age but was not significantly different from those observed in AGA infants of the same birth weight.

Early neonatal hypocalcemia has been reported in neonates under phototherapy.[25] Although the mechanism is not clear, it is possibly related to a disturbance in melatonin release.[26,27] The mechanism of early neonatal hypocalcemia in infants born to mothers with gestational anticonvulsant treatment may be related to phenobarbital or phenytoin-induction of the hepatic microsomal P450 oxidase activity which enhances metabolism of 25-OHD.[28–30] Decreased calcium intake,[31] transient neonatal hypoparathyroidism,[5,32] and abnormal vitamin D metabolism[33–36] are associated with early neonatal hypocalcemia. Neonatal hypocalcemia and congenital rickets have been described in infants born to mothers with abnormal vitamin D homeostasis: vitamin D deficiency osteomalacia may result from inadequate maternal dietary intake and sunlight exposure,[37–44] or intestinal malabsorption.[45] There is often an association of hypocalcemia with increased maternal parity and lower socio-economic status. Maternal chronic renal failure has been associated with neonatal hypocalcemia and congenital rickets.[46–49] Repeated administration of phosphate rectal enemas during pregnancy has been reported to cause congenital rickets and neonatal hypocalcemia[50] probably because of significant maternal hyperphosphatemia resulting in significant maternal and neonatal hypocalcemia and compensatory neonatal secondary hyperparathyroidism.

Maternal hyperparathyroidism and hypercalcemia may cause fetal hypercalcemia and suppression of the fetal parathyroid glands resulting in transient neonatal, or congenital, hypoparathyroidism with or without rickets.[51–53] Impaired secretion of PTH because of hypoparathyroidism or magnesium depletion results in hypocalcemia. At least 50% of infants born to hyperparathyroid mothers present with hypocalcemic tetany. However, the fact that some of these hypocalcemic infants had normal or elevated serum PTH concentrations,[54,55] suggests that other factors may be involved in the pathogenesis of hypocalcemia in these infants. Speculative explanations involve hypomagnesemia, defective calcitriol synthesis, or end-organ resistance to PTH.

Hypocalcemia may be a manifesting feature of abnormal vitamin D metabolism. Vitamin D deficiency may be caused by insufficient sunlight exposure, inadequate dietary intake, or malabsorption. Defective 25-hydroxylase activity may be associated with liver disease and may result in hypocalcemia, low serum 25-OHD concentration, and rickets.[56–58] Defective 1 alpha-hydroxylase activity may be caused by renal or parathyroid gland diseases. Renal hypophosphatemic rickets is a familial disorder characterized by decreased reabsorption of phosphate in the proximal renal tubules resulting in hypophosphatemia and rickets. It has an X-linked dominant mode of inheritance. Serum Ca concentration is either normal or low. Serum PTH concentration is either normal or increased. Serum 1,25(OH)2D concentration may be normal or low. Chronic renal failure is associated with hyperphosphatemia, hypocalcemia and depressed 1 alpha hydroxylase activity with low serum 1,25(OH)2D which results in secondary hyperparathyroidism.[59,60] Vitamin D-dependent rickets type I is a familial disorder with autosomal recessive inheritance pattern. It is characterized by depressed renal 1 alpha-hydroxylase activity, hypocalcemia, low serum 1,25(OH)2D concentration, and elevated serum PTH concentration.[61,62] Vitamin D-dependent rickets type II is a rare disease characterized by defective target organ response to 1,25(OH)2D which is attributed to a defect in the cellular and nuclear uptake of 1,25(OH)2D.[63] Receptors for 1,25(OH)2D are either absent or defective and bind abnormally to DNA (deoxyribonucleic acid) molecules because of the expression of a point mutation in the gene coding for these receptors.[64] Patients with this disease have hypocalcemia, elevated serum 1,25(OH)2D concentration and associated alopecia.

Primary hypoparathyroidism may present as neonatal hypocalcemia and may be sporadic or familial. Primary hypoparathyroidism is a chronic disease that requires supplementation with calcium and vitamin D metabolites to maintain eucalcemia and prevent osteopenia. Abnormalities in the gene coding for calcium sensing receptor have been linked to some cases of familial and sporadic symptomatic hypoparathyroidism.[65,66] Hypocalcemia and functional hypoparathyroidism may occur in critically ill children,[67] and ionized hypocalcemia may indicate greater severity of illness and higher mortality rate. The mechanism of hypocalcemia in sick children is poorly understood, but the finding of elevated serum calcitonin concentrations and an inverse correlation between serum CT and ionized calcium concentrations in these ill children, suggests that hypercalcitoninemia may play a significant role in the pathogenesis of hypocalcemia in these patients.[68] Tumors of mesenchymal origin (e.g., sarcomas, hemangiomas, giant cell tumors of bone, carcinoma of the breast)[69] and the epidermal nevus syndrome[70–72] may cause osteomalacia and hypocalcemia, which resolve after tumor ablation.[73] Most patients have marked hypophosphatemia because of excessive renal phosphate wasting and reduced proximal renal tubular reabsorption. The pathogenesis of the disease is attributed to the production of a phosphaturic substance by tumor cells that reduces renal tubular phosphate reabsorption and results in phosphate depletion. Rarely, vitamin D-resistant rickets has been observed in association with this syndrome.[74] Resistance to vitamin D results in decreased calcium absorption from the intestines and the kidney, which explains the associated hypocalcemia in these babies.

Late-onset hypocalcemia often presents as tetany by the end of the first week of life. The most common cause is excessive phosphorus intake from cow's milk formula,[75] phosphate-rich cereals[76] or phosphate-containing enemas. Hypocalcemia has also been described in a few infants born to hypercalcemic mothers with familial hypocalciuric hypercalcemia. The mechanism of hypocalcemia in these infants is possibly related to fetal parathyroid suppression by long-lasting maternal hypercalcemia.[77,78] Abnormal maternal vitamin D metabolism from suboptimal exposure to sunlight or dietary intake associated with advanced maternal age, multiparity and lower socioeconomic status, predisposes to late neonatal hypocalcemia.

Malignant infantile osteopetrosis,[79–81] a rare autosomal recessive disorder of osteoclastic function, is characterized by decreased resorption of calcified cartilage, abnormal mineralization of newly formed chondroid and osteoid tissues and persistent hypocalcemia requiring high dose calcium, phosphorus and 25-OHD supplements. It is believed to arise due to the failure of osteoclasts to resorb immature bone. This leads to abnormal bone marrow cavity formation and, clinically, to the signs and symptoms of bone marrow failure. Impaired bone remodeling associated with dysregulated activity of osteoclasts for such a condition may typically result in bony narrowing of the cranial nerve foramina, which typically results in cranial nerve (especially optic nerve) compression. Abnormal remodeling of primary woven bone to lamellar bone results in "brittle" bone that is prone to fracture. Thus, fractures, visual impairment, and bone marrow failure are the classical features of this disease.

Other risk factors include intestinal malabsorption of calcium,[82,83] hypomagnesemia,[15] and hypoparathyroidism.[32,64,84] Exchange transfusion with blood containing the anticoagulants citrate-dextrose or citrate-phosphate-dextrose can result in lower ionized serum calcium concentration because of Ca chelation by citrate.[85–88] Late-onset hypocalcemia has been reported in babies born to mothers who had excessive calcium carbonate consumption during pregnancy. Presumably excessive maternal calcium intake resulted in fetal hypercalcemia suppressing the fetal parathyroid glands and thus causing transient hypoparathyroidism after birth.[89] Hypocalcemia may also complicate the course of acute pancreatitis, phosphate therapy, or chemotherapy. Late hypocalcemia has been described in infants born to mothers with gestational exposure to anticonvulsant therapy.[29,30] The mechanism may be related to the effect of phenobarbital or phenytoin in enhancing accelerated metabolism of 25-OHD by hepatic microsomal P450 oxidase activity.[28] Rarely neonatal lupus erythematosus has been associated with transient late-onset hypocalcemia and seizures.[90]

Identification of neonatal hypocalcemia depends on its time of onset, clinical signs in the neonate, and maternal and family history. Early-onset neonatal hypocalcemia is usually asymptomatic and is detected only by biochemical measurements, particularly in very low birth weight (VLBW) (<1.5 kg) premature infants. It is a common practice to check serum Ca concentration in preterm newborns by 24 hours of life; in VLBW infants it may be necessary to check values at 12 hours of age. In contrast, late-onset neonatal hypocalcemia manifests clinically with neuromuscular twitching, seizures, laryngospasms, high-pitched cry, and positive Chvostek's and Trousseau's signs. A family history of metabolic Ca disorders (DiGeorge syndrome in a sibling) or maternal history of vitamin D deficiency, hyperparathyroidism, or drug ingestion is valuable in the

"work-up" of a hypocalcemic neonate. The circumstances of birth and delivery should be investigated for any coincident asphyctic/hypoxic insult.

Serum biochemical studies are helpful in the diagnosis of neonatal hypocalcemia; these include a serum total Ca, ionized Ca (a better physiologic indicator of Ca status), P, Mg, and 25-OHD. Hyperphosphatemia (>8 mg dL^{-1}) may be a clue to high dietary phosphate intake (cow's milk formula, cereal) or hypoparathyroidism. Hypomagnesemia (serum Mg <1.5 mg dL^{-1}) may be the etiologic factor for hypocalcemia in infants of diabetic mothers. Low serum 25-OHD (<10 ng mL^{-1}) points to vitamin D deficiency. Findings such as biochemical evidence of hypoparathyroidism with absence of the thymus on chest x-ray, cell-mediated immune defects, mucocutaneous candidiasis, and aortic arch anomalies are highly suggestive of DiGeorge syndrome. Measurements of corrected QT intervals on electrocardiograms may be of assistance in assessing the course of the hypocalcemia, but a prolonged QT interval is not necessarily indicative of a low serum ionized Ca. Early neonatal hypocalcemia can be prevented in neonates at risk by oral[31] and parenteral[91] Ca supplementation (75 mg elemental Ca kg day^{-1}). In some experimental trials,[34,35,92–94] prevention of neonatal hypocalcemia was achieved in large preterm infants with short-term use of moderately high doses of 1,25(OH)2D, the active metabolite of vitamin D (approximately 0.5 mcg kg^{-1}day^{-1} for 2 days).[35] However, VLBW neonates were responsive only at extremely high doses of 1,25(OH)2D (4 mcg kg^{-1} day^{-1}).[94]

Treatment of diagnosed hypocalcemia may be achieved by administration of oral or continuous intravenous Ca salts–usually Ca gluconate 10% solution; however, it is unclear whether asymptomatic hypocalcemia should be treated. Because Ca ions have a crucial physiologic role in the initiation of intracellular enzymatic processes, hypocalcemia, though asymptomatic, theoretically may have detrimental effects on cellular physiology. Administration of elemental Ca (as 10% Ca gluconate solution) at a dose of 75 mg kg^{-1} day^{-1} for 2 days usually achieves normocalcemia (ideally 8 to 10.5 mg dL^{-1}). Alternatively, Ca supplementation may be administered at gradually decreasing doses to allow a more physiologic Ca adaptation by the infant. For example, the first day's dose could be 75 mg kg^{-1}day^{-1}, followed by 38 mg kg^{-1}day^{-1} the next day and then 20 mg kg^{-1}day^{-1}.

Hypertonic Ca gluconate oral solutions, such as Neo-Calglucon (Sandoz Pharmaceuticals), have been associated with increased incidence of necrotizing enterocolitis[95] and should therefore be avoided. A daily oral dose of 10% Ca gluconate solution (for intravenous use) given in 4- to 6-hour intervals is well tolerated by low-birth-weight neonates with no significant side effects. Intravenous Ca gluconate administration is also an effective means to achieve normocalcemia. Continuous infusions are preferable to intermittent pulse infusions because the latter are associated with calciuria. Continuous infusions should be administered under strict cardiac monitoring because of the risk of bradycardia and even cardiac arrest associated with an accidental increase in the rate of the infusion. Intermittent intravenous boluses of 10% Ca gluconate should be given at a rate not exceeding 2 mL kg^{-1}10 min^{-1} and under simultaneous cardiac monitoring. In infants requiring alkali therapy, sodium bicarbonate therapy should not be given through the same intravenous line as Ca gluconate because of the risk of precipitate formation. Extravasation of Ca gluconate into cutaneous and subcutaneous tissues may be associated with skin burns and sloughing and therefore should be watched for and avoided by ensuring a patent intravenous line. Intra-arterial infusion of Ca salts is contraindicated because of the risk of necrosis of tissues supplied by the artery infused. Necrosis of intestinal tissue may occur following infusion of Ca salts into a mesenteric artery.[96] Hypocalcemia secondary to administration of high-phosphate milk formula is best treated by provision of a low-phosphate formula (such as PM60/40). Refractory hypocalcemia suggests the possibility of Mg deficiency or hypoparathyroidism. Alkalosis-related low serum concentrations of ionized Ca are best managed by avoiding excess alkali administration and hyperventilation of infants on respirators.

Maternal hypercalcemia

Maternal hypercalcemia causes an increase in transplacental calcium transfer from mother to fetus resulting in fetal hypercalcemia, which suppresses the fetal parathyroid glands resulting in neonatal hypocalcemia, once the fetus is delivered and the excessive maternal calcium supply is abruptly halted at birth.

Causes of maternal hypercalcemia are listed in Table 16.3. Primary hyperparathyroidism is a major cause of hypercalcemia. In 80%–85% of cases it is caused by parathyroid adenoma; in 15%–20% it results from parathyroid hyperplasia; and rarely, in 3%, it is caused by parathyroid carcinoma.[97] Hyperthyroidism is associated with increased bone turnover and hypercalcemia.[98] Hypercalcemia may occur in patients with untreated hypoadrenalism (Addison's disease). It is attributed to diminished renal excretion of calcium and volume depletion[99] or reduced secretion of corticosteroids.[100] Hypercalcemia and hyperparathyroidism are sometimes associated with pheochromocytoma or multiple endocrine

Table 16.3. Causes of maternal hypercalcemia

Endocrine
  Familial hypocalciuric hypercalcemia
  Hyperparathyroidism
    Congenital hyperparathyroidism
    Congenital hyperthyroidism
    Pheochromocytoma
  Abnormal vitamin D metabolism
    Granulomatous diseases (tuberculosis, sarcoidosis)
    Eosinophilic granuloma
    Infantile familial hypercalcemia, Williams syndrome
  Adrenal insufficiency
  Bartter's syndrome
  Hypophosphatasia
  VIPoma syndrome
Drugs
  Hypervitaminosis A or D
  Lithium toxicity
  Aluminum toxicity
  Excessive calcium intake
  Thiazides
  Milk alkali syndrome
Oncogenous
  Humoral hypercalcemia of malignancy
  Lymphoma
  Multiple myeloma
Miscellaneous
  Immobilization

neoplasia type II syndrome.[101] Familial hyperparathyroidism encompasses a spectrum of disorders including multiple endocrine neoplasia types 1 (MEN1) and 2A, hyperparathyroidism-jaw tumor syndrome (HPT-JT), familial hypocalciuric hypercalcemia (FHH), and familial isolated hyperparathyroidism (FIHP).[102] FHH is inherited in an autosomal dominant manner with 100% penetrance. It has been linked to mutations involving the gene encoding the calcium-sensing receptor[103] or autoantibodies directed to the calcium-sensing receptor.[104] Pancreatic VIPoma tumors secrete vasoactive intestinal peptide (VIP), which causes severe diarrhea. About 50% of the cases have hypercalcemia, possibly because of VIP-induced bone resorption.[105]

Hypercalcemia may be caused by drugs. Thiazides act directly to increase calcium release from the skeleton and promote renal tubular reabsorption of calcium.[106,107] Chronic lithium intake may cause hyperparathyroidism and mild hypercalcemia and hypermagnesemia.[108] Milk-alkali syndrome and hypercalcemia may be caused by excessive intake of calcium and phosphate in the form of milk and absorbable alkali, sodium carbonate, sodium bicarbonate, or calcium carbonate, usually for the treatment of peptic ulcer disease.[109] Bone resorption and hypercalcemia may be caused by vitamin D or vitamin A intoxication.

Hypercalcemia may be a feature of granulomatous diseases such as tuberculosis[110] and sarcoidosis[111] which are associated with abnormal vitamin D metabolism and increased circulating concentrations of 1,25(OH)2D in blood. Hypercalcemia may be associated with malignant tumors. The mechanism of hypercalcemia in malignancy may be due to production of parathyroid hormone related peptide (PTHrP) (humoral hypercalcemia of malignancy),[112] 1,25(OH)2D in lymphoma,[113] lymphotoxin in multiple myeloma[114] or other substances that cause bone resorption. Immobilization causes bone demineralization, osteoporosis, and secondary hypercalcemia because of increased bone resorption. Lactation causes a transient increase in bone resorption and secondary hypercalcemia, reversed by weaning.[115,116] Rarely, severe axial osteopenia with vertebral fractures can occur. Metabolic changes include elevated PTHrP with suppressed serum concentrations of PTH and calcitriol.[117] Elevated PTH activity may play a role in the recovery of bone mass after weaning by maintaining renal calcium conservation and by an anabolic action on bone.[118]

Neonatal hypercalcemia

Neonatal hypercalcemia is defined by a total serum Ca concentration > 11 mg dL^{-1} or serum ionized Ca concentration > 5.8 mg dL^{-1} as determined by the Radiometer ionized Ca electrode. Hypercalcemia may present early in the neonatal period or weeks or months later. Several factors can result in neonatal hypercalcemia including maternal, hereditary, or dietary factors (Table 16.4). Hypercalcemia in the neonate can be the result of prolonged maternal hypocalcemia from a multitude of causes (Table 16.1). Maternal hypoparathyroidism is most commonly postoperative due to inadvertent parathyroidectomy at thyroid surgery; less commonly it may be idiopathic or due to pseudohypoparathyroidism. Mechanistically, maternal hypocalcemia results in a decrease in placental calcium supply to the fetus despite a physiologically intact active transport system for calcium. As a result, fetal hypocalcemia stimulates the fetal parathyroid glands to normalize fetal serum Ca concentration. Consequently, a variable degree of congenital transient hyperparathyroidism results.[119–125] Infants with transient secondary hyperparathyroidism are described to have a spectrum of manifestations that depend on the severity of the maternal homeostatic disturbance: at one end of the

Table 16.4. Causes of neonatal hypercalcemia

Endocrine
  Hyperparathyroidism
    Congenital hyperparathyroidism
    Transient hyperparathyroidism secondary to maternal
      hypoparathyroidism
    Congenital hypothyroidism
    Pheochromocytoma
  Abnormal vitamin D metabolism
    Granulomatous diseases (tuberculosis, sarcoidosis)
    Eosinophilic granuloma
    Infantile hypercalcemia
    Subcutaneous fat necrosis
  Adrenal insufficiency
  VIPoma syndrome
Renal
  Familial hypocalciuric hypercalcemia
  Thiazides
  Bartter's syndrome
  Milk alkali syndrome
Bone Resorption
  Hypophosphatasia
  Hyperthyroidism
  Aluminum toxicity
Oncogenous
  Congenital nephroblastoma
Miscellaneous
  Hypervitaminosis A or D
  Lithium toxicity
  Excessive calcium intake
  Phosphorus deficiency syndrome

spectrum are normal infants; at the other end are infants with severe hyperparathyroidism with elevated cord blood PTH concentration, severe congenital bone demineralization and intrauterine fractures with clinical and radiological bowing of the long bones. Fortunately, the manifestations of secondary hyperparathyroidism improve rapidly after birth, once these infants are provided with adequate amounts of Ca, P, and vitamin D.

Primary neonatal hyperparathyroidism is an important cause of hypercalcemia, which may occur sporadically or have a familial basis. This entity may be inherited in an autosomal dominant[126] or recessive manner.[127] Neonates with congenital hyperparathyroidism may present soon after birth with respiratory distress, hypotonia, feeding difficulties, and bone deformities. Laboratory findings include hypercalcemia, hypophosphatemia, and elevated alkaline phosphatase and plasma parathyroid hormone concentrations. X-rays may show gross demineralization with metaphyseal fractures, erosions, and subperiosteal reaction along the bones, which usually resolve following parathyroidectomy and subsequent maintenance therapy with 1-alpha-hydroxycholecalciferol.[128]

Neonatal hyperparathyroidism may be associated with familial hypocalciuric hypercalcemia (FHH),[129] which is inherited in an autosomal dominant manner with high penetrance at all ages.[130–132] Genetic analysis of families with FHH has shown that some cases of neonatal severe hyperparathyroidism may be the expression of a homozygous form of FHH.[133–135] FHH is characterized by a variable degree of hypercalcemia associated with decreased renal clearance of calcium. Clinically, the spectrum of the disease ranges from the asymptomatic heterozygous person (heterozygous calcium receptor gene mutation),[136] with mild hypercalcemia detected by blood testing, to the homozygous (homozygous calcium receptor gene mutation)[137] subject with neonatal hyperparathyroidism and severe life-threatening hypercalcemia.[138] In several families of patients with neonatal hyperparathyroidism, other family members have FHH.[131,139] Also several patients who underwent parathyroidectomy in infancy were diagnosed with FHH later in life.[129,140,141] Recently, a self-limited form of neonatal hyperparathyroidism and hypercalcemia has been reported in a family of three siblings, in association with hypercalciuria, and renal tubular acidosis.[142]

Infants with congenital agoitrous hypothyroidism have also been described to be hypercalcemic. These infants possibly have congenital absence or dysfunction of the parafollicular calcitonin-producing C-cells; therefore they cannot mount a CT response to a Ca load.[143–145] Adults with congenital hypothyroidism have also been reported to have calcitonin deficiency.[146] They also were found to have reduced bone density,[146] which could be attributed to deficiency in both thyroid hormone and calcitonin.

Excessive maternal ingestion of vitamin D[147] or vitamin A[148] metabolites may result in bone resorption, and maternal and neonatal hypercalcemia. The same outcome may occur in infants of mothers who have prolonged hypercalcemia because of thyrotoxicosis[149] or chronic thiazides therapy.[150] It is possible that the fetal parathyroid gland threshold for PTH secretion becomes higher, or the glands themselves become "tolerant" to chronic maternal and fetal hypercalcemia.

Neonatal hypercalcemia and phosphorus deficiency syndrome have been reported in preterm infants fed human milk.[151,152] These infants become phosphorus-depleted because of insufficient dietary phosphate intake from human milk to keep up with mineral requirements for optimal bone mineralization. Secondarily they have suboptimal bone mineralization and hypercalcemia because calcium is not well incorporated into new bone hydroxy-

apatite crystals. Neonatal hypercalcemia is a basic feature of the severe infantile form of hypophosphatasia,[153] a rare disorder characterized by severe bone demineralization most pronounced at growth plates, low serum alkaline phosphatase concentrations, and elevated urine phosphoethanolamine concentrations.[153,154] The severe form of the disease is inherited in an autosomal recessive manner. Because of alkaline phosphatase deficiency, bone mineralization is severely depressed and most of the body's calcium is transferred to the circulation resulting in severe hypercalcemia, hypercalciuria, and nephrocalcinosis. Severely affected infants may die in utero or shortly after birth because of impaired skeletal support of the thorax and skull.

A subgroup of Bartter's syndrome,[155,156] which is an autosomal recessive disorder characterized by hypokalemic metabolic alkalosis, hyperreninemia and hyperaldosteronism, may be associated with infantile hypercalcemia[157,158] and prostaglandin-mediated hypercalciuria, the hyperprostaglandin E syndrome (HPS).[158] Molecular genetics has facilitated antenatal diagnosis of HPS by demonstrating mutations in the furosemide-sensitive Na-K-2Cl cotransporter or in the renal potassium channel encoding gene ROMK.[159–161] The mechanism of hypercalcemia in these infants is attributed to increased intestinal Ca absorption enhanced by elevated serum $1,25(OH)2D$ concentration, serum 25-OHD concentration being normal. It is thought that increased $1,25(OH)2D$ synthesis is mediated by prostaglandin E2 which has been demonstrated to stimulate renal 1-alpha hydroxylase activity in vivo in thyroparathyroidectomized rats[162] and in vitro in chick[163] and rat[164] kidney cells. In patients with this syndrome, serum $1,25(OH)2D$ concentrations correlate significantly with urinary PGE2 concentrations. Therapy with prostaglandin synthesis inhibitors such as indomethacin lowers serum calcitriol concentration, urinary PGE2 and calcium concentration, and improves the associated nephrocalcinosis.[157,165]

From recent evidence,[166] children with neonatal Bartter syndrome (NBS), who have hypercalciuria, nephrocalcinosis, and osteopenia, have increased circulating angiotensin II. Also a complex of basic-fibroblast growth factor (b-FGF) and a naturally occurring glycosaminoglycan has been identified in the serum and urine of these patients. This complex increases bone resorption in a bone disc bioassay system. Angiotensin II increases the synthesis of b-FGF by cultured endothelial cells and significantly decreased calcium uptake into bone discs. Adding b-FGF monoclonal antibody or indomethacin neutralized this effect. This decrease in calcium uptake in the bone disc bioassay system can be abrogated by antibody to b-FGF or prostaglandin synthetase inhibition. The authors suggest that in children with NBS, elevated levels of angiotensin II stimulate local skeletal b-FGF synthesis, with a resultant increase in bone resorption via a prostaglandin-dependent pathway.

Idiopathic hypercalcemia may occur in infancy.[167] The basic defect in this disease is still obscure. A subgroup of infants with idiopathic hypercalcemia have the "Williams Syndrome" which is characterized by elfin facies, short stature, mild mental retardation, hyperacusis, and congenital heart disease (commonly supravalvular aortic stenosis).[168] The hypercalcemia in these infants is associated with hypersensitivity to the effect of vitamin D metabolites manifesting as increased intestinal absorption of calcium. Defects in vitamin D[169–172] or calcitonin[173] metabolism have been suggested.

Newborns, especially large infants, who had difficult vaginal deliveries may develop subcutaneous fat necrosis over areas subjected to increased pressure such as the shoulders, back, upper arms, and outer thighs.[174] The condition is associated with indurated, erythematous or purple-erythematous nodules and plaques in the skin. Histology of affected skin shows granulomatous necrosis in the subcutaneous layer with radial crystals in lipocytes and giant cells.[175] Light microscopy may reveal adipocyte necrosis, lymphohistiocytic infiltration, and needle-shaped clefts within adipocytes and macrophages. Ultrastructurally, there may be aggregations of electron-lucent spaces in the form of spindles and needles arranged in parallel within altered adipocytes; macrophages surround these cells or their fragments and invade fat lobules.[176] Affected infants may develop transient hypercalcemia days or weeks later, probably because of calcium mobilization from necrotic tissues.[177,178] Although Veldhuis reported normal vitamin D concentrations, other authors suggested extrarenal production of calcitriol by macrophages within the inflammatory reaction to fat necrosis.[174,179–181] Although the natural history of this condition is spontaneous resolution of panniculitis,[182,183] close monitoring is required because severe life-threatening hypercalcemia requiring aggressive treatment has been reported. Prolonged hypercalcemia may also be complicated by nephrocalcinosis and nephrolithiasis.[184] Cold panniculitis has been reported following surface cooling to alleviate the sequelae of hypoxic ischemic encephalopathy,[185] following hypothermic cardiac surgery,[186,187] and following prolonged exposure to cold weather.[188] Rarely the condition may be complicated by calcifications in the liver, the inferior vena cava, and the atrial septum of the heart.[189] Treatment of hypercalcemia may include hydration with isotonic saline solu-

tion followed by diuresis with furosemide, corticosteroids, calcitonin, low calcium and vitamin D diet[190] or even oral bisphosphonates.[191–193]

Infants with miliary tuberculosis may develop hypercalcemia possibly because of extrarenal production of calcitriol.[194] Rarely, hypercalcemia may be an associated feature of congenital renal tumors, particularly mesoblastic nephroma.[195–199] The cause of hypercalcemia in these neoplasms is due to the production of ectopic PTH[200] or prostaglandin E by tumor cells.[201,202] In most cases, extirpation of the tumor corrects the hypercalcemia and recurrence is rare. Signs and symptoms of hypercalcemia in the neonatal period are generally nonspecific and may include lethargy, poor feeding, vomiting, irritability, polyuria, dehydration, constipation, and failure to thrive. Hypertension, nephrocalcinosis, and corneal and conjunctival calcifications are rarely noted in neonates. The presence of "elfin facies" and congenital heart disease suggest the diagnosis of Williams syndrome. Family history for hereditary disorders of Ca and P is important in the diagnosis of hypercalcemia in the neonatal period (e.g., familial hyperparathyroidism, familial hypocalciuric hypercalcemia, hypophosphatasia). Maternal dietary and drug history is also helpful in the work-up of neonatal hypercalcemia (excessive vitamin A and D intake).

Biochemical studies should include serum Ca (total and ionized); P; alkaline phosphatase and calciotropic hormones; and urinary Ca, P, and cyclic adenosine monophosphate (cAMP) concentrations. Renal wasting with hypercalcemia and elevated urine cAMP concentration may be a clue to the possibility of hyperparathyroidism. Radiological examination of the hands and wrists revealing subperiosteal resorption, in addition to hypercalcemia and hypophosphatemia, suggest the diagnosis of hyperparathyroidism. Therapy of neonatal hypercalcemia depends on the underlying cause. Excessive maternal ingestion of vitamins A and D should be discontinued, and vitamin D and Ca should be reduced in the diet. Hypercalcemia related to human milk feeding of preterm infants indicates a deficiency of P, and supplementation with P is required. However, in this instance there is usually concomitant Ca deficiency; therefore, the appropriate treatment is supplementation with both P and Ca.

Severe hypercalcemia results in major polyuric water loss and requires prompt repletion of extracellular fluids. Volume expansion is achieved by 10–20 ml kg^{-1} body weight of 0.9% normal saline solution, followed by administration of a calciuretic diuretic (furosemide, 1–2 mg kg^{-1} per dose) to increase the clearance of Ca in urine. Sodium ethylene diamine tetra acetic acid (EDTA) may be administered parenterally in severe cases to chelate Ca and increase its urinary excretion. Calcitonin has been used in severe cases, but is not usually recommended because of limited experience in neonates and development of antibodies to nonhuman calcitonin preparations. In chronic hypercalcemia, prednisone (2 mg kg^{-1}day^{-1}) may be used to decrease intestinal absorption of Ca, and bisphosphonates have been used successfully in cases of subcutaneous fat necrosis. Virtually all cases of primary hyperparathyroidism require subtotal or total parathyroidectomy, since the hypercalcemia may become life threatening and does not respond to medical management.[140] Finally, as mentioned earlier, indomethacin therapy decreases the hypercalciuria and nephrocalcinosis in a number of patients.[157]

Disorders of phosphate homeostasis

Neonatal hypophosphatemia

Moderate hypophosphatemia is defined as a serum phosphorus concentration between 2.5 and 1 mg dL^{-1} in adults, and is usually asymptomatic. Severe hypophosphatemia is defined as serum inorganic phosphorus concentration below 1.0 mg dL^{-1}. In children, serum phosphorus concentrations below 4 mg dL^{-1} are often considered abnormal. Hypophosphatemia may be caused by (1) decreased intestinal absorption of phosphate, (2) increased urine losses of phosphate, and an endogenous shift of inorganic phosphorus from extracellular to intracellular fluid compartments. Causes of hypophosphatemia are listed in Table 16.5.

Hypophosphatemia occurs in low birth weight babies who were fed human milk exclusively[203,204] and is an early sign of impending rickets or osteopenia. Phytates in soy formulas may complex with minerals and decrease intestinal absorption of Ca and P.[205] Soy formulas should be avoided in preterm infants less than 1800 g in birth weight. Preterm infants who weighed from 1500–1800 g and were fed methionine-supplemented soy protein-based formulas demonstrated significantly less weight gain, less length gain, and lower serum albumin levels than that achieved with cow milk-based formulas. In studies of preterm infants, serum phosphorus concentration was lower in preterm infants fed soy protein-based formula and serum alkaline phosphatase concentration was higher.[206,207] The incidence of osteopenia of prematurity was increased in low birth weight infants receiving soy protein-based formulas.[208,209] Even with supplemental calcium and vitamin D, radiographic evidence of increased osteopenia was present in 32% of preterm infants fed soy protein-based formula.[209] Researchers reported lower BMC determined by SPA in infants fed old formulations of

Table 16.5. Causes of hypophosphatemia

Endocrine
  Hyperparathyroidism
  Abnormal vitamin D metabolism
    Vitamin D deficiency
    Vitamin D resistant rickets type I
    Vitamin D resistant rickets type II
Renal Losses
  Tubular disorders
    Primary
      Fanconi syndrome
      Renal tubular acidosis
      Hypophosphatemia
        Familial
        Non-familial
    Secondary
      Diuretics
      Volume expanders
      Hypercalciuria
      Glucosuria
      Hypomagnesemia
Gastrointestinal
  Decreased dietary intake
  Decreased absorption
    Malabsorption
    Antacids
Others
  Mesenchymal tumors
  Metabolic acidosis
  Respiratory alkalosis
  Thermal burns
  Gram-negative sepsis

soy formulas compared with infants fed cow milk-based formulas.[210,211] However, newer soy formulas have higher Ca and P content and bioavailability, and infants fed these modified soy formulas had no difference in bone mineral content compared with infants fed cow-milk based formulas.[212]

Studies in term infants documented normal growth and development in neonates fed methionine-supplemented isolated soy protein-based formulas.[213–215] Average energy intakes in infants receiving soy protein formulas were equivalent to those achieved with cow milk formula. The serum albumin concentration, as a marker of nutritional adequacy, was normal, and bone mineralization also was equivalent to that documented with cow milk-based formula.[210,211,216–218] Hypophosphatemia and rickets may be associated with X-linked recessive nephrolithiasis, which is a rare hereditary form of progressive renal failure characterized by proximal renal tubular dysfunction and low molecular weight proteinuria, hypercalciuria with nephrocalcinosis and nephrolithiasis.[219] The syndrome may be due to a mutation involving CLCN5 gene, which maps to chromosome Xp11.22 and encodes a putative chloride channel expressed throughout the renal tubule. Mutations in the CLCN5 gene have been detected in Dent's disease and its phenotypic variants (X-linked recessive nephrolithiasis, X-linked recessive hypophosphatemic rickets, and idiopathic low-molecular-weight proteinuria of Japanese children). Dent's disease is a tubular disorder characterized by low-molecular-weight proteinuria, and nephrolithiasis associated with nephrocalcinosis and hypercalciuria.[220] Excessive renal losses of phosphate, phosphate depletion and rickets occur in Fanconi Syndrome and X-linked hypophosphatemic rickets. Hypophosphatemia may be a manifestation of familial benign hypercalcemia, or hypocalciuric hypercalcemia, which is a dominantly inherited disorder of calcium and magnesium metabolism, characterized by lifelong hypercalcemia and hypermagnesemia (both of variable degree), that usually is not associated with any symptoms, physical signs, reduced vitality, or ill health.[221]

Prolonged administration of aluminum-containing antacids, which reduce gastrointestinal phosphate absorption, has been associated with phosphate depletion and infantile rickets.[222] Phosphate-chelating antacids sequester phosphate in the gut lumen and markedly decrease intestinal absorption. Phosphate depletion may be associated with distal renal tubular acidosis. Hypophosphatemic rickets has been described in association with mesenchymal tumors, and epidermal nevus syndrome. Biochemically, most patients present with significant hypophosphatemia due to renal phosphate wasting, normal serum calcium, elevated serum alkaline phosphatase, and low serum calcitriol concentrations. The pathogenesis of rickets in these tumors is attributed to the production of phosphaturic factors by tumor cells resulting in total body phosphate depletion. Surgical excision of these tumors reverses the biochemical and radiological rachitic changes.

Neonatal hyperphosphatemia

Hyperphosphatemia is most often the result of decreased renal excretion of phosphate anions as encountered in acute or chronic renal failure, particularly when glomerular filtration rate is reduced to less than 25% of normal (Table 16.6). Hyperphosphatemia could also be the result of increased body phosphate load from phosphate-containing laxatives and enemas, blood transfusions, hyperalimentation, and is also a major component of

Table 16.6. Causes of hyperphosphatemia

Endocrine
Hypoparathyroidism
Idiopathic
Transient
Pseudohypoparathyroidism
Hyperthyroidism
Growth hormone excess
Vitamin D toxicity
Renal
Renal failure
Volume depletion
Increased load
Enteral
Cow milk feeding
Rectal enemas
Parenteral
Hyperalimentation
Blood transfusion
Tumor lysis syndrome
Rhabdomyolysis
Malignant hyperthermia

the tumor lysis syndrome secondary to cell lysis by cytotoxic therapy, and tissue injuries (hyperthermia, hypoxia or crush injuries) resulting in rhabdomyolysis and hemolysis. Increased renal tubular reabsorption of phosphate is responsible for hyperphosphatemia seen in hypoparathyroidism, hyperthyroidism, hypogonadism and growth hormone excess.

Neonatal hypoparathyroidism presents with hypocalcemia and hyperphosphatemia and decreased serum PTH concentrations.[223] Hyperphosphatemia may occur in infants of diabetic mothers due to transient neonatal hypoparathyroidism.[224] Neonatal pseudohypoparathyroidism causes hypocalcemia and hyperphosphatemia but serum PTH concentrations are elevated.[225,226] This condition may be transient and resolve within the first 6 months of life.[227] Transient neonatal pseudohypoparathyroidism and hyperphosphatemia has also been reported in babies born to mothers with hyperparathyroidism.[54] Neonatal and infantile hyperphosphatemia[228] with severe hypocalcemia and seizures[229] has been reported following administration of phosphate-containing enemas.

Disorders of magnesium homeostasis

The importance of optimal Mg homeostasis in the perinatal period is increasingly recognized. Pregnancy is associated

Table 16.7. Causes of maternal hypomagnesemia

Decreased intake
  Enteral or parenteral
  Malnutrition
  Alcoholism
Gastrointestinal disease
  Chronic diarrhea
  Chronic ulcerative colitis
  Crohn's disease
  Laxative abuse
  Villous adenoma
  Malabsorption
  Short bowel syndrome
  Gluten enteropathy
  Tropical sprue
  Familial magnesium malabsorption
Renal disorders
  Renal tubular acidosis
  Acute tubular acidosis (diuretic phase)
  Chronic pyelonephritis
  Chronic glomerulonephritis
  Familial and sporadic magnesium loss
  Diuretics (furosemide, thiazides, ethacrynic acid)
  Antibiotics (gentamicin, tobramicin, amphotericin)
  Cyclosporin
Endocrine disorders
  Hyperaldosteronism
  Hyperthyroidism
  Hypercalcemia
  Hyperparathyroidism
  Uncontrolled diabetes mellitus

Table 16.8. Causes of neonatal hypomagnesemia

Endocrine disorders
  Transient neonatal hypoparathyroidism
  Maternal hyperparathyroidism
    Maternal insulin-dependent diabetes mellitus
    Neonatal hypoparathyroidism
    Persistent neonatal hypoparathyroidism
      Congenital hypoplasia/aplasia of the parathyroid glands
      DiGeorge syndrome
    Hyperaldosteronism
    Hypercalcemia and hypervitaminosis D
    Hyperphosphatemia
Gastrointestinal
  Decreased enteral Mg intake
    Decreased intestinal absorption:
      Primary magnesium malabsorption
  Short bowel syndrome
  Enteropathy
    Increased intestinal losses
      Chronic diarrhea
      Fistulas, enterostomies
    Hepatobiliary disease
      Neonatal hepatitis
      Congenital biliary atresia
Renal losses
  Decreased renal tubular reabsorption
    Congenital
      Renal tubular acidosis
      Gitelman syndrome
    Acquired
      Acute tubular necrosis
      Diuretics (furosemide, thiazides)
      Antibiotics (gentamicin, amphotericin)
Miscellaneous
  Birth asphyxia
  Low Mg content in parenteral hyperalimentation
  Intrauterine growth retardation
  Exchange transfusion
  Zellweger syndrome

with increased renal excretion of magnesium, and a drop in serum Mg concentration, which may become more exaggerated if maternal dietary Mg intake is insufficient for optimal Mg homeostasis and fetal requirements. There are apparent benefits of maternal magnesium supplementation in reducing the incidence of preterm labor,[230] and allowing greater fetal growth. In one study,[231] a maternal Mg intake of 300 mg day^{-1} was associated with optimal birth weight, length, and head circumference.

Neonatal hypomagnesemia

Neonatal hypomagnesemia is defined as serum Mg concentration <1.5 mg dL^{-1}. However, tissue Mg deficiency may coexist with normal serum Mg concentrations.[232] Hypomagnesemia may cause hypocalcemia through several mechanisms: (1) decreased Mg-dependent adenylate cyclase-mediated secretion of PTH, (2) end-organ resistance to PTH, (3) decreased intestinal Ca absorption, or (4)

decreased heteroionic exchange of Ca for Mg at the bone surface.[233,234]

Hypomagnesemia is most commonly due to depletion of maternal body Mg stores, which leads to decreased transplacental Mg supply to the fetus. Causes of maternal hypomagnesemia are listed in Table 16.7. Etiologic factors in congenital hypomagnesemia are listed in Table 16.8 and include endocrine, familial, and hereditary disorders. Mothers with intestinal malabsorption were described in the literature to give birth to infants who develop hypomagnesemia.[235] Maternal hypomagnesemia may be caused by reduced Mg intake as in malnutrition or alcoholism, or increased intestinal Mg losses as in chronic diarrhea and malabsorption because of ulcerative colitis, Crohn's disease, celiac sprue, or gluten enteropathy. Maternal hypomagnesemia may result from excessive renal Mg losses because of acute tubular necrosis or chronic renal disease as in renal tubular acidosis, chronic pyelonephritis, or glomerulonephritis, or the use of nephrotoxic drugs (Foscarnet, Cisplatin, Cyclosporin), diuretics and antibiotics (Amphotericin, aminoglycosides). As described earlier, mothers with uncontrolled diabetes mellitus are often hypomagnesemic,[236] presumably because of hyperglycemia-induced hypermagnesuria (osmotic diuresis)[237] and deficient insulin-dependent cellular uptake of Mg.[238] Infants of diabetic mothers (IDM) may be secondarily magnesium-depleted and may develop hypomagnesemia, hypocalcemia, and hypoparathyroidism.[15,16] However, administration of intramuscular $MgSO_4$ to IDMs with cord magnesium <1.8 mg dL^{-1} does not reduce the incidence of hypocalcemia in infants of well-controlled diabetic mothers.[239] As described earlier, Mg is an intracellular cation and serum Mg concentration may not reflect total body Mg content. Therefore, tissue Mg deficiency may coexist with normomagnesemia.[232] Magnesium deficiency appears to have a significant impact on mineral homeostasis in insulin-dependent diabetes mellitus: it is associated with lower serum concentrations for calcium, PTH, calcitriol, and osteocalcin. Magnesium supplementation resulted in normalization of these biochemical perturbations in diabetic children.[240,241]

Familial hypomagnesemia is characterized by primary intestinal malabsorption or decreased renal tubular reabsorption of Mg. It is usually recognized in the neonatal period and predominantly occurs in males.[242–248] Shalev[249] reviewed the clinical presentation and long-term outcome of patients with autosomal recessive primary familial hypomagnesemia. The most common presenting events were generalized hypomagnesemic-hypocalcemic seizures at 4–5 weeks of age in 67%. The majority of infants who were treated soon after diagnosis with high dose enteral magnesium developed normally. Delay in establishing a diagnosis could lead to a convulsive disorder with permanent neurological impairment. The primary defect in renal tubular reabsorption of Mg may occur as an isolated or familial disease.[250–253]

The combination of hypomagnesemia and hypocalciuria is the phenotypic signature of two distinct genetic renal tubular transport disorders: Gitelman's syndrome (GS) and autosomal dominant isolated renal magnesium wasting.[254] The defective proteins involved in both diseases are located within the distal convoluted tubule, which plays an important role in active magnesium reabsorption in the nephron. In contrast to GS, autosomal dominant renal hypomagnesemia with hypocalciuria is not associated with hypokalemia and metabolic alkalosis. Gitelman syndrome (hypomagnesemia accompanied by hypocalciuria, hypokalemia and metabolic alkalosis) is an autosomal recessive familial disorder characterized by excessive renal magnesium and potassium losses requiring long-term supplementation,[252,255] hypocalciuria, and a defect in the gene encoding for the thiazide-sensitive sodium ion/chloride ion cotransporter.

The genetic basis and cellular defects of a number of primary magnesium wasting diseases have been elucidated over the past decade. Cole[256] reviewed the correlates of the clinical pathophysiology with the primary defect and secondary changes in cellular electrolyte transport. He described the following disorders: (1) hypomagnesemia with secondary hypocalcemia, an early onset, autosomal-recessive disease segregating with chromosome 9q12–22.2; (2) autosomal-dominant hypomagnesemia caused by isolated renal magnesium wasting, mapped to chromosome 11q23; (3) hypomagnesemia with hypercalciuria and nephrocalcinosis, a recessive condition caused by a mutation of the claudin 16 gene (3q27) coding for a tight junctional protein that regulates paracellular $Mg(2^+)$ transport in the loop of Henle; (4) autosomal-dominant hypoparathyroidism, a variably hypomagnesemic disorder caused by inactivating mutations of the extracellular $Ca(2^+)/Mg(2^+)$-sensing receptor, CASR: gene, at 3q13.3–21; and (5) Gitelman syndrome, a recessive form of hypomagnesemia caused by mutations in the distal tubular NaCl cotransporter gene, SLC12A3, at 16q13. The basis for renal magnesium wasting in this disease is not known. Hypomagnesemia may cause hypocalcemia either by decreased Mg-dependent adenylate cyclase-mediated secretion of PTH, or end-organ resistance to PTH, or by decreased heteroionic exchange of Ca for Mg at the bone surface.[234,257] Secondary hypocalcemia responds to magnesium supplementation.

Benigno[258] has reviewed the cardinal characteristics of primary hypomagnesaemia–hypercalciuria–nephrocalcinosis, which include renal magnesium wasting, marked hypercalciuria, renal stones, nephrocalcinosis, a tendency towards chronic renal insufficiency and sometimes even ocular abnormalities or hearing impairment.[258] This entity is inherited in an autosomal recessive mode. The molecular genetics of hereditary renal magnesium wasting has been reviewed by Konrad.[259,260]

Hypercalcemia of any cause (hyperparathyroidism, vitamin D intoxication),[261] hypercalciuria and hypophosphatemia[262] may cause excessive Mg losses in urine and hypomagnesemia. Renal tubulopathy and excessive Mg losses may be associated with administration of aminoglycosides[263] and amphotericin.[264] Also, the use of diuretics causes renal Ca and Mg wasting[265–267] potentially resulting in negative magnesium balance and secondary hyperparathyroidism.[268] The polyuric phase of acute renal failure or acute tubular necrosis is associated with hypermagnesemia, and may result in hypomagnesemia and other electrolyte disturbances.[261] Maternal hypomagnesemia is associated with preeclampsia.[269] Because most fetal Mg accretion occurs in the third trimester, preterm infants are at risk of developing hypomagnesemia if not supplied with enough Mg in their diet. GA infants frequently develop hypomagnesemia.[23,270] A proportion of these infants are born to hypomagnesemic preeclamptic mothers who may have placental insufficiency. Hyperaldosteronism is associated with excessive losses of magnesium in urine and feces and may result in hypomagnesemia and negative magnesium balance.

Maternal hyperparathyroidism and hyperthyroidism may be associated with negative Mg balance in the mother and fetus because of excessive maternal Mg losses in urine. Maternal hyperparathyroidism predisposes to transient neonatal hypoparathyroidism[54,271] manifesting as hypocalcemia and hypomagnesemia.[236,272] Neonatal hypoparathyroidism may be associated with neonatal hypomagnesemia.[15] Possible mechanisms involved are: decreased PTH-induced Mg release from bone, increased renal tubular Mg loss, and hyperphosphatemia.[273,274] Persistent congenital hypoparathyroidism may occur as an isolated or familial X-linked recessive or autosomal dominant entity as part of the DiGeorge syndrome (thymic aplasia and T-lymphocyte immunodeficiency, and aortic arch anomalies), as part of Zellweger syndrome (cerebrohepatorenal syndrome), or as an autoimmune disorder with mucocutaneous candidiasis. Neonatal cholestasis due to congenital biliary atresia or severe neonatal hepatitis may cause excessive intestinal Mg losses and magnesium depletion.[275] It is possible that decreased metabolism of aldosterone because of hepatocellular damage results in secondary hyperaldosteronism, which causes hypermagnesuria.[276] Excessive Mg losses and hypomagnesemia may occur in infants with short bowel syndrome following intestinal resection.[277–279]

Hypomagnesemia has been described in newborns with birth asphyxia but the pathogenesis is not clear.[15] Increased dietary phosphorus intake increases fecal losses of magnesium, and therefore decreases net absorption and retention of magnesium in VLBW infants.[280] Hypokalemia may be associated with hypomagnesemia because of increased potassium losses in the loop of Henle and cortical collecting tubules.[281] Hypomagnesemia may be asymptomatic or may present with intractable convulsions and coma. Because less than 1% of total body Mg is present in the blood and the remaining 99% is found intracellularly, serum Mg concentrations may not reflect tissue Mg deficiency.

Awareness of predisposing factors offers the best clinical clue to the diagnosis of hypomagnesemia, especially when the clinician is faced with a case of "intractable hypocalcemia." In fact, most cases of hypomagnesemia in the literature are first misdiagnosed as cases of hypoparathyroidism. Clinical signs of hypomagnesemia manifest with serum Mg concentrations less than 1.2 mg dL^{-1} [15] and are similar to those of hypocalcemia: tremors, irritability, hyperreflexia (with or without positive Chvostek and Trousseau signs), possibly muscle fasciculations and in severe cases, tetany and seizures. Often, biochemical testing reveals hypomagnesemia, secondary hypocalcemia, and possibly hypoparathyroidism.

The management of hypomagnesemia depends on the primary cause. Supplementation of Mg may be needed for prolonged periods in infants with congenital and hereditary, renal and hepatobiliary Mg-losing disorders. Infants with primary intestinal Mg malabsorption and those with intestinal resections and short gut syndrome require lifelong supply of high doses of Mg in their diet to prevent hypomagnesemia. Diet intake control, such as avoiding cow milk formulas in early infancy and adjusting Mg concentration in parenteral nutrition solutions, may prevent the occurrence of hypomagnesemia. Asymptomatic hypomagnesemia can be corrected with a 50% $MgSO_4$ solution given as an intramuscular injection of 0.2 g/kg body weight every 8–12 hours until serum Mg concentration is normal. In symptomatic infants, $MgSO_4$ solution is diluted to 5% or 10% solution and given as a slow intravenous infusion over 10 minutes under continuous cardiopulmonary monitoring because of the risk of sinoatrial or atrioventricular heart block, respiratory depression, and systemic hypotension.

Neonatal hypermagnesemia

Neonatal hypermagnesemia is defined by a serum Mg concentration above 2.5 mg dL^{-1}.[15] The most common cause of neonatal hypermagnesemia is maternal hypermagnesemia secondary to therapeutic magnesium sulfate administration for preeclampsia and preterm labor (Table 16.9).[15] Theoretically, high maternal serum Mg concentration may lead to transplacental Mg transfer to the fetus that exceeds the physiologic rate of Mg transport, resulting in fetal and neonatal hypermagnesemia. Administration of magnesium-containing enemas[15] or magnesium-containing antacids

Table 16.9. Causes of neonatal hypermagnesemia

Increased intake
   Hyperalimentation
   Maternal hypermagnesemia from $MgSO_4$ therapy
   Preeclampsia
   Tocolysis
      Mg-containing enemas
      Mg-containing antacids
Decreased renal excretion
   Oliguric renal failure
   Asphyxia neonatorum
   Prematurity

causes hypermagnesemia.[282] Reduced renal function and glomerular filtration due to prematurity,[283] birth asphyxia[284] or oliguric renal failure impairs Mg excretion and may result in elevated serum Mg concentrations.

Iatrogenic hypermagnesemia has been reported in neonates as a result of malfunction of an automated parenteral solution-mixing device[285] or from administration of an oral magnesium hydroxide laxative.[286] Use of magnesium sulfate infusions to prevent or alleviate the neurological sequelae of severe birth asphyxia is associated with hypermagnesemia.[287] Neonatal hypermagnesemia has been reported in severe primary hyperparathyroidism following parathyroidectomy and heterotopic autotransplantation.[288] Postoperatively, the infant had modest hypercalcemia, normal serum immunoreactive parathyroid hormone levels, hypermagnesemia, and relative hypocalciuria. The parents had familial hypocalciuric hypercalcemia. Rarely familial hypocalciuric hypercalcemia may be associated with hypermagnesemia.[221]

The main effects of hypermagnesemia are on the neuromuscular and cardiovascular systems. Excess Mg blocks transmission at the neuromuscular junction and the motor end plate, and antagonizes the effects of calcium. Therefore hypermagnesemia decreases skeletal and smooth muscle tone, resulting in variable degrees of hypotonia, vasodilatation, and hypotension.

Apgar scores, though lower in hypermagnesemic newborns, do not correlate with absolute serum Mg concentrations.[289] A significant correlation exists between neonatal neuromuscular depression and the duration of maternal therapy with Mg sulfate.[289] Elevated serum Mg concentrations suppress the parathyroid gland, resulting in low serum PTH concentrations.[290,291] However, serum Mg concentrations do not necessarily correlate with the clinical picture and may be of little diagnostic value.[292] Serum Ca concentrations may be normal or elevated in infants with hypermagnesemia[289] possibly due to heteroionic exchange of Ca for Mg at the blood–bone interface.[293]

Because of depressed muscular tone, hypermagnesemic neonates may present with meconium-plug syndrome.[294] In preterm newborns, immature renal function and delayed renal excretion of Mg predispose to more pronounced and prolonged hypermagnesemia. Severe hypermagnesemia causes parasympathetic blockade – including cutaneous flushing, hypotension, prolonged QT-interval, delayed intraventricular conduction, respiratory depression, neuromuscular blockade, and coma – and clinically mimics a central brainstem herniation syndrome. Hypotension, electrocardiographic changes, and evidence of sedation appear at serum magnesium concentrations of 3–8 mEq L^{-1}. Variable electrocardiographic changes (increased atrioventricular and ventricular conduction times) may be seen with serum Mg concentrations above 6 mg dL^{-1}. Disappearance of deep tendon reflexes, respiratory depression, weakness, and coma are reported at magnesium levels of 5–15 mEq L^{-1}; cardiac arrest is reported at serum magnesium levels of 20–30 mEq L^{-1}. Congenital bone demineralization and rickets have been described in reports of infants born to mothers who were treated with magnesium sulfate for preterm labor for a long period (up to 4 weeks).[295–297] Presumably, excess Mg enters the skeleton and displaces Ca into the circulation, thus distorting the mineral proportion (Ca, P, Mg) of the crystal lattice and resulting in bone demineralization.

Generally the treatment for neonatal mild hypermagnesemia consists of supportive care because it usually resolves spontaneously with adequate hydration as renal output increases significantly over the first few days of life. In infants who have severe hypermagnesemia presenting with significant hypotonia or EKG abnormalities, treatment with fluid resuscitation, diuresis, and calcium may be considered. Calcium ions counteract the effects of magnesium ions at the motor end plate and therefore might decrease the severity of hypotonia, and it will enhance renal excretion of magnesium ions. We recommend the use of 10% Ca gluconate infusions (0.2 to 0.3 ml kg^{-1} body weight) to counteract the inhibitory effect of Mg cations on neuromuscular excitability.[298] Loop diuretics (furosemide or ethacrinic acid) that increase Mg excretion may be given following adequate hydration. In cases of severe neuromuscular depression, hypotension and respiratory failure, maintenance of cardiopulmonary support (assisted ventilation, vasopressors) is of prime importance. Double volume "exchange" blood transfusions with citrated blood chelates Mg and helps decrease serum Mg concentrations in cases of life-threatening hypermagnesemia.[283] In patients with severe renal failure and markedly decreased urine output, severe hypermagnesemia should be treated with dialysis.

Disorders of vitamin D homeostasis

Vitamin D deficiency

Vitamin D deficiency in the pregnant woman may have drastic sequelae on bone mineralization of the fetus and newborn. Low dietary vitamin D intake, as in exclusively vegetarian women, and insufficient exposure to sunlight predispose to vitamin D deficiency manifesting as low serum concentration of 25-OHD and calcium, with or without rickets in the mother and the baby.[299–302] Congenital rickets, though rare, has been described in infants of mothers with severe vitamin D deficiency, severe intestinal malabsorption, or malnutrition. Vitamin D supplementation during pregnancy improves fetal skeleton growth in the rat.[38–40,45]

Vitamin D toxicity

Excessive dietary intake of vitamin D metabolites has been reported to cause hypercalcemia in both the mother and the newborn. Vitamin D and 25-OHD have a long half-life in the circulation. Transplacental transfer of excessive amounts of vitamin D or 25-OHD from mother to fetus may be responsible for prolonged hypercalcemia in the neonate. Hypervitaminosis D may result from drinking milk that is incorrectly and excessively fortified with vitamin D.[303] Infant formulas may be overfortified with vitamin D and theoretically might cause vitamin D toxicity.[304]

Rabbits fed a high vitamin D-containing diet develop soft tissue calcifications of arteries and kidneys.[305] In pregnant rabbits, excessive vitamin D administration resulted in offspring with supravalvular aortic stenosis and craniofacial and dental anomalies.[306] It is unclear how these findings may relate to the idiopathic hypercalcemia syndrome of infancy, in which hypersensitivity to vitamin D has been implicated and which includes craniofacial anomalies and supravalvular aortic stenosis.

Disorders of bone metabolism

Bone disease occurs when the balance between bone formation and resorption is perturbed. We have reviewed these disorders elsewhere.[307,308] Osteomalacia and rickets are primarily due to defective bone mineralization. Bone tissue is deficient in minerals, although the bone mass may be normal, decreased, or increased. The term rickets refers to changes in growing children at the cartilaginous growth plate (which is ossified in adults). The presence of the epiphyseal plate distinguishes rachitism of infancy and childhood from osteomalacia of adulthood. Rickets remains one of the most common bone disorders in infancy and childhood. A plethora of causative factors contribute to its pathogenesis. Osteomalacia refers to lack of bone calcification. While adults can have osteomalacia, both osteomalacia and rickets may coexist in children. A comprehensive list of causes of osteomalacia and rickets is reviewed elsewhere. In this section we limit the discussion to some disorders pertaining to neonates, infants, and children.

Vitamin D deficiency rickets[308,309]

Vitamin D deficiency rickets is "classical rickets" described since antiquity. The incidence of the disease has dropped markedly and generally, it is now rare in developed countries because basic food staples like milk and infant formulas are fortified with vitamin D. However, the disease is still encountered in less developed countries because of poverty, which entails insufficient sunshine exposure and dietary vitamin D intake. It is also encountered in exclusively human milk-fed infants and strict vegetarian adults even in developed countries who have limited sunshine exposure and who do not ingest milk and therefore have very limited sources of vitamin D. Pathophysiologically, vitamin D deficiency may be caused primarily by decreased sunshine exposure, compounded by decreased dietary vitamin D intake, or decreased intestinal absorption of vitamin D. It is debatable whether dark-skinned people have higher risk of vitamin D deficiency. The presence of a seemingly higher rate of rickets in dark-skinned infants in developed countries could relate directly to poor exposure to sunshine. Vitamin D is a fat-soluble vitamin and its intestinal absorption may be impaired by any intestinal disease process involving fat malabsorption. Increased intake of vegetables may decrease vitamin D availability to the body because they are poor sources of vitamin D and contain phytates and fiber, which bind dietary vitamin D and impair its intestinal absorption. The resulting vitamin D deficiency will result in decreased intestinal absorption of calcium and phosphorus and hypocalcemia. Consequently, the drop in serum calcium concentration will stimulate the parathyroid glands to synthesize and secrete PTH to normalize serum calcium concentration, therefore resulting in secondary hyperparathyroidism, which will demineralize bone unless the primary deficit of vitamin D is corrected.

Histopathologically, vitamin D deficiency rickets is characterized by excess osteoid formation with irregular bone-osteoid interface and marked decrease in bone cell activity.

Poor bone mineralization is reflected in the absence of the granular layer normally seen at bone-osteoid margin, and in disorganized epiphyseal overgrowth. Secondary hyperparathyroidism may be responsible for associated subperiosteal marrow fibrosis. Biochemically, the progression of vitamin D deficiency rickets occurs in three stages: (1) stage 1 is characterized by a drop in serum calcium concentration with normal serum phosphorus concentration; (2) stage 2 is characterized by a rise in serum PTH concentration in response to hypocalcemia, normocalcemia, hypophosphatemia secondary to PTH-induced hyperphosphaturia, aminoaciduria, and early rachitic bone disease on x-rays; (3) stage 3 is characterized by hypocalcemia despite elevated serum PTH concentration, more severe hypophosphatemia, hyperphosphaturia, aminoaciduria, and rachitic bone disease, and elevated serum alkaline phosphatase concentration. Although the mineralization defect is a generalized process, clinical rachitic bone disease is most prominent in rapidly growing bones such as costochondral junctions and long bone epiphyses. Rickets is most devastating during periods of life characterized by highest growth velocity in lifetime, namely infancy and childhood.

Clinically, the earliest rachitic features in infancy may be hypocalcemic tetany or seizures, particularly in vitamin D-unsupplemented, exclusively human milk-fed infants and infants with congenital rickets born to vitamin D-deficient osteomalacic mothers. Acute infections may precipitate hypocalcemic tetany possibly by mobilizing bone phosphate into the circulation and therefore decreasing serum calcium concentration. Rachitic bone changes evolve with the duration of the disease. In the first 6 months of life, craniotabes is the most common sign observed. Also, delayed closure of the posterior fontanelle, large anterior fontanelle, and bossing of frontal and parietal bones are often present. In the second part of infancy, epiphyseal changes are more florid. Epiphyseal widening occurs at the wrists, knees, ankles, and costochondral junctions (rachitic rosary). "Rachitic lungs" indicate rib cage weakening with secondary defective pulmonary ventilation. This feature occurs in the very young child, particularly among preterm infants. Harrison's sulcus is formed along the line of attachment of the diaphragm to the ribs, and a pectus carinatum (pigeon breast-like thoracic cage) may result from persistent sternal protrusion. Beyond infancy, increased weight bearing aggravates rachitic changes particularly in vertebral, pelvic, and lower limb bones resulting in spinal and pelvic deformities causing a waddling gait, and bowed legs or knock knees. Delayed teeth eruption, enamel hypoplasia, and dental caries may occur. Muscular weakness and hypotonia frequently involve proximal muscle groups in rickets, and contribute to waddling gait, protuberance of the abdomen, and inefficient lung ventilation in rachitic children. The muscular weakness is thought to be caused by decreased calcium uptake by myocytes. In developed countries, clinical diagnosis depends on the astute clinician encountering a dark-skinned infant who has been on prolonged breastfeeding and a questionable history of sun exposure without vitamin D supplementation.

Radiological signs correspond to clinical findings (Figure 16.1). The wrist and the knee are most useful in demonstrating even the earliest signs of rickets. Characteristic changes include diffuse decrease in bone density, pale and irregular ossification centers, bowing of long bones, cupping, fraying, widening of epiphyseal cartilage, decreased bone mineralization, and pathologic fractures with poor callus formation. Bone age may be delayed. In developed countries the diagnosis is often made incidentally when an x-ray of the infant is done for other reasons such as a possible chest infection.

Treatment of the disease is vitamin D. Prevention has been achieved in developed countries by vitamin D enrichment of common foods such as milk. Because human milk has low vitamin D content, human milk-fed infants who are sunshine-deprived may develop the disease if not supplemented with vitamin D.[310] We have found that human milk-fed infants require at least 30 minutes/week of sunlight (face and hands uncovered) to maintain serum 25-OHD within normal range (>11 ng ml^{-1}).[311] Standard formula-fed infants receive sufficient supplements of vitamin D in formula to prevent rickets. Intermittent high dose vitamin D prophylaxis against rickets (Stoss therapy) is used in less developed countries to ensure compliance. However, this regimen carries the risk of overdosage and hypercalcemia.[312]

Hepatic rickets

Hepatobiliary disease predisposes to rickets presumably because of decreased 25-hydroxylase activity, vitamin D malabsorption, and decreased enterohepatic circulation of 25-OHD. Malabsorption of vitamin D is probably of major impact in the pathogenesis of hepatic rickets.[308] Biochemically, serum 25-OHD and 1,25(OH)2D concentrations are low. Clinically, signs of rickets are superimposed on the primary hepatic disease. Infants with hepatitis and infants who required prolonged parenteral hyperalimentation may develop a variable degree of hepatic dysfunction and secondary rachitism.

Vitamin D-dependent rickets

Vitamin D-dependent rickets-I (VDDR-I) is inherited in an autosomal recessive pattern. The basic pathology in this disease is decreased renal 1-alpha-hydroxylase enzyme

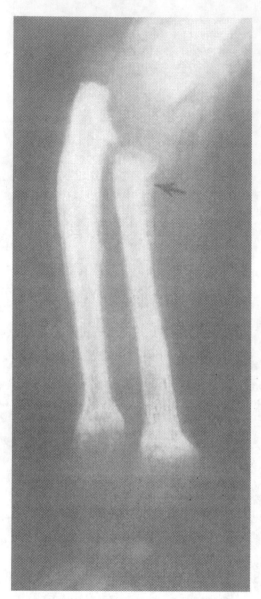

Figure 16.1. Florid rickets. Cupping and fraying of the metaphysic; increased distance between the distal radius metaphysic and its indistinct growth centers under mineralized cortices; fracture in proximal radius (dark arrow).

activity, which is necessary for the conversion of 25-OHD into calcitriol. Biochemically the disease is characterized by very low serum calcitriol concentrations in the face of normal serum 25-OHD concentration. Clinically, the disease presents before 2 years of age, most often in the first 6 months of life. A sporadic form of the disease has been described less often, and its onset is in late childhood and adolescence. Successful therapy of VDDR-I can be achieved with high doses of vitamin D or physiologic doses of calcitriol.

VDDR-II is usually inherited in an autosomal recessive pattern, with clustering of affected patients in the Mediterranean region. The hallmark of the disease is an end organ resistance to the effect of 1,25(OH)2D because of a defective calcitriol-receptor effector system, and mechanistically should be called calcitriol (1,25(OH)2D)-resistant rickets. Malloy *et al.* demonstrated a point mutation within the steroid-binding domain of the vitamin D receptor in seven Mediterranean families with the disease.[313,314] Clinically, the disease manifests as rickets and osteomalacia most commonly before 2 years of life. At least two-thirds of these patients have alopecia, and some have ectodermal anomalies: milia, epidermal cysts, and oligodontia. Occasionally, the disease may be associated with impetigo herpetiformis and ichthyosis.[315] Biochemically, these patients have low serum calcium and phosphorus concentrations, normal serum 25-OHD concentration, and elevated serum 1,25(OH)2D and PTH concentrations. Understanding the pathogenesis of this disease at the subcellular level reveals intracellular defects in the calcitriol receptor-effector system and permits classification into categories: (1) Hormone binding negative: this is the most common defect. It is characterized by a defect in hormone binding domain: calcitriol concentration is elevated but does not evoke a biochemical response. (2) Defect in hormone binding capacity: while hormone-binding affinity is normal, there is a reduced number of hormone binding sites (10% of normal). (3) Defect in hormone binding affinity: while the number of binding sites is normal (normal capacity), hormone binding affinity is reduced 20- to 30-fold. (4) Defective nuclear localization: in this form, calcitriol does not localize to the cell nucleus. (5) Decreased affinity of hormone-receptor complex to DNA. Intracellular defect categories 1, 2 and 5 do not respond to therapy with high vitamin D doses. In contrast, intracellular defects type 3 and 4 can be cured with high vitamin D doses. Prenatal diagnosis of this disease is now feasible and is indicated in high-risk families.[316]

Calcium deficiency rickets

The role of optimal dietary calcium intake in bone homeostasis has been stressed. Insufficient mineral intake predisposes children and young infants to rickets, particularly during rapid growth periods of infancy and childhood. Clinical evidence supports the theory that suboptimal calcium intake in childhood results in a lower peak bone mass, thus predisposing to adult osteoporosis. In rats, calcium deprivation may induce vitamin D deficiency and secondary hyperparathyroidism.[317]

In preterm infants optimal mineral retention for bone mineralization cannot be achieved with unfortified human milk or standard cow milk formulas. Before this fact was known a significant number of preterm infants had rachitic bone disease, which now appears to be ameliorated by fortification of preterm formulas and human milk fed to preterm infants. Increased calcium loss in urine is described with the use of loop diuretics (such as furosemide), and parenteral hyperalimentation, which theoretically aggravates osteopenia of prematurity.[318]

Calcium deficiency rickets has been reported in infants and toddlers fed low calcium diets[319] and in older black children from Africa.[320,321] These children are described to have suboptimal calcium intake in their diet. Pettifor found significant correlations between dietary calcium intake in these children and serum calcium and alkaline phosphatase concentrations, and urinary calcium excretion. Clinically, affected children have rachitic features with knock-knees, bowed legs, or wind-swept deformities (combined genu valgus and genu varus), but no muscular weakness. Radiological features correspond to clinical findings of rachitic changes. Osteopenia is described with or without features of secondary hyperparathyroidism (loss of lamina dura around teeth, but no subperiosteal cortical erosions in phalanges). Bone histology reveals features of osteomalacia and secondary hyperparathyroidism. Biochemical features of calciopenic rickets (hypocalcemia and hypocalciuria, normal serum 25-OHD, elevated serum alkaline phosphatase, elevated serum calcitriol and PTH concentrations) resolve after dietary calcium supplementation (1000 mg of elemental calcium day^{-1}).[321]

Children who are on strict vegetarian or high cereal diets are at risk of developing rickets. Some of these children have clinical and biochemical features of vitamin D deficiency, attributed to vitamin D binding by dietary phytates in the intestinal lumen. Impaired bone mineralization associated with the use of soy formulas has been attributed to several factors including (1) low methionine content, (2) the presence of phytates which chelate minerals in intestinal lumen and decrease retention of calcium and phosphorus, and (3) the absence of lactose which facilitates intestinal absorption of calcium.

Renal hypophosphatemic rickets ("Vitamin D resistant" rickets)

Renal hypophosphatemic rickets[322,323] is a familial disorder inherited in an autosomal or X-linked dominant fashion. The most frequent type is the X-linked dominant pattern and affects males. Outside the neonatal period, it is the most common form of rickets in childhood in the USA.

The disease is characterized by severe hypophosphatemia, decreased maximal tubular reabsorption of phosphate per volume of glomerular filtrate (TmP/GFR) and rickets. Pathophysiologically, the disease is caused by a congenital defect in phosphate reabsorption in proximal renal tubules, resulting in massive phosphaturia and hypophosphatemia. The defective gene responsible for this disease has been mapped to the short arm of the human X chromosome. Biochemically, serum phosphorus concentration is markedly decreased, while serum calcium concentration may be normal or decreased. Serum PTH concentration is either normal or increased and serum 1,25(OH)2D concentration is either normal or low. Clinically, rickets may manifest within a few months of life and is characterized by short stature, genu valgum, and coxa vara. It may also be associated with craniosynostosis, dental and periodontal abscesses, and intracerebral calcifications. Radiologically, two patterns of bone changes are described in this disease: Type A is characterized by bowing and prominent medial epiphyseal plate widening, especially in the lower limbs (mainly in the knees); type B is characterized by short bones and cortical thickening, and involvement of all limbs. In contrast to vitamin D deficiency rickets, craniotabes, rachitic rosary, amionoaciduria, secondary hyperparathyroidism and pelvic deformities are not features of familial hypophosphatemic rickets. Heterozygous females seem to have a milder disease presumably because of the normal allele on the unaffected X chromosome and random inactivation of the mutant X chromosome.

Treatment of this disease is a lifelong process. Best results are achieved by a combination of phosphate supplementation (40 mg kg^{-1}day^{-1} in five divided doses) and calcitriol (1,25(OH)2D). The goal of treatment is radiological healing of rachitic changes, and normophosphatemia without hypercalciuria. We recommend to start with an initial dose of 15 to 20 ng kg^{-1} day^{-1} (in two divided doses) and increase it to 30 to 60 ng kg^{-1} day^{-1} over several months to achieve normophosphatemia, and radiological healing of bone changes without hypercalciuria.[324,325] Calcitriol daily dosage is monitored by keeping the urine calcium to creatinine mg/mg ratio less than 0.2–0.3.[326]

Parenteral hyperalimentation induced osteopenia

Long-term parenteral alimentation (TPN) has been associated with osteopenia and bone demineralization.[327] The main feature seen in this metabolic bone disease is hypercalciuria (Table 16.10). Several factors have been implicated in the etiology of hypercalciuria including cyclic infusion of TPN solutions,[328] sulfur-containing acidic amino acids,[329–334] hypertonic dextrose infusions which

Table 16.10. Factors aggravating hypercalciuria in patients receiving TPN

Cyclic infusion of TPN solutions
Sulfur-containing acidic amino acids
Hypertonic dextrose infusions
Acidosis
Low phosphate in infused solutions
Aluminum contamination of TPN solutions

result in hyperinsulinemia and decreased tubular resorption of calcium, acidosis, and low phosphate in infused solutions.[327] Hypercalciuria may be ameliorated by phosphate supplementation.[328]

Aluminum-containing parenteral hyperalimentation solutions are responsible for causing a peculiar metabolic bone disease characterized by reduced bone formation. The degree of aluminum accumulation in bone correlates with decreased bone formation. Aluminum inhibits PTH secretion, and serum PTH concentration may be within normal limits. Also, aluminum directly impairs osteoblastic bone formation and mineralization processes. Histologically, the disease is characterized by osteomalacia with excess osteoid (unmineralized bone) and widened osteoid seams. Aluminum deposits are prominent within the mineralization front, where calcification of newly formed osteoid occurs.

Metabolic bone disease of prematurity (MBDP) or rickets/osteopenia of prematurity

The physical density of long bones such as the femoral diaphysis decreases by about 30% during the first six months of life. This is mostly due to an increase in marrow cavity size, which is faster than the increase in the cross sectional area of the bone cortex.[335] These postnatal adaptations of the skeletal system to extrauterine conditions also occur in premature infants, with the difference that they happen earlier than in term babies. The reasons for the postnatal adaptations of the skeleton are not entirely clear. However, the skeleton is exposed to different conditions before and after birth. In utero, regular mechanical stimulation by fetal kicks against the uterine wall represent an intrauterine form of resistance training. In the extrauterine life, the infant's movements occur with less resistance, thus putting smaller loads on the skeleton. Postnatally, the placental supply of estrogen and other hormones that stimulate bone formation has been cut off. Some authors question the validity of the aim to achieve intrauterine mineral accretion rates,

and suggest that the skeleton of these infants will adapt to the mechanical requirements, whether intrauterine calcium accretion rates are achieved or not.[335] An adequate supply of substrate (including minerals) is a prerequisite for the synthesis of bone tissue as well as to maintain the balance between bone formation and resorption. Bone formation may manifest in increase in bone length and increase in cross sectional bone strength (increase in bone width and cortical thickness, etc). Nutritional and mechanical factors have complementary roles in bone development. Thus, when the mechanical challenge posed by muscles is lacking, less new bone is added despite adequate supply of minerals and other substrates. We therefore emphasize that normal bone development requires the intricate interplay of several factors including the availability of optimal amount of minerals for deposition in the osteoid matrix as well as mechanical factors that are crucial for normal bone development.

Osteomalacia/rickets is a disorder of bone mineralization – that is, the incorporation of mineral into the organic bone matrix. In preterm infants, osteomalacia/rickets is generally due to a deficient supply or uptake of mineral.[336–338] When premature babies are fed human milk, the supply of both calcium and phosphorus is low, but the critical factor leading to osteomalacia/rickets is the lack of phosphorus.[339] Serum phosphate levels decrease and there is not enough substrate for incorporation into the organic bone matrix.

Osteopenia refers to a decreased amount of bone tissue, which manifests as decreased thickness or number of trabeculae and/or decreased thickness of the bone cortex. Osteopenia is caused by either insufficient deposition or increased resorption of organic bone matrix. In contrast with osteomalacia, the incorporation of calcium and phosphate into organic bone matrix is not affected. Osteopenia results from diminished synthesis and/or increased resorption of organic bone matrix. This can be caused by severe systemic disease, a drug side effect – for example, corticosteroids – or lack of mechanical stimulation ("disuse osteoporosis"). Evidence suggests that skeletal development may be driven by functional requirements.[338] This means that bone strength increases when and where it is required to maintain bone stability. Under physiological conditions, the largest challenges to bone stability result from muscle contraction and not just from passive gravity. Therefore, the stability of a bone must be adapted to local muscle force.

The importance of muscle–bone interaction is particularly obvious in newborns with muscular hypotonia of intrauterine onset, who often have fractures at birth.[340,341] Rodriguez investigated the effects of immobilization on fetal bone development through postmortem study of radiographs in newborns with congenital neuromuscular diseases (CNMD) of intrauterine onset. From their study they suggest that intrauterine immobilization induces a decrease in mechanical usage of bone, mainly influencing bone modeling and probably bone remodeling resulting in osteopenia and mechanical defects that predispose them to fractures.[340,341] They later demonstrated an impairment of the membranous (periosteal) ossification of long bones produced by immobilization and/or decrease of muscular strength.[342] However, lack of mechanical stimulation is not limited to these rare cases, but may be an important problem in neonatology.

Metabolic bone disease of prematurity (rickets or osteopenia of prematurity) is a disease of growing bone occurring primarily in preterm infants and is characterized by suboptimal mineralization of bone matrix resulting in fragile skeletal support and increased incidence of bone fracture with little mechanical stress. The incidence of this disease varies from 30%–70%. It is inversely related to the gestational age with highest incidence occurring in the VLBW infants (at least 30% in infants less than 1500 g birth weight).[343–348] In Callenbach's review a higher proportion of these infants were black, born in the spring, had a greater initial weight loss, and had a longer hospitalization. Some of these infants were fed soy formula, supplemented with calcium and vitamin D but not phosphorus. Soy isolate formula, as well as human milk does not provide sufficient calcium and phosphorus to keep pace with rates of intrauterine accretion. Steichen[349] and coworkers demonstrated lower bone mineral content using single photon absorptiometry in infants fed soy formula over the first year of life. The disease is even more aggravated in infants with chronic lung disease and significantly increased work of breathing and energy expenditure, with limited intake of minerals and exaggerated urinary mineral losses from chronic diuretic therapy.[350] Despite increasing awareness and institution of preventive measures by increasing mineral intake of preterm infants over the past 2 decades, there are no recent systematic studies of the incidence of the disease in infants who presumably received mineral supplementation that mimics intrauterine mineral supply.

The etiology of rickets of prematurity is multifactorial. Several pathophysiological explanations for this disease have been proposed. The major cause of metabolic bone disease in premature infants (MBDP) is insufficient intake of minerals (primarily calcium and phosphorus) short of the recommended intake for normal bone mineralization, remodeling, and growth. This results in deficient crystallization of Ca and phosphate in newly formed osteoid matrix. Human milk contains only approximately 25% of the amount of calcium and phosphorus needed for normal bone mineralization during postnatal growth of premature infants in the period equal to the third trimester, even when the infants are fed 200 ml kg^{-1} day^{-1}.[351–353] Even with a maximum oral intake of 200ml kg^{-1} day^{-1} and supplementation/fortification with calcium and phosphate, it is almost impossible to match the rate of intrauterine accretion of these two minerals in the third trimester (for Ca it is about 3.5 mmol kg^{-1} day^{-1} and for P it is about 2.7 mmol kg^{-1} day^{-1}).

Phosphorus deficiency rickets has been described in preterm infants fed human milk, which does not supply the minimum daily requirement of phosphorus for rapidly growing bones. Biochemically, these infants have low serum phosphate concentration, normal or elevated serum calcium concentration, increased tubular reabsorption of phosphorus, and elevated serum calcitriol concentrations. Clinically most patients are detected within the first 6 months of life with florid rachitic bone disease. Suboptimal caloric intake may additionally affect bone growth and modeling resulting in osteopenia in addition to rickets/osteomalacia.

From additional evidence it appears that increased bone resorption may also be a significant contributing factor to the pathogenesis of MBDP.[354,355] This is supported by the findings that urinary excretion of bone resorption markers like hydroxyproline, type 1 collagen telopeptide, and calcium and phosphorus is 3–4 times higher in preterm in comparison to term infants. Beyers et al.[354] noted that preterm infants at expected full-term age had significantly greater urine excretion of calcium (2.9x), phosphate (4.3x), and hydroxyproline (3.7x) compared with normal term infants. Serum alkaline phosphatase was twice as great (411 UL^{-1} v. 206 UL^{-1}) in preterm infants at expected full-term age compared with normal term infants. Moreover, radiological evaluation showed increased endosteal resorption in the preterm infants. Mora et al.[355] found that preterm infants (average gestational age of 33 weeks) had significantly higher blood levels of type 1 collagen telopeptide than term infants when both groups were studied at 4 weeks of age. Using osteocalcin and procollagen type 1 carboxyterminal propeptide as indices of bone formation, these investigators found lower concentrations of bone formation markers in the preterm infants than the term infants.

Miller proposed that biomechanical factors contribute significantly to the pathogenesis of MBDP. Increased bone resorption may be aggravated by a lesser degree of mechanical load on preterm bone following birth.[356] The effects of intrauterine kicking and bouncing have been stressed as important mechanical stimuli for bone formation in the last few weeks of pregnancy. Infants with this disease usually have normal serum vitamin D metabolites[346,347] and supplemental vitamin D administration does not improve the biochemical and radiological changes of this disease.

A significantly lower BMC in premature infants at term compared with term infants has been described in several studies.[357-360] The BMC was found to be around 50% lower at term in premature infants with birth gestational age < 32 weeks. The reduced rate of bone mineralization in premature infants may lead to complications, including risk of fractures[346,347] and high incidence of myopia because of the head flattening caused by osteopenia.[361] Other complications of the disease include defects in deciduous dentition.[362] The disease is aggravated by parenteral solution-induced cholestasis,[363] hypersulfatemia, and aluminum contamination of parenteral solutions.[364]

Aluminum (Al) impairment of bone matrix formation and mineralization may be mediated by its direct effect on bone cells or indirectly by its effect on parathyroid hormone and calcium metabolism.[364-366] Its toxic effects are proportional to the tissue Al load. Al contamination of nutrients depends on the amount of Al present naturally in chemicals or from the manufacturing process. Intravenous calcium, phosphorus, and albumin solutions have high Al (> 500 μg L^{-1}), whereas crystalline amino acid, sterile water, and dextrose water have low Al (< 50 μg L^{-1}) content. Enteral nutrients including human and whole cow milk have low Al, whereas highly processed infant formulas with multiple additives, such as soy formula, preterm infant formula, and formulas for specific disorders are heavily contaminated with Al. Healthy adults are in zero balance for Al. The intestinal mucosa of the gastrointestinal tract prevents the absorption of greater than 95% of dietary Al, and the kidney is the dominant organ for Al excretion. However, even with normal renal function, only 30%–60% of an Al load from parenteral nutrition is excreted in the urine, resulting in tissue accumulation of Al. The risk for Al toxicity is greatest in infants with chronic renal insufficiency, recipients of long-term parenteral nutrition, i.e., bypassing the gut barrier to Al loading, and preterm infants with decreased intestinal mucosal integrity. The rapid growth of the infant would theoretically potentiate Al toxicity in all infants, although the critical level of Al loading causing bone disorders is not known. To minimize tissue burden, Al content of infant nutrients should be similar to "background" levels, i.e., similar to whole milk (< 50 μg L^{-1}). The spectrum of the disease ranges from subclinical mild bone demineralization that resolves over several months[360,367] to overt rickets and nontraumatic fractures.[368] Approximately 10% of VLBW, preterm infants incur fractures within the first several months of life. The mean age of diagnosis of

fractures in one series of preterm infants with fractures was 76 days, and the types of fractures included long bone, rib, and metaphyseal fractures.[369]

Measurements of BMC are usually based on single photon absorptiometry applied to the forearm. This method has the limitation of measuring only a small part of the skeleton, and correction for body size, which is necessary to assess bone mineralization, is not used. Radiological examination of the skeleton has also been used, and a scale for grading the severity of metabolic bone disease has been developed.[370] A BMC < 50 % of the normal level is usually the detection limit for changes on radiographs, which significantly limits this method.

Probably, the most common clinical presentation of rickets of prematurity is subclinical rickets detected incidentally on radiological examination. The full-blown clinical picture of rickets comprises craniotabes, widening of costochondral junctions of the ribs (rachitic rosary) with or without respiratory distress (Figure 16.1),[371] and widening of the wrists and ankles. Preterm infants may present with skeletal fractures, usually of long bones and ribs. The most common age of presentation is between 2–4 months of life with a range from 4–20 weeks of postnatal life.

Biochemical changes of rickets are variable and depend on the severity of the disease, and compensatory mechanisms of the body: serum calcium concentration is commonly normal but may be low or even elevated; serum phosphorus concentration is often low but may be normal. The entity "phosphorus deficiency syndrome" is well described by Rowe and is a major cause of poor bone mineralization, hypercalciuria and calcium deficiency, and secondary rickets; serum 25-OHD concentration may be normal, low, or elevated; serum PTH may be normal or elevated if secondary hyperparathyroidism occurs as a compensatory mechanism to correct for hypocalcemia; serum 1,25(OH)2D concentration is typically elevated indicating renal compensatory activity to counteract the effects of mineral deficiency by decreasing excretion of calcium and phosphorus.[346,347] Serum alkaline phosphatase concentration is elevated, but is not specific for bone, because the enzyme is also produced in the liver. Bone specific alkaline phosphatase isoenzyme assay may be more reliable for follow up.

Kovar[372] used serum alkaline phosphatase in screening for rickets of prematurity and suggested a cut-off level of alkaline phosphatase activity above 5 times the upper limit of the normal adult reference rate (>1200 IU L^{-1}) as an indication of rickets. In another radiographic study Koo et al.[346,347] found a significant association between serum phosphate and bone mineralization. Though some photon absorptiometry studies[373,374] report an association between serum alkaline phosphatase or serum phosphate and BMC, others do not.[357,375] Ryan *et al.* found an association between serum alkaline phosphatase and phosphate and BMC, but the prediction of BMC was poor because the biochemical variables could only explain 7% of the variation in BMC. Abrams *et al.* found a significant positive association at 16 and 25 weeks of age between serum alkaline phosphatase and BMC measured by single photon absorptiometry (SPA), also when bone width was corrected for.

Lucas *et al.*[376] reported that a peak value of serum alkaline phosphatase >1200 IU L^{-1} was associated with reduced linear growth in the neonatal period and reduced height achievement at 18 months of age. They suggested that this may be due to metabolic bone disease, but did not measure BMC. Later Faerk[377] compared infants with high serum alkaline phosphatase (mean value >1200 U l^{-1}) with those with low values (mean value <600 U L^{-1}), and found no difference in BMC at term. They have also found a significant association between growth velocity and serum phosphate.[378] As serum phosphate is closely and negatively associated with serum alkaline phosphatase, it is likely that serum alkaline phosphatase is negatively associated with growth velocity, although this may not be due to a mineralization deficit, but rather to phosphorus deficiency.

Gross[379] found significantly lower serum phosphate and higher serum alkaline phosphatase concentrations in infants fed human milk alone compared with infants fed human milk supplemented with formula. MacMahon *et al.*[380] reported a significant association between high serum alkaline phosphatase concentration, low BMC assessed from radiographs, low serum phosphate concentration, and rickets. Two regional DEXA studies[380] report no association while others report an association between serum alkaline phosphatase and BMC or serum phosphate. Comparison of these studies is difficult because of inconsistency in the measurements of biochemical variables and BMC. Recently Faerk *et al.*[377] compared size-corrected BMC measured by DEXA with biochemical indicators of bone mineralization in premature infants. They found that serum alkaline phosphatase concentration was significantly and negatively associated with serum phosphate concentration in preterm infants.[377] Bone mineral content was not associated with mean or peak serum alkaline phosphatase, or mean serum phosphate concentrations at term.

The source of serum phosphate is a combination of phosphate coming out of bone due to bone resorption and dietary phosphate. Therefore, a high serum phosphate may indicate increased bone resorption leading to reduced BMC, and a low serum phosphate may be a marker of less bone resorption and thereby a normal BMC. In older children with rickets, bone resorption is associated with significant serum elevations of ICTP and osteocalcin[381] and serum ICTP concentration correlated with alkaline phosphate activity.

Prevention and therapy

Metabolic bone disease in the preterm infant has received increasing emphasis.[337,382] The increasing survival of extremely premature infants is associated with a rise in the number of subjects at high risk for rickets of prematurity, at least in the subclinical form. Ideally, these infants should receive sufficient amounts of minerals to meet the intrauterine mineral accretion rate required for adequate bone mineralization. Human milk and standard humanized cow milk formulas do not provide optimal Ca and P concentrations (Table 16.11) to meet the requirements of preterm infants. Formulas designed for preterm infants have a higher content of minerals to insure that dietary mineral intake can theoretically achieve fetal accretion rate. During the third trimester, daily net accretions for Ca and P range between 120 and 140 mg kg^{-1} and 60 to 75 mg kg^{-1}, respectively. Assuming that the intestinal absorptions for Ca and P in the preterm infant are 65% and 85%,[10] a daily intake of elemental Ca and P of 215 mg kg^{-1} and 90 mg kg^{-1}, respectively might be expected to provide sufficient mineral intake to meet intrauterine accretion rate in the preterm infant. The exclusive feeding of unfortified human milk in premature infants has been associated with poorer rates of growth and nutritional deficits during and beyond the period of hospitalization.[383–390] As a common goal for nutritional support is to meet the intrauterine rates of growth and nutrient retention, nutrient supplementation is necessary to optimize the use of human milk in the feeding of premature infants.[391]

The ideal Ca and P content of milk formulas to prevent rickets of prematurity is not known, especially in VLBW infants. However, with few exceptions[379,392] most studies demonstrated improvement in bone mineralization and biochemical measurements of rickets by Ca and P fortification of human milk or cow milk formulas fed to preterm infants.[391,393–399] Treatment with a formula supplemented with additional Ca and P, results in rapid improvement in bone mineralization with a concomitant decrease of 1,25(OH)2D to normal values, whereas 25-OHD values increase and parathyroid hormone values decrease.[347,400] MacMahon demonstrated that an increased mineral content in parenteral nutrition solutions reduces the severity of metabolic bone disease.[401]

Table 16.11. Calcium (Ca), Phosphorus (P), and magnesium (Mg) contents of Infant Formulas (units/100 kcal)*

	Ca (mg)	Ca:P	Mg(mg)	P(mg)
Human milk	38.89	2:1	4.86	19.44
Routine cow's milk formulas				
Enfamil (Mead Johnson)	69.00	1.5:1	7.80	47.00
PM 60/40 (Ross)	56.00	2:1	6.00	28.00
SMA (Wyeth)	63.00	1.5:1	7.00	42.00
Similac (Ross)	75.00	1.3:1	6.00	58.00
Preterm infant formulas				
Enfamil Premature (Mead Johnson)	117.00	2:1	4.90	59.00
Similac Special Care (Ross)	180.00	2:1	12.00	90.00
SMA Preemie (Wyeth)	90.00	1.8:1	8.60	50.00
Similac LBW (Ross)	90.00	1.3:1	10.00	70.00
Soy protein formulas				
ProSobee (Mead Johnson)	94.00	1.3:1	10.90	74.00
Isomil (Ross)	105.00	1.4:1	7.50	75.00
Isomil SF (Ross)	105.00	1.4:1	7.50	75.00
Nursoy (Wyeth)	90.00	1.4:1	10.00	63.00
Soyalac (Loma Linda)	94.00	1.7:1	12.00	55.00
i-Soyalac (Loma Linda)	102.00	1.4:1	11.00	71.00

*Adapted from data.[469]

The use of multinutrient fortifiers for human milk-fed premature infants has increased in neonatal centers. Mineral supplementation of unfortified human milk throughout hospitalization may improve linear growth and bone mineralization during and beyond the neonatal period.[391,402–404] Supplementation with both Ca and P also results in a normalization of biochemical indices of mineral status: serum Ca, P, and alkaline phosphatase activity; urinary excretion of Ca and P,[389,405] and bone density.[406]

Steichen[399] demonstrated that infants fed high-mineral concentration formula (120 mg calcium and 63 mg phosphate per 100 ml) achieved a BMC measured by SPA equal to the intrauterine levels. Infants fed the experimental high-mineral formula were already within the low normal intrauterine range at the start of the study (2 weeks) and increased their BMC by 58% to the average range during the following 10 weeks (Figures 16.2, 16.3). Modanlou[393] demonstrated that infants receiving fortified preterm human milk showed growth, biochemical status, and mineral status similar to those receiving high-caloric-density formula, but infants receiving fortified preterm human milk grew significantly faster, had higher serum protein, and tended to have better mineral status (higher serum calcium, lower alkaline phosphatase, and higher serum phosphorus, none individually significant) than infants receiving preterm human milk alone. Gross[379] showed no significant effect of early maternal milk supplementation with formula on bone mineralization by 44 weeks postconceptional age. Venkataraman[394] demonstrated that mineral supplementation of human milk resulted in higher bone mineral content. Holland et al.[397] found a significant effect of phosphorus supplementation on reducing the occurrence of rickets measured by x-ray in premature infants with birth weight <1250 g at 5 weeks of age. Lapillonne[398] demonstrated that mineral supplementation of human milk as well as feeding preterm formula result in better mineral retention and improved bone mineral content that is no different than that of term human infants by 6 months of age.

In striking contrast to previous reports, a recent Danish study[392] which examined the effect of different mineral supplements on bone mineral content at term in premature infants, found that when feeding 200 ml kg^{-1}day^{-1}, mineral supplementation of human milk or use of preterm formula did not significantly improve bone mineralization outcome at term. In this study infants received phosphate supplementation of human milk as recommended by the European Society of Pediatric Gastroenterology and Nutrition[407] or fortified supplementation with protein, calcium, and phosphorus or preterm formula as recommended by the American Academy of Pediatrics.[408] Interestingly neither phosphate, fortifier nor preterm formula supplementation had any significant effect on bone mineral content measured by DEXA scan at term compared with infants fed

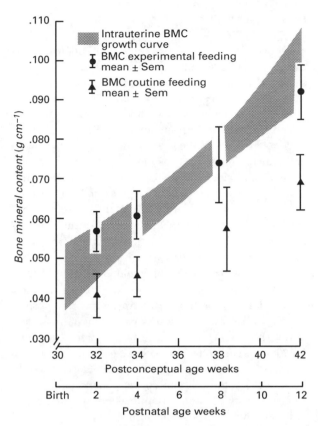

Figure 16.2. Postnatal bone mineral content (BMC) of infants born between 28 and 32 weeks gestation receiving experimental feeding (Ca and P fortified routine formula), compared with the intrauterine bone mineralization curve (IUBMC), and to postnatal BMC of infants born between 28 and 32 weeks gestation receiving routine formula (68 Kcal/100 ml). BMC in the experimental group is not different from the IUBMC and is significantly greater than MBC in the routine feeding group at 2, 4, and 12 weeks of postnatal age, respectively.

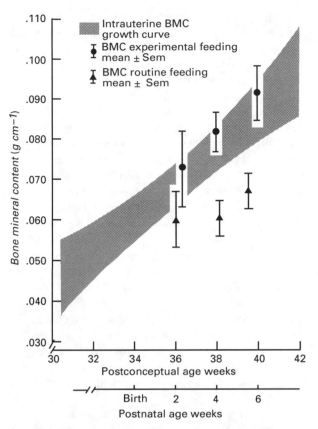

Figure 16.3. Postnatal bone mineral content (BMC) of infants born between 33 and 35 weeks gestation receiving experimental Ca and P fortified formula compared with the intrauterine bone mineralization curve (IUMBC) and to the postnatal BMC of routine formula-fed infants born between 33 and 35 weeks gestational age. BMC in the experimental group is not different from the IUMBC and is significantly greater than BMC in the routine feeding group at 4 and 6 weeks postnatal age.

their own mother's milk only. Infants fed preterm formula had a significantly higher weight at term compared with infants fed their own mother's milk only, but did not differ significantly in length or head circumference. The amount of supplemented phosphorus was significantly associated with weight at term. The lack of effect of mineral supplementation with either phosphate or a fortifier with both calcium and phosphate is surprising in comparison to many previously published results, and even more surprising is the finding that feeding with preterm formula does not significantly improve bone mineralization compared with feeding with their own mother's milk. The high volume of intake (200 ml kg^{-1}day^{-1}) increases mineral intake which may partly explain why infants fed their own mother's milk only were able to almost achieve the same BMC, length, and

head circumference as infants fed fortified human milk or preterm formula. It is not clear whether decreased intestinal mineral absorption or technical variation was responsible for the lack of detection of improved mineralization with mineral supplementation in this study.

Poor calcium absorption from certain cow milk-based formulas[409] could be due to the position of fatty acids in triacylglycerols.[410,411] In human milk, the most common fatty acid, palmitic acid, is placed in the sn-2 position, whereas in formulas, palmitic acid is often placed in the sn-1 or sn-3 position. Lipases hydrolyze the fatty acids in sn-1 and sn-3 positions and leave the fatty acid in the sn-2 position as monoacylglycerol. Palmitic acid in monoacylglycerol is well absorbed, whereas free palmitic acid is poorly absorbed and forms insoluble calcium soaps.

A significantly higher calcium and fat excretion in stools have been found in formula-fed infants compared with human milk-fed infants.[412,413] Koo *et al.*[414] recently demonstrated reduced bone mineralization in infants fed palm olein-containing formulas.

Treatment with furosemide contributes significantly to excessive urinary calcium losses and to the development of metabolic bone disease. Rowe[415] demonstrated that mineral supplementation of formula fed to infants receiving furosemide may promote bone mineralization and prevent the occurrence of secondary hyperparathyroidism. Treatment with high-dose dexamethasone for bronchopulmonary dysplasia in VLBW infants was associated with rapid and marked decrease in bone formation marker (PICP, BALP) concentrations, poor weight gain and lower extremity shrinkage.[416] The authors of this study report resolution of these biochemical changes during steroid weaning. The importance of physical activity in bone metabolism has become recognized.[417] Studies using SPA,[418] DEXA[419] and ultrasound techniques[420] have demonstrated that physical activity promotes better bone formation and density provided that a sufficient and balanced supply of energy, proteins, vitamins, calcium, phosphorus, and other essential nutrients for normal bone development are available.

Koo *et al.*[346,347] reported prospective longitudinal studies of the clinical course of fractures and rickets in VLBW infants during the first year of life: radiographic evidence of healing and remodeling occurred concurrently with increased enteral intake and physical growth, regardless of whether specific orthopedic treatment was initiated. Skeletal maturation as indicated by the development of ossification centers at the wrists was directly related to weight gain, and was similar to term infants by 1 year. No infant had skeletal deformities on follow-up examination. Therefore most VLBW infants with the disease can be managed "conservatively," with emphasis on nutritional intake to achieve weight gain. Fewtrell *et al.*[421] have reported on long-term follow-up of preterm children. They are shorter, lighter, and have lower bone mass than their peers at age 8–12 years.

Recommended enteral and parenteral mineral and vitamin D requirements

Determination of optimal nutrient requirement is based on several criteria including mineral balance studies that assess mineral accretion, biochemical indicators of bone and mineral homeostasis, and assessment of bone mineral content and density. Mineral as well as vitamin D deficiencies have been described earlier.

Parenteral nutrition

The indications, techniques, and complications of parenteral hyperalimentation are discussed elsewhere. This section is devoted to mineral components of currently utilized parenteral solutions in infants. The most current recommendations for mineral and vitamin D intake for infants are based on the results of metabolic studies in term and preterm infants, the goal sought being optimal bone and mineral homeostasis as indicated by normal serum minerals and vitamin D metabolites and relatively normal bone density. Currently, most parenteral solutions can provide minerals to meet 60%–70% of intrauterine mineral requirements. Tables 16.12 and 16.13 include recommended enteral and parenteral mineral intake for optimal bone and mineral homeostasis.

Parenteral mineral-containing solutions for LBW infants should be started soon after birth[422] to prevent excessive mineral loss and promote earlier resumption of postnatal growth. For the initiation of parenteral nutrition and during short-term therapy for less than 2 weeks' duration, LBW infants should receive parenteral nutrition solutions at rates of approximately 120–130 ml kg^{-1} day^{-1}, containing minerals at the following concentrations: Ca 15 mM, P 15 mM and Mg 2.5 mM. For optimal growth and nutrient utilization, however, LBW infants maintained on parenteral nutrition at rates of 120–130 ml kg^{-1} day^{-1} for 2 or more weeks should receive mineral concentrations of Ca 20 mM, P 20 mM, and Mg 2.5 mM.

When parenteral solutions were first utilized, a major problem was calcium and phosphate salts (mono and dibasic potassium phosphate) precipitation and therefore inability to deliver sufficient amounts of minerals to patients. Several remedies came about as a result of continuous research in this field.[423] The solubility of calcium and phosphate salts has been enhanced by several techniques including using appropriate Ca:P ratios[424] and optimal amounts of minerals, using organic calcium salts (calcium gluconate or gluceptate) and organic phosphate salts (sodium glycerophosphate or glucose monophosphate), decreasing the pH of the solution by using sulfur-containing acidic amino acids (L-cysteine hydrochloride), and mixing phosphate salts before addition of calcium salts.

Alternate day infusion of calcium and phosphate in VLBW infants is associated with excessive wasting of the infused minerals,[425] which increases the risk for nephrocalcinosis and nephrolithiasis.[426] Better mineral retention is achieved when calcium and phosphate are administered together rather than in separate solutions.[427] Hanning *et al.*[428] reported on the efficacy of the more soluble

Table 16.12. Mineral and vitamin D requirements for parenteral nutrition solutions*

	CA	P	MG	VITD	CA/P ratio
		$(\text{mg kg}^{-1}\text{day}^{-1})$		$(\text{IU kg}^{-1}\text{day}^{-1})$	By weight
Term	60	45	7	40–160	1.3:1–1.7:1
		$(\text{mmol kg}^{-1}\text{day}^{-1})$		(mcg per day)	Molar
	1.25–1.5	1.25–1.5	0.3	1.0–4.0	1:1–1.3:1
		$(\text{mg kg}^{-1}\text{day}^{-1})$		$(\text{IU kg}^{-1}\text{day}^{-1})$	By weight
Preterm	60–90	47–70	4.3–7.2	40–160	1.3:1–1.7:1
		$(\text{mmol kg}^{-1}\text{day}^{-1})$		(mcg day^{-1})	Molar
	1.5–2.25	1.5–2.25	0.18–0.3	1.0–4.0	1:1–1.3:1

Note: Ca and P concentrations are based on fluid intake of 120–150 ml kg^{-1}day^{-1}.
Precipitation may occur with concentrations above 60 mg dL^{-1} of calcium and 45 mg dL^{-1} of phosphate.
1.0 mmol of phosphate = 96 mg.
1 mEq of elemental calcium = 20 mg.
1 mcg of Vitamin D = 40 IU.
*Adapted from data.[466–468]

Table 16.13. Mineral and vitamin D requirements for enteral nutrition*

	CA	P	MG	VITD	CA/P ratio
		$(\text{mg kg}^{-1}\text{day}^{-1})$		(IU day^{-1})	By weight
Term	60	45	7	150–400	2:1
		$(\text{mmol kg}^{-1}\text{day}^{-1})$		$(\mu\text{g day}^{-1})$	Molar
	1.5–1.5	1.25–1.5	0.3	3.75–10	1:1
		$(\text{mg kg}^{-1}\text{day}^{-1})$		(IU day^{-1})	By weight
Preterm	120–200	70–120	7.2–9.6	150–400	2:1
		$(\text{mmol kg}^{-1}\text{day}^{-1})$		$(\mu\text{g day}^{-1})$	Molar
	3.0–5.0	2.0–3.5	0.3–0.4	3.75–10	1:1

*Adapted from data.[466–468]

calcium glycerophosphate in permitting larger mineral intake. Monobasic potassium phosphate salt improves the solubility of calcium and phosphorus in amino acid plus dextrose solutions, compared with mixtures of monobasic plus dibasic salts, and results in better retention of Ca and P.[429]

The use of parenteral solutions containing 60 mg dl^{-1} of calcium and 46mg dL^{-1} of phosphorus (a Ca:P ratio of 1.3:1 to 1.7:1 by weight and 1:1 molar ratio) has been associated with stable bone and mineral homeostasis and good mineral retention rates (88%–91% for Ca, 89%–97% for P) without increasing hypercalciuria.[430,431] For preterm

infants requiring PN, the use of PN solutions with a Ca content of 1.25–1.5 mmol dL^{-1} (50–60 mg dL^{-1}), a P content of 1.29–1.45 mmol dL^{-1} (40–45 mg dL^{-1}), and a Mg content of 0.2–0.3 mmol dL^{-1} (5–7 mg dL^{-1}) is supported by studies of mineral homeostasis with serial chemical and calciotropic hormone measurements, standard balance studies, and improved radiographic indices of bone mineralization.[432]

Based on the timing of development of fractures and rickets, changes in BMC, and skeletal growth data, the increased Ca and P intake should continue for at least 3 months after birth or until reaching a body weight of about 3.5 kg. In addition, nonnutritional factors may have the potential to increase mineral loss and disturb mineral homeostasis; chronic diuretic therapy increases mineral loss, and aluminum contamination of nutrients theoretically may compound any skeletal disorder. Thus, attention to the level of mineral intake and factors important in mineral loss and mineral metabolism should optimize mineral retention in small preterm infants.

Addition of the amino acid cysteine to parenteral solutions has been associated with greater solubility and concentrations of Ca and P and therefore greater delivery of minerals to patients. Tables 16.12 and 16.13 include recommended mineral intake for optimal bone and mineral homeostasis. In our practice we usually start with 70%–80% of our total goal of mineral delivery, and increase the amount of mineral delivered by 10% every day over 2–3 days to reach 100% of our goal. The rate of incremental increase is dictated by serum calcium and phosphorus concentrations which we advise to monitor daily or every other day for the first week and then weekly thereafter once these parameters are stable.

Prestridge et al.[433] demonstrated that increasing parenteral nutrition solution concentration of minerals from 1.25 mmol calcium and 1.5 mmol phosphorus per deciliter to 1.7 mmol calcium and 2.0 mmol phosphorus per deciliter over 3 weeks resulted in greater retention of these minerals during parenteral nutrition therapy and in greater bone mineral content after therapy. Serum calcium, magnesium, parathyroid hormone, 25-OHD, and osteocalcin concentrations did not change yet serum phosphorus concentration was significantly higher. Balance studies done by Schanler et al.[434] show that although urinary Ca, P, and Mg excretion increased after parenteral nutrition therapy was begun, net nutrient retention increased significantly above baseline for all nutrients. Average weekly nutrient retention was significantly below intrauterine estimates of nutrient accretion for Ca and P; and significantly exceeded those for Mg. Postnatal therapy with dexamethasone increased P excretion and decreased P retention. Therefore, positive mineral balance may be achieved early in the neonatal period. The magnitude of this effect may remain uniform during parenteral nutrition. Adjustments in parenteral nutrient intake are needed to provide nutrient intakes sufficient to support postnatal retention at rates similar to those of intrauterine accretion. Complications of TPN include disturbances in serum calcium, phosphorus, and magnesium and metabolic bone disease. However, with our current recommendations the incidence of these complications has been reduced markedly. One complication often cited is biliary sludge, which is best prevented and treated by initiation of trophic feedings and establishing enteral feedings.

The role of aluminum contamination of PN components and the potential role of aluminum in TPN-induced hepatocellular injury and cholestasis as well as in metabolic bone disease has been reviewed.[435,436] Aluminum remains a significant contaminant of total parenteral nutrition (TPN) solutions and may be elevated in bone, urine, and plasma of infants receiving TPN. Aluminum accumulation in tissues of uremic patients and adult TPN patients has been associated with low-turnover bone disease. Almost all components of PN solutions are contaminated with aluminum to a variable degree including vitamins and mineral solutions, amino acids, and to a lesser degree dextrose solutions and lipid emulsions. Though the degree of aluminum contamination of PN solutions has decreased over time, contamination still significantly exceeds levels that are safe for human neonates.[437] Currently, there is no evidence to indicate a safe level of aluminum exposure in neonates. The American Society of Clinical Nutrition/American Society of Enteral and Parenteral Nutrition Joint Commission recommends aluminum exposure in PN not to exceed 2 μg kg^{-1} day^{-1}.[438] The research of Klein[439] in animals demonstrates increased serum bile acids and alkaline phosphatase, and decreased bile flow that correlates inversely with increasing aluminum load and duration of exposure. Premature infants whose serum aluminum concentration exceeded 10 μg L^{-1},[440] demonstrated a significantly negative correlation between serum aluminum concentration and gestational age. Altogether, infants with high aluminum levels showed significantly more complications, especially bronchopulmonary dysplasia, necrotizing enterocolitis, cholestasis, and osteopenia.

Parenteral nutrition may be complicated by increased calcium and phosphorus urinary losses which are thought to be aggravated by excessive mineral load, excessive amino acid intake, increased sodium intake with resultant extracellular fluid expansion, increased vitamin D intake, increased glucose load, metabolic acidosis, and diuretic therapy. Hypercalciuria may be due to acidic sulfate solutions.[441] Research studies in the field of parenteral nutrition have been instrumental in demonstrating that vitamin D deficiency is rare in infants and children maintained on parenteral nutrition, and plays no role in the induction of metabolic bone disease or rickets of prematurity, which in fact is due primarily to decreased mineral retention secondary to inappropriate mineral ratio, and suboptimal delivery of minerals to patients with rapid growth rate. Investigators demonstrated normal mineral and vitamin D status in infants receiving 30–400 IU kg^{-1} day^{-1} of vitamin D in amino acid dextrose solution or 160–400 IU kg^{-1} day^{-1} in lipid emulsion. A low dose of vitamin D of 25 IU dL^{-1} of parenteral solution can maintain normal vitamin D status for as long as 6 months as indicated by normal serum 25-OHD concentrations, serum calcium, magnesium, phosphorus, alkaline phosphatase, creatinine (Cr), and vitamin D-binding protein concentrations or urinary Ca : Cr and Mg : Cr ratios.

Enteral nutrition

Balance studies demonstrated that variability in nutrient intake (mg kg^{-1} day^{-1}) accounted for 96% and 57% of the variability in phosphorus absorption and retention (mg kg^{-1} day^{-1}). Intake, birth weight, gestation, postnatal age, balance weight, and type of formula fed also accounted for a substantial part of the variability in calcium absorption and retention.[442] Using a 72-h balance technique, Bronner[443] evaluated the effect of calcium and vitamin D supplementation on net calcium absorption in low-birth-weight preterm infants. Net calcium absorption averaged 58% with an intake of 80 mg Ca kg^{-1} day^{-1}. Calcium absorption did not differ significantly, with neither vitamin D supplementation, nor supplementation with vitamin D and calcium, affecting per cent absorption significantly. Net calcium absorption was a linear function of calcium intake (40–130 mg Ca kg^{-1} day^{-1}), and vitamin D supplementation did not increase net calcium absorption. From these findings it appears that in preterm LBW infants, calcium absorption proceeds by a nonsaturable route, with the transcellular, vitamin D-regulated mechanism not yet expressed. Therefore in preterm infants fed human milk with mineral fortifier or preterm formula, calcium retention of 45–60 mg kg^{-1} day^{-1} can be achieved.[443,444] Human milk and standard cow milk formulas do not provide sufficient amount of minerals for optimal bone mineralization in preterm infants. Balance studies[445] demonstrated that although calcium and phosphorus intakes from standard cow milk formulas were higher than from human milk, retention of calcium and phosphorus in preterm infants fed either human milk or standard formula did not meet intrauterine retention rates, and hypophosphatemia developed in infants who received their mothers' milk.

Although the use of high mineral formula has been shown to increase bone mineral accretion and reduce the risk of osteopenia in preterm infants,[446–449] it has not eliminated it. Human milk-fed infants have lower bone accretion than formula-fed infants. The inclusion of palm olein oil in infant formula may reduce bone mineral accretion.[450] Bone accretion is not influenced by the timing of the introduction of weaning foods, despite higher serum PTH concentrations among infants who receive solids earlier.[450]

Pieltain[451] demonstrated that preterm formula-fed (PTF) infants showed a greater weight gain, fat mass deposition, bone mineral content gain, and increase in bone area compared with the fortified human milk-fed (FHM) infants. Growth and weight gain composition of the preterm infant during the first weeks of life differ from that of the fetus in utero. From birth to the time of discharge body weight and body-length growth deviate from intrauterine reference values[452] in the FHM infants and in the PTF infants. These findings are consistent with other studies[453,454] and may imply that there would be a long-term reduction in linear growth in these infants.[455,456] The difference in accretion of bone mineral content between the PTF and FHM fed infants disappeared when the data were adjusted for the weight gain difference, suggesting that the effect was largely caused by differences in bone matrix growth rate between the two groups.

Cooke[457] examined the effect of high protein and mineral intake on whole body composition in preterm infants after hospital discharge, using DEXA measurements over the first year of life. During the study, weight gain, and lean mass gain were greater in infants provided with higher protein and mineral intake. At 12 months, they also had greater weight, lean mass, fat mass, and bone mineral mass but not per cent fat mass or bone mineral density. In this study, increased weight gain primarily reflected an increase in lean mass. For infants requiring enteral nutrition (EN), an intake of approximately 4 mmol (200 mg) of Ca, 3.2 mmol (100 mg) of P, and 0.33 mmol (8 mg) of mg kg^{-1} day^{-1} based on an average retention rate of 64% for Ca, 71% for P, and 50% for Mg should be sufficient to meet the requirements of preterm infants in early infancy. This level of intake is supported by data from balance studies using standard and stable isotope techniques, changes in bone mineral content (BMC) measurements, and calciotropic hormone data.[432]

For human milk-fed LBW infants, as soon as enteral feeding is initiated in the first week of life, Ca and P should be supplied as fortifiers. Ca 2–3 mmol kg^{-1} day^{-1} and P 1.5–2.0 mmol kg^{-1} day^{-1} should be provided in addition to human milk. Magnesium supplementation of human milk is unnecessary. These recommendations assume that the intake of human milk is approximately 200 ml kg^{-1}day^{-1} and will decrease as more bioavailable mineral salts are found. For LBW infants fed commercial formula, the intake of Ca should be greater than 3.5 mmol kg^{-1} day^{-1}, P 2.5 mmol kg^{-1} day^{-1} and Mg 0.2 mmol kg^{-1} day^{-1}. These recommendations assume reported bioavailability of mineral salts. If more bioavailable sources are found, these recommendations will decrease.

Hillman et al.[458] studied the influence of variable protein intake on renal excretion of calcium and amino acids and on bone mineralization in preterm infants. Urinary calcium corrected for creatinine decreased as protein content increased. The authors suggested the high mineral content of premature formulas results in a higher growth rate and may increase protein requirements. Failure to meet protein requirements may result in underutilization of absorbed calcium and increased renal excretion of calcium. Therefore in preterm infants, higher protein intake probably supports rather than jeopardizes bone mineral accretion, and reduces rather than increases calciuria.

Giles et al.[459] demonstrated that increasing the calcium and phosphorus content of formulas for VLBW infants to the level required to decrease the incidence of rickets had a negative impact on magnesium balance. Using formulas variously supplemented with these minerals, they measured absorption and retention in two groups of preterm infants: (1) VLBW infants, less than 1500 g and at less than 32 weeks of gestational age, with 3-day mineral balances begun at days 10, 20, 30, and 40; (2) low birth weight infants appropriately grown and at 32–34 weeks of gestational age, with a single 3-day balance begun at day 10. Magnesium did not affect calcium balance in VLBW or LBW infants but promoted phosphorus retention in VLBW infants from day 20 onward. Absorption and retention of magnesium increased with postnatal age in VLBW infants, but this effect was obvious only when calcium or phosphorus intakes were low or when magnesium intake was high. Calcium and phosphorus supplementation further reduced magnesium absorption and retention in VLBW infants to the extent that they were in negative balance throughout the study; however, magnesium supplementation improved absorption and retention in VLBW infants. The LBW infants absorbed and retained more magnesium than VLBW infants at the same postnatal age whether or not magnesium was supplemented. Magnesium deficits occur at currently recommended intakes of 10 mg $kg^{-1}day^{-1}$ for VLBW infants with calcium and phosphorus intakes that allow retentions equivalent to in utero accretions; however, with magnesium intakes approaching 20 mg $kg^{-1}day^{-1}$, appropriate retention can be achieved.

Lapillonne[460] performed mineral metabolic balance studies in VLBW infants fed either pooled pasteurized human milk supplemented with calcium, phosphorus, and magnesium, or a preterm formula. Despite similar Ca, P, and Mg intake (100 mg $kg^{-1}day^{-1}$, 72 mg $kg^{-1}day^{-1}$ and 8 mg $kg^{-1}day^{-1}$, respectively), calcium and phosphorus retention was higher in infants fed fortified human milk than in those receiving a preterm formula (65 ± 14 and 62 ± 9 mg $kg^{-1}day^{-1}$ v. 55 ± 12 and 47 ± 7 mg $kg^{-1}day^{-1}$ respectively). Magnesium retention was similar in the two groups and averaged 3 mg $kg^{-1}day^{-1}$. Assessment of the whole body bone mineral content by DEXA at 3 and 6 months of age revealed low whole body BMCt at 3 months of age (theoretical term) compared with normal full-term newborns at birth. However this difference disappears at 6 months of age.

Koo et al.[461] randomized VLBW infants fed high-calcium and high-phosphorus infant formulas to one of three levels of vitamin D intake to approximate 200, 400, and 800 IU day^{-1} (with actual mean daily vitamin D intakes of 161, 361, and 766 IU, respectively). The study demonstrated that for VLBW infants fed high-calcium and high-phosphorus (10.74 and 6.93 mmol MJ^{-1}; 180 and 90 mg per 100 kcal, respectively) milk, an average daily vitamin D intake as low as 160 IU was sufficient to maintain normal and stable vitamin D status and normal physical growth, biochemical and hormonal indexes of bone mineral metabolism, and skeletal radiographs compared with infants receiving about 400 or 800 IU of vitamin D per day.

During the latter half of an infant's first year, adequate mineral and vitamin D intakes may be important not only for the prevention of rickets but also for the attainment of optimal adult peak bone mass. Ingestion of 400 IU vitamin D per day, either as a supplement or contained in formula or table milk, will result in normal serum concentrations of vitamin D,25-hydroxyvitamin D, and 1,25(OH)2D.[462] Human milk from a vitamin D-sufficient mother provides a marginal amount, less than 100 IU $L^{-1}day^{-1}$ of total vitamin D activity from the vitamin D and 25-OHD in milk. Infants exclusively fed human milk of vitamin D-deficient mothers, who do not receive adequate exposure to sunlight or additional vitamin D, are at significant risk for vitamin D-deficiency rickets. The low concentration of phosphorus in human milk is adequate for vitamin D-sufficient term infants but probably compounds any vitamin D deficiency when it occurs. Intake of phosphorus from formula or table milk is more than adequate, and the addition of baby foods increases this mineral's intake to generous levels. Calcium is well absorbed in human milk-fed term infants if vitamin D is sufficient. Hillman et al.[462] studied BMC and mineral homeostasis in term infants fed human milk (300 mg L^{-1} calcium), standard cow milk formula (440 mg L^{-1} calcium), or a soybean formula (600 mg L^{-1} calcium). All three types of feedings provided comparable bone mineralization and normal indicators of mineral homeostasis. Mean calcium retentions at 6 months, 9 months, and 12 months in all three groups were between 138 and 205 mg day^{-1}, substantially more than the 130 mg day^{-1} estimated to be needed from body composition data. Estimates for phosphorus were similarly generous.

Bone mineralization is an intricate and tightly regulated process. Calcium, magnesium, and phosphorus are the main minerals and play a principal role in skeletal mineralization. The large differences in Ca:P ratio between different formulas and between formulas and human milk suggest that within limits most healthy full-term infants can adjust to a wide range of Ca:P ratio in their diet. The differences in serum levels of minerals and of mineral-regulating hormones are rarely clinically significant and most probably reflect continued compensatory mechanisms activated in response to dietary differences to maintain these levels within clinically normal ranges. Thus in most cases, these compensatory mechanisms appear sufficient to reverse both short-term and long-term consequences and to prevent clinical disease. In the case of neonatal tetany, the compensatory mechanisms are overwhelmed, resulting in clinical signs and disease.

Vitamin D plays an essential role in bone mineralization. There are significant differences in vitamin D status in breast-fed infants with and without vitamin D supplementation and in infants fed various "humanized" formulas, whether cow milk-based or soy protein-based.[463] The major variables affecting bone mineralization are Ca:P ratio and mineral-regulating hormones. However, factors such as season, geography (i.e., sun exposure), race, and sex may have a significant long-term influence on bone mineralization and mineral metabolism. Some biological differences such as differences in serum vitamin D metabolite level may directly affect Ca:P absorption and retention and thus bone mineralization and growth. In a pilot study of preterm infants, retention of Ca and P was not improved by estradiol and progesterone to maintain intrauterine plasma concentrations of estradiol and progesterone,[464] although these preterm infants showed trends to higher bone mineral accumulation.[465]

REFERENCES

1 Crowder, J. A., Frieden, I. J., Price, V. H. Alopecia areata in infants and newborns. *Pediatr. Dermatol.* 2002;**19**:155–8.

2 Loughead, J., Mimouni, F., Tsang, R. Serum ionized calcium concentrations in normal neonates. *Am. J. Dis. Child.* 1988;**142**:516–18.

3 Rubin, L., Posillico, J., Anast, C., Brown, E. Circulating levels of biologically active and immunoreactive intact parathyroid hormone in human newborns. *Pediatr. Res.* 1991;**29**:201–7.

4 Venkataraman, P., Tsang, R., Chen, I., Sperling, M. Pathogenesis of early neonatal hypocalcemia: studies of serum calcitonin, gastrin and plasma glucagon. *J. Pediatr.* 1987;**110**:599–603.

5 Tsang, R., Chen, I., Friedman, M. *et al.* Neonatal parathyroid function: role of gestational age and postnatal age. *J. Pediatr.* 1973;**83**:728–38.

6 Tsang, R., Oh, W. Serum magnesium levels in low birth weight infants. *Am. J. Dis. Child.* 1970;**120**:44–8.

7 David, L., Salle, B., Chopard, P., Grafmeyer, D. Studies on circulating immunoreactive calcitonin in low birth weight infants during the first 48 hours of life. *Helv. Paediatr. Acta.* 1977;**32**:39–43.

8 Hillman, L., Rojanasathit, S., Slatopolsky, E., Haddad, J. Serial measurements of serum calcium, magnesium, parathyroid hormone, calcitonin, and 25-hydroxyvitamin D in premature and term infants during the first week of life. *Pediatr. Res.* 1977;**11**:739–44.

9 Romagnoli, C., Zecca, E., Tortorolo, G. *et al.* Plasma thyrocalcitonin and parathyroid hormone concentrations in early neonatal hypocalcemia. *Arch. Dis. Child.* 1987;**62**:580–4.

10 Mimouni, F., Loughead, J., Tsang, R. *et al.* The role of calcitonin (CT) in neonatal hypocalcemia (NHC) in infants of diabetic mothers (IDM's). *Pediatr. Res.* 1989;**25**:89A.

11 Mimouni, F., Mimouni, C., Loughead, J., Tsang, R. A case-control study of hypocalcemia in high-risk neonates: racial, but no seasonal differences. *J. Am. Coll. Nutr.* 1991;**10**:196–9.

12 Tsang, R. C., Chen, I., Hayes, W. *et al.* Neonatal hypocalcemia in infants with birth asphyxia. *J. Pediatr.* 1974;**84**:428–33.

13 Allgrove, J., Adami, S., Fraher, L. *et al.* Hypomagnesemia: studies of parathyroid hormone secretion and function. *Clin. Endocrinol.* 1984;**21**:435–49.

14 Noguchi, A., Eren, M., Tsang, R. Parathyroid hormone in hypocalcemic and normocalcemic infants of diabetic mothers. *J. Pediatr.* 1980;**97**:112–17.

15 Tsang, R., Kleinman, L., Sutherland, J. *et al.* Hypocalcemia in infants of diabetic mothers: studies in Ca, P and Mg metabolism and in parathyroid hormone responsiveness. *J. Pediatr.* 1972;**80**:384–95.

16 Tsang, R. Neonatal magnesium disturbances. *Am. J. Dis. Child.* 1972;**124**:282–93.

17 Bergman, L., Kjellmer, I., Seltam, U. Calcitonin and parathyroid hormone. Relation to early neonatal hypocalcemia in infants of diabetic mothers. *Biol. Neonate.* 1974;**24**:151–60.

18 Mimouni, F., Steichen, J. J., Tsang, R. C., Hertzberg, V., Miodovnik, M. Decreased bone mineral content in infants of diabetic mothers. *Am. J. Perinatol.* 1988;**5**:339–43.

19 Namgung, R., Tsang, R. C. Factors affecting newborn bone mineral content: in utero effects on newborn bone mineralizations. *Proc. Nutr. Soc.* 2000;**59**:55–63.

20 Lapillonne, A., Guerin, S., Braillon, P. *et al.* Whole body bone mineral content and body composition in infants of diabetic mothers. *J. Clin. Endocrinol. Metab.* 1997;**82**:3993–7.

21 Salle, B. L., Delvin, E. E., Lapillonne, A., Bishop, N. J., Glorieux, F. H. Perinatal metabolism of vitamin D. *Am. J. Clin. Nutr.* 2000;**71**:1317S–24S.

22 Tsang, R. C., Gigger, M., Oh, W., Brown, D. R. Studies in calcium metabolism in infants with intrauterine growth retardation. *J. Pediatr.* 1975;**86**:936–41.

23 Tsang, R. C., Oh, W. Neonatal hypocalcemia in low birth weight infants. *Pediatrics* 1970;**45**:773–81.

24 Lapillonne, A., Braillon, P., Claris, O. *et al.* Body composition in appropriate and in small for gestational age infants. *Acta Paediatr.* 1997;**86**:196–200.

25 Romagnoli, C., Polidori, G., Cataldi, L., Tortorolo, G., Segni, G. Phototherapy-induced hypocalcemia. *J. Pediatr.* 1979;**94**:815–16.

26 Hakanson, D. O., Bergstrom, W. H. Prevention of light-induced hypocalcemia by melatonin. In Norman, A. W., ed. *Vitamin D, Chemical, Biochemical and Clinical Endocrinology of Calcium Metabolism.* New York: Walter de Gruyter; 1982:1163–5.

27 Hakanson, D. O., Bergstrom, W. H. Pineal and adrenal effects on calcium homeostasis in the rat. *Pediatr. Res.* 1990;**27**:571–3.

28 Hahn, T. Drug-induced disorders of vitamin D and mineral metabolism. *Clin. Endocrinol. Metab.* 1980;**9**:107–29.

29 Markestad, T., Ulstein, M., Stanjord, R. Anticonvulsant drug in human pregnancy: effects on serum concentrations of vitamin D metabolites in maternal and cord blood. *Am. J. Obstet. Gynecol.* 1984;**150**:254–8.

30 Stamp, T. Effects of long-term anticonvulsant therapy on calcium and vitamin D metabolism. *Proc. R. Soc. Med.* 1979;**67**:64–8.

31 Brown, D. R., Tsang, R. C., Chen, I. Oral calcium supplementation in premature and asphyxiated neonates. *J. Pediatr.* 1976;**89**:973–7.

32 David, L., Anast, C. S. Calcium metabolism in newborn infants. The interrelationship of parathyroid function and calcium, magnesium, and phosphorus metabolism in normal, "sick," and hypocalcemic newborns. *J. Clin. Invest.* 1974;**54**:287–96.

33 Rosen, J. F., Roginsky, M., Nathenson, G., Finberg, L. 25-hydroxyvitamin D. Plasma levels in mothers and their premature infants with neonatal hypocalcemia. *Am. J. Dis. Child.* 1974;**127**:220–3.

34 Fleischman, A. R., Rosen, J. F., Nathenson, G. 25-Hydroxycholecalciferol for early neonatal hypocalcemia. Occurrence in premature newborns. *Am. J. Dis. Child.* 1978;**132**:973–7.

35 Chan, G. M., Tsang, R. C., Chen, I. W., DeLuca, H. F., Steichen, J. J. The effect of 1,25(OH)2 vitamin D3 supplementation in premature infants. *J. Pediatr.* 1978;**93**:91–6.

36 Hillman, L. S., Haddad, J. G. Perinatal vitamin D metabolism. II. Serial 25-hydroxyvitamin D concentrations in sera of term and premature infants. *J. Pediatr.* 1975;**86**:928–35.

37 Park, W., Paust, H., Kaufmann, H., Offermann, G. Osteomalacia of the mother – rickets of the newborn. *Eur. J. Pediatr.* 1987;**146**:292–3.

38 Sann, L., David, L., Frederick, A. *et al.* Congenital rickets. *Acta Paediatr. Scan.* 1977;**66**:323–7.

39 Moncrieff, M., Fadahunsi, T. Congenital rickets due to maternal rickets due to maternal vitamin D deficiency. *Arch. Dis. Child.* 1974;**49**:810–11.

40 Ford, J., Davidson, D., McIntosh, W., Fyfe, W. M., Dunnigan, M. G. Neonatal rickets in Asian immigrant population. *Br. Med. J.* 1973;**3**:211–2.

41 Teotia, M., Teotia, S. P., Nath, M. Metabolic studies in congenital vitamin D deficiency rickets. *Indian J. Pediatr.* 1995;**62**:55–61.

42 Anatoliotaki, M., Tsilimigaki, A., Tsekoura, T. *et al.* Congenital rickets due to maternal vitamin D deficiency in a sunny island of Greece. *Acta Paediatr.* 2003;**92**:389–91.

43 Maiyegun, S. O., Malek, A. H., Devarajan, L. V., Dahniya, M. H. Severe congenital rickets secondary to maternal hypovitaminosis D: a case report. *Ann. Trop. Paediatr.* 2002;**22**:191–5.

44 Mohapatra, A., Sankaranarayanan, K., Kadam, S. S. *et al.* Congenital rickets. *J. Trop. Pediatr.* 2003;**49**:126–7.

45 Begum, R., Coutinho, M., Dormandy, T., Yudkin, S. Maternal malabsorption presenting as congenital rickets. *Lancet* 1968;**1**:1048–52.

46 Al-Senan, K., Al-Alaiyan, S., Al-Abbad, A., LeQuesne, G. Congenital rickets secondary to untreated maternal renal failure. *J. Perinatol.* 2001;**21**:473–5.

47 Levin, T. L., States, L., Greig, A., Goldman, H. S. Maternal renal insufficiency: a cause of congenital rickets and secondary hyperparathyroidism. *Pediatr. Radiol.* 1992;**22**:315–16.

48 Wang, L. Y., Hung, H. Y., Hsu, C. H., Hih, S. L., Lee, Y. J. Congenital rickets: a patient report. *J. Pediatr. Endocrinol Metab.* 1997;**10**:437–41.

49 Kirk, J. Congenital rickets: a case report. *Aust. Pediatr. J.* 1982;**18**:291–3.

50 Rimensberger, P., Schubiger, G., Willi, U. Connatal rickets following repeated administration of phosphate enemas in pregnancy: a case report. *Eur. J. Pediatr.* 1992;**151**:54–6.

51 Wilson, R. D., Martin, T., Christensen, R., Yee, A. H., Reynolds, C. Hyperparathyroidism in pregnancy: case report and review of the literature. *Can. Med. Assoc. J.* 1983;**129**:986–9.

52 Ozsoylu, S., Bilginturan, N. Maternal hyperparathyroidism and neonatal rickets. *J. Pediatr.* 1989;**114**:508–9.

53 Hanukoglu, A., Chalew, S., Kowarski, A. Late-onset hypocalcemia, rickets, and hypoparathyroidism in an infant of a mother with hyperparathyroidism. *J. Pediatr.* 1988;**112**:751–4.

54 Monteleone, J., Lee, J., Tashjian, A., Cantor, H. Transient neonatal hypocalcemia, hypomagnesemia, and high serum parathyroid hormone with maternal hyperparathyroidism. *Ann. Intern. Med.* 1975;**82**:670–2.

55 Jacobson, B., Terslev, E., Lund, B., Sorensen, O. Neonatal hypocalcemia associated with maternal hyperparathyroidism. *Arch. Dis. Child.* 1978;**53**:308–11.

56 Kooh, S., Jones, G., Reilly, B. Pathogenesis of rickets in chronic hepatobiliary disease in children. *J. Pediatr.* 1979;**94**:870–4.

57 Long, R., Skinner, R., Wills, M. *et al.* Serum 25-hydroxyvitamin D in untreated parenchymal and cholestatic liver disease. *Lancet* 1976;**2**:650–2.

58 Yu, J., Walker-Smith, J., Burnard, E. Rickets, a common complication of neonatal hepatitis. *Med. J. Aust.* 1971;**1**:790–2.

59 Portale, A., Booth, B., Tsai, H., Morris, R. C. Jr. Reduced plasma concentration of 1,25-dihydroxyvitamin D in children

with moderate renal insufficiency. *Kidney Int.* 1982;**21**:627–32.

60 Chesney, R., Hamstra, A., Mazess, R., Rose, P., DeLuca, H. F. Circulating vitamin D metabolite concentration in childhood renal disease. *Kidney Int.* 1982;**21**:65–9.

61 Scriver, C., Reade, T., DeLuca, H., Hamstra, A. Serum 1,25-dihydroxyvitamin D levels in normal subjects and in patients with hereditary rickets or bone disease. *N. Engl. J. Med.* 1978;**299**:976–9.

62 Fraser, D., Kooh, S., Kind, H. *et al.* Pathogenesis of hereditary vitamin D-dependent rickets. An inborn error of vitamin D metabolism involving defective conversion of 25-hydroxyvitamin D to 1,25-dihydroxyvitamin D. *N. Engl. J. Med.* 1973;**289**:817–22.

63 Feldman, D., Chen, T., Cone, C. *et al.* Vitamin D resistant rickets with alopecia: cultured skin fibroblasts exhibit defective cytoplasmic receptors and unresponsiveness to 1,25(OH)2D3. *J. Clin. Endocrinol. Metab.* 1982;**55**:1020–2.

64 Anast, C., Winnacker, J., Forte, L., Burns, T. Impaired release of parathyroid hormone in magnesium deficiency. *J. Clin. Endocrinol. Metab.* 1976; **42**:707–17.

65 Baron, J., Winer, K. K., Yanovski, J. A. *et al.* Mutations in the Ca(2+)-sensing receptor gene cause autosomal dominant and sporadic hypoparathyroidism. *Hum. Mol. Genet.* 1996;**5**:601–6.

66 De Luca, F., Ray, K., Mancilla, E. E. *et al.* Sporadic hypoparathyroidism caused by de Novo gain-of-function mutations of the Ca(2+)-sensing receptor. *J. Clin. Endocrinol. Metab.* 1997;**82**:2710–15.

67 Cardenas-Rivero, N., Chernow, B., Stoiko, M., Nussbaum, S., Todres, D. Hypocalcemia in critically ill children. *J. Pediatr.* 1989;**114**:946–51.

68 Sanchez, G., Venkataraman, P., Pryor, R. *et al.* Hypercalcitoninemia and hypocalcemia in acutely ill children: studies in serum calcium, blood ionized calcium, and calcium-regulating hormones. *J. Pediatr.* 1989;**114**:952–6.

69 Weidner, N., Santa-Cruz, D. Phosphaturic mesenchymal tumors: a polymorphous group causing osteomalacia or rickets. *Cancer* 1987;**59**:1442–52.

70 Skovby, F., Svejgaard, E., Moller, J. Hypophosphatemic rickets in linear sebaceous nevus sequence. *J. Pediatr.* 1987;**111**:855–7.

71 Aschinberg, L., Solomon, L., Zeis, P. *et al.* Vitamin D resistant rickets associated with epidermal nevus syndrome: demonstration of a phosphaturic substance in the dermal lesions. *J. Pediatr.* 1977;**91**:56–60.

72 Olivares, J. L., Ramos, F. J., Carapeto, F. J., Bueno, M. Epidermal naevus syndrome and hypophosphataemic rickets: description of a patient with central nervous system anomalies and review of the literature. *Eur. J. Pediatr.* 1999;**158**:103–7.

73 Ryan, E., Reiss, E. Oncogenous osteomalacia. *Am. J. Med.* 1984;**77**:501.

74 Ivker, R., Resnick, S. D., Skidmore, R. A. Hypophosphatemic vitamin D-resistant rickets, precocious puberty, and the epidermal nevus syndrome. *Arch. Dermatol.* 1997;**133**:1557–61.

75 Venkataraman, P. S., Tsang, R. C., Greer, F. R. *et al.* Late infantile tetany and secondary hyperparathyroidism in infants fed humanized cow milk formula. Longitudinal follow-up. *Am. J. Dis. Child.* 1985;**139**:664–8.

76 Pierson, J. D., Crawford, J. D. Dietary dependent neonatal hypocalcemia. *Am. J. Dis. Child.* 1972;**123**:472–4.

77 Powell, B., Buist, N. Late presenting, prolonged hypocalcemia in an infant of a woman with hypocalciuric hypercalcemia. *Clin. Pediatr.* 1990;**29**:241–3.

78 Marx, S., Attie, M., Levine, M. The hypocalciuric or benign variant of familial hypercalcemia: clinical and biochemical features in fifteen kindreds. *Medicine* 1980;**60**:397–412.

79 Popp, D., Zieger, B., Schmitt-Graff, A., Nutzenadel, W., Schaefer, F. Malignant osteopetrosis obscured by maternal vitamin D deficiency in a neonate. *Eur. J. Pediatr.* 2000;**159**:412–15.

80 Chen, C. J., Lee, M. Y., Hsu, M. L., Lien, S. H., Cheng, S. N. Malignant infantile osteopetrosis initially presenting with neonatal hypocalcemia: case report. *Ann. Hematol.* 2003;**82**:64–7.

81 Srinivasan, M., Abinun, M., Cant, A. J. *et al.* Malignant infantile osteopetrosis presenting with neonatal hypocalcaemia. *Arch. Dis. Child Fetal Neonat. Edn.* 2000;**83**:F21–3.

82 Gribetz, D. Hypocalcemic states in infancy and childhood. *Am. J. Dis. Child.* 1957;**94**:301–12.

83 Mizrahi, A., London, R. D., Gribetz, D. Neonatal hypocalcemia – its causes and treatment. *N. Engl. J. Med.* 1968;**278**:1163–65.

84 Anast, C., Mohs, J., Kaplan, S., Burns, T. Evidence for parathyroid failure in magnesium deficiency. *Science* 1972;**177**:606–8.

85 Maisels, M. J., Li, T. K., Piechocki, J. T., Werthman, M. W. The effect of exchange transfusion on serum ionized calcium. *Pediatrics* 1974;**53**:683–6.

86 Wieland, P., Duc, G., Binswanger, U., Fischer, J. A. Parathyroid hormone response in newborn infants during exchange transfusion with blood supplemented with citrate and phosphate: effect of IV calcium. *Pediatr. Res.* 1979;**13**:963–8.

87 Dincsoy, M. Y., Tsang, R. C., Laskarzewski, P. *et al.* Serum calcitonin response to administration of calcium in newborn infants during exchange blood transfusion. *J. Pediatr.* 1982;**100**:782–6.

88 Dincsoy, M. Y., Tsang, R. C., Laskarzewski, P. *et al.* The role of postnatal age and magnesium on parathyroid hormone responses during "exchange" blood transfusion in the newborn period. *J. Pediatr.* 1982;**100**:277–83.

89 Robertson, W. C. Jr. Calcium carbonate consumption during pregnancy: an unusual cause of neonatal hypocalcemia. *J. Child. Neurol.* 2002;**17**:853–5.

90 Moudgil, A., Kishore, K., Srivastava, R. N. Neonatal lupus erythematosus, late onset hypocalcaemia, and recurrent seizures. *Arch. Dis. Child.* 1987;**62**:736–9.

91 Norvez, C. T., Shott, R. J., Bergstrom, W. H., Williams, M. L. Prophylaxis against hypocalcemia in low-birth-weight infants requiring bicarbonate infusion. *J. Pediatr.* 1975;**87**:439–42.

92 Venkataraman, P. S., Tsang, R. C., Steichen, J. J. *et al.* Early neonatal hypocalcemia in extremely preterm infants. High

incidence, early onset, and refractoriness to supraphysiologic doses of calcitriol. *Am. J. Dis. Child.* 1986;**140**:1004–8.

93 Salle, B. L., David, L., Glorieux, F. H. *et al.* Early oral administration of vitamin D and its metabolites in premature neonates. Effect on mineral homeostasis. *Pediatr. Res.* 1982;**16**:75–8.

94 Koo, W. W., Tsang, R. C., Poser, J. W. *et al.* Elevated serum calcium and osteocalcin levels from calcitriol in preterm infants. A prospective randomized study. *Am. J. Dis. Child.* 1986;**140**:1152–8.

95 Willis, D. M., Chabot, J., Radde, I. C., Chance, G. W. Unsuspected hyperosmolality of oral solutions contributing to necrotizing enterocolitis in very-low-birth-weight infants. *Pediatrics* 1977;**60**:535–8.

96 Book, L. S., Herbst, J. J., Stewart, D. Hazards of calcium gluconate therapy in the newborn infant: intra-arterial injection producing intestinal necrosis in rabbit ileum. *J. Pediatr.* 1978;**92**:793–7.

97 Habener, J., Potts, J. J. Primary hyperparathyroidism: clinical features. In DeGroot, L., ed. *Endocrinology*, vol. 2. Philadelphia, PA: W. B. Saunders; 1989:954.

98 Mundy, G., Shapiro, J., Bandelin, J. *et al.* Direct stimulation of bone resorption by thyroid hormones. *J. Clin. Invest.* 1976;**58**:529–34.

99 Muls, E., Bouillon, R., Boelaert, J. *et al.* Etiology of hypercalcemia in a patient with Addison's Disease. *Calcif. Tissue Int.* 1982;**34**:523–6.

100 Farrell, P., Rikkers, H., Moel, D. Cortisol dihydrotachysterol antagonism in a patient with hypoparathyroidism and adrenal insufficiency: apparent inhibition of bone resorption. *J. Clin. Endocrinol. Metab.* 1976;**42**:953–7.

101 Miller, S., Sizemore, G., Sheps, S., Tyce, G. Parathyroid function in patients with pheochromocytoma. *Ann. Intern. Med.* 1975;**82**:372–5.

102 Warner, J., Epstein, M., Sweet, A. *et al.* Genetic testing in familial isolated hyperparathyroidism: unexpected results and their implications. *J. Med. Genet.* 2004;**41**:155–60.

103 Speer, G., Toth, M., Niller, H. H. *et al.* Calcium metabolism and endocrine functions in a family with familial hypocalciuric hypercalcemia. *Exp. Clin. Endocrinol. Diabetes* 2003;**111**:486–90.

104 Kifor, O., Moore, F. D. Jr, Delaney, M. *et al.* A syndrome of hypocalciuric hypercalcemia caused by autoantibodies directed at the calcium-sensing receptor. *J. Clin. Endocrinol. Metab.* 2003;**88**:60–72.

105 Hohmann, E., Levine, L., Tashijian, A. H. Jr. Vasoactive intestinal peptide stimulates bone resorption via a cyclic adenosine 3′,5′-monophosphate- dependent mechanism. *Endocrinology* 1983;**112**:1233–9.

106 Duarte, C. G., Winnacker, J. L., Becker, K. L., Pace, A. Thiazide-induced hypercalcemia. *N. Engl. J. Med.* 1971;**284**:828.

107 Brickman, A., Massry, S., Coburn, J. Changes in serum and urinary calcium during treatment with hydrochlorothiazide: studies on mechnisms. *J. Clin. Invest.* 1972;**51**:945–54.

108 Mallette, L., Eichhorn, E. Effects of lithium carbonate on human calcium metabolism. *Arch. Intern. Med.* 1986;**146**:770–6.

109 Orwoll, E. The milk-alkali syndrome: current concepts. *Ann. Intern. Med.* 1982;**97**:242–8.

110 Bell, N., Shary, J., Shaw, S., Turner, R. Hypercalcemia associated with increased circulating 1,25-dihydroxyvitamin D in a patient with pulmonary tuberculosis. *Calcif. Tissue Int.* 1985;**37**:588–91.

111 Bell, N., Stern, P., Pantzer, E., Sinha, T. K., DeLuca, H. F. Evidence that increased circulating 1,25-dihydroxyvitamin D is the probable cause for abnormal calcium metabolism in sarcoidosis. *J. Clin. Invest.* 1979;**64**:218–25.

112 Suva, L., Winslow, G., Wettenhall, R. *et al.* A parathyroid hormone-related protein implicated in malignant hypercalcemia: cloning and expression. *Science* 1987;**237**:893–6.

113 Breslau, N., McGuire, J., Zerwekh, J., Frenkel, E. P., Pak, C. Y. Hypercalcemia associated with increased serum calcitriol levels in three patients with lymphoma. *Ann. Intern. Med.* 1984;**100**:1–6.

114 Garrett, I., Durie, B., Nedwin, G. *et al.* Production of the bone resorbing cytokine lymphotoxin by cultured human myeloma cells. *N. Engl. J. Med.* 1987;**317**:526–32.

115 Sowers, M. G., Hollis, B. W., Shapiro, B. *et al.* Elevated parathyroid hormone-related peptide associated with lactation and bone density loss. *J. Am. Med. Assoc.* 1996;**276**:549–54.

116 Specker, B., Tsang, R., Ho, M. Changes in calcium homeostasis over the first year postpartum: effect of lactation and weaning. *Obstet. Gynecol.* 1991;**78**:56–62.

117 Reid, I., Wattie, D., Evans, M., Budayr, A. Post-pregnancy osteoporosis associated with hypercalcemia. *Clin. Endocrinol.* 1992;**37**:298–303.

118 Kent, G., Price, R., Gutterdge, D. *et al.* Human lactation: forearm trabecular bone loss, increased bone turnover, and renal conservation of calcium and inorganic phosphate with recovery of bone mass following weaning. *J. Bone Min. Res.* 1990;**5**:361–9.

119 Stuart, C., Aceto, T. J., Kuhn, J., Terplan, K. Intrauterine hyperparathyroidism. *Am. J. Dis. Child.* 1979;**133**:67–70.

120 Bronsky, D., Kiamko, R., Moncada, R. *et al.* Intrauterine hyperparathyroidism secondary to maternal hypoparathyroidism. *Pediatrics* 1972;**42**:606–13.

121 Glass, E., Barr, D. Transient neonatal hyperparathyroidism secondary to maternal pseudohypoparathyroidism. *Arch. Dis. Child.* 1981;**56**:565–8.

122 Ozsoylu, S. Transient neonatal hyperparathyroidism secondary to maternal pseudohypoparathyroidism. *Arch. Dis. Child.* 1982;**57**:241.

123 Gradus, D., LeRoith, D., Karplus, M. *et al.* Congenital hyperparathyroidism and rickets secondary to maternal hypoparathyroidism and vitamin D deficiency. *Isr. J. Med. Sci.* 1981;**17**:705–8.

124 Landing, B., Kamoshita, S. Congenital hyperparathyroidism secondary to maternal hypoparathyroidism. *J. Pediatr.* 1970;**77**:842–7.

125 Loughead, J., Mughal, Z., Mimouni, F. *et al.* Spectrum and natural history of congenital hyperparathyroidism secondary to maternal hypocalcemia. *Am. J. Perinatol.* 1990;**7**:350–5.

126 Spiegel, A., Harrisson, H., Marx, S. *et al.* Neonatal primary hyperparathyroidism with autosomal dominant inheritance. *J. Pediatr.* 1977;**90**:269–72.

127 Goldbloom, R., Gillis, D., Prasad, M. Hereditary parathyroid hyperplasia: a surgical emergency of early infancy. *Pediatrics* 1972;**49**:514–23.

128 Dezateux, C. A., Hyde, J. C., Hoey, H. M. *et al.* Neonatal hyperparathyroidism. *Eur. J. Pediatr.* 1984;**142**:135–6.

129 Auwerx, J., Brunzell, J., Bouillon, R., Demedts, M. Familial hypocalciuric hypercalcemia-familial benign hypercalcemia: a review. *Postgrad. Med. J.* 1987;**63**:835–40.

130 Marx, S., Spiegel, A., Levine, M. *et al.* Familial hypocalciuric hypercalcemia: the relation to primary parathyroid hyperplasia. *J. Med.* 1982;**307**:416–26.

131 Marx, S., Attie, M., Spiegel, A. *et al.* An association between neonatal severe primary hyperparathyroidism and familial hypocalciuric hypercalcemia in three kindreds. *N. Engl. J. Med.* 1982;**306**:257–64.

132 Matsuo, M., Okita, K., Takemine, H., Fujita, T. Neonatal primary hyperparathyroidism in familial hypocalciuric hypercalcemia. *Am. J. Dis. Child.* 1982;**136**:728–31.

133 Schwarz, P., Larsen, N. E., Lonborg Friis, I. M. *et al.* Familial hypocalciuric hypercalcemia and neonatal severe hyperparathyroidism associated with mutations in the human Ca2$^+$-sensing receptor gene in three Danish families. *Scand. J. Clin. Lab. Invest.* 2000;**60**:221–7.

134 Cooper, L., Wertheimer, J., Levey, R. *et al.* Severe primary hyperparathyroidism in a neonate with two hypercalcemic parents: management with parathyroidectomy and heterotopic autotransplantation. *Pediatrics* 1986;**78**:263–8.

135 Steinmann, B., Gnehm, H. E., Rao, V. H., Kind, H. P., Prader, A. Neonatal severe primary hyperparathyroidism and alkaptonuria in a boy born to related parents with familial hypocalciuric hypercalcemia. *Helv. Paediatr. Acta.* 1984;**39**:171–86.

136 Pollak, M. R., Chou, Y. H., Marx, S. J. *et al.* Familial hypocalciuric hypercalcemia and neonatal severe hyperparathyroidism. Effects of mutant gene dosage on phenotype. *J. Clin. Invest.* 1994;**93**:1108–12.

137 Pearce, S. H., Trump, D., Wooding, C. *et al.* Calcium-sensing receptor mutations in familial benign hypercalcemia and neonatal hyperparathyroidism. *J. Clin. Invest.* 1995;**96**:2683–92.

138 Marx, S., Frazer, D., Rapoport, A. Familial hypocalciuric hypercalcemia: mild expression of the gene in heterozygotes and severe expression in homozygotes. *Am. J. Med.* 1985;**76**:15–22.

139 Fujita, T., Watanabe, N., Fukase, M. *et al.* Familial hypocalciuric hypercalcemia involving four members of a kindred including a girl with severe neonatal primary hyperparathyroidism. *Miner. Electrolyte Metab.* 1983;**9**:51–4.

140 Ross, A. J. 3rd, Cooper, A., Attie, M. F., Bishop, H. C. Primary hyperparathyroidism in infancy. *J. Pediatr. Surg.* 1986;**21**:493–9.

141 Sopwith, A. M., Burns, C., Grant, D. B. *et al.* Familial hypocalciuric hypercalcaemia: association with neonatal primary hyperparathyroidism, and possible linkage with HLA haplotype. *Clin. Endocrinol. (Oxf).* 1984;**21**:57–64.

142 Nishiyama, S., Tomoeda, S., Inoue, F., Ohta, T., Matsuda, I. Self-limited neonatal familial hyperparathyroidism associated with hypercalciuria and renal tubular acidosis in three siblings. *Pediatrics* 1990;**86**:421–7.

143 Carey, D., Jones, K., Parthemore, J., Deftos, L. Calcitonin secretion in congenital non-goitrous cretinism. *J. Clin. Invest.* 1980;**65**:892–5.

144 Carey, D., Jones, K. Hypothyroidism and hypercalcemia. *J. Pediatr.* 1987;**111**:155–6.

145 Tau, C., Garabedian, M., Farriaux, J. *et al.* Hypercalcemia in infants with congenital hypothyroidism and its relation to vitamin D and thyroid hormones. *J. Pediatr.* 1986;**109**:808–14.

146 Demeester-Mirkine, N., Bergmann, P., Body, J., Corvilain, J. Calcitonin and bone mass status in congenital hypothyroidism. *Calcif. Tissue Int.* 1990;**46**:222–6.

147 Marx, S., Swart, E., Hamstra, A. *et al.* Normal intrauterine development of the fetus of a woman receiving extraordinarily high doses of 1,25 dihydroxyvitamin D. *J. Clin. Endocrinol. Metab.* 1980;**51**:1138–42.

148 Fisher, G., Skillern, P. Hypercalcemia due to hypervitaminosis A. *J. Am. Med. Assoc.* 1974;**227**:1413–14.

149 Burman, K., Monchik, J., Earll, J., Wartofsky, L. Ionized and total serum calcium and parathyroid hormone in hyperthyroidism. *Ann. Intern. Med.* 1976;**84**:668–71.

150 Mahomadi, M., Bivins, L., Becker, K. Effect of thiazides on serum calcium. *Clin. Pharmacol. Ther.* 1979;**26**:390–4.

151 Sann, L., David, L., Loras, B. *et al.* Neonatal hypercalcemia in preterm infants fed with human milk. *Helv. Paediatr. Acta.* 1985;**40**:117–26.

152 Rowe, J., Carey, D. Phosphorus deficiency syndrome in very low birth weight infants. *Pediatr. Clin. N. Am.* 1987;**34**:997–1017.

153 Fraser, D. Hypophosphatasia. *Am. J. Med.* 1957;**22**:730–46.

154 Whyte, M. Heritable metabolic and dysplastic bone diseases. *Endocrinol. Metab. Clin. N. Am.* 1990;**19**:133–73.

155 Bartter, F., Pronove, P., Gill, J. *et al.* Hyperplasia of the juxtaglomerular complex with hyperaldosteronism and hypokalemic alkalosis: a new syndrome. *Am. J. Med.* 1962;**33**:811–28.

156 Stein, J. The pathogenetic spectrum of Bartter's syndrome. *Kidney Int.* 1985;**28**:85–93.

157 Restrepo deRovetto, C., Welch, T., Hug, G. *et al.* Hypercalciuria with Bartter syndrome: evidence for an abnormality of vitamin D metabolism. *J. Pediatr.* 1989;**115**:397–404.

158 Shoemaker, L., Welch, T., Bergstrom, W. *et al.* Calcium kinetics in the hyperprostaglandin E syndrome. *Pediatr. Res.* 1993;**33**:92–6.

159 Konrad, M., Leonhardt, A., Hensen, P., Seyberth, H. W., Kockerling, A. Prenatal and postnatal management of hyperprostaglandin E syndrome after genetic diagnosis from amniocytes. *Pediatrics* 1999;**103**:678–83.

160 Konrad, M., Vollmer, M., Lemmink, H. H. *et al.* Mutations in the chloride channel gene CLCNKB as a cause of classic Bartter syndrome. *J. Am. Soc. Nephrol.* 2000;**11**:1449–59.

161 Peters, M., Ermert, S., Jeck, N. *et al.* Classification and rescue of ROMK mutations underlying hyperprostaglandin E

syndrome/antenatal Bartter syndrome. *Kidney Int.* 2003;**64**: 923–32.

162 Yamada, M., Matsumoto, T., Takahashi, N. *et al.* Stimulatory effect of prostaglandin E2 on 1-alpha,25-dihydroxyvitamin D3 synthesis in rats. *Biochem. J.* 1983;**216**:237–40.

163 Wark, J., Taft, J., Michelangeli, V. *et al.* Biphasic action of prostaglandin E2 on conversion of 25-hydroxyvitamin D3 to 1,25-dihydroxyvitamin D3 in chick renal tubules. *Prostaglandins* 1984;**27**:453–63.

164 Kurose, H., Sonn, Y., Jafari, A. *et al.* Effects of prostaglandin E2 and indomethacin on 25-hydroxyvitamin D3-1-alpha-hydroxylase activity in isolated kidney cells of normal and streptozocin-induced diabetic rats. *Calcif. Tissue Int.* 1985;**37**:625–9.

165 Matsumoto, J., Kim Han, B., Restrepo deRovetto, C., Welch, T. Hypercalciuric Bartter syndrome: resolution of nephrocalcinosis with indomethacin. *Am. J. Radiol.* 1989;**152**:1251–53.

166 Schurman, S. J., Bergstrom, W. H., Shoemaker, L. R., Welch, T. R. Angiotensin II reduces calcium uptake into bone. *Pediatr. Nephrol.* 2004;**19**:33–5.

167 Martin, N., Snodgrass, G., Cohen, R. Idiopathic infantile hypercalcemia – a continuing enigma. *Arch. Dis. Child.* 1984;**59**:605–13.

168 Jones, K. L., Smith, D. W. The Williams elfin facies syndrome: a new perspective. *J. Pediatr.* 1975;**86**:718–23.

169 Aarskog, D., Aksnes, L., Markestad, T. Vitamin D metabolism in idiopathic infantile hypercalcemia. *Am. J. Dis. Child.* 1981;**135**:1021–4.

170 Chesney, R., DeLuca, H., Gertner, J. Increased plasma 1,25-dihydroxyvitamin D in infants with hypercalcemia and elfin facies. *N. Engl. J. Med.* 1985;**313**:889–90.

171 Garabedian, M., Jacqz, E., Guillozo, H. *et al.* Elevated plasma 1,25-dihydroxyvitamin D concentrations in infants with hypercalcemia and elfin facies. *N. Engl. J. Med.* 1985;**312**:948–52.

172 Taylor, A., Stern, P., Bell, N. Abnormal regulation of circulating 25-hydroxyvitamin D in the Williams syndrome. *N. Engl. J. Med.* 1982;**306**:972–5.

173 Culler, F., Jones, K., Deftos, L. Impaired calcitonin secretion in patients with Williams syndrome. *J. Pediatr.* 1985;**107**:720–3.

174 Hicks, M. J., Levy, M. L., Alexander, J., Flaitz, C. M. Subcutaneous fat necrosis of the newborn and hypercalcemia: case report and review of the literature. *Pediatr. Dermatol.* 1993;**10**:271–6.

175 Repiso-Jimenez, J. B., Marquez, J., Sotillo, I., Garcia-Bravo, B., Camacho, F. Subcutaneous fat necrosis of the newborn. *J. Eur. Acad. Dermatol. Venereol.* 1999;**12**:254–7.

176 Friedman, S. J., Winkelmann, R. K. Subcutaneous fat necrosis of the newborn: light, ultrastructural and histochemical microscopic studies. *J. Cutan. Pathol.* 1989;**16**:99–105.

177 Veldhuis, J., Kulin, H., Demers, L. *et al.* Infantile hypercalcemia with subcutaneous fat necrosis: endocrine studies. *J. Pediatr.* 1979;**95**:460–2.

178 Barltrop, D. Hypercalcemia associated with neonatal subcutaneous fat necrosis. *Arch. Dis. Child.* 1963;**38**:516–18.

179 Cook, J., Stone, M., Hansen, J. Hypercalcemia in association with subcutaneous fat necrosis of the newborn: studies of calcium-regulating hormones. *Pediatrics* 1992;**90**:93–6.

180 Finne, P., Sanderud, J., Aksnes, L., Bratlid, D., Aarskog, D. Hypercalcemia with increased and unregulated 1,25-dihydroxyvitamin D production in a neonate with subcutaneous fat necrosis. *J. Pediatr.* 1988;**112**:792–4.

181 Kruse, K., Irle, U., Uhlig, R. Elevated 1,25-dihydroxyvitamin D serum concentrations in infants with subcutaneous fat necrosis. *J. Pediatr.* 1993;**122**:460–3.

182 Burden, A. D., Krafchik, B. R. Subcutaneous fat necrosis of the newborn: a review of 11 cases. *Pediatr. Dermatol.* 1999;**16**:384–7.

183 Tran, J. T., Sheth, A. P. Complications of subcutaneous fat necrosis of the newborn: a case report and review of the literature. *Pediatr. Dermatol.* 2003;**20**:257–61.

184 Gu, L. L., Daneman, A., Binet, A., Kooh, S. W. Nephrocalcinosis and nephrolithiasis due to subcutaneous fat necrosis with hypercalcemia in two full-term asphyxiated neonates: sonographic findings. *Pediatr. Radiol.* 1995;**25**:142–4.

185 Wiadrowski, T. P., Marshman, G. Subcutaneous fat necrosis of the newborn following hypothermia and complicated by pain and hypercalcaemia. *Australas. J. Dermatol.* 2001;**42**:207–10.

186 Chuang, S. D., Chiu, H. C., Chang, C. C. Subcutaneous fat necrosis of the newborn complicating hypothermic cardiac surgery. *Br. J. Dermatol.* 1995;**132**:805–10.

187 Glover, M. T., Catterall, M. D., Atherton, D. J. Subcutaneous fat necrosis in two infants after hypothermic cardiac surgery. *Pediatr. Dermatol.* 1991;**8**:210–12.

188 Lee, S. K., Lee, J. H., Han, C. H. *et al.* Calcified subcutaneous fat necrosis induced by prolonged exposure to cold weather: a case report. *Pediatr. Radiol.* 2001;**31**:294–5.

189 Dudink, J., Walther, F. J., Beekman, R. P. Subcutaneous fat necrosis of the newborn: hypercalcaemia with hepatic and atrial myocardial calcification. *Arch. Dis. Child Fetal Neonat. Edn.* 2003;**88**:F343–5.

190 Barbier, C., Cneude, F., Deliege, R. *et al.* Subcutaneous fat necrosis in the newborn: a risk for severe hypercalcemia. *Arch. Pediatr.* 2003;**10**:713–15.

191 Hung, S. H., Tsai, W. Y., Tsao, P. N., Chou, H. C., Hsieh, W. S. Oral clodronate therapy for hypercalcemia related to extensive subcutaneous fat necrosis in a newborn. *J. Formos. Med. Assoc.* 2003;**102**:801–4.

192 Khan, N., Licata, A., Rogers, D. Intravenous bisphosphonate for hypercalcemia accompanying subcutaneous fat necrosis: a novel treatment approach. *Clin. Pediatr. (Phila).* 2001;**40**:217–19.

193 Bachrach, L. K., Lum, C. K. Etidronate in subcutaneous fat necrosis of the newborn. *J. Pediatr.* 1999;**135**:530–1.

194 Gerritsen, J., Knol, K. Hypercalcemia in a child with miliary tuberculosis. *Eur. J. Pediatr.* 1989;**148**:650–1.

195 Ferraro, E., Klein, S., Fakhry, J. *et al.* Hypercalcemia in association with mesoblastic nephroma: report of a case and review of the literature. *Pediatr. Radiol.* 1986;**16**:516–17.

196 Jayabose, S., Iqbal, K., Newman, L. *et al.* Hypercalcemia in childhood renal tumors. *Cancer* 1988;**62**:303–8.

197 Woolfield, N., Abbott, G., McRae, C. A mesoblastic nephroma with hypercalcemia. *Aust. Paediatr. J.* 1988;**24**:309–10.

198 Shanbhogue, L., Gray, E., Miller, S. Congenital mesoblastic nephroma of infancy associated with hypercalcemia. *J. Urol.* 1986;**135**:771–2.

199 Rousseau-Merck, M., Nogues, C., Roth, A. *et al.* Hypercalcemic infantile renal tumors: morphological, clinical, and biological heterogeneity. *Pediatr. Pathol.* 1985;**3**:155–64.

200 Rousseau-Merck, M., DeKeyzer, Y., Bourdeau, A. *et al.* PTH mRNA transcription analysis in infantile tumors associated with hypercalcemia. *Cancer* 1988;**62**:303–8.

201 Vido, L., Carli, M., Rizzoni, G., *et al.* Congenital mesoblastic nephroma with hypercalcemia: pathogenic role of prostaglandins. *Am. J. Pediatr. Hematol. Oncol.* 1986;**8**:149–52.

202 Calo, L., Cantaro, S., Bertazzo, L. *et al.* Synthesis and catabolism of PGE2 by a nephroblastoma associated with hypercalcemia without bone metastases. *Cancer* 1984;**54**:635–7.

203 Sagy, M., Birenbaum, E., Balin, A. *et al.* Phosphate-depletion syndrome in a premature infant fed human milk. *J. Pediatr.* 1980;**96**:683–5.

204 Hall, R. T., Wheeler, R. E., Montalto, M. B., Benson, J. D. Hypophosphatemia in breast-fed low-birth-weight infants following initial hospital discharge. *Am. J. Dis. Child.* 1989;**143**:1191–5.

205 American Academy of Pediatrics. Committee on Nutrition. Soy protein-based formulas: recommendations for use in infant feeding. *Pediatrics* 1998;**101**:148–53.

206 Naude, S. P., Prinsloo, J. G., Haupt, C. E. Comparison between a humanized cow's milk and a soy product for premature infants. *S. Afr. Med. J.* 1979;**55**:982–6.

207 Shenai, J. P., Jhaveri, B. M., Reynolds, J. W., Huston, R. K., Babson, S. G. Nutritional balance studies in very-low-birth-weight infants: role of soy formula. *Pediatrics* 1981;**67**:631–7.

208 Kulkarni, P. B., Hall, R. T., Rhodes, P. G. Rickets in very-low-birth-weight infants. *J. Pediatr.* 1980; **97**:249–52.

209 Callenbach, J. C., Sheehan, M. B., Abramson, S. J., Hall, R. T. Etiologic factors in rickets of very-low-birth-weight infants. *J. Pediatr.* 1981;**98**:800–5.

210 Steichen, J. J., Tsang, R. C. Bone mineralization and growth in term infants fed soy-based or cow milk-based formula. *J. Pediatr.* 1987;**110**:687–92.

211 Chan, G. M., Leeper, L., Book, L. S. Effects of soy formulas on mineral metabolism in term infants. *Am. J. Dis. Child.* 1987;**141**:527–30.

212 Bainbridge, R. R., Mimouni, F., Tsang, R. C. Bone mineral content of infants fed soy based formula. *J. Pediatr.* 1988;**113**:205–7.

213 Fomon, S. J., Ziegler, E. E. Soy protein isolates in infant feeding. In Wilcke, H. L., Hopkins, D. T., Waggle, D. H., eds. *Soy Protein and Human Nutrition*. New York: Academic Press Inc; 1979; 79–86.

214 Kohler, L., Meeuwisse, G., Mortensson, W. Food intake and growth of infants between six and twenty-six weeks of age on breast milk, cow's milk formula, or soy formula. *Acta Paediatr. Scand.* 1984;**73**:40–8.

215 Fomon, S. J., Ziegler, E. E. Isolated soy protein in infant feeding. In Steinke, F. H., Waggle, D. H., Volgarev, M. N., eds. *New Protein Foods in Human Health: Nutrition, Prevention, and Therapy*. Boca Raton, FL: CRC Press Inc; 1992:75–83.

216 Hillman, L. S., Chow, W., Salmons, S. S. *et al.* Vitamin D metabolism, mineral homeostasis, and bone mineralization in term infants fed human milk-based formula or soy-based formula. *J. Pediatr.* 1988;**112**:864–8.

217 Mimouni, F., Campaigne, B., Neylan, M., Tsang, R. C. Bone mineralization in the first year of life in infants fed human milk, cow-milk formula or soy-based formula. *J. Pediatr.* 1993;**122**:348–54.

218 Venkataraman, P. S., Luhar, H., Neylan, M. J. Bone mineral metabolism in full-term infants fed human milk, cow milk-based, and soy-based formulas. *Am. J. Dis. Child.* 1992;**146**:1302–5.

219 Langlois, V., Bernard, C., Scheinman, S. J. *et al.* Clinical features of X-linked nephrolithiasis in childhood. *Pediatr. Nephrol.* 1998;**12**:625–9.

220 Forino, M., Graziotto, R., Tosetto, E. *et al.* Identification of a novel splice site mutation of CLCN5 gene and characterization of a new alternative 5′ UTR end of ClC-5 mRNA in human renal tissue and leukocytes. *J. Hum. Genet.* 2004;**49**:53–60.

221 Heath, H. 3rd. Familial benign (hypocalciuric) hypercalcemia. A troublesome mimic of mild primary hyperparathyroidism. *Endocrinol. Metab. Clin. N. Am.* 1989;**18**:723–40.

222 Pivnick, E. K., Kerr, N. C., Kaufman, R. A., Jones, D. P., Chesney, R. W. Rickets secondary to phosphate depletion. A sequela of antacid use in infancy. *Clin. Pediatr. (Phila).* 1995;**34**:73–8.

223 Tseng, U. F. Shu, S. G., Chen, C. H., Chi, C. S. Transient neonatal hypoparathyroidism: report of four cases. *Acta Paediatr. Taiwan* 2001;**42**:359–62.

224 Tsang, R. C., Chen, I., Friedman, M. A. *et al.* Parathyroid function in infants of diabetic mothers. *J. Pediatr.* 1975;**86**:399–404.

225 Manzar, S. Transient pseudohypoparathyroidism and neonatal seizure. *J. Trop. Pediatr.* 2001;**47**:113–14.

226 Sajitha, S., Krishnamoorthy, P. N., Shenoy, U. V. Pseudohypoparathyroidism in newborn – a rare presentation. *Indian Pediatr.* 2003;**40**:47–9.

227 Minagawa, M., Yasuda, T., Kobayashi, Y., Niimi, H. Transient pseudohypoparathyroidism of the neonate. *Eur. J. Endocrinol.* 1995;**133**:151–5.

228 Soumoy, M. P., Bachy, A. Risk of phosphate enemas in the infant. *Arch. Pediatr.* 1998;**5**:1221–3.

229 Walton, D. M., Thomas, D. C., Aly, H. Z., Short, B. L. Morbid hypocalcemia associated with phosphate enema in a six-week-old infant. *Pediatrics* 2000;**106**:E37.

230 Spatling, L., Disch, G., Classen, H. G. Magnesium in pregnant women and the newborn. *Magnesium Res.* 1989;**2**:271–80.

231 Doyle, W., Crawford, M., Wynn, A., Wynn, S. Maternal magnesium intake and pregnancy outcome. *Magnesium Res.* 1989;**2**:205–10.

232 Harris, I., Wilkinson, A. Magnesium depletion in children. *Lancet* 1971;**2**:735–6.

233 Allen, D., Friedman, A., Greer, F., Chesney, R. W. Hypomagnesemia masking the appearance of elevated parathyroid hormone concentrations in familial pseudohypoparathyroidism. *Am. J. Med. Genet.* 1988;**31**:153–8.

234 Allgrove, J., Adami, S., Fraher, L. *et al.* Hypomagnesemia: studies of parathyroid hormone secretion and function. *Clin. Endocrinol.* 1984;**21**: 435–49.

235 Davis, J., Harvey, D., Yu, J. Neonatal fits associated with hypomagnesemia. *Arch. Dis. Child.* 1965;**40**:286–90.

236 Cruikshank, D., Pitkin, R., Reynolds, W. *et al.* Altered maternal calcium homeostasis in diabetic pregnancy. *J. Clin. Endocrinol. Metabol.* 1980;**50**:264–7.

237 Linderman, R., Adler, S., Yiengst, M., Beard, E. Influence of various nutrients on urinary divalent cation excretion. *J. Lab. Clin. Med.* 1967;**70**:236–45.

238 Aikawa, J. Effect of alloxan-induced diabetes on magnesium metabolism in rabbits. *Am. J. Physiol.* 1960;**199**:1084–6.

239 Mehta, K. C., Kalkwarf, H. J., Mimouni, F., Khoury, J., Tsang, R. C. Randomized trial of magnesium administration to prevent hypocalcemia in infants of diabetic mothers. *J. Perinatol.* 1998;**18**:352–6.

240 Saggese, G., Bertelloni, S., Baroncelli, G. I., Pelletti, A., Benedetti, U. Evaluation of a peptide family encoded by the calcitonin gene in selected healthy prenant women. A longitudinal study. *Horm. Res.* 1990;**34**:240–4.

241 Bertelloni, S. The parathyroid hormone-1,25-dihydroxyvitamin D endocrine system and magnesium status in insulin-dependent diabetes mellitus: current concepts. *Magnesium Res.* 1992;**5**:45–51.

242 Abdulrazzaq, Y. M., Smigura, F. C., Wettrell, G. Primary infantile hypomagnesaemia; report of two cases and review of literature. *Eur. J. Pediatr.* 1989;**148**:459–61.

243 Dudin, K. I., Teebi, A. S. Primary hypomagnesaemia. A case report and literature review. *Eur. J. Pediatr.* 1987;**146**: 303–5.

244 Friedman, M., Hatcher, G., Watson, L. Primary hypomagnesaemia with secondary hypocalcaemia in an infant. *Lancet* 1967;**1**:703–5.

245 Prebble, J. J. Primary infantile hypomagnesaemia: report of two cases. *J. Paediatr. Child Health.* 1995;**31**:54–56.

246 Paunier, L., Radde, I. C., Kooh, S. W., Conen, P. E., Fraser, D. Primary hypomagnesemia with secondary hypocalcemia in an infant. *Pediatrics* 1968;**41**:385–402.

247 Skyberg, D., Stromme, J. H., Nesbakken, R. *et al.* Congenital primary hypomagnesemia, an inborn error of metabolism. *Acta Paediatr. Scand.* 1967;**56**:26–7.

248 Stromme, J. H., Steen-Johnsen, J., Harnaes, K. *et al.* Familial hypomagnesemia – a follow up examination of three patients after 9 to 12 years of treatment. *Pediatr. Res.* 1981;**15**: 1134–9.

249 Shalev, H., Phillip, M., Galil, A., Carmi, R., Landau, D. Clinical presentation and outcome in primary familial hypomagnesaemia. *Arch. Dis. Child.* 1998;**78**:127–30.

250 Runeberg, L., Collan, Y., Jokinen, E. *et al.* Hypomagnesemia due to renal disease of unknown etiology. *Am. J. Med.* 1975;**59**:873–81.

251 Booth, B., Johanson, A. Hypomagnesemia due to renal tubular defect in reabsorption of magnesium. *J. Pediatr.* 1974;**85**: 350–4.

252 Gitelman, H., Graham, J., Welt, L. A new familial disorder characterized by hypokalemia and hypomagnesemia. *Trans. Assoc. Am. Physicians.* 1966;**79**:221–35.

253 Michelis, M., Drash, A., Linarelli, L. *et al.* Decreased bicarbonate threshold and renal magnesium wasting in a sibship with distal renal tubular acidosis. *Metabolism* 1972;**21**:905–20.

254 Knoers, N. V., de Jong, J. C., Meij, I. C. *et al.* Genetic renal disorders with hypomagnesemia and hypocalciuria. *J. Nephrol.* 2003;**16**:293–6.

255 Bettinelli, A., Metta, M., Perini, A., Basilico, E., Santeramo, C. Long-term follow-up of a patient with Gitelman's syndrome. *Pediatr. Nephrol.* 1993;**7**:67–8.

256 Cole, D. E., Quamme, G. A. Inherited disorders of renal magnesium handling. *J. Am. Soc. Nephrol.* 2000;**11**:1937–47.

257 Allen, D., Friedman, A., Greer, F., Chesney, R. W. Hypomagnesemia masking the appearance of elevated parathyroid hormone concentrations in familial pseudohypoparathyroidism. *Am. J. Med. Genet.* 1988;**31**:153–8.

258 Benigno, V., Canonica, C. S., Bettinelli, A. *et al.* Hypomagnesaemia–hypercalciuria–nephrocalcinosis: a report of nine cases and a review. *Nephrol. Dial. Transplant.* 2000;**15**:605–10.

259 Konrad Mand, S., Weber, S. Recent advances in molecular genetics of hereditary magnesium-losing disorders. *J. Am. Soc. Nephrol.* 2003;**14**:249–60.

260 Konrad, M., Schlingmann, K. P., Gudermann, T. Insights into the molecular nature of magnesium homeostasis. *Am. J. Physiol. Renal. Physiol.* 2004;**286**:F599–605.

261 Rude, R., Singer, F. Magnesium deficiency and excess. *Annu. Rev. Med.* 1981;**32**:245–59.

262 Dominguez, J., Gray, R., Lemann, J. Dietary phosphate deprivation in women and men: effects of mineral and acid balances, parathyroid hormone and the metabolism of 25-OH-Vitamin D. *J. Clin. Endocrinol. Metab.* 1976;**43**:1056–68.

263 Bar, R., Wilson, H., Mazzaferri, E. Hypomagnesemic hypocalcemia secondary to renal magnesium wasting. A possible consequence of high dose gentamicin therapy. *Ann. Int. Med.* 1975;**82**:646–9.

264 Barton, C., Pahl, M., Vaziri, N. *et al.* Renal magnesium wasting associated with Amphotericin B therapy. *Am. J. Med.* 1984;**77**:471–4.

265 Dyckner, T., Wester, P. Intracellular magnesium loss after diuretic administration. *Drugs* 1984;**28**:161–6.

266 Sheehan, J., White, A. Diuretic-associated hypomagnesemia. *Br. Med. J.* 1982;**285**:1157–9.

267 Ryan, M. Diuretics and potassium/magnesium depletion: directions for treatment. *Am. J. Med.* 1987;**82**:38–47.

268 Leary, W., Reyes, A. Diuretic-induced magnesium losses. *Drugs* 1984;**28**:182–7.

269 Seelig, M. Prenatal and neonatal mineral deficiencies: magnesium, zinc, and chromium. In Lifshitz, F., ed. *Pediatric Nutrition. Infant feedings – Deficiencies – Diseases. Clinical Disorders in Pediatric Nutrition, Vol. 2.* New York: Marcel Dekker Inc.;1982:167–96.

270 Jukarainen, E. Plasma magnesium levels during the first five days of life. *Acta Paediatr. Scand.* 1974;**222**:1–58.

271 Ertel, N., Reiss, J., Spergel, G. Hypomagnesemia in neonatal tetany associated with maternal hyperparathyroidism. *N. Engl. J. Med.* 1969;**50**:264–7.

272 Dooling, E., Stern, L. Hypomagnesemia with convulsions in a newborn infant. *Canad. Med. Assoc. J.* 1967;**97**:827–31.

273 MacIntyre, I., Boss, S., Troughton, V. Parathyroid hormone and magnesium homeostasis. *Nature* 1963;**198**:1058–60.

274 Jones, K., Fourman, P. Effects of infusions of magnesium and of calcium in parathyroid insufficiency. *Clin. Sci.* 1966;**30**:139–50.

275 Kobayashi, A., Shiraki, K. Serum magnesium level in infants and children with hepatic diseases. *Arch. Dis. Child.* 1967;**42**:615–18.

276 Cohen, M., McNamara, H., Finberg, L. Serum magnesium with cirrhosis. *J. Pediatr.* 1970;**76**:453–5.

277 Cowan, G., Luther, R., Sykes, T. Short bowel syndrome: causes and clinical consequences. *Nutr. Supp. Services.* 1984;**4**:25–32.

278 Weser, E. Nutritional aspects of malabsorption: short gut adaptation. *Am. J. Med.* 1979;**67**:1014–20.

279 Ziegler, M. Short bowel syndrome in infancy: etiology and management. *Clin. Perinatol.* 1986;**13**:163–73.

280 Rodder, S., Mize, C., Forman, L., Uauy, R. Effects of increased dietary phosphorus on magnesium balance in very low birth-weight babies. *Magnesium Res.* 1993;**5**:273–5.

281 Ryan, M. P. Interrelationships of magnesium and potassium homeostasis. *Mineral Electrolyte Metab.* 1993;**19**:290–5.

282 Brand, J., Greer, F. Hypermagnesemia and intestinal perforation following antacid administration in a premature infant. *Pediatrics* 1990;**85**:121–4.

283 Brady, J. P., Williams, H. C. Magnesium intoxication in a premature infant. *Pediatrics* 1967;**40**:100–3.

284 Engel, R. R., Elin, R. J. Hypermagnesemia from birth asphyxia. *J. Pediatr.* 1970;**77**:631–7.

285 Ali, A., Walentik, C., Mantych, G. J. *et al.* Iatrogenic acute hypermagnesemia after total parenteral nutrition infusion mimicking septic shock syndrome: two case reports. *Pediatrics* 2003;**112**:E70–2.

286 Mofenson, H. C., Caraccio, T. R. Magnesium intoxication in a neonate from oral magnesium hydroxide laxative. *Clin. Toxicol.* 1991;**29**:215–22.

287 Ichiba, H., Tamai, H., Negishi, H. *et al.* Randomized controlled trial of magnesium sulfate infusion for severe birth asphyxia. *Pediatr. Int.* 2002;**44**:505–9.

288 Cooper, L. Wertheimer, J., Levey, R. *et al.* Severe primary hyperparathyroidism in a neonate with two hypercalcemic parents: management with parathyroidectomy and heterotopic autotransplantation. *Pediatrics* 1986;**78**:263–8.

289 Donovan, E., Tsang, R., Steichen, J. *et al.* Neonatal hypermagnesemia: effect on parathyroid hormone and calcium homeostasis. *J. Pediatr.* 1980;**96**:305–10.

290 Buckle, R., Care, A., Cooper, C. The influence of plasma magnesium concentration on parathyroid hormone secretion. *J. Endocrinol.* 1968;**42**:529–34.

291 Massry, S. G., Coburn, J. W., Kleeman, C. R. Evidence for suppression of parathyroid gland activity by hypermagnesemia. *J. Clin. Invest.* 1970;**49**:1619–29.

292 Lipsitz, P. J. The clinical and biochemical effects of excess magnesium in the newborn. *Pediatrics* 1971;**47**:501–9.

293 MacManus, J., Heaton, F. W. The influence of magnesium on calcium release from bone in vitro. *Biochem. Biophys. Acta.* 1970;**215**:360–7.

294 Sokal, M., Koenigsberger, M., Rose, J. *et al.* Neonatal hypermagnesemia and the meconium-plug syndrome. *N. Engl. J. Med.* 1972;**286**:823–5.

295 Lamm, C., Norton, K., Murphy, R. *et al.* Congenital rickets associated with magnesium sulfate infusion for tocolysis. *J. Pediatr.* 1988;**113**:1078–82.

296 Holcomb, W. J., Shackelford, G., Petrie, R. Magnesium tocolysis and neonatal bone abnormalities: a controlled study. *Obstet. Gynecol.* 1991;**78**:611–14.

297 Cumming, W., Thomas, V. Hypermagnesemia: a cause of abnormal metaphyses in the neonate. *Am. J. Radiol.* 1989;**152**:1071–2.

298 Levine, B. S., Coburn, J. W. Magnesium, the mimic/antagonist of calcium. *N. Engl. J. Med.* 1984;**310**:1253–5.

299 Dent, C., Gupta, M. Plasma 25-hydroxyvitamin D levels during pregnancy in Caucasians and in vegetarian and non-vegetarian Asians. *Lancet* 1975;**2**:1057–60.

300 Heckmatt, J., Peacock, M., Davies, A. *et al.* Plasma 25-hydroxyvitamin D in pregnant Asian women and their babies. *Lancet* 1979;**2**:546–8.

301 Biale, Y., Shany, S., Levi, M. *et al.* 25-Hydroxycholecalciferol levels in Bedouin women in labor and in cord blood of their infants. *Am. J. Clin. Nutr.* 1979;**32**:2380–2.

302 Bassir, M., Laborie, S., Lapillonne, A. *et al.* Vitamin D deficiency in Iranian mothers and their neonates: a pilot study. *Acta Paediatr.* 2001;**90**:577–9.

303 Jacobus, C., Holick, M., Shao, Q. *et al.* Hypervitaminosis D associated with drinking milk. *N. Engl. J. Med.* 1992;**326**:1173–7.

304 Holick, M., Shao, Q., Liu, W., Chen, T. The vitamin D content of fortified milk and infant formula. *N. Engl. J. Med.* 1992;**326**:1178–81.

305 Zimmerman, T., Giddens, W., DiGiacomo, R., Ladiges, W. Soft tissue mineralization in rabbits fed a diet containing excess vitamin D. *Lab. Anim. Sci.* 1990;**40**:212–15.

306 Friedman, W., Mills, L. The relationship between vitamin D and the craniofacial and dental anomalies of the supravalvular aortic stenosis syndrome. *Pediatrics* 1969;**43**:12–18.

307 Itani, O., Tsang, R. C. Bone disease. In Kaplan, L. A., Pesce, A. J., eds. *Clinical Chemistry: Theory, Analysis and Correlation.* 4th edn. St. Louis: Mosby-Year Book;2003:507–34.

308 Bainbridge, R., Itani, O., Tsang, R. Rickets. In Carraza, F., Marcondes, E., eds. *Textbook of Clinical Nutrition in Pediatrics.* 1991:252–64.

309 David, L. Common vitamin D-deficiency rickets. In Glorieux, F., ed. *Rickets, Vol. 21.* New York, NY: Vevey/Raven Press;1991:107–22.

310 Chesney, R. Requirements and upper limits of vitamin D intake in the term neonate, infant, and older child. *J. Pediatr.* 1990;**116**:159–66.

311 Specker, B. L., Valanis, B., Hertzberg, V., Edwards, N., Tsang, R. C. Sunshine exposure and serum 25-hydroxyvitamin D concentrations in exclusively breast-fed infants. *J. Pediatr.* 1985;**107**:372–6.

312 Paunier, L. Prevention of rickets. In Glorieux, F., ed. *Rickets, Vol. 21.* New York, NY: Vevey/Raven Press;1991:263–72.

313 Malloy, P., Hochberg, Z., Tiosano, D. *et al.* The molecular basis of hereditary 1,25-dihydroxyvitamin D3 resistant rickets in seven related families. *J. Clin. Invest.* 1990;**86**:2071–80.

314 Malloy, P., Hochberg, Z., Wesley, R., Pike, J., Feldman, D. Abnormal binding of vitamin D receptors to deoxyribonucleic acid in a kindred with vitamin D- dependent rickets, type II. *J. Clin. Endocrinol. Metab.* 1989;**68**:263–9.

315 Holm, A., Goldsmith, L. Impetigo herpetiformis associated with hypocalcemia of congenital rickets. *Arch. Dermatol.* 1991;**127**:91–5.

316 Weisman, Y., Jaccard, N., Legum, C. *et al.* Prenatal diagnosis of vitamin D-dependent rickets, type II: response to 1,25-dihydroxyvitamin D in amniotic fluid cells and fetal tissues. *J. Clin. Endocrinol. Metab.* 1990;**71**:937–43.

317 Clements, M., Johnson, L., Fraser, D. A new mechanism for induced vitamin D deficiency in calcium deprivation. *Nature* 1987;**325**:62–5.

318 Senterre, J. Osteopenia versus rickets in premature infants. In Glorieux F., ed. *Rickets, Vol. 21,* New York: Vevey/Raven Press; 1991:145–54.

319 Legius, E., Proesmans, W., Eggermont, E. *et al.* Rickets due to dietary calcium deficiency. *Eur. J. Pediatr.* 1989;**148**:784–5.

320 Okonofua, F., Gill, D., Alabi, Z. *et al.* Rickets in Nigerian children: a consequence of calcium malnutrition. *Metabolism* 1991;**40**:209–13.

321 Pettifor, J. Dietary calcium deficiency. In Glorieux, F., ed. *Rickets, Vol. 21.* New York: Vevey/Raven Press;1991:123–43.

322 Balsan, S., Tieder, M. Linear growth in patients with hypophosphatemic vitamin D-resistant rickets: influence of treatment regimen and parental height. *J. Pediatr.* 1990;**116**:365–70.

323 Rivkees, S., El-Hajj-Fuleihan, G., Brown, E., Crawford, J. Tertiary hyperparathyroidism during high phosphate therapy of familial hypophosphatemic rickets. *J. Clin. Endocrinol. Metab.* 1992;**75**:1514–18.

324 Glorieux, F. Calcitriol treatment in vitamin D-dependent and vitamin D-resistant rickets. *Metabolism* 1990;**39**:10–12.

325 Hanna, J., Niimi, K., Chan, J. X-linked hypophosphatemia – Genetic and clinical correlates. *Am. J. Dis. Child.* 1991;**145**:865–70.

326 Verge, C., Lam, A., Simpson, J. *et al.* Effects of therapy in X-linked hypophosphatemic rickets. *N. Engl. J. Med.* 1991;**325**:1843–8.

327 Hurley, D., McMahon, M. Long-term parenteral nutrition and metabolic bone disease. *Endocrinol. Metab. Clin. N. Am.* 1990;**19**:113–31.

328 Wood, R., Bengoa, J., Sitrin, M., Rosenberg, I. Calciuretic effect of cyclic versus continuous total parenteral nutrition. *Am. J. Clin. Nutr.* 1985;**41**:614–19.

329 Pelegano, J., Rowe, J., Carey, D., *et al.* Effect of calcium/phosphorus ratio on mineral retention in parenterally fed premature infants. *J. Pediatr. Gastroenterol. Nutr.* 1991;**12**:351–5.

330 Block, G., Wood, R., Allen, L. A comparison of the effects of feeding sulfur amino acids and protein on urine calcium in man. *Am. J. Clin. Nutr.* 1980;**33**:2128–36.

331 Cole, D., Zlotkin, S. Increased sulfate as an etiological factor in the hypercalciuria associated with total parenteral nutrition. *Am. J. Clin. Nutr.* 1983;**37**:108–13.

332 Bengoa, J., Sitrin, M., Wood, R. Amino acid-induced hypercalciuria in patients on total parenteral nutrition. *Am. J. Clin. Nutr.* 1983;**38**:264–9.

333 Kaneko, K., Masaki, U., Aikyo, M. *et al.* Urinary calcium and calcium balance in young women affected by high protein diet of soy protein isolate and adding sulfur-containing amino acids and/or potassium. *J. Nutr. Sci. Vitaminol.* 1990;**36**:105–16.

334 Linkswiler, H., Zemel, M., Hegsted, M., Shuette, S. Protein-induced hypercalciuria. *Fed. Proc.* 1981;**40**:2429–33.

335 Rauch, F., Schoenau, E. Changes in bone density during childhood and adolescence: an approach based on bone's biological organization. *J. Bone Mineral Res.* 2001;**16**:597–604.

336 Rigo, J., De Curtis, M., Picltain, C. *et al.* Bone mineral metabolism in the micropremie. *Clin. Perinatol.* 2000;**27**:147–70.

337 Backstrom, M. C., Kuusela, A. L., Maki, R. Metabolic bone disease of prematurity. *Ann. Med.* 1996;**28**:275–82.

338 Greer, F. R. Osteopenia of prematurity. *Annu. Rev. Nutr.* 1994;**14**:169–85.

339 Bishop, N. Bone disease in preterm infants. *Arch. Dis. Child.* 1989;**64**:1403–9.

340 Rodriguez, J. I., Garcia-Alix, A., Palacios, J. *et al.* Changes in the long bones due to fetal immobility caused by neuromuscular disease. A radiographic and histological study. *J. Bone Joint Surg [Am].* 1988;**70**:1052–60.

341 Rodriguez, J. I., Palacios, J., Garcia-Alix, A. *et al.* Effects of immobilization on fetal bone development. A morphometric study in newborns with congenital neuromuscular diseases with intrauterine onset. *Calcif. Tissue Int.* 1988;**43**:335–9.

342 Rodriguez, J. I., Palacios, J., Ruiz, A. *et al.* Morphological changes in long bone development in fetal adinesia deformation sequence: an experimental study in curarized rat fetuses. *Teratology* 1992;**45**:213–21.

343 Callenbach, J. C., Sheehan, M. B., Abramson, S. J., Hall, R. T. Etiologic factors in rickets of very-low-birth-weight infants. *J. Pediatr.* 1981;**98**:800–5.

344 Masel, J. P., Tudehope, D., Cartwright, D., Cleghorn, G. Osteopenia and rickets in the extremely low birth weight infant – a survey of the incidence and a radiological classification. *Australas. Radiol.* 1982;**26**:83–96.

345 Lyon, A. J., McIntosh, N., Wheeler, K., Williams, J. E. Radiological rickets in extremely low birthweight infants. *Pediatr. Radiol.* 1987;**17**:56–8.

346 Koo, W. W., Sherman, R., Succop, P. *et al.* Fractures and rickets in very low birth weight infants: conservative management and outcome. *J. Pediatr. Orthop.* 1989;**9**:326–30.

347 Koo, W. W., Sherman, R., Succop, P., Ho, M., Buckley, D., Tsang, R. C. Serum vitamin D metabolites in very low birth weight infants with and without rickets and fractures. *J. Pediatr.* 1989;**114**:1017–22.

348 Msomekela, M. Manji, K., Mbise, R. L., Kazema, R., Makwaya, C. A high prevalence of metabolic bone disease in exclusively breastfed very low birthweight infants in Dar-es-Salaam, Tanzania. *Ann. Trop. Paediatr.* 1999;**19**:337–44.

349 Steichen, J. J., Tsang, R. C. Bone mineralization and growth in term infants fed soy-based or cow milk-based formula. *J. Pediatr.* 1987;**110**:687–92.

350 Campfield, T., Braden, G., Flynn-Valone, P., Powell, S. Effect of diuretics on urinary oxalate, calcium, and sodium excretion in very low birth weight infants. *Pediatrics* 1997;**99**:814–18.

351 Ziegler, E. E., O'Donnell, A. M., Nelson, S. E., Fomon, S. J. Body composition of the reference fetus. *Growth* 1976;**40**:329–41.

352 Lemons, J. A., Moye, L., Hall, D., Simmons, M. Differences in the composition of preterm and term human milk during early lactation. *Pediatr. Res.* 1982;**16**:113–17.

353 Butte, N. F., Garza, C., Johnson, C. A., Smith, E. O., Nichols, B. L. Longitudinal changes in milk composition of mothers delivering preterm and term infants. *Early Hum. Dev.* 1984;**9**:153–62.

354 Beyers, N., Alheit, B., Taljaard, J. F. *et al.* High turnover osteopenea in preterm infants. *Bone* 1994;**15**:5–13.

355 Mora, S., Weber, G., Bellini, A., Bianchi, C., Chiumello, G. Bone modeling alteration in preterm infants. *Arch. Ped. Adolesc. Med.* 1994;**148**:1215–17.

356 Miller, M. E. The bone disease of preterm birth: a biomechanical perspective. *Pediatr. Res.* 2003;**53**:10–15.

357 James, J. R., Congdon, P. J., Truscott, J., Horsman, A., Arthur, R. Osteopenia of prematurity. *Arch. Dis. Child.* 1986;**61**:871–6.

358 Horsman, A., Ryan, S. W., Congdon, P. J., Truscott, J. G., James, J. R. Osteopenia in extremely low birth weight infants. *Arch. Dis. Child.* 1989;**64**:485–8.

359 Horsman, A., Ryan, S. W., Congdon, P. J. *et al.* Bone mineral content and body size 56 to 100 weeks postconception in preterm and full term infants. *Arch. Dis. Child.* 1989;**64**:1579–86.

360 Congdon, P. J., Horsman, A., Ryan, S. W., Truscott, J. G., Durward, H. Spontaneous resolution of bone mineral depletion in preterm infants. *Arch. Dis. Child.* 1990;**65**:1038–42.

361 Pohlandt, F. Bone mineral deficiency as the main factor of dolichocephalic head flattening in very-low-birth-weight infants. *Pediatr. Res.* 1994;**35**:701–3.

362 Seow, W. K., Brown, J. P., Tudehope, D. A., O'Callaghan, M. Dental defects in the deciduous dentition of premature infants with low birth weight and neonatal rickets. *Pediatr. Dent.* 1984;**6**:88–92.

363 Toomey, F., Hoag, R., Batton, D., Vain, N. Rickets associated with cholestasis and parenteral nutrition in premature infants. *Radiology* 1982;**142**:85–8.

364 Koo, W. W., Kaplan, L. A., Horn, J., Tsang, R. C., Steichen, J. J. Aluminum in parenteral nutrition solution – sources and possible alternatives. *J. Parenter. Enter. Nutr.* 1986;**10**:591–5.

365 Koo, W. W., Kaplan, L. A. Aluminum and bone disorders: with specific reference to aluminum contamination of infant nutrients. *J. Am. Coll. Nutr.* 1988;**7**:199–214.

366 Koo, W. W. K. Parenteral nutrition-related bone disease. *J. Parenter. Enter. Nutr.* 1992;**16**:386–94.

367 Zuckerman, M., Pettifor, J. M. Rickets in very-low-birthweight infants born at Baragwanath Hospital. *S. Afr. Med. J.* 1994;**84**:216–20.

368 Koo, W. W. K., Bush, A. J., Walters, J., Carlson, S. E. Postnatal development of mineral status during infancy. *J. Am. Coll. Nutr.* 1998;**17**:65–70.

369 Dabezies, E. J., Warren, P. D. Fractures in very low birth weight infants with rickets. *Clin. Orthop.* 1997;**335**:233–9.

370 Koo, W. W. K., Gupta, J. M., Nayanar, V. V. *et al.* Skeletal changes in preterm infants. *Arch. Dis. Child.* 1982;**57**:447–52.

371 Glasgow, J. F., Thomas, P. S. Rachitic respiratory distress in small preterm infants. *Arch. Dis. Child.* 1977;**52**:268–73.

372 Kovar, I., Mayne, P., Barltrop, D. Plasma alkaline phosphatase activity: a screening test for rickets in preterm neonates. *Lancet* 1982;**i**:308–10.

373 Abrams, S. A., Schanler, R. J., Garza, C. Relation of bone mineralization measures to serum biochemical measures. *Am. J. Dis. Child.* 1988;**142**:1276–8.

374 Ryan, S. W., Truscott, J., Simpson, M. *et al.* Phosphate, alkaline phosphatase and bone mineralisation in preterm neonates. *Acta Paediatr.* 1993;**82**:518–21.

375 Bishop, N. J., King, F. J., Lucas, A. Increased bone mineral content of preterm infants fed with a nutrient enriched formula after discharge from hospital. *Arch. Dis. Child.* 1993;**68**:573–8.

376 Lucas, A., Brooke, O. G., Baker, B. A., Bishop, N., Morley, R. High alkaline phosphatase activity and growth in preterm neonates. *Arch. Dis. Child.* 1989;**64**:902–9.

377 Faerk, J., Peitersen, B., Petersen, S., Michaelsen, K. F. Bone mineralisation in premature infants cannot be predicted from serum alkaline phosphatase or serum phosphate. *Arch. Dis. Child Fetal Neonat. Edn.* 2002;**87**:F133–6.

378 Faerk, J., Petersen, S., Petersen, B. *et al.* Phosphorus intake is of major importance for growth velocity in premature infants. *Pediatr. Res.* 1999;**45**:915.

379 Gross, S. J. Bone mineralization in preterm infants fed human milk with and without mineral supplementation. *J. Pediatr.* 1987;**111**:450–8.

380 Tsukahara, H., Sudo, M., Umezaki, M. *et al.* Measurement of lumbar spine bone mineral density in preterm infants by dual-energy X-ray absorptiometry. *Biol. Neonate* 1993;**64**: 96–103.

381 Scariano, J. K., Walter, E. A., Glew, R. H. *et al.* Serum levels of the pyridinoline crosslinked carboxyterminal telopeptide of type I collagen (ICTP) and osteocalcin in rachitic children in Nigeria. *Clin. Biochem.* 1995;**28**:541–5.

382 Rigo, J., De Curtis, M., Pieltain, C. *et al.* Bone mineral metabolism in the micropremie. *Clin. Perinatol.* 2000;**27**: 147–70.

383 Atkinson, S. A., Bryan, M. H., Anderson, G. H. Human milk feeding in premature infants: protein, fat and carbohydrate balances in the first two weeks of life. *J. Pediatr.* 1981;**99**: 617–24.

384 Atkinson, S. A., Radde, I. C., Anderson, G. H. Macromineral balances in premature infants fed their own mothers' milk or formula. *J. Pediatr.* 1983;**102**:99–106.

385 Brooke, O. G., Onubogu, O., Heath, R., Carter, N. D. Human milk and preterm formula compared for effects on growth and metabolism. *Arch. Dis. Child.* 1987;**62**:917–23.

386 Cooper, P. A., Rothberg, A. D., Pettifor, J. M., Bolton, K. D., Devenhuis, S. Growth and biochemical response of premature infants fed pooled preterm milk or special formula. *J. Pediatr. Gastroenterol. Nutr.* 1984;**3**:749–54.

387 Kashyap, S., Schulze, K. F., Forsyth, M. *et al.* Growth, nutrient retention, and metabolic response of low-birth-weight infants fed supplemented and unsupplemented preterm human milk. *Am. J. Clin. Nutr.* 1990;**52**:254–62.

388 Stein, H., Cohen, D., Herman, A. A. B. Pooled pasteurized breast milk and untreated own mother's milk in the feeding of very low birth weight babies: a randomized controlled trial. *J. Pediatr. Gastroenterol. Nutr.* 1986;**5**:242–7.

389 Rowe, J. C., Wood, D. H., Rowe, D. W., Raisz, L. G. Nutritional hypophosphatemic rickets in a premature infant fed breast milk. *N. Engl. J. Med.* 1979;**300**:293–6.

390 Lucas, A., Brooke, O. G., Baker, B. A., Bishop, N., Morley, R. High alkaline phosphatase activity and growth in preterm neonates. *Arch. Dis. Child.* 1989;**64**:902–9.

391 Greer, F. R., McCormick, A. Improved bone mineralization and growth in premature infants fed fortified own mother's milk. *J. Pediatr.* 1988;**112**:961–9.

392 Faerk, J., Petersen, S., Peitersen, B., Michaelsen, K. F. Diet and bone mineral content at term in premature infants. *Pediatr. Res.* 2000;**47**:148–56.

393 Modanlou, H. D., Lim, M. O., Hansen, J. W., Sickles, V. Growth, biochemical status and mineral metabolism in very-low-birth-weight infants receiving fortified preterm human milk. *J. Pediatr. Gastroenterol. Nutr.* 1986;**5**:762–7.

394 Venkataraman, P. S., Blick, K. E. Effect of mineral supplementation of human milk on bone mineral content and trace element metabolism. *J. Pediatr.* 1988;**113**:220–4.

395 Chan, G. M., Mileur, L., Hansen, J. W. Calcium and phosphorus requirements in bone mineralization of preterm infants. *J. Pediatr.* 1988;**113**:225–9.

396 Horsmann, A., Ryan, S. W., Congdon, P. J., Truscott, J. G., Simpson, M. Bone mineral accretion rate and calcium intake in preterm infants. *Arch. Dis. Child.* 1989;**64**:910–18.

397 Holland, P. C., Wilkinson, A. R., Diez, J., Lindsell, D. R. Prenatal deficiency of phosphate, phosphate supplementation and rickets in very-low-birth weight infants. *Lancet* 1990;**335**: 697–701.

398 Lapillonne, A. A., Glorieux, F. H., Salle, B. L. *et al.* Mineral balance and whole body bone mineral content in very low-birth-weight infants. *Acta Paediatr. Suppl.* 1994;**405**:117–22.

399 Steichen, J. J., Cratton, T. L., Tsang, R. C. Osteopenia of prematurity: the cause and possible treatment. *J. Pediatr.* 1980;**96**:528–33.

400 Steichen, J. J., Tsang, R. C., Greer, F. R., Ho, M., Hug, G. Elevated serum 1,25 dihydroxyvitamin D concentrations in rickets of very low-birth-weight infants. *J. Pediatr.* 1981;**99**:293–8.

401 MacMahon, P., Blair, M. E., Treweeke, P., Kovar, I. Z. Association of mineral composition of neonatal intravenous feeding solutions and metabolic bone disease of prematurity. *Arch. Dis. Child.* 1989;**64**:489–93.

402 Wauben, I. P., Atkinson, S. A., Grad, T. L., Shah, J. K., Paes, B. Moderate nutrient supplementation of mother's milk for preterm infants supports adequate bone mass and short-term growth: a randomized, controlled trial. *Am. J. Clin. Nutr.* 1998;**67**:465–72.

403 Abrams, S. A., Schanler, R. J., Garza, C. Bone mineralization in former very low birth weight infants fed either human milk or commercial formula. *J. Pediatr.* 1988;**112**:956–62.

404 Abrams, S. A., Schanler, R. J., Tsang, R. C., Garza, C. Bone mineralization in former very low birth weight infants fed either human milk or commercial formula: one year follow-up observation. *J. Pediatr.* 1989;**114**:1041–4.

405 Schanler, R. J., Garza, C. Improved mineral balance in very low birth weight infants fed fortified human milk. *J. Pediatr.* 1987;**112**:452–6.

406 Pohlandt, F. Prevention of postnatal bone demineralization in very-low-birth-weight infants by individually monitored supplementation with calcium and phosphorus. *Pediatr. Res.* 1994;**35**:125–9.

407 Committee on Nutrition of the Preterm Infant, European Society of Paediatric Gastroenterology and Nutrition. *Nutrition and Feeding of Premature Infants.* Oxford: Blackwell Scientific Publications; 1987:117–32.

408 American Academy of Pediatrics. Nutritional needs of low-birth weight infants. *Pediatrics* 1985;**75**:976–86.

409 Bronner, F., Salle, B. L., Putet, G., Rigo, J., Senterre, J. Net calcium absorption in premature infants: results of 103 metabolic balance studies. *Am. J. Clin. Nutr.* 1992;**56**:1037–44.

410 Lien, E. L., Boyle, F. G., Yuhas, R., Tomarelli, R. M., Quinlan, P. The effect of triglyceride positional distribution on fatty acid absorption in rats. *J. Pediatr. Gastroenterol. Nutr.* 1997;**2**: 167–74.

411 Nelson, S. E., Rogers, R. R., Frantz, J. A., Zieger, E. E. Palm olein in infant formula: absorption of fat and minerals by normal infants. *Am. J. Clin. Nutr.* 1996;**64**:291–6.

412 Carnielli, V. P., Luijendijk, I. H. T., Van Goovener, J. B. *et al.* Structural position and amount of palmitic acid in infant formulas: effect on fat, fatty acid and mineral balance. *J. Pediatr. Gastroenterol. Nutr.* 1996;**23**:255–60.

413 Quinlan, P. T., Locker, J., Irwin, J., Lucas, A. The relationship between stool hardness and stool composition in breast- and formula-fed infants. *J. Pediatr. Gastroenterol. Nutr.* 1995;**20**:81–90.

414 Koo, W. W. K., Hammami, M., Margeson, D. P. *et al.* Reduced bone mineralization in infants fed palm olein-containing formula: a randomized, double-blinded, prospective trial. *Pediatrics* 2003;**111**:1017–23.

415 Rowe, J. C., Carey, D. E., Goetz, C. A., Adams, N. D., Horak, E. Effect of high calcium and phosphorus intake on mineral retention in very low birth weight infants chronically treated with furosemide. *J. Pediatr. Gastroenterol. Nutr.* 1989;**9**: 206–11.

416 Crofton, P. M., Stirling, H. F., Schonau, E. *et al.* Biochemical markers of bone turnover. *Horm. Res.* 1996;**45**:55–8.

417 Lemons, P. A daily physical activity programme increased the rate of weight gain and bone mass in preterm very low birth weight infants. *Evidence Based Nurs.* 2001;**4**:74.

418 Moyer-Mileur, L., Luetkemeler, M., Boomer, L., Chan, G. M. Effect of physical activity on bone mineralization in premature infants. *J. Pediatr.* 1995;**127**:620–5.

419 Moyer-Mileur, L. J., Brunstetter, V., McNaught, T. P., Gill, G., Chan, G. M. Daily physical activity program increases bone mineralization and growth in preterm very low birth weight infants. *Pediatrics* 2000;**106**:1088–92.

420 Litmanovitz, I., Dolfin, T., Friedland, O. *et al.* Early physical activity intervention prevents decrease of bone strength in very low birth weight infants. *Pediatrics* 2003;**112**: 15–19.

421 Fewtrell, M. S., Prentice, A., Jones, S. C. *et al.* Bone mineralization and turnover in preterm infants at 8–12 years of age: the effect of early diet. *J. Bone Mineral Res.* 1999;**14**: 810–20.

422 Schanler, R. J., Rifka, M. Calcium, phosphorus and magnesium needs for the low-birth-weight infant. *Acta Paediatr. Suppl.* 1994;**405**:111–16.

423 Pereira-da-Silva, L., Nurmamodo, A., Amaral, J. M. *et al.* Compatibility of calcium and phosphate in four parenteral nutrition solutions for preterm neonates. *Am. J. Health Syst. Pharm.* 2003;**60**:1041–4.

424 Pelegano, J. F., Rowe, J. C., Carey, D. E. *et al.* Simultaneous infusion of calcium and phosphorus in parenteral nutrition for premature infants: use of physiologic calcium/phosphorus ratio. *J. Pediatr.* 1989;**114**:115–19.

425 Hoehn, G. J., Carey, D. E., Rowe, J. C., Horak, E., Raye, J. R. Alternate day infusion of calcium and phosphate in very low birth weight infants: wasting of the infused mineral. *J. Pediatr. Gastroenterol. Nutr.* 1987;**6**:752–7.

426 Hoppe, B., Hesse, A., Neuhaus, T. *et al.* Urinary saturation and nephrocalcinosis in preterm infants: effect of parenteral nutrition. *Arch. Dis. Child.* 1993;**69**:299–303.

427 Kimura, S., Nose, O., Seino, Y. *et al.* Effects of alternate and simultaneous administrations of calcium and phosphorus on calcium metabolism in children receiving total parenteral nutrition. *J. Parenter. Enteral Nutr.* 1986;**10**: 513–16.

428 Hanning, R. M., Atkinson, S. A., Whyte, R. K. Efficacy of calcium glycerophosphate vs conventional mineral salts for total parenteral nutrition in low-birth-weight infants: a randomized clinical trial. *Am. J. Clin. Nutr.* 1991;**54**:903–8.

429 Chessex, P., Pineault, M., Brisson, G., Delvin, E. E., Glorieux, F. H. Role of the source of phosphate salt in improving the mineral balance of parenterally fed low birth weight infants. *J. Pediatr.* 1990;**116**:765–72.

430 Koo, W. W., Tsang, R. C., Steichen, J. J. *et al.* Vitamin D requirement in infants receiving parenteral nutrition. *J. Parenter. Enteral Nutr.* 1987;**11**:172–6.

431 Koo, W. W., Tsang, R. C., Steichen, J. J. *et al.* Parenteral nutrition for infants: effect of high versus low calcium and phosphorus content. *J. Pediatr. Gastroenterol. Nutr.* 1987;**6**:96–104.

432 Koo, W. W., Tsang, R. C. Mineral requirements of low-birth-weight infants. *J. Am. Coll. Nutr.* 1991;**10**:474–86.

433 Prestridge, L. L., Schanler, R. J., Shulman, R. J., Burns, P. A., Laine, L. L. Effect of parenteral calcium and phosphorus therapy on mineral retention and bone mineral content in very low birth weight infants. *J. Pediatr.* 1993;**122**: 761–8.

434 Schanler, R. J., Shulman, R. J., Prestridge, L. L. Parenteral nutrient needs of very low birth weight infants. *J. Pediatr.* 1994;**125**:961–8.

435 Koo, W. W. K. Parenteral nutrition-related bone disease. *J. Parenter. Enteral Nutr.* 1992;**16**:386–94.

436 Arnold, C. J., Miller, G. G., Zello, G. A. Parenteral nutrition-associated cholestasis in neonates: the role of aluminum. *Nutr. Rev.* 2003;**61**:306–10.

437 Popinska, K., Kierkus, J., Lyszkowska, M. *et al.* Aluminum contamination of parenteral nutrition additives, amino acid solutions, and lipid emulsions. *Nutrition* 1999;**15**:683–6.

438 ASCN/ASPEN Working Group on Standards for Aluminum Content of Parenteral Nutrition Solutions. Parenteral drug products containing aluminum as an ingredient or a contaminant: response to Food and Drug Administration notice of intent and request for information. *J. Parenter. Enteral Nutr.* 1991;**15**:194–8.

439 Klein, G. Aluminum in parenteral solutions revisited – again. *Am. J. Clin. Nutr.* 1995;**61**:449–56.

440 Von Stockhausen, H. B., Schrod, L., Bratter, P., Rosick, U. Aluminium loading in premature infants during intensive care as related to clinical aspects. *J. Trace Elem. Electrolytes Health Dis.* 1990;**4**:209–13.

441 Cole, D. E. C., Zlotkin, S. H. Increased sulfite as an etiological factor in the hypercalciuria associated with total parenteral nutrition. *Am. J. Clin. Nutr.* 1983;**37**:108–13.

442 Cooke, R. J., Perrin, F., Moore, J., Paule, C., Ruckman, K. Methodology of nutrient balance studies in the preterm infant. *J. Pediatr. Gastroenterol. Nutr.* 1988;**7**:434–40.

443 Bronner, F., Salle, B. L., Putet, G., Rigo, J., Senterre, J. Net calcium absorption in premature infants: results of 103 metabolic balance studies. *Am. J. Clin. Nutr.* 1992;**56**:1037–44.

444 Salle, B. L., Senterre, J., Putet, G. Calcium, phosphorus, magnesium, and vitamin D requirements in premature infants. In Salle, B. L., Swyer, P. R., eds. *Nutrition of the Low Birth Weight Infants*. New York, NY: Raven Press;1993:125–35.

445 Atkinson, S. A., Radde, I. C., Anderson, G. H. Macromineral balances in premature infants fed their own mothers' milk or formula. *J. Pediatr.* 1983;**102**:99–106.

446 Schanler, R. J., Abrams, S. A. Postnatal attainment of intrauterine macromineral accretion rates in low birth weight infants fed fortified human milk. *J. Pediatr.* 1995;**126**:441–7.

447 Schanler, R. J. Human milk fortification for premature infants. *Am. J. Clin. Nutr.* 1996;**64**:249–50.

448 Lucas, A., Fewtrell, M. S., Morley, R. *et al.* Randomized outcome trial of human milk fortification and developmental outcome in preterm infants. *Am. J. Clin. Nutr.* 1996;**64**:142–51.

449 Barrett Reis, B., Hall, R. T., Schanler, R. J. *et al.* Enhanced growth of preterm infants fed a new powdered human milk fortifier: a randomized, controlled trial. *Pediatrics* 2000;**106**:581–8.

450 Specker, B. Nutrition influences bone development from infancy through toddler years. *J. Nutr.* 2004;**134**:691S–5S.

451 Pieltain, C., De Curtis, M., Gérard, P., Rigo, J. Weight gain composition in preterm infants with dual energy x-ray absorptiometry. *Pediatr. Res.* 2001;**49**:120–4.

452 Usher, R., McLean, F. Intrauterine growth of liveborn Caucasian infants at sea level: standard obtained from measurements in 7 dimensions of infants born between 25 and 44 weeks of gestation. *J. Pediatr.* 1969;**74**:901–10.

453 Gill, A., Yu, V. Y., Bajuk, B., Astbury, J. Postnatal growth in infants born before 30 weeks' gestation. *Arch. Dis. Child.* 1986;**61**:549–53.

454 Hack, M., Weissman, B., Borawski-Clark, E. Catch-up growth during childhood among very low-birth-weight children. *Arch. Pediatr. Adolesc. Med.* 1996;**150**:1122–9.

455 Ross, G., Lipper, E. G., Auld, P. A. M. Growth achievement of very low birth weight premature children at school age. *J. Pediatr.* 1990;**117**:307–9.

456 Rigo, J., Boboli, H., Franckart, G., Pieltain, C., De Curtis, M. Surveillance de l'ancien prematuré: croissance et nutrition. *Arch. Pediatr.* 1998;**5**:449–53.

457 Cooke, R. J., McCormick, K., Griffin, I. J. *et al.* Feeding preterm infants after hospital discharge: effect of diet on body composition. *Pediatr. Res.* 1999;**46**:461–4.

458 Hillman, L. S., Salmons, S. S., Erickson, M. M. *et al.* Calciuria and aminoaciduria in very low birth weight infants fed a high-mineral premature formula with varying levels of protein. *J. Pediatr.* 1994;**125**:288–94.

459 Giles, M. M., Laing, I. A., Elton, R. A. *et al.* Magnesium metabolism in preterm infants: effects of calcium, magnesium, and phosphorus, and of postnatal and gestational age. *J. Pediatr.* 1990;**117**:147–54.

460 Lapillone, A. A., Glorieux, F. H., Salle, B. *et al.* Mineral balance and whole body bone mineral content in very-low-birth-weight infants. *Acta Pediatr. Suppl.* 1994;**405**:117–22.

461 Koo, W. W., Krug-Wispe, S., Neylan, M. *et al.* Effect of three levels of vitamin D intake in preterm infants receiving high mineral-containing milk. *J. Pediatr. Gastroenterol. Nutr.* 1995;**21**:182–9.

462 Hillman, L. S. Mineral and vitamin D adequacy in infants fed human milk or formula between 6 and 12 months of age. *J. Pediatr.* 1990;**117**:S134–42.

463 Steichen, J. J., Koo, W. W. Mineral nutrition and bone mineralization in full-term infants. *Monatsschr. Kinderheilkd.* 1992;**140**:S21–7.

464 Trotter, A., Maier, L., Pohlandt, F. Calcium and phosphorus balance of extremely preterm infants with estradiol and progesterone replacement. *Am. J. Perinatol.* 2002;**19**:23–9.

465 Trotter, A., Maier, L., Pohlandt, F. Management of the extremely preterm infant: is the replacement of estradiol and progesterone beneficial? *Paediatr Drugs.* 2001;**3**:629–37.

466 Koo, W. K., Tsang, R. C. Building better bones: calcium, magnesium, phosphorus and vitamin D. In Tsang, R. C., Zlotkin, S. H., Nichols, B. L., Hansen, J. W., eds. *Nutrition During Infancy*. Cincinnati, OH: Digital Educational Publishing. 1997:175–207.

467 Koo, W. K., Tsang, R. C. Calcium, magnesium, phosphorus and vitamin D. In Tsang, R., Lucas, A., Uauy, R., Zlotkin, S., eds. *Nutritional Needs of the Preterm Infant: Scientific Basis and Practical Guidelines*. Baltimore, MD: Williams & Wilkins; 1993:135–55.

468 Itani, O., Tsang, R. Calcium, phosphorus and magnesium in the newborn: pathophysiology and management. In Hay, W., ed. *Neonatal Nutrition and Metabolism*. St. Louis: Mosby-Year Book; 1991:171–202.

469 Koo, W. K., Tsang, R. C. Calcium, magnesium, and phosphorus. In Tsang, R. C., ed. *Nutrition in Infancy*. Philadelphia: Hanley and Belfus; 1988:419–24.

17

Trace minerals

K. Michael Hambidge

University of Colorado School of Medicine and The Children's Hospital, Denver, CO

Introduction

A trace element, by definition, contributes less than 0.01% to the total body weight. It is a term that, by common usage, applies to those elements that are consistently present in human tissues and have one or more definite, probable, or possible physiologic roles. The total body content of trace elements is small, but concentrations in individual tissues can range up to many parts per thousand. For example, the high iron concentration in erythrocytes results frequently, but mistakenly, in categorizing it as a major mineral. Trace elements that have a known or probable/possible role in human nutrition are listed in Table 17.1. This list may vary a little according to the author, reflecting the extent of current uncertainty, and it may not yet be complete. Since the publication of the last edition of this book, there has been progress, in some instances remarkable progress, in our understanding of the biology and clinical importance of those minerals that had already attracted clinical interest, while relatively little or no progress has been made with those of marginal or uncertain clinical relevance. Iron, zinc, and iodine and, to a lesser extent at this time, selenium and copper are the minerals that merit most attention in this chapter.

Though the trace elements are present in the human body in such small quantities, they are analogous to their organic counterparts, the vitamins, in that they have multiple, indispensable roles in a variety of important metabolic pathways. The activity of many enzymes is known to be dependent on one or another trace element, as is the integrity or biological activity of other proteins of cardinal importance in intermediary metabolism. The structure as well as the function of subcellular organelles is also dependent on optimal quantities of trace elements. Several of the trace elements have key roles in redox reactions and cell signaling is among other recognized roles. Several of these minerals have regulatory roles in gene expression. All of these biological functions are, of course, specific for individual elements.

Both deficiencies and excesses of the trace elements are causes of morbidity and mortality. The dose–response curve depicted in Figure 17.1 is applicable to all nutrients but has perhaps found special application with the trace elements because of long-recognized toxicity of overdoses of some of the essential trace elements, notably iron and copper, as well as the toxicity of non-essential elements such as mercury and aluminum. With the exception of iron, nutritional deficiencies of the trace elements in the general population of North America are quite subtle and frequently undetected. Trace element fortification of an ever-increasing number of products and the widespread use of mineral supplements has resulted in notably high intakes by many people at all stages of the life cycle, but marginal or low intakes for specific minerals still occur in North America. On a global basis, trace element deficiencies continue to be a major contributor to morbidity and mortality, especially in young children. Indeed, our awareness of the extent of this public health problem is currently increasing as the role of zinc deficiency in childhood morbidity and mortality is documented and the occurrence of selenium deficiency is also recognized while efforts to contain iron and iodine deficiency continue.

While the low birth weight infant (LBWI) will be the principal focus of this chapter, even the term infant merits special consideration with respect to trace element nutrition. Breast milk or/and neonatal stores usually assure

Neonatal Nutrition and Metabolism. Second Edition, ed. P. Thureen and W. Hay. Published by Cambridge University Press.
© Cambridge University Press 2006.

Table 17.1. Trace elements of biologic interest

Importance	Element
Identified human deficiencies	Iron, iodine, zinc, copper, selenium
Limited evidence for human deficiencies	Chromium, molybdenum, manganese
Pharmacologic value	Fluorine
Other trace elements of known biological importance in the human	Cobalt
Other trace elements of established biological importance in other mammalian species	Nickel, arsenic, vanadium, boron, silicon
Other trace elements of possible biologic importance in mammals	Beryllium, tin, cadmium, lead
Examples of trace elements of toxic importance only	Aluminum, mercury

Table 17.2. Overview of trace element homeostasis*

Element	Intestine		Storage	Liver biliary excretion	Kidney excretion in urine
	Fractional absorption	Endogenous excretion			
Iron	+ + + +		+ +		
Iodine			+ +		+ + +
Zinc	+ + +	+ +			+
Copper	+		+	+ + +	
Selenium					+ + +
Manganese	+ + +			+ + +	
Chromium	?				+
Molybdenum					+

* Plus signs indicate the relative importance on a scale of least (+) to most (+ + + +). No plus sign indicates no importance.

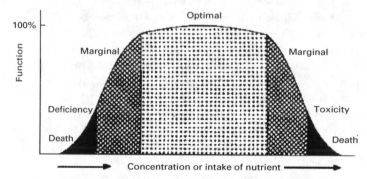

Figure 17.1. Dependence of biological function on tissue concentration of a nutrient (Used by permission .[98]).

adequate supply of bioavailable trace elements until 4–6 months of postnatal life. Subsequently, the provision of iron-fortified infant cereal may avert the risk of iron-deficiency in infants not receiving iron fortified formula, but the older exclusively breast-fed infant is at risk from suboptimal intake of zinc.[1] Meats, good sources of bioavailable iron and zinc, are to be encouraged as early complementary foods. The formula-fed term infant receives generous supplies of key trace minerals, though further research is warranted to refine these intakes. In addition to nutritional deficiencies, morbidity from genetic defects in trace element metabolism first becomes evident in infancy. Notable examples are *acrodermatitis enteropathica*[2] and Menke's Steely Hair Syndrome.[3] Other genetic defects, not specifically of trace element metabolism, may lead to clinically significant trace mineral deficiencies. Examples are malabsorption of zinc in cystic fibrosis[4] and excessive urine losses of zinc in biliary atresia.[5] Other genetic defects, notably hemachromatosis and hepatolenticular degeneration, both of which result in trace mineral toxicity, do not become clinically evident until later in development, though perinatal hemochromatosis has been described.[6]

It is helpful to have a working knowledge of trace element homeostasis, which varies widely for different minerals (Table 17.2). For some elements the gastrointestinal tract has the major or only role. For others excretion via the kidneys has the key role. Two minerals, copper and manganese, are excreted primarily via the bile and can accumulate in toxic excess with biliary obstruction.[7] One important cause of the latter, especially in the LBWI, is intravenous nutrition and the parenteral supply of these elements requires reduction in these circumstances.

The LBWI requires generous exogenous sources of trace minerals for two reasons. First, neonatal stores are low.

In addition to iron and copper, it is now known that this applies also to zinc.[8] Second, the relatively rapid growth of the LBWI, once this has started, increases the demand for trace elements. Other factors may also be invoked, including, possibly, immaturity of homeostatic mechanisms.[8] Therapeutic modalities, notably the use of erythropoietin, can also increase requirements, in this case of iron.[9]

Iron

Biological role

The most prominent role of iron is in oxygen transport, principally in hemoglobin. The iron is present in a porphyrin-heme complex and an adjacent histidine residue of the globin maintains the iron in the ferrous state, which facilitates a reversible association between iron and oxygen. Among the other known iron-proteins, cytochrome a, b, and c and cytochrome oxidase are the most prominent. These enzymes are essential for electron transport and have a central role in cellular energetics.[10]

Metabolism

Whole body iron homeostasis is dependent on regulation of absorption in the upper small intestine and normally there is very little excretion of this mineral.[11] Absorption of inorganic iron is limited not only by regulatory mechanisms but also by dietary factors that limit bioavailability. The high bioavailability of iron from human milk is of limited practical significance because of the very low iron concentrations. Factors associated with improved absorption of iron are the ferrous state and ascorbate. Dietary factors that contribute to the very high incidence of iron deficiency in older infants and young children in developing countries include low intakes of meat and high levels of dietary phytate from cereal grains.

The 28- and 40-week fetus contain 64 and 94 µg iron per gram of fat-free tissue respectively.[12] Almost 80% of the iron in the term neonate is present in hemoglobin. The physiological depression of erythropoiesis for approximately 2 months postnatally, together with progressive expansion of blood volume, results in about a 30% decline in hemoglobin concentration. The degradation of hemoglobin releases iron which is used by other tissues, including the brain, and, to some extent, initially increases stores resulting in serum ferritin levels at 1 month as high as 400 µg L^{-1}.[13] The acquisition of iron in utero is sufficient to meet the needs of the term breast-fed infant until at least 4 months postnatally, despite the very low levels of iron in human milk.

The special circumstances of the premature infant will be considered below under "requirements."

Deficiency

Early postnatal anemia is more pronounced in preterm than in the term infant. In contrast to the third-trimester fetus in utero, erythropoiesis decreases abruptly after birth in the premature infant, and the hemoglobin concentration declines at a rate of approximately 1 g dL^{-1} week^{-1}.[14] During the first 1–3 months of postnatal life, the extent of the early "anemia of prematurity" depends on the gestational age. This early decline is not affected by the administration of exogenous iron unless given in conjunction with erythropoietin. After 1–3 months, postnatal erythropoiesis commences and total body hemoglobin increases. Because of a rapidly expanding blood volume, this may not be reflected in an immediate increase in circulating hemoglobin concentrations. If adequate iron is not given postnatally, late anemia of prematurity will start to develop sometime after 2 months of postnatal life. Iron depletion will be reflected by a decrease in serum ferritin and disappearance of stainable iron from the bone marrow. Red cell protoporphyrin concentrations increase and mean cell volume will decrease. This will be followed by a decline in hemoglobin concentration.

Effects of iron deficiency are not limited to those of iron-deficiency anemia.[15] The long-term cognitive sequelae and shorter-term motor sequelae of iron deficiency are particularly notable.[16] These effects occur regardless of potentially confounding variables such as socio-economic status. Adverse effects on brain function occur before the development of anemia, which is a relatively late development in the progression of iron deficiency. There are variable reports on the reversibility of the neurocognitive sequelae of iron deficiency in the infant and toddler.[17,18]

The role of iron in resistance to infection is complex. On the one hand, free iron is essential for the multiplication of all bacteria and excess iron is thought to enhance the risk of gram-negative septicemia. On the other hand, iron is necessary for the normal development and functional integrity of the immune system. Other functional deficits resulting from iron deficiency include decreased exercise tolerance. Anorexia and failure to thrive are other possible complications of iron deficiency.

Toxicity

Iron is a strong oxidant and is very toxic in excess. Acute iron overload can cause fatal damage to the liver and other organs. The premature infant is at especially high risk from excess iron because of low serum iron-binding capacity and immaturity of anti-oxidant defenses.[19] Research that has linked the iron status of LBWI to retinopathy of prematurity or to bronchopulmonary dysplasia has been either negative or inconclusive. Concerns have related primarily to iron administered in packed red cell infusions. The preterm infant is capable of loading iron into ferritin when it is delivered more slowly as is the case with ingested iron. However, the possibility of damage from oxidative stress resulting from excessive intake of iron emphasizes the need for caution in providing excessive quantities of this mineral.[8]

Another putative concern of excess iron is the recognized interactions with other minerals, most notably zinc,[20] though a negative effect of iron on zinc bioavailability has been most convincingly demonstrated only when both are given simultaneously as inorganic supplements. Additional research is necessary to ensure that current recommendations for iron in preterm formulas do not have any negative effect on zinc bioavailability.

Iron requirements

Factors to be considered in determining iron requirements and the risk of iron deficiency in LBWI include:

1. Body weight: the quantity of body iron in the fetus is positively correlated with body weight. Because of the accumulation of adipose tissue, the quantity of iron per kg body weight remains fairly constant at 70–80 mg iron per kg body weight, despite the increase in concentration of iron in fat-free tissues as the third trimester progresses.
2. Gestational age: during the last trimester the fetus accumulates 1.7–2.0 mg iron per day.
3. Initial hemoglobin: the bulk of the fetal iron (approximately 80%) is present as hemoglobin. One gram of hemoglobin contains 3.4 mg Fe. Iron stores in the liver and spleen at birth amount to only approximately 10 mg kg^{-1}. The remaining body iron (7 mg kg^{-1}), is in the tissues. The initial hemoglobin value is lower in preterm infants, e.g., 9–11 g dL^{-1} at 30–34 weeks gestation.
4. High rate of postnatal growth and of expansion of blood volume leading to higher requirements.
5. Postnatal blood loss, especially that resulting from the need for repetitive laboratory assays.
6. Treatment with rhEpo which stimulates early erythropoiesis.
7. Infections. Even a mild infection can increase iron requirements.

Other factors tend to mitigate the extent of iron deficiency, i.e.,

8. Relatively high absorption of iron from formulas.[21] This may be related to either immature regulatory mechanisms in the gut or/and upregulation of absorption due to lower body iron.
9. A high incidence of exposure to iron-containing blood products which is, however, very variable. Packed RBCs usually have a hematocrit of 70% and a hemoglobin concentration of 25 g per 100ml. With a conversion factor of 3.4 mg elemental iron per g hemoglobin, 85 mg iron will be administered per 100 ml packed RBCs. A typical transfusion of 10–15 ml kg^{-1} provides 8–13 mg iron per kg body weight.

Premature infants weighing 1000 to 2000g require 2–3 mg supplemental Fe per kg body weight by approximately 2 weeks postnatal age. This iron may be administered either as ferrous sulfate or given in an iron-fortified formula. This level of iron intake should be continued for 12–15 months. If the birth weight is less than 1000 g, this supplement should be increased to 3 to 4 mg Fe kg^{-1} day^{-1}. Higher medicinal doses of iron (6 mg or more per day) are required with rhEpo therapy.

Recent recommendations for preterm infant formulas are a minimum of 1.7 mg Fe L^{-1} and a maximum of 3.0 mg Fe L^{-1}.[8]

Iron requirements for the intravenously fed premature infant have been calculated at 200 µg Fe kg^{-1} day^{-1}. Because of the uncertainties related to administration of parenteral iron it is not recommended to normally start adding iron to intravenous infusates before 2 months postnatal age.

Zinc

Biological roles

The ubiquity of zinc in biology, the crucial roles of this micronutrient in cellular growth and differentiation and the wealth of data from animal models attesting to the extraordinary importance of zinc in pre- and postnatal growth and development all serve to emphasize the extraordinary importance of this mineral to the LBWI.[22] Zinc has been favored in evolution for its exceptional ability to form strong but flexible and rapidly exchanging ligands with organic molecules,[23] especially proteins and nucleic acids. Zinc is also relatively safe, not having the oxidant properties of iron or copper, and can be transported and incorporated into biological systems relatively simply and safely. Zinc proteins account for 3% of the human genome that has been identified.[24] Prominent among the zinc proteins are proteins with the zinc

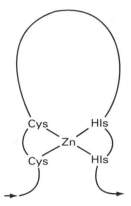

Figure 17.2. "Zinc fingers" binding to DNA.

finger motif (Figure 17.2), including those that are transcription proteins and those that serve at hormone receptor sites. Many enzymes are zinc metalloenzymes, with a zinc atom at the catalytic site, and others sometimes present with a structural role. Zinc has many other structural roles, for example, in biological membranes. Among other prominent recognized roles of zinc are those in gene expression[25] and those in signal transduction. In the brain, zinc is required for glutaminergic synaptic conduction.[26] All cells, tissues, and organs depend extensively on zinc for a wide range of biological roles, some quite generalized to most or all cells, others specific for specific tissues. Some of these have a specific role in early development of the conceptus.[27]

Metabolism

Physiologic quantities of zinc are absorbed primarily by a saturable transport mechanism.[28] Specific zinc transporters have been identified both at the brush border membrane[29] and at the basolateral membrane of enterocytes in the small intestine.[30] These can be upregulated in response to high zinc intakes, but the fraction of zinc absorbed varies inversely with the quantity of bioavailable zinc ingested. The intestinal tract, including the pancreas, is also the major site for secretion and subsequent partial excretion of endogenous zinc.[31] It appears that regulation of the quantity of endogenous zinc excreted via the intestine has the major role in the maintenance of whole body zinc homeostasis. The urine is a minor, though not entirely insignificant route of excretion of endogenous zinc. On a body weight basis, urine zinc excretion rates are unusually high (averaging about 35 μg Zn kg^{-1} day^{-1}) during the first 5 weeks of postnatal life.[32] These rates then decline quite rapidly to the adult range of $\leq$10 μg per kg body weight

day^{-1}. Integumental losses in the preterm infant are probably negligible.

The concentration of zinc in the fetal liver from 20 to 40 week's gestation ranges from ~100–300 g Zn per g wet weight, with a small decline as gestational age advances.[33] At term, hepatic zinc accounts for 20% of total term neonatal zinc compared with 2% in the adult.[8] These higher levels are associated with a larger fraction of hepatic zinc attached to metallothionein,[34] which probably serves as a readily available store in early postnatal life. The large percentage of body zinc is found in bone and muscle and most of this, at least in the adult, exchanges with zinc in plasma only slowly.[35] Though zinc concentrations vary to some extent between tissues and organs, unlike iron and iodide, zinc is not concentrated primarily in any one organ. Moreover, within individual cells zinc is present in all organelles. Thus it is a trace element in every sense of the word.

The premature infant absorbs approximately 25% of zinc from fortified formulas or fortified breast milk.[36] This is similar to the efficiency of absorption from high zinc intakes expected at any age. The size of the exchangeable zinc pool (EZP: the combined pools of zinc that exchange with zinc in plasma within 3 days) is positively correlated with net absorption which is consistent with the conclusion that zinc stores can be at least partially maintained/replenished in the very low birth weight infant (VLBWI) by good absorption of exogenous zinc postnatally. The EZP in VLBWI is relatively high, accounting for 50% or more of total body zinc. While some of this is attributable to labile hepatic neonatal stores, it is unclear whether a substantial amount of bone and/or muscle zinc is readily exchangeable in this population.

Zinc deficiency

Globally, zinc deficiency is widespread in infants and young children in developing countries, being a major cause of morbidity and mortality and of impaired growth.[37,38] It has been calculated recently that administration of adequate zinc is fourth among relatively simple putative preventive measures of any kind for reducing under 5-year childhood mortality.[39] Used as a preventive or treatment, intervention has been calculated to have the potential to achieve a reduction in deaths of 350 000 and 400 000 per year respectively. This reduction in mortality would be achieved principally by a reduction in deaths from diarrhea and from pneumonia and an even greater reduction in childhood morbidity would be achieved. The defects in zinc-dependent host-defense mechanisms that underlie the high prevalence and severity of zinc-responsive/preventable diarrhea and pneumonia include, but are not limited to, defects in both T-cell and B-cell function.[40]

There are special reasons for the high risk of zinc deficiency in the developing world, notably the poor intake of bioavailable zinc from transitional and later diets and excessive losses in diarrheal fluids. However, growth-limiting zinc deficiency, apparently of dietary origin has been quite extensively documented in infants and young children in North America within recent years,[41] studies that have been included in a recent meta-analysis of effects of zinc supplementation on physical growth worldwide.[42] Though data are still quite limited, brain growth and function can also be affected adversely by zinc deficiency in infants and young children, including cognitive and motor development.[43,44] Both physical growth and brain function have been demonstrated to improve in premature infants in North America when provided with additional zinc through the first year of postnatal life.[45] Special benefits from postnatal zinc supplementation starting quite early in infancy have been documented in those delivered small-for-gestational-age (SGA).[46,47] SGA infants in North America have been shown recently to have low zinc mass in the EZP even on a body weight basis, suggesting greater than typical needs for exogenous zinc in the young SGA infant.[48]

Severe zinc deficiency has been identified in term and/or premature infants in three main circumstances. These are:

1. Acquired severe deficiency states. Most, but not all of these, cases have been attributable at least in part to intravenous feeding without adequate addition of zinc to the infusate.[49] This problem has not been reported recently following the standard provision of adequate quantities of zinc in the infusates.

2. The rare, autosomal recessive inherited disorder, *acrodermatitis enteropathica*. A defect in one of the zinc transporters has been reported in this disorder[50] resulting in an impairment of the normal carrier-mediated intestinal absorption of zinc. It usually presents clinically by 2–3 months of age in the formula-fed infant, but clinical manifestations may be delayed until after weaning if the infant is breast-fed.

3. Failure of the mammary gland to secrete normal quantities of zinc into the milk even when the mother's zinc nutritional status is apparently normal. There have now been several case reports of this circumstance, which is analogous to the lethal milk mutation in mice which results from a defective zinc transporter in the mammary gland.[51] In the majority of reports the symptomatic infant has been born prematurely. An infant born at term and breast-fed for 6 months by one of the subjects

remained asymptomatic, whereas a premature infant fed by the same mother developed severe symptomatic zinc deficiency by 2–3 months postnatal age.[51,52]

The hallmark of severe zinc deficiency states is the skin rash with its characteristic acro-orificial distribution. The dermatitis also involves flexures and friction areas and may become more generalized. In premature infants, characteristic changes in the anterior neck fold may occur at an early stage, with a poorly marginated erythema in the depth of the fold which becomes well demarcated and scaling within 5 days.[49] Exematoid, psoriaform, vesiculobullous, and pustular lesions may be present. Mucous membranes are characteristically involved at an early stage with dermatitis, glossitis, and conjunctivitis. Histologically, the early lesions are characterized by loss of the granular layer of the epidermis and replacement of this layer by clear cells and focal parakeratosis. If untreated, the epidermis becomes increasingly psoriaform and the parakeratosis becomes more and more confluent. Pallor of the upper part of the epidermis, attributable to the formation of balloon cells with pyknotic nuclei, is the single most typical histologic finding.

Alopecia becomes prominent in poorly treated *acrodermatitis enteropathica*. The majority of patients exhibit diarrhea. Characteristically, there is cessation of weight gain with onset of the rash. If untreated, failure to thrive will be progressive. Depressed mood is a consistent and notable feature of severe zinc deficiency. Premature infants exhibit excessive crying and difficulty in consolation. Susceptibility to bacterial and candida infections is evident with evidence of impaired lymphocyte, especially T-cell function. Leukocyte function is also zinc-dependent and has been found to be impaired in *acrodermatitis enteropathica*. In the pre-zinc era, *acrodermatitis enteropathica* typically had a downhill course, with a fatal outcome in later infancy or early childhood.

The severe acute presentation of zinc deficiency is clinically quite dramatic. In contrast, "milder" degrees of zinc deficiency are clinically nonspecific and cannot be diagnosed by clinical exam. Recent experience in the developing world, however, has demonstrated that these "milder" presentations can be fatal in conjunction with inadequately treated infections of the respiratory and gastrointestinal systems.

Diagnosis of zinc deficiency

Diagnosis of the severe acute zinc deficiency syndromes is based on clinical exam supported by the finding of a very low plasma zinc concentration, i.e., less than 55 µg dL^{-1}. In the milder cases of zinc deficiency, plasma zinc may be in a normal range or only slightly depressed (<70 µg dL^{-1}). Appropriate suspicion of the diagnosis is then based on a combination of clinical findings, e.g., unexplained slowing of physical growth, and likely clinical and, especially, nutritional circumstances. Plasma zinc concentrations are unusually high during the first week or two of postnatal life in the premature infant, averaging 100–110 µg Zn dL^{-1}. Subsequently, these fall quite rapidly to adult levels or often considerably lower.[53] The extent of this decline varies with the type of feeding and may be related primarily to variations in zinc nutritional status rather than to temporary physiologic changes or to low levels of serum albumin. In our own experience, there appears to be little effect of changes in serum albumin on plasma zinc until albumin levels fall to 3 g dL^{-1}, below which plasma zinc may drop about 10 µg dL^{-1} for every 1 g dL^{-1} decline in serum albumin.[5] Another factor that may have an important effect on circulating zinc concentrations in this population is bone reabsorption. Plasma zinc concentrations have been found to be higher in premature infants with osteopenia and bone fractures than in infants matched for postconceptional age who have no evidence of rickets.[54] Zinc concentrations in erythrocytes are unusually low in early postnatal life because the great majority of erythrocyte zinc is accounted for by the zinc present in carbonic anhydrase. Erythrocyte carbonic anhydrase activity is especially low in the premature infant.[55]

Zinc requirements

Based on a factorial approach, dietary zinc requirements have recently been calculated to be 2.0, 1.7, and 1.3 mg kg^{-1} day^{-1} for very young but growing infants with weights of less than 1000 g, 1000–2000 g, and 2000–3500 g respectively.[8] These calculations assume that the VLBWI and LBWI have no need to accumulate the same stores of zinc that are accumulated by the fetus during the third trimester; they also assume that the stores that have been accumulated in the second trimester and up until delivery in the third trimester are available for utilization during the first 2 postnatal months. They were based on 30% absorption, which it now appears is too high.[36] Using a figure of 25%,[36] these figures need revision to 2.4, 2.0, and 1.6 mg Zn kg^{-1} day^{-1}. The calculations for retention required have been based on remarkably high data for fetal accumulation rates for zinc that have never been subjected to formal peer review or independently verified. Nor is this type of analysis likely to be repeated. Another substantial uncertainty is the minimal loss of endogenous zinc via the intestine. Further research is required to determine if the relatively high losses reported recently[36] result from regu-

latory mechanisms to maintain homeostasis when intake and the quantity absorbed are both higher than needed or from lack of regulation in the VLBWI leading to excessive losses.

Factorial calculations for the intravenously fed infant are a little simpler.[56] Fecal losses average 25 µg Zn kg^{-1} day^{-1} in the intravenously fed infant,[57] though it is possible that, as in the adult, gastrointestinal losses may be much higher in the presence of abnormal gastrointestinal fluid losses. Urine zinc losses have been found to vary very substantially depending on the commercial source of amino acids used in the infusate. Such losses make a very substantial difference to estimated requirements, and these are difficult to account for until more complete data on the effect of different amino acids infusates are available. The recommended figure of 400 µg Zn per kg body weight[56] provides some margin for excessive urine zinc losses. The results of studies based on balance data and on plasma zinc data give some support to this factorial calculation. Thus, premature infants were found to retain 240 µg Zn kg^{-1} day^{-1} when given 450 µg Zn kg^{-1} day^{-1} intravenously.[57] Low-birth-weight premature infants were also found to have a decrease in plasma zinc with intakes of 200 µg kg^{-1} day^{-1} of zinc, but this was not observed with intravenous intakes of 400 µg kg^{-1} day^{-1}.[58]

Treatment of zinc deficiency

A standard recommendation for treatment of suspected mild zinc deficiency is 1–2 mg kg^{-1} day^{-1} of zinc. One milligram of the zinc ion (Zn^{++}) is equivalent to 4.5 mg zinc sulfate (ZnSO$_4$). In cases of severe zinc deficiency attributable to a defect in mammary zinc secretion, human milk can be supplemented with 2–4 mg kg^{-1} day^{-1} of zinc. Increase this dose if necessary. Skin rash should resolve in 2–3 days. Zinc supplements can be discontinued when other zinc-containing foods are introduced into the diet. However, in the treatment of classic *acrodermatitis enteropathica*, permanent zinc therapy is necessary to achieve and maintain a complete clinical remission. Doses of 20–30 mg zinc per day are likely to be needed in infants with *acrodermatitis enteropathica*.

Toxicity

Zinc does interfere with copper absorption at the level of the intestinal mucosal cell.[59] The quantities of zinc used in the treatment of severe zinc deficiency states may be sufficient to at least mildly impair copper status.[60] Monitoring of serum copper or ceruloplasmin concentrations is recommended.

Selenium

Biologic role

Selenium is an essential component of glutathione peroxidase (GSHPx), which catalyzes the reduction of hydrogen peroxide to water by the addition of reducing equivalents derived from glutathione.[61] This enzyme is also capable of catalyzing the reduction of a wide range of lipid hydroperoxides to the corresponding hydroxy acids. This becomes important when peroxides of unsaturated fatty acids are released from the cell membrane by the action of phospholipase A_2. In the absence of dietary selenium when GSHPx levels are low, accumulation of fatty acid peroxide will lead to the formation of fatty acid peroxyl radicals or oxy radicals under the catalytic activity of iron. Thus selenium is an important nutrient in the body's defenses against free radicals.[62] Four types of GSHPx have been identified. Thioredoxin reductase and three iodothyronine deiodinases are among the other selenoproteins that have been identified.[63]

Selenium metabolism/homeostasis

Fractional absorption of dietary selenium is relatively high, averaging about 60%.[64] From some foods, for example, human milk, absorption is as high as 80%. Absorption and bioavailability depend on the chemical form. For example, when selenium is added as a supplement to formula, bioavailability is greatest from selenite and least favorable from selenomethionine and selenocysteine;[65] in contrast, in the postabsorptive state, absorption of selenomethionine is greater. Distribution of selenomethionine within the body is different, with a considerably greater percentage being taken up by skeletal muscle. As the biologic significance of this difference in distribution is poorly understood, it is advisable to use the selenite or selenate form both enterally and intravenously.[63] Homeostasis of selenium metabolism is controlled by the kidney. Urine selenium excretion reflects recent selenium intake. Highest body selenium concentrations are found in liver, tooth enamel, and nails, but the majority of selenium is in skeletal muscle. The total adult body content of selenium in North America is about 15 mg, but in New Zealand, where selenium intakes are lower, body content is only about 6 mg.

Selenium deficiency

Selenium deficiency is now recognized as the major etiologic factor in Keshan disease, an often fatal dilated (congestive) cardiomyopathy, affecting children and young women in a large geographic area from the northeast toward the southwest of China.[66] Histologically, there are focal areas of myocyte loss and fibrous replacement scattered throughout the ventricular sub-epicardium. The incidence and severity of Keshan disease have been dramatically reduced following public health measures to provide selenium supplementation in the affected geographic areas.[67] A few similar case reports concern patients maintained on long-term intravenous nutrition in North America.[68] Skeletal myopathies have also been attributable to selenium deficiency in these circumstances.[69] Milder cases of selenium deficiency have been reported recently in parenterally fed infants and children.[70] Clinical manifestations were a macrocytosis and loss of hair pigment. Selenium deficiency may also have been an important cause of morbidity in some infants suffering from protein energy malnutrition.[71]

In the quite recent past, selenium intakes of formula-fed infants have been notably lower than those of breast-fed infants. These low levels have been associated with low serum selenium levels, but have not had any detectable clinical consequences. In contrast, low selenium intake in preterm infants was linked to hemolytic anemia a quarter of a century ago.[72] Selenium concentrations in serum and erythrocytes from cord blood of preterm infants do not differ from those of infants born at term. However, in VLBWI, selenium concentrations dropped very rapidly within 72 hours of delivery.[73] Particularly, low plasma selenium concentrations, which persist for many weeks, have been found in premature infants who develop bronchopulmonary dysplasia. As a component of GSHPx, selenium functions as an antioxidant[63] and thus could be protective from the high level of oxidative stress to which low birth weight infants are exposed. In a prospective study in New Zealand, where selenium intakes are low, the extent of the decline in plasma selenium of preterm infants postnatally was associated with the extent of respiratory morbidity and those with oxygen dependency at 28 days had significantly lower selenium levels.[74] However, it remains uncertain to what extent selenium deficiency may contribute to the onset or severity of the disease processes resulting from oxygen damage in the very low birth weight premature infant. Nor is it known if suboptimal selenium intake may impair thyroid function in preterm infants secondary to impaired conversion of thyroxin to tri-iodothyronine.

Diagnosis

Whole blood, erythrocyte, and plasma (serum) selenium concentrations are depressed in selenium deficiency states. Activity of GSHPx in erythrocytes and serum is also reduced. These laboratory parameters of selenium status vary widely according to age and geographical location (i.e., geochemical environments). Though average adult blood selenium levels in North America vary by 100% between populations with "medium" and "high" selenium exposure, whole blood GSHPx activity is the same because selenium intake is adequate to assure maximal activity of this enzyme in all subjects. On the other hand, GSHPx activity is lower in New Zealand, where it is positively correlated with blood selenium.[75] Plasma selenium in cord blood averages 40–50 ng mL^{-1} (0.5–0.63 μM). In breast-fed infants, or in infants fed a formula containing a similar quantity of selenium (i.e., about 20 μg L^{-1}) in North America, levels increase to an average of 75–100 mg mL^{-1} by 6–12 months.[64,76] However, in some countries, selenium intake and selenium levels are much lower[77] and GSHPx activity correlates with plasma selenium levels.[78] Many plasma selenium levels below 40 ng mL^{-1} and even below 10 ng mL^{-1} have been documented in subjects who have had no overt signs of selenium deficiency. However, selenium levels below 40 ng mL^{-1} and especially below 10 ng mL^{-1} have also been associated with clinical evidence of selenium deficiency.

Toxicity

Although excess selenium can cause serious economic consequences in agriculture, chronic toxicity of selenium does not appear to be a major problem in humans. Loss of hair, brittleness of fingernails, garlic odor, a high incidence of dental caries, increased fatigue, and irritability were reported to be signs of selenosis in an early survey of South Dakota in which urinary selenium excretion was elevated.

Requirements

Selenium requirements have been especially difficult to define in adults because of the outstanding extent to which long-term adaptation can take place to low selenium intakes. Thus, adults in New Zealand, though exhibiting lower blood selenium levels, have no recognized ill-effects from selenium intakes that are extremely low by standards in most parts of the world, including North America. It has been calculated that North Americans require about 70 μg Se day^{-1}, whereas only 20 μg Se day^{-1} is needed to maintain balance in young New Zealand women. However, from studies in China including measurements of glutathione peroxidase activity, it has been concluded that the minimal requirement for adults is 50 μg Se day^{-1}.[79] In infants, requirements have been calculated at 2.5–3.0 μg^{-1}

Se kg day^{-1}. The minimum concentration recommended for preterm formulas is 1.8 mg per 100 kcal.[8]

Because of the high absorption of selenium, estimates for intravenous requirements are only a little lower than those for oral requirements. Recommendations for infants fed intravenously are 2 μg Se kg^{-1} day^{-1}. If renal function is impaired, it may be judicious to lower this level. Selenate is probably the chemical form of choice for intravenous administration.

Copper

Biologic role

Copper has a major role in aerobic metabolism as an essential component of cytochrome oxidase, the terminal oxidase in the electron transport chain which plays a crucial role in the electron shuttle of aerobic metabolism. Cytochrome oxidase catalyzes the oxidation of reduced cytochrome C by molecular oxygen, which is itself reduced to water. This enzyme is thus necessary for the production of most of the energy of metabolism. Copper-containing monoamine oxidases, including lysyl oxidase, are necessary for the cross-linking of collagen and elastin. Lysyl oxidase catalyzes the oxidative deamination of epsilon amino groups of lysine, a necessary step in the synthesis of desmosine. Dopamine beta hydroxylase is another copper-containing enzyme necessary for the synthesis of catecholamines. Tyrosinase, which catalyzes the first two steps in the oxidation of tyrosine to melanin, is another example of an oxidative cuproenzyme. Both mitochondrial and cytosolic superoxide dismutase enzymes contain copper. These enzymes catalyze the dismutation of superoxide free radical ions with the formation of molecular oxygen and hydrogen peroxide. Thus, while the cupric ion and some copper enzymes are pro-oxidant, others are very important physiologic antioxidants.

Because it is so highly reactive, copper must be transported through the circulation tightly bound to ceruloplasmin, a glycoprotein that contains six copper atoms per molecule (0.32% copper).[80] Ceruloplasmin also appears to have several other roles including ferroxidase activity. In this capacity, ceruloplasmin and another copper enzyme, ferroxidase 2, catalyzes the oxidation of stored ferrous iron to ferric iron, a step that is necessary before binding to transferrin for transport to the bone marrow.

Absorption, metabolism and excretion of copper

In the adult, approximately one-third of ingested copper is absorbed in the stomach and small intestine.[81] Percentage absorption is inversely related to the quantity ingested and is increased in copper deficiency states. Fractional absorption also depends on the chemical form and on other dietary constituents. Ascorbic acid inhibits copper absorption, probably by reducing cupric ions to cuprous ions. Copper absorption is enhanced by fructose. Zinc, iron, and cadmium can interfere with copper absorption at the level of the intestinal mucosa. Absorbed copper is transported in the portal circulation attached to albumin and is taken up by the hepatocytes, in which it may be temporarily stored attached to metallothionein. Large hepatic stores of copper are accumulated by the fetus during the third trimester.[82] Within the hepatocytes, copper is used for the synthesis of cuprous proteins, especially ceruloplasmin, which is released 3 days later into the systemic circulation. Because of its chemical reactivity, it appears that copper must be transported in the circulation tightly bound to this cuproprotein. The rate of ceruloplasmin synthesis is low in the term neonate, gradually increasing to an adult level by about 3 months of age. Circulating levels of ceruloplasmin, and hence of plasma copper, are correspondingly low. Synthesis of ceruloplasmin in the premature infant is exceptionally low and increases only slowly so that at 40 weeks postconception, circulating levels of copper and ceruloplasmin are similar to those at delivery in the term infant. In order for copper to be released when ceruloplasmin attaches to its peripheral receptor sites, cupric ions must be reduced to cuprous ions, primarily by ascorbic acid. This may be the reason why the bone lesions of scurvy are so similar to those of copper deficiency. The term neonate contains about 17 mg copper, of which one-half to two-thirds is in the liver.[83] Neonatal hepatic copper concentrations are of the order of ~200–400 μg Cu per g dry weight or 10–20 times that of the adult liver. Two-thirds of the neonatal hepatic copper is in a special storage form attached to metallothionein.[83] During the third trimester, the fetus accumulates 50 μg Cu per kg body weight day^{-1}. Two-thirds of this copper is located in the liver. The major route of excretion of endogenous copper is the bile. Copper is complexed in a form that renders it unavailable for reabsorption. Copper excretion in urine of the premature infant is less than 5 μg Cu kg^{-1} day^{-1}.

Copper deficiency

The premature infant is at risk from copper deficiency because of the limited hepatic copper stores. Clinical manifestations of copper deficiency may be evident by 2–3 months following delivery.[84,85] The risk of copper deficiency in premature infants in North America appears to

have been greatly diminished by steps to provide adequate copper supplements in formulas consumed by premature infants. Several case reports have cited clinical copper deficiency in infants fed intravenously without the addition of copper to the infusate.[86] Chronic diarrhea or fat malabsorption aggravates the risk of copper deficiency.

The principal features of copper deficiency are a hypochromic anemia that is unresponsive to iron therapy, neutropenia, and osteoporosis. The bone marrow exhibits megaloblastic changes and vacuolization of the erythroid series. Iron deposits may be seen by electron microscopy in mitochondria and in some of the cytoplasmic vacuoles in red blood cell precursors. Iron stores in the intestinal mucosa, reticuloendothelial system, and liver are increased. The anemia is initially hypoferremic, but later becomes hyperferremic because of a decreased uptake of transferrin-bound iron by the developing erythrocytes. Anemia is attributed in part to lack of copper-containing ferroxidases, including ceruloplasmin. There is maturation arrest of the granulocytic series. The third major feature of copper deficiency is the bone lesions[87] attributed to a lack of copper-containing amine oxidases necessary for the cross-linking of bone collagen. Early radiologic findings are osteoporosis and retarded bone age. Findings in the established case are increased density of the provisional bone of calcification and cupping, with sickle-shaped spurs in the metaphyseal region. Other features include periosteal layering and sub-metaphyseal and rib fractures. Reported clinical findings of copper deficiency in premature infants also include pallor, decreased pigmentation of skin and hair, prominent superficial veins, skin lesions similar to those of seborrheic dermatitis, failure to thrive, diarrhea, and hepatosplenomegaly. Features suggestive of central nervous system involvement are hypotonia, a lack of interest in outside surroundings, psychomotor retardation, lack of visual responses, and apneic episodes.

In Menke's Steely Hair Syndrome, there is an inherited defect in the intracellular transport of copper, affecting most if not all tissues apart from the liver.[3] This results in a profound copper deficiency disorder that cannot be corrected by the parenteral administration of copper. These infants, typically delivered prematurely, have severe and progressive neurologic disease, which becomes clinically apparent by about the second month of postnatal life. Both the neurologic disease and hypothermia have been attributed to decreased activity of cytochrome oxidase. A variety of defects of connective tissue are also apparent, including aneurysms of the aorta and bladder diverticular. For unexplained reasons, anemia and neutropenia are not characteristic features.

Diagnosis

The differential diagnosis of copper deficiency includes findings of scurvy, rickets, and nonaccidental trauma. With more advanced skeletal changes, copper deficiency can be differentiated from rickets by the increased density of the provisional zone of calcification and the absence of metaphyseal fraying. Differentiation of the metaphyseal fractures of copper deficiency from those of nonaccidental trauma includes the symmetric nature of the fractures of copper deficiency and other radiologic signs.

Laboratory confirmation of suspected copper deficiency in the premature infant is problematic. Erythrocyte superoxide dismutase activity remains a research tool at this time. Plasma copper concentrations are normally very low in the premature infant, averaging about $\sim$35 μg dL^{-1} prior to 35 weeks' postconception, 40–45 μg dL^{-1} for 35–38 weeks; 50–59 μg dL^{-1} from 39–42 weeks; 65 μg dL^{-1} at 43–44 weeks, and 75 μg dL^{-1} at 45 weeks. Levels that are even lower than these may be seen in association with copper deficiency.[80]

Copper requirements

Calculations of copper requirements in early postnatal life are complicated by inadequate understanding of the rate of release and efficiency of utilization of neonatal hepatic copper stores.[89] These stores are effective in protecting the term infant from copper deficiency for several months even when intake is very low. The lower the gestational age at delivery, the smaller are the hepatic stores. However, even at 26–28 week's gestation 2 mg of hepatic storage copper is probably present, and the very premature infant does not appear to be at any risk of copper deficiency until 2 months of postnatal age. Because of the more limited copper stores in the premature infant and because of evidence of poor absorption (10%–15%) of copper from formulas, it is recommended that the premature infant receive 100–120 μg Cu kg^{-1} day^{-1}. The premature infant fed with own mother's milk will probably ingest only 30–40 μg Cu kg^{-1} day^{-1}. However, because of superior absorption, this is quite adequate.

Calculations of intravenous copper requirements for the premature infant are given in Table 17.3.[56] The major uncertainty is again the amount of copper supplied from hepatic stores. In practice, however, 20 μg kg^{-1} day^{-1} appears to be quite adequate, and should be reduced or withheld in the presence of cholestatic disease. Once again, the cupric ion is a highly reactive pro-oxidant which, when given in the intravenous infusate, is introduced into the systemic circulation without being tightly bound to ceruloplasmin. Hence, there should be considerable caution with the administration of intravenous copper. Nutritional copper deficiency in premature infants can be treated with 200–600 μg Cu day^{-1} provided as a 1% solution of copper sulfate.

Table 17.3. Estimate of intravenous copper requirement for premature infants (μg Cu kg^{-1} day^{-1})

Copper accumulation by fetus in utero[a]	60
Copper stored in liver[a]	40
Therefore requirements for growth[a]	20
Urine losses = 5	
Fecal losses = 10[b]	
Total endogenous losses[c]	15
Physiological requirement (20 + 15)[c]	35
Assumed minimal supply from fetal hepatic stores[d]	15

[a] During third trimester.

[b] Higher in cases of biliary drainages or jejunostomy.

[c] Estimated, for example, as follows: 26-week fetal liver contains 3 mg copper; assumed that two-thirds is storage copper which is released over 2-month period and that there is 5% utilization of released copper. This particular example would provide 17 μg Cu^{-1} day^{-1}.

[d] Intravenous Cu requirement.

Copper toxicity

Acute ingestion of quantities of copper that are 1000 times the daily requirement can have a fatal outcome. Copper intoxication has occurred from consumption of contaminated drinking water with a copper concentration of 2–8 mg L^{-1}. Contamination of cow's milk with copper from brass containers has been cited as the major environmental factor in the cause of Indian childhood cirrhosis. It has been calculated that cow's milk stored in brass utensils would supply approximately 400 μg kg^{-1} day^{-1} of copper to an infant. This disease may be an example of a genetic–nutrient interaction. Acute copper poisoning has toxic effects on the liver, kidneys, heart, and central nervous system, and causes intravascular hemolysis. These changes may all be attributable to oxidative damage from the free cupric ion. Chronic copper toxicity may cause cirrhosis.

Formulas providing 300 μg Cu per 100 kcal have been fed to premature infants without evidence of adverse effects. However, it is advisable to restrict the copper content of formulas to no more than 200 μg per 100 kcal.[8] In practice, this is considerably more than is ever needed.

Table 17.4. Features in neurologic and hypothyroid cretinism

Feature	Neurologic cretin	Hypothyroid cretin
Mental retardation	Present, often severe	Present, often severe
Deaf-mutism	Usually present	Absent
Cerebral diplegia	Often present	Absent
Stature	Usually normal, occasionally slight growth retardation	Severe growth retardation
General features	No physical signs of hypothyroidism	Coarse dry skin, protuberant abdomen with umbilical hernia; large tongue
Reflexes	Excessively brisk	Delayed relaxation
Electrocardiogram	Normal	Small voltage QRS complexes and other abnormalities of hypothyroidism
X-ray limbs	Normal	Epiphyseal dysgenesis
Effect of thyroid hormones	No effect	Improvement

Iodide

Biologic role

The only clearly demonstrated role for iodine is as a component of the thyroid hormones. Iodide may have a direct role in early fetal development; however, effects thought to be attributable to iodide may be attributable to maternal thyroid hormones.[90] The physiologic effects of the thyroid hormones are primarily due to T_3. Most of the T_3 that appears in plasma is derived from peripheral deiodination of T_4.

Iodine metabolism

Iodine is rapidly reduced to iodide in the gut, and at least 50% of iodide is absorbed in the upper small bowel. Absorbed iodide is cleared from the plasma primarily by the thyroid gland and the kidney. In the thyroid gland, iodide is oxidized and is attached to tyrosyl residues of thyroglobulin. Monoiodotyrosine and diiodotyrosine are converted to iodothyronine through another oxidative step. The thyroid gland normally stores enough hormones to last several months. In conditions of iodide deficiency, secretion of thyrotropic hormone (TSH) by the pituitary is increased. This promotes iodide uptake by the thyroid and may lead to hyperplasia and hypertrophy of the gland. Shortly after birth, circulating levels of TSH temporarily increase and, in response, levels of T_4 and T_3 also increase. Levels of T_4 and T_3 are lower in the cord blood of the premature infant, and these postnatal changes are of smaller magnitude. Levels remain in the hypothyroid range in the first weeks of postnatal life and then increase, corresponding to increased synthesis of thyroid-binding globulin. Iodide is excreted via the kidneys.

Iodide deficiency

Maternal iodine deficiency during pregnancy can have a spectrum of adverse effects on fetal development that can be prevented by treating maternal iodine deficiency prior to pregnancy. Endemic goiter occurs in the offspring when maternal iodine intake is <20 μg day^{-1}. Some cases of endemic goiter have evidence of classic endemic cretinism. Maternal iodine excretion (intake) is <15 μg day^{-1} for this to occur. There are two well-defined clinical presentations of endemic cretinism, neurological and hypothyroid or myxedematous (Table 17.4). The myxedematous form is typically seen in Zaire and used to be seen in various European countries. Some cases in China are of this type.[91] In a number of other geographic areas, deaf-mutism and cerebral diplegia occur as characteristic manifestations of the neurologic form. Milder impairment of brain development, especially motor function, is much more common in areas of endemic goiter than is frank endemic cretinism. The pathogenesis of the neurologic disorder remains unclear, and the possibility of a direct effect of iodine deficiency on the fetus during the third trimester has been considered. Endemic cretinism no longer exists in North America, but on a global basis is still a major public health problem. It occurs especially in isolated mountainous regions where the iodine has been leached from the soil. China, Indonesia, the Indian subcontinent, and certain South American countries are prominent among those that have still not developed adequate preventive programs.

Neonatal hypothyroidism

In regions of endemic goiter, milder degrees of iodine deficiency in utero and after delivery may have detrimental effects on growth and intellectual development. Levels of T_3 and T_4 are lower in young infants from endemic goiter areas than from nonendemic goiter areas even when there is no evidence of goiter. Levels in the preterm infant are lower than those of the term infant, both in endemic goiter and nonendemic goiter areas.

Neonatal primary hypothyroidism can sometimes be transient. This condition appears to be extremely rare in North America but is a good deal more common in several European countries where iodide intakes are not as high as those in North America. The majority of the isolated case reports in North America have been secondary to the administration of maternal antithyroid drugs or of iodine medications. Maternal iodine overload is a recognized cause of neonatal hypothyroidism. Temporary neonatal hypothyroidism occurs most commonly in premature infants, especially those who are acutely ill with the respiratory distress syndrome. In European studies, serum levels of TSH and of thyroid hormone were normal in core blood. Hormonal levels dropped quickly after birth, however, together with markedly elevated TSH concentrations. This appears to be a multifactorial syndrome resulting both from immaturity of the newborn thyroid gland and from external factors including iodine deficiency or iodine excess. It is recommended that if this condition is diagnosed it should be treated promptly with iodide and T_3 therapy. In Germany, it has been reported that T_4 and T_3 administration on admission to the neonatal intensive care unit significantly lowered mortality rates.[92] This was thought to result from accelerated production of surfactant in the lungs.

Requirements

Oral requirements of iodide in the infant, including the premature infant, are no more than 2–4 μg iodide day^{-1}. Both human milk and cow's milk in North America contain very substantial quantities of iodide, and neither breast-fed nor formula-fed premature infants are at risk from iodide deficiency. When hypothyroidism occurs it is due to a metabolic abnormality in the thyroid gland rather than to iodine deficiency. Hence, while thyroid replacement therapy may be required in some neonates, iodine supplements are not indicated.

In general, it appears that the intravenously fed infant acquires sufficient iodide accidentally from dressings, antiseptic lotions used on the skin, and so forth. However, biochemical evidence of iodide deficiency has been reported in an infant on long-term parenteral nutrition, and it is advisable to supplement the intravenous infusate with 1–2 μg iodide per kg body weight day^{-1}.

Toxicity

Though iodide intakes of up to 1000 μg day^{-1} in children have been found to be devoid of harmful effects, there has been recent concern about the potential dangers of excess iodide. It appears that 4% of individuals are particularly sensitive to iodide excess, which can cause hypothyroidism.

Fluoride

Fluoride is of established value in the prevention of dental caries and may also have a beneficial effect on the skeletal system. No specific recommendations for fluoride supplementation have been made for premature infants. However, prematurity is associated with an increased incidence of dental caries, and there appears to be particular reason for ensuring adequate fluoride supplementation in premature infants. It is not clear to what extent, if any, that fluoride will exert a beneficial effect on nonerupted teeth, or what, if any, benefits can be conferred by systemic fluoride as opposed to the local effect in the oral cavity. However, it is prudent to provide 0.1 mg fluoride per kg body weight day^{-1} up to a maximum of 0.25 mg fluoride day^{-1} to premature infants,[93] other than those who are fed with formula that has been made up with water in a fluoridated area. Infant formulas and packaged water marketed for making up powdered formula provide less than 0.3 mg fluoride L^{-1}.

Manganese

Physiologic role

Mitochondrial superoxide dismutase and pyruvate carboxylase are manganese metalloenzymes. Manganese is required for the synthesis of mucopolysaccharides through the manganese-dependent enzymes polymerase and galactotransferrase. Manganese deficiency in various animal species leads to impaired skeletal development and ataxia. The latter is due to defective formation of the otoliths in fetal life. Abnormalities in carbohydrate and liver metabolism have also been documented.

Metabolism

Adults absorb only about 3% of an ingested dose of isotopically labeled $MnCl_2$ and this low level does not change when the quantity of carrier is altered. Ten days later 1.5% of the ingested dose is retained by adults, but newborns retain

8% and premature infants 16%.[94] Manganese absorption is especially high in very early postnatal life in the mouse, and little manganese is excreted at that stage.[95] Dietary manganese absorption does depend on the level of manganese intake and also on the type of diet. When various milks and infant formulas are fed to adults, the percentage absorption ranged from 1% when given with soy formula up to 9% with human milk. Absorption from cow's milk and from humanized cow's milk formulas ranged from 3–6% but dropped to 1.5% with iron-fortified formulas.[96] Much higher percentage absorption of manganese from milks and formulas has been observed in rat pups with manganese retention from human milk exceeding 80%. Comparable data for the human infant are lacking.

Manganese is excreted almost entirely through the bile. When manganese intake is increased, there is a decrease in the percentage absorption and an increase in biliary excretion. Intestinal mucosa and the liver together provide effective homeostatic control of manganese status in normal circumstances, although it is not clear that this pertains to premature infants.

Manganese deficiency

Human manganese deficiency has not been described convincingly apart from a case of one volunteer on an experimental synthetic diet from which manganese was inadvertently omitted. Features attributed to manganese deficiency in this case were hypercholesterolemia, depressed levels of clotting proteins in the plasma, weight loss, and slow growth of hair and nails. The lack of evidence of manganese deficiency in circumstances in which many other trace elements have been identified, especially intravenous nutrition, may be attributable to the widespread use of manganese supplements from an early stage in the history of synthetic diets and formulas. No established laboratory criteria are available for the assessment of manganese status. Low serum manganese levels have been reported in some diabetic and epileptic children, and a negative manganese balance has been observed in children with pancreatic insufficiency. The clinical significance of these observations is obscure.

Manganese requirements

Manganese intake of the fully breast-fed infant is approximately 0.5 µg Mn kg^{-1} day^{-1}.[97] Because of differences in fractional absorption it is likely that the manganese requirements of the formula-fed infant are an order of magnitude higher than this. Many formulas provide even more manganese, and this applies especially to soy formulas with which a higher concentration of manganese is naturally associated. Soy formulas are likely to provide approximately 50 µg Mn kg^{-1} day^{-1}. Though no toxic effects have been observed on these higher intakes, no careful examination of the safety of such intakes in premature infants has been reported. In view of the evidence for a higher fractional absorption in premature infants and the indications from an animal model that excretion may be very limited, considerable care is recommended in providing manganese to VLBW premature infants. Pending further information, a maximum figure of 50 µg kg^{-1} day^{-1} from a soy formula and 10 µg kg^{-1} day^{-1} from a cow's milk-based formula is suggested.

A supplement sufficient to provide 1 µg Mn kg^{-1} day^{-1} intravenously appears to be adequate for patients fed parenterally. Larger quantities than this are discouraged in the premature infant. In parenterally fed patients who develop cholestatic liver disease marked hypermanganesemia has been documented.[7] In the face of cholestatic liver disease, suspension of intravenous manganese supplement is recommended. The background manganese contamination in the infusate is sufficient to maintain serum manganese concentrations over a period of many months.

Chromium

Trace quantities of chromium in rat diets were found in the 1960s to be necessary for normal glucose tolerance. The results of subsequent research were consistent with the hypothesis that chromium acted as a cofactor for insulin while facilitating the initial attachment of insulin to peripheral receptors. However, chromium has not been detected in these receptors.

The results of several studies in the 1960s and 1970s suggested that human chromium deficiency may be a cause of impaired glucose tolerance, especially in the elderly and in patients on prolonged parenteral nutrition. Chromium deficiency was also reported in infants with protein energy malnutrition. In general, more recent studies have failed to confirm earlier observations, and the importance of chromium in human nutrition remains uncertain.

Results of earlier tissue analyses indicated that tissue chromium concentrations are relatively high in the term neonate and decrease progressively during the life cycle. Relatively low chromium concentrations were observed in the plasma and hair of infants born prematurely and those with intrauterine growth retardation. More recent advances in analytical techniques for the measurement of chromium in biologic samples have led to major revisions in normal values for tissue chromium concentrations. Unfortunately, no data are available for the premature infant or on changes in tissue chromium concentrations through the life cycle using modern analytic methodology.

There have been two careful studies of zinc concentrations in human milk with modern analytic techniques. The concentration averaged $0.3\ \mu g\ Cr\ L^{-1}$, and the range is quite small. Thus the chromium intake of the breast-fed infant is approximately $0.05\ \mu g\ Cr\ kg^{-1}\ day^{-1}$. In reaching tentative estimates of chromium requirements of the formula-fed infant, it is advisable to assume that absorption is considerably less than from human milk. Thus, the recommended intake is $2.5\ \mu g\ Cr\ kg^{-1}\ day^{-1}$.

Molybdenum

Molybdenum (Mo) enzymes that have been identified in the human are xanthine oxidase, which is involved in purine metabolism, and sulfite oxidase. One case of human molybdenum deficiency has been described in an adult on long-term total parenteral nutrition. Features included tachycardia, tachypnea, vomiting, and central scotomas, with rapid progression to coma. There was intolerance to infused amino acids, and methionine levels were elevated. Serum uric acid and urine excretion of sulphate were decreased. The clinical and biochemical response to $2.5\ \mu g$ Mo $kg^{-1}\ day^{-1}$ in the infusate was excellent.

The concentration of molybdenum in human milk is about $2\ \mu g\ L^{-1}$. Thus the infant receiving human milk has an intake of approximately $0.3\ \mu g\ Mo\ kg^{-1}\ day^{-1}$. This level of intake is probably adequate for the premature infant as well as the term infant. However, data on tissue concentration and fetal accumulation are inadequate. Intravenously, an intake of $0.25\ \mu g\ Mo\ kg^{-1}\ day^{-1}$ is probably adequate. Intravenous molybdenum supplements are recommended only with long-term intravenous nutrition.

REFERENCES

1 Krebs, N. F., Westcott, J. Zinc and breastfed infants: if and when is there a risk of deficiency? In Davis, M. K., Isaacs, C. E., Hanson, L. A., Wright, A. L., eds. *Integrating Population Outcomes, Biological Mechanisms and Research Methods in the Study of Human Milk and Lactation.* New York, NY: Kluwer Academic/Plenum Press; 2002:69–76.

2 Hambidge, K. M., Walravens, P. A. Disorders of mineral metabolism. *Clin. Gastroenterol.* 1982;**11**:87–117.

3 Danks, D. M. Heredity disorders of copper metabolism in Wilson's disease and Menkes' disease. In Stanbury, J. B., Wyngaarden, J. B., Frederickson, D. S. *et al.*, eds. *The Metabolic Basis of Inherited Disease.* 5th edn. New York, NY: McGraw-Hill Book Co; 1983:1251–6.

4 Easley, D., Krebs, N., Jefferson, M. *et al.* Effect of pancreatic enzymes on zinc absorption in cystic fibrosis. *J. Pediatr. Gastroenterol. Nutr.* 1998;**26**:136–9.

5 Hambidge, K. M., Krebs, N. F., Lilly, J. R., Zerbe, G. O. Plasma and urine zinc in infants and children with extrahepatic biliary atresia. *J. Pediatr. Gastroenterol. Nutr.* 1987;**6**:872–7.

6 Knisely, A. S., O'Shea, P. A., Stocks, J. F., Dimmick, J. E. Oropharyngeal and upper respiratory tract mucosal-gland siderosis in neonatal hemochromatosis: an approach to biopsy diagnosis. *J. Pediatr.* 1988;**113**:871–4.

7 Hambidge, K. M., Sokol, R. J., Fidanza, S. J., Goodall, M. A. Plasma manganese concentrations in infants and children receiving parenteral nutrition. *J. Parenter. Enteral. Nutr.* 1989;**13**:168–71.

8 Klein, C. J. Nutrient requirements for preterm infant formulas. *J. Nutr.* 2002;**132**:1395S–7S.

9 Bader, D., Blondheim, O., Jonas, R. *et al.* Decreased ferritin levels, despite iron supplementation, during erythropoietin therapy in anaemia of prematurity. *Acta Paediatr.* 1996;**85**:496–501.

10 Dallman, P. R. Biochemical basis for the manifestations of iron deficiency. *Annu. Rev. Nutr.* 1986;**6**:13–40.

11 Beard, J. L., Dawson, H., Pinero, D. J. Iron metabolism: a comprehensive review. *Nutr. Rev.* 1996;**54**:295–317.

12 Dallman, P. R. Nutritional anemia of infancy: iron, folic acid, and vitamin B12. In Tsang, R. C., Nicholas, B. L., eds. *Nutrition during infancy.* Philadelphia, PA: Hanley & Belfus, Inc; 1988:216–35.

13 Rios, E., Hunter, R. E., Cook, J. D., Smith, N. J., Finch, C. A. The absorption of iron as supplements in infant cereal and infant formulas. *Pediatrics* 1975;**55**:686–93.

14 Oski, F. A. Iron requirements of the premature infant. In Tsang, R. C., ed. *Vitamin and Mineral Requirements in Preterm Infants.* New York, NY: Marcel Dekker; 1985:9–22.

15 Vyas, D., Chandra, R. K. Functional implications of iron deficiency. In Stekel, A., ed. *Iron Nutrition in Infancy and Childhood.* New York, NY: Raven Press; 1984:45–59.

16 Nokes, C., van den Bosch, C., Bundy, D. *The Effects of Iron Deficiency and Anemia on Mental and Motor Performance, Educational Achievement, and Behavior in Children. A Report of the INACG.* Washington, DC: International Life Sciences Institute; 1998.

17 Lozoff, B., Jimenez, E., Wolf, A. W. Long-term developmental outcome of infants with iron deficiency. *N. Engl. J. Med.* 1991;**325**:687–94.

18 Pollitt, E. Iron deficiency and cognitive function. *Annu. Rev. Nutr.* 1993;**13**:521–37.

19 Chockalingam, U., Murphy, E., Ophoven, J. C., Georgieff, M. K. The influence of gestational age, size for dates, and prenatal steroids on cord transferrin levels in newborn infants. *J. Pediatr. Gastroenterol. Nutr.* 1987;**6**:276–80.

20 Whittaker, P. Iron and zinc interactions in humans. *Am. J. Clin. Nutr.* 1998;**68**:442S–6S.

21 Ehrenkranz, R. A., Gettner, P. A., Nelli, C. M. *et al.* Iron absorption and incorporation into red blood cells by very low birth weight infants: studies with the stable isotope 58Fe. *J. Pediatr. Gastroenterol. Nutr.* 1992;**15**:270–8.

22 Hambidge, K. M., Krebs, N. F. Zinc in the fetus and the neonate. In Polin, R. A., Fox, W. W., Abman, S. H., eds. *Fetal and Neonatal Physiology.* 3rd edn. Philadelphia, PA: W. B. Saunders; 2003:342–7.

23 Williams, R. J. P. An introduction to the biochemistry of zinc. In Mills, C. F., ed. *Zinc in Human Biology.* London: Springer-Verlag; 1989:15–31.

24 Maret, W. Editorial. *Biometals* 2001;**14**:187–90.

25 Cousins, R. J., Blanchard, R. K., Moore, J. B. *et al.* Regulation of zinc metabolism and genomic outcomes. *J. Nutr.* 2003;**133**:1521S–6S.

26 Frederickson, C. J., Bush, A. I. Synaptically released zinc: physiologic functions and pathologic effects. *Biometals* 2001;**14**:335–66.

27 Falchuk, K. H., Montorzi, M. Zinc physiology and biochemistry in oocytes and embryos. *Biometals* 2001;**14**:385–95.

28 Steele, L., Cousins, R. J. Kinetics of zinc absorption by luminally and vascularly perfused rat intestine. *Am. J. Physiol.* 1985;**248**:G46–53.

29 Cragg, R. A., Christie, G. R., Phillips, S. R. *et al.* A novel zinc-regulated human zinc transporter, hZTL1, is localized to the enterocyte apical membrane. *J. Biol. Chem.* 2002;**277**:22789–97.

30 Cousins, R. J., McMahon, R. J. Integrative aspects of zinc transporters. *J. Nutr.* 2000;**130**:1384S–7S.

31 Hambidge, K. M., Krebs, N. F., Miller, L. Evaluation of zinc metabolism with use of stable-isotope techniques: implications for the assessment of zinc status. *Am. J. Clin. Nutr.* 1998;**68**:410S–13S.

32 Krebs, N. F., Hambidge, K. M. Zinc requirements and zinc intakes of breast-fed infants. *Am. J. Clin. Nutr.* 1986;**43**:288–92.

33 Widdowson, E. M., Southgate, D. A. T., Hey, E. Fetal growth and body composition. In Lindblad, B. S., ed. *Perinatal Nutrition.* New York, NY: Academic Press;1998:3–14.

34 Zlotkin, S. H., Cherian, M. G. Hepatic metallothionein as a source of zinc and cysteine during the first year of life. *Pediatr Res.* 1988;**24**:326–9.

35 Wastney, M. E., Angelus, P., Barnes, R. M., Subramanian, K. N. Zinc kinetics in preterm infants: a compartmental model based on stable isotope data. *Am. J. Physiol.* 1996;**271**:R1452–9.

36 Jalla, S., Krebs, N. F., Rodden, D. J., Hambidge, K. M. Zinc homeostasis in premature infants does not differ between those fed preterm formula or fortified human milk. *Pediatr. Res.* 2004; **56**:615–20.

37 Black, M. M. Zinc deficiency and child development. *Am. J. Clin. Nutr.* 1998;**68**:464S–9S.

38 Hambidge, M. Human zinc deficiency. *J. Nutr.* 2000;**130**: 1344S–49S.

39 Jones, G., Steketee, R. W., Black, R. E., Bhutta, Z. A., Morris, S. S. How many child deaths can we prevent this year? *Lancet* 2003;**362**:65–71.

40 Ibs, K. H., Rink, L. Zinc-altered immune function. *J. Nutr.* 2003;**133**:1452S–6S.

41 Hambidge, K. M. Mild zinc deficiency in human subjects. In Mills, C., ed. *Zinc in Human Biology.* London: Springer-Verlag; 1989.

42 Brown, K. H., Peerson, J. M., Rivera, J., Allen, L. H. Effect of supplemental zinc on the growth and serum zinc concentrations of prepubertal children: a meta-analysis of randomized controlled trials. *Am. J. Clin. Nutr.* 2002;**75**:1062–71.

43 Black, M. M. The evidence linking zinc deficiency with children's cognitive and motor functioning. *J. Nutr.* 2003;**133**:1473S–6S.

44 Sandstead, H. H., Penland, J. G., Alcock, N. W. *et al.* Effects of repletion with zinc and other micronutrients on neuropsychological performance and growth of Chinese children. *Am. J. Clin. Nutr.* 1998;**68**:470S–5S.

45 Friel, J. K., Andrews, W. L., Matthew, J. D. *et al.* Zinc supplementation in very-low-birth-weight infants. *J. Pediatr. Gastroenterol. Nutr.* 1993;**17**:97–104.

46 Castillo-Duran, C., Rodriguez, A., Venegas, G., Alvarez, P., Icaza, G. Zinc supplementation and growth of infants born small for gestational age. *J. Pediatr.* 1995;**127**:206–11.

47 Sazawal, S., Black, R. E., Menon, V. P. *et al.* Zinc supplementation in infants born small for gestational age reduces mortality: a prospective, randomized, controlled trial. *Pediatrics* 2001;**108**:1280–86.

48 Krebs, N. F., Bartlett, A., Westcott, J. E. *et al.* Exchangeable zinc pool size is smaller at birth in small for gestational age infants. *Pediatr. Res.* 2003;**53**:394A.

49 Arlette, J. P., Johnston, M. M. Zinc deficiency dermatosis in premature infants receiving prolonged parenteral alimentation. *J. Am. Acad. Dermatol.* 1981;**5**:37–42.

50 Wang, K., Zhou, B., Kuo, Y. M., Zemansky, J., Gitschier, J. A novel member of a zinc transporter family is defective in acrodermatitis enteropathica. *Am. J. Hum. Genet.* 2002;**71**:66–73.

51 Huang, L., Gitschier, J. Novel gene involved in zinc transport is deficient in the lethal milk mouse. *Nat. Genetics.* 1997;**17**:292–7.

52 Zimmerman, A. W., Hambidge, K. M., Lepow, M. L. *et al.* Acrodermatitis in breast-fed premature infants: evidence for a defect of mammary zinc secretion. *Pediatrics* 1982;**69**:176–83.

53 Hambidge, K. M. Zinc deficiency in the premature infant. *Pediatr. Rev.* 1985;**6**:209–16.

54 Koo, W. W., Succop, P., Hambidge, K. M. Serum alkaline phosphatase and serum zinc concentrations in preterm infants with rickets and fractures. *Am. J. Dis. Child.* 1989;**143**:1342–5.

55 Kleinman, L. I., Petering, H. G., Sutherland, J. M. Blood carbonic anhydrase activity and zinc concentration in infants with respiratory-distress syndrome. *N. Engl. J. Med.* 1967;**277**:1157–61.

56 Greene, H. L., Hambidge, K. M., Schanler, R., Tsang, R. C. Guidelines for the use of vitamins, trace elements, calcium, magnesium, and phosphorus in infants and children receiving total parenteral nutrition: report of the Subcommittee on Pediatric Parenteral Nutrient Requirements from the Committee on Clinical Practice Issues of the American Society for Clinical Nutrition. *Am. J. Clin. Nutr.* 1988;**48**:1324–42.

57 Zlotkin, S. H., Buchanan, B. E. Meeting zinc and copper intake requirements in the parenterally fed preterm and full-term infant. *J. Pediatr.* 1983;**103**:441–6.

58 Lohman, T. G., Roche, A. F., Martorell, R. *Anthropometric Standardization Reference Manual.* Champaign, IL: Human Kinetics Books; 1988.

59 Festa, M. D., Anderson, H. L., Dowdy, R. P., Ellersieck, M. R. Effect of zinc intake on copper excretion and retention in men. *Am. J. Clin. Nutr.* 1985;**41**:285–92.

60 Hambidge, K. M., Walravens, P. A., Neldner, K. H. Zinc, copper and fatty acids in acrodermatitis enteropathica. In Kirchgessner, M., ed. *International Symposium on Trace Element Metabolism in Man and Animals.* 3rd edn. Freising-Weihenstephan, Germany: Arbeitskreis für Tierenahrungsforschung, Institut für Ernährungsphysiologie, Technische Universität München; 1978:413–17.

61 Hoekstra, W. G. Biochemical function of selenium and its relation to vitamin E. *Fed Proc.* 1975;**34**:2083–9.

62 Machlin, L. J., Bendich, A. Free radical tissue damage: protective role of antioxidant nutrients. *FASEB J.* 1987;**1**:441–5.

63 Levander, O. A., Burk, R. F. Selenium. In *Present Knowledge in Nutrition.* 7th edn. Washington, DC: ILSI Press; 1996: 320–8.

64 Levander, O. A. The importance of selenium in total parenteral nutrition. *Proceedings: Working Conference on Parenteral Trace Elements 2.* New York, NY: New York Academy of Science; 1984:144–55.

65 McGuire, M. K., Burgert, S. L., Picciano, M. F. *et al.* Selenium nutriture of infants fed human milk or bovine milk-based formula with or without selenium. *FASEB J.* 1989;**3**:1309.

66 Keshan Disease Research Group. Epidemiologic studies on the etiologic relationship of selenium and Keshan disease. *Chin. Med. J. (Engl).* 1979;**92**:477–82.

67 Keshan Disease Research Group. Observations of effects of sodium selenite in prevention of Keshan disease. *Chin. Med. J. (Engl).* 1979;**92**:471–6.

68 Johnson, R. A., Baker, S. S., Fallon, J. T. *et al.* An occidental case of cardiomyopathy and selenium deficiency. *N. Engl. J. Med.* 1981;**304**:1210–12.

69 Kien, C. L., Ganther, H. E. Manifestations of chronic selenium deficiency in a child receiving total parenteral nutrition. *Am. J. Clin. Nutr.* 1983;**37**:319–28.

70 Vinton, N. E., Dahlstrom, K. A., Strobel, C. T., Ament, M. E. Macrocytosis and pseudoalbinism: manifestations of selenium deficiency. *J. Pediatr.* 1987;**111**:711–17.

71 Golden, M. H. N., Ramdath, D. Free radicals in the pathogenesis of kwashiokor. In Taylor, T. G., Jenkins, N. K., eds. *Proceedings of the XIII Congress of International Nutrition.* London: Libbey, J; 1985:597–8.

72 Gross, S. Hemolytic anemia in premature infants: relationship to vitamin E, selenium, glutathione peroxidase, and erythrocyte lipids. *Semin. Hematol.* 1976;**13**:187–99.

73 Lombeck, I., Kasperek, K., Harbisch, H. D. *et al.* The selenium state of children. II. Selenium content of serum, whole blood, hair and the activity of erythrocyte glutathione peroxidase in dietetically treated patients with phenylketonuria and maple-syrup-urine disease. *Eur. J. Pediatr.* 1978;**128**:213–23.

74 Darlow, B. A., Inder, T. E., Graham, P. J. *et al.* The relationship of selenium status to respiratory outcome in the very low birth weight infant. *Pediatrics* 1995;**96**:314–19.

75 Lockitch, G., Jacobson, B., Quigley, G., Dison, P., Pendray, M. Selenium deficiency in low birth weight neonates: an unrecognized problem. *J. Pediatr.* 1989;**114**:865–70.

76 Whanger, P. D., Beilstein, M. A., Thomson, C. D., Robinson, M. F., Howe, M. Blood selenium and glutathione peroxidase activity of populations in New Zealand, Oregon, and South Dakota. *FASEB J.* 1988;**2**:2996–3002.

77 Kumpulainen, J., Salmenpera, L., Siimes, M. A. *et al.* Formula feeding results in lower selenium status than breast-feeding or selenium supplemented formula feeding: a longitudinal study. *Am. J. Clin. Nutr.* 1987;**45**:49–53.

78 van Caillie-Bertrand, M., Degenhart, H. J., Fernandes, J. Influence of age on the selenium status in Belgium and The Netherlands. *Pediatr. Res.* 1986;**20**:574–6.

79 Yang, G. Q., Ge, K. Y., Chen, J. S., Chen, X. S. Selenium-related endemic diseases and the daily selenium requirement of humans. *World Rev. Nutr. Diet.* 1988;**55**:98–152.

80 Frieden, E. Ceruloplasmin – a multifunctional cupro-protein of vertebrate plasma. In Sorenson, J., ed. *Inflammatory Diseases and Copper.* Clifton, NJ: Humana Press; 1982:159–69.

81 Solomons, N. W. Biochemical, metabolic, and clinical role of copper in human nutrition. *J. Am. Coll. Nutr.* 1985;**4**: 83–105.

82 Widdowson, E. M. Trace elements in foetal and early postnatal development. *Proc. Nutr. Soc.* 1974;**33**:275–84.

83 Bakka, A., Webb, M. Metabolism of zinc and copper in the neonate: changes in the concentrations and contents of thionein-bound Zn and Cu with age in the livers of the newborn of various mammalian species. *Biochem. Pharmacol.* 1981;**30**:721–5.

84 Seely, J. R., Humphrey, G. B., Matter, B. J. Copper deficiency in a premature infant fed on iron-fortified formula. *N. Engl. J. Med.* 1972;**286**:109–10.

85 al-Rashid, R. A., Spangler, J. Neonatal copper deficiency. *N. Engl. J. Med.* 1971;**285**:841–3.

86 Tokuda, Y., Yokoyama, S., Tsuji, M. *et al.* Copper deficiency in an infant on prolonged total parenteral nutrition. *J. Parenter. Enteral Nutr.* 1986;**10**:242–4.

87 Ashkenazi, A., Levin, S., Djaldetti, M., Fishel, E., Benvenisti, D. The syndrome of neonatal copper deficiency. *Pediatrics* 1973;**52**:525–33.

88 Sutton, A. M., Harvie, A., Cockburn, F., Farquharson, J., Logan, R. W. Copper deficiency in the preterm infant of very low birth-weight. Four cases and a reference range for plasma copper. *Arch. Dis. Child.* 1985;**60**:644–51.

89 Casey, C. E., Hambidge, K. M. Trace element requirements. In Tsang, R., ed. *Vitamin and Mineral Requirements of Preterm Infants.* New York, NY: Marcel Dekker; 1985:153–84.

90 Escobar del Rey, F., Pastor, R., Mallol, J., Morreale de Escobar, G. Effects of maternal iodine deficiency on the L-thyroxine and 3,5,3'-triiodo-L-thyronine contents of rat embryonic tissues before and after onset of fetal thyroid function. *Endocrinology* 1986;**118**:1259–65.

91 Report of the Subcommittee for the Study of Endemic Goitre and Iodine Deficiency of the European Thyroid Association. Goitre and iodine deficiency in Europe. *Lancet* 1985;**1**:1289–93.

92 Schonberger, W., Grimm, W., Emmrich, P., Gempp, W. Thyroid administration lowers mortality in premature infants. *Lancet* 1979;**2**:1181.

93 Committee on Nutrition. Fluoride supplementation: revised dosage schedule. *Pediatrics* 1979;**63**:150–2.

94 Mena, L. Manganese. In Bronner, F., Coburn, J. W., eds. *Disorders of Mineral Metabolism.* New York, NY: Academic Press; 1981:223–70.

95 Miller, S. T., Cotzias, G. C., Evert, H. A. Control of tissue manganese: initial absence and sudden emergence of excretion in the neonatal mouse. *Am. J. Physiol.* 1975;**229**:1080–4.

96 Davidson, L., Sederblad, A., Lonnerdal, B. *et al.* Manganese absorption from human milk, cow's milk and infant formulas. In Hurley, L. S., ed. *Trace Elements in Man and Animals.* 6th edn. New York, NY: Plenum Publishing; 1988:511–12.

97 Casey, C. E., Hambidge, K. M., Neville, M. C. Studies in human lactation: zinc, copper, manganese and chromium in human milk in the first month of lactation. *Am. J. Clin. Nutr.* 1985;**41**:1193–200.

98 Mertz, W. The essential trace elements. *Science.* 1981;**213**:1330.

18

Iron

Michael K. Georgieff

Department of Pediatrics and Child Development, University of Minnesota, Minneapolis, MN

Overview

Iron is a ubiquitous element required by virtually all cells for normal growth and metabolism. Rapidly growing and differentiating cells have particularly high iron requirements.[1] Since preterm and term human infants have high growth rates (on a per-weight basis), it is not surprising that these infants also have high iron needs. Term infants typically acquire adequate iron stores during the last trimester of gestation, but preterm infants are relatively compromised in this respect.[2] This fact, combined with their higher postnatal growth rates in the first year, renders preterm infants at higher risk than their term counterparts for iron deficiency and iron-deficiency anemia.[3,4] This increased risk could theoretically be avoided by administering large doses of iron to the preterm infant, were it not for the concern of iron toxicity; iron plays an important catalytic role in the Fenton reaction, which creates radical oxygen species that peroxidate the lipids in cell membranes. The concern is relevant particularly in the premature infant whose plasma total iron-binding capacity (TIBC) is low and whose antioxidant defense system is immature.[5,6] Thus, iron can be considered a highly necessary element with a narrow therapeutic window where both deficiency and overload contribute to significant morbidity.

Iron balance in the fetus and neonate

Iron is classically seen as an integral part of the hemoglobin molecule, and iron deficiency is thus frequently assumed to be synonymous with anemia. Although most of the total body iron is found in the red blood cell mass,[2] iron-containing proteins are found throughout the body and are involved in processes as basic as cellular proliferation, mitochondrial electron transport/oxidative phosphorylation, detoxification, neurotransmitter synthesis and muscle oxygen transport. The total iron load of the third trimester fetus and the neonate is approximately 75 mg per kg of body weight distributed through three compartments.[2] The red cell mass contains 75% of this endowment in the form of hemoglobin. Another 15% is found in storage pools, primarily bound to ferritin in the liver and spleen. Humans are born with relatively large iron stores, and cord serum ferritin concentrations are high (>60 ng ml^{-1}).[7] The final 10% represents non-heme, non-storage-tissue iron. Although this is the smallest pool, depletion of tissue iron is responsible for many of the symptoms of iron deficiency.[8] It is a classic misconception that the symptoms of iron deficiency are due solely to anemia. During periods when iron supply does not meet iron demand, an interorgan redistribution occurs. Iron is prioritized to the red cells first (at the expense of the storage pool), and then to the non-heme-tissue pool.[9] Within the latter, the skeletal muscle compartment is compromised before the heart and brain.

Iron status at birth is a function of fetal iron accretion and birth events. Common factors that can alter neonatal iron status are listed in Table 18.1.

On a worldwide scale, maternal iron deficiency is the most common cause of compromised fetal and neonatal iron status. Up to 30% of pregnancies in developing countries are complicated by iron deficiency to a degree that will affect fetal iron status at birth. The newborn's low iron status can be further complicated by a postnatal diet that is low in iron, such as the use of low-iron formula or breast milk from

Neonatal Nutrition and Metabolism. Second Edition, ed. P. Thureen and W. Hay. Published by Cambridge University Press.
© Cambridge University Press 2006.

Table 18.1. Factors altering neonatal iron status

Event	Cause	Effect
Fetal events		
Maternal iron deficiency (maternal Hgb < 8.5 g/dl)	Decreased maternal iron supply; affects up to 30% of pregnancies in developing countries	Reduced total body iron
Placental insufficiency (IUGR)	Reduced placental iron transport; affects up to 10% of pregnancies; 50% of infants affected	Reduced total body iron; shift of iron from storage and tissues into red cells; can cause brain iron deficiency
Maternal glucose intolerance (Type I or gestational)	Increased fetal iron demand and decreased placental iron transport capacity; affects up to 10% of pregnancies; 40%–65% of infants affected	Close to normal total body iron; shift of iron from storage and tissues into red cells; can cause brain iron deficiency
Maternal cigarette smoking	Chronic fetal hypoxia	Reduced fetal iron stores with shift of iron into expanded red cell mass
Congenital hemochromatosis	Unknown, but likely genetic defect of proteins involving placental iron transport	Fetal iron overload with severe cardiac and hepatic dysfunction
Perinatal events		
Premature birth	Lack of fetal iron accretion in third trimester	Normal total body iron for size; decreased total iron endowment for first postnatal year's growth
Delayed cord clamping	Increased delivery of placental blood (up to 20 cc per kg body weight)	Increased total body iron – all in red cell mass initially; risk of polycythemia; positive effect on hemoglobin concentration at 2 months
Fetal-maternal/placental hemorrhage/ cord accident	Acute loss of hemoglobin iron	Decreased total body iron – all in red cell mass initially; probably earlier mobilization of iron stores postnatally
Perinatal infection	Sequestration of iron	Elevated cord ferritin concentration

an iron-deficient mother. Intrauterine growth retardation is also common in developing countries, and complicates up to 10% of pregnancies in developed countries. Maternal malnutrition is the most common cause in developing countries; maternal hypertension during gestation is the most common cause in developed countries. In the latter case, mothers are usually iron sufficient, but maternal–fetal iron delivery is apparently restricted by the diseased placenta. Approximately 50% of infants demonstrate low cord serum ferritin concentrations (<60 ng ml^{-1}).[10] Their total body iron is likely to be low, although some loss of storage iron can be accounted for in the elevated hemoglobin concentration of these infants who were chronically hypoxic during fetal life. Infants with severe intrauterine growth retardation (IUGR) can be iron deficient, up to a 33% loss of brain iron.[11] Infants born to mothers who smoked during pregnancy are born with low iron stores.[12] The mechanism is likely related to a redistribution of iron from the storage pool to the red cell mass. The effect does not appear to be

as severe as that found with maternal hypertension and IUGR.

Diabetes during gestation induces a complex pathology that results in neonatal liver, heart, and brain iron deficiency.[13] The severity of the iron imbalance is inversely related to maternal glycemic control.[14] The effects are seen in Type I and gestational diabetes since both can be complicated by maternal hyperglycemia that results in fetal hyperglycemia, islet cell hyperplasia and hyperinsulinemia. Fetal hyperglycemia and hyperinsulinemia increase fetal oxygen consumption by approximately 30% in a relatively oxygen-limited environment.[15,16] The subsequent state of chronic intrauterine hypoxia results in release of fetal erythropoietin and expansion of the hemoglobin mass by 30%.[17,18] Each gram of newly synthesized hemoglobin requires an additional 3.47 mg of elemental iron, which can initially be supplied by mobilization of fetal iron stores. The placenta is responsive to the apparent loss of storage iron and responds by increasing transferrin receptor expression on its apical (maternal-facing) surface.[19] However, the affinity of the receptor for maternal transferrin is decreased, possibly due to hyperglycosylation of the oligosaccharides found in the binding domain.[20] The net result is an insufficient compensatory attempt to increase placental iron transport[19] and a subsequent channeling of available fetal iron to the red cells and away from the liver, heart, and brain.[13] Up to 65% of infants of diabetic mothers (IDM) are affected, and approximately 25% are at risk for brain and heart iron deficiency.[10,14] The most severe cases demonstrate a 40% loss of brain iron and a 55% loss of heart iron.[13] The potential physiologic consequences are discussed below.

Iron can also be acutely lost through hemorrhage. Blood can be lost to the placenta (e.g., fetal–placental hemorrhage or holding the infant above the perineum prior to cord clamping) or externally (e.g., cord accident). The result is a loss of total body iron. Without replacement, iron stores will be mobilized earlier to support the subsequent reticulocytosis. Tissue iron status will be largely unaffected because of the relatively large iron stores, but infants with significant iron loss through hemorrhage at birth may be at increased risk for iron deficiency after 6 months of age.

Total body iron overload is an unusual event in the fetal/neonatal period. Congenital hemochromatosis is an exceedingly rare disease, most likely of genetic origin, that results in massive iron overload of the fetal organs.[21] Infants usually die of heart and liver failure secondary to iron overload in the neonatal period, although aggressive chelation has reportedly been successful. It has been postulated that the pathophysiology involves abnormalities of regulation of iron transport proteins in the placenta, although no candidate molecule has been identified. The mutation is not the same as that found in hereditary hemochromatosis.[22]

Neonatal iron status also can be augmented by delayed cord clamping.[23] Holding the infant below the perineum prior to clamping increases placental–fetal transfusion and may approach a volume of 70 mL of blood. The effect of delayed cord clamping on long-term iron status is unclear. One study reports an increase in hemoglobin concentration of 0.7 g dL^{-1} at 2 months of age, following delayed cord clamping with the infant held at the level of the perineum.[23] The advantage of this increase in iron status must be weighed against the risks of polycythemia and its attendant hyperviscosity in the neonatal period.

Postnatal iron balance

Postnatal iron balance in the term infant is largely determined by the growth rate of the infant and by the expansion

Table 18.2. Postnatal factors that result in positive or negative iron balance in preterm infants

Factors contributing to negative iron balance
  Low neonatal iron stores
  High growth rate
  Uncompensated phlebotomy
  Restrictive transfusion policy
  Recombinant erythropoietin therapy
  Low iron delivery

Factors contributing to positive iron balance or iron overload
  Multiple red cell transfusions
  High-dose iron therapy (intravenous or enteral)

of the red cell mass associated with this growth. Initially, the term infant is well protected from iron deficiency by a higher hemoglobin concentration than is necessary for extrauterine life, and by relatively high iron stores. These factors endow the term infant with enough iron for the first 4 postnatal months. However, if not provided with a source of dietary iron, the term infant will deplete available iron stores by that age and will be at risk for subsequent iron deficiency.[24] Most term infants are healthy and thus are not excessively phlebotomized or transfused. Their greatest risk for subsequent iron deficiency relates to low dietary iron intake or excessive gastrointestinal iron loss (e.g., due to parasitic diseases). Although all infant formula in the USA provides sufficient iron to support the typical term infant, the rate of iron deficiency in formula-fed term infants remains around 8%.[25]

In contrast to the term infant, the preterm infant is at high risk for negative iron balance and subsequent iron deficiency, and also at risk for iron overload. The increased risk of abnormal iron balance relates closely to the degree of illness encountered in the newborn period. Table 18.2 lists the postnatal factors that alter iron balance in the preterm infant.

The fetus maintains a constant 75 mg of iron per kg body weight. Therefore, premature delivery followed by a lack of iron intake matching intrauterine accretion rates will result in a negative iron balance. The majority of the term infant's birth weight is achieved after 28 weeks gestation as the fetus goes from a mean weight of 1 kg to a weight of 3 kg. The blood volume and the need for iron to support red cell hemoglobin synthesis expand proportionately. Premature birth arrests this process. Initially, while the premature infant is in a catabolic transitional phase and is not growing, there is no need for supplemental iron. As the infant ventures further through the "premie grower" phase, however, maintaining iron sufficiency becomes more important, though the timing of this transition and the consequent age at which supplementation should begin has not been precisely determined.[26]

The process toward negative iron balance in the premature neonate will be hastened by uncompensated phlebotomy, restrictive transfusion policies intended to limit blood donor exposure, and the use of recombinant human erythropoietin to stimulate erythropoiesis. The preterm infant is expected to undergo a process termed "the anemia of prematurity," which initially was described as an exaggeration of the "physiologic anemia" observed in term infants.[27] There are, however, likely substantive differences between the two processes. Because there is little need for the preterm infant to maintain as high a hemoglobin concentration in the "normoxic" ex utero environment as in the "hypoxic" in utero environment, a decline in the hemoglobin concentration during the first 2 months of postnatal life is expected. The severe nadir and the poor growth often associated with the lower end of the range of hemoglobin concentration at this age (e.g., 6 to 8 g dL^{-1}) suggest that this process is not "physiologic." On the other hand, whether this early anemia has a component of iron deficiency remains debatable. Some studies have shown that this anemia is not responsive to iron therapy shortly after birth,[28] while others have documented elevated Zn protoporphyrin levels consistent with a deficiency of available iron for hemoglobin synthesis.[29] In any case, compared with less restrictive policies, restrictive transfusion policies result in a lower total body iron pool since red cells contain a large amount of iron. While the use of recombinant human erythropoietin has no impact on total body iron, it does result in a shift of iron into the red cells at the expense of storage and potentially non-heme tissue pools. Whether aggressive erythropoiesis during a major growth phase in a relatively iron-restricted environment results in tissue-level iron deficiency remains to be determined. The current recommendations to increase the amount of supplemental iron during treatment with erythropoietin seems prudent.[30]

As discussed below, the timing and route of iron supplementation may contribute to negative or positive iron balance. The American Academy of Pediatrics (AAP) and multiple other organizations currently recommend that premature infants receive 2–4 mg of elemental iron per kg body weight enterally each day beginning between 2 weeks and 2 months of postnatal age.[27,31] Both later onset of supplementation and smaller doses of iron result in a higher risk of subsequent iron deficiency.[3,4] Parenteral iron appears to be more bioavailable for erythropoeisis than enteral iron.[32]

Premature infants also are at risk for iron overload, as evidenced by several studies that demonstrated high ferritin levels (>500 ng mL^{-1}) at the end of the neonatal intensive care unit (NICU) hospitalization.[33–35] Not surprisingly, these infants tend to have had very unstable hospital courses, requiring multiple red blood cell transfusions. Both the number of red cell transfusions and the serum ferritin concentration have been correlated with an increased incidence of chronic diseases associated with oxidant injury, including retinopathy of prematurity (ROP) and bronchopulmonary dysplasia (BPD).[33–35] The causal relationship to iron itself, however, has been more difficult to determine because these are often high-risk infants who have been mechanically ventilated longer, who have been exposed to more oxygen, and who have had more septic episodes than the lower-risk premature infant with normal ferritin levels.

Besides the cumulative risk of multiple red cell transfusions on iron status over the entire hospitalization, premature infants are also at risk for potential iron toxicity early in their neonatal course because their antioxidant systems remain immature. Vitamin E concentrations are low, and the ability to absorb this fat-soluble vitamin from the intestine is poor until close to 34 weeks gestation.[36] The vitamin C system, vital for scavenging free radicals, is immature until 2 weeks of postnatal age.[37] Premature infants can be deficient in superoxide dismutase.[38] An early oxidant challenge, such as a serum iron concentration greater than the total iron-binding capacity, may result in tissue damage due to unquenched free radicals. This would most likely occur in the setting of intravenous iron therapy or in hemolysis after red cell transfusions. Because of these risks, the AAP and other organizations do not recommend dosing with iron prior to 2 weeks of postnatal age.[31]

Potential consequences of early iron deficiency

The term newborn infant is not likely to present with classic iron-deficiency anemia unless born to an extremely iron-deficient mother. Most anemia in the newborn is due to intrauterine hemolysis or acute blood loss at birth, and therefore does not result in loss of storage and non-heme iron. In many intrauterine conditions that cause tissue-level iron deficiency (e.g., intrauterine growth retardation and diabetes during pregnancy), the hemoglobin will be normal or elevated. Non-heme tissue iron deficiency should be suspected when the newborn serum ferritin concentration is less than 30 ng mL^{-1}, even if the hemoglobin concentration is normal.[39]

The immediate consequences of early iron deficiency in the term infant may not be inherently obvious. However, many of the symptoms of iron deficiency are due to loss of non-heme tissues such as the heart, and brain. A review of the symptomatology common to IUGR and IDM infants reveals the possibility of a contributing role for tissue-level iron deficiency. These infants tend to be more medically fragile and to not tolerate illnesses such as respiratory distress. Perinatal iron deficiency decreases cytochrome c concentrations in skeletal muscle, heart, and brain.[40,41] This finding may in part explain the symptoms of metabolic "crippling" apparent in these patients, including their higher rates of cardiac dysfunction and lethargy. The immediate consequences of anemia (and perhaps co-incident iron deficiency) in the premature infant are poor growth, lethargy, and myopathy.

The long-term consequences of early iron deficiency relate primarily to neurodevelopment and the risk of later-onset iron-deficiency anemia. Iron-containing enzymes are central to myelination,[42] neurotransmitter synthesis,[43] cell proliferation[44] and neuronal energetics.[45] Postnatal iron deficiency as early as 6 months of age has an adverse effect on the central nervous system (CNS).[46] Arguably, the faster-growing and more immature brain of the preterm and term infant is at even greater risk. The greatest concern is that early iron deficiency affects cognition not only during the period of iron deficiency, but up to 10 years after iron repletion.[47] Animal models strongly support an important role for iron in the developing brain. A recent study in humans confirmed that term infants born with ferritin concentrations in the lowest quartile are at a higher risk for neurocognitive sequelae at school age than are infants born with ferritins in the middle quartiles.[48]

Gestational iron deficiency in animal models results in hypomyelination,[42] alterations in dopamine metabolism,[43] and selective areas of decreased neuronal metabolism.[45] It is interesting to note that IDMs have abnormal cognitive functioning at birth while they are iron deficient,[49] persistence of these abnormalities once iron status has been restored,[50,51] and compromised cognitive outcomes at school age.[52] Although both diabetes during pregnancy and intrauterine growth restriction are characterized by multiple neurocognitive risks (e.g., hypoxia, hypoglycemia), one cannot discount the potential role of iron deficiency in inducing long-lasting structural and metabolic defects in important cognitive structures such as the hippocampus and the striatum. Given the concerns surrounding the potential contribution of iron deficiency to the anemia of prematurity and the role of iron in brain development, it is surprising that no studies to date have addressed the relationship between neurodevelopmental status and long-term outcome of premature infants with abnormal iron indices.

As discussed earlier, premature infants are at increased risk for iron deficiency at an earlier age than term infants, particularly if iron supplementation is delayed until 2 months of postnatal age, or if the daily dose of iron is less than $2 \, mg \, kg^{-1}$ of body weight.[3,4] There are few data on the long-term hematologic outcomes of term infants born with low iron status. A small follow-up study of infants born with abnormally low ferritins demonstrated that the infants had normal iron status at 9 months but that their iron stores were still significantly lower than control.[53] Whether this confers a risk for iron deficiency in the second year of life remains to be determined.

Potential consequences of early iron overload

The neonate in general and the preterm infant in particular is at high risk for the toxic sequelae of iron overload. Although the setting in which iron overload occurs is usually not a "nutritional" issue in the classic sense, the involvement of iron in chemical reactions that generate potentially deleterious oxygen free-radical species is worth considering in this chapter. Studies in human adults and in neonatal animal models demonstrate that free (non-protein bound) iron has a central role in free radical generation through the Fenton reaction (shown below). The Fenton reaction equation:

$$2O_2^- + 2H^+ \rightarrow H_2O_2 + O_2$$
$$Fe^{2+} + H_2O_2 \rightarrow Fe^{3+} + OH^- + OH$$

The Fenton reaction is most likely to occur in two clinical situations: tissue reperfusion after hypoxic–ischemic injury[54,55] and rapid introduction of iron into the serum resulting in saturation of iron-binding capacity. The latter is most likely to happen with parenteral iron therapy or with hemolysis following red blood cell transfusion. High doses of oral iron may result also in transient increases in free iron, although this appears to be a rare event, and at this point the physiologic significance is still a matter of active research.[33] The fetus and preterm neonate are at particularly high risk because of the factors listed in Table 18.3. The risk of free radical injury appears to remain high, at least through the first postnatal week.[34] This may be related in part to lack of maturation of the vitamin C system until after 2 weeks of age.[37]

The role of free iron in the pathogenesis of specific neonatal diseases is, based on animal models, biologically plausible. For example, Palmer et al. demonstrated significant iron deposition in multiple brain structures over a 3-week period following hypoxia–ischemia in the neonatal rat.[56]

Table 18.3. Predisposing fetal and neonatal factors for toxicity from iron overload

High incidence of pre-, peri- and postnatal hypoxic–ischemic events with reperfusion
Immature antioxidant systems (e.g., vitamin E, selenium, superoxide dismutase)
Low serum levels of iron-binding proteins (e.g., transferrin)
Increased sensitivity of rapidly growing tissues to free radicals

The effects were preventable or lessened by pre-treatment with the iron chelator, desferroxiamine.[57] Reactive oxygen species, whose production is stimulated by free iron, are responsible for activating tissue cytokines, initiating arachidonic acid cascades, damaging mitochondrial DNA and promoting apoptotic events.[50,59,60] Proposed target organs that have been studied include the intestine,[61] the lung,[62] the red blood cells,[63] the retina,[64] and the brain.[56]

The evidence in human neonates is more indirect and remains difficult to quantify. Reviews by Perrone *et al.*[65] and by Jansson[6] summarize the role of iron in free radical injury, especially as it relates to developing brain structures. Bracci *et al.* have shown clear evidence of free-iron-induced stress to neonatal red blood cell membranes.[63] Others have epidemiologically linked the risk of neonatal diseases thought to be mediated by oxidant stress to the number of red blood cell transfusions (and, by analogy, exposure to iron). The risk of BPD in preterm infants has been associated with the number of blood transfusions and to free-iron levels,[35] although lipid peroxidation has not been demonstrated. Similarly, it has been noted that infants with severe ROP also have high ferritin concentrations.[36] It remains unclear whether this association is due to free iron toxicity or to the fact that sicker, more premature infants are more likely to get retinopathy and to receive more transfusions. Furthermore, elevated ferritin concentrations are a sign of inflammation, a likely contributory factor to both ROP and BPD. In summary, studies in immature animals demonstrate plausible biological mechanisms for iron toxicity in developing organ systems. Further research in neonatal humans will be needed.

Iron requirements

Term infants require approximately 1 mg kg^{-1} of elemental iron daily if they are formula-fed.[66] Infants consuming their mother's milk receive far less than this amount, but the iron is more bioavailable.[67] Absorption rates of iron from human milk average 50%, compared with 7–12% from infant formula.

At this time, treatment with iron beyond the normal recommended amounts does not appear warranted for term infants born with low iron stores. A small follow-up study of term and near-term infants born with low iron stores from various causes revealed that none had iron deficiency (ferritin <10 ng mL^{-1}) or iron-deficiency anemia (hemoglobin <10.5 g dL^{-1}) at 9 months of age. The infants were fed predominantly breast milk and most were given vitamins with iron,[54] but did not receive additional iron supplementation. Nevertheless, the ferritin concentrations of this group were significantly lower than those of a group of control infants born with normal iron stores. Therefore, these infants can be considered at increased risk for iron deficiency in their second postnatal year.

Preterm infants require substantially more iron on a per kg body weight basis than term infants. The AAP recommends 2–4 mg kg^{-1} of enteral iron daily, depending on the degree of prematurity, beginning between 2 weeks and 2 months after birth.[31] Premature infants should be maintained on these higher doses after discharge from the hospital. Infants treated with rhEpo will require more iron in order to spare their meager iron stores.[30] Enteral doses of 6 mg kg^{-1} day^{-1} appear adequate to sustain modest erythropoiesis in these infants.[30]

Intravenous iron should be used very cautiously because of the risk of overwhelming the TIBC. Since human infants are born with enough iron stores to meet their demands for the first 2 months, delaying iron delivery until the infant is able to tolerate enteral iron may be prudent. If prolonged parenteral nutrition is anticipated, parenteral iron can be utilized at 100–200 µg kg^{-1} day^{-1}.[27]

REFERENCES

1 Kuhn, L., Schulman, H. M., Ponka, P. Iron-transferrin requirements and transferrin receptor expression in proliferating cells. In Ponka, P., Schulman, H. M., Woodworth, R. C., eds. *Iron Transport and Storage*. Boca Raton, FL: CRC Press; 1990:149–92.

2 Oski, F. A., Naiman, J. L. The hematologic aspects of the maternal–fetal relationship. In Oski, F. A., Naiman, J. L., eds. *Hematologic Problems in the Newborn*. 3rd edn. Philadelphia: WB Saunders;1982:32–55.

3 Hall, R. T., Wheeler, R. E., Benson, J., Harris, G., Rippetoe, L. Feeding iron-fortified premature formula during initial hospitalization to infants less than 1800 grams birth weight. *Pediatrics* 1993;**92**:409–14.

4 Friel, J. K., Andrews, W. L., Aziz, K. *et al.* A randomized trial of two levels of iron supplementation and developmental

outcome in low birth weight infants. *J. Pediatr.* 2001;**139**: 254–60.

5 Chockalingam, U., Murphy, E., Ophoven, J. C., Georgieff, M. K. The influence of gestational age, size for dates, and prenatal steroids on cord transferrin levels in newborn infants. *J. Pediatr. Gastroenterol. Nutr.* 1987;**6**:276–80.

6 Jansson. L. T. Iron, oxygen stress, and the preterm infant. In Lonnerdal, B., ed. *Iron Metabolism in Infants.* Boca Raton, FL: CRC Press;1990:73–85.

7 Rios, E., Lipschitz, D. A., Cook, J. D., Smith, N. J. Relationship of maternal and infant iron stores as assessed by determination of plasma ferritin. *Pediatrics* 1975; **55**:694–9.

8 Dallman, P. R. Biochemical basis for the manifestations of iron deficiency. *Ann. Rev. Nutr.* 1986;**6**:13–40.

9 Guiang, S. F., III, Georgieff, M. K., Lambert, D. J., Schmidt, R. L., Widness, J. A. Intravenous iron supplementation effect on tissue iron and hemoproteins in chronically phlebotomized lambs. *Am. J. Physiol.* 1997;**273**:R2124–31.

10 Chockalingam, U., Murphy, E., Ophoven, J. C., Weisdorf, S. A., Georgieff, M. K. Cord transferrin and ferritin levels in newborn infants at risk for prenatal uteroplacental insufficiency and chronic hypoxia. *J. Pediatr.* 1987;**111**:283–6.

11 Georgieff, M. K., Petry, C. D., Wobken, J. D., Oyer, C. E. Liver and brain iron deficiency in newborn infants with bilateral renal agenesis (Potter's syndrome). *Pediatr. Pathol. Lab. Med.* 1996;**16**:509–19.

12 Sweet, D. G., Savage, G., Tubman, T. R., Lappin, T. R., Halliday, H. L. Study of maternal influences on fetal iron status at term using cord blood transferrin receptors. *Arch. Dis. Child Fetal Neonatal. Edn.* 2001;**84**:F40–3.

13 Petry, C., Eaton, M. A., Wobken, J. D. *et al.* Iron deficiency of liver, heart, and brain in newborn infants of diabetic mothers. *J. Pediatr.* 1992;**121**:109–14.

14 Georgieff, M., Landon, M. B., Mills, M. M. *et al.* Abnormal iron distribution in infants of diabetic mothers: spectrum and maternal antecedents. *J. Pediatr.* 1990;**117**:455–61.

15 Philipps, A. F., Porte, P. J., Strabinsky, S., Rosenkranz, T. S., Raye, J. R. Effects of fetal hyperglycemia upon oxygen consumption in the ovine uterus and conceptus. *J. Clin. Invest..* 1984;**74**:279–86.

16 Milley, J. R., Papacostas, J. S., Tabata, B. K. Effect of insulin on uptake of metabolic substrates by the fetus. *Am. J. Physiol.* 1986;**251** (*Endocrinol. Metab. 14*): E349–59.

17 Widness, J. A., Susa, J. B., Garcia, J. F. *et al.* Increased erythropoiesis and elevated erythropoietin in infants born to diabetic mothers and in hyperinsulinemic rhesus fetuses. *J. Clin. Invest.* 1981;**67**:637–42.

18 Georgieff, M. K., Widness, J. A., Mills, M. M., Stonestreet, B. S. The effect of prolonged intrauterine hyperinsulinemia on iron utilization in fetal sheep. *Pediatr. Res.* 1989; **26**:467–9.

19 Petry, C., Eaton, M. A., Wobken, J. D. *et al.* Placental transferrin receptor in diabetic pregnancies with increased iron demand. *Am. J. Physiol.* 1994;**121**:109–14.

20 Georgieff, M. K., Petry, C. D., Mills, M. M., McKay, H., Wobken, J. D. Increased N-glycosylation and reduced transferrin-binding capacity of transferrin receptor isolated from placentae of diabetic women. *Placenta* 1997;**18**:563–8.

21 Cox, T. M., Halsall, D. J. Hemochromatosis–neonatal and young subjects. *Blood Cells Mol. Dis.* 2002; **29**:411–17.

22 Butler, E. The HFE Cys282Tyr mutation as a necessary but not sufficient cause of clinical hereditary hemochromatosis. *Blood* 2003;**101**:3347–50.

23 Grajeda, R., Perez-Escamilla, R., Dewey, K. G. Delayed clamping of umbilical cord improves hematologic status of Guatemalan infants at 2 months of age. *Am. J. Clin. Nutr.* 1997;**65**:425–31.

24 Fomon, S. J., Nelson, S. E., Ziegler, E. E. Retention of iron by infants. *Annu. Rev. Nutr.* 2000; **20**:273–90.

25 American Academy of Pediatrics Committee on Nutrition. Iron deficiency. In Kleinman, R. E., ed. *Pediatric Nutrition Handbook.* 4th Edn. Elk Grove Village, IL: American Academy of Pediatrics; 1998:233–46.

26 Ehrenkranz, R. A. Iron requirements of preterm infants. *Nutrition* 1994;**10**:77–8.

27 Dallman, P. R., Siimes, M. A. Iron deficiency in infancy and childhood: a report for the international nutritional anemia consultative group. Washington, DC: The Nutrition Foundation, 1979.

28 Ehrenkranz, R. A. Iron, folic acid, and vitamin B12. In Tsang, R. C., Lucas, A., Uauy, R., Zlotkin, S. eds. *Nutritional Need of the Preterm Infant.* 2nd Edn. Baltimore, MD: Williams & Wilkins; 1993:177–94.

29 Winzerling, J., Kling, P. Iron-deficient erythropoiesis in premature infants measured by blood zinc protoporphyrin/heme. *J. Pediatr.* 2001;**139**:134–6.

30 Carnielli, V. P., Da Riol, R., Montini, G. Iron supplementation enhances response to high doses of recombinant human erythropoietin in preterm infants. *Arch. Dis. Child Fetal Neonatal Edn.* 1998;**79**:F44-8.

31 American Academy of Pediatrics Committee on Nutrition. Nutritional needs of preterm infants. In Kleinman, R. E., ed. *Pediatric Nutrition Handbook.* Elk Grove Village, IL: American Academy of Pediatrics; 1998:55–87.

32 Pollak, A., Hayde, M., Hayn, M. *et al.* Effect of intravenous iron supplementation on erythropoiesis in erythropoietin-treated premature infants. *Pediatrics* 2001;**107**:78–85.

33 Inder, T. E., Clemett, R. S., Austin, N. C., Graham, P., Darlow, B. A. High iron status in very low birth weight infants is associated with an increased risk of retinopathy of prematurity. *J. Pediatr.* 1997;**131**:541–4.

34 Romagnoli, C., Zecca, E., Gallini, F., Girlando, P., Zuppa, A. A. Do recombinant human erythropoietin and iron supplementation increase the risk of retinopathy of prematurity? *Eur. J. Pediatr.* 2000;**159**:627–8.

35 Cooke, R. W., Drury, J. A., Yoxall, C. W., James, C. Blood transfusion and chronic lung disease in preterm infants. *Eur. J. Pediatr.* 1997;**156**:47–50.

36 Baydas, G., Karatas, F., Gursu, M. F. *et al.* Antioxidant vitamin levels in term and preterm infants and their relation to maternal vitamin status. *Arch. Med. Res.* 2002;**33**:276–80.

37 Berger, T. M., Polidori, M. C., Dabbagh, A. *et al.* Antioxidant activity of vitamin C in iron-overloaded human plasma. *J. Biol. Chem.* 1997;**272**:15656–60.

38 Davis, J. M. Role of oxidant injury in the pathogenesis of neonatal lung disease. *Acta. Paediatr. Suppl.* 2002;**91**:23–5.

39 Saarinen, U. M., Siimes, M. A. Serum ferritin in assessment of iron nutrition in healthy infants. *Acta. Paediatr. Scand.* 1978;**67**:745–51.

40 Georgieff, M. K., Schmidt, R. L., Mills, M. M., Radmer, W. J., Widness, J. A. Fetal iron and cytochrome c status after intrauterine hypoxemia and erythropoietin administration. *Am. J. Physiol.* 1992;**262**:R485–91.

41 Guiang, S. F. III, Widness, J. A., Flanagan, K. B. *et al.* The relationship between fetal arterial oxygen saturation and heart and skeletal muscle myoglobin concentrations in the ovine fetus. *J. Dev. Physiol.* 1993;**19**:99–104.

42 Connor, J. R., Menzies, S. L. Relationship of iron to oligodendrocytes and myelination. *Glia* 1996;**17**:83–93.

43 Nelson, C., Erikson, K., Piñero, J., Beard, J. L. In vivo dopamine metabolism is altered in iron-deficient anemic rats. *J. Nutr.* 1997;**127**:2282–8.

44 Thelander, L. Ribonucleotide reductase. In Ponka, P., Schulman, H. M., Woodworth, R. C., eds. *Iron Transport and Storage.* Boca Raton, FL: CRC Press; 1990:193–200.

45 de Ungria, M., Rao, R., Wobken, J. D. *et al.* Perinatal iron deficiency decreases cytochrome c oxidase activity in selected regions of neonatal rat brain. *Pediatr. Res.* 2000;**48**: 169–76.

46 Roncagliolo, M., Garrido, M., Walter, T., Peirano, P., Lozoff, B. Evidence of altered central nervous system development in infants with iron deficiency anemia at 6 mo: delayed maturation of auditory brainstem responses. *Am. J. Clin. Nutr.* 1998;**68**:683–90.

47 Algarin, C., Peirano, P., Garrido, M., Pizarro, F., Lozoff, B. Iron deficiency anemia in infancy: long-lasting effects on auditory and visual system functioning. *Pediatr. Res.* 2003;**53**:217–23.

48 Tamura, T., Goldberg, R. L., Hou, J. *et al.* Cord serum ferritin concentrations and mental and psychomotor development of children at five years of age. *J. Pediatr.* 2002;**140**:165–70.

49 deRegnier, R. A., Nelson, C. A., Thomas, K., Wewerka, S., Georgieff, M. K. Neurophysiologic evaluation of auditory recognition memory in healthy newborn infants and infants of diabetic mothers. *J. Pediatr.* 2000;**137**:777–84.

50 Nelson, C. A., Wewerka, S., Thomas, K. M. *et al.* Neurocognitive sequelae of infants of diabetic mothers. *Behav. Neurosci.* 2000;**114**:950–6.

51 Nelson, C. A., Wewerka, S., Borscheid, A. J., deRegnier, R.-A., Georgieff, M. K. Electrophysiologic evidence of impaired cross-modal recognition memory in 8-month-old infants of diabetic mothers. *J. Pediatr.* 2003;**142**:575–82.

52 Rizzo, T. A., Metzger, B. E., Dooley, S. L. & Cho, N. H. Early malnutrition and child neurobehavioral development: insights from the study of children of diabetic mothers. *Child Dev.* 1997;**68**:26–38.

53 Georgieff, M. K., Wewerka, S. W., Nelson, C. A., deRegnier, R.-A. Iron status at 9 months of infants with low iron stores at birth. *J. Pediatr.* 2002;**141**:405–9.

54 Liu, P. K. Ischemia-reperfusion-related repair deficit after oxidative stress: implications of faulty transcripts in neuronal sensitivity after brain injury. *J. Biomed. Sci.* 2003;**10**:4–13.

55 Buonocoare, G., Perrone, S., Longini, M. *et al.* Oxidative stress in preterm babies at birth and on the seventh day of life. *Pediatr. Res.* 2003;**52**:46–9.

56 Palmer, C., Menzies, S. L., Roberts, R. L., Pavlick, G., Connor, J. R. Changes in iron histochemistry after hypoxic-ischemic brain injury in the neonatal rat. *J. Neurosci. Res.* 1999;**56**:60–71.

57 Palmer, C., Roberts, R. L., Bero, C. Deferoxamine posttreatment reduces ischemic brain injury in neonatal rats. *Stroke* 1994;**25**:1039–45.

58 Hagberg, H., Gilland, E., Bona, E. *et al.* Enhanced expression of interleukin (IL)-1 and IL-6 messenger RNA and bioactive protein after hypoxia-ischemia in neonatal rats. *Pediatr. Res.* 1996;**40**:603–9.

59 Mishra, O. P., Delivoria-Papadopoulos, M. Cellular mechanisms of hypoxic injury in the developing brain. *Brain Res. Bull.* 1998;**25**:766–70.

60 Akhtar, W., Ashraf, Q. M., Zanelli, S. A., Mishra, O. P., Delivoria-Papadopoulos, M. Effect of graded hypoxia on cerebral cortical genomic DNA fragmentation in newborn piglets. *Biol. Neonate* 2001;**79**:187–93.

61 Hsueh, W., Caplan, M. S., Qu, X. W. *et al.* Neonatal necrotizing enterocolitis: clinical considerations and pathogenetic concepts. *Pediatr. Dev. Pathol.* 2003;**6**:6–23.

62 Saugstad, O. D. Bronchopulmonary dysplasia-oxidative stress and anti-oxidants. *Semin. Neonatol.* 2003;**8**:39–49.

63 Bracci, R., Perrone, S., Buonocore, G. Oxidant injury in neonatal erythrocytes during the perinatal period. *Acta Paediatr. Suppl.* 2002;**438**:S130–4.

64 Hirano, K., Morinobu, T., Kim, H. *et al.* Blood transfusion increases radical promoting non-transferrin bound iron in preterm infants. *Arch. Dis. Child. Fetal Neonatal Edn* 2001;**84**:F188–93.

65 Perrone, S., Bracci, R., Buonocore, G. New biomarkers of fetal-neonatal hypoxic stress. *Acta Paediatr. Suppl.* 2002: **438**:S135–8.

66 American Academy of Pediatrics. Iron fortification of infant formulas. *Pediatrics* 1999;**104**:119–23.

67 Fomon, S. J., Ziegler, E. E., Nelson, S. E. Erythrocyte incorporation of ingested 58Fe by 56 day old breast-fed and formula-fed infants. *Pediatr. Res.* 1993;**33**:573–6.

19

Conditionally essential nutrients: choline, inositol, taurine, arginine, glutamine, and nucleotides

Jane Carver

Department of Pediatrics, University of South Florida College of Medicine, Tampa, FL

Introduction

The term "conditionally essential" has been used to describe the role of choline, inositol, taurine, arginine, glutamine, and nucleotides in human nutrition. The biochemical pathways to synthesize these nutrients are present, and their absence from the diet does not lead to a classical clinical deficiency syndrome. However, under certain conditions, the biosynthetic capacity may be below functional metabolic demands. The conditions under which these nutrients may become essential include prematurity, certain disease states, periods of limited nutrient intake or rapid growth, and the presence of regulatory or developmental factors that interfere with full expression of the endogenous synthetic capacity. Under these conditions, dietary intake of the nutrient may optimize tissue function.[1]

Several of the conditionally essential nutrients are present in significantly higher quantities in human milk versus infant formulas, and several are added to term and/or preterm formulas. On-going research will help to clarify their roles in neonatal nutrition and metabolism.

Choline

Choline was classified in 1998 as an essential nutrient for humans by the Food and Nutrition Board of the Institute of Medicine of the National Academy of Sciences. The Board recognized that fetal development and infancy constitute periods of increased demand for choline.[2] The classification of choline as an essential nutrient will likely stimulate renewed interest and research in its role in the developing infant.

Choline has a variety of biological functions. It is a precursor for the neurotransmitter acetylcholine, and for two signaling lipids, platelet-activating factor and sphingosylphosphorylcholine. Choline can be enzymatically oxidized to betaine, a source of labile methyl groups used in the resynthesis of methionine from homocysteine, thus providing methionine for protein synthesis and transmethylation reactions. Choline is also the precursor of phosphatidylcholine and sphingomyelin, phospholipids that serve as components of biological membranes.[2,3]

During development, large amounts of choline are delivered to the fetus via placental transport systems that pump it against a concentration gradient. Plasma concentrations are 6- to 7-fold higher in the fetus and neonate than in the adult, with levels decreasing during the first weeks of life. The high neonatal levels presumably ensure enhanced availability of choline to tissues.[2–4]

The mammary gland actively synthesizes choline, and concentrations in milk can be as high as sixty times those found in maternal plasma. Choline and choline ester concentrations are highest in colostrum and transitional milk (150 μmol/dl) and are lower in mature milk (75–110 μmol/dl). An infant consuming 150 ml/kg per day of human milk ingests a level of choline that is 2–3 times that ingested by the adult human. Cow's milk-based infant formulas contain 40–150 μmol/dl, depending on the protein source, and soy formulas contain about 120 μmol/dl. Relative concentrations of free choline and choline-containing compounds differ between human milk and formulas, with unesterified choline concentrations in mature milk being significantly lower than bovine milk or infant formulas.[3,5]

Neonatal Nutrition and Metabolism. Second Edition, ed. P. Thureen and W. Hay. Published by Cambridge University Press.
© Cambridge University Press 2006.

Zeisel[4] speculates that these differences may affect the relative balance of choline used by tissues, and recommends that they be considered when modifications are made to infant formulas.

Amino acid–glucose solutions used in parenteral nutrition contain no choline, while intravenous lipid emulsions contain 1.2% egg phospholipid, providing 117 mg choline per dL. Malnourished patients and those receiving choline-free parenteral nutrition solutions have decreased plasma and erythrocyte choline concentrations, they lose less betaine in urine, and they may develop liver dysfunction.[6–8] Chronic ingestion of a choline-deficient diet results in fatty infiltration of the liver and hepatic dysfunction,[9] and choline deficient animals are more likely to develop liver cancers.[10] The cholinergic-dependent aspects of these effects are reversible by the addition of choline to the diet, or by the use of intravenous lipids with choline containing soy or egg phospholipid. The likely mechanism for the hepatocyte lipid accumulation is deficient liver phospholipid synthesis, which is necessary for lipoprotein assembly and extrusion of very low density lipoprotein from hepatocytes.[6] There is also a relationship between choline and carnitine metabolism. Rats fed choline-free diets have reduced tissue levels of carnitine, which has been attributed to a deficiency of available methyl groups required for carnitine synthesis.[11] Dodson and Sachan[12] demonstrated that supplementary choline reduced urinary carnitine excretion in human subjects.

There is increasing evidence that choline plays a role in early brain development. The capacity of the brain to extract choline from blood is greatest during the neonatal period, and choline concentrations in neonatal rat brain are 2-fold higher than adult brain. Provision of supplemental choline during the perinatal period further increases levels of choline and choline metabolites in the brains of offspring.[4] There appear to be two sensitive pre- and postnatal periods in the rat during which supplementation with choline results in significant long-lasting facilitation of spatial memory. These periods correlate with formation of cholinergic neurons (neurogenesis; prenatal) and with formation of nerve-nerve connections (synaptogenesis; postnatal).[4] Meck and Williams[13,14] reported that offspring of dams that received choline supplementation during pregnancy were more adept at tasks that measured spatial and temporal memory and attention, while those of dams fed no choline had impairments in attentional and certain memory tasks. The effects persisted beyond 2 years of age, when a rat is developmentally old. These data suggest that choline's effects on brain organization and function are permanent.[15]

Choline availability during brain development alters the timing of mitosis, apoptosis and early commitment to neuronal differentiation by progenitor cells in the brain septum and hippocampus – two brain regions known to be associated with learning and memory.[16,17] Other studies suggested that supplemental choline influences neuronal transmembrane signaling, accelerates the synthesis and release of acetylcholine by neurons, and mediates changes in brain levels of choline metabolites such as betaine and phosphocholine.[2,4,5]

Although the functional effects of choline supplementation on the central nervous system in humans are unknown, oral administration of either free choline or phosphatidyl-choline (lecithin) may have application in human disease, particularly those involving brain functions that involve cholinergic neurons.[18–20] Choline and lecithin have been studied as potential memory enhancers in patients with Alzheimer disease, however, the results have been disappointing. It was suggested that the choice of patient groups may be a factor, since investigations have primarily been made in subjects with chronic, degenerative nervous system diseases.[19]

The European Society for Pediatric Gastroenterology and Nutrition and the American Academy of Pediatrics Committee on Nutrition have made no specific recommendations for choline. The Life Sciences Research Office (LSRO) of the American Society for Nutritional Sciences recommended a minimum content of 7 mg per 100 kcal for both term and preterm formulas, and a maximum content of 30 and 23 mg per 100 kcal for term and preterm infant formulas, respectively.[21,22] The maximum level of 23 mg per 100 kcal for preterm formula is closer to the upper level of choline reported in human milk.[21]

Inositol

Inositol is a six-carbon sugar alcohol present in biological systems primarily as *myo*-inositol. Inositol and phospho-inositides mediate transmembrane signaling, activate cell surface enzymes and receptors, serve as growth factors for human cell lines, are lipotropic factors that promote lipid synthesis, and they serve as a source of arachidonic acid for the synthesis of eicosanoids.[23–25] Inositols are readily synthesized by many tissues including the brain, testis, liver and kidney, with the kidney serving as the main site of biosynthesis. Serum inositol levels are dependent on the balance between biosynthesis, intake, renal clearance, and catabolism.[26,27] Despite the capacity for endogenous synthesis, tissue concentrations are sensitive to fluctuations in dietary intake.[26,28]

No human deficiency syndrome has been described for inositol, and inositol is not listed as an essential nutrient for humans. However, it was recognized over 40 years ago that inositol can prevent hepatic or intestinal fat accumulation in several adult animal species fed inositol-depleted diets. Rats fed inositol-deficient diets also develop markedly elevated triacyglycerol and esterified cholesterol levels.[23,26,29] The fatty liver and intestine are thought to be due to limited lipoprotein secretion induced by low liver phosphoinositides, promotion of the expression of a fatty acid synthetic enzyme, or mobilization of fatty acids from adipose tissue.[26,30] These effects were not observed in neonatal animals fed inositol depleted diets, suggesting that newborn animals may be able to maintain proper cellular and organ function in spite of a dietary deficiency.[29]

Several clinical conditions, including diabetes mellitus and renal failure, are associated with impaired inositol metabolism.[23,31,32] Inositol administration reverses the altered growth, renal and nerve function, and the lower inositide synthesis seen in diabetic animals.[33,34] More recently, van Straaten and Copp determined that inositol supplementation prevented folic-acid-resistant neural tube defects in a rodent model, which may be due to increased action of protein kinase C.[35]

Human milk inositol levels range from 1500 to over 4000 $\mu M/l$, with higher levels in colostrum.[28,36] Most infant formulas contain <400 $\mu M/l$, and total parenteral solutions contain <100 $\mu M/l$.[36] Consequently, human milk-fed infants have higher serum inositol levels than formula-fed and parenterally fed infants.[28,36] Levels in human milk-fed preterm infants have been reported to increase up to 3 weeks after birth and then decline, or to decrease from birth onward. Levels decline more rapidly in formula-fed and parenterally fed infants.[28,36–39] However, Carver et al.[40] reported that feeding formula with high levels of inositol did not prevent the postnatal decline in serum levels. Inositol levels declined in preterm infants despite feedings with formula containing 1110 $\mu M/l$, a level nearly six times higher than most preterm formulas and closer to reported human milk levels. The number of days of parenteral nutrition was the most important determinant of inositol levels at the time of achieving full enteral feedings, with lower levels associated with prolonged parenteral nutrition.

Although the role of dietary inositol in infant development is unclear, studies indicate that provision of supplemental inositol may be beneficial for infants born prematurely. Serum inositol levels are high during neonatal life and decline to adult levels by approximately 8 weeks of age.[27] Levels in fetal and preterm infant blood are significantly higher than in term infant blood.[27,36,41] Preterm infant cord blood levels are reported to be more than twice those of term infants, and three times higher than maternal levels.[27,36,40,41] The relatively high levels in early life may be due to low renal catabolism and a high rate of synthesis.[27] Hallman et al.[38] suggested that low serum inositol in some preterm infants is a consequence of negative inositol balance which results from low inositol feedings or renal "wastage" of inositol.

A potential benefit of inositol supplementation on surfactant production and lung development has been reported in both animals and preterm infants.[42] Serum myo-inositol levels influence the metabolism of lung surfactant in the newborn, which may relate to inositol's role in potentiating the glucocorticoid-induced acceleration of the differentiation of lung surfactant.[41,43] Hallman et al. reported that preterm infants supplemented with inositol had an increased saturated phosphatidylcholine/sphingomyelin ratio in tracheal aspirates[38] and required less mechanical ventilation.[44] In a subsequent study[39] preterm infants with respiratory distress who were supplemented with intravenous inositol had increased survival without bronchopulmonary dysplasia.

While the role of inositol in development of the retina is unknown, two studies suggest that inositol supplementation may protect against the development of retinopathy of prematurity. In the study of Hallman et al.,[39] preterm infants supplemented with intravenous inositol had a lower incidence of retinopathy of prematurity. Friedman et al.[37] fed low birth weight (LBW) infants feedings containing one of three different inositol concentrations: 2500, 710, or 242 $\mu M/l$. Infants who received the high inositol formula and who had higher serum inositol concentrations had a significantly lower incidence of severe retinopathy.

Howlett and Ohlsson[42] conducted a meta-analysis of the studies of inositol supplementation for the prevention of respiratory distress syndrome in preterm infants (Table 19.1). They concluded that inositol supplementation resulted in statistically significant and clinically important reductions in important short-term adverse neonatal outcomes, and suggested that a multi-center randomized clinical trial of appropriate size is justified to confirm these findings.

The relatively high inositol levels in cord blood and in preterm infants suggest that inositol plays an important role in prenatal and neonatal development. The LSRO recommended a minimum content of inositol in term infant formulas of 4 mg per 100 kcal, and a maximum content of 40 and 44 mg per 100 kcal for term and preterm infant formulas, respectively.[21,22]

Table 19.1. A summary of results from three randomized clinical trials of inositol supplementation in preterm infants[42]

	Relative risk (95% C. I.)	Risk difference (95% C. I.)
Bronchopulmonary dysplasia at 28 days	0.68 (0.45, 1.02)	−0.085 (−0.172, 0.003)
Retinopathy of prematurity, stage 4	0.09 (0.01, 0.67)	−0.078 (−0.128, −0.027)
Intraventricular hemorrhage, grade III or VI	0.55 (0.32, 0.95)	−0.090 (−0.170, −0.010)
Death	0.48 (0.28, 0.80)	−1.31 (−0.218, −0.043)

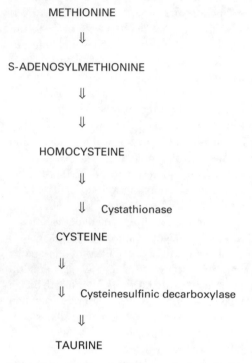

Figure 19.1. An abbreviated schematic of taurine biosynthesis.

Taurine

Taurine is a β-amino sulfonic acid that is formed endogenously from cysteine in many mammalian tissues. It is not a component of structural proteins, but is the most predominant intracellular free amino acid in mammals. A number of functions have been identified for taurine, including detoxification of retinol, iron, and xenobiotics, calcium transport, and osmotic regulation in the brain and kidney. Taurine also serves as a bile acid conjugate, and it plays a critical role in visual development.[21,45] It is synthesized de novo from methionine (Figure 19.1), however, under certain conditions the biosynthetic capacity may not be sufficient to meet physiologic needs.

Human milk taurine levels range from 34 to 80 mg/l, while cow's milk levels are about 1.25 mg/l. As a result, tau-

rine concentrations are very low in formula based on cow's milk proteins, especially casein. Taurine bile acid conjugates predominate in the serum and urine of breast-fed infants,[46,47] and plasma and urinary levels of taurine are higher in preterm and term infants fed human milk versus infant formulas with low taurine levels.[48,45] Rassin *et al.* reported that in preterm infants fed unsupplemented cow's milk formula, taurine was the only plasma amino acid that was present at lower concentrations than in infants fed human milk.[49] The low taurine levels may be due, in part, to low activity of cystathionase, the enzyme that catalyzes the formation of cysteine from methionine. Cystathionase activity is low in humans, and may be absent in term and preterm infant liver.[50] Children who receive taurine-free TPN are reported to have normal plasma levels of methionine and cysteine, but low levels of taurine, suggesting low activity of cysteine sulfinic acid decarboxylase, the enzyme that catalyzes the synthesis of taurine from cysteine.[51]

Taurine is a dietary requirement for cats due to low biosynthetic activity of cysteine sulfinic decarboxylase, and cats fed taurine-free diets develop a dilated cardiomyopathy and retinal degeneration.[45] Neuringer and colleagues[52,53] demonstrated loss of visual acuity and morphological changes in the photoreceptors of rhesus monkeys fed taurine-free formula from birth to 3 months of age. Additional studies demonstrated that infant monkeys are dependent on dietary taurine to maintain normal retinal structure until at least 6 months of age.[54,55] Infants, children, and adults develop reduced plasma taurine levels when maintained on TPN solutions devoid of taurine. Retinal and electroretinogram abnormalities have been reported in children maintained on these solutions for extended periods of time.[56,57] The low taurine levels are normalized by adding taurine to the TPN solution.[51,56,58,59]

The low plasma taurine levels that develop in preterm infants maintained on taurine-free TPN may relate to renal immaturity. Helms *et al.*[60] reported that the fractional excretion of taurine was inversely proportional to birth weight in preterm infants receiving TPN. Zelikovic *et al.*[61] reported that LBW infants maintained on taurine-free parenteral nutrition had low plasma taurine levels and markedly increased mean fractional excretion of taurine compared with healthy, term infants fed human milk or taurine-supplemented formula. Levels increased to normal once oral feeding was started. The authors concluded that the limited ability of the immature kidney to adapt to low taurine intake by increasing tubular reabsorption may result in depleted taurine body pools during the first weeks of life in preterm infants. The taurine reabsorption adaptive response has been localized to the renal proximal tubule brush border membrane, and the molecular signals for the renal conservation of taurine have recently been identified.[62]

Taurine is found in high concentrations in the brain, where it plays a role in osmoregulation. Levels are significantly higher in neonatal versus adult neural tissues.[21,45,63] In vitro studies have demonstrated that taurine enhances neuron extension, proliferation, and survival.[64] Tyson et al.[65] reported that preterm infants who were supplemented with taurine had more mature auditory evoked responses, however, results from this study have been criticized as being inconclusive.[45] Chesney et al.[45] suggested that, due to taurine's osmoregulatory role in the brain and to limited renal taurine conservation, immature infants deprived of taurine may be unable to respond well to hyper- or hypo-osmolar stress without large changes in neuronal volume. They further suggested that the high brain levels of taurine at birth may be a protective feature or compensation for renal immaturity.

Dietary taurine levels affect bile acid synthesis. Taurine-conjugated bile acids favor the formation of mixed micelles, and they promote cholesterol and fatty acid absorption. Taurine deficiency may contribute to the development of cholestasis by increasing levels of the less soluble glycine conjugates of bile acids.[66,67] Okamoto et al.[68] reported that total duodenal bile salt concentration correlated positively with taurine status in preterm infants, and that infants fed taurine-supplemented formula had lower duodenal cholesterol concentrations, suggesting increased conversion to bile acids. Wasserhess et al.[69] reported that preterm infants fed taurine-supplemented formula had lower rates of cholesterol synthesis, and higher bile acid excretion and fatty acid absorption. The lower incidence of cholestasis seen in neonates today is likely due, in part, to the addition of taurine to most pediatric TPN solutions.[21,45]

Other reported effects of taurine supplementation include prevention of hyperaminoacidemia in term infants fed high-protein cow's milk formula,[70] and better vitamin D absorption in preterm infants.[71] Taurine may also influence immune responsiveness. Taurine protects lymphocytes against oxidant-induced injury, and it is reported to be effective in ameliorating endothelial cell cytotoxicity and defective phagocyte and proinflammatory cell microbicidal capacity.[72]

The FDA approved the addition of taurine to infant formulas in 1984, and it is now added to most infant formulas and to pediatric parenteral nutrition solutions. The Expert Panel of the LSRO found no compelling evidence to mandate the addition of taurine to formulas for term infants, but did recommend a maximum content of 12 mg per 100 kcal for term formulas, a value similar to the upper limit reported for human milk.[22] The LSRO considered taurine to be conditionally essential for preterm infants, and recommended minimum and maximum levels of 5 mg per 100 kcal and 12 mg per 100 kcal, respectively, for preterm infant formulas.[21]

Arginine

Recent studies have demonstrated the vital and versatile roles that arginine plays in nutrition and metabolism. Arginine serves as a precursor for the synthesis of nitric oxide (NO), ornithine, urea, polyamines, proline, creatine, glutamine and glutamate. It plays important roles in gastrointestinal, immune, pulmonary, liver, renal, cardiovascular and reproductive function.[21,73]

Preterm infants appear to have higher dietary requirements for arginine than term infants.[21] In early life, arginine plays a role in priming the urea cycle and in the activation of carbamoyl phosphate synthetase (Figure 19.2). In 1972,

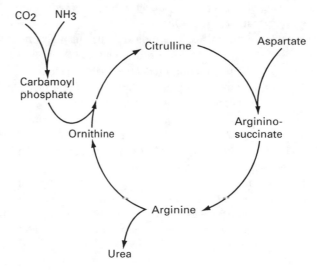

Figure 19.2. Urea cycle showing arginine. Reprinted with permission.[1]

Heird *et al.*[74] reported that hyperammonemia in preterm infants receiving TPN could be effectively treated by intravenous administration of L-arginine, suggesting that this condition resulted from hypoarginemia rather than from an insufficiency of urea cycle enzymes. Current hyperalimentation solutions may have inadequate levels of arginine for preterm infants.[73,75]

Plasma levels of arginine reportedly do not vary between breast versus formula-fed infants born at term.[21] Among preterm infants, however, plasma levels of arginine are significantly lower in infants fed preterm formula versus expressed breast milk.[76,77] Brooke *et al.* reported that no other amino acid was significantly lower in the plasma of formula- versus breast-fed infants.[76]

Much of the interest in arginine relates to its role as a precursor to NO. NO, an intracellular signal that leads to smooth muscle relaxation, is synthesized from L-arginine by NO synthases. In the intestine, NO is an anti-inflammatory chemical mediator and vasodilator that is involved in the maintenance of mucosal integrity, intestinal barrier function, intestinal blood flow regulation, and the inhibition of platelet and leukocyte adhesion during inflammation or injury.[73,78,79] In animal models of necrotizing enterocolitis (NEC), inhibition of NO synthesis increases intestinal damage, while exogenous sources of NO attenuate injury.[80–82]

Decreased blood levels of arginine may relate to the development of NEC in preterm infants. Zamora *et al.*[83] reported that plasma arginine levels were significantly lower at the time of diagnosis in infants with NEC compared with control infants. Plasma ammonia concentrations were elevated, and they decreased with postnatal age and with increasing plasma arginine concentrations. Becker *et al.*[84] reported that preterm infants with NEC have selective amino acid deficiencies, including arginine, that may predispose to the illness. More recently, Amin *et al.*[85] reported that arginine supplementation decreased the incidence of NEC. In a randomized, double-blind study, 152 preterm infants were assigned to receive either supplemental arginine or placebo with their oral feeds/parenteral nutrition during the first 28 days of life. NEC developed in 6.7% of the infants in the supplemented group, versus 27.3% in the unsupplemented group (p < 0.001). Plasma arginine concentrations were lower in both groups at the time of diagnosis of NEC. The authors speculated that low levels of de novo arginine synthesis in immature bowel tissues may lead to a relative arginine deficiency and low tissue levels of NO, and that the resulting vasoconstriction and ischemia-reperfusion injury may predispose to the development of NEC. They further commented that the low plasma arginine

concentrations may result from an increased metabolic demand for arginine in an effort to maintain gastrointestinal blood flow. While much of the protective effect of arginine supplementation is likely mediated through its effects on NO production, Neu[86] remarked that arginine is also the precursor for other amino acids that play important roles in intestinal metabolism, including glutamine and glutamate.

Arginine may also protect against the development of neonatal pulmonary disease. Zamora *et al.*[87] reported that plasma arginine was decreased on the third day of life in preterm infants with respiratory distress. There was an inverse correlation between the oxygenation index and arginine concentration, suggesting that arginine was consumed by the production of large amounts of NO in the pulmonary vasculature. Alternatively, the authors speculated that there was a relative lack of arginine that interfered with NO production, thus contributing to increased severity of respiratory distress syndrome. Castillo *et al.*[88] reported an association between whole body arginine metabolism and NO synthesis in newborns with persistent pulmonary hypertension.

Other reported effects of dietary arginine include prevention of maternal hypoxia-induced fetal growth restriction in the rat[89] and reversal of fetal growth restriction induced by inhibition of NO synthesis.[90] Arginine has also been identified as an "immunonutrient." Enteral arginine administration is reported to upregulate immune function, reduce the incidence of postoperative infection, and to enhance wound healing in children.[91,92] Arginine may also have antiatherogenic effects, which may be mediated through NO effects on vascular tone, or through NO-independent effects.[93,94] Studies in adults have demonstrated that L-arginine administration under pathologic conditions can reverse or attenuate vasoconstriction.[95,96]

While relative arginine deficiency may play a role in the etiology of certain neonatal diseases, the administration of excessive levels of arginine can have adverse effects, which may relate to an increase in inducible NO synthase.[97] In addition, hyperargininemia caused by congenital hepatic arginase deficiency is associated with growth failure and neurological abnormalities.[21]

The LSRO recommended 86 mg/kg per day as a level of arginine intake that can help to prevent the hyperammonemia associated with arginine deficiency in preterm infants. The committee recommended a minimum level for preterm formula of 72 mg per 100 kcal, and a maximum level of 104 mg per 100 kcal.[21] The LSRO made no specific recommendations for arginine levels in term infant formulas.[22]

Glutamine

Glutamine is the most abundant amino acid in the body, accounting for about 20% of free amino acids and about 60% of skeletal muscle. Glutamine plays many diverse roles. It is a major fuel for the enterocyte, a substrate for purine and pyrimidine nucleotide synthesis, a regulator of protein synthesis, and it also plays a role in immune responsiveness and the development and maintenance of the intestinal mucosal system.[98–100] Under most circumstances, glutamine is synthesized in sufficient amounts to meet the needs of the growing infant. However, glutamine may be important under conditions of physiologic stress, including low energy and protein reserves, and treatment with catabolic glucocorticoids.[101] These conditions may be particularly relevant for preterm infants who frequently receive TPN but minimal enteral nutrition in the first few weeks of life. Human milk and infant formulas contain glutamine; however, parenteral nutrition solutions do not.

Glutamine supplementation may be beneficial in the prevention of infection and sepsis. Severe infection causes marked derangements in the flow of glutamine among organs, and the intracellular glutamine pool becomes depleted. Cells of the immune system are major glutamine consumers during inflammation, when cell proliferation is increased. Under these conditions, glutamine availability may become rate limiting for key cell functions such as phagocytosis and antibody production.[102] Several studies in critically ill adults have reported that glutamine supplementation was associated with decreased hospital acquired sepsis, decreased hospital costs, and decreased mortality.[103–106]

Glutamine's beneficial effects on sepsis prevention may relate, in part, to effects on the gastrointestinal tract. Studies in humans have demonstrated that parenteral and enteral administration of glutamine can increase the growth and absorptive capacity of intestinal mucosa following malnutrition, improve gastrointestinal recovery following starvation-induced atrophy, enhance the structure and function of transplanted small intestine, reduce bacterial translocation, and increase protein synthesis in the intestinal mucosa.[104,106–108] The precise mechanisms by which glutamine exerts its beneficial effects on the gastrointestinal system have not been determined. However, glutamine plays a regulatory role in intestinal metabolism, and it serves as a precursor to substances that play an important role in intestinal growth and maturation. For example, the amide nitrogen of glutamine is required for the synthesis of purine and pyrimidine nucleotides, which are utilized by the rapidly proliferating cells of the neonatal intestine.[101,109] He et al.[110] demonstrated that glutamine and nucleotides may act synergistically in intestinal epithelial proliferation and differentiation. The amide nitrogen of glutamine is also critical for the synthesis of hexosamines, which are components of glycoproteins and amino sugars that play a role in maintenance of absorptive and gut barrier functions.[109] In vitro and animal studies have demonstrated that glutamine deprivation can alter the luminal mucus gel, break down small intestinal inter-epithelial junctional integrity, increase bacterial translocation, and cause sloughing of microvilli.[109,111] These findings may relate to the low serum levels of glutamine reported in infants who develop NEC.[84]

Several studies in preterm infants have demonstrated beneficial effects of glutamine administration. Lacey et al.[112] reported that infants with birth weights < 800 g who received glutamine-supplemented versus standard TPN required fewer days of hyperalimentation, had shorter length of time to full feeds, and required less time on the ventilator. Neu et al.[113] reported that very low birth weight infants (VLBW) fed glutamine-supplemented versus non-supplemented formula had significantly lower rates of hospital-acquired sepsis, and better tolerance to enteral feedings. Glutamine supplementation was also associated with a blunting of the rise in HLA-DR$^+$ and CD16$^+$ lymphocytes, which the authors speculated may relate to decreased stimulation of the immune response secondary to less bacterial translocation. A subsequent publication demonstrated that the enteral glutamine supplementation was associated with decreased hospital costs.[114] Des Roberts et al.[115] reported that intravenous glutamine had an acute protein-sparing effect in VLBW, as demonstrated by suppressed leucine oxidation and protein breakdown. Others have investigated whether glutamine might reverse the catabolic effects of glucocorticoids, however, the results have been varied.[109]

Two large multi-center studies of glutamine supplementation in preterm infants have recently been completed. In a study conducted by the NICHD Neonatal Research Network, preterm infants with birth weights 401–1000 g were randomized to receive either TPN or an isonitrogenous solution with 20% glutamine. Data for 1352 patients revealed no effect upon survival rates, the incidence of late-onset sepsis or NEC, mortality rates, days to full enteral feeds, or length of hospital stay.[116] Vaughn et al.[117] randomized 649 VLBWI to receive enteral glutamine supplementation or water placebo for 28 days. There was no difference in the number of infants who developed proven or suspected sepsis, however, a secondary outcome

Table 19.2. Reported effects of dietary nucleotides in humans and in animals

	Human	Animal
Promotion of small intestinal growth		+
Increased small intestinal disaccharidase activity		+
Protection against diarrheal disease	+	+
Effects on intestinal blood flow	+	
Effects on stool flora	+/−	
Enhanced cellular immunity	+	+
Effects on blood lipids	+/−	+/−

analysis showed that fewer infants treated with glutamine had gastrointestinal dysfunction or severe neurological sequelae.

The LSRO did not make specific recommendations regarding the addition of glutamine to term or preterm infant formulas. Interest in the role of glutamine in intestinal growth and maturation, and its potential role in decreasing the incidence of sepsis continues.

Nucleotides

Nucleotides (NT) and their related metabolic products play key roles in many biological processes. They serve as nucleic acid precursors, physiological mediators, components of coenzymes, and sources of cellular energy. NT consist of a nitrogenous base, a pentose sugar and one or more phosphate groups. The purine and pyrimidine bases can be synthesized de novo, or they can be salvaged during metabolism. However, these are metabolically costly processes, and utilization of dietary NT is more efficient.[1, 118,119] The results of studies in human infants and in animals support their role as conditionally essential nutrients (Table 19.2).

NT are a component of the nonprotein nitrogen fraction of milk. NT levels are low in cow's milk and in unsupplemented cow's milk-based formulas.[120] A wide range of NT concentrations, from 3 to over 7 mg/dl, has been reported for human milk.[121–123] Human milk contains polymeric NT, monomeric NT, nucleosides, and NT adducts, which account for 48%, 36%, 8%, and 9%, respectively, of the amount potentially available.[122] The metabolic fate of these compounds in the breast-fed infant is unknown; however, investigations in animals suggest that nucleosides are the primary form by which NT are absorbed. The relative quantities of the individual NT vary in human milk, although

cytidine is usually reported to be present in the highest concentrations.[121,122]

Dietary NT are degraded in the intestine, and most are absorbed into the enterocyte where they are rapidly degraded, and the catabolic products are excreted in the urine and intestine. However, studies in animals have demonstrated that a portion of dietary NT are incorporated into tissue pools, primarily within the small intestine, liver, and skeletal muscle. As the level of dietary nucleic acids increases, the amount of dietary NT that are utilized increases.[118,119]

Dietary NT are reported to play a role in growth and differentiation of gastrointestinal tissues.[121,124] In animal studies, dietary NT supplementation was associated with increased mucosal protein, DNA, villus height, and disaccharidase activities,[125] and increased small bowel weight and protein synthesis.[126] In animal models of bowel injury, dietary NT supplementation increased tissue DNA content and disaccharidase activities, promoted small bowel ulcer healing, and inhibited endotoxin-induced bacterial translocation in mice fed a protein-free diet.[121] LeLeiko *et al.*[127] reported that feeding NT-free diets to rats was associated with altered gene expression of intestinal enzymes, and with significant decreases in total RNA and protein in the gastrointestinal tissues. In vitro, exogenous NT increased the normal growth and maturation of enterocytes, and reduced their dependence on exogenous glutamine.[128] Tanaka *et al.*[129] suggested that AMP may play an important role in cellular turnover in the developing human small intestine.

Dietary NT also affect gastrointestinal function in infants. In three studies, infants fed NT-supplemented formula had a significantly lower incidence of diarrhea compared with infants fed unsupplemented formula.[130–132] There are contradictory reports regarding dietary NT effects on the microbial pattern in stool.[133,134] Superior mesenteric artery blood flow velocity was reported to be significantly higher in term[135,136] and preterm[137] infants following a feeding with NT-supplemented versus unsupplemented formula. While the significance of these findings is unclear, dietary NT effects on the gastrointestinal tract may relate to alterations in intestinal blood flow.

Dietary NT are also reported to affect immune responsiveness. Feeding NT-supplemented versus NT-free diet to rodents was associated with increases in the following immune responses: graft versus host disease mortality, delayed cutaneous hypersensitivity, alloantigen and mitogen-induced lymphoproliferation, natural killer cell activity, resistance to microbial challenge, macrophage phagocytic capacity, spleen cell production of interleukin-2, peripheral blood total leukocyte counts, and neutrophil numbers following infection.[119,121] Dietary NT may up-regulate the Th1 response in systemic immunity, which could enhance tolerance to antigen challenge.[138,139]

Dietary NT affect immune responsiveness in infants. Pickering *et al.*[131] reported that term infants fed NT-supplemented versus unsupplemented formula had significantly higher antibody responses following vaccination with *Haemophilus influenzae* type b. Increased levels of natural killer cell activity,[140] higher serum concentrations of IgG antibody to β-lactoglobulin[141] and higher plasma levels of IgM and IgA[142] were reported in infants fed NT-supplemented versus unsupplemented formula. Although the mechanism of dietary NT effects on immunity is unknown, dietary NT effects on peripheral immunity may be mediated, in part, through effects on gut-associated lymphoid tissues.[121]

Other reported effects of dietary NT supplementation of infant formula include increased catch-up growth in small-for-gestational-age (SGA) infants,[143] and modulation of lipoprotein and fatty acid metabolism.[144,145] The effects on lipid metabolism have been refuted by other investigators.[146,147] In rodents, dietary nucleotide supplementation affected hepatic composition and histology.[118,126]

NT are added to most formulas for term infants, however, they are not added to preterm formulas marketed in the US. The LSRO made no recommendations regarding minimal levels of NT for term[22] or preterm formulas.[21] They recommended a maximum level of 16 mg per 100 kcal of NT and NT precursors, and recommended that levels not exceed 20% of the total nonprotein nitrogen.[21] Continued research on dietary NT, including long-term, large-scale clinical trials, was strongly encouraged.[22]

REFERENCES

1 Uauy, R., Greene, H., Heird, W. Conditionally essential nutrients: cysteine, taurine, tyrosine, arginine, glutamine, choline, inositol, and nucleotides. In Tsang, R., Lucas, A., Uauy, R., Zlotkin, S., eds. *Nutritional Needs of the Preterm Infant*. Pawling, NY: Caduceus Medical Publishers; 1993:267–80.

2 Blusztajn, J. K. Choline, a vital amine. *Science* 1998;**281**:794–5.

3 Zeisel, S. H. Choline: an essential nutrient for humans. *Nutrition* 2000;**16**:669–71.

4 Zeisel, S. H. Choline: essential for brain development and function. In Barness, L. A., ed. *Advances in Pediatrics*. Chicago, IL: Mosby-Year Book; 1997:263–95.

5 Zeisel, S. H. Choline: needed for normal development of memory. *J. Am. Coll. Nutr.* 2000;**19**:528S-31S.

6 Buchman, A. L., Ament, M. E., Sohel, M. *et al.* Choline deficiency causes reversible hepatic abnormalities in patients receiving parenteral nutrition: proof of a human choline requirement: a placebo-controlled trial. *J. Parenter. Enteral Nutr.* 2001;**25**:260–8.

7 Chawla, R. K., Wolf, D. C., Kutner, M. H., Bonkovsky, H. L. Choline may be an essential nutrient in malnourished patients with cirrhosis. *Gastroenterology* 1989;**97**:1514–20.

8 Sheard, N., Tayek, J., Bistrian, B., Blackburn, G., Zeisel, S. H. Plasma choline concentrations in humans fed parenterally. *Am. J. Clin. Nutr.* 1986;**43**:219–24.

9 Kaminski, D. L., Adams, A., Jellinek, M. The effect of hyperalimentation on hepatic lipid content and lipogenic enzyme activity in rats and man. *Surgery* 1980;**88**:93–100.

10 Chandar, N., Lombardi, B. Liver cell proliferation and incidence of hepatocellular carcinomas in rats fed consecutively a choline-devoid and a choline-supplemented diet. *Carcinogenesis* 1988;**9**:259–63.

11 Buchman, A. Relation between choline and carnitine homeostasis. *Am. J. Clin. Nutr.* 1997;**65**:574–5.

12 Dodson, W., Sachan, D. Choline supplementation reduces urinary carnitine excretion in humans. *Am. J. Clin. Nutr.* 1996;**63**:904–10.

13 Meck, W. H., Williams, C. L. Perinatal choline supplementation increases the threshold for chunking in spatial memory. *Neuroreport* 1997;**8**:3053–9.

14 Meck, W. H., Williams, C. L. Characterization of the facilitative effects of perinatal choline supplementation on timing and temporal memory. *Neuroreport* 1997;**8**:2831–5.

15 Meck, W. H., Williams, C. L. Choline supplementation during prenatal development reduces proactive interference in spatial memory. *Brain Res. Dev. Brain Res.* 1999;**118**:51–9.

16 Albright, C. D., Friedrich, C. B., Brown, E. C., Mar, M. H., Zeisel, S. H. Maternal dietary choline availability alters mitosis, apoptosis and the localization of TOAD-64 protein in the developing fetal rat septum. *Brain Res. Dev. Brain Res.* 1999;**115**:123–9.

17 Albright, C. D., Mar, M. H., Friedrich, C. B. *et al.* Maternal choline availability alters the localization of p15Ink4B and p27Kip1 cyclin-dependent kinase inhibitors in the developing fetal rat brain hippocampus. *Dev. Neurosci.* 2001;**23**:100–6.

18 Cohen, E., Wurthman, R. Brain acetylcholine: control by dietary choline. *Science* 1976;**191**:561–2.

19 Fernstrom, J. D. Can nutrient supplements modify brain function? *Am. J. Clin. Nutr.* 2000;**71**:1669S-75S.

20 Klein, J., Koppen, A., Loffelholz, K. Regulation of free choline in rat brain: dietary and pharmacological manipulations. *Neurochem. Intl.* 1998;**32**:479–85.

21 Klein, C. J., ed. Nutrient requirements for preterm infant formulas. A report from the American Society for Nutritional Sciences, Life Sciences Research Office. *J. Nutr.* 2002;**132**:1431S–49S.

22 Raiten, D., Talbot, J., Waters, J. eds. Assessment of nutrient requirements for infant formulas. A report from the American Society for Nutritional Sciences, Life Sciences Research Office. *J. Nutr.* 1998;**128**:2059S–293S.

23 Holub, B. J. The nutritional importance of inositol and the phosphoinositides. *N. Engl. J. Med.* 1992;**326**:1285–7.

24 Holub, B. J. The cellular forms and functions of the inositol phospholipids and their metabolic derivatives. *Nutr. Rev.* 1987;**45**:65–71.

25 Kirk, C. J., Maccallum, S. H., Michell, R. H., Barker, C. J. Inositol phosphates in receptor-mediated cell signaling: metabolic origins and interrelationships. *Biotechnol. Appl. Biochem.* 1990;**12**:489–95.

26 Holub, B. J. Metabolism and function of myo-inositol and inositol phospholipids. *Ann. Rev. Nutr.* 1986;**6**:563–97.

27 Lewin, L. M., Melmed, S., Passwell, J. H. *et al.* Myoinositol in human neonates: serum concentrations and renal handling. *Pediatr. Res.* 1978;**12**:3–6.

28 Bromberger, P., Hallman, M. Myoinositol in small preterm infants: relationship between intake and serum concentration. *J. Pediatr. Gastroenterol. Nutr.* 1986;**5**:455–8.

29 Burton, L. E., Ray, R. E., Bradford, J. R. *et al.* Myo-inositol metabolism in the neonatal and developing rat fed a myo-inositol-free diet. *J. Nutr.* 1976;**106**:1610–16.

30 Beach, D. C., Flick, P. K. Early effect of myo-inositol deficiency on fatty acid synthetic enzymes of rat liver. *Biochim. Biophys. Acta.* 1982;**711**:452–9.

31 Clements, R. S., Jr., Vourganti, B., Kuba, T., Oh, S. J., Darnell, B. Dietary myo-inositol intake and peripheral nerve function in diabetic neuropathy. *Metabolism* 1979;**28**:477–83.

32 Haneda, M., Kikkawa, R., Arimura, T. *et al.* Glucose inhibits myo-inositol uptake and reduces myo-inositol content in cultured rat glomerular mesangial cells. *Metabolism* 1990;**39**:40–5.

33 Pugliese, G., Tilton, R. G., Speedy, A. *et al.* Modulation of hemodynamic and vascular filtration changes in diabetic rats by dietary myo-inositol. *Diabetes* 1990;**39**:312–22.

34 Kim, J., Kyriazi, H., Greene, D. A. Normalization of $Na^{(+)}-K^{(+)}$-ATPase activity in isolated membrane fraction from sciatic nerves of streptozocin-induced diabetic rats by dietary myo-inositol supplementation in vivo or protein kinase C agonists in vitro. *Diabetes* 1991;**40**:558–67.

35 Van Straaten, H. W., Copp, A. J. Curly tail: a 50-year history of the mouse spina bifida model. *Anat. Embryol. (Berl).* 2001;**203**:225–37.

36 Pereira, G. R., Baker, L., Egler, J., Corcoran, L., Chiavacci, R. Serum myoinositol concentrations in premature infants fed human milk, formula for infants, and parenteral nutrition. *Am. J. Clin. Nutr.* 1990;**51**:589–93.

37 Friedman, C. A., McVey, J., Borne, M. J. *et al.* Relationship between serum inositol concentration and development of retinopathy of prematurity: a prospective study. *J. Pediatr. Ophthalmol. Strabismus* 2000;**37**:79–86.

38 Hallman, M., Arjomaa, P., Hoppu, K. Inositol supplementation in respiratory distress syndrome: relationship between serum concentration, renal excretion, and lung effluent phospholipids. *J. Pediatr.* 1987;**110**:604–10.

39 Hallman, M., Bry, K., Hoppu, K., Lappi, M., Pohjavuori, M. Inositol supplementation in premature infants with respiratory distress syndrome. *N. Engl. J. Med.* 1992;**326**:1233–9.

40 Carver, J. D., Stromquist, C. I., Benford, V. J. *et al.* Postnatal inositol levels in preterm infants. *J. Perinatol.* 1997;**17**:389–92.

41 Hallman, M., Saugstad, O. D., Porreco, R. P., Epstein, B. L., Gluck, L. Role of myoinositol in regulation of surfactant phospholipids in the newborn. *Early Hum. Dev.* 1985;**10**:245–54.

42 Howlett, A., Ohlsson, A. Inositol for respiratory distress syndrome in preterm infants. *Cochrane Database Syst Rev.* 2000:CD000366.

43 Hallman, M., Slivka, S., Wozniak, P., Sills, J. Perinatal development of myoinositol uptake into lung cells: surfactant phosphatidylglycerol and phosphatidylinositol synthesis in the rabbit. *Pediatr. Res.* 1986;**20**:179–85.

44 Hallman, M., Jarvenpaa, A. L., Pohjavuori, M. Respiratory distress syndrome and inositol supplementation in preterm infants. *Arch. Dis. Child.* 1986;**61**:1076–83.

45 Chesney, R. W., Helms, R. A., Christensen, M. *et al.* An updated view of the value of taurine in infant nutrition. *Adv. Pediatr.* 1998;**45**:179–200.

46 Boehm, G., Braun, W., Moro, G., Minoli, I. Bile acid concentrations in serum and duodenal aspirates of healthy preterm infants: effects of gestational and postnatal age. *Biol. Neonate.* 1997;**71**:207–14.

47 Strandvik, B., Wahlen, E., Wikstrom, S. A. The urinary bile acid excretion in healthy premature and full-term infants during the neonatal period. *Scand. J. Clin. Lab. Invest.* 1994;**54**:1–10.

48 Gaull, G. E., Rassin, D. K., Raiha, N. C., Heinonen, K. Milk protein quantity and quality in low-birth-weight infants. III. Effects on sulfur amino acids in plasma and urine. *J. Pediatr.* 1977;**90**:348–55.

49 Rassin, D. K., Gaull, G. E., Jarvenpaa, A. L., Raiha, N. C. Feeding the low-birth-weight infant: II. Effects of taurine and cholesterol supplementation on amino acids and cholesterol. *Pediatrics.* 1983;**71**:179–86.

50 Sturman, J. A., Gaull, G., Raiha, N. C. Absence of cystathionase in human fetal liver: is cysteine essential? *Science* 1970;**169**:74–6.

51 Vinton, N. E., Laidlaw, S. A., Ament, M. E., Kopple, J. D. Taurine concentrations in plasma, blood cells, and urine of children undergoing long-term total parenteral nutrition. *Pediatr. Res.* 1987;**21**:399–403.

52 Neuringer, M., Palackal, T., Sturman, J. A., Imaki, H. Effects of postnatal taurine deprivation on visual cortex development in rhesus monkeys through one year of age. *Adv. Exp. Med. Biol.* 1994;**359**:385–92.

53 Neuringer, M., Sturman, J. Visual acuity loss in rhesus monkey infants fed a taurine-free human infant formula. *J. Neurosci. Res.* 1987;**18**:597–601.

54 Imaki, H., Jacobson, S. G., Kemp, C. M. *et al.* Retinal morphology and visual pigment levels in 6- and 12-month-old rhesus monkeys fed a taurine-free human infant formula. *J. Neurosci. Res.* 1993;**36**:290–304.

55 Imaki, H., Neuringer, M., Sturman, J. Long-term effects on retina of rhesus monkeys fed taurine-free human infant formula. *Adv. Exp. Med. Biol.* 1996;**403**:351–60.

56 Geggel, H. S., Ament, M. E., Heckenlively, J. R., Martin, D. A., Kopple, J. D. Nutritional requirement for taurine in patients receiving long-term parenteral nutrition. *N. Engl. J. Med.* 1985;**312**:142–6.

57 Vinton, N. E., Heckenlively, J. R., Laidlaw, S. A. *et al.* Visual function in patients undergoing long-term total parenteral nutrition. *Am. J. Clin. Nutr.* 1990;**52**:895–902.

58 Kopple, J. D., Vinton, N. E., Laidlaw, S. A., Ament, M. E. Effect of intravenous taurine supplementation on plasma, blood cell, and urine taurine concentrations in adults undergoing long-term parenteral nutrition. *Am. J. Clin. Nutr.* 1990;**52**: 846–53.

59 Vinton, N. E., Laidlaw, S. A., Ament, M. E., Kopple, J. D. Taurine concentrations in plasma and blood cells of patients undergoing long-term parenteral nutrition. *Am. J. Clin. Nutr.* 1986;**44**:398–404.

60 Helms, R. A., Christensen, M. L., Storm, M. C., Chesney, R. W. Adequacy of sulfur amino acid intake in infants receiving parenteral nutrition. *J. Nutr. Biochem.* 1995;**6**:462–6.

61 Zelikovic, I., Chesney, R. W., Friedman, A. L., Ahlfors, C. E. Taurine depletion in very low birth weight infants receiving prolonged total parenteral nutrition: role of renal immaturity. *J. Pediatr.* 1990;**116**:301–6.

62 Han, X., Patters, A. B., Chesney, R. W. Transcriptional repression of taurine transporter gene (TauT) by p53 in renal cells. *J. Biol. Chem.* 2002;**277**:39266–73.

63 Sturman, J. A., Messing, J. M., Rossi, S. S., Hofmann, A. F., Neuringer, M. D. Tissue taurine content and conjugated bile acid composition of rhesus monkey infants fed a human infant soy-protein formula with or without taurine supplementation for 3 months. *Neurochem. Res.* 1988;**13**:311–16.

64 Lima, L., Obregon, F., Cubillos, S., Fazzino, F., Jaimes, I. Taurine as a micronutrient in development and regeneration of the central nervous system. *Nutr. Neurosci.* 2001;**4**:439–43.

65 Tyson, J. E., Lasky, R., Flood, D. *et al.* Randomized trial of taurine supplementation for infants less than or equal to 1,300-gram birth weight: effect on auditory brainstem-evoked responses. *Pediatrics* 1989;**83**:406–15.

66 Howard, D., Thompson, D. F. Taurine: an essential amino acid to prevent cholestasis in neonates? *Ann. Pharmacother.* 1992;**26**:1390–2.

67 Tazawa, Y., Yamada, M., Nakagawa, M., Konno, Y., Tada, K. Unconjugated, glycine-conjugated, taurine-conjugated bile acid nonsulfates and sulfates in urine of young infants with cholestasis. *Acta Paediatr. Scand.* 1984;**73**:392–7.

68 Okamoto, E., Rassin, D. K., Zucker, C. L., Salen, G. S., Heird, W. C. Role of taurine in feeding the low-birth-weight infant. *J. Pediatr.* 1984;**104**:936–40.

69 Wasserhess, P., Becker, M., Staab, D. Effect of taurine on synthesis of neutral and acidic sterols and fat absorption in preterm and full-term infants. *Am. J. Clin. Nutr.* 1993;**58**:349–53.

70 Raiha, N. C., Fazzolari-Nesci, A., Boehm, G. Taurine supplementation prevents hyperaminoacidemia in growing term infants fed high-protein cow's milk formula. *Acta Paediatr.* 1996;**85**:1403–7.

71 Zamboni, G., Piemonte, G., Bolner, A. *et al.* Influence of dietary taurine on vitamin D absorption. *Acta Paediatr.* 1993;**82**:811–15.

72 Redmond, H. P., Stapleton, P. P., Neary, P., Bouchier-Hayes, D. Immunonutrition: the role of taurine. *Nutrition* 1998;**14**:599–604.

73 Wu, G., Meininger, C., Knabe, D., Baze, F., Rhoads, J. Arginine nutrition in development, health and disease. *Curr. Opin. Clin. Nutr. Met. Care* 2000;**3**:59–66.

74 Heird, W., Nicholson, J., Driscoll, J., Schullinger, J., Winters, R. Hyperammonemia resulting from intravenous alimentation using a mixture of synthetic l-amino acids: a preliminary report. *J. Pediatr.* 1972;**81**:162–5.

75 Brunton, J. A., Ball, R. O., Pencharz, P. B. Current total parenteral nutrition solutions for the neonate are inadequate. *Curr. Opin. Clin. Nutr. Metab. Care* 2000;**3**:299–304.

76 Brooke, O. G., Onubogu, O., Heath, R., Carter, N. D. Human milk and preterm formula compared for effects on growth and metabolism. *Arch. Dis. Child.* 1987;**62**:917–23.

77 Tikanoja, T., Simell, O., Viikari, M., Jarvenpaa, A. L. Plasma amino acids in term neonates after a feed of human milk or formula. II. Characteristic changes in individual amino acids. *Acta Paediatr. Scand.* 1982;**71**:391–7.

78 Alican, I., Kubes, P. A critical role for nitric oxide in intestinal barrier function and dysfunction. *Am. J. Physiol.* 1996;**270**:G225–37.

79 Wu, G. Intestinal mucosal amino acid catabolism. *J. Nutr.* 1998;**128**:1249–52.

80 Caplan, M. S., Hedlund, E., Hill, N., MacKendrick, W. The role of endogenous nitric oxide and platelet-activating factor in hypoxia-induced intestinal injury in rats. *Gastroenterology* 1994;**106**:346–52.

81 Kubes, P. Ischemia-reperfusion in feline small intestine: a role for nitric oxide. *Am. J. Physiol.* 1993;**264**:G143–9.

82 MacKendrick, W., Caplan, M., Hsueh, W. Endogenous nitric oxide protects against platelet-activating factor-induced bowel injury in the rat. *Pediatr. Res.* 1993;**34**:222–8.

83 Zamora, S. A., Amin, H. J., McMillan, D. D. *et al.* Plasma L-arginine concentrations in premature infants with necrotizing enterocolitis. *J. Pediatr.* 1997;**131**:226–32.

84 Becker, R. M., Wu, G., Galanko, J. A. *et al.* Reduced serum amino acid concentrations in infants with necrotizing enterocolitis. *J. Pediatr.* 2000;**137**:785–93.

85 Amin, H., Zamora, S., McMillan, D. *et al.* Arginine supplementation prevents necrotizing enterocolitis in the premature infant. *J. Pediatr.* 2002;**140**:425–31.

86 Neu, J. Arginine supplementation and the prevention of necrotizing enterocolitis in very low birth weight infants. *J. Pediatr.* 2002;**140**:389–92.

87 Zamora, S. A., Amin, H. J., McMillan, D. D. *et al.* Plasma L-arginine concentration, oxygenation index, and systemic

blood pressure in premature infants. *Crit. Care Med.* 1998; **26**:1271–6.

88 Castillo, L., DeRojas-Walker, T., Yu, Y. M. *et al.* Whole body arginine metabolism and nitric oxide synthesis in newborns with persistent pulmonary hypertension. *Pediatr. Res.* 1995;**38**:17–24.

89 Vosatka, R., Hassoun, P., Harvey-Wilkes, K. Dietary L-arginine prevents fetal growth restriction in rats. *Am. J. Obstet. Gynecol.* 1998;**178**:242–6.

90 Helmbrecht, G. D., Farhat, M. Y., Lochbaum, L. *et al.* L-arginine reverses the adverse pregnancy changes induced by nitric oxide synthase inhibition in the rat. *Am. J. Obstet. Gynecol.* 1996;**175**:800–5.

91 Envoy, D., Lieberman, M., Fahey, T., Daly, J. Immunonutrition: the role of arginine. *Nutrition* 1998;**14**:611–17.

92 Yu, Y.-M., Sheridan, R., Burke, J. *et al.* Kinetics of plasma arginine and leucine in pediatric burn patients. *Am. J. Clin. Nutr.* 1996;**64**:60–6.

93 Cooke, J. P., Tsao, P. Arginine: a new therapy for atherosclerosis? *Circulation* 1997;**95**:311–12.

94 Wu, G., Meininger, C. J. Arginine nutrition and cardiovascular function. *J. Nutr.* 2000;**130**:2626–9.

95 Creager, M. A., Gallagher, S. J., Girerd, X. J. *et al.* L-arginine improves endothelium-dependent vasodilation in hypercholesterolemic humans. *J. Clin. Invest.* 1992;**90**:1248–53.

96 Drexler, H., Fischell, T. A., Pinto, F. J. *et al.* Effect of L-arginine on coronary endothelial function in cardiac transplant recipients. Relation to vessel wall morphology. *Circulation* 1994;**89**:1615–23.

97 Peters, H., Border, W. A., Ruckert, M. *et al.* l-Arginine supplementation accelerates renal fibrosis and shortens life span in experimental lupus nephritis. *Kidney Int.* 2003;**63**:1382–92.

98 Andrews, F., Griffiths, R. Glutamine: essential for immune nutrition in the critically ill. *Br. J. Nutr.* 2002;**87**:S3–8.

99 Burrin, D. G., Stoll, B. Key nutrients and growth factors for the neonatal gastrointestinal tract. *Clin. Perinatol.* 2002;**29**:65–96.

100 Reeds, P. J., Burrin, D. G. Glutamine and the bowel. *J. Nutr.* 2001;**131**:2505S–8S; discussion 2523S–24S.

101 Neu, J., DeMarco, V., Li, N. Glutamine: clinical applications and mechanisms of action. *Curr. Opin. Clin. Nutr. Met. Care* 2002;**5**:69–75.

102 Karinch, A. M., Pan, M., Lin, C. M., Strange, R., Souba, W. W. Glutamine metabolism in sepsis and infection. *J. Nutr.* 2001;**131**:2535S–8S.

103 Andrews, F., Griffiths, R. Glutamine-enhanced nutrition in the critically ill patient. *Hosp. Med.* 2002;**63**:144–7.

104 Boelens, P. G., Nijveldt, R. J., Houdijk, A. P., Meijer, S., van, Leeuwen, P. A. Glutamine alimentation in catabolic state. *J. Nutr.* 2001;**131**:2569S–77S.

105 Houdijk, A. P., Rijnsburger, E. R., Jansen, J. *et al.* Randomised trial of glutamine-enriched enteral nutrition on infectious morbidity in patients with multiple trauma. *Lancet* 1998;**352**:772–6.

106 Novak, F., Heyland, D. K., Avenell, A., Drover, J. W., Su, X. Glutamine supplementation in serious illness: a systematic review of the evidence. *Crit. Care Med.* 2002;**30**:2022–9.

107 Duggan, C., Gannon, J., Walker, W. A. Protective nutrients and functional foods for the gastrointestinal tract. *Am. J. Clin. Nutr.* 2002;**75**:789–808.

108 Kudsk, K. A. Effect of route and type of nutrition on intestine-derived inflammatory responses. *Am. J. Surg.* 2003;**185**:16–21.

109 Neu, J. Glutamine in the fetus and critically ill low birth weight neonate: metabolism and mechanism of action. *J. Nutr.* 2001;**131**:258S–9S.

110 He, Y., Chu, S. H., Walker, W. A. Nucleotide supplements alter proliferation and differentiation of cultured human (Caco-2) and rat (IEC-6) intestinal epithelial cells. *J. Nutr.* 1993;**123**:1017–27.

111 Postic, B., Holliday, N., Lewis, P. *et al.* Glutamine supplementation and deprivation: effect on artificially reared rat small intestinal morphology. *Pediatr. Res.* 2002;**52**:430–6.

112 Lacey, J. M., Crouch, J. B., Benfell, K. *et al.* The effects of glutamine-supplemented parenteral nutrition in premature infants. *J. Parenter. Enteral Nutr.* 1996;**20**:74–80.

113 Neu, J., Roig, J., Meetze, W. *et al.* Enteral glutamine supplementation for very low birth weight infants decreases morbidity. *J. Pediatr.* 1997;**131**:691–9.

114 Dallas, M., Bowling, D., Roig, J., Auestad, N., Neu, J. Enteral glutamine supplementation for very-low-birth-weight infants decreases hospital costs. *J. Parenter. Enteral Nutr.* 1998;**22**:352–6.

115 des Robert, C., Le Bacquer, O., Piloquet, H., Roze, J. C., Darmaun, D. Acute effects of intravenous glutamine supplementation on protein metabolism in very low birth weight infants: a stable isotope study. *Pediatr. Res.* 2002;**51**:87–93.

116 Poindexter, B., Ehrenkranz, R. A., Stoll, B. J. *et al.* Parenteral glutamine supplementation in ELBW infants: a multicenter randomized clinical trial. *Pediatr. Res.* 2002;**51**:317A.

117 Vaughn, P., Thomas, P., Clark, R., Neu, J. Enteral glutamine supplementation and morbidity in low-birth-weight infants. *Pediatr. Res.* 2003;**53**:437A.

118 Carver, J., Walker, W. The role of nucleotides in human nutrition. *J. Nutr. Biochem.* 1995;**6**:58–72.

119 Rudolph, F. B. The biochemistry and physiology of nucleotides. *J. Nutr.* 1994;**124**:124S–7S.

120 Janas, L. M., Picciano, M. F. The nucleotide profile of human milk. *Pediatr. Res.* 1982;**16**:659–62.

121 Carver, J. D. Dietary nucleotides: effects on the immune and gastrointestinal systems. *Acta Paediatrica.* 1999;**430**:83–8.

122 Leach, J. L., Baxter, J. H., Molitor, B. E., Ramstack, M. B., Masor, M. L. Total potential available nucleosides of human milk by stage of lactation. *Am. J. Clin. Nutr.* 1995;**61**:1224–30.

123 Thorell, L., Sjöberg, L. B., Hernell, O. Nucleotides in human milk: sources and metabolism by the newborn infant. *Pediatr. Res.* 1996;**40**:845–52.

124 Walker, W. A. Exogenous nucleotides and gastrointestinal immunity. *Transplant Proc.* 1996;**28**:2438–41.

125 Uauy, R., Stingel, G., Thomas, R., Quan, R. Effect of dietary nucleosides on growth and maturation of the developing gut in the rat. *J. Pediatr. Gastroenterol. Nutr.* 1990;**10**: 497–503.

126 López-Navarro, A. T., Ortega, M. A., Peragón, J. *et al.* Deprivation of dietary nucleotides decreases protein synthesis in the liver and small intestine in rats. *Gastroenterology* 1996;**110**:1760–9.

127 LeLeiko, N. S., Walsh, M. J., Abraham, S. Gene expression in the intestine: the effect of dietary nucleotides. In Barness, L., DeVivo, D., Kaback, M. *et al.*, eds. *Advances in Pediatrics*. St. Louis, MO: Mosby-Year Book; 1995:145–69.

128 Sanderson, I. R., He, Y. Nucleotide uptake and metabolism by intestinal epithelial cells. *J. Nutr.* 1994;**124**:131S–7S.

129 Tanaka, M., Lee, K., Martinez-Augustin, O. *et al.* Exogenous nucleotides alter the proliferation, differentiation and apoptosis of human small intestinal epithelium. *J. Nutr.* 1996;**126**:424–33.

130 Brunser, O., Espinoza, J., Araya, M., Cruchet, S., Gil, A. Effect of dietary nucleotide supplementation on diarrhoeal disease in infants. *Acta Paediatrica* 1994;**83**:188–91.

131 Pickering, L. K., Granoff, D. M., Erickson, J. R. *et al.* Modulation of the immune system by human milk and infant formula containing nucleotides. *Pediatrics* 1998;**101**:242–9.

132 Yau, K. T., Huang, C., Chen, W. *et al.* Effect of nucleotides on diarrhea and immune responses in healthy term infants in Taiwan. *J. Pediatr. Gastr. Nutr.* 2003;**36**:37–43.

133 Balmer, S., Hanvey, L., Wharton, B. Diet and faecal flora in the newborn: nucleotides. *Arch. Dis. Child.* 1994;**70**: F137–40.

134 Gil, A., Corral, E., Martinez, A., Molina, J. Effects of dietary nucleotides on the microbial pattern of faeces in the at term newborn infants. *J. Clin. Nutr. Gastroent.* 1986;**1**:127–32.

135 Carver, J. D., Sosa, R., Zaritt, J., Siktberg, M. R., Meyer, L. Dietary nucleotide effects on superior mesenteric artery blood flow in term infants. *Pediatr. Res.* 2000;**45**:284A.

136 Özkan, H., Ören, H., Erdag, N., Çevik, N. Breast milk versus infant formulas: effects on intestinal blood flow in neonates. *Indian J. Pediatr.* 1994;**61**:703–9.

137 Carver, J. D., Saste, M., Sosa, R. *et al.* The effects of dietary nucleotides on intestinal blood flow in preterm infants. *Pediatr. Res.* 2002;**52**:425–9.

138 Jyonouchi, H., Sun, S., Winship, T., Kuchan, M. J. Dietary ribonucleotides increase antigen-specific type 1 T-helper cells in the regional draining lymph nodes in young BALB/cJ mice. *Nutrition* 2003;**19**:41–6.

139 Nagafuchi, S., Hachimura, S., Totsuka, M. *et al.* Dietary nucleotides can up-regulate antigen-specific Th1 immune responses and suppress antigen-specific IgE responses in mice. *Intl. Arch. Aller. Immunol.* 2000;**122**:33–41.

140 Carver, J. D., Pimentel, B., Cox, W. I., Barness, L. A. Dietary nucleotide effects in formula-fed infants. *Pediatrics* 1991;**88**:359–63.

141 Martinez-Augustin, O., Boza, J. J., Del Pino, J. I. *et al.* Dietary nucleotides might influence the humoral immune response against cow's milk proteins in preterm neonates. *Biol. Neonate.* 1997;**7**:215–23.

142 Navarro, J., Maldonado, J., Narbona, E. *et al.* Influence of dietary nucleotides on plasma immunoglobulin levels and lymphocyte subsets of preterm infants. *Biofactors* 1999;**10**:67–76.

143 Cosgrove, M., Davies, D. P., Jenkins, H. R. Nucleotide supplementation and growth of term small for gestational age infants. *Arch. Dis. Child.* 1996;**74**:F122–5.

144 Pita, M., Fernández, M., De-Lucchi, C. *et al.* Changes in the fatty acids pattern of red blood cell phospholipids induced by type of milk, dietary nucleotide supplementation, and postnatal age in preterm infants. *J. Pediatr. Gastr. Nutr.* 1988;**7**: 740–7.

145 Sánchez-Pozo, A., Ramírez, M., Gil, A. *et al.* Dietary nucleotides enhance plasma lecithin cholesterol acyl transferase activity and apolipoprotein A-IV concentration in preterm newborn infants. *Pediatr. Res.* 1995;**37**:328–33.

146 Henderson, T., Homosh, M., Mehta, N., Angclus, P., Hamosh, P. Red blood cell phospholipid docosahexaenoic acid and arachidonic acid concentrations in very low birth weight infants are not affected by nucleotide supplementation of premie formula and are lower than mother's own milk. *Pediatr. Res.* 1994;**35**:313A.

147 Woltil, H. A., van Beusekom, C. M., Siemensma, A. D. *et al.* Erythrocyte and plasma cholesterol ester long-chain polyunsaturated fatty acids of low-birth-weight babies fed preterm formula with and without ribonucleotides: comparison with human milk. *Am. J. Clin. Nutr.* 1995;**62**:943–9.

20

Intravenous feeding

William C. Heird

Department of Pediatrics, Children's Nutrition Research Center and Baylor College of Medicine, Houston, TX

Total parenteral nutrition as practiced today was not a part of modern medicine until the late 1960s. Having demonstrated that normal growth of puppies could be achieved solely with parenterally administered nutrients,[1] Dudrick *et al.* adapted the technique used in animals for clinical use.[2] Shortly thereafter, Wilmore and Dudrick[3] described use of this new technique in treatment of an infant who had virtually no remaining small intestine and, therefore, was totally dependent upon parenterally delivered nutrients. Although the infant eventually succumbed, normal growth and development was maintained for several months solely with parenterally delivered nutrients.

This successful attempt to deliver sufficient nutrients parenterally was preceded by centuries of unsuccessful attempts beginning shortly after description of the circulatory system in the early seventeenth century and the realization that ingested nutrients reached the circulation.[4,5] These attempts included infusion of wine, ale, olive oil, and milk. As easily predicted today, most were disasters. However, two of three patients who received milk infusions for treatment of cholera in the early 1800s survived but whether this was because of, or despite, the milk infusions is not clear. Since the practice was not continued, the latter seems more likely.

By the late 1800s the potentially deleterious effects of catabolism and starvation were recognized, rekindling interest in ability to provide nutrients parenterally. This resulted in development of products that could be delivered parenterally and, by the early 1940s, glucose and protein hydrolysates that could be delivered safely by the parenteral route were available.[5]

The first report of successful use of parenteral nutrition in the clinical management of a pediatric patient appeared in 1944.[6] The patient, a 5-month-old male with severe marasmus secondary to Hirschsprung's disease, received alternate peripheral vein infusions of a mixture of 50% glucose and 10% casein hydrolysate and a noncommercial homogenate of olive oil and lecithin providing 130 kCal kg^{-1} day^{-1} and a total volume of 150 ml kg^{-1} day^{-1}. The infusions were stopped after 5 days because of inability to maintain venous access. At the end of this period, according to the authors, "... the fat pads of the cheeks had returned, the ribs were less prominent, and the general nutritional status was much improved."[6] The eventual fate of the child is unknown.

Inability to maintain venous access for more than a few days plagued attempts to administer nutrients parenterally for the next 25 years. For a brief period, there was some enthusiasm for the use of ethanol and various polyalcohols (e.g., sorbitol, xylitol) as alternative parenteral energy sources. Although peripheral vein infusion of a mixture of protein hydrolysate, glucose, and ethanol along with electrolytes, minerals, and vitamins was shown to result in weight gain and general improvement in nutritional and clinical status,[7] maintenance of the infusion required considerable effort and, eventually, could not be continued. In addition, the amount of ethanol tolerated by individual infants was both variable and unpredictable. Infusion of large volumes of less concentrated mixtures of glucose and protein hydrolysate, even with administration of diuretics to prevent fluid overload, also enjoyed a brief period of popularity but was soon abandoned because of the severe plasma electrolyte and acid base disturbances that frequently ensued. The availability in the 1960s of a cottonseed oil emulsion as a concentrated energy source helped somewhat but the emulsion was unstable and was associated

Neonatal Nutrition and Metabolism. Second Edition, ed. P. Thureen and W. Hay. Published by Cambridge University Press.
© Cambridge University Press 2006.

with so many problems that it was withdrawn within a decade of its introduction.

The technique described by Wilmore and Dudrick in 1968[3] overcame the problem of maintaining venous access by infusing the hypertonic nutrient infusate via a catheter inserted into the superior vena cava. The rapid flow in this vessel immediately diluted the hypertonic mixture of glucose, protein hydrolysate, minerals, electrolytes, and vitamins. Since acceptable lipid emulsions still were not available, periodic plasma infusions were given to provide essential fatty acids and trace minerals. It soon became apparent, however, that these were not adequate.

By the early 1970s, the technique was being used extensively in infants and children with congenital or acquired surgically correctable lesions of the gastrointestinal tract[8,9] and in infants with intractable diarrhea.[9,10] Use of the technique in nutritional management of low birth weight infants (LBWI) soon followed.[9,11,12] Currently, more than 1% of all infants born in the USA (i.e., those who weigh less than 1500 g at birth) receive parenterally delivered nutrients as their major source of nutrition for the first several days to weeks of life. Between August 1994 and August 1995, for example, parenteral nutrition infusates provided more than 75% of the total fluid volume of infants weighing between 500–700 g at birth for ~21 days; even those weighing between 1200 and 1500 g at birth received at least 75% of total fluid volume as a parenteral nutrition infusate for ~5 days.[13]

Since the endogenous nutrient stores of LBWI are limited and their rate of ongoing energy expenditure is relatively high, these infants are at great risk for rapid development of malnutrition or actual starvation.[14] The available endogenous nutrient stores of the 1000 g infant, for example, are not sufficient to support survival without exogenous nutrients for more than about 5 days. However, the extent to which the increasing use of parenteral nutrition in LBWI over the past 2 decades has contributed to the concurrent dramatic improvement in survival of these infants is not clear.[15] During this time, there also have been improvements in other aspects of neonatal care and, in the absence of controlled studies, it is impossible to distinguish between the contribution of the ability to provide nutrients exogenously v. improvements in other aspects of care. Nonetheless, parenteral delivery of nutrients obviously is a firmly established part of the care of LBWI, particularly VLBWI.

Despite the widespread use of parenteral nutrition in VLBWI, a number of aspects of the technique remain poorly understood and limit use of the technique in additional infants who might benefit from better nutritional management. This chapter is intended to enhance understanding of all aspects of parenteral nutrition. Practical aspects of the therapy that may enhance its efficacy and safety as well as a variety of unsolved problems are discussed.

Techniques of parenteral nutrition therapy

The basic concept of parenteral nutrition therapy as described by Wilmore and Dudrick in 1968[3] was infusion of the necessarily hypertonic nutrient solution at a constant rate into a vessel with rapid blood flow. In their original patient, the solution was infused through an indwelling catheter placed through a surgical cutdown in the external jugular vein. The distal tip of the catheter ended in the superior vena cava just above the right atrium and the proximal portion was tunneled subcutaneously to exit on the anterior chest where it was covered by an occlusive dressing. Channeling of the catheter to a point distant from the phlebotomy site was thought to protect the catheter from both inadvertent dislodgement and contamination by microorganisms. It also makes maintenance and care of the catheter exit site easier.

The inferior vena cava also is a large vessel with rapid flow and catheters placed in this vessel just below the right atrium appear to be equally effective.[16] In theory, however, introduction of a catheter through a cutdown in the groin area may increase the risk of infection and for this reason, inferior vena cava catheters have never been as popular as superior vena cava catheters. On the other hand, such catheters, tunneled subcutaneously to an exit site on the abdominal wall or the thigh, may represent no greater risk with respect to infection than the usual superior vena cava catheters. Unfortunately, no firm data are available to substantiate this possibility.

Because polyvinyl catheters have a tendency to become very rigid once they have been in place for a short period of time, silastic catheters which remain soft and pliable for some time are preferred. Catheters with a polyvinyl cuff on the portion that is tunneled subcutaneously are often used. The cuff promotes fibroblast proliferation which helps secure the catheter in place, thereby increasing the life of a single catheter. Such catheters are particularly useful for home parenteral nutrition.

Radiographic confirmation of correct catheter position prior to infusing the nutrient mixture is mandatory. Otherwise, the hypertonic nutrient infusate may be infused into an undesired site. Regular and meticulous care of the central vein catheter also is essential for prolonged, safe, complication-free use. Attention to this detail seems to be particularly important in preventing infection. The usual recommendation is that the occlusive dressing at the catheter exit site be changed at least every other day. Each time, the skin area should be cleaned with a defatting as well as an antiseptic agent and an antiseptic ointment as well as a fresh occlusive dressing should be applied. Use of the catheter for purposes other than delivery of the nutrient infusate, particularly for blood transfusions and blood sampling, should be discouraged. With meticulous care, a single catheter can be used safely for months.

Although the complications of central vein delivery of concentrated nutrient mixtures (see below) can be reduced to an acceptable level, doing so requires considerable effort, personnel, and expense. Thus, parenteral nutrition regimens that can be infused by peripheral vein have largely replaced regimens that must be delivered by central vein catheters, particularly for LBWI. Of necessity, the glucose concentration of such regimens cannot be much greater than 10%; thus, the nutrient intake that can be delivered by peripheral vein without excessive fluid intake is somewhat limited. Use of parenteral lipid emulsions helps compensate for this drawback but, if fluid intake is limited to a total volume of $150 \, \mathrm{ml \, kg^{-1} \, day^{-1}}$ and intravenous lipid intake is limited to $3 \, \mathrm{g \, kg^{-1} \, day^{-1}}$, the maximum energy intake that can be delivered is approximately $80 \, \mathrm{kCal \, kg^{-1} \, day^{-1}}$. Obviously, the growth achievable with such an intake is less than that achievable with conventional central vein regimens that can easily deliver up to 50% more energy. However, as discussed below, the additional weight gain achievable with the higher energy intake is likely to be primarily fat. Thus, since peripheral vein regimens can supply the same intake of amino acids as central vein regimens, they are beneficial for most infants.

Currently, use of small silastic or polyurethane catheters inserted into the superior vena cava through a needle placed percutaneously into a peripheral vein[17] is quite popular. To date, the advantages and disadvantages of this technique v. those of conventional central and/or peripheral vein techniques of nutrient delivery have not been evaluated extensively. Available data suggest that these catheters may not remain functional as long as central catheters placed in the conventional manner[18] but that they can be used for a much longer period than can a single peripheral vein site.[19] Moreover, they appear to be as safe as conventional central vein catheters.[20] Since they allow infusion of a more concentrated nutrient infusate, they permit delivery of more nutrients without excessive fluid intake.

Evidence that delivery of parenteral nutrients by peripheral vein is easier and less time-consuming than successful delivery by central vein is not available. The supervision required for successful peripheral vein delivery is somewhat less than that required for successful central vein delivery. However, since a single infusion site rarely lasts for more than 24 hours, considerable time and effort are required to maintain peripheral vein infusions. Finally, although the complications associated with the two routes of delivery differ in nature and severity, the number of complications per day of therapy does not appear to differ.[21] Thus, it seems reasonable to base the choice of delivery route for parenteral nutrients on an individual patient's clinical condition and nutritional needs rather than on the perceived ease or difficulty of a particular technique.

Indications for parenteral nutrition

Any infant who is unable to tolerate sufficient enteral feedings for a significant period of time is a candidate for parenterally delivered nutrients. However, there is considerable disagreement about the definition of "significant period of time" and the indications for central v. peripheral vein delivery. A reasonable approach is to gauge the extent to which an infant's endogenous nutrient stores are likely to be eroded if nutrient intake is inadequate. A large infant who is intolerant of enteral feedings for only a few days is unlikely to experience serious erosion of endogenous nutrient stores whereas a small infant, particularly one with pre-existing nutritional depletion, may experience considerable further depletion of already limited endogenous stores with even a few days of inadequate nutrient intake.

Since peripheral vein parenteral nutrition regimens can maintain existing body composition, this route of delivery is a reasonable choice for a normally nourished infant who is likely to tolerate an adequate enteral regimen within a week to 10 days. On the other hand, central vein delivery using a catheter placed either conventionally or percutaneously is a more reasonable choice for an infant who is unlikely to tolerate enteral feedings right away. This distinction is based largely on the practical consideration of the difficulty in maintaining peripheral vein infusions for more than about a week.

Infants rarely require parenteral nutrients as their sole source of nutrition for more than 2–3 weeks. While it was formerly thought that a period of complete "bowel rest" was an important contributor to the success of parenteral nutrition, this concept no longer seems valid. Rather, delivery of at least some nutrients by the enteral route appears to be desirable. Most VLBWI now receive parenteral nutrients as well as about $1 \, \mathrm{mL \, kg^{-1} \, h^{-1}}$ of breast milk or formula for the first 10–14 days of life. This enteral intake contributes minimally to nutrient needs but has been shown to have favorable effects, including earlier achievement of full enteral feeding.[22–24]

Table 20.1. Composition of a nutrient infusate suitable for central vein infusion and peripheral vein infusion

Component	Central vein (Amount/ (kg d^{-1}))	Peripheral vein (Amount/ (kg d^{-1}))
Crystalline amino acids (g)	3–4	2.5–3.0
Glucose (g)	20–30	15
Lipid emulsion (g)	0.5–3.0	0.5–3.0
Sodium (mEq)	3–4	3–4
Potassium[a] (mEq)	2–4	2–4
Calcium (mg)	40–80	40–80
Magnesium (mEq)	0.25	0.25
Chloride (mEq)	3–4	3–4
Phosphorus[a] (mMoles)	1.4	1.4
Zinc (μg)	200	200–400
Copper (μg)	20	
Iron[b]		
Other trace minerals[c]		
Vitamins (MVI^R-Pediatric)[d]		
Total Volume (ml)	120–130	150

[a] Hyperphosphatemia frequently develops if phosphorus intake exceeds 1.4 mMoles/(kg d^{-1}), the amount given with a daily potassium intake of 2 mEq kg^{-1} as a mixture of KH_2PO_4 and K_2HPO_4; if a potassium intake of more than 2 mEq kg^{-1}day^{-1} is required, the additional potassium should be given as KCl.

[b] Iron Dextran (Imferon^R, Fisons Corp., Bedford, MA) can be added to the infusate of patients requiring prolonged parenteral nutrition therapy; but the dose should be limited to 0.1 mg/(kg day^{-1}). Alternatively, the indicated intramuscular dose can be used intermittently, either as the sole source of iron or as an additional dose.

[c] See text and Table 20.4.

[d] MVI^R-Pediatric (Armour Pharmaceutical Co., Chicago, IL) is a lyophilized product. When reconstituted, as directed, 5 ml added to the daily nutrient infusate provides 80 mg vitamin C, 700 μg vitamin A, 10 μg vitamin D, 1.3 mg thiamine, 1.4 mg riboflavin, 1.0 mg pyridoxine, 17 mg niacin, 5 mg pantothenic acid, 7 mg vitamin E, 20 μg biotin, 140 μg folic acid, 1 μg vitamin B_{12}, and 200 μg vitamin K_1.

Infusate composition and delivery

The parenteral nutrition infusate, whether delivered by central or peripheral vein, should include a nitrogen source as well as adequate energy, electrolytes, minerals, and vitamins. Suitable peripheral and central vein infusates for most pediatric patients are shown in Table 20.1. One of several crystalline amino acid mixtures (Table 20.2) is usually used as the nitrogen source. The amount of amino acids

provided ranges from less than 2.0 to 4 g kg^{-1} day^{-1}; an intake of 2.5–3.0 g kg^{-1} day^{-1} results in nitrogen retention comparable to that observed in enterally fed, normal term infants but a higher intake is required to achieve a rate of nitrogen retention equal to the intrauterine rate, the usual minimal recommendation for LBWI.

Glucose is the major energy source of most parenteral nutrition regimens. An intake greater than 10 g kg^{-1} day^{-1}, about 40 kcal kg^{-1} day^{-1}, rarely is tolerated by any infant on the first day of therapy and VLBWI often tolerate even less. However, intake usually can be increased by 2–5 g kg^{-1} day^{-1} until the desired intake is achieved. Since any patient who receives a fat-free parenteral nutrition regimen will develop essential fatty acid deficiency within a relatively short period (preterm and nutritionally depleted infants do so within days, particularly if growth is rapid),[25,26] a sufficient amount of a parenteral lipid emulsion to prevent this deficiency (i.e., 0.5–1.0 g kg^{-1} day^{-1}) is indicated. The maximum intake usually recommended for the LBWI is 3 g kg^{-1}day^{-1} [27] but some routinely provide at least 4 g kg^{-1} day^{-1}.

Convenient additive preparations of electrolytes, minerals, and vitamins have been available for some time. Since the requirements for these nutrients vary considerably among infants, the amounts shown in Table 20.1 cannot be interpreted as absolute requirements. The amount of calcium suggested almost certainly is inadequate for optimal skeletal mineralization but inclusion of more calcium without decreasing the amount of phosphate (and risking development of hypophosphatemia) is likely to result in precipitation of calcium phosphate. The amounts of vitamins listed in Table 20.1 are particularly tenuous but can be provided conveniently using currently available products. Since zinc deficiency develops relatively quickly, this mineral should be added to the infusate of any infant likely to require parenteral nutrients exclusively for up to a week. Inclusion of other essential trace minerals (e.g., copper,[28] chromium,[29] selenium,[30] and molybdenum[31]) should be considered if exclusive or near-exclusive parenteral nutrition is required for more than a week.

The most recent recommendations for parenteral vitamin and trace mineral intakes (no longer quite so recent) are summarized in Tables 20.3 and 20.4.

The nutrient infusate should be delivered at a constant rate using one of several available constant infusion pumps. Use of a 0.22 μ-membrane filter between the catheter and the administration tubing is considered unnecessary by some but failure to do so increases the likelihood of infusing particulate matter or any contaminating organisms.

Table 20.2. Composition of available parenteral amino acid mixtures (mMoles per 2.5g)

Amino acid	Aminosyn (Abbott)	Aminosyn-PF (Abbott)	FreAmineIII (B. Braun)	Neopham (Cutter)	Travasol (Travenol)	TrophAmine (B. Braun)
Threonine	1.090	1.080	0.840	1.160	0.910	0.883
Valine	1.710	1.390	1.420	1.180	0.980	1.675
Leucine	1.795	2.267	1.730	2.050	1.180	2.671
Isoleucine	1.375	1.458	1.325	0.930	0.910	1.567
Lysine	1.235	1.156	1.740	1.475	0.790	1.396
Methionine	0.670	0.300	0.890	0.335	0.970	0.571
Cysteine	0	0	0.050	0.410	0	0.050
Histidine	0.485	0.510	0.455	0.520	0.705	0.771
Phenylalanine	0.665	0.650	0.855	0.630	0.935	0.729
Tyrosine	0.120	0.088	0	0.110	0.055	0.333[a]
Tryptophan	0.195	0.220	0.185	0.265	0.220	0.246
Arginine	1.410	1.760	1.361	0.910	1.490	1.742
Serine	1.000	1.181	1.400	1.395	0	0.904
Proline	1.870	1.789	2.430	1.875	0.945	1.492
Glycine	4.265	1.280	4.667	1.075	6.910	1.200
Alanine	3.595	1.966	1.985	2.720	5.820	1.517
Aspartate	0	1.000	0	1.190	0	0.608
Glutamate	0	1.411	0	1.860	0	0.854
Taurine	0	0.171	0	0	0	0.057

[a] Mixture of L-tyrosine and N-acetyl-L-tyrosine.

Many patients tolerate the same infusate for the total duration of parenteral nutrition. Others, however, require frequent adjustment of the intake of one or more nutrients. For this reason, ability to change the composition of the infusate in response to clinical and chemical monitoring or to increase the volume in response to diarrheal and other ongoing losses is important.

Rationale for recommended parenteral nutrient intakes

The parenteral requirements for various nutrients depend upon the endpoints to be achieved with the parenteral nutrition regimen and any peculiarities of metabolism of specific nutrients incident to route of administration. The requirements for normal growth, and certainly those for normal growth plus catch-up growth, are considerably greater than the requirements for merely preserving existing body composition but the specific requirements for achieving either goal have not been studied extensively; further, these are likely to vary considerably from infant to infant. Very little information is available concerning any special requirements imposed by parenteral v. enteral delivery of nutrients.

Amino acids

According to Zlotkin et al.,[32] the parenteral amino acid intake required to reproduce the intrauterine rate of nitrogen accretion (i.e., ~300 mg kg^{-1} day^{-1}) is approximately 3 g kg^{-1} day^{-1}, provided energy intake is at least 80 kCal kg^{-1} day^{-1}. This combination of amino acid and energy intakes also supports the intrauterine rate of weight gain (i.e., approximately 15 g kg^{-1} day^{-1}). An even higher rate of nitrogen retention, but not weight gain, was achieved with an amino acid intake of 4 g kg^{-1} day^{-1} and the same energy intake. The rates of both nitrogen retention and weight gain of infants who received amino acid intakes of 3 and 4 g kg^{-1} day^{-1} with an energy intake of 50 kCal kg^{-1} day^{-1} v. 80 kCal kg^{-1} day^{-1} were lower than intrauterine rates.

About 20 years ago, Anderson et al.[33] reported that LBWI who received a parenteral regimen providing 60 kCal kg^{-1} day^{-1} and an amino acid intake of 2.5 g kg^{-1} day^{-1} during the first week of life were in positive nitrogen balance (178 mg kg^{-1} day^{-1}) whereas control infants who received the same energy intake with no amino acids were in negative balance (−132 mg kg^{-1} day^{-1}).

Similar findings have been reported over the past decade in smaller, sicker, more immature infants.[34–39] These also show that infants who receive no amino acid intake during

Table 20.3. Suggested parenteral intakes of vitamins[49]

Vitamin	Preterm infants (Amount (kg day^{-1}))[a]	Term infants and children (Amount day^{-1})[b]
Vitamin A (μg)	280	700
Vitamin E (mg)	2.8	7
Vitamin K (μg)	80	200
Vitamin D (μg)	4	10
Ascorbic acid (mg)	25	80
Thiamin (mg)	0.48	1.2
Riboflavin (mg)	0.56	1.4
Pyridoxine (mg)	0.4	1.0
Niacin (mg)	6.8	17
Pantothenate (mg)	2.0	5
Biotin (μg)	8.0	20
Folate (μg)	56	140
Vitamin B$_{12}$ (μg)	0.4	1.0

[a] Total daily dose should not exceed that recommended for term infants and children. A dose of 2 ml of reconstituted MVI^R-Pediatric provides the recommended amount (kg day^{-1}) of all vitamins except ascorbic acid.

[b] These amounts are provided by 5 ml of reconstituted MVI^R-Pediatric (Armour Pharmaceutical Co.).

Table 20.4. Recommended parenteral intakes of trace minerals[a][49]

Trace Mineral	Preterm Infants (μg/kg day^{-1})	Term infants (μg/kg day^{-1})
Zinc	400	250[b]
Copper	20	20
Selenium	2.0	2.0
Chromium	0.20	0.20
Manganese	1.0	1.0
Molybdenum	0.25	0.25
Iodide	1.0	1.0

[a] If parenteral nutrients are used as a supplement for tolerated enteral feedings or as the sole source of nutrients for <4 weeks, only zinc is needed.

[b] 100 mg (kg^{-1} day^{-1}) for infants >3 mo of age.

the first week of life are in negative nitrogen balance (130–180 mg kg^{-1} day^{-1}). Since these nitrogen losses undoubtedly reflect tissue breakdown, infants who receive no nitrogen intake for the first few days of life lose from 0.8–1.1 g kg^{-1} day^{-1} of endogenous protein, or about 1% of total endogenous protein stores per day. This can be prevented by providing an amino acid intake slightly in excess of endogenous protein losses (e.g., 1–1.5 g kg^{-1} day^{-1}) but a higher intake is necessary to achieve a significantly positive nitrogen balance. These recent studies in small, sick LBWI show that a parenteral amino acid intake of 2–2.5 g kg^{-1} day^{-1} with an energy intake as low as 35–50 kCal kg^{-1} day^{-1} consistently results in positive nitrogen retention without significant metabolic abnormalities.[38,39] However, nitrogen retention is only approximately a third of the intrauterine rate of accretion.

The quality of the parenteral amino acid intake has not been studied extensively but obviously is important. Duffy et al.[40] found that infants who received a regimen containing a crystalline amino acid mixture retained a greater percentage of the nitrogen intake than those who received a regimen containing casein hydrolysate. In addition, protein synthesis accounted for a greater percentage of the total nitrogen flux of those who received the crystalline amino acid regimen. Helms et al.[41] observed that infants who received a regimen containing a parenteral amino acid mixture designed for infants retained 78% of the amino acid intake whereas infants who received an isocaloric and isonitrogenous regimen containing an older parenteral amino acid mixture designed for adults retained only 66% of intake.

Neither of these studies provides insight into the reason one regimen was utilized better than the other. The more efficiently utilized regimen studied by Helms et al.[41] contained more cyst(e)ine and tyrosine.[42] Thus, since both are considered indispensable amino acids for the infant, the investigators suggested that provision of more optimal intakes of these two amino acids improved nitrogen retention. This is a logical suggestion although perhaps not a valid explanation. For example, the less efficiently utilized nitrogen source studied by Duffy et al.[40] provided more cysteine and tyrosine than the more efficiently utilized source.

Cysteine and tyrosine are insoluble and cysteine is unstable in aqueous solution; hence, no currently available parenteral amino acid mixture contains appreciable amounts of either amino acid. Consequently, plasma cysteine and tyrosine concentrations of infants receiving cysteine- and tyrosine-free amino acid mixtures are quite low.[43] Moreover, greater intakes of the precursors, methionine and phenylalanine, do not result in greater plasma concentrations, respectively, of cysteine and tyrosine although they do result in higher plasma concentrations of the precursors.[43–45]

Hepatic activity of cystathionase, which is required for endogenous conversion of methionine to cysteine, is absent or low throughout gestation and for some time postnatally.[46,47] This developmental deficit, although not apparent in all nonhepatic tissues,[47] is an acceptable explanation for the low plasma cysteine concentration of infants receiving cysteine-free parenteral nutrition regimens. Since there appears to be no developmental delay in the hepatic activity of phenylalanine hydroxylase which converts phenylalanine to tyrosine,[48] the low plasma tyrosine concentration of infants receiving tyrosine-free parenteral nutrition regimens is not explicable on this basis. Moreover, plasma cysteine and tyrosine concentrations also are low in adults receiving conventional parenteral nutrition.[49]

Cysteine hydrochloride is soluble and also is reasonably stable in aqueous solution for up to 48 hours; thus, it is possible to supplement parenteral nutrition infusates with cysteine hydrochloride, as was done in the study of Helms et al.[41] However, trials of cysteine supplementation[50,51] have not shown a beneficial effect of parenteral cysteine intake on nitrogen retention, perhaps because the tyrosine content of the control regimens of these studies also was low and any beneficial effect of cysteine intake on nitrogen retention was masked by concurrent tyrosine deficiency.

Some of the newer parenteral amino acid mixtures contain N-acetyl-L-tyrosine (Table 20.2), which is soluble but the absolute efficacy of this tyrosine derivative is questionable.[42,52] Although infants receiving a parenteral amino acid mixture containing this soluble tyrosine salt have higher plasma tyrosine concentrations than infants receiving mixtures without it,[42] N-acetyl-L-tyrosine also was present in plasma and urinary excretion of N-acetyl-L-tyrosine was considerable. A recent study suggests that a dipeptide (i.e., glycyltyrosine) is a more efficacious source of tyrosine.[53] If so, it should be possible to define the need for both tyrosine and cysteine in infants requiring parenteral nutrition.

Glutamine, one of the most abundant amino acids in plasma as well as in human milk, is an effective energy source for cells with rapid turnover.[54] Further, in small studies in both infants and adults, supplementation of parenteral nutrition infusates with this amino acid has been associated with lower rates of sepsis and mortality.[55] Thus, it is thought by many to be a conditionally essential amino acid. However, like cysteine, it is unstable in aqueous solution and, therefore, is not a component of any parenteral amino acid mixture. Hence, until recently there were very little firm data concerning the importance of including glutamine in parenteral nutrition regimens, particularly those for VLBWI.

A large randomized placebo-controlled trial of parenteral glutamine supplementation of VLBWI was recently completed.[56,57] This trial showed that glutamine supplementation (20% of total amino acid intake) was safe but was not accompanied by clinical benefits. Specifically, rates of death, late-onset sepsis, and necrotizing enterocolitis (NEC) did not differ between supplemented and placebo groups. Further, the times required to achieve full enteral feedings and to regain birthweight as well as length of hospital stay were identical in the two groups. Thus, it appears that the absence of glutamine in parenteral amino acid mixtures is not a major concern.

Energy

Theoretically, if amino acid intake is adequate, an energy intake approximating resting energy expenditure is sufficient for maintenance (i.e., prevention of weight loss) but not for supporting weight gain. However, because of genetic differences as well as differences in other factors affecting energy expenditure, the resting energy requirement varies considerably from infant to infant. Thus, the total energy intake necessary to produce a specific rate of weight gain will be greater in infants with higher resting energy expenditures. For example, the resting energy expenditure of infants with bronchopulmonary dysplasia is 10–30% greater than that of infants without bronchopulmonary dysplasia.[58] Hence, for the same rate of weight gain, infants with bronchopulmonary dysplasia require a greater energy intake than infants without this condition. Whether the same is true for infants with other chronic or acute clinical conditions is not clear.

As discussed above, LBWI who receive an energy intake of 80 kCal kg^{-1} day^{-1} with a concomitant amino acid intake of 3 g $kg^{-1}day^{-1}$ gain weight at a rate approximating the intrauterine rate.[32] Theoretically, those who receive a greater energy intake will experience an even greater rate of weight gain. However, this greater rate of weight gain most likely will represent primarily deposition of additional adipose tissue. Hence, if the rate of weight gain of a LBWI receiving 80 kCal kg^{-1} day^{-1} is at or near the intrauterine rate, it is unlikely that a greater energy intake will be particularly desirable unless it is accompanied by a greater amino acid intake thereby supporting greater rates of deposition of both protein and adipose tissue.

The relationship between energy intake and nitrogen utilization also must be considered. The usual concept, developed primarily in animals and adults, is that an increase in energy intake increases utilization of any single adequate protein intake.[59] One of the few such studies of this issue in parenterally nourished LBWI is that of Zlotkin et al.[32] documenting greater retention of amino acid intakes of both 3 and 4 g kg^{-1} day^{-1} with a concomitant energy intake of 80 v. 50 kCal kg^{-1} day^{-1}. In another such study, Pineault *et al.*[60] observed only a small additional effect of an energy intake of 80 v. 60 kCal kg⁻¹ day⁻¹ on nitrogen retention of LBWI receiving an amino acid intake of 2.7 g kg⁻¹ day⁻¹. These two sets of data suggest that an energy intake greater than 60 kCal kg⁻¹ day⁻¹ will not appreciably enhance retention of an amino acid intake of 2.7 g kg⁻¹ day⁻¹ but that an energy intake greater than 50 kCal kg⁻¹ day⁻¹ will enhance retention of the slightly greater amino acid intake of 3 g kg⁻¹ day⁻¹.

The distribution of energy intake between glucose and lipid also may be important with respect to amino acid utilization. In general, the nitrogen sparing effect of carbohydrate in the absence of nitrogen intake is not shared by fat, but the effect of parenterally administered glucose v. lipid on utilization of concomitantly administered amino acids is less well understood. In infants, Pineault *et al.*,[60] studying the effects of parenteral lipid intakes of 3 v. 1 g kg⁻¹ day⁻¹ at total energy intakes of 60 and 80 kCal kg⁻¹ day⁻¹, found that the higher carbohydrate regimens, regardless of total energy intake, resulted in somewhat lower plasma concentrations of most amino acids. This suggests that the amino acid intake was used more efficiently by infants who received the greater carbohydrate intakes; however, the rates of nitrogen retention with the two regimens at each energy intake did not differ significantly. Another study shows no effect of the quality of energy intake on nitrogen utilization and suggests that inclusion of lipid, in fact, may be preferable.[61]

The foregoing data suggest that utilization of the amino acid content of a parenteral nutrition infusate with an amino acid:energy ratio similar to the lower energy infusates studied by Pineault *et al.*[60] i.e., 4.5 g amino acid per 100 kCal will be acceptable, although perhaps not maximal. While not tested extensively in clinical studies, this suggestion is not refuted by the available data. In practical terms, it implies that an infant who can tolerate an energy intake of only 30 kCal kg⁻¹ day⁻¹ should easily utilize an amino acid intake of 1.35 g kg⁻¹ day⁻¹. Since the nitrogen content of this intake is somewhat greater than expected urinary nitrogen losses, it should result in nitrogen equilibrium, perhaps a minimally positive nitrogen balance. This does not mean necessarily that an infant who is receiving only 30 kCal kg⁻¹ day⁻¹ will not tolerate a somewhat greater amino acid intake; in fact, an amino acid intake of 2–2.5 g kg⁻¹ day⁻¹ appears to be utilized quite well at a concomitant energy intake of 30–35 kCal kg⁻¹ day⁻¹.[38,39] Nor does it mean that an amino acid intake as low as 1.35 g kg⁻¹ day⁻¹ will not be utilized somewhat more efficiently at an energy intake above 30 kCal kg⁻¹ day⁻¹ but, at this low amino acid intake, an increase in energy intake is not likely to be nearly as effective in promoting nitrogen retention as

Table 20.5. Composition (amount/liter) of representative parenteral lipid emulsions

Component	Soybean oil emulsion[a]	Soybean/Safflower oil emulsion[b]
Soybean oil (g)	100[c]	50[c]
Safflower oil (g)	–	50[c]
Egg yolk phospholipid (g)	12	up to 12
Glycerol (g)	22.5	25
Fatty acids (% of total)		
16:0	10	8.8
18:0	3.5	3.4
18:1	26	17.7
18:2	50	65.8
18:3	9	4.2
Particle size (microns)	0.5	0.4

[a] Intralipid[R], Kabi-Vitrum, Sweden.
[b] Liposyn II[R], Abbott Laboratories, N. Chicago, IL.
[c] 20% emulsions also are available; these contain twice as much of the oils but roughly the same amounts of all other ingredients.

an increase in amino acid intake or an increase in amino acid and energy intakes.

Although gradually increasing amino acid intake over the first several days of parenteral nutrition is often advocated, there is no evidence that this increases tolerance of amino acids. Rather, this practice seems to be a "holdover" from the early days of parenteral nutrition when full strength parenteral infusates were diluted (e.g., to one-fourth or half strength) to prevent hyperglycemia.

Parenteral lipid intakes

Parenteral lipid emulsions containing either soybean oil or a mixture of safflower and soybean oils are currently available in the USA (Table 20.5). The emulsifying agent of both is egg yolk phospholipid and the emulsion particles of both are roughly the size of chylomicrons or VLDL. After infusion, the triglyceride portion of these particles is hydrolyzed by endothelial lipoprotein lipase and the released free fatty acids and glycerol are metabolized by the usual pathways.[62] The ability to hydrolyze the infused emulsion particles increases with increasing gestational age and, at any gestational age, the capacity for hydrolysis is greater in the infant whose size is appropriate v. small-for-gestational-age (SGA).[63] A number of clinical conditions (e.g., infection, surgical stress, malnutrition) adversely affect the hydrolysis step[62] but less information is available concerning the factors that affect metabolism of free fatty acids and glycerol.

If the lipid emulsion is infused at a rate equal to or less than the rate of hydrolysis, a dramatic change in plasma triglyceride concentration reflecting accumulation of the infused triglyceride emulsion is unlikely. However, if the rate of infusion exceeds the rate of hydrolysis, plasma triglyceride concentration will rise resulting in the known adverse effects of elevated triglyceride concentrations on pulmonary diffusion[64,65] and polymorphonuclear leukocyte function.[66,67] If, instead, the rate of hydrolysis exceeds the rate at which the released free fatty acids are oxidized, the plasma concentration of free fatty acids will increase. Since free fatty acids displace bound bilirubin from albumin,[68] this possibility is of some concern in infants with hyperbilirubinemia. Unfortunately, the concentration of free fatty acids likely to result in displacement of albumin-bound bilirubin in vivo is not known.[62] Limiting the amount of parenteral lipid emulsion to 0.5–1.0 g kg^{-1} day^{-1} in infants with a serum bilirubin concentration in excess of 8–10 mg dL^{-1}, as is common practice, should circumvent this potential problem.

It has been suggested that low plasma carnitine concentrations, commonly observed in infants and adults receiving carnitine-free parenteral nutrition regimens,[69,70] may inhibit fatty acid oxidation. However, most trials of carnitine supplementation have shown little, if any, effect of supplemental carnitine on fatty acid oxidation.[71,72] One exception is a study in which carnitine supplementation following a prolonged period of carnitine-free parenteral nutrition improved fatty acid oxidation.[73] It seems wise, therefore, to provide modest amounts of carnitine in order to prevent deficiency. Large amounts have been associated with adverse effects[74] and should be avoided.

The amount of soybean oil emulsion necessary to prevent linoleic acid deficiency is approximately 0.5 g kg^{-1} day^{-1}, a dose that is likely to be tolerated by all infants. Since the linoleic acid content of safflower oil is approximately 50% higher than that of soybean oil, an even smaller dose of the safflower plus soybean oil emulsion should provide the linoleic acid requirement. A previously available emulsion of safflower oil, which contained little or no α-linolenic acid, was associated with α-linolenic acid deficiency[75,76] but, so far as is known, both types of emulsions currently available in the USA contain an adequate amount of α-linolenic acid (see below).

A prudent approach for use of the currently available lipid emulsions in LBWI is to limit intake initially to 0.5–1.0 g kg^{-1} day^{-1}, particularly in infants who are likely to experience difficulties hydrolyzing the emulsions and in those with hyperbilirubinemia. Subsequently, as tolerance of the emulsion is demonstrated and/or hyperbilirubinemia resolves, the amount can be increased. This approach is common in clinical practice but it appears to be based on the false assumption that slow introduction of the lipid emulsion increases the recipient infant's ability to utilize the infused lipid. Rather, as shown some time ago by Brans et al.,[77] plasma triglyceride and free fatty acid concentrations of LBWI receiving parenteral lipid emulsions, regardless of the method or duration of lipid infusion, are a function of the amount of emulsion administered and the time over which it is administered. In this study, plasma triglyceride and free fatty acid concentrations remained at acceptable levels so long as the dose of emulsion did not exceed 2–3 g kg^{-1} day^{-1}.

Although there appears to be little physiological reason to gradually increase the dose of lipid emulsion over several days to induce tolerance, gradual introduction is more prudent in the smaller infant, the SGA infant or the infant who is infected or experiencing other complications associated with delayed triglyceride hydrolysis. In such infants, gradual increases permit assessment of lipid tolerance before the next increase in dose.

Parenteral intakes of other nutrients

The electrolyte content of parenteral nutrition regimens has always been the same as that of maintenance parenteral fluid regimens (i.e., approximately 3 mMoles kg^{-1} day^{-1} of sodium and chloride and approximately 2 mMoles kg^{-1} day^{-1} of potassium) and these intakes seem to be appropriate for most stable, growing infants. Very small LBWI, however, may require lesser or greater intakes of sodium to maintain a normal plasma sodium concentration and nutritionally depleted infants may require greater potassium intakes as well as greater intakes of other intracellular nutrients (e.g., phosphorus and magnesium) to maintain normal plasma concentrations of these nutrients. In all infants, frequent monitoring of plasma electrolyte concentrations and appropriate reformulation of the nutrient infusate in order to maintain normal plasma electrolyte concentrations is recommended, particularly during the first few days of parenteral nutrition.

The recommended parenteral intakes of phosphorus, i.e., 1.4–2.0 mMoles kg^{-1} day^{-1}, and magnesium, i.e., 3–6 mg kg^{-1} day^{-1}, were established largely by trials of various intakes. These intakes, too, appear to maintain "normal" plasma phosphorus and magnesium concentrations in most infants. However, frequent monitoring of the plasma concentration of both and appropriate reformulation of the infusate, if indicated, are recommended.

Because of the insolubility of calcium phosphate, most commonly used parenteral nutrition regimens, although they maintain "normal" plasma concentrations of calcium and phosphorus, do not provide an adequate calcium intake. Hence, osteopenia, rickets, and collapsed vertebra have been reported in both LBW and term infants receiving parenteral nutrition as their sole source of nutrient intake for prolonged periods.[78,79] The fetus deposits ~100 mg (2.5 mMoles kg^{-1} day^{-1}) of calcium[80] during the last trimester of gestation but, until recently, it was impossible to provide more than half this amount, i.e., 40–60 mg (1–1.5 mMoles kg^{-1} day^{-1}) parenterally unless the phosphorus intake was lowered sufficiently to result in hypophosphatemia.

The lower pH of infusates containing some of the available parenteral amino acid mixtures and of infusates containing cysteine-HCl permits administration of more calcium without sacrificing phosphorus intake. Koo et al.[81] studied the effects of regimens containing 25 IU dL^{-1} of vitamin D and either 0.5 or 1.5–2.0 mMoles dL^{-1} of both calcium and phosphorus. Serum 1,25-dihydroxy-D concentrations of the high calcium/phosphorus group were stable and within the normal range; tubular reabsorption of phosphorus also was stable and consistently less than 90%. Serum 1,25-dihydroxy-D concentrations of the low calcium/phosphorus group, on the other hand, were high and tubular reabsorption of phosphorus was consistently greater than 90%. Thus, it appears that delivery of calcium and phosphorus intakes approaching those required to achieve intrauterine accretion rates exerts less stress on calcium and phosphorus homeostatic mechanisms than delivery of smaller intakes. A recent study[82] suggests that higher parenteral calcium and phosphorus intakes also result in more optimal skeletal mineralization although, interestingly, serum alkaline phosphatase activity of the two groups did not differ.

Calcium phosphate, unlike most salts, is more soluble at low v. high temperatures. This raises serious concerns about the overall safety of the frequently advocated "three-in-one" or "complete" parenteral nutrition infusates i.e., infusates containing glucose, amino acids, and the lipid emulsion along with electrolytes, minerals, and vitamins in the same bottle or bag. Since these infusates must be administered without an in-line filter, or with a larger pore filter than usually used, and since the presence of the lipid in the infusate obscures any precipitate of calcium phosphate that may occur either upon removal of the infusate from refrigeration and warming prior to administration or during the time of infusion, their use in LBWI seems unwise. This is particularly true while attempting to maximize calcium and phosphate intakes.

Vitamin mixtures for parenteral use have been available since the early days of parenteral nutrition and have been used to formulate parenteral nutrition infusates. Hence, the amounts provided, to a large extent, have been determined by the preparations available.

During the early years of parenteral nutrition, it was thought that frequent plasma and/or blood transfusions provided needed trace minerals. However, reports of zinc[83] and copper deficiencies,[28] even in infants who had received these transfusions, quickly demonstrated the inadequacy of this approach and led to the availability of zinc and copper additives. Today, additives of all trace minerals for which a deficiency has been demonstrated are available.

Little definitive information is available concerning the parenteral requirements of either trace minerals or vitamins. Research concerning the parenteral requirements of these nutrients by infants has been and is still hindered by the difficulties both of measuring plasma concentrations of the nutrients using small volumes of plasma and of interpreting the physiological significance of plasma concentrations. Accurate studies of the retention of these nutrients also are notoriously difficult. The current recommendations for parenteral vitamin and trace mineral intakes (Tables 20.3 and 20.4), although not revised recently, are based on the most reliable information available, much of it theoretical rather than based on data from randomized trials of various intakes.[84] Nonetheless, the recommended intakes appear to prevent deficiencies and also appear to be safe.

Strategies for improving tolerance of parenterally delivered nutrients

Many LBWI, particularly smaller infants and infants with a variety of medical problems are unable to tolerate appreciable amounts of many nutrients. However, even during the first several days of life, most will tolerate an amino acid intake of at least 2 g kg^{-1} day^{-1}, a glucose intake of 5–10 g kg^{-1} day^{-1} and a lipid intake of 1 g kg^{-1} day^{-1}. While this intake may be less than required for positive energy balance, it almost certainly will result in nitrogen equilibrium and, probably, nitrogen retention. A 5–10% glucose and electrolyte infusion, on the other hand, will definitely result in negative nitrogen balance equivalent to a daily loss of about 1% of endogenous protein stores.[33–39] Equally important, neither marked hyperaminoacidemia nor azotemia is likely with the suggested regimen containing amino acids.

According to Collins et al.,[85] the glucose intolerance of most VLBWI can be alleviated by careful intravenous administration of insulin, thus permitting delivery of considerably greater intakes of glucose. Moreover, in these investigator's hands, insulin administration did not result in hypoglycemia or other problems. Understandably, even though use of insulin may be safe, the advisability of using it routinely to circumvent what can best be described as physiological insulin resistance rather than insulin deficiency has been questioned. Moreover, a recent study in VLBWI showed that euglycemic hyperinsulinemia was accompanied by a 3-fold increase in plasma lactate concentration and metabolic acidosis.[86]

Infusion of 20% v. 10% lipid emulsions lessens the likelihood of hyperlipidemia.[87] The mechanism appears to be related, at least in part, to the lower phospholipid/triglyceride ratio of the 20% v. the 10% emulsion and, hence, less inhibition of lipoprotein lipase activity secondary to infused phospholipid.[88] Although not available in the USA, emulsions containing medium chain triglycerides are being used with increasing frequency in other parts of the world. Since the triglycerides of these emulsions are hydrolyzed more rapidly by lipoprotein lipase[89] and the medium chain fatty acids released are oxidized more rapidly,[90] they may permit safe administration of larger parenteral doses of lipid than is possible with conventional emulsions.

For most LBWI, it is relatively easy, using some combination of the strategies discussed above, to achieve reasonable intakes of most nutrients within the first 24 hours of life. This undoubtedly is preferable to the common practice of ignoring nutritional needs for the first several days after birth.

Complications of parenteral nutrition

The complications of total parenteral nutrition are usually classified into two general categories – those related to the technique (infusion-related complications) and those related to composition of the infusate (metabolic complications).

The major infusion-related complication with central vein delivery is infection. Although many of the infusate components support growth of various microorganisms,[91,92] a contaminated infusate rarely is the underlying cause of infection. Rather, most infections appear to result either from improper care of the catheter, particularly failure to follow meticulously the requirement for frequent changes of the exit site dressing or frequent use of the catheter for purposes other than delivery of the nutrient infusate. Other complications related to this infusion technique include malposition or dislodgment of the catheter and thrombosis, including superior (or inferior) vena cava thrombosis. Malposition of the catheter can be avoided by radiographic confirmation of the location of the catheter tip prior to infusion of the hypertonic nutrient infusate

and reconfirmation as indicated thereafter. The other complications in this category cannot be completely avoided; however, careful attention to all procedures involving the catheter will reduce them to an acceptable level.

Infusion-related complications associated with peripheral vein delivery of nutrients include thrombophlebitis as well as skin and subcutaneous sloughs secondary to infiltration of the hypertonic infusate. Infection appears to be much less common with peripheral than with central vein delivery, probably because infusion sites must be changed so frequently.

The metabolic complications of parenteral nutrition include those related to the patient's limited metabolic tolerance of the various components of the infusate, those related to the infusate per se, and those related to the fact that nutrients are administered by vein rather than by the gastrointestinal tract. These are summarized in Table 20.6.

The metabolic complications related to the patient's metabolic tolerance of the infusate components are likely to be less with the less-concentrated peripheral vein regimens. Certainly, glucose intolerance is less frequent with peripheral vein delivery which limits glucose intake to about 15 g kg^{-1} day^{-1}. Electrolyte and mineral disorders usually result from provision of either too much or too little of the particular nutrient although electrolyte disorders also can result from osmotic diuresis secondary to hyperglycemia.

Since the infusates delivered by central vein and peripheral vein are qualitatively similar, the metabolic complications related to the infusate are similar with the two routes of delivery. One concern in this category is the fact that none of the currently available amino acid mixtures results in a completely normal plasma amino acid pattern.[43] In part, this concern is based on the long-recognized coexistence of elevated plasma concentrations of specific amino acids in patients with inborn errors of metabolism (e.g., hyperphenylalaninemia in patients with phenylketonuria) and mental retardation. However, in patients receiving parenteral nutrition, the plasma concentration of many amino acids is low rather than high, suggesting that the intake of these amino acids may be inadequate. As discussed above, plasma concentrations of the conditionally indispensable amino acids cysteine and tyrosine are often quite low, presumably because these amino acids, which are either unstable or insoluble in aqueous solution, are not present in appreciable amounts in available parenteral amino acid mixtures.

The low plasma concentrations of these amino acids are of concern because they may limit utilization of all amino acids for protein synthesis. Another theoretical concern is the relationship between plasma concentrations of specific

Table 20.6. Metabolic complications of parenteral nutrition and their most common cause

Disorder	Most common cause
Disorders related to metabolic capacity of patient	
Hyperglycemia	Excessive intake (either excessive concentration or excessive infusion rate, e.g., pump dysfunction); change in metabolic state (e.g., infection)
Hypoglycemia	Sudden cessation of infusion
Azotemia	Excessive nitrogen intake
Electrolyte, mineral (major and trace) and vitamin disorders	Excessive or inadequate intake
Disorders related to infusate composition	
Abnormal plasma aminograms	Amino acid pattern of nitrogen source
Hypercholesterolemia/phospholipidemia	Characteristics of lipid emulsion
Abnormal fatty acid pattern	Characteristics of lipid emulsion or its route of metabolism
Hepatic disorders	Unknown

amino acids and concentrations of various neurotransmitters within the central nervous system (CNS), e.g., plasma tryptophan concentration and CNS serotonin; plasma tyrosine concentration and CNS catecholamines; plasma concentrations of amino acids that may function as neurotransmitters and CNS concentration of that amino acid. Unfortunately, this latter area has not been studied sufficiently to warrant major concern or to allay fears.

Many of the metabolic problems related to use of available parenteral lipid emulsions are better understood than those related to available parenteral amino acid mixtures.[62] Perhaps the most pressing concern is related to the fatty acid pattern of these emulsions. Although both emulsions available in the USA contain adequate amounts of linoleic and α-linolenic acids, the parent fatty acids, respectively, of the n-6 and n-3 fatty acids, they do not contain the longer-chain, more unsaturated fatty acids of either series (Table 20.5) and the plasma concentrations of these long-chain, polyunsaturated fatty acids are low.[93] Since infants, including preterm infants, can convert the parent fatty acids to the longer-chain, polyunsaturated fatty acids,[94–97] the reasons for this are not obvious.

Appreciable amounts of long-chain, polyunsaturated ω-3 and ω-6 fatty acids accumulate in the developing central nervous system during development,[98,99] particularly docosahexaenoic (22:6 ω-3) and arachidonic acid (20:4 ω-6). Thus, the possibility that adequate amounts of the parent fatty acids are not converted to the longer-chain, more unsaturated derivatives gives rise to concern regarding the fatty acid pattern of tissue lipids. Indeed, the long-chain, polyunsaturated fatty acid contents of both the liver and brain of infants who succumb after receiving only parenteral nutrition are low compared with that of normal

infants.[99] Whether such an abnormal pattern is associated with functional abnormalities remains unknown. However, some recent studies in enterally fed infants suggest that neurodevelopmental indices and visual acuity are lower in infants fed formulas containing only the parent fatty acids than in infants fed the same formula supplemented with long-chain, polyunsaturated fatty acids.[100]

Some of the elongated, desaturated derivatives of linoleic and α-linolenic acid are precursors of various eicosanoid series. Thus, if these precursors cannot be formed or are formed in inappropriate ratios to each other, infants receiving available lipid emulsions may develop derangements in eicosanoid metabolism secondary to specific long-chain, polyunsaturated fatty acid deficiencies. Indeed, the arachidonic acid content of serum lipids decreases in infants receiving the available soybean oil emulsion and, in these infants, urinary excretion of a stable metabolite of prostaglandin E, which is synthesized from arachidonic acid, is very low.[101] Although these abnormalities have not been associated with clinical abnormalities, they are disturbing. To date, however, they have received little attention. Emulsions containing fish oil which is rich in long chain polyunsaturated ω-3 fatty acids, although not available in the USA, are available in other countries. To date, published experience with these emulsions is inadequate to permit a thorough evaluation of either their safety or their efficacy in infants.

The final subcategory of metabolic problems resulting from parenteral nutrition is related to the fact that the gastrointestinal tract is bypassed. Since the one unquestioned clinical indication for use of parenteral nutrition is to maintain or restore the nutritional status of patients with deranged gastrointestinal function, there has been considerable interest in the consequences of this therapy with respect to gastrointestinal function. In normal animals, parenteral nutrition, like starvation, results in an appreciable decrease in enteric mucosal mass.[102, 103] It has been suggested that this interferes with the normal barrier function and allows translocation of bacteria from the lumen to the blood stream.[104] If so, this could contribute to the high rate of infection in infants requiring prolonged parenteral nutrition. It also has been suggested that bypassing the gastrointestinal tract diminishes release of the various enteric hormones.[105]

The effect of parenteral nutrition on mucosal enzyme activities is unclear. Some studies suggest that the specific activity of some disaccharidases decreases relative to that of control animals[106] while others show no difference in specific activity of these enzymes between control animals and animals receiving parenteral nutrition.[107] These discrepancies may be related to the nature of the diet consumed by the control animals of the different studies. Interestingly, while many animal studies have shown a decrease in mucosal mass as well as mucosal protein and DNA content with parenteral nutrition, none of the available clinical studies of the effects of parenteral nutrition on intestinal tract structure and function demonstrate morphological involution.[108, 109] However, disaccharidase activities, which usually are low when parenteral nutrition begins, are not fully restored until enteral intake is reinstituted.[109]

One of the more illuminating studies of this issue, at least in piglets, was published recently by Burrin *et al.*[110] In this study, groups of 3-week-old piglets were maintained on either enteral or parenteral nutrients for 6 days. The following day, all animals were given an enteral feeding followed by continuous intraduodenal infusion of formula and measurement of net portal absorption of various nutrients. At the end of the study, the animals were killed and the small intestine was removed for weighing and determination of protein and DNA concentrations as well as the activity of various enzymes. Intestinal weight and DNA content as well as the specific activity of several digestive enzymes, including lactase, were about 50% lower in the group that had received only parenteral nutrients for 6 days prior to study. Lactose digestion, hexose transport and net portal balance of several amino acids also were lower in this group. Thus, this study documents both structural and functional effects of parenteral v. enteral nutrition on the small intestine. However, the question of how long these changes persist remains unanswered.

Many infants maintained solely on parenteral nutrition develop typical clinical and histological findings of cholestasis.[111] Whether this results from a toxic effect of some component of the parenteral nutrition infusate or

simply from bypassing the gastrointestinal tract is not clear. A number of studies, none rigorously controlled, suggest a variety of etiologies. Some suggest that the cholestasis is related to parenteral amino acid intake.[112, 113] In an uncontrolled study, infants receiving one of the pediatric parenteral amino acid mixtures had a lower-than-expected incidence of cholestasis.[42] However, a randomized controlled study with this mixture v. another pediatric amino acid mixture showed no difference in incidence of cholestasis between the two groups.[114] A randomized trial of the effects of the same amount of amino acids with or without taurine revealed no effects of taurine on liver function during the first 10 days of life;[115] however, none of the infants in either group developed hepatic dysfunction. Other trials[116] suggest that cholestasis can be reduced by minimal enteral feeding; thus, since the release of a number of gastrointestinal hormones appears to be delayed by exclusive parenteral nutrition,[105] it might be particularly informative to determine if parenteral nutrition affects the release of cholecystokinin, which stimulates contraction of the gall bladder, and if development of cholestasis is related to the pattern of cholecystokinin release.

Owens *et al.*[117] recently addressed the question of the amount of enteral feeding necessary to maintain intestinal mass and motility of newborn puppies. While as little as 10% of total nutrient requirements by the enteral route had positive effects on motility, at least 40% of total nutrient requirements by the enteral route was required to maintain enteric mass. This implies that the positive effects of minimal enteral feeding, which usually provides only about 15% of nutrient requirements, are related to maintenance of the enteric humoral system.

Minimizing the complications of parenteral nutrition

Many of the complications of parenteral nutrition can be minimized by a monitoring system that permits early detection of both infusion-related and metabolic complications. It also is important to monitor the actual intake of specific nutrients as well as the clinical results of the intake carefully if the full potential of the technique is to be realized. Adequate clinical monitoring to prevent infiltration of infusates delivered by peripheral vein and to assure long-term function of the central vein catheters usually requires considerable time as well as personnel who are familiar with the intricacies of the intravenous infusion apparatus, including the many varieties of constant infusion pumps that are an absolute necessity both for central vein and peripheral vein delivery.

Table 20.7. Suggested monitoring schedule during parenteral nutrition

| Variables to be monitored | Suggested frequency (per week)[a] | |
	Initial period	Later period
Growth variables		
Weight	7	7
Length	1	1
Head circumference	1	1
Metabolic variables		
Blood or plasma		
Electrolytes	2–4	1
Ca, Mg, P	2	1
Acid Base Status	2	1
Urea Nitrogen	2	1
Albumin	1	1
Liver Function Studies	1	1
Lipids[b]		
Hemoglobin	2	1
Urine Glucose	2–6/day	2/day
Prevention and detection of infection		
Clinical observations (activity, temperature)	Daily	Daily
White Blood Cell count and differential	As indicated	As indicated
Cultures	As indicated	As indicated

[a] "Initial period" refers to the time before full intake is achieved as well as any period during which metabolic instability is present or suspected (i.e., postoperative period, presence of infection). "Later period" refers to the time during which the patient is in a metabolic steady state.
[b] See text.

A suggested schedule for chemical monitoring is shown in Table 20.7. This schedule allows detection of metabolic complications in sufficient time for correction by altering the infusate. It differs somewhat from other suggested schedules. Instead of routinely monitoring blood glucose concentration, as often suggested, checking the urine regularly for the presence of glucose (at least three times daily during the first few days when the glucose content of the infusates is being increased) and determining blood glucose concentrations only when glucosuria is present should be adequate. The suggested monitoring schedule also omits determinations of plasma osmolality which, in the absence of hyperglycemia, can be estimated sufficiently accurately as twice the plasma sodium concentration. In addition, routine monitoring of the plasma amino acid pattern, which is predictable from the pattern of the mixture of amino acids used,[43] is omitted as is routine monitoring of the leukocyte count and routine blood cultures.

The monitoring required to ensure safe and efficacious use of intravenous fat emulsions is somewhat problematic. The common clinical practice of periodic visual or nephelometric inspection of the plasma for presence of lipemia is not reliable for detecting elevated plasma concentrations of both triglycerides and free fatty acids.[118] However, since microtechniques for measuring plasma triglyceride and free fatty acid concentrations are not routinely available, such monitoring often is not practical. A reasonable compromise is to inspect the plasma frequently, either visually or by nephelometry, and determine actual triglyceride and free fatty acid concentrations weekly. More frequent monitoring is necessary during the first few days of parenteral nutrition and when the patient develops a clinical condition likely to interfere with triglyceride hydrolysis. Other serum lipid abnormalities associated with use of parenteral lipid emulsions (hypercholesterolemia, hyperphospholipidemia, deranged free fatty acid patterns of serum and tissue lipids) are predictable and/or of uncertain clinical relevance; thus, monitoring to detect these is not necessary. Samples for visual or nephelometric inspection as well as those for measuring triglyceride and free amino acid concentrations should be obtained during infusion of the lipid emulsion rather than 2–4 hours after stopping the infusion as is sometimes suggested. The latter practice helps assure normal values even though the concentration of triglyceride and/or free fatty acids may have been elevated during the previous 20–22 hours of infusion.

Other considerations

Some of the questions most commonly asked concerning parenteral nutrition include: When should the therapy be started? How long should it be continued? When should enterally delivered nutrients be introduced? Unfortunately, there are few definitive data concerning any of these questions. Thus, it is not surprising that some nurseries routinely start parenteral nutrition soon after birth and continue this form of nutritional management exclusively or as the major source of nutrition support for several days to weeks while others start parenteral nutrition much later, with or without enterally delivered nutrients, and discontinue it as soon as possible.

The question of when to start parenteral nutrients is reasonably easy to address. As discussed above, preterm infants who receive only glucose lose at least 1% of endogenous nitrogen stores daily whereas those who receive an isocaloric infusate providing at least $1.5 \, g \, kg^{-1} \, day^{-1}$ of amino acids are in nitrogen equilibrium or slightly positive balance. Moreover, higher intakes are unlikely to result in marked hyperaminoacidemia or azotemia. Thus, for preterm infants, it is difficult to argue against a policy of starting a parenteral nutrition regimen containing amino acids as soon after birth as feasible, preferably within the first 24 hours.

Because of the concern that lack of enteral nutrients depresses secretion of gastrointestinal hormones and might impair intestinal tract development (see above), the practice of minimal enteral feeding, i.e., infusion of $\sim 1 \, ml \, kg^{-1} \, h^{-1}$ of human milk or a standard preterm infant formula (about 16% of total nutrient requirement) during the early days to weeks of life, when the bulk of nutrient intake is supplied by parenteral nutrients, has become quite popular. Indeed, this practice appears to result in earlier tolerance of full enteral intakes and a lower incidence of cholestasis without a higher incidence of NEC.[119] Whether a slow increase in volume instead of maintaining the same small volume for 10–14 days would be equally or even more efficacious has not been addressed.

Currently, it is impossible to recommend a single strategy for use of parenteral nutrition in LBW neonates. On the one hand, the concern that early enteral feeding may contribute to development of NEC cannot be totally discounted. On the other, the concern that prolonged use of exclusive parenteral feeding may contribute to development of the troubling problem of cholestasis also is valid. Perhaps the most appropriate strategy is to individualize the early nutritional management of each infant. Those with a number of predisposing factors for development of NEC might receive parenteral nutrients primarily until some of these factors resolve while those deemed to be less likely to develop NEC might be started on enteral feedings much earlier. Although many nurseries have standard policies for increasing the volume of enteral intake of all infants, this aspect of feeding also is one that might best be determined on an individual basis.

Regardless of the method chosen for early nutritional management, there inevitably is a period during which infants receive a combination of parenterally and enterally delivered nutrients. During this period, careful monitoring of the intake of each major nutrient received by each route is crucial if nutrient imbalances are to be avoided. Differences in likely retention of nutrients delivered parenterally v. enterally also must be considered.

When to stop parenteral nutrition also is frequently debated. Usually this is done when sufficient enteral intake to supply fluid requirements ($>100 \, ml \, kg^{-1} \, day^{-1}$) is tolerated. Although this practice may result in nutrient intake being less than optimal for a few days, it seems acceptable, particularly if nutrient intake prior to this time was reasonable.

There is a major void in knowledge concerning the advantages, disadvantages, and costs of the various ways parenteral nutrition is managed at individual institutions. Currently, these range from strict control, i.e., only a few individuals supervise the parenteral nutrition program for all patients, to virtually no control, i.e., any physician is allowed to order any regimen desired for any patient, with or without an assessment of the patient's need for parenteral nutrition and with or without requirements for monitoring either the efficacy or the safety of the particular regimen ordered. A system in which one of a few standard parenteral nutrition infusates can be ordered by any physician represents a common intermediate system for management of parenteral feeding.

In the one randomized controlled study addressing this issue,[120] neonates requiring parenteral feeding were assigned alternately to receive either a standardized formulation or an individualized formulation monitored by a clinical pharmacist. The group assigned to the individualized formulation with pharmacist monitoring received higher intakes of amino acids (2.2 v. $1.9 \, g \, kg^{-1} \, day^{-1}$), lipid (2 v. $1.5 \, g \, kg^{-1} \, day^{-1}$) and total energy (63 v. $53 \, kCal \, kg^{-1} \, day^{-1}$); this group also had a greater rate of weight gain (11.8 v. $4.9 \, g \, day^{-1}$). The total cost of the individualized system was approximately 40% greater but the cost per gram of weight gain was approximately 40% less. Moreover, this cost analysis included neither the cost of wasted solutions, which was greater for the standardized group, nor the cost of nursing time, which also was greater for the standardized group. The results of this study confirm earlier impressions that a centralized system of managing parenteral nutrition is most likely to maximize benefits and minimize risks of the technique.[9] Nonetheless, more such studies are needed.

In fact, randomized, controlled studies assessing every aspect of parenteral nutrition are needed. Without the information that such studies can provide, decisions concerning many aspects of the therapy (e.g., catheter A v. catheter B; pump A v. pump B; amino acid mixture A v. amino acid mixture B; Policy A v. Policy B, etc.) will continue to be made, frequently by administrators rather than health professionals, on the basis of cost or some other factor rather than on the basis of efficacy or safety. Obviously, this situation must change before the technique of parenteral nutrition can be improved beyond its current status. It no longer is sufficient to view the technique simply as one that permits provision of nutrients to infants who cannot be fed; rather, it must be viewed as a method of nutrient delivery that permits better nutritional management than was possible 35 years ago but one that, undoubtedly, can be improved further. Additional data from carefully conducted, randomized trials are crucial for these badly needed further improvements.

REFERENCES

1 Dudrick, S. J., Wilmore, D. W., Vars, H. M. Long term total parenteral nutrition with growth in puppies and positive nitrogen balance in patients. *Surg. Forum.* 1967;**18**:356.

2 Dudrick, S. J., Wilmore, D. W., Vars, H. M., Rhoads, J. E. Long term parenteral nutrition with growth, development, and positive nitrogen balance. *Surgery* 1968;**64**:134–42.

3 Wilmore, D. M., Dudrick, S. J. Growth and development of an infant receiving all nutrients by vein. *J. Am. Med. Assoc.* 1968;**203**:860–4.

4 Wretlind, A. Total parenteral nutrition. *Surg. Clin. N. Am.* 1978;**58**:1055–70.

5 Wilmore, D. W. The history of parenteral nutrition. In Baker, R. D., Baker, S. S., Davis, A. M., eds. *Pediatric Parenteral Nutrition.* New York, NY: Chapman and Hall; 1997:1–6.

6 Helfrick, F. W., Abelson, N. M. Intravenous feeding of a complete diet in a child: a report of a case. *J. Pediatr.* 1944;**25**:400–3.

7 Heird, W. C. Parenteral nutrition. In Grand, R. J., Sutphen, J. L., Dietz, W. H., Jr, eds. *Pediatric Nutrition: Theory and Practice.* Boston, MA: Butterworths; 1987:747–61.

8 Filler, R. M., Eraklis, A. J., Rubin, V. G., Das, J. B. Long-term parenteral nutrition in infants. *N. Engl. J. Med.* 1969; **281**: 589–94.

9 Heird, W. C., Winters, R. W. Total parenteral nutrition: the state of the art. *J. Pediatr.* 1975;**86**:2–16.

10 Keating, J. P., Ternberg, J. L. Amino acid-hypertonic glucose treatment for intractable diarrhea in infants. *Am. J. Dis. Child.* 1971;**122**:226–8.

11 Driscoll, J. M. Jr, Heird, W. C., Schullinger, J. N., Gongaware, R. D., Winters, R. W. Total intravenous alimentation in low birth weight infants: a preliminary report. *J. Pediatr.* 1972;**81**:145–53.

12 Peden, V. H., Karpel, J. T. Total parenteral nutrition in premature infants. *J. Pediatr.* 1972;**81**:137–44.

13 Ehrenkrantz, R. A., Younes, N., Lemons, J. A. *et al.* Longitudinal growth of hospitalized very low birth weight infants. *Pediatrics* 1999;**104**:280–9.

14 Heird, W. C. Nutritional support of the pediatric patient. In Winters, R. W., Greene, H. L., eds. *Nutritional Support of the Seriously Ill Patient.* New York, NY: Academic Press; 1983:157–79.

15 Heird, W. C. Parenteral feeding. In Sinclair, J. C., Bracken, M. B., eds. *Effective Care of the Newborn Infant.* Oxford: Oxford University Press; 1992:141–60.

16 Mulvihill, S. J., Fonkalsrud, E. W. Complication of superior versus inferior vena cava occlusion in infants receiving central Total Parenteral Nutrition. *J. Pediatr. Surg.* 1984;**19**:752.

17 Shaw, J. C. L. Parenteral nutrition in the management of sick low birth weight infants. *Pediatr. Clin. N. Am.* 1973;**20**:333–58.

18 Shulman, R. J., Pokorny, W. J., Martin, C. G., Petitt, R., Baldaia, L., Roney, D. Comparison of percutaneous and surgical placement of central venous catheters in neonates. *J. Pediatr. Surg.* 1986;**21**:348–50.

19 Nakamura, K. T., Sato, Y., Erenberg, A. Evaluation of a percutaneously placed 27-gauge central venous catheter in neonates weight <1200 grams. *J. Parenter. Enteral Nutr.* 1990;**14**:295–9.

20 Chathas, M. K., Paton, J. B., Fisher, D. E. Percutaneous central venous catheterization. *Am. J. Dis. Child.* 1990;**144**:1246–50.

21 Jacobowski, D., Ziegler, M. D., Perreira, G. Complications of pediatric parenteral nutrition: central versus peripheral administration. *J. Parenter. Enteral Nutr.* 1979;**3**:29.

22 Dunn, L., Hulman, S., Weiner, J., Kliegman, R. Beneficial effects of early hypocaloric enteral feeding on neonatal gastrointestinal function: preliminary report of a randomized trial. *J. Pediatr.* 1988;**112**:622–9.

23 Slagle, T. A., Gross, S. J. Effect of early low-volume enteral substrate on subsequent feeding tolerance in very low birth weight infants. *J. Pediatr.* 1988;**113**:526–31.

24 Meetze, W. H., Valentine, C., McGuigan, J. E. *et al.* Gastrointestinal priming prior to full enteral nutrition in very low birth weight infants. *J. Pediatr. Gastroenterol. Nutr.* 1992;**15**:163–70.

25 Friedman, Z., Danon, A., Stahlman, M. T., Oates, J. A. Rapid onset of essential acid deficiency in the newborn. *Pediatrics* 1976;**58**:640–9.

26 Friedman, Z., Frolich, C. Essential fatty acids and the major urinary metabolites of the E prostaglandins in thriving neonates and infants receiving parenteral fat emulsions. *Pediatr. Res.* 1979;**13**:932–6.

27 Committee on Nutrition, American Academy of Pediatrics. Use of intravenous fat emulsions in pediatric patients. *Pediatrics* 1981;**68**:738–43.

28 Heller, R. M., Kirchner, S. G., O'Neill, J. A. Jr, *et al.* Skeletal changes of copper deficiency in infants receiving prolonged total parenteral nutrition. *J. Pediatr.* 1978;**92**:947–9.

29 Jeejeebhoy, K. N., Chu, R. C., Marliss, E. B., Greenberg, G. R., Bruce-Robertson, A. Chromium deficiency, glucose intolerance, and neuropathy reversed by chromium supplementation, in a patient receiving long-term total parenteral nutrition. *Am. J. Clin. Nutr.* 1977;**30**:531–8.

30 Kien, C. L., Ganther, H. E. Manifestations of chronic selenium deficiency in a child receiving total parenteral nutrition. *Am. J. Clin. Nutr.* 1983;**37**:319–28.

31 Abumrad, N. N., Schneider, A. J., Steel, D., Rogers, L. S. Amino acid intolerance during prolonged total parenteral nutrition reversed by molybdate therapy. *Am. J. Clin. Nutr.* 1981;**34**:2551–9.

32 Zlotkin, S. H., Bryan, M. H., Anderson, G. H. Intravenous nitrogen and energy intakes required to duplicate in utero nitrogen accretion in prematurely born human infants. *J. Pediatr.* 1981;**99**:115–20.

33 Anderson, T. L., Muttart, C., Bieber, M. A., Nicholson, J. F., Heird, W. C. A controlled trial of glucose *vs* glucose and amino acids in premature infants. *J. Pediatr.* 1979;**94**:947–51.

34 Saini, J., MacMahon, P., Morgan, J. B., Kovar, I. Z. Early parenteral feeding of amino acids. *Arch. Dis. Child.* 1989;**64**:1362–6.

35 Mitton, S. G., Garlick, P. J. Changes in protein turnover after the introduction of parenteral nutrition in premature infants: comparison of breast milk and egg protein-based amino acid solutions. *Pediatr. Res.* 1992;**32**:447–54.

36 Rivera, A., Bell, E. F., Bier, D. M. Effect of intravenous amino acids on protein metabolism of preterm infants during the first three days of life. *Pediatr. Res.* 1993;**33**:106–11.

37 Van Goudoever, J. B., Colen, T., Wattimena, J. L. D. *et al.* Immediate commencement of amino acid supplementation in preterm infants: effect on serum amino acid concentrations and protein kinetics on the first day of life. *J. Pediatr.* 1995;**127**:458–65.

38 Thureen, P. J., Melara, D., Fennessey, P. V., Hay, W. W. Jr. Effect of low versus high intravenous amino acid intake on very low birth weight infants in the early neonatal period. *Pediatr. Res.* 2003;**53**:24–32.

39 Kashyap, S., Heird, W.C. Protein requirements of low birthweight, very low birthweight, and small for gestational age infants. In Räihä, N. C. R., ed. *Nestle Nutrition Workshop Series: Protein Metabolism During Infancy.* New York, NY: Nestec Ltd., Vevey/Raven Press;1994:133–51.

40 Duffy, B., Gunn, T., Collinge, J., Pencharz, P. The effect of varying protein quality and energy intake on the nitrogen metabolism of parenterally fed very low birth weight (1600 g) infants. *Pediatr. Res.* 1981;**15**:1040–4.

41 Helms, R. A., Christensen, M. L., Mauer, E. C., Storm, M. C. Comparison of a pediatric versus standard amino acid for-

mulation in preterm neonates requiring parenteral nutrition. *J. Pediatr.* 1987;**110**:466–72.

42 Heird, W. C., Hay, W., Helms, R. A. *et al.* Pediatric parenteral amino acid mixture in low birth weight infants. *Pediatrics* 1988;**81**:41–50.

43 Winters, R. W., Heird, W. C., Dell, R. B., Nicholson, J. F. Plasma amino acids in infants receiving parenteral nutrition. In Greene, H. L., Holliday, M. A., Munro, H. N., eds. *Clinical Nutrition Update: Amino Acids.* Chicago, IL: American Medical Association; 1977:147–54.

44 Roberts, S. A., Ball, R. O., Filler, R. M., Moore, A. M., Pencharz, P. B. Phenylalanine and tyrosine metabolism in neonates receiving parenteral nutrition differing in pattern of amino acids. *Pediatr. Res.* 1998;**44**:907–14.

45 Wykes, L. J., House, J. D., Ball, R. O., Pencharz, P. B. Aromatic amino acid metabolism of neonatal piglets receiving TPN: effect of tyrosine precursors. *Am. J. Physiol.* 1994;**267**:E672–9.

46 Sturman, J. A., Gaull, G. A., Räihä, N. C. R. Absence of cystathionase in human liver: is cystine essential? *Science* 1970;**169**:74–6.

47 Zlotkin, S. H., Anderson, G. H. The development of cystathionase activity during the first year of life. *Pediatr. Res.* 1982;**16**:65–8.

48 Räihä, N. C. R. Phenylalanine hydroxylase in human liver during development. *Pediatr. Res.* 1973;**7**:1–4.

49 Chawla, R. K., Berry, C. J., Kutner, M. H., Rudman, D. Plasma concentrations of transsulfuration pathway products during nasoenteral and intravenous hyperalimentation of malnourished patients. *Am. J. Clin. Nutr.* 1985;**42**:577–84.

50 Zlotkin, S. H., Bryan, M. H., Anderson, G. H. Cysteine supplementation to cysteine-free intravenous feeding regimens in newborn infants. *Am. J. Clin. Nutr.* 1981;**34**:914–23.

51 Malloy, M. H., Rassin, D. K., Richardson, C. J. Total parenteral nutrition in sick preterm infants: effects of cysteine supplementation with nitrogen intakes of 240 & 400 mg/kg/d. *J. Pediatr. Gastroenterol. Nutr.* 1984;**3**:239–44.

52 Van Goudoever, J. B., Sulkers, E. J., Timmerman, M. Amino acid solutions for premature infants during the first week of life: the role of N-acetyl-L-cysteine and N-acetyl-L-tyrosine. *J. Parenter. Enteral Nutr.* 1994;**18**:404–8.

53 Roberts, S. A., Ball, R. O., Moore, A. M., Filler, R. M., Pencharz, P. B. The effect of graded intake of glycyl-L-tyrosine on phenylalanine and tyrosine metabolism in parenterally fed neonates with an estimation of tyrosine requirement. *Pediatr. Res.* 2001;**49**:111–19.

54 Souba, W. W., Austgen, T. R. Interorgan glutamine flow following surgery and infection. *J. Parenter. Enteral Nutr.* 1990;**14**:90S–3S.

55 Lacey, J. M., Wilmore, D. W. Is glutamine a conditionally essential amino acid? *Nutr. Rev.* 1990;**48**:297–309.

56 Poindexter, B. B., Ehrenkranz, R. A., Stoll, B. J. *et al.* Effect of parenteral glutamine supplementation on plasma amino acid concentrations in extremely low-birth-weight infants. *Am. J. Clin. Nutr.* 2003;**77**:737–43.

57 Poindexter, B. B., Ehrenkrantz, R. A., Stoll, B. J. *et al.* Parenteral glutamine supplementation in ELBW infants: a multicenter randomized clinical trial. *Pediatr. Res.* 2002;**51**:317A.

58 Weinstein, M. R., Oh, W. Oxygen consumption in infants with bronchopulmonary dysplasia. *J. Pediatr.* 1981;**99**:958–61.

59 Munro, H. N. General aspects of the regulation of protein metabolism by diet and hormone. In Munro, H. N., ed. *Mammalian Protein Metabolism, Vol. I. Biochemical Aspects of Protein Metabolism.* New York, NY: Academic Press; 1964:381–481.

60 Pineault, M., Chessex, P., Bisaillon, S., Brisson, G. Total parenteral nutrition in the newborn: impact of the quality of infused energy on nitrogen metabolism. *Am. J. Clin. Nutr.* 1988;**47**:298–304.

61 Bresson, J. L., Bader, B., Rocchiccioli, F. *et al.* Protein-metabolism kinetics and energy-substrate utilization in infants fed parenteral solutions with different glucose-fat ratios. *Am. J. Clin. Nutr.* 1991;**54**:370–6.

62 Heird, W. C. Lipid metabolism in parenteral nutrition. In Fomon, S. J., Heird, W. C., eds. *Energy and Protein Needs During Infancy.* New York, NY: Academic Press; 1986:215–29.

63 Andrew, G., Chan, G., Schiff, D. Lipid metabolism in the neonate. I. The effect of intralipid infusion on plasma triglyceride and free fatty acid concentrations in the neonate. *J. Pediatr.* 1976;**88**:273–8.

64 Greene, H. L., Hazlett, D., Demaree, R. Relationship between intralipid-induced hyperlipidemia and pulmonary function. *Am. J. Clin. Nutr.* 1976;**29**:127–35.

65 Pereira, G. R., Fox, W. W., Stanley, C. A., Baker, L., Schwartz, J. G. Decreased oxygenation and hyperlipidemia during intravenous fat infusions in premature infants. *Pediatrics* 1980;**66**:26–30.

66 Loo, L. S., Tang, J. P., Kohl, S. The inhibition of leukocyte cellular cytotoxicity to herpes simplex virus in vitro and in vivo by intralipid. *J. Infect. Dis.* 1982;**146**:64–70.

67 Cleary, T. C., Pickering, L. K. Mechanisms of intralipid effect on polymorpho-nuclear leukocytes. *J. Clin. Lab. Immunol.* 1983;**11**:21–6.

68 Odell, G. B., Cukier, J. O., Ostrea, E. M. Jr, Maglalang, A. C., Poland, R. L. The influence of fatty acids on the binding of bilirubin to albumin. *J. Lab. Clin. Med.* 1977;**89**:295–307.

69 Penn, D., Schmidt-Sommerfeld, E., Pascu, F. Decreased carnitine concentration in newborn infants receiving total parenteral nutrition. *Early Hum. Dev.* 1979;**4**:23–8.

70 Schmidt-Sommerfeld, E., Penn, D., Wolf, H. Carnitine deficiency in premature infants receiving total parenteral nutrition: effect of L-carnitine supplementation. *J. Pediatr.* 1983;**102**:931–5.

71 Orzali, A., Donzelli, F., Enzi, G., Rubaltelli, F. F. Effect of carnitine on lipid metabolism in the newborn. I. Carnitine supplementation during total parenteral nutrition in the first 48 hours of life. *Biol. Neonate.* 1983;**43**:186–90.

72 Christensen, M. L., Helms, R. A., Mauer, E. C., Storm, M. C. Plasma carnitine concentration and lipid metabolism in infants receiving parenteral nutrition. *J. Pediatr.* 1989;**115**:794–8.

73 Helms, R. A., Whitington, P. F., Mauer, E. C. *et al.* Enhanced lipid utilization in infants receiving oral L-carnitine during long-term parenteral nutrition. *J. Pediatr.* 1986;**109**:984–8.

74 Sulkers, E. J., Lafeber, H. N., Degenhart, H. J. *et al.* Effects of high carnitine supplementation on substrate utilization in low-birth-weight infants receiving total parenteral nutrition. *Am. J. Clin. Nutr.* 1990;**52**:889–94.

75 Holman, R. T., Johnson, S. B., Hatch, T. F. A case of human linolenic acid deficiency involving neurological abnormalities. *Am. J. Clin. Nutr.* 1982;**35**:617–23.

76 Bjerve, K. S., Fischer, S., Alme, K. Alpha-linolenic acid deficiency in man: effect of ethyl linolenate on plasma and erythrocyte fatty acid composition and biosynthesis of prostanoids. *Am. J. Clin. Nutr.* 1987b;**46**:570–6.

77 Brans, Y. W., Andrew, D. S., Carrillo, D. W. *et al.* Tolerance of fat emulsions in very-low-birth-weight neonates. *Am. J. Dis. Child.* 1988;**142**:145–52.

78 Koo, W. W. K., Tsang, R. C. Bone mineralization in infants. *Prog. Food Nutr. Sci.* 1984;**8**:229–302.

79 Koo, W. W. K., Tsang, R. C. Rickets in infants. In Nelson, N. M., ed. *Current Therapy in Neonatal Perinatal Medicine.* Philadelphia, PA: BC Decker; 1985:299–304.

80 Ziegler, E. E., O'Donnell, A. M., Nelson, S. E., Fomon, S. J. Body composition of the reference fetus. *Growth* 1976;**40**:329–41.

81 Koo, W. W. K., Tsang, R. C., Steichen, J. J. *et al.* Parenteral nutrition for infants: effect of high versus low calcium and phosphorus content. *J. Pediatr. Gastroenterol. Nutr.* 1987;**6**:96–104.

82 Prestridge, L. L., Schanler, R. J., Shulman, R. J., Burns, P. A., Laine, L. L. Effect of parenteral calcium and phosphorus therapy on mineral retention and bone mineral content in very low birth weight infants. *J. Pediatr.* 1993;**122**:761–8.

83 Arakaw, T., Tamura, T., Igarasi, Y., Suzuki, M., Sandstead, M. M. Zinc deficiency in two infants during total parenteral alimentation for diarrhea. *Am. J. Clin. Nutr.* 1976;**29**:197–204.

84 Greene, H. L., Hambidge, K. M., Schanler, R., Tsang, R. C. Guidelines for the use of vitamins, trace elements, calcium, magnesium, and phosphorus in infants and children receiving total parenteral nutrition: report of the subcommittee on pediatric parenteral nutrient requirements from the committee on clinical practice issues of the American Society for Clinical Nutrition. *Am. J. Clin. Nutr.* 1988;**48**:1324–42.

85 Collins, J. W. Jr, Hoope, M., Brown, K. *et al.* A controlled trial of insulin infusion in parenteral nutrition in extremely low birth weight infants with glucose intolerance. *J. Pediatr.* 1991;**118**:921–7.

86 Poindexter, B. B., Karn, C. A., Denne, S. C. Exogenous insulin reduces proteolysis and protein synthesis in extremely low birth weight infants. *J. Pediatr.* 1998;**132**:948–53.

87 Haumont, D., Deckelbaum, R. J., Richelle, M. *et al.* Plasma lipid and plasma lipoprotein concentrations in low birth weight infants given parenteral nutrition with 20% compared to 10% Intralipid. *J. Pediatr.* 1989;**115**:787–93.

88 Fielding, C. J. Human lipoprotein lipase inhibition of activity by cholesterol. *Biochim. Biophys. Acta* 1970;**218**:221–6.

89 Deckelbaum, R. J., Hamilton, J., Moser, A. *et al.* Medium chain versus long chain triacylglycerol emulsion hydrolysis by lipoprotein lipase and hepatic lipase: implications for the mechanisms of lipase action. *Biochemistry* 1990;**29**:1136–42.

90 Park, W., Paust, H., Brösicke, M. S., Knoblach, G., Helge, H. Impaired fat utilization in parenterally fed low-birth-weight infants suffering from sepsis. *J. Parenter. Enteral Nut.* 1986;**10**:627–30.

91 Goldman, D. A., Martin, W. T., Worthington, J. W. Growth of bacteria and fungi in total parenteral nutrition solutions. *Am. J. Surg.* 1973;**126**:314–18.

92 McKee, K. T. Jr, Melly, M. A., Greene, H. L., Schaffner, W. Gram-negative bacillary sepsis associated with use of lipid emulsion in parenteral nutrition. *Am. J. Dis. Child.* 1979;**133**:649–50.

93 Sosenko, I. R. S., Rodriguez-Pierce, M., Bacalari, E. Effect of early initiation of intravenous lipid administration on the incidence and severity of chronic lung disease in premature infants. *J. Pediatr.* 1993;**123**:975–82.

94 Carnielli, V. P., Wattimena, J. D. L., Luijendijk, I. H. *et al.* The very-low-birth-weight premature infant is capable of synthesizing arachidonic and docosahexaenoic acid from linoleic and linolenic acid. *Pediatr. Res.* 1996;**40**:169–74.

95 Salem, Jr. N., Wegher, B., Mena, P., Uauy, R. Arachidonic and docosahexaenoic acids are biosynthesized from their 18-carbon precursors in human infants. *Proc. Natl. Acad. Sci. USA* 1996;**93**:49–54.

96 Sauerwald, T. U., Hachey, D. L., Jensen, C. L. *et al.* Intermediates in endogenous synthesis of C22:6ω3 and C20:4ω6 by term and preterm infants. *Pediatr. Res.* 1997;**41**:183–7.

97 Uauy, R., Mena, P., Wegher, B., Nieto, S., Salem, N. Jr. Long chain polyunsaturated fatty acid formation in neonates: effect of gestational age and intrauterine growth. *Pediatr. Res.* 2000;**47**:127–35.

98 Clandinin, M. T., Chappell, J. E., Leong, S. *et al.* Intrauterine fatty acid accretion rates in human brain: implications for fatty acid requirements. *Early Hum. Dev.* 1980;**4**:121–9.

99 Martinez, M., Ballabriga, A. Effect of parenteral nutrition with high doses of linoleate on the developing human liver and brain. *Lipids* 1987;**22**:133–8.

100 Heird, W. C. The role of essential fatty acids in development. In Hay, W. W., Thureen, P., eds. *Neonatal Nutrition and Metabolism.* 2005.

101 Friedman, Z., Frolich, J. C. Essential fatty acids and the major urinary metabolites of the E prostaglandins in thriving neonates and in infants receiving parenteral fat emulsions. *Pediatr. Res.* 1979;**13**:926–32.

102 Feldman, E. J., Dowling, R. H., McNaughton, J., Peters, T. J. Effects of oral versus intravenous nutrition on intestinal adaptation after small bowel resection in the dog. *Gastroenterology* 1976;**70**:712–9.

103 Johnson, L. R., Copeland, E. M., Dudrick, S. J., Lichtenberger, L. M., Castro, G. A. Structural and hormonal alterations in the gastrointestinal tract of parenterally fed rats. *Gastroenterology* 1975;**68**:1177–83.

104 Lipman, T. O. Bacterial translocation and enteral nutrition in humans: an outsider looks in. *J. Parenter. Enteral Nutr.* 1995;**19**:156–65.

105 Lucas, A., Bloom, S. R., Aynsley-Green, A. Metabolic and endocrine effects of depriving preterm infants of enteral nutrition. *Acta Paediatr. Scand.* 1983;**72**:245–9.

106 Levine, G. M., Deren, J. J., Steiger, E., Zinno, R. Role of oral intake in maintenance of gut mass and disaccharidase activity. *Gastroenterology* 1974;**67**:975–82.

107 Castro, G. A., Copeland, E. M., Dudrick, S. J., Johnson, L. R. Intestinal disaccharidase and peroxidase activities in parenterally nourished rats. *J. Nutr.* 1975;**105**:776–81.

108 Shwachman, H., Lloyd-Still, J. D., Khaw, K. T., Antonowicz, I. Protracted diarrhea of infancy treated with intravenous alimentation. II. Studies of small intestinal biopsy results. *Am. J. Dis. Child.* 1973;**125**:365–8.

109 Greene, H. L., McCabe, D. R., Merenstein, G. B. Intractable diarrhea and malnutrition in infancy: changes in intestinal morphology and disaccharidase activities during treatment with total intravenous nutrition or oral elemental diets. *J. Pediatr.* 1975;**87**:695–704.

110 Burrin, D. G., Stoll, B., Chang, X. *et al.* Parenteral nutrition results in impaired lactose digestion and hexose absorption when enteral feeding is initiated in infant pigs. *Am. J. Clin. Nutr.* 2003;**78**:461–70.

111 Merritt, R. J. Cholestasis associated with total parenteral nutrition. *J. Pediatr. Gastroenterol. Nutr.* 1980;**5**:9–22.

112 Black, D. D., Suttle, E. A., Whitington, P. F., Whitington, G. L., Korones, S. D. The effect of short-term total parenteral nutrition on hepatic function in the human neonate: a prospective randomized study demonstrating alteration of hepatic canalicular function. *J. Pediatr.* 1981;**99**:445–9.

113 Brown, M. R., Thunberg, B. J., Golub, L. *et al.* Decreased cholestasis with enteral instead of intravenous protein in the very low-birth-weight infant. *J. Pediatr. Gastroenterol. Nutr.* 1989;**9**:21–7.

114 Forchielli, M. L., Gura, K. M., Sandler, R., Lo, C. Aminosyn PF or trophamine: which provides more protection from cholestasis associated with total parenteral nutrition? *J. Pediatr. Gastroenterol. Nutr.* 1995;**21**:374–82.

115 Cooke, R. J., Whitington, P. F., Kelts, D. Effect of taurine supplementation on hepatic function during short-term parenteral nutrition in the premature infant. *J. Pediatr. Gastroenterol. Nutr.* 1984;**3**:234–8.

116 Tyson, J. E., Kennedy, K. A., Cochrane Neonatal Group. Minimal enteral nutrition for promoting feeding tolerance and preventing morbidity in parenterally fed infants. *Cochrane Database Syst. Rev.* 2000;**2**:CD000504.

117 Owens, L., Burrin, D. G., Berseth, C. L. Minimal enteral feeding induces maturation of intestinal motor function but not mucosal growth in neonatal dogs. *J. Nutr.* 2002;**132**:2717–22.

118 Schreiner, R. L., Glick, M. R., Nordschow, C. D. *et al.* An evaluation of methods to monitor infants receiving intravenous lipids. *J. Pediatr.* 1979;**94**:197–200.

119 Schanler, R. J., Shulman, R. J., Lau, C., Smith, E. O., Heitkemper, M. Feeding strategies for preterm infants: randomized trial of time of initiation and method of feeding. *Pediatrics* 1999;**103**:434–9.

120 Dice, J. E., Burckart, G. J., Woo, J. T., Helms, R. A. Standardized versus pharmacist-monitored individualized parenteral nutrition in low-birth-weight infants. *Am. J. Hosp. Pharm.* 1981;**38**:1487–9.

21

Enteral amino acid and protein digestion, absorption, and metabolism

David K. Rassin and Karen E. Shattuck

Department of Pediatrics, University of Texas Medical Branch at Galveston, Galveston, TX

Introduction

The amino acid requirements of neonates continue to be an area of investigation despite numerous studies, due to the complexity of determining these requirements within the ever-changing biochemical environment of the developing infant. In the following discussion some of the issues related to digestibility and absorption, special aspects of development as they impact on requirements – including amino acid metabolism and infant responses to amino acid variations in the diet – will be addressed.

Protein is often assessed for its function in infant nutrition based on its role in supporting growth. However, protein is responsible for supplying some 20 individual amino acids with a variety of specific functions, as well as serving as precursors for a number of biologically active proteins (for example enzymes, cytokines, and immunoglobulins) that have more complex roles than to merely supply the amino acid building blocks for the body's proteins.[1] The major conundrum in determining protein requirements for infants is that human milk proteins are fundamentally different than the proteins supplied in various substitution formulas. Human milk is perfectly satisfactory nutrition for the healthy term infant (and is also usually satisfactory for preterm infants when supplemented with additional nutrients to support the greater requirements of these infants). Thus, the determination of infant protein requirements is often an exercise in comparing human milk protein nutriture to various possible substitutes (adapted cow milk or soy proteins, usually). Human milk is a dynamic form of nutrition that changes during lactation (protein declines and the content of bioactive components change) and also includes greater proportions of nonprotein nitrogen constituents than do available substitutes.

Protein digestibility and absorption

The indices of protein digestibility have been comprehensively reviewed,[2] including discussions of the weaknesses of the various methods. The basic measure of protein quality for use in infant formulas is the protein efficiency ratio or PER. This method is based upon comparing the effects of proteins to be studied to a control protein, usually casein, upon the growth of weanling rats.[3] A True Protein Digestibility Index, also determined in rats, was proposed to better account for fecal excretion of nitrogen.[4] A protein digestibility-corrected amino acid score has been proposed to take into account the limiting essential amino acid in a given protein.[5,6] This latter method permits the use of human milk protein as a reference protein.

The net conclusion of applying these various methods to protein products commonly used in infants was that they are highly bioavailable,[6,7] as are those proteins in human milk. Thus, either cow-milk protein-based or soy-milk protein-based formulas supply proteins that the infant may utilize efficiently for growth. This latter statement does need to be qualified with the fact that a variety of treatments that are used during the preparation of substitute formulas may change this bioavailability. Formula constituents are heated, spray-dried, electrophoresed, acid extracted and stored, all factors that may and do change composition. Even the physical form of the formula (powder versus

Neonatal Nutrition and Metabolism. Second Edition, ed. P. Thureen and W. Hay. Published by Cambridge University Press.
© Cambridge University Press 2006.

liquid) may influence digestibility due to differences in preparation methodologies.[8]

Both human milk and currently available formulas are efficiently digested and absorbed by the infant. The efficiency by which human milk proteins, which are present in lower concentrations (compared with formulas), support growth may reflect the presence of other factors that promote nutrient absorption.[9]

The above evaluations of protein digestibility lead to the conclusion that human milk is the preferred reference for feeding healthy term infants, however as human milk contains less protein than infant formulas and changes in content occur during lactation, perhaps formulas should contain less protein than they do currently. Human milk appears to progress from a high of 1.6 g of protein dL^{-1} during early lactation to a low of 0.7 g dL^{-1} by 6 months.[10] Most infant formulas contain 1.5 g of protein dL^{-1} (matching human milk only during early lactation). This difference has been the impetus for considering the use of "step-down" formulas with lower protein content for older infants. Such preparations appear to adequately support growth and biochemical development.[11]

Amino acid requirements

Amino acid requirements have generally been presented in terms of "essential" or "indispensable" amino acids. This subgroup of amino acids has been defined by growth and nitrogen-balance studies, but in infants has been modified by the addition of a number of amino acids that have been called "semi-essential" or "conditionally essential" based upon the special biochemical developmental state of such infants.[12] The application of newer methodologies, such as stable isotope studies, has contributed to the modification of the classical list of essential amino acids. When the "quality" of proteins is discussed, it is really their ability to deliver an optimal mixture of amino acids to the baby that is being presented. Such an optimal mixture would appear to include all the amino acids ("indispensable" and "dispensable"). Indeed, it has been noted that in 1954 eight amino acids were classified as indispensable and twelve as dispensable, while by 1994 nine were considered indispensable, seven conditionally indispensable, and only five as dispensable.[13] It seems only a matter of time until all are considered indispensable to the infant (Table 21.1).

In this vein, it is clear that it would not be acceptable to feed a protein that only contained essential amino acids (if such could be constructed). Indeed, even total parenteral nutrition mixtures made up of individual amino

Table 21.1. Amino acid content of human milk

Clinically indispensable amino acids	Conditionally indispensable	Not yet defined as indispensable
Valine	Arginine	Alanine
Isoleucine	Cysteine	Asparagine
Leucine	Glutamine	Aspartate
Lysine	Glycine	Glutamate
Methionine	Histidine	Serine
Phenylalanine	Proline	
Threonine	Taurine*	
Tryptophan	Tyrosine	

* Not a protein constituent.

acids, include most of the dispensable amino acids and only exclude amino acids due to issues of stability, solubility, or proposed toxicity.[14] Given this situation it would seem that the most appropriate amino acid requirements would be those patterned on the overall content of human milk proteins (begging the issue of the potential use of bioactive proteins for nutritional support).

Several investigations have presented the amino acid content of human milk proteins (Table 21.2), and these data may serve as a sound basis for modifying the protein content of substitute feedings. An examination of the variability of these data indicates a quite consistent delivery of amino acids, including their amounts relative to one another (Table 21.3). The consistency of these data is remarkable given that they were reported by 15 different investigators over a 47-year period using a variety of different methodologies. Data are also presented relative to the content of histidine (Table 21.3), one of the least variable amino acids in content in human milk. Thus, one can appreciate that the pattern from report to report stays remarkably consistent. Human milk substitute amino acid composition is invariably different, reflecting differences in the fundamental amino acid composition of the proteins used in these preparations (Table 21.4). Methionine is typically high and cysteine low in these preparations. Phenylalanine tends to be high in casein-predominant formulas while threonine tends to be high in whey-predominant formulas (Table 21.4).

It should be noted that the glutamine content of human milk and formulas is rarely given; it is generally converted to glutamate in the process of hydrolysis. Formula preparation may well convert glutamine to glutamate, thus it is possible that human milk-fed infants receive more glutamine relative to glutamate than do formula-fed infants. This difference may have implications for the development of the

Table 21.2. Human milk amino acid content

Amino acid	N	Mean	Standard deviation	Minimum	Maximum	Coefficient of variation
Isoleucine	20	54.62	8.17	41.00	77.50	14.96
Leucine	20	98.78	8.41	75.80	116.10	8.52
Valine	20	53.80	8.78	41.10	72.50	16.33
Methionine	19	13.69	3.07	9.40	22.00	22.42
Cystine	14	20.59	4.61	10.10	26.00	23.38
Phenylalanine	19	37.03	6.16	29.50	52.80	16.65
Tyrosine	17	40.35	9.27	28.50	61.50	22.98
Threonine	20	44.75	4.22	38.00	55.60	9.44
Tryptophan	15	16.93	3.19	11.90	22.00	18.89
Lysine	20	69.16	9.72	55.40	98.00	14.06
Glutamate	17	172.28	21.13	128.80	198.50	12.26
Aspartate	17	88.67	6.74	79.00	102.90	7.60
Serine	17	46.88	9.98	38.80	79.90	21.30
Glycine	17	23.11	2.73	19.40	30.60	11.83
Alanine	15	37.88	3.60	31.60	45.00	9.52
Proline	17	81.68	12.89	61.30	100.20	15.78
Arginine	19	39.26	7.17	29.00	59.70	18.25
Histidine	20	22.35	2.77	17.80	28.00	12.42

Amino acids are presented in mg g^{-1} of protein.[11,17,52–67]

Table 21.3. Human milk amino acid composition expressed relative to histidine content

Amino acid	N	Mean	Standard deviation	Minimum	Maximum	Coefficient of variation
Isoleucine	20	2.47	0.42	1.77	3.49	17.29
Leucine	20	4.46	0.51	3.51	5.44	11.54
Valine	20	2.42	0.35	1.76	3.06	14.82
Methionine	19	0.62	0.13	0.42	0.93	21.93
Cysteine	15	1.56	0.20	1.07	2.01	13.33
Phenylalanine	19	1.67	0.20	1.21	2.08	12.15
Tyrosine	18	3.43	0.50	2.70	4.49	14.55
Threonine	20	2.02	0.22	1.49	2.41	11.09
Tryptophan	15	0.76	0.12	0.42	0.92	16.70
Lysine	20	3.13	0.54	2.09	4.10	17.23
Glutamate	17	7.77	0.86	5.79	9.28	11.11
Aspartate	17	4.01	0.40	3.10	4.77	10.10
Serine	17	2.11	0.42	1.47	3.46	20.15
Glycine	17	1.04	0.10	0.92	1.32	9.75
Alanine	15	1.66	0.14	1.45	1.99	8.92
Proline	17	3.66	0.37	2.80	4.13	10.11
Arginine	19	1.78	0.29	1.26	2.58	16.70
Histidine	20	1.00	0.00	1.00	1.00	0.00

Amino acids concentrations were calculated relative to the histidine content of each published data set.[11,17,52–67]

Table 21.4. Amino acid composition of selected human milk substitutes

Amino acid	Casein predominant		Whey predominant		Soy	
	mg g^{-1}	Relative to histidine	mg g^{-1}	Relative to histidine	mg g^{-1}	Relative to histidine
Isoleucine	49	2.33	54	2.70	49	1.88
Leucine	94	4.48	101	5.05	82	3.15
Valine	54	2.57	56	2.80	50	1.92
Methionine	28*	1.33	25*	1.25	13	0.50
Cysteine	9*	0.43	17	0.85	13*	0.50
Phenylalanine	49*	2.33	33	1.65	52*	2.00
Tyrosine	44	2.10	34	1.70	38	1.46
Threonine	43	2.05	60*	3.00	38	1.46
Tryptophan	13	0.62	12	0.60	13	0.50
Lysine	71	3.38	81	4.05	63	2.42
Glutamate	206*	9.81	187	9.35	191	7.35
Aspartate	77	3.67	98	4.90	116*	4.46
Serine	55	2.62	55	2.75	52	2.00
Glycine	19	0.90	19	0.95	42	1.62
Alanine	32	1.52	43	2.15	43	1.65
Proline	97*	4.62	78	3.90	51*	1.96
Arginine	31	1.48	30	1.50	76*	2.92
Histidine	21	1.00	20	1.00	26	1.00

Compiled from various sources of composition of commercial products. The asterisks indicate a deviation from human milk content that may influence infant status.

intestine, as glutamine appears to have an important role in this process.[15]

Role of amino acid metabolism

Many of the issues related to the development of amino acid metabolism were described in detail in the previous edition of this book.[12] The special metabolism of the developing infant has been a major stimulus to our understanding of neonatal amino acid requirements. The list of amino acids in Table 21.1, and especially the growing list of "conditionally indispensable" amino acids speaks to our growing appreciation of neonatal metabolism.

The pathways that seem especially important during early development involve the urea cycle (especially arginine), the aromatic amino acids (phenylalanine and tyrosine), and the sulfur-containing amino acids (methionine, cysteine, and taurine). In addition, there appear to be special methodologic issues related to determining the nutrition and metabolism of cysteine[16] and tryptophan.[17]

Infants depend upon arginine availability for protection against hyperammonemia,[18] especially if fed parenterally.[19] This dependence appears due to the slow maturation of the enzyme argininosuccinate synthetase.[20, 21]

The phenylalanine metabolic pathway has hepatic enzyme activities considerably lower in the fetus than in the adult.[22, 23] The phenylalanine to tyrosine (catalyzed by phenylalanine hydroxylase) conversion appears to be more robust than the catabolism of tyrosine.[24] Thus, the occurrence of a buildup of tyrosine in the blood of infants fed proteins enriched in aromatic amino acids occurs.[25] However, in parenterally fed infants there appears to be a paradoxical failure to maintain tyrosine concentrations[26] in spite of the apparent availability of sufficient enzyme activity and precursor phenylalanine. This paradoxical response occurs despite stable isotope evidence that phenylalanine is converted to tyrosine in these infants.[27] These latter investigators have suggested that the apparent low concentrations of plasma tyrosine may be explained by the activation of alternative metabolic pathways of phenylalanine in parenterally fed infants.

The sulfur amino acid pathway first became of major interest when it was demonstrated that human fetal liver lacked the protein cystathionase, responsible for catalyzing cysteine synthesis.[28, 29] This finding has led to numerous attempts to define cysteine requirements in both preterm and term infants. These investigations have been complicated by the difficulty in accurately determining cysteine. It exists as the disulfide cystine, as the sulfhydryl cysteine, and as a disulfide bound to plasma proteins.[16] There is also some portion of the molecule bound as a disulfide to other sulfhydryls such as homocysteine and glutathione. These various forms of cysteine will change with storage, especially if samples are not kept frozen and are in the presence of plasma proteins.[16] Most published investigations (with a few exceptions such as Picone *et al.*, and Malloy *et al.*)[11,17,30] have only measured the disulfide form, cysteine, as this form of the compound can be determined readily by automated amino acid analysis.

As cysteine is also a component of the intracellular antioxidant glutathione, there has been interest in its role in protecting the neonate against oxidative stress. Glutathione is dependent upon cysteine availability for synthesis,[31] and so nutritional regimens, such as total parenteral nutrition, which do not readily supply cysteine (due to its lack of stability and to the insolubility of its disulfide form in parenteral nutrition solutions) may place infants at risk for insults from oxidative stress.

The sulfur amino acid pathway also supplies the amino acid taurine, which is not readily synthesized by humans.[32] This amino acid is not normally present in protein and has to be added to infant formulas as a supplement (it is present in human milk). While taurine has been implicated in visual and brain development,[33,34] its most documented role in human nutrition is as a bile acid conjugator. When present in infant feeding regimens the taurine conjugates of bile salts predominate, and when not present, as in unsupplemented formulas, the glycine conjugate predominates.[35] This finding may be one explanation for the improved absorption of nutrients in human milk compared with formula-fed infants.

Infant responses

The gross endpoints for adequate absorption and digestion of proteins by the infant have always been growth and nitrogen balance. However, these endpoints give little information about the true quality of the proteins being fed. While stable isotope studies have held great promise for determining amino acid requirements, they have often appeared to generate more controversy than answers.[36] Thus, if formulas and human milk support adequate growth and nitrogen balance the only other consistent measure of the quality of such nutrition has been plasma amino acid patterns.

By 72 hours of life the plasma amino acid patterns of healthy term infants reflect the type of feeding (human milk or formulas with differing protein composition) that they have received.[37] The norm for such patterns is that of the healthy breastfed term infant. Suggestions that cord blood concentrations might be an appropriate goal can be disabused just by examining the dramatic changes that occur in the concentrations of amino acids such as threonine and lysine immediately after birth. Also, the relative amounts of glutamate to glutamine (shifts from high to low) change and may reflect the more anerobic milieu of the fetus compared with the newborn infant.[37]

The fact that bovine casein proteins stimulate increased aromatic amino acid concentrations[25] has been well documented. In addition, Kashyap *et al.*[38] have shown that most plasma amino acids reflect the amount of protein intake. As most infant formulas provide greater concentrations of protein than human milk, it is clear why most formula-fed infants have greater plasma amino acid concentrations than infants fed human milk. The consequences of these differing amino acid concentrations are not fully understood, but as amino acids serve as both neurotransmitters and neurotransmitter precursors, it is quite possible that the development of the brain is influenced.[39] Indeed, the amount of protein in infant formulas appears to be associated with behavioral responses in preterm infants.[40]

Clinical perspectives on infant enteral feeding

These findings regarding amino acid absorption have supported general clinical practice regarding infant feeding. The superiority of human milk feeding has been conclusively demonstrated in the term infant.[41,42] If human milk is not available, or is contraindicated, satisfactory commercial formulas have been developed with cow milk as the protein source. Most formulas commonly used in the USA, including Enfamil (Mead Johnson, Evansville, IN) and generic store brands (formerly Wyeth's, Radnor, PA SMA) have a 60:40 whey-casein ratio. Improved Similac (Ross Laboratories, Columbus, OH) has a 50:50 whey-casein ratio.[43] However, no study has demonstrated that whey predominant formulas are nutritionally advantageous to casein-predominant formulas in the term infant.[42,44]

Thus, for the term infant, the clinician should advise breast-feeding unless contraindicated, and may recommend commercial formulas based upon individual preferences. The contraindications to breast-feeding include maternal use of specific medications, maternal herpetic breast lesions, maternal infection with HIV (in the USA), HTLV-I, HTLV-II, or active tuberculosis, or infant galactosemia.[42,43,45–51]

Enteral feeding of the preterm infant is far more problematic. Ideally, breast milk should be fed, but it is not completely adequate for the special nutritional needs of

Table 21.5. Serum protein and albumin concentrations in term and preterm infants

		Week 1	Week 4	Week 8
Total protein (g dL^{-1}, mean $\pm$ SD)	Term	5.58 ± 0.4	5.41 ± 0.32	5.64 ± 0.24
	Preterm	4.80 ± 0.1	4.5 ± 0.1	4.2 ± 0.1
Albumin (g dL^{-1}, mean $\pm$ SD)	Term	3.54 ± 0.29	3.82 ± 0.24	4.09 ± 0.24
	Preterm	3.1 ± 0.1	2.9 ± 0.1	3.0 ± 0.1

All infants were fed breast milk. Term infants were demand-fed, and preterm infants (28–36 weeks at the time of recruitment) were fed 170 ml kg^{-1}day^{-1}. Data were obtained from the same laboratory. Term data from Järvenpää et al.[59,60] Preterm data from Räihä et al.[63]

the preterm infant less than 34 weeks' gestation. Fortified human milk or a 24-calorie per ounce, calcium-enriched, whey-predominant preterm formula is the preferred feeding.[42] This enteral feeding is often supplemented initially with parenteral nutrition due to the immaturity of the preterm gut.

There is a surprising lack of evidence that this standard approach is satisfactory, and some indirect evidence that it is not very effective, particularly with regard to the protein status of the infant. Measurements of serum albumin of term infants, but not those of preterms, increase in the first 2 months of life (Table 21.5). Measurements of total protein are stable in term babies, but decline in preterms, even in those who are apparently healthy (Table 21.5). Clinical experience demonstrates that the rates of weight gain of preterms are slower after birth than in utero, particularly in the last trimester. Unfortunately, other than weight gain, no simple ways to monitor nutritional status have been developed for standardized use. Preterm infants remain smaller compared with their term-born peers for years into childhood, an effect which increases with decreasing gestational age at birth. Most preterm babies at hospital discharge are smaller, more edematous, and appear to have less "baby fat" than term newborns, despite the fact that they are at term postconceptual age.

The reasons for these disparities have not been addressed. One possible contributing factor is the high caloric concentrations of glucose and fat, with relatively low protein content, used in parenteral nutrition. Parenteral nutrition has customarily been tailored to simulate the nutrient needs of the term infant or adult and to avoid metabolic abnormalities such as hyperglycemia, hyperammonemia, and uremia. In contrast, the placental transfer of nutrients to the fetus consists mostly of glucose and protein.

In summary, despite considerable advances in both enteral and parenteral nutrition, the preterm baby at term postconceptual age often weighs less and may look malnourished compared with the term newborn. The long-term effects of these frequently observed, but poorly documented, differences are unknown. Further studies are needed to improve the nutritional assessment and protein status of the preterm infant.

Conclusion

There are a variety of methods for determining digestibility of proteins for use in infant nutrition. Most of these methods are based upon animal (rat) models. Infant requirements for amino acids have gradually been determined to include almost all the amino acids, and nobody really promotes feeding proteins that only include "essential" amino acids. Infants have immature metabolic pathways that further emphasize their special amino acid requirements. Infants respond to their protein nutrition with changes in their plasma milieu that are specific to the proteins being fed. The net result of all these observations is that human milk provides the optimal protein nutrition for the healthy term neonate (and with some modifications for the preterm infant). Alterations in the amino acid milieu of the infant may have implications for the brain development of the infant[39] in much the same way that it has been proposed that long chain polyunsaturated fatty acids (docosahexaenoic and arachidonic acids) may be responsible for the cognitive advantages that have been noted in human milk-fed compared with formula-fed infants.

REFERENCES

1 Rassin, D. K., Garofalo, R., Ogra, P. L. Human milk. In Remington, J. S., Klein, J. O., eds. *Infectious Diseases of the Fetus and Newborn Infant.* 5th edn. Philadelphia, PA: WB Saunders;2001:169–203.

2 Raiten, D. J., Talbot, J. M., Waters, J. H., eds. Assessment of nutrient requirements for infant formulas. *J. Nutr.* 1998;**128**:2110s–27s.

3 Association of Official Analytical Chemists. Protein efficiency ratio. In Helrich, K., ed. *Official Methods of Analysis of the Association of Official Analytical Chemists*. 15th edn. Arlington, VA: Association of Official Analytical Chemists; 1990:1095–6.

4 FAO/WHO. Expert Consultation. Protein Quality Evaluation. *Report of a Joint FAO/ WHO Expert Consultation*. Rome, Italy: Food and Agriculture Organization; 1990.

5 Fomon, S. J. Protein. In Craven, L., ed. *Nutrition of Normal Infants*. St. Louis, MO: Mosby-Year Book; 1993:121–46.

6 Sarwar, G., Botting, H., Peace, R. W. Amino acid rating method for evaluating protein adequacy of infant formulas. *J. Assoc. Official Analyt. Chem.* 1989a;**72**:622–6.

7 Sarwar, G., Peace, R. W., Botting, H. G. Differences in protein digestibility and quality of liquid concentrate and powder forms of milk-based infant formulas fed to rats. *Am. J. Clin. Nutr.* 1989b;**49**:806–13.

8 Lönnerdal, B., Hernell, O. Effects of feeding ultrahigh-temperature (UHT) treated infant formula with different protein concentrations or powdered formula as compared with breast-feeding, on plasma amino acids, hematology, and trace element status. *Am. J. Clin. Nutr.* 1998;**68**:350–6.

9 Lönnerdal, B. Nutritional and physiologic significance of human milk proteins. *Am. J. Clin. Nutr.* 2003;**77**:1537s–43s.

10 Lönnerdal, B., Forsum, E., Hambraeus, L. A longitudinal study of the protein, nitrogen, and lactose contents of human milk from Swedish well-nourished mothers. *Am. J. Clin. Nutr.* 1976;**29**:1127–33.

11 Picone, T. A., Benson, J. D., Maclean, W. C. Jr, Sauls, H. S. Amino acid metabolism in human-milk and formula-fed term infants. In Atkinson, S. A., Lonnerdal, B., eds. *Protein and Non-Protein Nitrogen in Human Milk*. Boca Raton, FL: CRC Press;1989: 173–86.

12 Rassin, D. K. Amino acid and protein metabolism in the premature and term infant. In Hay, W. W., Jr, ed. *Neonatal Nutrition and Metabolism*. St. Louis, MO: Mosby Year Book; 1991:110–21.

13 Dupont, C. Protein requirements during the first year of life. *Am. J. Clin. Nutr.* 2003;**77**:1544s–9s.

14 Stegink, L. O. Amino acids in pediatric parenteral nutrition. *J. Dis. Child.* 1983;**137**:1008.

15 Potsic, B., Holliday, N., Lewis, P. *et al.* Glutamine supplementation and deprivation: effect on artificially reared rat small intestinal morphology. *Ped. Res.* 2002;**52**: 430–6.

16 Malloy, M. H., Rassin, D. K., Gaull, G. E. A method for measurement of free and bound plasma cyst(e)ine. *Analyt. Biochem.* 1981;**113**:407–15.

17 Picone, T. A., Benson, J. D., Moro, G. *et al.* Growth, serum biochemistries, and amino acids of term infants fed formulas with amino acid and protein concentrations similar to human milk. *J. Pediatr. Gastroenterol. Nutr.* 1989;**9**:351–60.

18 Czarnecki, G. L., Baker, D. H. Urea cycle function in the dog with emphasis on the role of arginine. *J. Nutr.* 1984;**114**:581–90.

19 Anderson, T. L., Heird, W. C., Winters, R. W. Clinical and physiological consequences of total parenteral nutrition in the pediatric patient. In Greef, M. 3rd, Soeterz, B., Wesdorp, R. I. C., Fischer, J. B., eds. *Current Concepts in Parenteral Nutrition*. The Hague, Netherlands: Martinus Nijhoff; 1977:111–27.

20 Räihä, N. C. R., Suihkonen, J., Development of urea-synthesizing enzymes in human liver. *Acta Paediatr. Scand.* 1968a;**57**:121–4.

21 Räihä, N. C. R., Suihkonen, J., Factors influencing the development of urea-synthesizing enzymes in rat liver. *Biochem. J.* 1968b;**107**:793–7.

22 Kretchmer, N., Levine, S. Z., McNamara, H., Barnett, H. L. Certain aspects of tyrosine metabolism in the young, 1. The development of the tyrosine oxidizing system in human liver. *J. Clin. Invest.* 1956;**35**:236–44.

23 Kretchmer, N., Levine, S. Z., McNamara, H. The in vitro metabolism of tyrosine and its intermediates in the liver of the premature infant. *J. Dis. Child.* 1957;**93**:19–20.

24 Del Valle, J. A., Greengard, O. Phenylalanine hydroxylase and tyrosine aminotransferase in human fetal and adult liver. *Pediatr. Res.* 1976;**11**:2–5.

25 Rassin, D. K., Gaull, G. E., Räihä, N. C. R., Heinonen, K. Milk protein quantity and quality in low birth-weight infants. IV. Effects on tyrosine and phenylalanine in plasma and urine. *J. Pediatr.* 1977;**90**:356–60.

26 Bell, E. F., Filer, L. J. Jr, Wong, A. P., Steginx, L. D. Effects of a parenteral nutrition regimen containing dicarboxylic amino acids on plasma, erythrocyte, and urinary amino acid concentrations of young infants. *Am. J. Clin. Nutr.* 1983;**37**:99–107.

27 Roberts, S. A., Ball, R. O., Filler, R. M., Moore, A. M., Pencharz, P. B. Phenylalanine and tyrosine metabolism in neonates receiving parenteral nutrition differing in pattern of amino acids. *Pediatr. Res.* 1998;**44**:907–14.

28 Sturman, J. A., Gaull, G. E., Räihä, N. C. R. Absence of cystathionase in human fetal liver. Is cysteine essential? *Science* 1970;**169**:74–6.

29 Pascal, T. A., Gillam, B. M., Gaull, G. E. Cystathionase: immunochemical evidence for absence from human fetal liver. *Pediatr. Res.* 1972;**6**:773–8.

30 Malloy, M. H., Rassin, D. K., Richardson, C. J. Total parenteral nutrition in sick preterm infants: the effects of cysteine supplementation with nitrogen intakes of 240 and 400 mg/kg. *J. Pediatr. Gastroenterol. Nutr.* 1984;**3**:239–44.

31 Meister, A. New aspects of glutathione biochemistry and transport-selective alteration of glutathione metabolism. *Nutr. Res.* 1984;**42**:397–410.

32 Gaull, G. E., Rassin, D. K., Räihä, N. C. R., Heinonen, K. Milk protein quantity and quality in low-birth-weight infants, III. Effects on sulfur-containing amino acids in plasma and urine. *J. Pediatr.* 1977;**90**:348–55.

33 Sturman, S. A., Won, G. V., Wisnlewski, H. M., Neurlnger, M. D. Retinal degeneration in primates raised on a synthetic human infant formula. *Int. J. Dev. Neurosci.* 1984;**2**:121–9.

34 Sturman, S. A., Moretz, H. C., French, I. H., Wisniewski, H. M. Postnatal taurine deficiency in the kitten results in a persistence of the cerebellar external granule cell layer: correction by taurine feeding. *J. Neurosci. Res.* 1985;**13**:521–8.

35 Watkins, J. B., Järvenpää, A.-L., Szczepanik-Van Leeuwen, P. *et al.* Feeding the low-birth weight infant: V. Effects of taurine, cholesterol, and human milk on bile acid kinetics. *Gastroenterology* 1983;**85**:793–800.

36 Kurpad, A., Young, V. R., What is apparent is not always real: lessons from lysine requirement studies in adult humans. *J. Nutr.* 2003;**133**:1227–30.

37 Cho, F., Bhatia, J., Rassin, D. K. Amino acid responses to dietary intake in the first 72 hours of life. *Nutrition* 1990;**6**:449–55.

38 Kashyap, S., Schulze, K. F., Abildskov, K., Ramakrishnan, R., Heird, W. C. Effect of protein (P) and energy (E) intakes on plasma amino acid concentrations (AA) of low birth weight (LBW) infants. *Pediatr. Res.* 2003;**53**:442A.

39 Rassin, D. K. Essential and non-essential amino acids in neonatal nutrition. In Räihä, N. C. R., ed. *Protein Metabolism during Infancy.* New York, NY: Raven Press; 1994:183–92.

40 Bhatia, J., Rassin, D. K., Cerreto, M. C., Bee, B. F. Effect of protein/energy ratio on growth and behavior of premature infants: preliminary findings. *J. Pediatr* 1991;**119**:103–10.

41 American Academy of Pediatrics Work Group on Breastfeeding. Breast feeding and the use of human milk. *Pediatrics* 1997;**100**:1035–9.

42 Sapsford, A. L. Human milk and enteral nutrition products. In Groh-Wargo, S., Thompson, M., Cox, J. H., eds. *Nutritional Care for High-Risk Newborns.* 3rd edn. Chicago, IL: Precept Press; 2000:265–302.

43 American Academy of Pediatrics. Formula feeding of term infants. In Kleinman, R. E., ed. *Pediatric Nutrition Handbook.* 4th edn. Elk Grove Village, IL: American Academy of Pediatrics; 1998:29–42.

44 Harrison, G. G., Graver, E. J., Vargas, M., *et al.* Growth and adiposity of term infants fed whey-predominant or casein-predominant formulas or human milk. *J. Pediatr. Gastroenterol. Nutr.* 1987;**6**:739–47.

45 American Academy of Pediatrics Committee on Pediatric AIDS. Human milk, breastfeeding and transmission of human immunodeficiency virus in the United States. *Pediatrics* 1995;**96**:977–9.

46 American Academy of Pediatrics Committee on Infectious Diseases. Recommendations for care of children in special circumstances: human milk. In *2003 Red Book: Report of the Committee on Infectious Diseases.* 26th edn. Elk Grove Village, IL: American Academy of Pediatrics; 2003:118–20.

47 American Academy of Pediatrics Committee on Drugs. The transfer of drugs and other chemicals into human milk. *Pediatrics* 1994;**93**:137–50.

48 Bailey, B., Ito, S., Breast-feeding and maternal drug use. *Pediatr. Clin. N. Am.* 1997;**44**:41–54.

49 Howard, C. R., Lawrence, R. A. Drugs and breastfeeding. *Clin. Perinatol.* 1999;**26**:447–78.

50 Lawrence, R. A., Howard, C. R. Given the benefits of breastfeeding: are there any contraindications? *Clin. Perinatol.* 1999;**26**:479–90.

51 World Health Organization. Consensus statement from the WHO/UNICEF consultation on HIV transmission and breast feeding. Geneva, Switzerland; April 20–May 1, 1992.

52 Atkinson, S. A., Hanning, R. A. Amino acid metabolism and requirements of the premature infant: is human milk the "Gold Standard"? In Atkinson, S. A., Lonnerdal, B., eds. *Protein and Non-Protein Nitrogen in Human Milk.* Boca Raton, FL: CRC Press; 1989:187–209.

53 Cheung, M. W., Pratt, E. L., Fowler, D. I. Total amino acid composition in mature human milk. *J. Pediatr.* 1953;**12**: 353–7.

54 Davis, T. A., Nguyen, H. V., Garcia-Bravo, R. *et al.* Amino acid composition of human milk is not unique. *J. Nutr.* 1994;**124**:1126–32.

55 Diehm, K., ed. *Documenta Geigy: Scientific Tables.* 6th edn. Ardsley, NY: Geigy Pharmaceuticals; 1962:514.

56 FAO/WHO/UNU. Expert Consultation. *Energy and Protein Requirements.* Geneva, Switzerland: WHO; 1985.

57 Janas, L. M., Picciano, M. F. Quantities of amino acids ingested by human milk-fed infants. *J. Pediatr.* 1986;**109**:802–7.

58 Janas, L. M., Picciano, M. F., Hatch, T. F. Indices of protein metabolism in term infants fed either human milk or formulas with reduced protein concentration and various whey/casein ratios. *J. Pediatr.* 1987;**110**:838–48.

59 Järvenpää A.-L., Räihä, N. C. R., Rassin, D. K., Gaull, G. E. Milk protein quantity and quality in the term infant. I. Metabolic responses and effects on growth. *Pediatrics* 1982;**70**: 214–20.

60 Järvenpää, A.-L., Räihä, N. C. R., Rassin, D. K., Gaull, G. E. Milk protein quantity and quality in the term infant. II. Effects on acidic and neutral amino acids. *Pediatrics* 1982;**70**: 221–30.

61 Macy, I. G. Composition of human colostrum and milk. *Am. J. Dis. Child.* 1949;**78**:589–603.

62 Miller, S., Ruttinger, V. Essential amino acids in mature human milk. *Proc. Soc. Exp. Biol. Med.* 1951;**77**:96–9.

63 Räihä, N. C. R., Heinonen, K., Rassin, D. K., Gaull, G. E. Milk protein quantity and quality in low-birthweight infants. I. Metabolic responses and effects on growth. *Pediatrics* 1976;**57**:659–74.

64 Roberts, S. A., Ball, R. O., Filler, R. M., Moore, A. M., Penchar, P. B. Phenylalanine and tyrosine metabolism in neonates receiving parenteral nutrition differing in pattern of amino acids. *Pediatr. Res.* 1998;**44**:907–14.

65 Sarwar, G., Darling, P., Ujiie, M., Botting, H. G., Pencharz, P. B. Use of amino acid profiles of preterm and term human milks in evaluating scoring patterns for routine protein quality assessment of infant formulas. *J. Assoc. Official Analyt. Chem. int.* 1996;**79**:498–502.

66 Soupart, P., Moore, S., Bigwood, E. J., Amino acid composition of human milk. *J. Biochem.* 1954;**206**:699–704.

67 Svanberg, U., Gebre-Medhin, M., Ljungqvist, B., Olsson, M. Breast milk composition in Ethiopian and Swedish mothers. III. Amino acids and other nitrogenous substances. *Am. J. Clin. Nutr.* 1977;**30**:499–507.

22

Enteral carbohydrate assimilation

C. Lawrence Kien

Department of Pediatrics, University of Texas Medical Branch at Galveston, Galveston, TX

Introduction

Glucose is an important, if not the sole, source of energy metabolism in the fed state for brain and other nervous tissue, red blood cells, renal medulla, and retina.[1-4] Assimilation of diet-derived glucose is necessary to provide glucose per se for these tissues, to serve as a source of nonprotein energy, and to stimulate normal rates of insulin secretion required to adequately suppress protein degradation and excessive lipolysis, and to stimulate protein synthesis. Carbohydrate contributes approximately 40% of the energy intake in infants ingesting human milk or cow milk-based formulas, and lactose provides perhaps the sole source of diet-derived glucose in human milk[5,6] and about 50% of the diet-derived glucose in preterm formulas.

Dietary carbohydrate is assimilated via the intestine and colon in humans of all ages, but in the preterm newborn or young infant with defective function of the small intestine, bacterial fermentation of dietary carbohydrate is an especially quantitatively important metabolic pathway for enteral carbohydrate assimilation. This process may have both beneficial and adverse effects on the infant.[7] Figure 22.1 summarizes carbohydrate assimilation by the gut. Lactose, like other dietary sugars fed to newborn infants (such as glucose polymer), is digested in the small intestine but also may undergo some fermentation in the colon. Glucose and galactose, derived from lactose digestion, are absorbed in the small intestine, enter the portal vein, and then undergo uptake by the liver, where galactose is almost quantitatively removed by the combined processes of conversion to glucose or incorporation into glycogen. Human milk oligosaccharides are depicted in Figure 22.1 because human milk is an important source of nutrition for both preterm and term infants. As discussed below, these oligosaccharides are almost entirely fermented in the colon (in a similar fashion as a fraction of dietary starch and some chemical forms of fiber in older infants and children). Short chain fatty acids (SCFA) produced via bacterial fermentation are almost entirely absorbed in the colon and then are metabolized by the colonic mucosa to a lesser (e.g., acetic acid) or greater extent (e.g., butyric acid). SCFA then enter the liver where further metabolism occurs.

Besides its overall role as a source of glucose and energy, carbohydrate may have a number of important biological effects of possible clinical significance: function of the intestine and colon via the stimulatory effects of SCFA on cell proliferation and ion absorption;[8,9] insulin secretion with its associated effects on urinary sodium excretion (inhibits natriuresis) and metabolism and growth;[10-16] peripheral deiodination of thyroxine to triiodothyronine;[17-19] metabolic response to growth hormone;[20] calcium absorption;[21-28] respiratory quotient (RQ, the relative proportion of CO_2 generated per mole of ATP produced or oxygen consumed).[29]

Glucose metabolism

Glucose metabolism will be discussed in much more detail elsewhere in this book and has been reviewed by the author elsewhere.[5] However, certain principles of glucose metabolism are relevant to further consideration of the biological relevance of bacterial fermentation of carbohydrate since SCFA, such as acetate or butyrate, probably cannot be converted, in a net sense, to glucose, although there is some evidence of a biochemical pathway for this.[30,31]

Neonatal Nutrition and Metabolism. Second Edition, ed. P. Thureen and W. Hay. Published by Cambridge University Press.
© Cambridge University Press 2006.

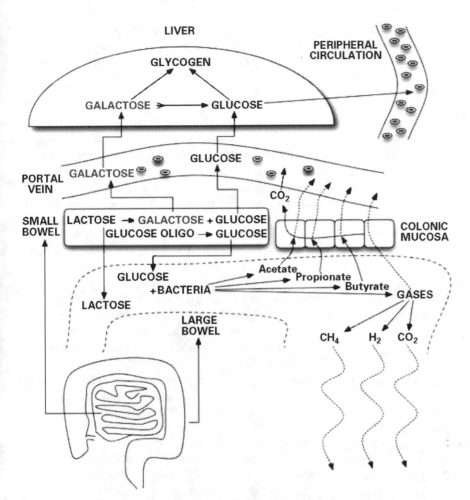

Figure 22.1. Graphemic summary of carbohydrate assimilation by the gut.

It has been estimated that the neonatal brain consumes about 11.5 g glucose kg^{-1} day^{-1}.[32,33] In human milk and preterm infant formulas, there is approximately 9–11 g carbohydrate per 100 kcal. At an energy intake of 120 kcal kg^{-1} day^{-1}, this "requirement" for glucose would be minimally satisfied by 100% absorption of the glucose or galactose derived from lactose or from the glucose polymers present in infant formulas,[5,32] but if a substantial fraction of dietary carbohydrate were fermented in the colon to SCFA, there could be effects on the fuel consumption of the brain. Apart from ketone metabolism by the brain, some of the potential deficit in the "glucose requirement" of the brain could be met by endogenous glucose production, which has been estimated to range from about 7 g kg^{-1} day^{-1} in term infants to 11–13 g kg^{-1} day^{-1} in preterm infants.[5,32–44] However, while temporarily stored glycogen can provide this endogenous glucose, under chronic conditions of both marginal metabolizable glucose intake (i.e., defective carbohydrate digestion in the intestine) and incomplete adaptation to starvation, these body glucose needs would be met by gluconeogenesis from amino acids, with its attendant effects on protein accretion. Therefore, in theory, brain glucose metabolism, protein accretion, and growth could be affected in those infants who manifest defective digestion of lactose.[45–47] Thus, an understanding of how enteral carbohydrates are assimilated by the gut is important not only to the "health" of the intestine and colon[7,9] but also to the overall nutritional status and wellbeing of the infant.

Carbohydrates in human milk and preterm infant formulas

In human milk, lactose is probably the sole carbohydrate providing metabolizable glucose, but recent studies suggest that human milk also contains oligosaccharides that are formed from the addition of monosaccharides (such as fucose and galactose) to lactose.[48,49] The concentration of these oligosaccharides ranges from about 2.0 g dL^{-1} in colostrum to 1.6 g dL^{-1} at 90 days of age.[32,49] The lactose content of mature human milk has been reported as 6.8 g dL^{-1} or 9.1 g per 100 kcal (0.022 g kJ^{-1})[50] and 7.4 g dL^{-1}.[51] The calculated values for carbohydrate concentration of preterm milk are 6.99 g dL^{-1} after a 26–31 week gestation and 6.24 g dL^{-1} after 32–36 weeks' gestation.[52] Lactose concentration in term human milk is about 7.37 g dL^{-1}.[51] Term formulas may contain 100% of the carbohydrate as lactose or none. In most preterm infant formulas, lactose and glucose polymers each constitute approximately 50% of the carbohydrate content, and the total carbohydrate concentration is about 8.7 g dL^{-1} in the concentrated form of the formulas (i.e., 0.8 kcal mL^{-1}). The glucose polymers of these formulas are mostly medium length (approximately five glucose units) and are prepared from partially hydrolyzed cornstarch.[53]

Fetal development of carbohydrate digestion and absorption

Lactose is hydrolyzed in the small intestine by β-galactosidase (lactase) present on the brush border at the villus tip. Sucrase-isomaltase, present both at the midvillus zone and at its tip, hydrolyses sucrose and maltose (disaccharide of two glucose molecules released during glucose polymer digestion).[8] Starch or glucose polymers can be digested by salivary and pancreatic amylase, α-amylase present in human milk, and by intestinal mucosal hydrolases.[8] Intestinal sucrase-isomaltase and maltase activities rise slowly from 10–26 weeks, and then rise more rapidly; by 34 weeks, the activities are 70% those of term infants.[54] Intestinal lactase is detectable as early as 12 weeks but accumulates more slowly so that by 34 weeks, the activities are only 30% those of term infants, and by 35–38 weeks, 70% those of term infants.[54] The presence of amylase in fetal pancreas is controversial.[8,55–57]

There are not much data on monosaccharide absorption in the fetus.[8] In the human fetus, glucose transport is more developed in the jejunum than in the ileum, and it appears that the capacity for jejunum transport of glucose is present at 10 weeks and increases substantially from 10 weeks to 16–19 weeks. The time when glucose transport reaches "term" levels is not clear.[8,58,59]

Post-natal development of capacity to digest and absorb carbohydrates

Digestion of starch and glucose oligosaccharides

As noted above, human milk contains oligosaccharides.[32,49] Hydrogen is produced by gut bacteria during fermentation of carbohydrate; this hydrogen is partially absorbed and excreted in the breath and has been used as an index of how much carbohydrate is fermented in the colon.[7,45] Comparisons have been made of breath H_2 concentration during feeding with human milk oligosaccharides and lactulose (a disaccharide of galactose and fructose that cannot be digested by mammalian enzymes and is quantitatively fermented). Based on these studies, it appears that these oligosaccharides also are quantitatively fermented and not digested in the small intestine.[6] These results might explain why human milk-fed term infants manifest elevated breath H_2 concentrations.[60]

Starch is not often fed to newborn infants, except in situations where cornstarch is used to maintain blood glucose concentrations in infants with glucose-6-phosphatase deficiency or fatty acid oxidation disorders or where cereal is used to thicken formulas of infants with gastroesophageal reflux. However, polymers of glucose are often fed to newborn term and preterm infants as constituents of commercial formulas. The number of glucose molecules in such polymers is variable but usually about 6–10. Pancreatic amylase does not appear to contribute substantially to starch or glucose polymer digestion in newborn infants. Rather, glucose polymer digestion is effected by salivary amylase and mucosal glucoamylases and sucrase-α-dextrinase (sucrase-isomaltase).[8,53,61–63] The blood glucose and insulin responses of preterm infants fed test doses of glucose polymers were similar to those of term infants.[53] Using a duodenum/proximal jejunum perfusion technique, Shulman et al.[64] compared the absorption of lactose and glucose polymers in preterm infants. Disappearance of glucose polymers from the lumen (presumably absorption) correlated with postnatal age.

Clinical responses to lactose in preterm infants: growth and feeding tolerance

As indicated above, there is evidence for low lactase activity in the fetus and, by implication, in preterm infants.[54,65–67] Certain types of data, reviewed below, favor the concept that postnatally, preterm infants acquire a relatively efficient capacity to hydrolyze lactose in the small intestine (e.g., $\geq$ 80% digested at that site) at an apparently earlier developmental stage than in utero. Preterm infants (< 32 weeks' gestation) ingesting human milk or formulas containing lactose as the sole carbohydrate do seem to thrive, excrete in the feces only minimal energy derived from lactose, and generally do not exhibit osmotic diarrhea.[64,68,69] In several small studies comparing formulas that were 100% lactose to 50% lactose/50% glucose polymer, we did observe slight differences, albeit statistically nonsignificant, in the ratio between rate of weight gain and energy intake (apparently lower in the 100% lactose group).[47]

One study has suggested that elimination of lactose from formula ameliorates feeding intolerance.[46] These investigators carried out a prospective, randomized double-masked controlled trial in 306 preterm infants. This trial was a comparison of two whey-predominant, cow-protein formulas that differed in the type of carbohydrate. The carbohydrate in the control formula was 41% lactose and 59% corn syrup solids whereas the carbohydrate in the experimental formula ("low lactose formula") was 35.1% maltose, 64% corn syrup solids, and less than 1% lactose. The infants were studied on one of these formulas for an average of 4 weeks (J. W. Hansen, Personal Communication). The intention-to-treat groups and treatment-received groups were distinguished by the fact that despite assignment to one of the two formulas, the former also received some human milk feeding or only human milk. In both the intention-to-treat and treatment-received groups, markedly reducing (effectively eliminating) the lactose from the formula resulted in trends of increased weight gain and formula intake and a reduction in the average gastric residuals (mL day^{-1}) as well as the number of days to reach full enteral feedings ("115 kcal kg^{-1} day^{-1}"), but none of these individual outcome variables were statistically significant between formula groups. However, using the multivariate, rank sum test to analyze all these outcome variables (as well as some additional variables), there was a statistically significant improvement in "feeding outcome" in the infants receiving the low lactose formula. Shulman et al.[70] also found that the time to full enteral feedings was inversely correlated with lactase activity measured using an indirect method. We have speculated[71] that impaired motility in the esophagus, stomach, and small intestine (and impaired tolerance of ingested volume of feedings) in preterm infants might be mediated by the hormone, peptide YY (PYY) secreted by cells in the distal ileum and colon in response to undigested sugar, SCFA, fat, and protein.[72–75] It is difficult to balance the clinical significance of the multivariate statistic reported by Griffin and Hansen[46] against the many years of successful feeding of preterm infants using human milk or cow-milk formulas containing lactose.

Lactose digestion and fermentation

Controversy exists in the literature over the extent to which lactose fed to preterm infants is hydrolyzed to glucose and galactose (digestion) or is fermented. Data on lactose digestion in the preterm infant is derived from studies based on measurements of blood glucose concentration ("tolerance tests"), breath H_2 concentration, studies of the disappearance of perfused lactose from the small intestinal lumen, measurements of the relative rates of appearance of glucose and lactose-derived glucose into the peripheral circulation (stable isotope studies), and assessment of the relative amount of lactulose v. lactose in the urine. Lactose tolerance tests in preterm infants indicate that blood glucose concentration rises equally after meals containing lactose, glucose, and glucose polymers.[76–78] While it is impossible to determine without a tracer to what extent compensatory increased hepatic output can maintain blood glucose concentration during such tolerance tests, the results do suggest that glucose is either absorbed or produced in response to the lactose-containing meal. On the other hand, one study comparing "added lactose" to "added sucrose" formulas did show a relative increase in the incidence of diarrhea and metabolic acidosis during the first week of life with the former type of formula.[79] Moreover, studies of breath H_2 concentration support the view that lactose is not efficiently hydrolyzed in the small intestine in the preterm infant and instead reaches the colon where it undergoes extensive fermentation.[68,80,81] Breath H_2 concentration also correlates with lactose intake in preterm infants.[68,81] These findings are consistent with the hypothesis that a significant proportion of dietary lactose reaches the colon in the preterm infant.[63,68,81] The broad range of estimates of the percent of dietary lactose not hydrolyzed and reaching the colon, 66–100% (assuming adult colon absorption rates of H_2)[81] or 12–19% (based on actual measurements of absorption in six infants)[82] lead one to question the biological relevance of high breath H_2 concentration in preterm infants as an index of the capacity for lactose hydrolysis.

Intestinal perfusion with unlabeled lactose allows one to estimate "absorption" in the classical sense: disappearance from the lumen. Using this technique, Shulman et al.[64] found that absorption of lactose was less efficient than absorption of glucose polymers. However, fetal lactase activity, although fairly uniformly distributed along the small intestine, is lower in the duodenum where these perfusion studies were carried out.[65,66] Moreover these studies are indirect and measure what is left in the intestine. If there were any small intestinal fermentation of lactose, lactose disappearances would not equate exactly to digestion. In preterm infants who develop necrotizing enterocolitis, H_2 is found within the intestinal wall, implying that fermentation can occur in the small intestinal lumen.[9]

We have developed a stable isotope method that can assess directly the relative appearance rate into the lumen of labeled glucose from lactose and glucose tracers respectively.[83] Thus, this method allows for the first time a direct measurement of lactose digestion. In the initial application of the method,[83] we reported the fraction of lactose digested in five preterm infants. In four of five infants, lactose digestion was approximately 100% and was 80% in one infant. However, in all infants interval measurements of breath H_2 concentration suggested significant carbohydrate fermentation in the colon which raised the question about whether glucose and/or galactose malabsorption was the explanation for the fermentation activity. In a larger study of infants >32 weeks postconceptional age,[45] we found that lactose digestion averaged 73%. In four infants, less than 80% of lactose was digested.

Lactulose quantitatively reaches the colon, where a small percentage is absorbed intact and excreted in the urine.[84] The excretion of this compound in the urine is thought to be a marker for the nonspecific absorption of carbohydrate in the colon. Lactose reaching the colon also may be absorbed intact.[85,86] Thus, measurements of the ratio of urine lactose to lactulose in preterm infants fed both sugars in a constant ratio are thought to provide insight into how much lactose escapes intestinal digestion; such studies suggest that intestinal lactase activity is adequate to fully digest dietary lactose shortly after birth.[84]

Intestinal absorption of monosaccharides

Glucose absorption capacity in preterm infants is about three-fourths that in term infants and seems to increase during the first 3 weeks of life but then declines somewhat after that.[8,59] Glucose and galactose derived from lactose and glucose derived from sucrose or glucose polymer are absorbed via the same specific transporter. The absorption of glucose by preterm infants has been examined using a perfusion technique.[87] There was a positive correlation between the maximum rate of absorption and both the gestational age at birth and the postnatal age of the infants at the time of study. The rate of glucose absorption was not correlated with the $mL\,kg^{-1}\,day^{-1}$ of the feeding that the infants were receiving. However, interestingly, at the same glucose infusion rate, glucose absorption was greater when the concentration of glucose in the infusate was lower.[87] This observation would seem to have relevance to the debate that clinicians have had for years over whether formula tolerance is better when the formulas are given as higher volume, lower strength feedings or as lower volume, full strength feedings. This study also suggested that intrapartum steroids given to the mother appeared to enhance glucose absorption.

Special aspects of dietary carbohydrate assimilation: calcium absorption, colonic fermentation, and role of galactose

Calcium absorption

Data from studies in rats, which cannot digest lactose, suggest that lactose promotes calcium absorption.[25] The promoting effect of sugars on calcium absorption in the jejunum may be related to the process of sugar absorption and thus water absorption, resulting in an increase in calcium concentration at the site of its absorption.[26] In lactose-tolerant normal healthy adults, lactose, when administered as an aqueous solution, has been found to have a positive effect[25] or no effect on calcium absorption[88] (determined, respectively, using a dual radiolabeled calcium technique or a stable strontium loading test). However, in healthy, young adults, characterized as lactase deficient based on breath H_2 testing, the administration of lactose in an aqueous solution reduced calcium absorption,[25] whereas lactose administered as a milk formula increased calcium absorption in similar subjects.[24]

As with data from studies in adults, the data in term human newborns also are conflicting with respect to the effect of lactose on calcium absorption. In term infants fed soy formula and studied during the first few months of life, Ziegler and Fomon[21] found that lactose promoted calcium absorption. However, the mean calcium intake was significantly higher and fecal excretion of calcium only "somewhat less" (61 ± 30 v. 66 ± 25 mg kg^{-1} day^{-1}, mean $\pm$ SD) in the infants fed formula containing lactose than in the infants fed formula containing sucrose and cornstarch hydrolysate. Moya et al.[27] also showed improvement (20%) in fractional calcium absorption in term infants when lactose, as opposed to glucose polymers, was the source of carbohydrate in a cow-milk formula. In a similar, later study designed apparently to evaluate a new lactose-free formula, Moya et al.[89] did not observe a significant effect of lactose on calcium absorption. Although in this later study, calcium retention was actually greater on the lactose-free formula, this difference was ascribed by the authors to the higher calcium concentration of the lactose-free formula (and thus higher calcium intake). Based on stable calcium isotope studies, calcium absorption was higher in preterm infants fed glucose polymers than with a similar amount of lactose.[28] Calcium absorption correlated positively with water and carbohydrate absorption, but the authors did not indicate whether lactose impaired calcium absorption in those infants who may have had relatively more efficient lactose absorption (i.e., equivalent to glucose polymer absorption). In this study, the authors used a catheter perfusion technique and only measured calcium absorption in the proximal intestine; the absorption in the distal gut was not quantified. During fetal life, lactase activity is higher in the jejunum than in the duodenum.[65,66] Moreover, lactose affects calcium absorption by the non vitamin D-dependent, paracellular uptake process, which is thought to be facilitated by unhydrolyzed lactose and to occur throughout the small intestine, especially distal to the duodenum.[88] Wirth *et al.*[22] found no effect on mineral absorption of increasing the lactose content of a "standard" preterm infant formula (from 50% to 100%).

Possible clinical significance of carbohydrate fermentation

As noted above, all dietary carbohydrate is not digested in the small intestine and thus is fermented in the colon, where some of the constituent energy can be retrieved or "salvaged" via the avid absorption of SCFA.[7] The absorption of SCFA appears to be necessary for normal absorption of sodium and water by the colon, and the removal of unabsorbed carbohydrates by fermentation also decreases the osmolarity in the colon lumen, which then facilitates net water absorption.[90] Among the SCFA produced during fermentation are acetate, propionate, and butyrate. The latter two are removed almost quantitatively from the circulation via combined, sequential uptake by the colon and liver.[91–94]

SCFA in the colon have trophic effects on the small intestine via an apparent neural pathway.[95] Butyric acid has a potential special role in the colon as a preferential substrate for colonocytes.[96] In adults, diversion of the fecal stream from a segment of colon markedly reduces fermentation and thus SCFA production in the segment, which tends to undergo a process of chronic, intractable inflammation and mucosal atrophy. This condition in humans can be treated with instillation of SCFA into the diverted segment.[97] Obviously, one could argue that lactose malabsorption or the ingestion of nondigestible oligosaccharides in human milk serves a beneficial, "fiber-like" function for preterm infants undergoing rapid intestinal and colonic development. However, butyric acid also has pro-inflammatory effects when rapidly infused into the rumen,[98] and high luminal concentrations of acetate can lead to local irritant effects and even ulceration of the colon.[99] It has been suggested that butyric acid may be a factor in the etiology of necrotizing enterocolitis.[100,101] Further concern about the possibility that fermentation of carbohydrate could be linked etiologically to necrotizing enterocolitis comes from studies suggesting that rapid feeding and

elevation of breath H_2 may be a risk factor for necrotizing enterocolitis.[9] Indeed, pneumatosis intestinalis is fundamentally a condition in which H_2 cannot escape the intestinal mucosa because of intestinal ischemia.[9] The presence of H_2 in the small intestinal bowel wall implies that fermentation is occurring in the small intestine, possibly because of motility defects that also could relate to ischemia or inflammation per se. This raises the suspicion that fermentation does not cause necrotizing enterocolitis primarily but that ischemia in the small intestine or colon may be correlated with fermentation activity. Human milk feeding to term neonates tends to stimulate colonization of the gut with bifidobacteria species and suppresses colonization by clostridia, one of the proposed causes for both experimental necrotizing enterocolitis and increased butyric acid production rates.[100,102] Thus, it is possible that feeding human milk, with its high lactose concentration compared with preterm infant formulas, represents a special case where lactose malabsorption could play a lesser role in causing gut toxicity or inflammation. This also would be consistent with the notion that human milk, which contains mostly lactose as the carbohydrate source, lessens, not increases, the risk of necrotizing enterocolitis.[103]

Galactose

Galactose represents 50% of the monosaccharide present in lactose and thus is an important energy source in milk and an important metabolite of small intestinal digestion of lactose. Except for the inborn error, galactosemia, little research emphasis has been given to this important nutrient.[104] One can speculate that galactose may have an essential role in the synthesis of glycoproteins.[104] After digestion of lactose by lactase, glucose and galactose are readily absorbed by the same carrier mechanism.[105] The fate of galactose in the enterocyte is not entirely understood, but it is assumed that more than 90% of the absorbed glucose and galactose reach the portal vein.[105] The systemic concentration of galactose in normal infants is generally quite low (< 30 mg L^{-1}), and the liver removes most of the dietary galactose on first pass principally by converting it to glucose or glycogen.[105–109] Galactose may not directly stimulate insulin secretion, but through conversion to glucose and via stimulation of the secretion of gastric inhibitory peptide by enterally administered galactose, feeding this sugar may ultimately result in some insulin secretion, although the response may be slightly less than that for glucose.[105,106,110,111] Experimental galactose feeding, compared with glucose, seems to result in a preferential utilization of galactose for glycogen synthesis.[105,108–111] Also, a 50% substitution of galactose for glucose in a parenteral infusion in preterm infants resulted in a lower blood glucose concentration, the elimination of glucosuria, and prompted an increase in the carbohydrate infusion rate.[105,112] Thus, it is possible that galactose administration as a component of lactose could have theoretical, comparative advantages, relative to glucose polymer feeding in terms of suppression of hepatic output of glucose, control of hyperglycemia, and increased glycogen synthesis. However, it is unclear whether less insulin secretion would necessarily be advantageous (and it is not clear that this would be a definite outcome).

Acknowledgment

The work described in this paper attributed to the author was supported in part by NIH Grants HD 19773 and DK 61775.

REFERENCES

1 Cowett, R. M. Pathophysiology, diagnosis, and management of glucose homeostasis in the neonate. *Curr. Probl. Pediatr.* 1985;**15**:1–47.

2 Ferre, P., Decaux, J. F., Issad, T., Girard, J. Changes in energy metabolism during the suckling and weaning period in the newborn. *Reprod. Nutr. Develop.* 1986;**26**:619–31.

3 Cremer, J. E. Substrate utilization and brain development. *J. Cereb. Blood Flow Metab.* 1982;**2**:394–407.

4 Doyle, L. W., Nahmias, C., Firnau, G. *et al.* Regional cerebral glucose metabolism of newborn infants measured by positron emission tomography. *Dev. Med. Child Neurol.* 1983;**25**:143–51.

5 Kien, C. L. Carbohydrates. In *Nutritional Needs of the Preterm Infant: Scientific Basis and Practical Guidelines.* In Tsang, R. C., Zlotkin, S. H., Lucas, A., Uauy, R., eds. Patterson, NY: Caduceus Med Pub; 1993:47–63.

6 Brand-Miller, J. C., McVeagh, P., McNeil, Y., Messer, M. Digestion of human milk oligosaccharides by healthy infants evaluated by the lactulose hydrogen breath test. *J. Pediatr.* 1998;**133**:95–8.

7 Kien, C. L. Digestion, absorption, and fermentation of carbohydrates in the newborn. *Clin Perinatol.* 1996;**23**:211–28.

8 Kien, C. L., Heitlinger, L. A., Li, B. U., Murray, R. D. Digestion, absorption, and fermentation of carbohydrates. *Semin. Perinat.* 1989;**13**:78–87.

9 Kien, C. L. Colonic fermentation of carbohydrate in the premature infant: possible relevance to necrotizing enterocolitis. *J. Pediatr.* 1900;**117**:S52–8.

10 Rocchini, A. P., Key, J., Bondie, D. *et al.* The effect of weight loss on the sensitivity of blood pressure to sodium in obese adolescents. *N. Engl. J. Med.* 1989;**321**:580–5.

11 DeHaven, J., Sherwin, R., Hendler, R., Felig, P. Nitrogen and sodium balance and sympathetic-nervous-system activity in obese subjects treated with a low-calorie protein or mixed diet. *N. Engl. J. Med.* 1980;**302**:477–82.

12 Fukagawa, N. K., Minaker, K. L., Rowe, J. W. *et al.* Insulin-mediated reduction of whole body protein breakdown: dose-response effects on leucine metabolism in post-absorptive men. *J. Clin. Invest.* 1985;**76**:2306–11.

13 Abumrad, N. N., Jefferson, L. S., Rannels, S. R. *et al.* Role of insulin in the regulation of leucine kinetics in the conscious dog. *J. Clin. Invest.* 1981;**70**:1031–41.

14 Flakoll, P. J., Kulaylat, M. Frexes-Steed, M. *et al.* Amino acids augment insulin's suppression of whole body proteolysis. *Am. J. Physiol.* 1989;**257**:E839–47.

15 Millward, D. J., Odedra, B., Bates, P. C. The role of insulin, corticosterone and other factors in the acute recovery of muscle protein synthesis on refeeding food-deprived rats. *Biochem. J.* 1983;**216**:583–7.

16 McNurlan, M. A., Garlick, P. J. Influence of nutrient intake on protein turnover. *Diabetes Metab. Rev.* 1989;**5**:165–89.

17 Balsam, A., Ingbar, S. H. The influence of fasting, diabetes, and several pharmacological agents on the pathways of thyroxine metabolism in rat liver. *J. Clin. Invest.* 1978;**62**:415–24.

18 Azizi, F. Effect of dietary composition on fasting-induced changes in serum thyroid hormones and thyrotropin. *Metabolism* 1978;**27**:935–42.

19 Otten, M. H., Hennemann, G., Docter, R., Visser, T. J. The role of dietary fat in peripheral thyroid hormone metabolism. *Metabolism* 1980;**29**:930–5.

20 Snyder, D. K., Clemmons, D. R., Underwood, L. E. Dietary carbohydrate content determines responsiveness to growth hormone in energy-restricted humans. *J. Clin. Endocrinol. Metab.* 1989;**69**:745–52.

21 Ziegler, E. E., Fomon, S. J. Lactose enhances mineral absorption in infancy. *J. Ped. Gastroenterol. Nutr.* 1983;**2**:288–94.

22 Wirth, F. H. Jr, Numerof, B., Pleban, P., Neylan, M. J. Effect of lactose on mineral absorption in preterm infants. *J. Pediatr.* 1990;**117**:283–7.

23 Griessen, M., Speich, P. V., Infante, F. *et al.* Effect of absorbable and nonabsorbable sugars on intestinal calcium absorption in humans. *Gastroenterology* 1989;**96**:864–72.

24 Griessen, M., Cochet, B., Infante, F. *et al.* Calcium absorption from milk in lactase-deficient subjects. *Am. J. Clin. Nutr.* 1989;**49**:377–84.

25 Cochet, B., Jung, A., Griessen, M. *et al.* Effects of lactose on intestinal calcium absorption in normal and lactase-deficient subjects. *Gastroenterology* 1983;**84**:935–40.

26 Schuette, S. A., Knowles, J. B., Ford, H. E. Effect of lactose or its component sugars on jejunal calcium absorption in adult man. *Am. J. Clin. Nutr.* 1989;**50**:1084–7.

27 Moya, M., Cortes, E., Ballester, M. I., Vento, M., Juste, M. Short-term polycose substitution for lactose reduces calcium absorption in healthy term babies. *J. Pediatr. Gastroenterol. Nutr.* 1992;**14**:57–61.

28 Stathos, T. H., Shulman, R. J., Schanler, R. J., Abrams, S. A. Effect of carbohydrates on calcium absorption in premature infants. *Pediatr. Res.* 1996;**39**:666–70.

29 Askanazi, J., Rosenbaum, S. H., Hyman, A. I. *et al.* Respiratory changes induced by the large glucose loads of total parenteral nutrition. *J. Am. Med. Assoc.* 1980;**243**:1444–7.

30 Hillman, R. E., Ege, M., Hillman, L. S. Increase in oxalate excretion with lipid infusion-evidence for the presence of the glyoxylate shunt in humans. *Pediatr. Res.* 1991;**29**:296A.

31 Davis, W. L., Jones, R. G., Farmer, G. R., Matthews, J. L., Goodman, D. B.. Glyoxylate cycle in the epiphyseal growth plate: isocitrate lyase and malate synthase identified in mammalian cartilage. *Anat. Rec.* 1989;**223**:357–62.

32 Klein, C. J. Nutrient requirements for preterm infant formulas. *J. Nutr.* 2002;**132**:1395S–577S.

33 Kalhan, S. C., Kilic, I. Carbohydrate as nutrient in the infant and child: range of acceptable intake. *Eur. J. Clin. Nutr.* 1999;**53**:S94–100.

34 Cowett, R. M., Oh, W., Schwartz, R. Persistent glucose production during glucose infusion in the neonate. *J. Clin. Invest.* 1983;**71**:467–75.

35 Lafeber, H. N., Sulkers, E. J., Chapman, T. E., Sauer, P. J. J. Glucose production and oxidation in preterm infants during total parenteral nutrition. *Pediatr. Res.* 1990;**28**:153–7.

36 Bougneres, P. F., Castano, L., Rocchicioli, F. *et al.* Medium-chain fatty acids increase glucose production in normal and low birth weight newborns. *Am. J. Physiol.* 1989;**256**: E692–7.

37 Kalhan, S. C., Bier, D. M., Savin, S. M., Adam, P. A. Estimation of glucose turnover and 13C recycling in the human newborn by simultaneous [1-13C] glucose and [6,6-2H2] glucose tracers. *J. Clin. Endocrinol. Metab.* 1980;**50**:456–60.

38 Bier, D. M., Leake, R. D., Haymond, M. W. *et al.* Measurement of "true" glucose production rates in infancy and childhood with 6,6-dideuteroglucose. *Diabetes* 1977;**26**:1016–23.

39 Denne, S. C., Kalhan, S. C. Glucose carbon recycling and oxidation in human newborns. *Am. J. Physiol.* 1986;**251**: E71–7.

40 Kalhan, S. C., Oliven, A., King, K. C., Lucero, C. Role of glucose in the regulation of endogenous glucose production in the human newborn. *Pediatr. Res.* 1986;**20**:49–52.

41 Kalhan, S. C., Savin, S. M., Adam, P. A. Measurement of glucose turnover in the human newborn with glucose 1-13C. *J. Clin. Endocrinol. Metab.* 1976;**43**:704–7.

42 Zarlengo, K. M., Battaglia, F. C., Fennessey, P., Hay, W. W. Relationship between glucose utilization rate and glucose concentration in preterm infants. *Biol. Neonate.* 1986;**49**:181–9.

43 Cowett, R. M., Susa, J. B., Oh, W., Schwartz, R. Glucose kinetics in glucose-infused small for gestational age infants. *Pediatr. Res.* 1984;**18**:74–9.

44 Cowett, R. M., Andersen, G. E., Maguire, C. A., Oh, W. Ontogeny of glucose homeostasis in low birth weight infants. *J. Pediatr.* 1988;**112**:462–5.

45 Kien, C. L., McClead, R. E., Cordero, L. Jr. In vivo lactose digestion in preterm infants. *Am. J. Clin. Nutr.* 1996;**64**:700–5.

46 Griffin, M. P., Hansen, J. W. Can the elimination of lactose from formula improve feeding tolerance in premature infants? *J. Pediatr.* 1999;**135**:587–92.

47 Kien, C. L. Lactose in formulas for preterm infants. *J. Pediatr.* 2001;**138**:148–9.

48 Miller, J. B., McVeagh, P. Human milk oligosaccharides: 130 reasons to breast-feed. *Br. J. Nutr.* 1999;**82**:333–5.

49 Coppa, G. V., Pierani, P., Zampini, L. *et al.* Oligosaccharides in human milk during different phases of lactation. *Acta Paediatr. Suppl.* 1999;**88**:89–94.

50 Fomon, S. J., Filer, L. J. Milks, and formulas. In Fomon, S. J., ed. *Infant Nutrition.* Philadelphia, PA: W. B. Saunders Co., 1974: 359–407.

51 Committee on Nutrition of the Preterm Infant, ESPGN. *Nutrition and Feeding of Preterm Infants.* Oxford: Blackwell Scientific; 1987:62–7.

52 Lepage, G., Collet, S., Bougle, D. *et al.* The composition of preterm milk in relation to the degree of prematurity. *Am. J. Clin. Nutr.* 1984;**40**:1042–9.

53 Williams, P. R. Comparison of glucose tolerance and insulin response of full-term and preterm infants fed glucose polymers. In Sauls, H. S., Benson, J. D., eds. *Meeting Nutritional Goals for Low-Birth-Weight Infants, Proceedings of the Second Ross Clinical Research Conference.* Columbus, OH: Ross Laboratories; 1982:87–9.

54 Antonowicz, I., Lebenthal, E. Developmental pattern of small intestinal enterokinase and disaccharidase activities in the human fetus. *Gastroenterology.* 1977;**72**:1299–303.

55 Keene, M. F. L., Hewer, E. E. Digestive enzymes of the human fetus. *Lancet* 1929;**1**:767–9.

56 Track, N. S., Creutzfeldt, C., Bockermann, M. Enzymatic, functional and ultrastructural development of the exocrine pancreas. *Comp. Biochem. Physiol.* 1975;**51**:95–100.

57 Davis, M. M., Hodes, M. E., Munsick, R. A. Pancreatic amylase expression in human development. *Hybridoma* 1986;**5**:137–45.

58 Jirsova, V., Koldovsky, O., Heringova, A. The development of the functions of the small intestine of the human fetus. *Biol. Neonate.* 1965;**9**:44–9.

59 McNeish, A. S., Mayne, A., Ducker, D. A., Hughes, C. A. Development of D-glucose absorption in the perinatal period. *J. Ped. Gastroenterol. Nutr.* 1983;**2**:S222–6.

60 Barr, R. G., Hanley, J., Patterson, D. K., Wooldridge, J. Breath hydrogen excretion in normal newborn infants in response to usual feeding patterns: evidence for "functional lactase insufficiency" beyond the first month of life. *J. Pediatr.* 1984;**104**:527–33.

61 Gray, G. M. Starch digestion and absorption in nonruminants. *J. Nutr.* 1992;**122**:172–7.

62 Tucker, N. T., Hodge, C., Choi, T. *et al.* Postprandial glucose and insulin responses to glucose polymers by premature infants. *Biol. Neonate.* 1987;**52**:198–204.

63 Kien, C. L., Sumners, J. E., Stetina, J. S., Heimler, R., Grausz, J. P. A method for assessing carbohydrate energy absorption and its application to premature infants. *Am. J. Clin. Nutr.* 1982;**36**:910–6.

64 Shulman, R. J., Feste, A., Ou, C. Absorption of lactose, glucose polymers, or combination in premature infants. *J. Pediatr.* 1995;**127**:626–31.

65 Auricchio, S., Rubino, A., Murset, G. Intestinal glycosidase activities in the human embryo, fetus, and newborn. *Pediatrics* 1963;**35**:944–54.

66 Antonowicz, I., Chang, S. K., Grand, R. J. Development and distribution of lysosomal enzymes and disaccharidases in human fetal intestine. *Gastroenterology* 1974;**67**:51–8.

67 Mobassaleh, M., Montgomery, R. K., Biller, J. A., Grand, R. J. Development of carbohydrate absorption in the fetus and neonate. *Pediatrics* 1985;**75**:160–6.

68 Kien, C. L., Liechty, E. A., Myerberg, D. Z., Mullett, M. D. Dietary carbohydrate assimilation in the premature infant: evidence for a nutritionally significant bacterial ecosystem in the colon. *Am. J. Clin. Nutr.* 1987;**46**:456–60.

69 Kien, C. L., Liechty, E. A., Mullett, M. D. Effects of lactose intake on nutritional status in premature infants. *J. Pediatr.* 1990;**116**:446–9.

70 Shulman, R. J., Schanler, R. J., Lau, C. *et al.* Early feeding, feeding tolerance, and lactase activity in preterm infants. *J Pediatr.* 1998;**133**:645–9.

71 Kien, C. L., McClead, R. E., Cordero, L. Jr. Effects of lactose intake on lactose digestion and colonic fermentation in preterm infants. *J. Pediatr.* 1998;**133**:401–5.

72 Layer, P., Peschel, S., Schlesinger, T., Goebell, H. Human pancreatic secretion and intestinal motility: effects of ileal nutrient perfusion. *Am. J. Physiol. Gastrointest. Liver Physiol.* 1990;**258**:G196–201.

73 Wen, J., Phillips, S. F., Sarr, M. G., Kost, L. J., Holst, J. J. PYY and GLP-1 contribute to feedback inhibition from the canine ileum and colon. *Am. J. Physiol. Gastrointest. Liver Physiol.* 1995;**269**:G945–52.

74 Longo, W. E., Ballantyne, G. H., Savoca, P. E. *et al.* Short-chain fatty acid release of peptide YY in the isolated rabbit distal colon. *Scand. J. Gastroenterol.* 1991;**26**:442–8.

75 Piche, T., Zerbib, F., Varannes, S. B. *et al.* Modulation by colonic fermentation of LES function in humans. *Am. J. Physiol. Gastrointest. Liver Physiol.* 2000;**278**:G578–84.

76 Cicco, R., Holzman, I. R., Brown, D. R., Becker, D. J. Glucose polymer tolerance in premature infants. *Pediatrics* 1981;**67**:498–501.

77 Boellner, S. W., Beard, A. G., Panos, T. C. Impairment of intestinal hydrolysis of lactose in newborn infants. *Pediatrics.* 1965;**36**:542–9.

78 Jarrett, E. C., Holman, G. H. Lactose absorption in the premature infant. *Arch. Dis. Child.* 1966;**41**:525–7.

79 Fosbrooke, A. S., Wharton, B. A. 'Added lactose' and 'added sucrose' cow's milk formulae in nutrition of low birthweight babies. *Arch. Dis. Child.* 1975;**50**:409–18.

80 Kien, C. L., Liechty, E. A., Myerberg, D. Z., Mullett, M. D. Effects in premature infants of normalizing breath H_2 concentrations with CO_2: increased H_2 concentration and reduced interaliquot variation. *J. Pediatr. Gastroenterol. Nutr.* 1987;**6**:286–89.

81 MacLean, W. C. Jr, Fink, B. B. Lactose malabsorption by premature infants: magnitude and clinical significance. *J. Pediatr.* 1980;**97**:383–8.

82 Modler, S., Kerner, J. A. Jr, Castillo, R. O., Vreman, H. J., Stevenson, D. K. Relationship between breath and total body hydrogen excretion rates in neonates. *J. Pediatr. Gastroenterol. Nutr.* 1988;**7**:554–8.

83 Kien, C. L., Ault, K., McClead, R. E. In vivo estimation of lactose hydrolysis in premature infants using a dual stable tracer technique. *Am. J. Physiol.* 1992;**263**:E1002–9.

84 Weaver, L. T., Laker, M. F., Nelson, R. Neonatal intestinal lactase activity. *Arch. Dis. Child.* 1986;**61**:896–9.

85 Murray, R. D., Ailabouni, A. H., Powers, P. A. *et al.* Absorption of lactose from the colon of newborn piglet. *Am. J. Physiol.* 1991;**261**:G1–8.

86 Kien, C. L., Murray, R. D., Ailabouni, A. H., Habash, D. L., Powers, P. A. Measurement of the rate of entry of intact colon-derived lactose into the circulation: a model for assessing gut uptake of molecules not endogenously synthesized. *J. Pediatr. Gastroenterol. Nutr.* 1997;**25**:68–73.

87 Shulman, R. J. In vivo measurements of glucose absorption in preterm infants. *Biol. Neonate* 1999;**76**:10–18.

88 Zittermann, A., Bock, P., Drummer, C. *et al.* Lactose does not enhance calcium bioavailability in lactose-tolerant, healthy adults. *Am. J. Clin. Nutr.* 2000;**71**:931–6.

89 Moya, M., Lifschitz, C., Ameen, V., Euler, A. R. A metabolic balance study in term infants fed lactose-containing or lactose-free formula. *Acta Paediatr.* 1999;**88**:1211–15.

90 Saunders, D. R., Wiggins, H. S. Conservation of mannitol, lactulose, and raffinose by the human colon. *Am. J. Physiol.* 1981;**241**:G397–402.

91 Reilly, K. H., Rombeau, J. L. Metabolism and potential clinical applications of short-chain fatty acids. *Clin. Nutr.* 1993;**12**:97–105.

92 Bergman, E. N., Wolff, J. E. Metabolism of volatile fatty acids by liver and portal-drained viscera in sheep. *Am. J. Physiol.* 1971;**221**:586–92.

93 Cummings, J. H. Short chain fatty acids in the human colon. *Gut* 1981;**22**:763–79.

94 Bugaut, M., Bentejac, M. Biological effects of short-chain fatty acids in nonruminant mammals. *Ann. Rev. Nutr.* 1993;**13**:217–41.

95 Frankel, W. L., Zhang, W., Singh, A. *et al.* Mediation of the trophic effects of short-chain fatty acids on the rat jejunum and colon. *Gastroenterology* 1994;**106**:375–80.

96 Roediger, W. E. Utilization of nutrients by isolated epithelial cells of the rat colon. *Gastroenterology* 1982;**83**:424–9.

97 Harig, J. M., Soergel, K. H., Komorowski, R. A., Wood, C. M. Treatment of diversion colitis with short-chain-fatty acid irrigation. *N. Engl. J. Med.* 1989;**320**:23–8.

98 Sakata, T., Tamate, H. Rumen epithelial cell proliferation accelerated by rapid increase in intraruminal butyrate. *J. Dairy Sci.* 1978;**61**:1109–13.

99 Argenzio, R. A., Meuten, D. J. Short-chain fatty acids induce reversible injury of porcine colon. *Dig. Dis. Sci.* 1991;**36**:1459–68.

100 Butel, M. J., Roland, N., Hibert, A. *et al.* Clostridial pathogenicity in experimental necrotising enterocolitis in gnotobiotic quails and protective role of bifidobacteria. *J. Med. Microbiol.* 1998;**47**:391–9.

101 Szylit, O., Maurage, C., Gasqui, P. *et al.* Fecal short-chain fatty acids predict digestive disorders in premature infants. *J. Parenter. Enteral Nutr.* 1998;**22**:136–41.

102 Mackie, R. I., Sghir, A., Gaskins, H. R. Developmental microbial ecology of the neonatal gastrointestinal tract. *Am. J. Clin. Nutr.* 1999;**69**:1035S–45S.

103 Schanler, R. J., Shulman, R. J., Lau, C. Feeding strategies for premature infants: beneficial outcomes of feeding fortified human milk versus preterm formula. *Pediatrics* 1999;**103**:1150–7.

104 Martin, A., Rambal, C., Berger, V., Perier, S., Louisot, P. Availability of specific sugars for glycoconjugate biosynthesis: a need for further investigations in man. *Biochimie* 1998;**80**:75–86.

105 Kliegman, R. M., Sparks, J. W. Perinatal galactose metabolism. *J. Pediatr.* 1985;**107**:831–41.

106 Hay, W. W. Fetal and neonatal glucose homeostasis and their relation to the small for gestational age infant. *Semin. Perinatol.* 1984;**8**:101–16.

107 Kaempf, J. W., Li, H.-Q, Groothuis, J. R. *et al.* Galactose, glucose, and lactate concentrations in the portal venous and arterial circulations of newborn lambs after nursing. *Pediatr. Res.* 1988;**23**:598–602.

108 Kliegman, R. M., Morton, S. Sequential intrahepatic metabolic effects of enteric galactose alimentation in newborn rats. *Pediatr Res.* 1988;**24**:302–7.

109 Kunst, C., Kliegman, R., Trindade, C. The glucose-galactose paradox in neonatal murine hepatic glycogen synthesis. *Am. J. Physiol.* 1989;**257**:E697–703.

110 Kliegman, R. M., Miettinen, E. L., Kalhan, S. C., Adam, P. A. J. The effect of enteric galactose on neonatal canine carbohydrate metabolism. *Metabolism* 1981;**30**:1109–18.

111 Kliegman, R. M., Miettinen, E. L., Morton, S. Potential role of galactokinase in neonatal carbohydrate assimilation. *Science* 1983; **220**:302–4.

112 Sparks, J. W., Avery, G. B., Fletcher, A. B., Simmons, M. A., Glinsmann, W. H. Parenteral galactose therapy in the glucose-intolerant premature infant. *Pediatrics* 1982;**100**:255–9.

23

Enteral lipid digestion and absorption

Margit Hamosh

Georgetown University Medical Center, Washington DC, 20057

Fats are vital for normal growth and development, and are the main energy source of the newborn infant. In addition to providing 40%–50% of the total calories in human milk or formula, fats are an integral part of all cell membranes, provide fatty acids necessary for brain development, and are the sole vehicle for fat-soluble vitamins and hormones in milk.[1] Furthermore, these energy-rich lipids can be stored in the body in nearly unlimited amounts, in contrast to the limited storage capacity for carbohydrates and proteins. Before birth, glucose is the major energy source for the fetus, with the fetal requirement for fatty acids supplied mainly as free fatty acids from the maternal circulation. After birth, fat is supplied chiefly in the form of milk or formula triglycerides.[2]

Lipids are nonpolar or amphipathic substances that are insoluble in aqueous media (Figure 23.1). Absorption of fat permits the efficient assimilation of a great number of hydrophobic (fat-soluble) chemicals, some beneficial (such as the fat-soluble vitamins) and some detrimental (such as hydrophobic xenobiotics, drugs, and food additives).[3]

Major lipids in infant nutrition

The major lipid classes are glycerides, phospholipids, sterols (cholesterol), and free fatty acids (Figure 23.1).

Glycerides are nonphosphorus-containing lipids that result from the esterification of glycerol and fatty acids (Figure 23.1). Triglycerides (neutral fat) are the most abundant lipids in animal tissue and serve as an important energy source. In triglycerides all three of the carbon molecules of glycerol are esterified with fatty acids. Monoglycerides

and diglycerides are compounds resulting from ester links between glycerol and one or two fatty acids, respectively.

Phospholipids, phosphorus-containing lipid compounds, may be subdivided into three classes: derivatives of glycerol-3-phosphate (phosphatidyl choline, phosphatidyl ethanolamine, phosphatidyl serine, and phosphatidyl inositol), sphingosine, and the glycolipids. Phospholipids are found as structural components of all biologic membranes. They are important in oxidative phosphorylation, in transport across cell membranes, in electron transport reactions and intracellular signaling. They are also the main components of pulmonary surfactant.

Sterols are alcohols with the cyclopentanoperhydrophenanthrene skeletal structure. The principal sterol is cholesterol, the parent compound of the steroids, including the adrenocortical, ovarian, and testicular hormones. The bile acids, degradative products of cholesterol, are important in gastrointestinal absorptive processes.

Fatty acids of animal origin are usually unbranched, monocarboxylic acids containing an even number of carbon atoms, varying from 2 to 24 in chain length. The fatty acid chains may be either saturated or unsaturated (Table 23.1). Most biologically important fatty acids are esterified with glycerol; a small portion is linked with other compounds or is free. The functions of the lipid classes discussed are summarized in Table 23.2.

Fat composition of human milk

Mature human milk has a 2.5%–4.5% fat content. The fat in milk is contained within membrane-enclosed milk fat

Neonatal Nutrition and Metabolism. Second Edition, ed. P. Thureen and W. Hay. Published by Cambridge University Press.
© Cambridge University Press 2006.

Table 23.1. Structure of fatty acids[11]

Descriptive name	Systematic name	Carbon atoms	Double bonds	Position of double bonds	Fatty acid class
Acetic	–	2	0	–	–
Butyric	–	4	0	–	–
Caproic	Hexanoic	6	0	–	–
Caprylic	Octanoic	8	0	–	–
Capric	Decanoic	10	0	–	–
Lauric	Dodecanoic	12	0	–	–
Myristic	Tetradecanoic	14	0	–	–
Palmitic	Hexadecanoic	16	0	–	–
Palmitoleic	Hexadecaenoic	16	1	9	n-7
Stearic	Octadecanoic	18	0	–	–
Oleic	Octadecaenoic	18	1	9	n-9
Linoleic	Octadecadienoic	18	2	9, 12	n-6
Linolenic	Octadecatrienoic	18	3	9, 12, 15	n-3
Linolenic	Octadecatrienoic	18	3	6, 9, 12	n-6
Homolinolenic	Eicosatrienoic	20	3	8, 11, 14	n-6
Arachidonic	Eicosatetraenoic	20	4	5, 8, 11, 14	n-6
EPA	Eicosapentaenoic	20	5	5, 8, 11, 14, 17	n-3
DHA	Docosahexaenoic	22	6	4, 7, 10, 12, 19, 21	n-3

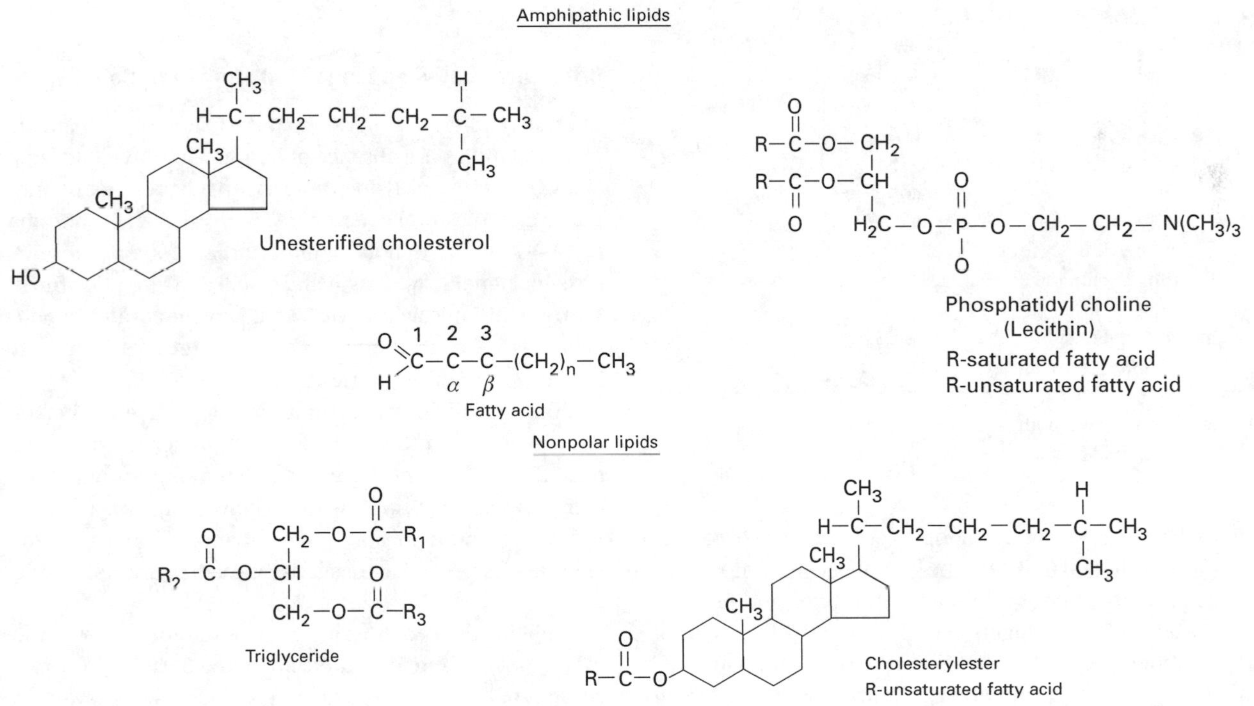

Figure 23.1. Principal dietary lipid components.[94]

Table 23.2. Function of lipids in mammals[1]

Lipid class	Function
Glycerides	Fatty acid storage, metabolic intermediates
Phospholipids sterols	Membrane structure, lung surfactant
Cholesterol	Membrane and lipoprotein structure
	Precursors of steroid hormones
	Degradation products are bile salts important in fat digestion and absorption
Cholesteryl ester	Storage and transport
Fatty acids	Major energy source
	Components of most lipids
	Precursors of prostaglandins
	Essential for normal brain and retina development

Table 23.3. Composition of human milk fat[4a]

Glycerides	3.0–4.5 g^{-1} dL
Triglycerides	98.7%[b] Major component of the core of milk fat globules
Monoglycerides	0
Diglycerides	0.01%
Free fatty acids	0.08%
Cholesterol	10–15 mg^{-1} dL. Major component of milk fat globules
Phospholipids	10–15 mg^{-1} dL. Major component of milk fat globules
Sphingomyelin	37%[b]
Phosphatidylcholine	28%
Phosphatidylserine	9%
Phosphatidylinositol	6%
Phosphatidylethanolamine	19%

[a] Mature milk from mothers of term infants.
[b] Percent in lipid class.

globules.[4] The core of the globules consists of triglycerides (98%–99% of total milk fat); the globule membrane is composed mainly of phospholipids, cholesterol, and proteins (Table 23.3). The packaging of triglyceride within the core of the globules permits the dispersion of these nonpolar lipids in the aqueous environment of milk and also protects them from hydrolysis by milk lipases.[5,6]

Milk fat content and composition change during lactation.[7] These changes are most pronounced during early lactation (colostrum), and again during weaning. Mature milk, however, maintains a constant fat composition.

Total fat content increases gradually from colostrum (2.0%) to mature milk (3.5%–4.5%).[7] Cholesterol content is highest in colostrum and decreases to lower levels in mature milk, it is distributed as 87% free cholesterol and 13% cholesteryl ester (see Table 23.3). Phospholipids show a similar decrease from high levels in colostrum to lower levels in mature milk. The decline in phospholipid and cholesterol levels agrees well with an increase in the fat globule size, and thus, a decrease in the amount of membrane lipids (containing about 60% of milk phospholipid and 85% of milk cholesterol).[8]

Over 98% of the fat in human milk is present in 11 major fatty acids from C10:0 to C22:6n3 (Table 23.4). Saturated fatty acids constitute 42%, and unsaturated fatty acids 57% of total lipid in human milk. Essential fatty acid contents are higher in colostrum than in mature milk.[7] Long-chain polyunsaturated fatty acids derived from linoleic acid (20:2n6, 20:3, 20:4, 22:5n6) and from linolenic acid (20:5, 22:5n3, 22:6n3) show a similar decrease throughout lactation (Table 23.5). The level of these fatty acids is significantly higher in colostrum and milk of mothers of preterm infants than mothers of full-term infants.[7,9]

Differences between human milk and formula fat

The major differences between the fat in human milk and in infant formulas are absence of long-chain polyenoic fatty acids greater than C18 in formulas and the presence of only traces of cholesterol as compared with an average amount of 10–16 mg dL^{-1} cholesterol in human milk. Because of possible benefits to growth and visual and cognitive function, arachidonic acid (AA, C20:4n6) and docosahexaenoic acid (DHA, C22:6n3) are now added to term and preterm formulas in many countries.[10]

Although milk AA concentrations are relatively constant and do not seem to vary widely with maternal nutrition, milk DHA levels show great variety among populations, being lowest in countries with a relatively high meat intake (i.e., USA), and highest where most animal foods are provided as fish (Far East, Nigeria, Canadian Inuits) (Table 23.6).[11]

While formulas deliver a constant amount of fat to the infant during each feed, there are marked variations in fat content of human milk, fat concentrations being lowest in fore milk and gradually increasing to highest levels in hind milk. In addition, fat content rises during the day, early morning milk having the lowest fat content.

Table 23.4. Fatty acid composition (%) of human milk[7]

Fatty acid	Structure	VPT 26–30 weeks	PT 31–36 weeks	T 37–40 weeks
Capric	10:0	1.37+0.17	1.27+0.18	0.97+0.28
Lauric	12:0	7.47+0.72	6.55+0.77	4.46+1.17
Myristic	14:0	8.41+0.83	7.55+0.89	5.68+1.36
	15:0	0.23+0.04	0.27+0.05	0.31+0.07
Palmitic	16:0	20.13+1.40	23.16+1.49	22.20+2.28
Palmitoleic	16:1	2.56+1.40	2.92+0.26	3.83+0.39
	17:0	0.34+0.22	0.60+0.24	0.49+0.36
Stearic	18:0	7.24+1.13	7.25+1.21	7.68+1.85
Oleic	18:1	33.41+1.67	33.74+1.79	35.51+2.73
Linoleic	18:2	15.75+1.22	13.83+1.20	15.58+1.99
Linolenic	18:3	0.76+0.13	0.76+0.14	1.03+0.21
	20:0	0.17+0.07	0.09+0.08	0.32+0.11
	20:2	0.35+0.13	0.33+0.13	0.18+0.20
Homolinolenic	20:3	0.51+0.09	0.43+0.10	0.53+0.15
Arachidonic	20:4	0.55+0.18	0.58+0.19	0.60+0.29
	20:5	0.04+0.05		
	21:0	0.05+0.07	0.07+0.08	0.17+0.12
	22:4	0.13+0.10	0.24+0.11	0.07+0.16
	22:5n6	0.11+0.05	0.04+0.05	0.03+0.08
EPA	22:5n3	0.42+0.09	0.12+0.10	0.11+0.15
DHA	22:6n3	0.24+0.09	0.21+0.09	0.23+0.14

VPT, very preterm; PT, preterm; T, term; milk was collected at 6 weeks of lactation. Data are means + SEM.

Table 23.5. Effect of length of lactation on DHA and AA in human milk[11]

Lactation	Bitmam (1983)	Boersma (1991)	Spear (1992)	Spear (1992)	Luukkainen (1994)	Henderson (1996)
Docosahexaenoic acid						
Colostrum	0.31	1.10	0.34	0.32	0.44	
1–3 weeks		0.88	0.20		0.38	
1–3 months	0.18	0.56	0.15		0.25	0.20
6 months					0.18	0.08
12 months						0.08
Arachidonic acid						
Colostrum	0.78	1.60	0.84	1.20	0.60	
1–3 weeks		0.84	0.76		0.46	
1–3 months	0.57	0.54	0.52		0.40	0.54
6 months					0.28	0.43
12 months						0.39

Data are percent of milk fatty acids. The number of subjects in each study varied from 2–31.
Table references can be located in the source reference.[11]

Table 23.6. DHA and AA in mature human milk: geographic variations[11]

Country	Authors	Year of publication	DHA%	AA%
USA	Putnam *et al.*	1982	0.10	0.60
	Dodson *et al.*	1992	0.16	0.53
	Bitman *et al.*	1983	0.18	0.57
	Tomarelli	1988	0.25	0.46
	Jackson *et al.*	1994	0.21	0.71
Hungary	Sas *et al.*	1986	0.10	0.50
Germany	Koletzko *et al.*	1988	0.22	0.36
	Harzer *et al.*	1983	0.16	0.39
Sweden	Jansson *et al.*	1981	0.30	0.40
England	Hall	1979	0.29	0.19
	Sanders *et al.*	1978	0.59	0.54
Spain	Villacampa *et al.*	1982	0.30	0.57
	de la Presa-Owens *et al.*	1996	0.34	0.50
	de Lucchi *et al.*	1988	0.40	0 80
South Africa	van der Westhuyzen *et al.*	1988	0.20	0.60
Tanzania	Muskiet *et al.*	1987	0.27	0.60
Gambia	Prentiss *et al.*	1989	0.39	0.31
Nigeria	Koletzko *et al.*	1991	0.93	0.82
St. Lucia	Boersma *et al.*	1991	0.56	0.58
China	Kneebone *et al.*	1985	0.71	0.64
Malaysia	Kneebone *et al.*	1985	0.90	0.47
India	Kneebone *et al.*	1985	0.90	0.57
Canada Inuit	Innis *et al.*	1988	1.40	0.60

Three–forty subjects per study. Milk collected 0.5–8 months after delivery.
Data are percent of total milk fatty acids. DHA, docosahexaenoic acid; AA, arachidonic acid.
Table references can be located in the source reference.[11]

Minerals, trace elements, and enzymes associated with the cream fraction of milk have similar diurnal variations.

In contrast to the changes in fat concentration, the fat composition of mature human milk is remarkably constant. Only drastic changes in the diet, such as consumption of excessively large amounts of polyunsaturated fats, or carbohydrates, or severe limitations of total food intake, result in the increase of linoleic acid, medium-chain fatty acids, and palmitic acid, respectively.[12] Recent studies show that the amounts of trans fatty acids (geometric isomers of cis fatty acids, formed during partial hydrogenation of fat) rises markedly in milk of women who consume large amounts of hydrogenated fats.[13,14] The greatest increase in milk trans fatty acids occurred in women who were

Table 23.7. Factors that affect milk fat content and composition[24]

Variable	Change
Gestation	LC-PUFA higher in preterm[a] and transitional milk
Lactation	Phospholipid, cholesterol higher in colostrum (preterm > term) LC-PUFA decrease during lactation (3 mo–1 y) in term milk, but remain constant in preterm milk for 6 months
Parity	P10 +: lower endogenous synthesis of FA $(C_6–C_{16})$
Volume	Low milk fat concentration associated with high volume
Feed	Fat: fore < mid < hind milk
Diet	
High CHO intake	Increase in endogenous synthesis of FA$(C_6–C_{16})$
Low caloric intake	Increase in palmitic acid (C_{16})
High margarine	Increase in trans FA
Pregnancy weight gain	Positively associated with milk fat content

[a] Preterm, term refer to milk or colostrum of women who delivered prematurely or at term. LC-PUFA, long chain polyunsaturated fatty acids; FA, fatty acids; CHO, carbohydrate.

losing weight and consuming hydrogenated fat.[14] From these data it appears that trans fatty acids from the diet and from the mother's fat depots contribute to milk trans fatty acids. Parity has been reported to affect mammary gland de novo synthesis of medium chain fatty acids (Table 23.7).[15]

Milk fat composition is also markedly affected by maternal diseases[16] such as cystic fibrosis,[17] diabetes[18] and hyperlipemia.[19]

Fat digestion

More than 95% of dietary fat (including that in human milk and infant formula) is triglyceride (Figure 23.1, Table 23.3). For efficient fat digestion, the infant depends on mechanisms that are different from the adult. Fat absorption, however, seems to be very efficient even in premature infants. Because much progress has been made recently in our understanding of the enzymes responsible for fat digestion[20] in the newborn,[21,22] this aspect will be discussed in greater detail than the topic of fat absorption.

Table 23.8. Lipases in the newborn and their contribution to fat digestion[24]

Lipase	Site of action	Cofactors	Substrate	Contribution
Gastric lipase	Stomach	None	Triglyceride	Moderate to high[a]
Pancreas				
Colipase-dependent lipase (CDL)	Intestine duodenum	Colipase Bile salts	Triglyceride phospholipids	Low
Carboxylester lipase (CEL)	Intestine duodenum	Bile salts	Triglyceride, other esters	Unknown to high[b]
Pancreatic lipase related proteins (PLRP[1] and PRLP[2])	Intestine	?	Phospholipids, triglyceride	Unknown
Milk bile salt dependent lipase (BSDL)	Intestine	Bile salts	Triglyceride > other esters	Moderate to high[c]

[a] Activity level depends on species; [b] High in rat, shark (activity in humans unknown); [c] Moderate in human and carnivores, high in ferrets.

Luminal phase

Fat digestion requires adequate lipase activity and bile salt concentrations, the former for the breakdown of triglycerides and the latter for emulsification of fat prior to and during lipolysis.[3] The significant lipases for fat digestion are listed in Table 23.8. Fat digestion begins in the stomach with the action of lingual or gastric lipase.[21,23] Further digestion takes place in the small intestine through the action of pancreatic lipase and, in the breast-fed infant, of milk bile salt dependent lipase (BSDL) (Table 23.8).[24]

The stomach

Initial hydrolysis of fat in the stomach leads to the formation of partial glycerides and free fatty acids.[25] This critical step is necessary for efficient fat absorption in the adult with adequate pancreatic function.[25] In the newborn and especially the preterm infant, pancreatic lipase and intraduodenal bile acid concentrations (the major components of intestinal fat digestion) are low.[26] Therefore, efficient fat absorption in the newborn depends on alternate mechanisms for the digestion of dietary fat.

Of special importance is intragastric lipolysis in which lingual and gastric lipases compensate for low pancreatic lipase (Table 23.8). In addition, the products of intragastric lipolysis (fatty acids and monoglycerides) compensate for low bile salt concentrations by emulsifying the lipid mixture.[27]

The digestion of fat starts in the stomach. It is catalyzed by three enzymes of similar structure and characteristics, but depending upon the species of different origin.[21,25] The enzymes originate either in the lingual serous glands (lingual lipase), the glossoepiglottic area (pre-gastric esterase), or the gastric mucosa (gastric lipase).

Rat lingual lipase[28] and human gastric lipase,[29] have been cloned and expressed in *Escherichia coli* or yeast. They are glycoproteins of an approximate molecular weight of 52 kD and consist of 377 and 379 kD amino acid residues and an un-glycosylated molecular weight of 42.56 kD and 43.16 kD for lingual and gastric lipase, respectively.[28,29] The amino acid sequence of the two enzymes has an overall homology of 78%.[30,31] De-glycosylation does not reduce catalytic activity; however, the terminal tetrapeptide, in particular lysine-4, is essential for enzyme binding to the lipid-water interface.[32] Rabbit and human gastric lipases have been crystallized recently.[30] Low pH optimum (2.5–6.5), absence of requirements for specific cofactors or bile salts, and stability to pepsin enables these enzymes to act in the stomach, and in certain diseases associated with pancreatic insufficiency (cystic fibrosis and chronic alcoholism)[21,23,25,32,33] also in the intestine (Table 23.8).

Substrate selectivity is relevant to specific aspects of neonatal digestion. Fatty acid and site selectivity (that is, position of the fatty acid on the triglyceride molecule) of gastric lipase result in release of the fatty acids at the Sn3 position.[34] Long-chain polyunsaturated fatty acids of milk are located mainly at this position and are efficiently released by gastric lipase. Similar location of medium-chain fatty acids (MCFA) in milk fat leads also to their preferential release in the stomach[34] an observation that started the erroneous belief that gastric lipase is specific for MCFA. This site specificity indicates that fatty acids essential for infant development such as LC-PUFA, necessary for brain and retinal development (DHA, C22:6n3) and infant growth

(AA, C20:4n6) as well as MCFA, an easily available energy source, are preferentially released.

In vitro studies that simulate the gastric milieu have shown strong product inhibition that limits lipolysis to 10–20%,[21,25,35,36] however, in vivo studies that have actually measured the extent of lipolysis show that this process is extensive.[35–38]

The extent of gastric digestion of fat has been studied most extensively with mother's milk as the substrate. Depending upon species, fat digestion in the stomach can account for 25%–60% of total lipid digestion.[37–39] In the infant, although gastric function and expression of gastric lipase are unaffected by diet, the extent of fat digestion is significantly greater in preterm infants fed mother's milk (25%) than formula (14%).[40] This difference is probably due to the structural differences in substrate presentation, that is, triglyceride within the milk fat globules or within formula fat particles. Indeed, recent studies show that during the hydrolysis of lipid emulsions by purified human gastric lipase, free fatty acid-rich clusters are formed at the surface of the lipid droplets.[35] Colocalization of gastric lipase with free fatty acids within these clusters indicates that the lipase is bound to fatty acids and perhaps trapped within these fatty acid-rich particles that are generated during lipolysis at the droplet interface, thereby preventing further hydrolysis of the substrate.[37]

The accessibility of triglyceride, the main energy source of the newborn, to the other lipases that affect lipid digestion, has been examined. Earlier in vitro studies have shown that pancreatic colipase-dependent lipase cannot penetrate into milk fat globules and therefore is unable to hydrolyze the core triglyceride.[38,39] These studies have also shown that gastric lipase[38] and lingual lipase[39] can hydrolyze the triglyceride within milk fat globules. Access to the core triglyceride is probably facilitated by the hydrophobic nature of lingual and gastric lipases, as well as by the fact that these enzymes do not hydrolyze the acyl bond of phospholipids,[21,25] or cholesteryl ester[25] major components of the milk fat globule membrane.[41]

More recently, it became apparent that the milk bile salt-dependent lipase is also unable to penetrate into milk fat globules and that its activity in the hydrolysis of milk fat depends upon initial partial hydrolysis by gastric lipase.[34,42] One can conclude that the phospholipid-protein membrane of milk fat globules is not an obstacle to the action of pre-duodenal lipases. Phospholipids are a major barrier to triglyceride hydrolysis by milk bile salt-dependent lipases,[42] and a mixture of proteins and phospholipids prevents triglyceride hydrolysis by pancreatic colipase-dependent lipase.[38,43,44] Indeed, the hydrolysis of milk fat globule triglyceride by either of these enzymes depends upon the initial predigestion by gastric lipase.[34,38,39]

Recent electron microscopy studies of milk fat globules at the end of 50 minutes of gastric digestion in infants show that the globules maintain their initial shape, and that the products of lipolysis are contained within the particles.[40] Similar milk fat globule-contained lipolysis products were previously reported during in vitro incubation of milk fat globules with lingual lipase and visualization by phase contrast or freeze-etching techniques.[45] The free fatty acids and monoglycerides produced are more polar than the globule core triglyceride and migrate to the polar membrane. At this site, they might destabilize the membrane, which facilitates its breakdown in the intestine and subsequent action by pancreatic and milk lipases. Breaking of the milk fat globule membrane is also aided by bile salts, even at very low concentrations.[46] Thus, contrary to the minimal contribution of the stomach to protein digestion, the stomach is essential to fat digestion not only because (depending on the species) 30%–60% of milk fat is digested at this site in the newborn, but also because partial hydrolysis in the stomach is a prerequisite for the subsequent intestinal digestion of fat. Furthermore, recent studies show that lipase activity and output in preterm infants is equal to that of healthy adults kept on a high fat diet (23 ± 5 v. 23 ± 3 U kg^{-1} body weight, respectively) and is higher than in adults consuming a low fat diet (5.2 ± 1.3 U kg^{-1}).[47] The regulation of gastric lipase expression by dietary fat[47] combined with the high fat consumption in infancy might explain the high gastric lipase activity even in very preterm infants. Gastric lipolysis might also be of considerable importance during the transition from total parenteral nutrition (TPN) to gavage feeding because, contrary to intestinal and pancreatic digestive enzymes whose activity decreases during TPN,[48,49] gastric lipase activity is unaffected by mode of feeding.[50]

The ontogeny of gastric lipase has been studied by quantifying enzyme activity in gastric aspirates taken at birth in infants of gestational age 25–40 weeks[51] and more recently in gastric explants from 10–20 weeks gestation fetuses.[52]

In gastric aspirates, lipase activity is high already at 25 weeks gestation; activity remains constant up to 34 weeks, when it increases about 40% above the prior level and decreases again slightly before term delivery.[51] In fetal gastric explants, lipase expression is evident at 10–13 weeks gestation and the adult distribution (that is, mainly in the body, with only traces of activity in the antrum) is established at 15 weeks' gestation. Contrary to pepsin, the secretion mechanism of lipase seems well developed at this time.[52]

Table 23.9. Function of preduodenal lipolysis in infants[23]

Gastric lipolysis of milk fat is extensive, i.e. 30%–60%

Penetration into milk fat globules and initial lipolysis is a prerequisite for hydrolysis by pancreatic lipase and milk bile salt-dependent lipase

Long-chain polyunsaturated fatty acids located at the sn-3 position of milk triglyceride are preferentially released in the stomach

Medium-chained fatty acids released in the stomach are absorbed through the gastric mucosa

Gastric lipase activity, contrary to that of pancreatic lipase, is fully retained during prolonged total parenteral nutrition

Gastric lipolysis is a significant compensatory mechanism for low pancreatic and hepatic function

There are marked differences in the ontogeny of the two main enzymes secreted by the gastric mucosa. Although in the human pepsin and gastric lipase are located at the same site, in the chief cells of the gastric mucosa,[53] the enzymes do not develop in parallel fashion. Thus, whereas pepsin activity and output are much lower in infants[40] than in adults,[47] gastric lipase activity and output are equal in infants and adults.[40,47]

A recent survey of the ontogeny of pepsin and lipase in the ferret, a species very similar to the human in its digestion of fat (gastric lipase is the principal preduodenal lipase,[27] pancreatic lipase activity is low in the newborn, and milk bile salt dependent lipase (BSDL) is high in the jill's (female ferret) milk),[54,55] shows a similar nonparallel development of gastric proteolytic and lipolytic enzymes. Indeed, in the newborn pepsin amounts to only 0.3% of adult activity, as compared with 20% for gastric lipase.[56] Furthermore, at the end of the nursing period (4 weeks of age) pepsin amounts to only 30% of adult activity, whereas lipase is at a level higher than in the adult (153%).[56] A similar picture is seen in the human, where at 4 weeks of age pepsin amounts to only 18% of adult activity, but lipase activity is equal to the adult. The function of gastric lipolysis in infants is summarized in Table 23.9.

The intestine

Several lipases can participate in the intestinal digestion of dietary fat: pancreatic colipase-dependent lipase (CDL), carboxyl ester lipase (CEL), and in the breast-fed infant, milk BSDL. The latter two lipases are identical and are expressed in the pancreas (CEL) and in the mammary gland (BSDL). We will describe briefly the characteristics of CDL and will discuss BSDL (identical to CEL) in greater detail (Table 23.8).

Numerous investigators have reported the very slow development of CDL in the newborn,[57,58] and have suggested that the efficient digestion of fat is probably accomplished by other lipases.[25] The "classical" CDL has a molecular weight of 48 kD, is glycosylated, has a serine at the catalytic site, and has a signal peptide that comprises the first 16 amino acids.[59] The preferred substrates of CDL are emulsions of triglycerides or insoluble micelles.[59,60] Water-soluble esters are hydrolyzed at much lower rates. Colipase-dependent lipase is inhibited by bile salts in concentrations found in the duodenum. This inhibition is reversed by pancreatic colipase, a 10-kD, 86-amino acid protein that is secreted as procolipase and is activated to colipase by trypsin through the cleavage of a pentapeptide activation peptide.[61] Pancreatic lipase (which has no activation peptide) activity might be regulated by the balance between colipase and procolipase.[59] The three-dimensional structure of pancreatic lipase has been determined and shows the presence of two domains: an amino terminal domain (residues 1–335) containing the active site, and a carboxyl-terminal domain (336–449).[62] Procolipase binds to the C-terminal domain of the lipase.[62] Lipase activity is regulated by a "lid," a surface helix covering the catalytic triad that moves, and thereby changes the hydrophobicity around the active site. This explains the interfacial activation of pancreatic lipase: that is, the increase in activity in the presence of a water-lipid interface. Site-specific mutagenesis has recently been used to clarify further the function of colipase. These studies have established that colipase has a function in lipolysis in addition to anchoring lipase to an interface: namely, to stabilize the lid domain of lipases in the open conformation, thereby facilitating lipolysis.[63] Pancreatic lipase has lower activity on triglycerides containing LC-PUFA probably because of the proximity of the double bond to the carboxyl end of the fatty acid,[64,65] but is still able to hydrolyze menhaden oil, rich in LC-PUFA.[66] There is a six-fold difference between the best (oleic acid) and worst (docosahexaenoic acid) substrates.

Lower lipase activity, as compared with trypsin activity in small-for-gestational age (SGA) than in appropriate-for-gestational age (AGA) premature infants,[62] suggests that pancreatic lipase might be more susceptible to nutrient deprivation in utero than are proteolytic enzymes.

In contrast to gastric and lingual lipase, expression of pancreatic lipase and phospholipase A_2 is not detected in the early stages of gestation. Enzyme activity is $< 0.02\%$ of the adult level at 20 weeks and 20% at birth, in association with a low level of lipase mRNA.[70] The reason for this low level of pancreatic lipase at birth is not known. One possibility is that, at this age, pancreatic acinar cells may lack the receptors for ligands that affect lipase synthesis.[71]

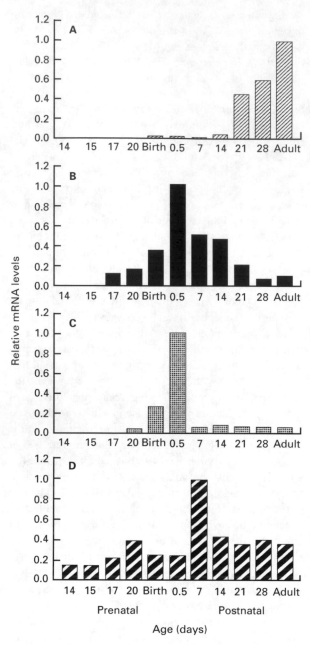

Figure 23.2. Developmental patterns of pancreatic lipase (A), PLRP1 (B), PLRP2 (C), and colipase (D) mRNA in the rat. Data are average of 2–3 separate determinations.[70]

For example, in infants <1 month old, the pancreas does not respond to secretin,[72] a hormone that stimulates lipase synthesis.

Another lipase, the carboxylester lipase (CEL), a 100kD glycoprotein, amounts to 4% of total protein in adult pancreatic juice.[73] As indicated above, this lipase is identical to the milk BSDL.

In contrast to pancreatic lipase, CEL develops early and the CEL gene is detected as early as 6 weeks of gestation in the human fetus,[74] however, little is known about the contribution of CEL to digestion in the newborn. It is proposed that its main function might be the hydrolysis of fat-soluble vitamins and cholesterol esters[75] and possibly of triglycerides in the newborn.

CEL is well represented among other species: it is the only pancreatic lipase in the shark[76] and is the main pancreatic lipase in the suckling rat,[77] before the development of CDL.

The pancreas also secretes a group of pancreatic lipase-related proteins (PLRP1 and PLRP2),[78] whose characteristics differ from those of CDL by exhibiting high phospholipase activity, absence of interfacial activation and absence of colipase effect in maintaining activity at high bile salt concentrations.[78] These pancreatic lipase-related proteins are under investigation in the human,[78] as well as in several animal species.[79–81] There is high homology between PLRP1 and PLRP2 and still remarkable but somewhat lower homology between these pancreatic proteins and CDL. Because of their high phospholipase activity and inhibition by bile salts (that cannot be overcome by colipase), it has recently been suggested that they function mainly as phospholipases.[81] The potential role of these additional members of the lipase gene family, especially PLRP1, which is present in high amounts only during the suckling period, in neonatal fat digestion is currently unknown.

Although the similarities between these proteins and CDL (25% and 68% amino acid identity with CDL) suggest that the three proteins are related, the differences prove that the proteins are encoded by different genes of the growing lipase gene family.[81] There are differences among PLRPs of different species.[81] Thus, the inactivation by bile salts and procolipase dependence of rat PLRP2 are in contrast to the properties reported for human and mouse PLRP2.[81] Rat PLRP1 has little activity against triolein, and could act on other substrates, possibly phospholipids, cholesterol esters, or vitamin esters.[82] Mutations in the 178–181 domain have recently been shown to convert PLRP1 to an active form, possibly through conformational changes in the lid domain resulting in access of fat to the active site of the enzyme.[71] There are also marked developmental differences between PLRP1 and PLRP2 (Figure 23.2). Rat PLRP1 and PLRP2 mRNA is abundant before birth, contrary to rat CDL mRNA. Pancreatic lipase-related protein 1 mRNA, however, remains high until weaning, whereas PLRP2 mRNA decreases sharply after birth.[82] Payne *et al.* suggest that the genes for the rat PLRPs are under different regulatory controls during development than is the rat CDL gene. Procolipase mRNA differs from that of CDL mRNA; the former is present during fetal and neonatal development contrary to the absence of the latter until the weaning period (Figure 23.2).[82] PLRP1 and 2 may be important in the digestion of colostrum and milk in the absence of CDL.[82] Whereas a substrate has not yet been identified for PLRP1, the activity of PLRP1 against triglycerides, phospholipids, and galactolipids suggests that it could be important in the hydrolysis of milk fat globules, which contain a phospholipid-rich membrane in addition to the triglyceride core.[82] The tight association of PLRP2 and the pancreatic zymogen granule,[83] suggests it may also be active in the release of zymogen granule contents.

There is indirect evidence that the milk bile salt-dependent lipase (BSDL) improves fat absorption in the newborn,[84,85] and a greater body of evidence gathered from in vitro studies that the enzyme remains active in the infant's gastrointestinal tract[85-88] and, therefore, might contribute significantly to fat digestion. Milk lipolytic activity was discovered early[89] and has been extensively studied.[88,90]

Great progress has been made recently in our understanding of this enzyme's origin, structure, enzymology, species distribution, and possible function. The enzyme is identical to carboxylester hydrolase, a pancreatic enzyme of wide species distribution that is involved in the intestinal absorption of dietary cholesteryl esters and fat-soluble vitamins.[91,19] In human and carnivore species this enzyme is also expressed in the mammary gland.[54,55] The BSDL cDNA sequence has been cloned from several species,[90] human, rat, cow, rabbit, salmon, and mouse. In all species except mouse and human the BSDL cDNA has been cloned from pancreas only. The enzyme has recently been cloned from ferret lactating mammary gland.[93] The characterization of this enzyme as distinct from lipoprotein lipase (an enzyme present in the milk of many species, but with no function in the process of fat digestion),[94] first in human[95] and then in gorilla[96] milk, led to the assumption that this enzyme is a "newcomer" present only in the milk of high primates.[97]

In mature human milk BSDL activity is higher than in colostrum,[98] and is present in prepartum mammary secretions collected during the last 2 months of pregnancy as well.[99] Other milk enzymes, including lipoprotein lipase, appear first only during the colostral phase.[99]

There is good evidence that BSDL may be a constitutive enzyme of the mammary gland because it is independent of milk volume, activity being similar before the onset of lactation[99] and during weaning. This assumption is also supported by the high concentration of this lipase protein (1% of total milk protein) in human and carnivore milk.[54,100] Although activity varies among women, it seems to remain constant within each woman,[98] a characteristic shared

with the other milk digestive enzyme, amylase.[101] During the first 3 months of lactation, activity levels are similar irrespective of length of gestation,[98] although it has been reported that in the initial colostrum stage lipase activity is higher in the milk of mothers of premature infants.[102]

Recent studies have elucidated the gene organization and expression of BSDL.[90,93] The amino acid sequence of the N-terminal domain is highly conserved among species and the C-terminal tail of 11 amino acid residues is also well conserved. There is, however, great variability for repeated sequence units of 11 amino acids rich in proline, glutamic acid, serine, and threonine, from none in salmon to 39 in gorilla. While these repeats do not affect BSDL activity, they are responsible for the marked differences in molecular weight among species.[54,90]

Enzyme characteristics are identical in milk from mothers of preterm and full-term infants.[103] Activity in milk is constant and does not change diurnally or within a feeding.[54] Bile salt-dependent lipase activity is also remarkably stable during prolonged storage (1–2 years) at either $-20\,^\circ$C or $-70\,^\circ$C[105] and during short-term storage (at least 24 hours) at higher temperatures (15–38 $^\circ$C).[106] Thus, banked human milk stored frozen maintains its fat-digesting capacity for long periods, as does the milk of working women or of mothers of sick or LBW infants who might have to keep the milk at suboptimal conditions for short periods after collection and during transport.

Bile salt-dependent lipase acts at a pH optimum of 7.5–9.0 and has an absolute dependence on primary bile salts.[98] Thus, the enzyme's action is limited to the intestine, where it continues the digestive process started in the stomach by gastric lipase. Indeed, as discussed earlier in this chapter, partial digestion by gastric lipase is a prerequisite for the subsequent hydrolysis of milk fat by BSDL.[34,35]

Bile salt-dependent lipase has no positional or fatty acid specificity and, therefore, can catalyze the complete hydrolysis of milk triglyceride. This is an important aspect of this enzyme's function, because neither gastric nor pancreatic lipase completely hydrolyzes triglycerides; the former produces mainly diglycerides, and the latter monoglycerides.[24] It is of great physiologic importance that BSDL hydrolyzes diglyceride (the product of gastric lipolysis) at higher rates than triglyceride,[107] whereas monoglyceride (the product of intestinal lipolysis by pancreatic lipase) hydrolysis does not require the presence of bile salts.[108] The lipolysis product of BSDL, free fatty acids, is more readily absorbed than monoglycerides[24] at the low-bile salt concentrations found in the newborn.[109] Indeed, fat absorption in breast-fed, contrary to formula-fed infants, is not correlated with bile salt levels.[109] The low substrate specificity of milk lipase is probably the reason for hydrolysis of retinyl palmitate.[110] Recent studies indicate an even broader spectrum for BSDL.[71] Amidase activity against lipoyl 4-amidobenzoate is not bile salt dependent, but is enhanced by some (trihydroxy) bile salts. Ceramidase activity, as well as hydrolysis of galactolipids, has also been reported.

The high extent of intragastric lipolysis indicates that the combined action of gastric lipase and BSDL could accomplish the process of milk fat digestion in the presence of very little or even in the absence of pancreatic lipase.[23,25] There may be distinct advantages for the newborn in having digestion at this stage depend mainly on gastric and milk lipases. Pancreatic lipase release of LC-PUFA, especially docosahexaenoic acid (22:6n3), is inefficient because of the proximity of the double bond to the carboxyl group, which interferes with the hydrolytic activity of this enzyme.[64-66] As discussed previously, gastric lipase readily releases these fatty acids from milk lipids,[34,35] as does BSDL.[111] The sequential release of fatty acids from milk triglyceride as well as the complete hydrolysis of the triglyceride molecule, catalyzed only by BSDL, probably explain the excellent fat absorption in breast-fed preterm infants (Table 23.9).[44]

Data are conflicting with regard to the effect of maternal nutrition on the activity of BSDL. Although an earlier study reported similar activity levels in the milk of well-nourished and undernourished women,[112] two later studies indicate that the milk of malnourished women has lower digestive lipase levels[113,114] which decrease by 80–90% during the first 4 months of lactation,[114] contrary to the constant activity levels in the milk of well-nourished women,[114] even after prolonged lactation.[22] This low lipase activity could adversely affect infants in undernourished areas or during periods of malnutrition. Not only would mother's milk provide insufficient digestive lipase, which might be needed even more than during normal conditions because of the malnutrition-induced decrease in pancreatic digestive function, but it could also affect the infant's resistance to infection, since free fatty acids and monoglycerides (the products of fat digestion) have anti-infective properties.[115]

Fat absorption

Fat absorption seems to be well developed in the newborn[20] since premature infants fed human milk or formula absorb 95 and 93% of dietary fat, respectively.[44] The topic of fat absorption is actively investigated, and although there are still many questions, recent research has added much to our understanding of this complex function.[116-120] The main steps involved are: solubilization of fat during digestion by bile salts, uptake of the free fatty acids through the brush border membrane (BBM), transport within the enterocyte, re-esterification into triglyceride or phospholipid, incorporation into chylomicrons and release from the enterocyte through the lymphatics into the circulation. Short and some medium chain fatty acids are taken up as free fatty acids (bound to albumin) into the liver through the portal vein.

Bile acids are synthesized from cholesterol in the liver and secreted within bile into the intestine. In the terminal ileum, the luminal bile acids are actively reabsorbed by enterocytes and are returned to the liver via the portal circulation. This process, known as the enterohepatic circulation, is the major factor in the maintenance of the bile acid pool.[121] Both components of this mechanism, synthesis in the liver[25] and uptake in the ileum[122] are not well developed at birth, especially in premature infants. Furthermore, the Na^+ dependent ileal BBM bile acid transport,[123] appears only during weaning in the rat ileum and is absent during the period of high fat intake associated with suckling.[124] In the adult, micellar solubilization of LCFA by bile salt increases their luminal concentration 100–1000-fold.[116]

FA uptake at the brush border membrane

The unstirred water-layer in the immediate proximity of the brush border membrane (BBM) has a lower pH than the intestinal lumen.[116,119,120] This acid microclimate, specific to enterocytes, is the result of trapping of hydrogen ions in the glycoprotein network of mucus and BBM glycocalyx, and the presence of Na^+/H^+ exchangers in the BBM. This acidic environment reduces FA solubility in micelles causing their release at the BBM. The efficiency of FA uptake by the enterocytes is dependent upon this acid microclimate. Indeed, inactivation of the Na^+/H^+ exchanger by amyloride markedly decreases oleic acid uptake by rat jejunal sheets or rabbit BBM vesicles.[125] The LCFA cross the enterocyte membrane by two mechanisms, passive diffusion and protein-mediated transport.[118,119,126,127] While the quantitative aspects of these two mechanisms are not known, the high capacity, low-affinity of the former ensure that FA uptake is not rate limiting for intestinal fat absorption.[119] Four membrane lipid binding proteins (LPB) provide a low-capacity, high-affinity fatty acid uptake mechanism, probably most important when intestinal lipid levels are low.[119] The main characteristics of the four plasma membrane LPBs are listed in Table 23.10.

Transport of FA within the enterocyte is facilitated by two 14–15 kDa cytosolic fatty acid binding proteins I-FABP and L-FABP found in the intestine only, or in both liver and intestine, respectively.[128,129] Their expression in the intestine and physiologic characteristics are listed in

Table 23.10. Plasma membrane lipid-binding proteins (LBP) expressed in the small intestine

LBP	Structure	Tissue expression	Ligand(s)	Biochemical characteristics
FABPpm/AspAT fatty acid-binding protein	43-kDa peripheral protein, associated with plasma membrane	Small intestine, adipose tissue, muscles, liver, placenta	LCFA, LPC, CS	Plasma membrane isoform of the mitochondrial aspartate aminotransferase (AspAT)
Caveolin-1	22-kDa integral plasma membrane protein	Small intestine, adipose tissue, heart	LCFA, CS	Marker of caveolae. Putative interaction with various signaling molecules
FAT/CD 36 Fatty acid Translocase	53- to 88-kDa transmembrane protein	Small intestine, adipose tissue, skeletal muscle, heart	LCFA	Highly glycosylated, found caveolae, putative palmitoylation, homo/heterodimerization, and association with Src-kinases
FATP1 Fatty acid transport protein	63-kDa multimembrane-spanning protein	Small intestine, adipose tissue, skeletal muscle, heart	LCFA	Acts in coordination with ACS, contains a sequence of ATP binding

LCFA, long-chain fatty acids; LPC, lysophosphatidyl-choline; CS, cholesterol; ACS, acyl-CoA synthetase.
Cited with permission from Besnard, P. and Niot, I., Ref. 119.

Figure 23.3. Their main functions are desorption of LCFA from the plasma membrane, facilitation of intracellular diffusion, FA targeting to the TG synthesis pathway (I-FABP) or the phospholipid pathway (L-FABP), and protection against the cytotoxic effects of free fatty acids.[119] Polymorphism in the I-FABP gene such as one base substitution causing substitution of Ala[54] by Thr[54] leads to a 2-fold higher affinity for LCFA (112) and greater TG synthesis that result in higher plasma TG levels, insulin resistance, and an increase in body mass index.[119,130]

Re-esterification of FA and release of TG-rich lipoproteins

The first step in the cellular metabolism of LCFA is their activation to acyl-CoA by acyl-CoA synthetase (ACS).[131] ACS are expressed in many organ cells, but little is known about their regulation.[119] Acyl CoAs are transported by a specific 100 kDa, 86 amino acid binding protein (ACBP), with FA-binding affinity proportional to FA chain length, C14–22, but unrelated to number of double bonds.[119,132,133] This protein, which is highly conserved in nature, is probably involved in the control of lipid metabolism.[119,132] Re-esterification takes place in the endoplasmic reticulum to triglyceride, phospholipid or cholesterylester. The newly synthesized triglyceride is transferred to the cysternae of the endoplasmic reticulum by the microsomal triglyceride transfer protein (MTP)[134] for incorporation into chylomicrons (Figure 23.4).

MTP, a heterodimer, consisting of a 55 kDa multifunctional protein domain and a 97 kDa protein domain which provides the lipid transfer activity of the heterodimer, plays a critical role in the assembly and secretion of apo B-containing lipoproteins (chylomicrons and VLDL). Mutations in the gene encoding for the 97 kDa unit lead to absence of functional MTP in the duodenum and abetalipoproteinemia.[135] Indeed, bulk transfer of triglyceride into the lumen of the endoplasmic reticulum is impaired in MTP knock-out mice.[136]

Transport of TG-rich particles out of the endoplasmic reticulum to the Golgi apparatus and interstitium is facilitated by acquisition of apo B.[137] Chylomicrons are released through the basolateral enterocyte membrane into the lacteals and from there into the blood. Apoprotein 48 mRNA appears at 10 weeks gestation and reaches a level of 80% by the end of the second trimester of gestation.[138]

In the enterocyte, there are two major mechanisms of fatty acids re-esterification, both of which ultimately yield chylomicrons, the monoglyceride and the phosphatidic acid pathway. The former is of primary importance in dietary fat absorption, while the latter gives rise to either triglyceride or phospholipid. The monoglyceride pathway, associated primarily with the smooth endoplasmic reticulum is the major mechanism for postprandial triglyceride synthesis within the enterocyte.[139] The phosphatidic acid pathway, on the other hand, is active when 2-monoglyceride is unavailable, i.e., during fasting, and is confined largely to the rough endoplasmic reticulum membranes.

While as much as 70% of absorbed fat is transported to the blood through the lymph, short and medium chain fatty acids are absorbed mainly through the portal vein, unless they are esterified at the Sn2 position of the glycerol molecule.[140] C4 and C6 fatty acids are not absorbed

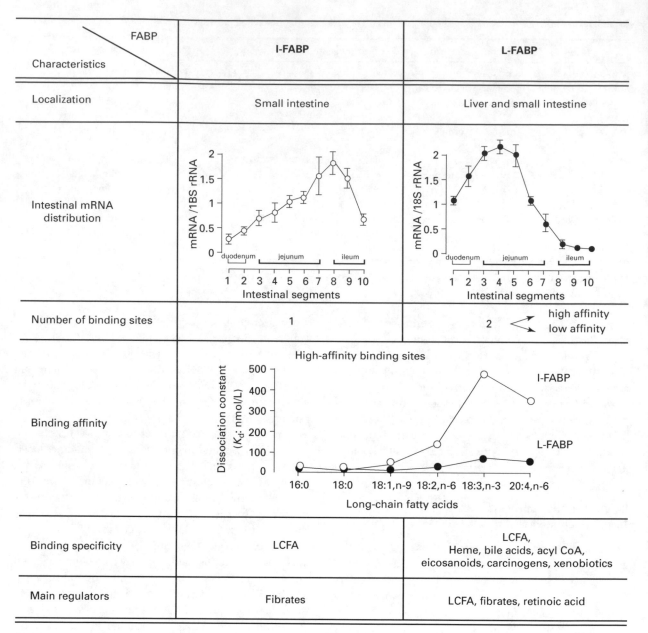

Characteristics \ FABP	I-FABP	L-FABP
Localization	Small intestine	Liver and small intestine
Intestinal mRNA distribution		
Number of binding sites	1	2 (high affinity / low affinity)
Binding affinity		
Binding specificity	LCFA	LCFA, Heme, bile acids, acyl CoA, eicosanoids, carcinogens, xenobiotics
Main regulators	Fibrates	LCFA, fibrates, retinoic acid

Figure 23.3. Main differences in the distribution, regulation, and binding characteristics of the two fatty acid binding proteins (FABP) expressed in the small intestine. I-FABP: intestinal fatty acid binding protein; L-FABP: liver fatty acid binding protein; LCFA: long chain fatty acids.[119] Cited with permission from Besnard, P. and Niot, I., Ref. 119.

through the lymphatic route, whereas C8, 10, and 12 were recovered in lymph triglycerides in 20%, 60%, and 100% yield, respectively.[141]

The possibility of TG hydrolysis within the enterocyte before transport out of the cell has been suggested[142] because TG particles accumulated in the intestine during fat absorption appeared to be too large for secretion as chylomicrons. The recent reports of lipases within liver microsomal membranes[143] and Caco-2 cells[144] suggests that such restructuring of triglyceride might occur in the intestine.[145]

The topic of chylomicron assembly has been reviewed recently.[146] Apo B-48 synthesized in the intestine is smaller (48%) than apo B-100 synthesized in the liver. Very low density lipoproteins (VLDL) contain one molecule of apo B-100, whereas chylomicrons (large particles 1–6 mm in

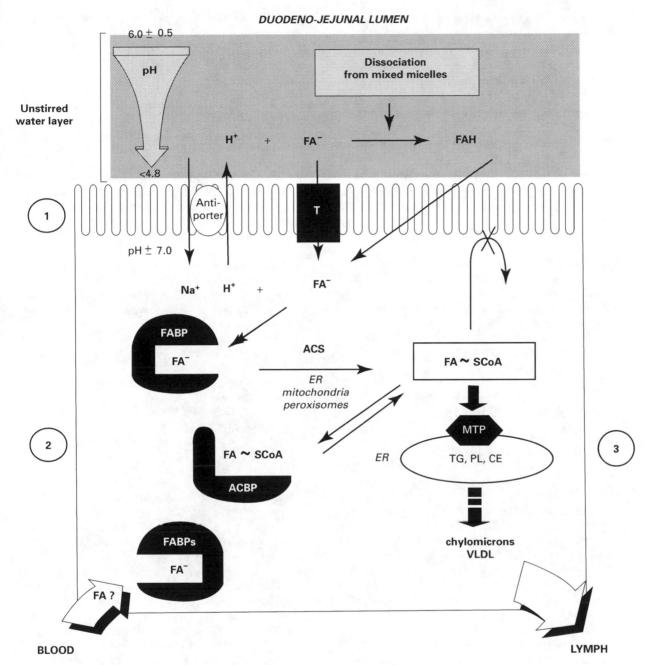

Figure 23.4. Role of lipid-binding protein (in black) in the uptake and metabolic fate of long-chain fatty acids (LCFA) in the small intestine. The main steps of the absorption are shown as follows: (1) Transport of LCFA across the apical membrane of enterocytes by both passive diffusion and protein mediated transport (T). (2) Binding of LCFA and acyl-CoA to cytoplasmic fatty acid-binding proteins (FABP) and acyl-CoA-binding protein (ACBP), respectively. (3) Involvement of the microsomal transfer protein (MTP) in the structure of lipoprotein. Abbreviations: FA−, ionized fatty acids; FAH, protonated fatty acids; ACS, acyl-CoA synthetase; TG, triglycerides; PL, phospholipids; CE, cholesterol esters; ER, endoplasmic reticulum; VLDL, very-low-density lipoproteins.[119] Cited with permission from Besnard, P. and Niot, I.[119]

diameter) may contain two or more apo B-48 molecules.[145] Intestinal VLDL structure and composition is identical to that of chylomicrons, except that they are smaller. VLDL and chylomicrons acquire additional apoproteins (AI, CII, CIII$_0$, CIII$_3$, A-IV, and E) from plasma lipoproteins. Apo B is nontransferable. Apo B-48, a translational product of the apo B gene is essential for the assembly of chylomicrons. Its synthesis is regulated by biliary lipids and not dietary triglyceride, whereas synthesis rate correlates with microsomal triglyceride content.[145] During active TG absorption, the enterocyte increases the size, but not the number of chylomicrons.[147]

REFERENCES

1   Hamosh, M. Fat needs for term and preterm infants. In Tsang, R. C., Nichols, B. L., eds. *Nutrition during Infancy*. Philadelphia, PA: Hanley & Belfus; 1988:133–59.

2   Hamosh, M. Lipid metabolism in premature infants. *Biol. Neonat.* 1987;**52**:50–64.

3   Patton, J. S. Gastrointestinal lipid digestion. In Johnson, L. R., ed. *Physiology of the Gastrointestinal Tract*. New York, NY: Raven Press; 1981:1123–46.

4   Hamosh, M., Bitman, J., Wood, D. L. *et al.* Lipids in milk and the first steps in their digestion. *Pediatrics* 1985;**75**:146–50.

5   Mehta, N. R., Jones, J. B., Hamosh, M. Lipases in human milk: ontogeny and physiologic significance. *J. Pediatr. Gastroenterol. Nutr.* 1982;**1**:317–26.

6   Hamosh, M. Physiological role of human milk lipase. In Lebenthal, E., ed. *Gastrointestinal Development and Infant Nutrition*. New York, NY: Raven Press; 1981:473–82.

7   Bitman, J., Wood, D. L., Hamosh, M. *et al.* Comparison of the lipid composition of breast milk from mothers of term and preterm infants. *Am. J. Clin. Nutr.* 1983;**38**:300–13.

8   Ruegg, M., Blanc, B. The fat globule size distribution in human milk. *Biochim. Biophys. Acta* 1981;**666**:7–13.

9   Luukkainen, P., Sato, M. K., Nikkari, T. Changes in fatty acid composition of preterm and term milk from 1 week to 6 months of lactation. *J. Pediatr. Gastroenterol. Nutr.* 1994;**18**:355–60.

10 Raiten, D. J., Talbot, J. M., Naters, J. H. LSRO Report: Assessment of nutrient requirements for infant formulas. *J. Nutr.* 1998;**128**:20595–22938.

11 Hamosh, M., Salem, N. Jr. Long-chain polyunsaturated fatty acids. *Biol. Neonate.* 1998;**74**:106–20.

12 Hamosh, M. Nutrition during lactation. *Bibl. Nutr. Diet* 1996;**53**:23–36.

13 Craig-Schmidt, M. C., Weete, J. D., Faircloth, S. A. *et al.* The effect of hydrogenated fat in the diet of nursing mothers on lipid composition and prostaglandin content of human milk. *Am. J. Clin. Nutr.* 1984;**39**:778–86.

14 Chappell, J. E., Clandinin, M. T., Kearney-Volpe, C. Trans fatty acids in human milk lipids: influence of maternal diet and weight loss. *Am. J. Clin. Nutr.* 1985;**42**:49–56.

15 Prentice, A., Jarjou, L. M., Drury, P. J. *et al.* Breastmilk fatty acids of rural Gambian mothers: effect of diet and maternal parity. *J. Pediatr. Gastroenterol. Nutr.* 1989;**8**:486–90.

16 Hamosh, M., Bitman, J. Human milk in diseases: lipid composition. *Lipids* 1992;**27**:848–57.

17 Bitman, J., Hamosh, M., Wood, D. L. *et al.* Lipid composition of milk from mothers with cystic fibrosis. *Pediatrics* 1987;**80**:927–32.

18 Bitman, J., Hamosh, M., Hamosh, P. *et al.* Milk composition and volume during the onset of lactation in a diabetic mother. *Am. J. Clin. Nutr.* 1989;**50**:1364–9.

19 Wang, C. S., Illingworth, D. R. Lipid composition and lipolytic activities in milk from a patient with homozygous familial hypobetalipoproteinemia. *Am. J. Clin. Nutr.* 1987;**45**:730–6.

20 Flores, C. A., Hing, S. A., Wells, M. A. *et al.* Rates of triolein absorption in suckling and adult rats. *Am. J. Physiol.* 1989;**257**:G823–8.

21 Hamosh, M. Gastric and lingual lipases. In Johnson, L. R., ed. *Physiology of the Gastrointestinal Tract*. 3rd edn. New York, NY: Raven Press; 1994:1239–53.

22 Hamosh, M. Digestion in the premature infant: the effects of human milk. *Semin. Perinatol.* 1994;**18**:485–94.

23 Hamosh, M. Preduodenal fat digestion. In Christophe, A. B., De Vriese, S., eds. *Fat Digestion and Absorption*. Champaign, IL: AOCS Press; 2000:1–12.

24 Hamosh, M. Digestion in the neonate. *Clin. Perinatol.* 1996;**23**:191–209.

25 Hamosh, M. *Lingual and Gastric Lipase: their Role in Fat Digestion*. Boca Raton, FL: CRC Press; 1990.

26 Watkins, J. B. Mechanism of fat absorption and the development of gastrointestinal function. *Pediatr. Clin. N. Am.* 1975;**22**:721–30.

27 Hamosh, M., Klaeveman, H. L., Wolf, R. O. *et al.* Pharyngeal lipase and digestion of dietary triglycerides in man. *J. Clin. Invest.* 1975;**55**:908–13.

28 Docherty, A. J. P., Bodmer, M. W., Angal, S. *et al.* Molecular cloning and nucleotide sequences of rat lingual lipase rDNA. *Nucleic Acids Res.* 1985;**13**:891–903.

29 Bodmer, M. W., Angal, S., Yarraton, C. T. *et al.* Molecular cloning of a human gastric lipase and expression of the enzyme in yeast. *Biochim. Biophys. Acta.* 1987;**902**:237–44.

30 Moreau, H., Gargouri, Y., Lecat, D. *et al.* Purification, characterization and kinetic properties of the rabbit gastric lipase. *Biochim. Biophys. Acta.* 1988;**960**:286–93.

31 Bernback, S., Blackberg, L. Human gastric lipase. The N-terminal peptide is essential for lipid binding and lipase activity. *Eur. J. Biochem.* 1989;**182**:495–9.

32 Abrams, C. K., Hamosh, M., Dutta, S. K. *et al.* Lingual lipase in cystic fibrosis. Quantitation of enzyme activity in the upper small intestine of patients with exocrine pancreatic insufficiency. *J. Clin. Invest.* 1984;**73**:374–82.

33 Abrams, C. K., Hamosh, M., Dutta, S. K. Role of non-pancreatic lipolytic activity in exocrine pancreatic insufficiency. *Gastroenterology* 1987;**92**:125–9.

34 Hamosh, M., Iverson, S. J., Kirk, C. L. *et al.* Milk lipids and neonatal fat digestion: relationships between fatty acid

composition and endogenous and exogenous digestive enzymes and digestion of milk fat. *World Rev. Nutr. Diet.* 1994;**75**:86–91.

35 Iverson, S. J., Kirk, C. L., Hamosh, M. *et al.* Milk lipid digestion in the neonatal dog: the combined actions of gastric and bile salt stimulated lipases. *Biochim. Biophys. Acta* 1991;**1083**: 109–19.

36 Hamosh, M., Hamosh, P. Development of secreted digestive enzymes. In Sanderson, I. R., Walker, W. A., eds. *Development of the Gastrointestinal Tract.* Hamilton, ONT: Decker Inc. Publ.; 2000:261–77.

37 Parfumi, Y., Lairon, D., Lechen de la Porte P. *et al.* Mechanism of inhibition of triacylglycerol hydrolysis by human gastric lipase. *J. Biol. Chem.* 2002;**277**:28070–9.

38 Cohen, M., Morgan, G. R. H., Hofmann, A. F. Lipolytic activity of human gastric and duodenal juice against medium and long-chain triglycerides. *Gastroenterology* 1971;**60**:1–15.

39 Plucinski, T. M., Hamosh, M., Hamosh, P. Fat digestion in the rat: role of lingual lipase. *Am. J. Physiol.* 1979;**237**:E541–7.

40 Reugg, M., Blanc, B. Structure and properties of the particulate constituents of human milk. A review. *Food Microstructure* 1982;**1**:25–40.

41 Bernback, S., Blackberg, L., Hernell, O. The complete digestion of human milk triacylglycerol in vitro requires gastric lipase, pancreatic colipase-dependent lipase and bile salt stimulated lipase. *J. Clin. Invest.* 1990;**85**:1221–6.

42 Lindstrom, M. B., Sternby, B., Borgstrom, B. Concerted action of human carboxyl ester lipase and pancreatic lipase during lipid digestion in vitro: importance of the physio-chemical state of the substrate. *Biochim. Biophys. Acta* 1988;**959**: 178–89.

43 Lindstrom, M. B., Persson, J., Thurn, L. *et al.* Effect of pancreatic phospholipase A2 and gastric lipase on the action of pancreatic carboxylester lipase against lipid substrate in vitro. *Biochim. Biophys. Acta* 1991;**1084**:194–7.

44 Armand, M., Hamosh, M., Mehta, N. R. *et al.* Effect of human milk or formula on gastric function and fat digestion in the premature infant. *Pediatr. Res.* 1996;**40**:439–47.

45 Patton, J. S., Rigler, M. W., Liao, T. H. *et al.* Hydrolysis of triacylglycerol emulsions by lingual lipase – a microscopic study. *Biochim. Biophys. Acta* 1982;**712**:400–7.

46 Patton, S., Borgstrom, B., Stemberger, B. H. *et al.* Release of membrane from milk fat globules by conjugated bile salts. *J. Pediatr. Gastroenterol. Nutr.* 1986;**5**:262–7.

47 Armand, M., Hamosh, M., DiPalma, J. S. *et al.* Dietary fat modulates gastric lipase activity in healthy humans. *Am. J. Clin. Nutr.* 1995;**61**:74–80.

48 Levine, G. M., Deren, J. J., Steiger, E. *et al.* Role of oral intake in maintenance of gut mass and disaccharidase activity. *Gastroenterology* 1974;**67**:975–82.

49 Rossi, T. M., Lee, P. C., Lebenthal, E. Total parenteral nutrition in infancy affects amylase and lipase but not trypsin secretion. *Pediatr. Res.* 1987;**21**:276A.

50 Mehta, N. R., Liao, T. H., Hamosh, M. *et al.* Effect of total parenteral nutrition on lipase activity in the stomach of very low birth weight infants. *Biol. Neonate.* 1988;**53**:261–6.

51 Hamosh, M., Scanlon, J. W., Ganot, D. *et al.* Fat digestion in the newborn: characterization of lipase in gastric aspirates of premature and term infants. *J. Clin. Invest.* 1981;**67**:838–46.

52 Menard, D., Monfils, E., Tremblay, E. Ontogeny of human gastric lipase and pepsin activities. *Gastroenterology* 1995;**108**:1650–6.

53 Moreau, H., Bernadac, A., Gargouri, Y. *et al.* Immunocytolocalization of human gastric lipase in chief cells of the fundic mucosa. *Histochemistry* 1989;**91**:419–23.

54 Ellis, L. A., Hamosh, M. Bile salt stimulated lipase: comparative studies in ferret milk and lactating mammary gland. *Lipids* 1992;**27**:917–22.

55 Sbarra, V., Mas, E. Henderson, T. R. *et al.* Digestive lipases of the newborn ferret: compensatory role of milk bile salt dependent lipase. *Pediatr. Res.* 1996;**40**:263–8.

56 Hamosh, M., Henderson, T. R., Hamosh, P. Gastric lipase and pepsin activities in the developing ferret: nonparallel development of the two gastric digestive enzymes. *J. Pediatr. Gastroenterol. Nutr.* 1998;**26**:162–8.

57 Zoppy, G., Andreotti, G., Payno-Ferrara, F. *et al.* Exocrine pancreatic function in premature and full-term neonates. *Pediatr. Res.* 1972;**6**:88–94.

58 Lebenthal, E., Lee, P. C. Development and functional response in human exocrine pancreas. *Pediatrics* 1980;**66**:556–60.

59 Lowe, M. E. The structure and function of pancreatic enzymes. In Johnson, L. R., ed. *Physiology of the Gastrointestinal Tract.* 3rd edn. New York, NY: Raven Press; 1994:1531–42.

60 Lowe, M. E. Structure and function of pancreatic lipase and colipase. *Ann. Rev. Nutr.* 1997;**17**:141–58.

61 Erlanson-Albertson, C. Pancreatic colipase. Structural and physiological aspects. *Biochim. Biophys. Acta* 1992;**1124**: 1–7.

62 Van Tilbeurgh, H., Sarda, L., Verger, R. *et al.* Structure of the pancreatic lipase-procolipase complex. *Nature* 1992;**359**: 159–62.

63 Lowe, M. E. Colipase stabilizes the lid domain of pancreatic triglyceride lipase. *J. Biol. Chem.* 1997;**272**:9–12.

64 Brockerhoff, H. Substrate specificity of pancreatic lipase: influence of the structure of fatty acids on the reactivity of esters. *Biochim. Biophys. Acta* 1979;**212**:92–101.

65 Savary, P. The action of pure pancreatic lipase upon esters of long-chain fatty acids and short-chain primary alcohols. *Biochim. Biophys. Acta* 1971;**159**:296–303.

66 Yang, L.-Y., Kuksis, A., Myher, J. J. Lipolysis of menhaden oil triacylglycerols and the corresponding fatty acid alkyl esters by pancreatic lipase in vitro: a reexamination. *J. Lipid Res.* 1990;**31**:137–48.

67 Lowe, M. E. Molecular mechanisms of rat and human pancreatic triglyceride lipase. *J. Nutr.* 1997;**127**:549–57.

68 Boehm, G., Bierback, U., Senger, H. *et al.* Activities of lipase and trypsin in duodenal juice of infants small for gestational age. *J. Pediatr. Gastroenterol. Nutr.* 1991;**12**:324–7.

69 Bokerman, M., Track, N. S., Creutzfelt, C., *et al.* Biochemical and ultrastructural changes in human pancreas during fetal development. In Kaiser, D., ed. *Approaches to Cystic Fibrosis.* Heilbronn, Germany: Thunert and Bofinger; 1983:221–9.

70 Payne, R. M., Sims, H. F., Jennens, M. L. *et al.* Rat pancreatic lipase and two related proteins: enzymatic properties and mRNA expression during development. *Am. J. Physiol.* 1994;**266**:G914–21.

71 Duan, R. D. Enzymatic aspects of fat digestion in the gastrointestinal tract. In Christophe, A. B., De Vriese, S., eds. *Fat Digestion and Absorption.* Champaign, IL: AOCS Press; 2000:25–46.

72 Rausch, A., Rudiger, K., Vasiloudes, P. *et al.* Lipase synthesis in the rat pancreas is regulated by secretin. *Pancreas* 1986;**1**: 522–8.

73 Lombardo, D., Guy, O., Figarella, C. Purification and characterization of a carboxyl ester hydrolase from human pancreatic juice. *Biochim. Biophys. Acta* 1978;**527**:142–9.

74 Roudani, S., Miralles, F., Margotat, A. *et al.* Bile salt dependent lipase transcripts in human fetal tissues. *Biochim. Biophys. Acta* 1995;**1264**:141–50.

75 Howles, P. N., Carter, C. P., Hui, D. Y. Dietary free and esterified cholesterol absorption in cholesterol esterase (bile salt stimulated lipase) genetically targeted mice. *J. Biol. Chem.* 1996;**271**:7196–202.

76 Patton, J. S., Warner, T. G., Benson, A. A. Partial characterization of the bile salt-dependent triacylglycerol lipase from the leopard shark pancreas. *Biochim. Biophys. Acta* 1977;**486**: 322–30.

77 Bradshaw, W. S., Rutter, W. J. Multiple pancreatic lipases. Tissue distribution and pattern of accumulation during embryological development. *Biochemistry* 1972;**11**:1517–28.

78 Giller, T., Buchwald, P., Blum-Kaelin, D. *et al.* Two novel human pancreatic lipase related proteins, hPLRP1 and hPLRP2. *J. Biol. Chem.* 1992;**267**:16509–16.

79 Thirstrup, K., Verger, R., Carriere, F. Evidence for a pancreatic lipase subfamily with new kinetic properties. *Biochemistry* 1994;**33**:2748–56.

80 Carriere, F., Thirstrup, K., Hjiorth, S. *et al.* Cloning of the classical guinea pig pancreatic lipase and comparison with the lipase related protein 2. *FEBS Lett.* 1994;**338**:63–8.

81 Cygler, M., Schrog, J. D., Sussman, J. L. *et al.* Relationship between sequence conservation and three-dimensional structure in a large family of esterases, lipases and related proteins. *Protein Sci.* 1993;**2**:366–82.

82 Payne, R. M., Sims, H. F., Jennens, M. L. *et al.* Rat pancreatic lipase and two related proteins: enzymatic properties and mRNA expression during development. *Am. J. Physiol.* 1994;**266**:G914–21.

83 Wishart, M. J., Andrews, P. C., Nichols, R. *et al.* Identification and cloning of GP-3 from rat pancreatic acinar zymogen granules as a glycosylated membrane-associated lipase. *J. Biol. Chem.* 1993;**268**:10303–11.

84 Williamson, S., Finucane, E., Ellis, H. *et al.* Effect of heat treatment of human milk on absorption of nitrogen, fat, sodium, calcium, and phosphorus by preterm infants. *Arch. Dis. Child.* 1978;**53**:555–63.

85 Alemi, B., Hamosh, M., Scanlon, J. W. *et al.* Fat digestion in very low birth weight infants: effect of addition of human milk to low birth weight formula. *Pediatrics* 1981;**68**:484–9.

86 Hamosh, M. Lingual and breast milk lipase. *Adv. Pediatr.* 1982;**29**:33–67.

87 Hamosh, M. Enzymes in human milk: their role in nutrient digestion, gastrointestinal function and nutrition in infancy. In Lebenthal, E., ed. *Textbook of Gastroenterology and Nutrition in Infancy.* 2nd edn. New York, NY: Raven Press;1989: 121–34.

88 Hamosh, M. Enzymes in human milk. In Jensen, R. G., ed. *Handbook of Milk Composition.* San Diego, CA: Academic Press; 1995:388–427.

89 Marfan, A. B. Allaitment naturel et allaitment artificiel. *Presse Med.* 1901;**9**:13–19.

90 Lombardo, D. Bile salt dependent lipase: its pathophysiological implications. *Biochim. Biophys. Acta* 2001;**1533**:1–28.

91 Lombardo, D., Fauvel, J., Guy, O. Studies on the substrate specificity of a carboxyl ester hydrolase from human pancreatic juice. I. Action on carboxyl esters, glycerides and phospholipids. *Biochim. Biophys. Acta* 1980;**611**:135–46.

92 Lombardo, D., Guy, O. Studies on the substrate specificity of a carboxyl ester hydrolase from human pancreatic juice. II. Action on cholesterol esters and lipid soluble vitamin esters. *Biochim. Biophys. Acta* 1980;**611**:147–55.

93 Sbarra, V., Bruneau, N., Mas, E. *et al.* Molecular cloning of the bile salt dependent lipase of ferret lactating mammary gland: an overview of functional residues. *Biochim. Biophys. Acta* 1998;**1393**:80–9.

94 Hamosh, M., Hamosh, P. Lipoprotein lipase, its physiological and clinical significance. *Mol. Aspects Med.* 1983;**6**: 199–289.

95 Freudenberg, E. Die Frauenmilch-lipase. Basel, Switzerland: Karger; 1953.

96 Freudenberg, E. A lipase in the milk of gorilla. *Experientia* 1966;**22**:317.

97 Blackberg, L., Hernell, O., Olivecrona, T. *et al.* The bile salt stimulated lipase in human milk is a newcomer derived from a non-milk protein. *FEBS Lett.* 1980;**112**:51–4.

98 Freed, L. M., Berkow, S. E., Hamosh, P. *et al.* Lipase in human milk: effect of gestational age and length of lactation on enzyme activity. *J. Am. Coll. Nutr.* 1989;**8**:143–50.

99 Hamosh, M. Enzymes in human milk. In Howell, R. R., Morris, F. H., Pickering, L. K., eds. *Human Milk in Infant Nutrition and Health.* Springfield, IL: Charles C. Thomas; 1986: 66–97.

100 Blackberg, L., Angquist, K. A., Hernell, O. Bile salt stimulated lipase in human milk: evidence for its synthesis in the lactating mammary gland. *FEBS Lett.* 1987;**217**:37–42.

101 Jones, J. B., Mehta, N. R., Hamosh, M. α-Amylase in preterm human milk. *J. Pediatr. Gastroenterol. Nutr.* 1982;**1**:43–8.

102 Pamblanco, M., Ten, A., Conin, J. Bile salt stimulated lipase activity in human colostrum from mothers of infants of different gestational age and birth weight. *Acta Paediatr. Scand.* 1987;**76**:328–31.

103 Freed, L. M., York, C. M., Hamosh, P. *et al.* Bile salt stimulated lipase of human milk: characteristics of the enzyme in the milk of mothers of premature and full-term infants. *J. Pediatr. Gastroenterol. Nutr.* 1987;**6**:598–604.

104 Freed, L. M., Neville, M. C., Hamosh, P. *et al.* Diurnal and within-feed variations in lipase activity and triglyceride content of human milk. *J. Pediatr. Gastroenterol. Nutr.* 1986;**5**: 938–42.

105 Berkow, S., Freed, L. M., Hamosh, M. *et al.* Lipase and lipids in human milk: effects of freeze thawing and storage. *Pediatr. Res.* 1984;**18**:1257–63.

106 Hamosh, M., Henderson, T. R., Ellis, L. A. *et al.* Digestive enzymes in human milk: stability at suboptimal storage temperatures. *J. Pediatr. Gastroenterol. Nutr.* 1997;**24**:38–43.

107 Wang, C. S., Hartstruck, J. A., Downs, D. Kinetics of acylglycerol sequential hydrolysis by human milk bile salt activated lipase and effect of taurocholate as fatty acid acceptor. *Biochemistry* 1988;**27**:4234–40.

108 Hernell, O., Blackberg, L. Digestion of human milk lipids: physiological significance of sn-2 monoacylglycerol hydrolysis by bile salt-stimulated lipase. *Pediatr. Res.* 1982;**16**: 882–5.

109 Signer, E., Murphy, G. M., Edkins, S. *et al.* Role of bile salts in fat malabsorption of premature infants. *Arch. Dis. Child.* 1974;**49**:174–80.

110 Frederikzon, B., Hernell, O., Blackberg, L. *et al.* Bile salt stimulated lipase in human milk: evidence of activity in vivo and of a role in the digestion of milk retinol esters. *Pediatr. Res.* 1978;**12**:1048–52.

111 Hernell, O., Blackberg, L., Chen, O. Does the bile salt stimulated lipase of human milk have a role in the use of the milk long-chain polyunsaturated fatty acids? *J. Pediatr. Gastroenterol. Nutr.* 1993;**16**:425–31.

112 Hernell, O., Gebre-Medhin, M., Olivecrona, T. Breast milk composition in Ethiopian and Swedish mothers. IV. Milk lipase. *Am. J. Clin. Nutr.* 1977;**30**:508–11.

113 Ginder, J., Nwankwo, M. U., Omene, J. A. *et al.* Breast milk composition and bile salt stimulated lipase in well nourished and undernourished Nigerian mothers. *Eur. J. Pediatr.* 1987;**146**:184–6.

114 Dupuy, P., Sauniere, J. F., Vis, H. L. *et al.* Change in bile salt dependent lipase in human breast milk during extended lactation. *Lipids* 1991;**26**:134–8.

115 Hamosh, M. Fatty acids and monoglycerides: anti-infective agents produced during the digestion of milk fat by the newborn. *Adv. Exp. Med. Biol.* 1991;**310**:151–8.

116 Tso, P. Intestinal lipid absorption. In Johnson, L. R., ed. *Physiology of the Gastrointestinal Tract.* New York, NY: Raven Press 1994:1867–907.

117 Levy, E. The 1991 Borden Award Lecture. Selected aspects of intraluminal and intracellular bases of intestinal fat absorption. *Can. J. Physiol. Pharmacol.* 1992;**70**:413–19.

118 Hamilton, J. A. Fatty acid transport: difficult or easy? *J. Lipid Res.* 1998;**29**:467–81.

119 Besnard, P., Niot, I. Role of lipid binding proteins in intestinal absorption of long-chain fatty acids. In Christophe, A. B., De Vries, S., eds. *Fat Digestion and Absorption.* Champaign, IL: AOCS Press; 2000:96–118.

120 Clandinian, M. T., Thomson, A. B. R. Intestinal absorption of lipids: a view toward the millennium. In Christophe, A. B., De Vriese, S., eds. *Fat Digestion and Absorption.* Champaign, IL: AOCS Press; 2000:298–324.

121 Montagnani, M., Aldini, R., Roda, A. *et al.* New insights in the physiology and molecular basis of the intestinal bile acid absorption. *Ital. J. Gastroenterol. Hepatol.* 1998;**30**:435–40.

122 Little, G. M., Lester, R. Ontogenesis of intestinal bile salt absorption in the neonatal rat. *Am. J. Physiol.* 1980;**239**: G319–23.

123 Wong, M. H., Oelkers, P., Craddock, A. L. *et al.* Expression, cloning and characterization of the hamster ileal sodium-dependent bile acid transporter. *J. Biol. Chem.* 1994;**269**: 1340–7.

124 Cristie, D. M., Dawson, P. A., Thevananther, S. *et al.* Comparative analysis of the ontogeny of a sodium-dependent bile acid transporter in rat kidney and ileum. *Am. J. Physiol.* 1996;**271**:G377–83.

125 Schoeller, C., Keelan, M., Mulvey, G. *et al.* Oleic acid uptake into rat and rabbit brush border membrane. *Biochim. Biophys. Acta* 1995;**1236**:51–64.

126 Berk, P. D. How do long-chain fatty acids cross cell membrane? *Proc. Soc. Exp. Biol. Med.* 1996;**212**:1–4.

127 McArthur, M. J., Atshaves, B. P., Frolov, A. *et al.* Cellular uptake and intracellular trafficking of long-chain fatty acids. *J. Lipid Res.* 1999;**40**:1371–83.

128 Bernlohr, D. A., Simpson, M. A., Hertzel, A. V. *et al.* Intracellular lipid-binding proteins and their genes. *Ann. Rev. Nutr.* 1997;**17**:277–303.

129 Ribarik Coe, N., Bernlohr, D. A. Physiological properties of intracellular fatty acid binding proteins. *Biochim. Biophys. Acta* 1998;**1391**:287–306.

130 Boier, L. J., Socchettini, J. C., Knowler, W. C. *et al.* An amino acid substitution in the human intestinal fatty acid binding protein is associated with increased fatty acid binding, increased fat oxidation, and insulin resistance. *J. Clin. Invest.* 1995;**95**: 1281–7.

131 Fujino, T., Kang, M.-J., Suzuki, H. *et al.* Molecular characterization and expression of rat acyl-CoA synthetase. *J. Biol. Chem.* 1996;**271**:16748–52.

132 Knudsen, J., Jensen, M. V., Hansen, J. K. *et al.* Role of acyl-CoA binding protein in acyl CoA transport, metabolism and cell signaling. *Mol. Cell Biochem.* 1999;**192**:95–103.

133 Frolov, A., Schroeder, F. Acyl coenzyme A binding protein. *J. Biol. Chem.* 1998;**273**:11049–55.

134 Lim, M. C. M., Arbeeny, C., Berquist, K. *et al.* Cloning and regulation of hamster microsomal triglyceride transfer protein. *J. Biol. Chem.* 1994;**269**:29138–45.

135 Wettereau, J. R., Aggerbeck, L. P., Bouma, M. E. *et al.* Absence of microsomal triglyceride transfer protein in individuals with abetalipoproteinemia. *Science* 1993;**258**:999–1001.

136 Raabe, M., Veniant, M. M., Sullivan, M. A. *et al.* Analysis of the role of microsomal triglyceride transfer protein in liver of specific knockout mice. *J. Clin. Invest.* 1999;**103**: 1287–98.

137 Hamilton, R. L., Wong, J. S., Cham, C. M. *et al.* Chylomicron-sized lipid particles are formed in the setting of apolipoprotein B deficiency. *J. Lipid Res.* 1998;**49**:1543–57.

138 Patterson, A. P., Tennyson, G. E., Hoegg, J. M. *et al.* Onto-genic regulation of apolipoprotein B mRNA editing during human and rat development in vivo. *Arterioscler. Thromb.* 1992;**12**:468–73.

139 Lehner, R., Kuksis, A. Biosynthesis of triacylglycerols. *Prog. Lipid Res.* 1996;**35**:169–201.

140 Bezard, L., Bugant, M. Absorption of glycerides containing short, medium and long-chain fatty acids. In Kuksis, A., ed. *Fat Absorption, v1.* Boca Raton, FL: CRC Press; 1986:119–58.

141 Yang, L. Y., Kuksis, A., Myher, J. J. *et al.* Absorption of short chain triacylglycerides from butter and coconut oil. *INFORM* 1992;**3**:551.

142 Mansbach, C. M., Arnold, A., Garrett, M. Effect of chloro-quine on intestinal lipid metabolism. *Am. J. Physiol.* 1987;**253**: G673–8.

143 Lehner, R., Cui, Z., Vance, D. E. Subcellular localization, devel-opmental expression and characterization of a liver triacyl-glycerol hydrolase. *Biochem. J.* 1999;**338**:761–8.

144 Spalinger, J. H., Seidman, E. G., Menard, D. *et al.* Endogen-ous lipase activity in Caco-2 cells. *Biochim. Biophys. Acta* 1998;**1393**:119–27.

145 Kuksis, A. Biochemistry of glycerolipids and formation of chy-lomicrons. In Christophe, A. B., DeVriese, S., eds. *Fat Digestion and Absorption.* Champaign, IL: AOCS Press; 2000:119–81.

146 Van Greevenbroek, M. M. J., de Bruin, T. W. A. Chylomicron synthesis by intestinal cells in vitro and in vivo. *Atherosclerosis* 1998;**141**:S9–16.

147 Hoyoshi, H., Fujimoto, K., Cordelli, J. A. *et al.* Fat feeding increases size, but not number of chylomicrons produced by the small intestine. *Am. J. Physiol.* 1990;**259**: G709–19.

24

Minimal enteral nutrition

Josef Neu and Hilton Bernstein

Department of Pediatrics, University of Florida, Gainesville, FL

Introduction

As the field of neonatal intensive care began to emerge in the mid-1960s, efforts were made to save prematurely born babies that were previously thought to be nonviable. Many of these infants were considered to be "too unstable" to feed. They were provided neither enteral feedings nor intravenous glucose, essentially being starved for several days after birth.[1,2] Some investigators recognized that this caused catabolism with subsequent endogenous tissue breakdown and introduced the practice of providing intravenous glucose to sick premature infants, which unsurprisingly reduced catabolism and improved survival.[3] Although we have made progress in the past 40 years, the practice of withholding enteral support to sick infants remains prevalent. The provision of parenteral support with lipids, amino acids, vitamins, minerals, and trace elements likewise, is frequently delayed and/or interrupted for poorly substantiated reasons. As a result, most of these infants experience a significant delay in the growth they would have attained in utero (Figure 24.1).[4] Although many of these individuals catch up in somatic growth to their nonpremature peers over a period of years, it should be recognized that optimum nutrition for the rapidly developing neonate should be aimed at goals beyond simply improved weight gain. The short- and long-term effects of undernutrition during a critical window of susceptibility to several illnesses, as well as the potential for poor neurodevelopment, should not be underestimated.[5,6] Furthermore, poor nutrition during these critical periods could result in chronic health problems, many of which may be more devastating than those seen with in utero growth retardation.[7]

What is the reason behind our slow progress in providing nutritional support to critically ill very low birth weight (VLBW) infants? In the 1970s, along with the aggressive support measures provided to increase survival in premature infants, previously rare diseases began to emerge. The most prominent of these, which led to the practice of withholding enteral nutrition, is necrotizing enterocolitis (NEC). Prior to the development of modern neonatology, this disease was quite rare. Currently, NEC is the most common serious gastrointestinal problem in the neonate and affects approximately 5%–10% of VLBW neonates.[8] Because enteral feeding has been associated with the pathogenesis of NEC, the avoidance of gastrointestinal feedings for prolonged periods, occasionally several weeks after birth, became a prevalent practice. Table 24.1 lists some common "excuses" often given to not provide nutrients by the enteral route because they could predispose to NEC. Although these are all based on credible theoretical considerations, prevention of NEC by avoiding the enteral route completely based on these factors is supported by neither epidemiological nor experimental studies.

On the other hand, over the past two decades, evidence has emerged in animal models and humans that a lack of nutrients in the intestinal lumen results in detrimental effects. These include mucosal atrophy, digestive-absorptive dysfunction, immune deficits, and exacerbation of inflammatory responses that may result in pathology to organs outside the gastrointestinal tract. In addition to their requirement for growth, most of these infants are critically ill. They are at high risk for lung damage, sepsis, neurological injury, and several other pathologic entities associated with inflammation. The

Neonatal Nutrition and Metabolism. Second Edition, ed. P. Thureen and W. Hay. Published by Cambridge University Press.
© Cambridge University Press 2006.

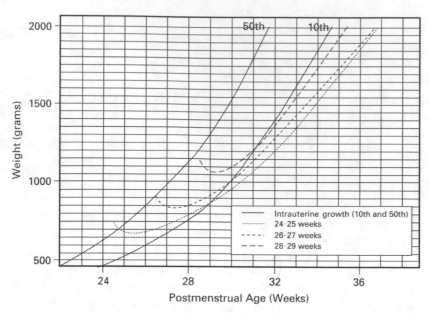

Figure 24.1. Growth deficits in low birthweight infants.[4]

Table 24.1. Excuses to withhold enteral "feedings"

Low Apgar scores
Umbilical catheters
Apnea and bradycardia
Mechanical ventilation
CPAP
Vasoactive drugs

CPAP, continuous positive airway pressure.

underdeveloped gastrointestinal tract lies at the crux of these problems because it is the major immune organ of the body. Thus the amount and composition of what is provided enterally to these infants may fit a model beyond that of mere provision of nutrients but also the inclusion of immuno- and/or pharmaconutrients.

This chapter will focus on potential problems associated with inappropriate use or lack of use of the enteral route for nutrition. The response of the intestine to enteral nutrients in terms of human milk/commercially available formulas, intestinal trophic hormone production, immunonutrients, intestinal growth, adaptation to stress, and mucosal immunity will be discussed. We will also discuss rational approaches to minimal enteral nutrition for the critically ill VLBW infant (VLBWI).

Problems associated with aggressive enteral feeding

Transition from intrauterine to extrauterine enteral nutrition

Not providing enteral nutrition to VLBWI is nonphysiologic when one considers that the fetus swallows about 150 ml kg^{-1} day^{-1} of amniotic fluid during the last trimester of fetal development. This amniotic fluid provides about 0.5 g kg^{-1} day^{-1} of protein, 0.3 g kg^{-1} day^{-1} of carbohydrate and 0.03 g kg^{-1} day^{-1} of lipid.[9] This occurs without the development of NEC in utero. Thus, the presentation of relatively high volumes of physiologic iso-osmolar fluid is nonharmful to the fetal gastrointestinal tract. If similar volumes of full strength human milk or formula could be safely fed to VLBWI shortly after birth, a majority of the infant's nutritional needs could rapidly be met using this route. However, two major variables between intra- and extrauterine life that result in differences in intestinal damage susceptibility are the absence of microbial colonization in the fetus and the concentration and composition of the fluid entering the gastrointestinal tract in prenatal versus postnatal life. In the postnatal environment, the interaction of relatively large volumes of concentrated feedings to an immature intestine in a host who is highly stressed is poorly tolerated. An intestine with poor motility receiving high volumes of food that it is not mature enough to adequately digest and absorb, which is also colonized with pathogenic microorganisms indigenous to neonatal intensive care units, is highly prone to bacterial overgrowth and the NEC-inciting inflammatory cascade. These pathogenic mechanisms are discussed in detail elsewhere.[10]

Fear of NEC and feeding intolerance

As previously mentioned, the fear of NEC is the most prevalent reason provided to withhold enteral feedings in neonates. Although NEC occasionally occurs in infants who have never been fed, it most frequently occurs in premature infants whose enteral intakes are being aggressively increased.[10] Despite one study that suggests sick VLBWI can tolerate greater quantities,[11] other studies suggest that the advancement of enteral feedings at rates greater than 20 kcal $kg^{-1}day^{-1}$ are associated with an increase in the incidence of NEC.[12,13]

Although not quite as dramatic as, but often seen as a precursor to NEC that precludes enteral feedings is "feeding intolerance," a term that has no uniform definition. The manifestations of feeding intolerance vary and are based on pre-feed gastric residual volumes, their color, and associated clinical manifestations including abdominal distension, emesis, the presence of blood in the stool, and apnea and bradycardia. Using the criteria established by Bell et al.,[14] these are similar manifestations to those described for "Stage I NEC," a term that has led to considerable confusion because of its lack of specificity. These signs and symptoms are most commonly due to immaturity of gastric emptying and gastrointestinal motility. Whether these are predictive of serious disease, such as Stage II or III NEC, a delayed ability to achieve full enteral alimentation, or merely a physiologic expectation when feeding VLBWI are issues that still need to be addressed.

Problems associated with the lack of enteral feeding

Several of the problems associated with a lack of nutrients in the lumen of the GI tract are seen in Figure 24.2. Here we will describe these in greater detail.

Loss of mucosal mass

Several studies in animals have demonstrated that lack of enteral feedings and TPN is associated with mucosal atrophy of the gastrointestinal mucosa. Potential dangers of

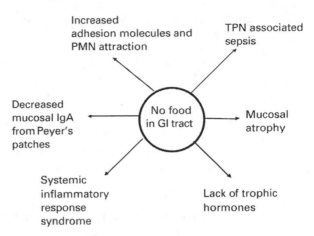

Figure 24.2. Results of no food in gastrointestinal tract.

avoidance of all enteral feedings began to emerge with the early studies of Widdowson,[15,16] who demonstrated in piglets that early enteral feeding was associated with a huge increase in intestinal mucosal mass and that lack of feeding resulted in lack of mucosal growth. Subsequent studies in other species have supported this finding.[17,18] How much enteral feeding is necessary to significantly increase mucosal mass in humans is not known. A study by Burrin et al.[19] examined this question by using a term neonatal piglet model provided with both enteral and parenteral nutrition. These results suggested that an enteral intake of at least 40% of total nutrient intake (based on total needs) is required to increase intestinal mucosal mass. A similar study done in dog pups that were fed through both the enteral and parenteral routes showed that giving 10% of nutrition in the form of enteral feeds increased intestinal motility. However, enteral feeding volumes of greater than 30% of fluid intake (based on total needs) were required to stimulate mucosal growth.[20] Since these studies were done in term, relatively nonstressed animals, it is difficult to extrapolate whether similar quantities of nutrients are required for mucosal growth in human neonates, but it is likely these percentages would represent a minimum needed for mucosal growth in highly stressed, VLBWI. Nevertheless, it is clear that very small quantities of enteral nutrients (in both animal models and human neonates) can induce other significant physiologic effects.

Effect on gastrointestinal hormone secretion

Several studies in term and preterm neonates demonstrated that gastrointestinal hormone increases do not occur if enteral feeding is withheld.[21–24] One study by Lucas *et al.*[23] showed that as little as 12 ml kg^{-1} over 6 days produced significant increases in enteroglucagon, gastrin, and gastric inhibitory polypeptide (GIP) concentrations. Surges in motilin with enteral feedings may improve feeding tolerance by stimulating the appearance of migrating motor complexes and enhancing the flow of nutrients through the intestine.[25] It may also decrease bacterial overgrowth and stasis in the intestine that may contribute to intestinal pathology.[9]

TPN and sepsis

The intestine comprises the largest surface area of the body and is also the largest immune organ of the body. One layer of epithelial cells that is lined by a thin layer of mucous is all that separates the internal milieu of the body from huge quantities of microbes. Although the vast majority of microorganisms are located in the colon and distal small intestine in the healthy individual, there are factors that can increase the bacterial load as well as the type of bacteria in the colon and more proximal small intestine. These include poor motility, the use of pharmacologic agents that inhibit the killing of microorganisms by acid[26] in the upper GI tract and the lack of food-dependent motility-inducing hormonal surges.[21-23]

Total parenteral nutrition is associated with a significant increase in neonatal hospital-acquired sepsis.[27] Many investigators have studied potential mechanisms underlying the septic complications associated with TPN and lack of enteral stimulation. One hypothesis involves bacterial translocation where lack of intraluminal stimulation leads to a loss of integrity of intestinal mucosal defenses, which in turn allows bacterial translocation from the intestinal lumen into the gut lymphatic and blood stream to seed distant sites.[28] Most of this work has been done in rats where a lack of enteral feeding produces a rapid atrophy in the proximal gut mucosa to approximately 50%–60% of normal. Several studies suggest that enteral feedings, especially in the very critically ill patient with severe burns,[29] trauma,[30] and VLBWI[31] are associated with a lower incidence of sepsis. However, the lack of direct evidence linking extra-intestinal infections to luminal bacteria in the human GI tract makes hospital-acquired sepsis due to intestinal bacterial translocation controversial.[32] Other mechanisms such as an increased propensity to inflammation in an immature intestine that is exacerbated by TPN are also likely to play a role.

Effect on intestinal inflammation

The intestinal immune/inflammatory response also appears to be affected significantly by nutrients in the

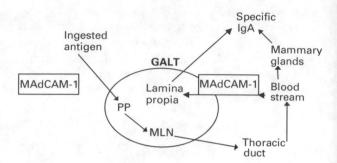

Figure 24.3. The relationship of enteral nutrients to the mucosal immune system. GALT, gut-associated lymphoid tissue; MAdCAM-1, mucosal addressin adhesion molecule-1; PP, Peyer's patches; MLN, mesenteric lymph nodes.

gastrointestinal tract. Figure 24.3 shows a diagram of the gut-associated lymphoid tissue (GALT), which is a major component of the mucosal immune system.[33] The afferent limb of this system consists of Peyer's patches (PP) and mesenteric lymph nodes. Intraluminal antigen is taken up by M cells overlying the PP, processed by antigen-presenting cells that then interact with naïve T and B-lymphocytes which enter the PP via interaction with mucosal addressin adhesion molecule-1 (MAdCAM-1). These sensitized cells are distributed via the thoracic duct drainage and the vascular system to various submucosal locations where they contribute to the efferent limb of the GALT. The lamina propria is one effector site where such activated T and B-lymphocytes accumulate and produce IgA after conversion of the B cells to plasma cells. This IgA, after transport into the lumen by the overlying epithelial cells, prevents adherence of bacteria, viruses, and other toxic molecules to the mucosal surface.

It is known that continued intraluminal antigenic stimulation maintains an immunologic barrier to microbial invasion. In the mouse, lack of enteral feeding for 72 hours quickly leads to a dramatic reduction in PP, lamina propria, and intraepithelial lymphocytes.[34] A mechanism thought to be responsible for this change relates to MAdCAM-1, which directs unsensitized lymphocytes to the Peyer's patches and sensitized lymphocytes to the lamina propria.[35] Within hours of parenteral nutrition alone, PP MAdCAM-1 expression drops but recovers rapidly with enteral refeeding.[36]

Lack of enteral feeding also alters the balance of cytokines controlling lymphocyte maturation. The CD4 : CD8 ratio decreases with a consequent decrease in IL-4 and IL-10. Both IL-4 and IL-10 upregulate IgA production.[37] Studies using mouse models have consistently shown decreases in both intestinal and nasotracheal IgA levels within 3 days of "gut starvation" with TPN.[34,38] Mice intranasally immunized against *Pseudomonas* accumulate antigenic-specific IgA in their respiratory tracts. When immunized animals are challenged with a bacterial load 5 days after initiating a parenteral diet, their mortality rate is over 70% higher than chow-fed animals, comparable to the mortality rate of nonimmunized animals, reflecting a loss in established antibacterial immunity[39] with a lack of enteral feeding.

Effect on vascular inflammatory responses

The alterations in the mucosa-associated immune system associated with lack of enteral nutrition may also contribute to noninfectious mediated multiple organ failure by augmenting inflammatory responses to subsequent stresses. The vascular bed of the GI tract has the capacity to prime polymorphonuclear neutrophils (PMN), which, once activated, respond to subsequent insults by causing further tissue destruction, which may extend beyond the GI tract. This has been especially well documented in the lungs.[40] PMNs are involved in the acute, nonspecific inflammatory response where they adhere to the capillary endothelium, migrate across the endothelial wall and can cause destruction of both invasive microbes and body tissues by releasing destructive enzymes and toxic oxygen radicals. Such tissue destruction can contribute to eventual multiple organ failure.

Lack of enteral feeding and TPN induces priming of PMNs by recruiting PMNs to the GI tract. As previously mentioned, the expression of IL-4 and IL-10 are reduced by TPN.[41,42] These are important inhibitors of intracellular adhesion molecule-1 (ICAM-1) expression. ICAM-1 on endothelial cells binds to the CD11/18 integrins on PMNs. TPN also increases expression of P-selectin in the GI tract and E-selectin in the lungs.[43] These adhesion molecules expressed on the surface of endothelial cells trigger leukocyte rolling along the endothelium of post capillary venules as a precursor to adhesion through CD11/18-ICAM-1 interaction. TPN increases the expression of P-selectin in the GI tract and E-selectin in the lungs.[44] Myeloperoxidase (MPO) becomes elevated because of the accumulation of PMNs associated with increased adhesion molecule expression.[45] Reinstitution of an oral diet returns MPO and ICAM-1 levels back to normal within 4 days.

Thus, even though mucosal atrophy with TPN and lack of enteral feedings has not been clearly demonstrated in humans, enteral feeding initiates intestinal hormonal release, which provides physiologic benefits. The capability of enteral nutrients to upregulate IgA production and downregulate the intestinal inflammatory response may play a major role in protection of not only the intestine, but

Table 24.2. Results from studies of minimal enteral nutrition

Improved feeding tolerance and growth
Less need for phototherapy
Decreased cholestasis
Decreased osteopenia
Gastrointestinal trophic hormone surges
Improved motility
No increase in complications (e.g. necrotizing enterocolitis)

is likely to also benefit other organs such as the lung and brain.

Minimal enteral nutrition

Definition and purpose

As previously mentioned, with the advent of neonatal TPN and problems associated with aggressive enteral feeding, neonatologists began to withhold all enteral feedings during the time the infants were critically ill. In the early 1980s studies by Lucas and colleagues suggested that very small amounts of enteral feedings in premature infants could provide benefits. These were termed "minimal enteral feedings."[21-23] Since these early trials, several additional studies of minimal enteral nutrition have been completed in VLBWI.[24,46-51] Overall, these have shown benefit without adverse consequences (Table 24.2). One problem in interpretation and application of these studies to clinical care in the neonatal intensive care unit is that most used somewhat different techniques of "minimal enteral feedings." Intakes ranged from approximately 1–20 kcal kg^{-1} day^{-1} starting from day 1–7 of life. In order to translate these studies to clinical care, we first need to consider a general definition of minimal enteral nutrition. Studies in both animals and humans suggest that enteral intakes of less than about 20–30 kcal kg^{-1} day^{-1} elicit beneficial changes in the GI tract without providing optimal overall nutrition. The parenteral route provides the remainder of the nutritional needs. Hence, we will define minimal enteral nutrition as relatively small amounts of enteral intakes, usually < 25 ml kg^{-1} day^{-1} (<20 kcal kg^{-1} day^{-1} in the neonate), of human milk or formula, which are not intended to be the primary source of nutrition. They are intended to provide the previously described beneficial physiologic effects that can be derived by having small volumes of food in the intestinal tract.

The use of minimal enteral nutrition should at least partially alleviate the anxiety clinicians have in providing enteral nutrients to critically ill patients. Minimal enteral nutrition provides a safe means to stimulate and maintain digestive-absorptive, immunologic, and neuroendocrine functions of the GI tract, while allowing the parenteral route to provide the major overall route of nutritional support.

Methods of minimal enteral nutrition delivery

Suggested approach

Figure 24.4 shows a generalized schema that provides guidelines for minimal enteral feedings in VLBWI. These guidelines are presented in an attempt to correlate minimal enteral nutrition with physiologic development of the GI tract and to aid in the standardization of feeding methods. One needs to remember that no single method of minimal enteral nutrition delivery has been found to be the most efficacious.

Because of individual characteristics of each patient, specific feeding protocols or guidelines cannot be used for all infants. How quickly should we advance enteral feedings? Clinical judgment based on available scientific data and experience presently appears to be the best criteria upon which we should base our feeding practices. Note that none of the "excuses" in Table 24.1 preclude minimal enteral nutrition in this scheme. There is also no evidence supporting withholding minimal enteral nutrition if the infant has a patent ductus arteriosus or is receiving indomethacin. Most of the available studies utilized minimal enteral feedings for 5–10 days before initiating more aggressive advancement.

The choice of minimal enteral feeding composition is primarily between expressed breast milk and formula. Breast milk compared with formula appears to be advantageous for protection against infection, the development of allergies, and NEC.[52,53] Dilute formula or breast milk does not stimulate GI motor activity as well as full-strength formula or breast milk.[25]

Whether bolus or continuous feeds are advantageous remains controversial. In a study of 171 infants < 30 weeks' gestation, infants randomized to bolus feeding (over 20 minutes) had less feeding intolerance than those on continuous feedings.[51] Another study suggested that intermittent "slow bolus" administration produces a better duodenal motility pattern than "rapid bolus" feedings given over 15 minutes.[54] Nevertheless, most "minimal enteral feeding" regimens involve such small volumes that the bolus versus continuous feeding argument is moot.

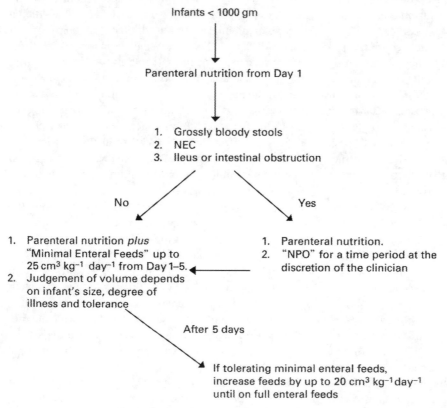

Figure 24.4. Guidelines for minimal enteral nutrition. NEC, necrotizing enterocolitis. NPO, nothing per os (nil by mouth).

Summary

Early minimal enteral nutrition refers to a small enteral intake of $< 25\ \text{ml kg}^{-1}\ \text{day}^{-1}$ (providing about 20 kcal kg^{-1} day^{-1}), either in the form of breast milk or preterm formula, started within the first few days after birth. This has been found to induce trophic hormone release, induce anti-inflammatory changes, promote immunity, and increase intestinal motility. Although many of the studies are limited, these suggest that minimal enteral nutrition is safe and provides several additional benefits including a reduction in the incidence of late-onset sepsis by reducing the period spent receiving parenteral nutrition and therefore the use of IV lines. Minimal enteral nutrition also prevents the colonization of harmful bacteria and allows normal flora to colonize the gut and in this way helps to develop the innate immune system of the GI tract. Although it provides benefits, minimal enteral nutrition combined with parenteral nutrition still does not meet all the requirements of the critically ill VLBW infants. Much still needs to be learned about adjunctive therapies that provide certain individual nutrients or other factors that can be used to prevent both long- and short-term morbidity during the period of time when the infant cannot receive full enteral nutrition.

REFERENCES

1 Cone, T. E. Jr. *History of the Care and Feeding of the Premature Infant.* Boston, MA: Little, Brown; 1985.

2 Brown, E. G., Sweet, A. Y. Neonatal necrotizing enterocolitis. *Pediatr. Clin. N. Am.* 1982;**29**:1149–70.

3 Krauss, A. N., Auld, P. A. Metabolic requirements of low-birth-weight infants. *J. Pediatr.* 1969;**75**:952–6.

4 Ehrenkranz, R. A., Younes, N., Lemons, J. A. *et al.* Longitudinal growth of hospitalized very low birth weight infants. *Pediatrics.* 1999;**104**:280–9.

5 Lucas, A. Programming by early nutrition: an experimental approach. *J. Nutr.* 1998;**128**:401S–6S.

6 Waterland, R. A., Garza, C. Potential mechanisms of metabolic imprinting that lead to chronic disease. *Am. J. Clin. Nutr.* 1999;**69**:179–97.

7 Godfrey, K. M., Barker, D. J. Fetal nutrition and adult disease. *Am. J. Clin. Nutr.* 2000;**71**:1344S–52S.

8 Stoll, B. J. Epidemiology of necrotizing enterocolitis. *Clin. Perinatol.* 1994;**21**:205–18.

9 Abbas, T. M., Tovey, J. E. Proteins of the liquor amnii. *Br. Med. J.* 1960;**5171**:476–9.

10 Neu, J. Necrotizing enterocolitis: the search for a unifying pathogenic theory leading to prevention. *Pediatr. Clin. N. Am.* 1996;**43**:409–32.

11 Rayyis, S. F., Ambalavanan, N., Wright, L., Carlo, W. A. Randomized trial of "slow" versus "fast" feed advancements on the incidence of necrotizing enterocolitis in very low birth weight infants. *J. Pediatr.* 1999;**134**:293–7.

12 Anderson, D. M., Kliegman, R. M. The relationship of neonatal alimentation practices to the occurrence of endemic necrotizing enterocolitis. *Am. J. Perinatol.* 1991;**8**:62–7.

13 Zabielski, P. B., Groh-Wargo, S. L., Moore, J. J. Necrotizing enterocolitis: feeding in endemic and epidemic periods. *J. Parenter. Enteral Nutr.* 1989;**13**:520–4.

14 Bell, M. J., Ternberg, J. L., Feigin, R. D. *et al.* Neonatal necrotizing enterocolitis: therapeutic decisions based upon clinical staging. *Ann. Surg.* 1978;**187**:1–6.

15 Stoddart, R. W., Widdowson, E. M. Changes in the organs of pigs in response to feeding for the first 24 h after birth. III. Fluorescence histochemistry of the carbohydrates of the intestine. *Biol. Neonate* 1976;**29**:18–27.

16 Hall, R. A., Widdowson, E. M. Response of the organs of rabbits to feeding during the first days after birth. *Biol. Neonate.* 1979;**35**:131–9.

17 Berseth, C. L. Effect of early feeding on maturation of the preterm infant's small intestine. *J. Pediatr.* 1992;**120**:947–53.

18 Heird, W. C., Schwarz, S. M., Hansen, I. H. Colostrum-induced enteric mucosal growth in beagle puppies. *Pediatr. Res.* 1984;**18**:512–15.

19 Burrin, D. G., Stoll, B., Jiang, R. *et al.* Minimal enteral nutrient requirements for intestinal growth in neonatal piglets: how much is enough? *Am. J. Clin. Nutr.* 2000;**71**:1603–10.

20 Owens, L., Burrin, D. G., Berseth, C. L. Minimal enteral feeding induces maturation of intestinal motor function but not mucosal growth in neonatal dogs. *J. Nutr.* 2002;**132**:2717–22.

21 Lucas, A., Adrian, T. E., Christofides, N., Bloom, S. R., Aynsley-Green, A. Plasma motilin, gastrin, and enteroglucagon and feeding in the human newborn. *Arch. Dis. Child.* 1980;**55**:673–7.

22 Lucas, A., Bloom, S. R., Aynsley-Green, A. Postnatal surges in plasma gut hormones in term and preterm infants. *Biol. Neonate* 1982;**41**:63–7.

23 Lucas, A., Bloom, S. R., Aynsley-Green, A. Gut hormones and "minimal enteral feeding." *Acta Paediatr. Scand.* 1986;**75**:719–23.

24 Meetze, W. H., Valentine, C., McGuigan, J. E. *et al.* Gastrointestinal priming prior to full enteral nutrition in very low birth weight infants. *J. Pediatr. Gastroenterol. Nutr.* 1992;**15**:163–70.

25 Berseth, C. L., Nordyke, C. Enteral nutrients promote postnatal maturation of intestinal motor activity in preterm infants. *Am. J. Physiol.* 1993;**264**:G1046–51.

26 Beck-Sague, C. M., Azimi, P., Fonseca, S. N. *et al.* Bloodstream infections in neonatal intensive care unit patients: results of a multicenter study. *Pediatr. Infect. Dis. J.* 1994;**13**:1110–16.

27 Sohn, A. H., Garrett, D. O., Sinkowitz-Cochran, R. L. *et al.* Prevalence of nosocomial infections in neonatal intensive care unit patients: results from the first national point-prevalence survey. *J. Pediatr.* 2001;**139**:821–7.

28 Alverdy, J. C., Aoys, E., Moss, G. S. Total parenteral nutrition promotes bacterial translocation from the gut. *Surgery* 1988;**104**:185–90.

29 Mainous, M. R., Block, E. F., Deitch, E. A. Nutritional support of the gut: how and why. *New Horiz.* 1994;**2**:193–201.

30 Alpers, D. H. Enteral feeding and gut atrophy. *Curr. Opin. Clin. Nutr. Metab. Care.* 2002;**5**:679–83.

31 Stoll, B. J., Hansen, N., Fanaroff, A. A. *et al.* Late-onset sepsis in very low birth weight neonates: the experience of the NICHD Neonatal Research Network. *Pediatrics* 2002;**110**:285–91.

32 Lichtman, S. M. Bacterial translocation in humans. *J. Pediatr. Gastroenterol. Nutr.* 2001;**33**:1–10.

33 Kudsk, K. A. Current aspects of mucosal immunology and its influence by nutrition. *Am. J. Surg.* 2002;**183**:390–8.

34 Li, J., Kudsk, K. A., Gocinski, B. *et al.* Effects of parenteral and enteral nutrition on gut-associated lymphoid tissue. *J. Trauma* 1995;**39**:44–52.

35 Streeter, P. R., Berg, E. L., Rouse, B. T., Bargatze, R. F., Butcher, E. C. A tissue-specific endothelial cell molecule involved in lymphocyte homing. *Nature* 1988;**331**:41–6.

36 Fukatsu, K., Zaraur, B. L., Johnson, C. D. *et al.* Decreased MAdCAM-1 expression in Peyer patches: a mechanism for impaired mucosal immunity during lack of enteral nutrition. *Surg. Forum* 2000;**51**:211–14.

37 Lebman, D. A., Coffman, R. L. Cytokines in the mucosal immune system. In Ogra, P. L., ed. *Handbook of mucosal immunology.* San Diego, CA: Academic Press; 1994:243–9.

38 Kudsk, K. A., DeWitt, R. C., Tolley, E. A., Li, J. Route and type of nutrition influence IgA-mediating intestinal cytokines. *Ann. Surg.* 1999;**229**:662–7.

39 King, B. K., Kudsk, K. A., Li, J., Wu, Y., Renegar, K. B. Route and type of nutrition influence mucosal immunity to bacterial pneumonia. *Ann Surg.* 1999;**229**:272–8.

40 Moore, E. E., Moore, F. A., Franciose, R. J. *et al.* The postischemic gut serves as a priming bed for circulating neutrophils that provoke multiple organ failure. *J. Trauma* 1995;**37**:881–7.

41 Fukatsu, K., Kudsk, K. A., Zarzaur, B. L. *et al.* TPN decreases IL-4 and IL-10 mRNA expression in lipopolysaccharide stimulated intestinal lamina propria cells but glutamine supplementation preserves the expression. *Shock* 2001;**15**:318–22.

42 Renkonen, R., Mattila, P., Majuri, M. L., Paavonen, T., Silvennoinen, O. IL-4 decreases IFN-gamma-induced endothelial ICAM-1 expression by a transcriptional mechanism. *Scand. J. Immunol.* 1992;**35**:525–30.

43 Imhof, B. A., Dunon, D. Leukocyte migration and adhesion. *Adv. Immunol.* 1995;**58**:345–416.

44 Fukatsu, K., Lundberg, A. H., Hanna, M. K. *et al.* Increased expression of intestinal P-selectin and pulmonary E-selectin during intravenous total parenteral nutrition. *Arch. Surg.* 2000;**135**:1177–82.

45 Fukatsu, K., Lundberg, A. H., Hanna, M. K. *et al.* Route of nutrition influences intercellular adhesion molecule-1 expression and neutrophil accumulation in intestine. *Arch. Surg.* 1999;**134**:1055–60.

46 Ostertag, S. G., LaGamma, E. F., Reisen, C. E., Ferrentino, F. L. Early enteral feeding does not affect the incidence of necrotizing enterocolitis. *Pediatrics* 1986;**77**:275–80.

47 Slagle, T. A., Gross, S. J. Effect of early low-volume enteral substrate on subsequent feeding tolerance in very low birth weight infants. *J. Pediatr.* 1988;**113**:526–31.

48 Dunn, L., Hulman, S., Weiner, J., Kliegman, R. Beneficial effects of early hypocaloric enteral feeding on neonatal gastrointestinal function: preliminary report of a randomized trial. *J. Pediatr.* 1988;**112**:622–9.

49 Troche, B., Harvey-Wilkes, K., Engle, W. D. *et al.* Early minimal feedings promote growth in critically ill premature infants. *Biol. Neonate.* 1995;**67**:172–81.

50 McClure, R. J., Newell, S. J. Randomised controlled study of clinical outcome following trophic feeding. *Arch. Dis. Child. Fetal Neonatal Ed.* 2000;**82**:F29–33.

51 Schanler, R. J., Shulman, R. J., Lau, C., Smith, E. O., Heitkemper, M. M. Feeding strategies for premature infants: randomized trial of gastrointestinal priming and tube-feeding method. *Pediatrics* 1999;**103**:434–9.

52 Schanler, R. J. The use of human milk for premature infants. *Pediatr. Clin. N. Am.* 2001;**48**:207–19.

53 Lucas, A., Cole, T. J. Breast milk and neonatal necrotising enterocolitis. *Lancet* 1990;**336**:1519–23.

54 Baker, J. H., Berseth, C. L. Duodenal motor responses in preterm infants fed formula with varying concentrations and rates of infusion. *Pediatr. Res.* 1997;**42**:618–22.

25

Milk secretion and composition

Margaret C. Neville[1] and James L. McManaman[2]

[1]Departments of Physiology and Biophysics and
[2]Department of Obstetrics and Gynecology, University of Colorado School of Medicine, Denver, CO 80220

Introduction

The secretion of milk depends on the cellular coordination of a host of synthetic and secretory processes that combine to produce a fluid rich in lipid, carbohydrate, proteins, minerals, vitamins, growth factors, and protective substances. In humans, this fluid is capable of providing the full-term human infant all the nutrients required for the first 4–5 months of life as well as offering significant protection against infectious disease.[1,2] Milk delivery to the infant depends on two separate processes, milk secretion and milk ejection. Milk is secreted more or less continuously by specialized epithelial cells that line the lumina of the breast alveoli (or acini). Prolactin, secreted by the anterior pituitary, is the major hormone that regulates the synthesis and secretion of milk products by mammary alveolar cells.[3] The alveoli are surrounded by myoepithelial cells that contract in response to oxytocin to force the milk out of the alveoli into the milk ducts and thence to the nipple. This process, called the "let-down reflex," is brought about by episodic secretion of oxytocin secreted from the posterior pituitary. To make clear how these processes work, in this article the anatomy of the secretory apparatus will be described, followed by a brief description of human milk composition and a discussion of the mechanisms and regulation of both secretion and let-down. We will then summarize the initiation of lactation, a process that requires a series of carefully programmed functional changes in the breast that take place during the first week postpartum and transform a prepared, but nonsecretory gland, into a fully functioning organ. Most lactation problems arise during this period. Additional information on the hormonal regulation of mammary development and lactation can be found in an excellent on-line chapter by Wysolmerski and Van Houten.[4] The protective elements of human milk are well summarized in the chapter by Schanler in this volume.[5]

The anatomy of the breast

The lobes of the breast, shown in historic nineteenth century images by the renowned British surgeon, Sir Astley Cooper, in Figure 25.1. are formed from a tubulo-alveolar parenchyma embedded in a connective and adipose tissue stroma. Unlike many mammals, in which a single collecting duct brings the milk to the nipple, in humans 10–15 branching ducts each lead to a tree-like pattern of secondary ducts that extend to the edges of a specialized fat pad on the anterior wall of the thorax. These lobules comprise a duct with a small number of branching ductules terminating in acini that will become the milk secreting unit (Figures 25.1B and 25.1C). The stylized diagram of the milk secreting unit is shown in Figure 25.1C. The epithelial cell layer responsible for milk secretion is shown surrounded by supporting structures that include the contractile myoepithelial cells responsible for milk ejection and a connective tissue stroma composed of connective tissue, a large bed of adipocytes, and a copious blood supply. Plasma cells that collect in the interstitial space during lactation are responsible for the secretion of immunoglobulins into milk.

Milk composition

Milk is a complex fluid composed of several phases that can be separated by centrifugation.[7] With short-term low-speed centrifugation, membrane-bound globules (the

Neonatal Nutrition and Metabolism. Second Edition, ed. P. Thureen and W. Hay. Published by Cambridge University Press.

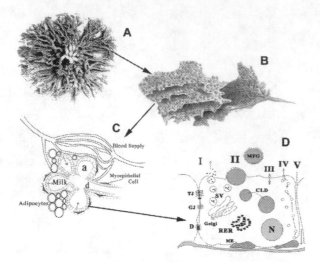

Figure 25.1. The anatomy of the milk-secreting organ. A. Wax-injected breast shows lobes with ducts terminating at the nipple.[91] B. Single lobe of a wax injected breast from a pregnant woman showing acinar clusters, the site of milk secretion, and the ducts leading to the nipple. Milk must be ejected from the acini to the collecting duct to arrive at the nipple for the suckling infant.[91] C. Diagram of the alveolus (a) showing the duct (d), the myoepithelial cells that contract to expel milk and the surrounding adipocytes and blood supply. D. Cartoon of a mammary alveolar cell showing the five pathways (I–V) for the secretion of milk components. Tj, tight junctions; GJ, gap junctions; D, desmosome; ME, myoepithelial cell process; RER, rough endoplasmic reticulum; SV, secretory vesicle containing casein micells; CLD, cytoplasmic lipid droplet; N, nucleus; MFG, milk fat droplet in the lumen of the gland. Redrawn with permission.[92]

milk fat globules) containing the milk lipids rise to the surface where they form the "cream" layer overlying the skim milk. In human and cow's milk the fat accounts for about 4% of milk volume[8] and also contains such milk components as cholesterol, phospholipids, steroid hormones, etc. Cellular components, mostly sloughed epithelial cells, macrophages, neutrophils, and lymphocytes account for a very small fraction of the total milk volume. Casein micelles form a separate phase that can be pelleted by high speed centrifugation or acidification. The aqueous fraction of milk, often called whey, is a true solution that contains all the milk sugar as well as the major milk proteins lactoferrin, α-lactalbumin, and secretory immunoglobulin A (sIgA), the monovalent ions sodium, potassium, and chloride, citrate, calcium, free phosphate and most of the water-soluble minor components of milk. The casein fraction from cow's milk, usually obtained by rennin precipitation, is used in cheese-making while the whey finds a multiplicity of uses, most notably as the base for infant formula.

Table 25.1. Comparison of the macronutrient contents of human and bovine milk[89]

Component	Human milk	Bovine milk
Carbohydrates		
Lactose	$7.3\,\mathrm{g/dL^{-1}}$	$4.0\,\mathrm{g/dL^{-1}}$
Oligosaccharides	$1.2\,\mathrm{g/dL^{-1}}$	$0.1\,\mathrm{g/dL^{-1}}$
Proteins		
Caseins	$0.2\,\mathrm{g/dL^{-1}}$	$2.6\,\mathrm{g/dL^{-1}}$
α-lactalbumin	$0.2\,\mathrm{g/dL^{-1}}$	$0.2\,\mathrm{g/dL^{-1}}$
Lactoferrin	$0.2\,\mathrm{g/dL^{-1}}$	trace
Secretory IgA	$0.2\,\mathrm{g/dL^{-1}}$	trace
β-lactoglobulin	0	$0.5\,\mathrm{g/dL^{-1}}$
Milk lipids		
Triglycerides	4.0%	4.0%
Phospholipids	0.04%	0.04%
Minerals and other ionic constituents		
Sodium	5.0 mM	15 mM
Potassium	15.0 mM	43 mM
Chloride	15.0 mM	24 mM
Calcium	7.5 mM	30 mM
Magnesium	1.4 mM	5 mM
Phosphate	1.8 mM	11 mM
Bicarbonate	6.0 mM	5 mM

The composition of mature human milk is fairly constant, varying only slightly for most components with stage of lactation and, for some constituents such as fatty acids, somewhat more with diet.[9] A few milk components such as the B vitamins[10] and selenium[11] are profoundly affected by diet. In general, sufficient milk of adequate composition is available to the infant even in periods of inadequate food intake by the mother. In species where lactation uses substantial body reserves, such as rodents and dairy cows, dietary restriction does alter milk production, so that, in this respect, these species are not good models for human lactation.

The major macronutrients in milk are the sugar, lactose – a disaccharide unique to milk, milk fat – mainly in the form of triglyceride, proteins including casein, lactoferrin, secretory immunoglobulin A (sIgA), α-lactalbumin, and many others present at lower concentration, and minerals including sodium, potassium, chloride, calcium, and magnesium. The secretion mechanisms for most of these components are well understood. The function and secretion mechanism of many minor components including enzymes, vitamins, oligosaccharides, trace elements, and growth factors are less well-understood. The concentrations of the major components of human milk are compared with bovine milk in Table 25.1.

Cellular mechanisms for milk synthesis and secretion

Solutes enter milk through both transcellular and paracellular routes that can be divided into five general pathways as shown in the cartoon of a lactating mammary alveolar cell in Figure 25.1D. Most of the components of the aqueous fraction of milk including casein, α-lactalbumin, lactoferrin, lactose, oligosaccharides, citrate, phosphate, and calcium are secreted via an exocytotic pathway (pathway I) similar to exocytotic secretory pathways found in other types of cells.[12,13] Lipids are secreted by a pathway unique to the mammary epithelium (Pathway II).[14] Fat droplets consisting largely of triglycerides surrounded by coat proteins are synthesized in the mammary alveolar cell and transported to the apical pole of the cell where they are secreted as membrane enveloped structures called milk fat globules (MFG). The transcytotic pathway (pathway III) transports a wide range of macromolecular substances derived from serum or stromal cells, including serum proteins such as immunoglobulins and albumin,[6,15] protein hormones such as insulin and prolactin,[15,16] and stromal derived agents such as IgA, cytokines, and lipoprotein lipase.[16] In addition, various membrane transport pathways (pathway IV) exist for the transfer of ions and small molecules, such as glucose and amino acids, and water.[18] Finally, a paracellular pathway (V) provides a direct route for entry of serum and interstitial substances into milk.[19] Transport through these pathways is affected by the functional state of the mammary gland and regulated by direct and indirect actions of hormones and growth factors. The compounds secreted by these various pathways as well as certain aspects of their secretion are summarized next.

Exocytosis

Pathway I (Figure 25.1D), like the exocytotic pathway in all cells, ultimately begins in the nucleus with the synthesis of mRNA molecules specific for milk proteins. The mature mRNA serve as templates for protein synthesis. The protein molecules are transported into the endoplasmic reticulum where they are folded and transported through the Golgi system to take part in secretory vesicle formation. Secretory vesicles move continuously to the apical membrane where they discharge their contents into the alveolar lumen by exocytosis.

A number of specialized reactions take place in the Golgi compartment utilizing proteins synthesized as described above. An important reaction is the synthesis of lactose.[20] The enzyme β-galactosidase with α-lactalbumin acting as a cofactor adds glucose to UDP-galactose both of which have entered from the cytoplasm using specific transporters.[21,22] As lactose accumulates, water is drawn into the Golgi vesicles, which take on the swollen appearance characteristic of the lactating mammary cell. Casein micelle formation begins in the terminal Golgi with condensation of casein molecules, which are simultaneously phosphorylated.[23] Addition of calcium, possibly in the secretory vesicle, leads to maturation of the casein micelles into particles sufficiently dense to be seen in the electron microscope. This particle thus delivers an efficient package of protein, calcium, and phosphate that provides the nutrients necessary for bone growth, among other things. The difference in casein content between human and bovine milk, 0.2 v. 2.6 g dL^{-1} undoubtedly reflects the different needs of the relatively slow-growing human infant compared with the rapidly growing calf.

Lipid synthesis and secretion

Milk lipid is an important source of both calories and essential fatty acids to the newborn.[14,24] It is synthesized and secreted by a unique process that puts the lactating mammary gland among the most active triglyceride synthesizing organs. The fatty acids for triglyceride synthesis are synthesized within the gland from glucose or derived from plasma triglycerides or nonesterified fatty acids (NEFA) (Figure 25.2). For endogenous fatty acid synthesis glucose enters the mammary alveolar cell via a glucose transporter. It passes through the glycolytic chain to be converted through a number of steps to malonyl CoA which is then utilized by fatty acid synthase to produce fatty acids.[25] The chain length of the fatty acids in the mammary gland is controlled by a special enzyme, thioesterase II, which terminates fatty acid synthesis at 12, 14, or 16 carbons to produce medium chain saturated triglycerides.[26,27] Plasma triglycerides in the form of chylomicrons or very low density lipoproteins (VLDL) are broken down by lipoprotein lipase in the capillary to glycerol and fatty acids for transport into the cell. In the fasting state the concentration of nonesterified fatty acids (NEFA) rises considerably allowing transfer of lipid from body stores through the plasma bound to albumin and thence to the alveolar cell.[24] These substrate transfers have been best studied in the lactating goat[28] although studies in women using stable isotopes are also available.[29] Once available in the mammary alveolar cells fatty acids are activated by combination with Coenzyme A and joined with glycerol-3-phosphate to form triglycerides.

In the fully lactating woman secreting 800 ml of milk containing 4% fat per day, the mammary gland synthesizes about 32 g of triglyceride daily or nearly 6 kg, 10% of the

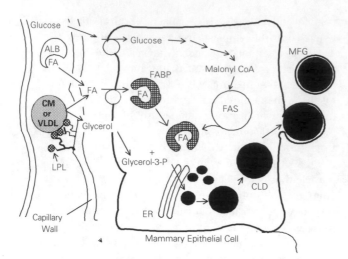

Figure 25.2. Lipid synthesis in the mammary epithelial cell. Fatty acids (FA), held by fatty acid binding protein (FABP), combine with glycerol-3-phosphate in the endoplasmic reticulum (ER) to form the triglycerides that make up the cytoplasmic lipid droplets (CLD). These droplets move to the apical membrane of the cell where they are engulfed in plasma membrane and budded into the lumen as the milk fat globule (MFG). Fatty acids are either synthesized in the alveolar cell from glucose or taken up from the plasma. Free fatty acids arrive in the capillary lumen bound to albumin and can be taken up directly into the cell. Triglycerides arrive either in the form of chylomicra (CM) from the intestine or VLDL from the liver. They are hydrolyzed by lipoprotein lipase bound to the capillary wall and the resulting fatty acids and glycerol are taken up to be re-esterified in the cell. Modified with permission.[24]

weight of the woman, in a typical 6-month lactation. There is a considerable diversity in the fatty acid composition of milk triglycerides (Table 25.2), for which a number of factors are responsible. The proportion of medium chain (C_{8-14}) fatty acids is defined both by species and diet, with humans having 15%–35%.[8,24] Medium chain fatty acids are synthesized only in the mammary gland using glucose (or acetate in ruminants) as substrate. Synthesis of this class of fatty acids varies with the lipid content of the diet.[30] For example, the milks of Nigerian women who have a high carbohydrate diet contain significantly more lauric and myristic acid. In Western women up to 85% of the fatty acids in milk are derived from dietary lipid or fat depots.[31,32] While long chain fatty acids (C_{16} and above) can be synthesized in the mammary gland, they also enter the alveolar cell from the plasma and can be derived either from the diet in the fed state or lipid stores in the fasting state. In ruminants[33] and mice,[34] and presumably humans, the mammary alveolar cell contains a 9 desaturase that converts 18:0 (stearic acid) and other unsaturated fatty acids to 18:1 (oleic acid) and

other mono-unsaturated fatty acids. Polyunsaturated fatty acids (PUFA) and the long chain polyunsaturated fatty acids (LC-PUFA), thought to be extremely important in neural development in the neonate,[35,36] are found at relatively high concentrations in human milk (Table 25.2; compare human and cow's milk). Although human mammary cells possess the elongases and desaturases necessary for the synthesis of LC-PUFA,[37] it is not clear how much is synthesized in the mammary epithelium and how much in the liver. These fatty acids can also originate in the diet as shown by a comparison of the T-3 fatty acids in the milks of Western women and Nigerian women in Table 25.2. The latter have a diet high in fish oils, an important source of T-3 fatty acids.

The mechanism for fat secretion by the mammary gland is not duplicated in any other organ.[14] Triglycerides coalesce into cytoplasmic lipid droplets (CLD) that travel to the apex of the cell where they bulge against the membrane and are finally budded off as membrane bound lipid droplets known as milk fat globules (MFG).

Transport of small molecules across the apical membrane

In contrast to the other pathways for milk secretion, the pathways for the direct transport of substances across the apical membrane of the mammary alveolar cell are poorly understood (Pathway III, Figure 25.2).[18] Linzell and Peaker[12] devised a clever technique to determine what molecules could utilize this pathway, infusing isotopes of small molecules up the teat of a goat and calculating how much of the substance left the milk and entered the blood. They found that sodium, potassium, chloride, and certain monosaccharides as well as water directly permeated this membrane but calcium, phosphate, and citrate did not. Although the mechanisms are not understood it is clear that apical membrane transport pathways are limited to a modest number of small molecules that also include glucose and possibly amino acids.

Transcytosis of interstitial molecules

Intact proteins in the interstitial space can cross the mammary epithelium in two possible ways: by transcytosis and through the paracellular pathway. Since the paracellular pathway is closed during lactation, plasma proteins must enter milk via transcytosis (Pathway IV, Figure 25.3).[15] The best-studied molecule in this regard is immunoglobulin A (IgA).[6] IgA is synthesized by plasma cells in the interstitial spaces of the mammary gland or elsewhere in the body. It has been shown to bind to receptors on the basal surface

Table 25.2. Major fatty acids of human and bovine milks (wt%)

Fatty acid		Human milk		Bovine milk
		western diet[a]	low fat diet[b]	
Saturated fatty acids				
Intermediate and medium chain (formed in mammary gland)				
8:0	Octanoic acid	0.46	–	1.3
10:0	Decanoic acid	1.03	0.54	2.7
12:0	Lauric acid	4.40	8.34	3.0
14:0	Myristic acid	6.27	9.57	10.6
Long chain				
16:0	Palmitic acid	22.00	23.35	28.2
18:0	Stearic acid	8.06	10.15	12.6
Mono-unsaturated fatty acids (MUFA)				
16:1 n-7 (cis)	Palmitoleic acid	3.29	0.91	1.6
18:1 n-9 (cis)	Oleic acid	31.30	18.52	21.4
Polyunsaturated fatty acids (PUFA) (essential fatty acids)				
18:2 n-6	Linoleic acid	10.76	11.06	2.9
18:3 n-3	Linolenic acid	0.81	1.41	0.3
Long chain PUFA (n-6)				
18:3 n-6	-linolenic acid	0.16	0.12	2.9
20:2 n-6		0.34	0.26	0.03
20:3 n-6	Dihomo--Linolenic acid	0.26	0.49	0.10
20:4 n-6	Arachidonic acid	0.36	0.82	0.2
Long chain PUFA (n-3)				
20:5 n-3	Eicosapentaenoic acid	0.04	0.48	0.08
22:5 n-3		0.17	0.39	NA
22:6 n-3	Docosahexaenoic acid	0.22	0.93	0.09

[a] Data from ref.[90]

[b] Data from Nigerian women who also had a diet high in fish, as reflected in the n-3 LC-PUFA.

of the mammary alveolar cell; the entire IgA-receptor complex is endocytosed and transferred to the apical membrane where the extracellular portion of the receptor is cleaved and secreted together with the IgA. The cleaved receptor portion is known as the secretory component and the secreted product is thus secretory IgA or sIgA. The many proteins, hormones, and growth factors that find their way into milk from the plasma are also thought to be secreted by a similar, but much less well-studied, mechanism. Among these molecules are serum albumin, insulin, prolactin, IGF-1, and probably any molecule that enters the interstitial space.

The role of the paracellular pathway in milk secretion

Pathway V (Figure 25.1D) involves passage of substances between epithelial cells, rather than through them, and for this reason is designated the paracellular pathway. During full lactation the passage of even small molecular weight substances between alveolar cells is impeded by a gasket-like structure called the tight junction that joins the epithelial cells tightly, one to another.[38] Although immune cells apparently can pass between epithelial cells to reach the milk,[39] the junctions seal tightly behind them leaving no permanent gap. During pregnancy, with mastitis and after involution the tight junctions become leaky and allow components of the interstitial space to pass unimpeded into the milk. At the same time milk components can enter the plasma. This leakiness is useful during pregnancy since the products of prepartum secretion are allowed to leave the gland. During mastitis inflammatory cells can enter the alveolar space to attack pathogens. Opening of the junctions during involution may reflect loss of epithelial cells. When the junctions are open the mammary secretion has a high concentration of sodium and chloride, a fact that is sometimes useful in diagnosing breast-feeding problems.[40]

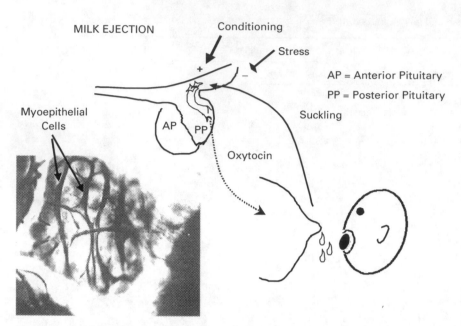

Figure 25.3. Milk ejection is a conditioned neuroendocrine reflex. Sucking sends an afferent impulse to the central nervous system that stimulates neurons in the hypothalamus whose axon processes course to the posterior pituitary. Oxytocin is coordinately released by these neurons into the blood stream where it travels to the myoepithelial cells that surround the mammary alveolus. Contraction of these cells leads to milk expulsion. Inset: A mammary alveolus from a goat, stained to show the basket-work of myoepithelial cells that contract to force out the milk.[57] AP, anterior pituitary; PP, posterior pituitary.

The regulation of milk synthesis, secretion, and ejection

Milk is synthesized and secreted continuously into the alveolar lumen where it is stored until milk removal from the breast is initiated. This means that two levels of regulation must exist: regulation of the rate of synthesis and secretion and regulation of milk ejection. Although both processes ultimately depend on sucking by the infant or other stimulation of the nipple, the mechanisms involved, both central and local, are very different. Prolactin mediates the central nervous system regulation of milk synthesis and secretion, but its influence is greatly modified by local factors that depend on milk removal from the breast. Oxytocin, the stimulus for the let-down reflex on the other hand, is the effector in a neuroendocrine reflex, activating contraction of the myoepithelial cells that surround the alveoli and ducts. When these cells contract, milk is forced out of the alveoli to the nipple, becoming available to the suckling infant. If the letdown reflex is inhibited, milk cannot be removed from the breast and local mechanisms lead to inhibition of milk synthesis and secretion, as will be explained in more detail below.

Milk volume production in lactating women

A meta-analysis of the mean volume of milk secreted by women exclusively breast-feeding a single infant at 6 months postpartum was remarkably constant at about 800 mL day^{-1} in populations throughout the world.[7] However, this figure in no way represents the maximal capacity of the breast to secrete milk. Mothers of twins, and occasionally even triplets, are able to produce volumes of milk sufficient for complete nutrition of their multiple infants.[41] Studies of wet nurses, completed in the 1930s, show that at least some women are capable of producing up to 3.5 liters of milk per day.[42] Women with very low body fat secrete milk with a lower lipid content resulting in a decrease in caloric density of up to 15%.[43] Surprisingly, milk volume is increased 5%–15% in such women so that caloric intake by their infants remains constant. It is thought that the mechanism involves increased sucking by the infant resulting in increased emptying of the breast, which, in turn, brings about increased milk production. On the other hand, if infants are supplemented with foods other than breastmilk, milk secretion is proportionately reduced. For example, in countries like Peru and the Gambia where infants are customarily supplemented with small amounts of food at mealtimes, but given several breast-feeds a day, the daily milk production remains at about 600 mL day^{-1} for 12 months or longer.[44–46] These observations all illustrate the important principle that the volume of milk secretion in lactating women is regulated by infant demand.

Prolactin secretion in lactating women

Prolactin is secreted episodically with peaks of up to 75 minutes in duration that occur 7–20 times a day.[47] For this reason, accurate measurement requires frequent sampling intervals, as close as 15–20 minutes. The prolactin peaks appear to be superimposed upon a continuous background level of secretion whose magnitude depends on the physiological condition.[48] During pregnancy serum prolactin levels increase steadily from about 10 ng mL^{-1} in the prepregnant state to about 200 ng mL^{-1} at term.[49] After parturition the basal prolactin levels decrease, returning to prepregnancy values at 2–3 weeks in the woman who is not breast-feeding.[50] In the lactating woman suckling usually leads to a rapid rise in prolactin secretion.[51] The rise is greatest in the immediate postpartum period increasing as much as 150 ng mL^{-1} above the basal level; the rise is much less apparent after 6 months, amounting to only 5–10 ng mL^{-1}. The prolactin rise induced by suckling is dependent on activity of the afferent innervation of the nipple as demonstrated by the fact that it is inhibited by application of Xylocaine or surgical intervention.[52] The prolactin rise was doubled when two infants were put to the breast simultaneously,[52] suggesting that prolactin release is directly related to the intensity of nipple stimulation.

Despite the fact that plasma prolactin is related to the suckling stimulus, it is unlikely that plasma prolactin concentration directly controls the volume of milk produced. Although prolactin levels are consistently above basal values for the duration of lactation,[53] they are not proportional to milk volume secretion. Thus, while prolactin is necessary for milk synthesis and secretion and probably for alveolar cell survival, plasma prolactin concentrations do not directly regulate milk synthesis and secretion. This function is thought to reside in local regulatory mechanisms.

Local regulation of milk volume production

Two local mechanisms have been implicated in the regulation of milk volume production. Peaker and Wilde[54] have summarized the extensive evidence for the existence of a feedback inhibitor of lactation in milk (FIL). This factor is thought to build up as milk accumulates in the lumen of the mammary gland and inhibits milk secretion. The other candidate for local regulation is stretching of the alveoli. Indirect evidence suggests that stretch of mammary alveolar cells alters their capacity to secrete milk.[55,56] Understanding this regulation may be very important in helping women to increase their milk supply, particularly in the postpartum period and, therefore, increased research is badly needed.

Oxytocin and milk ejection

Milk removal from the breast is accomplished by the let-down reflex, a coordinated contraction of myoepithelial cells whose processes form a basket-like network around the alveoli where milk is stored (Figure 25.3, inset).[57] When the infant is suckled, afferent impulses from sensory stimulation of nerve terminals in the areolus travel to the central nervous system where they promote the release of oxytocin from the posterior pituitary. This neuroendocrine reflex can be conditioned, and in the woman oxytocin release is often associated with such stimuli as the sight or sound, or even the thought, of the infant. The oxytocin is carried through the blood-stream to the mammary gland, where it interacts with specific receptors on myoepithelial cells, initiating their contraction and expelling milk from the alveoli into the ducts and sub-areolar sinuses. The passage of milk through the ducts is facilitated by longitudinally arranged myoepithelial cell processes whose contraction shortens and widens the ducts, allowing free flow of milk to the nipple. To reiterate, this process is essential to milk removal from the lactating breast.

During correct suckling the nipple and much of the areola are drawn well into the mouth so that a long teat reaching nearly to the infant's soft palate is formed.[58] The terminal ducts extend into this teat where milk is removed, not so much by suction, as by the stripping motion of the tongue again the hard palate. This motion carries milk through the teat into the baby's mouth. The large ducts continue to fill as the continued action of oxytocin forces milk from the alveoli into the ducts.

Newton and Newton showed in 1948 that psychological stress or pain decreased milk output.[59] Recently the basis for this finding was shown by Aono and colleagues[60] to be inhibition of oxytocin release. In relaxed, undisturbed women suckling their infants oxytocin release begins with the onset of suckling, or even prior to suckling,[53] when the infant cries or becomes restless. When the suckling women were asked to carry out difficult mental calculations while nursing the infant or fed traffic noise through earphones the number of oxytocin pulses was significantly reduced.

The prolactin response to suckling was not impaired by the psychological stress.

Ethyl alcohol is a potent inhibitor of oxytocin release. Chronic ethanol ingestion by lactating rats led to both a decrease in milk production and a change in milk composition, with decreased lactose and increased lipid content.[61] An elegant, early study in women in which intramammary pressure was measured in response to suckling by the infant demonstrated that ethanol inhibited milk ejection in a dose-dependent manner.[62] In this study Cobo found that doses of alcohol up to 0.45 g kg^{-1}, doses that produce a blood level less than 0.1%, had no effect on intramammary pressure.

Initiation of lactation

The initiation of lactation or lactogenesis has two stages:
1. Secretory differentiation. This phase, sometimes called lactogenesis 1, takes place in the last half of pregnancy when the breast develops the capacity to secrete milk components. Secretion is held in check by the high circulating concentrations of progesterone. Regulation of this stage is complex and poorly understood. The interested reader is referred to a recent review on the subject.[3]
2. Secretory activation, the onset of copious milk secretion. This phase, sometimes called lactogenesis 2, normally takes place during the first 5 days postpartum. It is characterized by a substantial increase in milk volume starting on day 2 or 3 after parturition and is accompanied by a set of carefully programmed changes in milk composition that lead, after 4 days, to a mammary secretion product with a composition close to that of mature milk.[63]

Milk transfer to the infant during secretory activation

Figure 25.4 A shows the individual rates of milk transfer to the infant during the first 8 days postpartum in 11 multiparous middle-class Caucasian women who weighed their infants before and after every feed.[64] Although there is considerable variation between individuals the general pattern emerges when the average milk transfer is plotted (Figure 25.4B). Milk transfer, originally between 0 and 200 mL per day, began to increase about 36 hours postpartum, continued dramatically upward for about 48 hours and then leveled off after about 4 days at volumes between 400 and 800 mL per day. By 1 month postpartum mean infant intake was 770 mL (range 495–1144). A similar pattern has been observed in other careful studies of

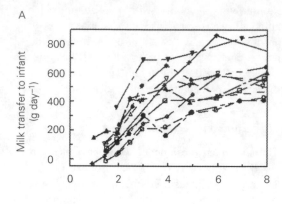

A

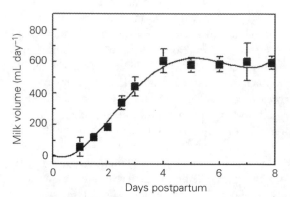

B

Figure 25.4. Initiation of lactation. A. Eleven multiparous women weighed their infants before and after every feed for 7–8 days postpartum. Milk output was averaged by 0.5 day intervals for the first 3 days and then daily for the remainder of the experiment. All women had successfully breast-fed at least one previous infant. Note the extensive variation in the volumes of milk produced. All these women breast-fed successfully for at least 6 months. B. Mean output in the women shown in A.[64] Graphs used with permission.[93]

disease-free women delivering term infants by the vaginal route.[64–66]

Changes in milk composition

Figure 25.5 shows the changes in the concentrations of certain milk components over the same time interval. Sodium and chloride concentrations begin to decline immediately after birth accompanied by an increase in the lactose concentration (Figure 25.2A). These modifications were largely complete by 72 hours postpartum and are consistent with changes seen by others.[67,68] They preceded the onset of the increase in milk volume by at least 24 hours and can be explained by closure of the tight junctions that block the

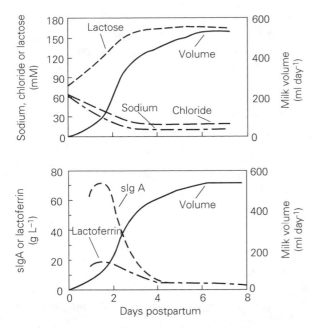

Figure 25.5. Changes in milk composition during the first week postpartum. A. Time course of changes in the lactose, chloride, and sodium concentrations contrasted with the mean milk volume transfer to the infant.[88] Changes in these milk components begin immediately postpartum and are complete at least 24 hours prior to the achievement of a steady state in milk volume. As described in the text, the decrease in sodium and chloride and increase in lactose concentration reflect closure of the tight junctions between the mammary epithelial cells. B. Changes in the concentration of secretory IgA and lactoferrin during the onset of lactation in women.[69] Figure modified with permission.[94]

paracellular pathway. With closure of the tight junctions, lactose, made by the epithelial cells, can no longer pass between the epithelial cells into the plasma, and sodium and chloride can no longer pass from the interstitial space into the lumen of the mammary alveolus and must be secreted by the cellular route (Figure 25.1D).

The next changes to occur are increases in the concentrations of sIgA and lactoferrin.[69] These two important protective proteins remain high for the first 48 hours after birth, the two together comprising as much as 10% by weight of the milk (Figure 25.5B). Their concentrations fall rapidly after day 2, both as a consequence of dilution as milk volume secretion increases and of an actual decrease in the rate of secretion, particularly of immunoglobulins (inset). By 8 days postpartum these protective proteins together make up less than 1% of the total weight of the milk; however, the secretion rate is still substantial, amounting to 2–3 g day^{-1} for each protein. Concentrations of

oligosaccharides in milk are also high in the early secretion product of the mammary gland – about 20 g L^{-1} or 2% of milk weight on day 4,[70] falling significantly to a level of about 14 g L^{-1} on day 30. These complex sugars are also considered to have substantial protective effect against a variety of infections.[71]

Finally, at about 36 hours postpartum milk secretion began in earnest in these multiparous women who initiated breast feeding on the first day after birth and a 10-fold increase in volume from about 50 mL day^{-1} to 500–600 mL day^{-1} occurred over the subsequent 36 hours (Figure 25.4). This volume increase is perceived by the parturient woman as the "coming in" of the milk and reflects a massive increase in the rates of synthesis and/or secretion of almost all the components of mature milk including but not limited to lactose, protein (mainly casein),[72] lipid, calcium, sodium, magnesium, citrate, glucose, and free phosphate.

In a recent study by Chen et al.,[72] milk volumes of primiparous women delivering both vaginally and by Cesarean section were determined only on day 5, the onset of casein secretion was determined by daily measurements, and the time at which milk was observed to "come in" was also noted. In these women milk volumes on day 5 were significantly greater in multiparous women and signs of copious milk secretion appeared somewhat earlier.

Hormonal requirements

With respect to the breast the hormones of pregnancy have a dual job: to maintain and promote the pregnancy and produce a developed mammary epithelium that is poised to secrete milk, but does not do so. From animal studies it has now become clear that both progesterone[73] and prolactin[74] (or possibly its congener, placental lactogen) are involved in alveolar development. Further, it has been clear for nearly three decades that the major inhibitor of milk production during pregnancy is progesterone.[75] A developed mammary epithelium, the continuing presence of levels of prolactin near 200 ng mL^{-1} and a fall in progesterone are necessary for the onset of copious milk secretion following parturition. In humans, removal of the placenta, the source of progesterone during pregnancy in this species, has long been known to be necessary for the initiation of milk secretion.[76] Further, retained placental fragments with the potential to secrete progesterone were reported to delay milk secretion in humans.[77] The conundrum that progesterone does not inhibit established lactation was solved when Haslam and Shyamala showed that progesterone receptors are lost in lactating mammary tissues.[78] Bromocriptine and other analogs of dopamine, drugs that effectively prevent prolactin secretion, inhibit secretory activation when given in appropriate doses (reviewed elsewhere[79]).

In all in vitro mammary systems, insulin and corticoids, in addition to prolactin, are necessary to maintain synthesis of milk components.[80] Further, cortisol replacement is required for maintenance of milk production in adrenalectomized animals.[81,82] An early notion that a surge of glucocorticoids is the initiator of lactogenesis is likely to be incorrect since the rise in cortisol seen in unanesthetized women associated with the stress of labor is over by the time that milk volume begins to increase to any extent. Further increased cortisol, particularly in cord blood, was associated with a delay in lactogenic markers.[72] Because lactogenesis proceeds at parturition in severely diabetic rats,[83] a role for insulin in lactogenesis as opposed to metabolic adjustments during lactation seems improbable.

In summary, the most reasonable interpretation of the data available from both animal and human studies is that the hormonal trigger for lactogenesis is a fall in progesterone in the presence of maintained prolactin. Postpartum prolactin levels are similar in both breast-feeding and nonbreast-feeding women so that the basic process occurs whether breast-feeding is initiated or not. The caveat is, of course, that the mammary epithelium must be sufficiently prepared by the hormones of pregnancy to respond with milk synthesis.

Delays in secretory activation

A delay in the onset of milk secretion is a problem for the initiation of breast feeding in a significant fraction of parturient women. The timing of secretory activation has been determined carefully from milk volume or composition in a few studies of middle-class women of Caucasian descent.[3] Most of the data are in reasonable accord but some do suggest that either parity or previous lactation experience may influence the timing of secretory activation. A number of pathological conditions have been reported to delay secretory activation in women including Cesarean section, diabetes, obesity,[84] and stress during parturition.[72] The role of Cesarian section is controversial, no effect having been found in a large study from the laboratory of Peter Hartmann;[67] a small effect, statistically significant, was found in a more recent study where breast fullness and the appearance of casein in the secretion were measured.[72]

Women with poorly controlled diabetes, studied in both the USA[85] and Australia,[66] often had a delay in secretory activation. In a recent, well-controlled study, stress during parturition, accompanied by an increase in cord blood glucose, had the same result and milk production on day 5 postpartum was significantly decreased. Another apparent

cause of delayed milk secretion, obesity, has only come to our attention recently. In studies reviewed by Rasmussen[84] women with a high prepartum body mass index had more difficulty initiating lactation.

Delays in secretory activation have been classified as preglandular, glandular, and postglandular.[40] The delays described above would be classified as preglandular, as they are a result of some aberrant physiological situation in the mother. Glandular delay might result from insufficient mammary tissue due to a genetic defect or possibly breast surgery.[86] Such problems may or may not be permanent. Postglandular delay would result from insufficient milk removal, either by an infant with a weak suck or inappropriate latch-on or, in the case of the mother of a premature infant, from too few pumping regimens per day. In most cases, except permanent damage to the pituitary gland or vastly deficient mammary tissue, the situation can often be remedied by more frequent milk removal either by the infant or an effective breast pump or judicious use of both.[87]

REFERENCES

1 Whitehead, R. G. For how long is exclusive breast-feeding adequate to satisfy the dietary energy needs of the average young baby. *Pediatr. Res.* 1995;**37**:239–43.

2 Anonymous. Breastfeeding and the use of human milk. American Academy of Pediatrics. Work Group on Breastfeeding. *Pediatrics* 1997;**100**:1035–9.

3 Neville, M. C., McFadden, T. B., Forsyth, I. A. Hormonal regulation of mammary differentiation and lactation. *J. Mammary Gland Biol. Neoplasia* 2002;**7**:49–66.

4 Wysolmerski, J. J., Van Houten, J. N. Normal mammary development and disorders of breast development and function. In: Burrow, G., ed. *Endotext.com.* Endotext.org. 2002.

5 Schanler, R. J. Rationale for breastfeeding. In: Thureen, P. J., Hay, W. W., Jr, eds. *Neonatal Nutrition and Metabolism.* 2nd edn. Cambridge University Press; 2006.

6 Kraehenbuhl, J. P., Hunziker, W. Epithelial transcytosis of immunoglobulins. *J. Mammary Gland Biol. Neoplasia* 1998; **3**:289–304.

7 Neville, M. C. Sampling and storage of human milk. In: Jensen, R. G., ed. *Handbook of Milk Composition.* San Diego: Academic Press, 1995:63–79.

8 Jensen, R. G. The lipids in human milk. In: *Anonymous Progress in Lipid Research.* Amsterdam: Elsevier;1996:53–92.

9 Genzel-Boroviczeny, O., Wahle, J., Koletzko, B. Fatty acid composition of human milk during the 1st month after term and preterm delivery. *Eur. J. Pediatr.* 1997;**156**:142–7.

10 Picciano, M. F. Water soluble vitamins in milk. In: Jensen, R. G., ed. *Handbook of Milk Composition.* San Diego, CA: Academic Press; 1995.

11 Mannan, S., Picciano, M. F. Influence of maternal selenium status on human milk selenium concentration and glutathione peroxidase activity. *Am. J. Clin. Nutr.* 1987;**46**:95–100.

12 Linzell, J. L., Peaker, M. Mechanism of milk secretion. *Physiolog. Rev.* 1971;**51**:564–97.

13 Neville, M. C. Anatomy and physiology of lactation. *Ped. Clin. N. Am.* 2001;**48**:1–34.

14 Mather, I. H., Keenan, T. S. Origin and secretion of milk lipids. *J. Mammary Gland Biol. Neoplasia* 1998;**3**:259–74.

15 Monks, J. A., Neville, M. C. Trancytosis of proteins across the mammary epithelium into milk. *J. Women's Cancer* 2001;**2**:193–200.

16 Ollivier-Bousquet, M. Transferrin and prolactin trancytosis in the lactating mammary epithelial cell. *J. Mammary Gland Biol. Neoplasia* 1998;**3**:303–13.

17 Goldman, A. S. Evolution of the mammary gland defense system and the ontogeny of the immune system. *J. Mammary Gland Biol. Neoplasia* 2001;**7**:277–89.

18 Shennan, D. B., Peaker, M. Transport of milk constituents by the mammary gland. *Physiol. Rev.* 2000;**80**:925–51.

19 Nguyen, D.-A. D., Neville, M. C. Tight junction regulation in the mammary gland. *J. Mammary Gland Biol. Neoplasia* 1998;**3**:233–46.

20 Bussmann, L. E., Ward, W., Kuhn, N. J. Lactose and fatty acid synthesis in lactating-rat mammary gland. *Biochem. J.* 1984;**219**:173–80.

21 Nemeth, B. A., Tsang, S. W. Y., Geske, R. S., Haney, P. M. Golgi targeting of the GLUT1 glucose transporter in lactating mouse mammary gland. *Pediatr. Res.* 2000;**47**:444–50.

22 Toma, L., Pinahl, M. A., Dietrich, C. P., Nader, H. B., Hirschberg, C. B. Transport of UDP-galactose into the Golgi lumen regulates the biosynthesis of proteoglycans. *J. Biol. Chem.* 1996;**271**:3897–901.

23 Kakalis, L. T., Kumosinski, T. F., Farrell, H. M. Jr. A multinuclear, high-resolution NMR study of bovine casein micelles and submicelles. *Biophys. Chem.* 1990;**38**:87–98.

24 Neville, M. C., Picciano, M. F. Regulation of milk lipid secretion and composition. *Annu. Rev. Nutr.* 1997;**17**:159–83.

25 Smith, S. The animal fatty acid synthase: one gene, one polypeptide, seven enzymes. *FASEB J.* 1994;**8**:1248–59.

26 Smith, S., Pasco, D., Nandi, S. Biosynthesis of medium-chain fatty acids by mammary epithelial cells from virgin rats. *Biochem. J.* 1983;**2112**:155–9.

27 Buchbinder, J. L., Witkowski, A., Smith, S., Fletterick, R. J. Crystallization and preliminary diffraction studies of thioesterase II from rat mammary gland. *Proteins* 1995;**22**:73–5.

28 West, C. E., Bickerstaffe, R., Annison, E. F., Linzell, J. L. Studies on the mode of uptake of blood triglycerides by the mammary gland of the lactating goat. The uptake and incorporation into milk fat and mammary lymph of labeled glycerol, fatty acids and triglycerides. *Biochem. J.* 1972;**126**:477–90.

29 Demelmair, H., Baumheuer, M., Koletzko, B., Dokoupil, K., Kratl, G. Investigation of long-chain polyunsaturated fatty acid metabolism in lactating women by means of stable isotope techniques. *Adv. Exp. Med. Biol.* 2001;**501**:169–77.

30 Insull, W. Jr, Hirsch, J., James, T., Ahrens, E. H. The fatty acids of human milk. II. Alterations produced by manipulation of caloric balance and exchange of dietary fats. *J. Clin. Invest.* 1958;**38**:443–50.

31 Jensen, R. G., Bitman, J., Carlson, S. E. *et al.* Milk lipids: human milk lipids. In: Jensen, R. G., ed. *Handbook of Milk Composition.* San Diego, CA: Academic Press, 1995:495–542.

32 Hachey, D. L., Thomas, M. R., Emken, E. A. *et al.* Human lactation: maternal transfer of dietary triglycerides labeled with stable isotopes. *J. Lipid Res.* 1987;**28**:1185–92.

33 Dils, R. R. Milk fat synthesis. In: Mepham, T. B., ed. *Biochemistry of Lactation.* Amsterdam: Elsevier; 1983:141–57.

34 Rao, G. A., Abraham, S. Fatty acid desaturation by mammary gland microsomes from lactating mice. *Lipids* 1974;**9**: 269–71.

35 Koletzko, B. Importance of dietary lipids. In: Tsang, R., ed. *Nutrition during Infancy: Birth to Two Years.* New York, NY: Academic Press; 1996.

36 Larque, E., Demmelmair, H., Koletzko, B. Perinatal supply and metabolism of long-chain polyunsaturated fatty acids: importance for the early development of the nervous system. *Ann. NY Acad. Sci.* 2002;**967**:299–310.

37 Grammatikos, S. I., Subbaiah, P. V., Victor, T. A., Miller, W. M. *n*-3 and *n*-6 fatty acid processing and growth effects in neoplastic and non-cancerous human mammary epithelial cell lines. *Br. J. Cancer* 1994;**70**:219–27.

38 Nguyen, D.-A. D., Beeman, N., Neville, M. C. Regulation of tight junction permeability in the mammary gland. In: Cerejido, M., Anderson, J. M., eds. *Tight Junctions.* 2nd edn. New York, NY: CRC Press; 2001:395–414.

39 Seelig, L. L. Jr, Beer, A. E. Transepithelial migration of leukocytes in the mammary gland of lactating rats. *Biol. Reprod.* 1981;**22**:1157–63.

40 Morton, J. A. The clinical usefulness of breast milk sodium in the assessment of lactogenesis. *Pediatrics* 1994;**93**:802–6.

41 Saint, L., Maggiore, P., Hartmann, P. E. Yield and nutrient content of milk in eight women breast-feeding twins and one woman breast-feeding triplets. *Br. J. Nutr.* 1986;**56**:49–58.

42 Macy, I. G., Hunscher, H. A., Donelson, E., Nims, B. Human milk flow. *Am. J. Dis. Child.* 1930;**6**:492–515.

43 Butte, N. F., Villalpando, S., Wong, W. W. *et al.* Human milk intake and growth faltering of rural Mesoamerindian infants. *Am. J. Clin. Nutr.* 1992;**55**:1109–16.

44 Brown, K. H., Stallings, R. Y., Creed de Kanashiro, H., Lopez de Romaña, G., Black, R. E. Effects of common illnesses on infants' energy intakes from breast milk and other foods during longitudinal community-based studies in Huascar (Lima), Peru. *Am. J. Clin. Nutr.* 1990;**52**:1005–13.

45 Neville, M. C. Volume and caloric density of human milk. In: Jensen, R. G., ed. *Handbook of Milk Composition.* San Diego, CA: Academic Press 1995:101–13.

46 Prentice, A. M., Paul, A., Prentice, A. *et al.* Cross-cultural differences in lactational performance. In: Hamosh, M., Goldman, A. S., eds. *Human Lactation: Maternal and Environmental Factors.* New York, NY: Plenum Press, 1986:13–50.

47 Madden, J. D., Boyar, R. M., MacDonald, P. C., Porter, J. C. Analysis of secretory patterns of prolactin and gonadotropins during twenty-four hours in a lactating woman before and after resumption of menses. *Am. J. Obstet. Gynecol.* 1997;**132**: 436–41.

48 Frantz, A. G. Rhythms in prolactin secretion. In: Krieger, D. T., ed. *Endocrine Rhythms*. New York, NY: Raven Press; 1979:175–85.

49 Rigg, L. A., Lein, A., Yen, S. S. Pattern of increase in circulating prolactin levels during human gestation. *Am. J. Obstet. Gynecol.* 1977;**129**:454–6.

50 Martin, R. H., Glass, M. R., Chapman, C., Wilson, G. D., Woods, K. L. Human alpha-lactalbumin and hormonal factors in pregnancy and lactation. *Clin. Endocrinol.* 1980;**13**:223–30.

51 Howie, P. W., McNeilly, A. S., McArdle, T., Smart, L., Houston, M. The relationship between suckling-induced prolactin response and lactogenesis. *J. Clin. Endocrinol. Metab.* 1980;**50**:670–3.

52 Tyson, J. E. Nursing and prolactin secretion: principal determinants in the mediation of puerperal infertility. In: Crosignani, P. G., Robyn, C., eds. *Prolactin and Human Reproduction*. New York, NY: Academic Press; 1977:97–108.

53 McNeilly, A. S., Robinson, I. C., Houston, M. J., Howie, P. W. Release of oxytocin and prolactin in response to suckling. *Br. Med. J. Clin. Res.* 1983;**286**:257–9.

54 Peaker, M., Wilde, C. J. Feedback control of milk secretion from milk. *J. Mammary Gland Biol. Neoplasia* 1996;**1**:307–15.

55 Millar, I. D., Barber, M. C., Lomax, M. A., Travers, M. T., Shennan, D. B. Mammary protein synthesis is acutely regulated by the cellular hydration state. *Biochem. Biophys. Res. Commun.* 1997;**230**:351–5.

56 Sudlow, A. W., Burgoyne, R. D. A hypo-osmotically induced increase in intracellular Ca^{2+} in lactating mouse mammary epithelial cells involving Ca^{2+} influx. *Pflugers Arch.* 1997;**433**:609–16.

57 Richardson, K. C. Contractile tissue in the mammary gland with special reference to the myoepithelium in the goat. *Proc. R. Soc. Lond. Ser. B.* 1949;**136**:30–45.

58 Ardran, G. M., Kemp, F. H., Lind, J. A cineradiographic study of breast feeding. *Br. J. Radiol.* 1958;**31**:156–62.

59 Newton, M., Newton, N. R. The let-down reflex in human lactation. *J. Pediatr.* 1948;**33**:698–704.

60 Ueda, T., Yokoyama, Y., Irahara, M., Aono, T. Influence of psychological stress on suckling-induced pulsatile oxytocin release. *Obstet. Gynecol.* 1994;**84**:259–62.

61 Vilaro, S., Vinas, O., Remesar, X., Herrera, E. Effects of chronic ethanol consumption on lactational performance in rat: mammary gland and milk composition and pups' growth and metabolism. *Pharmacol. Biochem. Behav.* 1987;**27**: 333–9.

62 Cobo, E. Effect of different doses of ethanol on the milk ejection reflex in lactating women. *Am. J. Obstet. Gynecol.* 1973;**115**:817–21.

63 Neville, M. C., Allen, J. C., Archer, P. C. *et al.* Studies in human lactation: milk volume and nutrient composition during weaning and lactogenesis. *Am. J. Clin. Nutr.* 1991;**54**:81–92.

64 Neville, M. C., Keller, R. P., Seacat, J. *et al.* Studies in human lactation: milk volumes in lactating women during the onset of lactation and full lactation. *Am. J. Clin. Nutr.* 1988;**48**:1375–86.

65 Saint, L., Smith, M., Hartmann, P. E. The yield and nutrient content of colostrum and milk of women from giving birth to one month postpartum. *Br. J. Nutr.* 1984;**52**:87–95.

66 Arthur, P. G., Smith, M., Hartmann, P. Milk lactose, citrate and glucose as markers of lactogenesis in normal and diabetic women. *J. Ped. Gastroenterol. Nutr.* 1989;**9**:488–96.

67 Kulski, J. K., Smith, M., Hartmann, P. E. Normal and Caesarean section delivery and the initiation of lactation in women. *Aust. J. Exp. Biol. Med. Sci.* 1981;**59**:405–12.

68 Aperia, A., Broberger, O., Herin, P., Zetterstroem, R. Salt content in human breast milk during the first three weeks after delivery. *Acta Paed. Scand.* 1979;**68**:441–2.

69 Lewis-Jones, D. I., Lewis-Jones, M. S., Connolly, R. C., Lloyd, D. C., West, C. R. Sequential changes in the antimicrobial protein concentrations in human milk during lactation and its relevance to banked human milk. *Pediatr. Res.* 1985;**19**:561–5.

70 Coppa, G. V., Pierani, P., Zambini, L. *et al.* Oligosaccharides in human milk during different phases of lactation. *Acta Paediatr. Suppl.* 1999;**88**:89–94.

71 Newburg, D. S. Oligosaccharides and glycoconjugates of human milk: their role in host defense. *J. Mammary Gland Biol. Neoplasia* 1996;**1**:271–83.

72 Chen, D. C., Nommsen-Rivers, L., Dewey, K. G., Lonnerdal, B. Stress during labor and delivery and early lactation performance. *Am. J. Clin. Nutr.* 1998;**68**:335–44.

73 Humphreys, R. C., Lydon, J., O'Malley, B. W., Rosen, J. M. Use of PRKO mice to study the role of progesterone in mammary gland development. *J. Mammary Gland Biol. Neoplasia* 1997;**2**:343–54.

74 Ormandy, C. J., Binart, N., Kelly, P. A. Mammary gland development in prolactin receptor knockout mice. *J. Mammary Gland Biol. Neoplasia* 1997;**2**:355–63.

75 Kuhn, N. J. Progesterone withdrawal as the lactogenic trigger in the rat. *J. Endocrinol.* 1969;**44**:39–54.

76 Halban, J. Die innere Secretion von Ovarium und Placenta und ihre Bedeutung fur die Function der Milchdruse. *Arch. Gynaekol.* 1905;**75**:353–441.

77 Neifert, M. R., McDonough, S. L., Neville, M. C. Failure of lactogenesis associated with placental retention. *Am. J. Obstet. Gyn.* 1981;**140**:477–8.

78 Haslam, S. Z., Shyamala, G. Effect of oestradiol on progesterone receptors in normal mammary glands and its relationship with lactation. *Biochem. J.* 1979;**182**:127–31.

79 Neville, M. C., Walsh, C. T. Effects of drugs on milk secretion and composition. In: Bennett, P. N., edn. *Drugs and Human Lactation*. 2nd edn. Amsterdam: Elsevier; 1996:15–45.

80 Topper, Y. J., Freeman, C. S. Multiple hormone interactions in the developmental biology of the mammary gland. *Physiol. Rev.* 1980;**60**:1049–106.

81 Cowie, A. T., Lyons, W. R. Mammogenesis and lactogenesis in hypophysectomized, ovariectomized, adrenalectomized rats. *J. Endocrinol.* 1959;**19**:29–32.

82 Cowie, A. T. General hormonal factors involved in lactogenesis. In: Reynolds, M., Folley, S. J., eds. *Lactogenesis, the Initiation of Milk Secretion at Parturition*. Philadelphia, PA: University of Pennsylvania Press; 1969:157–69.

83 Kyriakou, S. Y., Kuhn, N. J. Lactogenesis in the diabetic rat. *J. Endocrinol.* 1973;**59**:199–200.

84 Rasmussen, K. M., Hilson, J. A., Kjolhede, C. L. Obesity may impair lactogenesis II. *J. Nutr.* 2001;**131**:3009–11.

85 Neubauer, S. H., Ferris, A. M., Chase, C. G. *et al.* Delayed lactogenesis in women with insulin-dependent diabetes mellitus. *Am. J. Clin. Nutr.* 1993;**58**:54–60.

86 Neifert, M., DeMarzo, S., Seacat, J. *et al.* The influence of breast surgery, breast appearance, and pregnancy-induced breast changes on lactation sufficiency as measured by infant weight gain [see comments]. *Birth* 1990;**17**:31–8.

87 Neifert, M. R. Clinical aspects of lactation. Promoting breast-feeding success. *Clin. Perinatol.* 1999;**26**:281–306.

88 Allen, J. C., Keller, R. P., Archer, P. C., Neville, M. C. Studies in human lactation: 6. Milk composition and daily secretion rates of macronutrients in the first year of lactation. *Am. J. Clin. Nutr.* 1991;**54**:69–80.

89 Neville, M. C. Physiology of lactation. *Clin. Perinatol.* 1998;**26**:251.

90 Jensen, R. G. *Handbook of Milk Composition*. San Diego, CA: Academic Press; 1995.

91 Cooper, A. *The Anatomy and Diseases of the Breast*. Philadelphia, PA: Lea and Blanchard;1845.

92 Neville, M. C., Allen, J. C., Watters, C. The mechanisms of milk secretion. In: Neville, M. C., Neifert, M. R., eds. *Lactation: Physiology, Nutrition and Breast-Feeding*. New York, NY: Plenum Press; 1983:50.

93 Neville, M. C. Lactogenesis in women: a cascade of events revealed by milk composition. In: Jensen, R. D., ed. *The Composition of Milks*. San Diego, CA: Academic Press;1995: 87–98.

94 Neville, M. C., Morton, J., Umemora, S. Lactogenesis: the transition from pregnancy to lactation. *Pediatr. Clin. Am.* 2001;**48**:35–52.

26

Rationale for breastfeeding

Richard J. Schanler

Neonatal–Perinatal Medicine, Schneider Children's Hospital at North Shore, North Shore University Hospital, Manhasset, NY
and Pediatrics, Albert Einstein College of Medicine, Bronx, NY

Introduction

Both governmental and medical professional organizations have strongly recommended breastfeeding for all infants.[1-3] Human milk is recommended as the exclusive nutrient source for feeding full-term infants for approximately the first 6 months after birth and should be continued, with the addition of solid foods, for at least 12 months, and thereafter for as long as mutually desired.[1] The recommendation for human milk feeding arises because of its acknowledged benefits with respect to infant nutrition, gastrointestinal function, host defense, and psychological wellbeing. It is important to note that favorable outcomes of breastfeeding are reported both for infants and mothers. The unique species-specificity of human milk should be considered in any discussion of the merits of breastfeeding. The incidence of breastfeeding in the USA increased during the 1970s and peaked in the mid-1980s. Nationwide figures for 1983 indicated that 62% of women chose to breastfeed their newborns.[4] Recent data suggest that rates of initiation and maintenance of breastfeeding are continuing to increase at a rate of 2% per year.[5,6] To meet the challenge imposed by this increased awareness, physicians desire to expand their knowledge to understand the reasons why breastfeeding is so vital to health and wellbeing.[7] This chapter describes the rationale behind the current recommendations for breastfeeding, including the effects of breastfeeding on infants, mothers, and society.

Milk composition

The milk produced in the first few days is colostrum, a relatively denser milk characterized by high concentrations of protein and antibodies. The transition to mature milk occurs around days 3 to 5, with mature milk appearing by about day 10. Key to understanding how breastfeeding benefits infants and mothers is an appreciation for the quality and quantity of nutritional and non-nutritional components in the milk. Many of the components in human milk have dual roles, one as a nutrient source or to facilitate nutrient absorption, and the other as an enhancer of host defense or gastrointestinal function.

Nutritional aspects

The nutrient composition of human milk is remarkable for its variability, as the content of some nutrients change during lactation, throughout the day, or differ among women, while the contents of other nutrients remain relatively constant through lactation.[8] The variability in component composition probably adapts the nutrient composition to specifically meet the needs of the infant, while the lack of monotonous diet possibly stimulates sensory development, allowing better acceptance of new flavors and foods.[9]

Protein (nitrogen)

In the first 2–4 weeks after birth, the total nitrogen content of milk from mothers who deliver premature infants is greater than milk obtained from women delivering full-term infants.[10-13] Usually beyond 4 weeks of lactation, the total nitrogen content in both milks declines to levels that are similar and remain relatively unchanged thereafter.[12,13] Despite a decline in content, protein status of breastfed term infants is normal at 1 year of age.[14]

Neonatal Nutrition and Metabolism. Second Edition, ed. P. Thureen and W. Hay. Published by Cambridge University Press.
© Cambridge University Press 2006.

Approximately 20% of the total nitrogen is in the form of nonprotein nitrogen-containing compounds, such as free amino acids and urea, in contrast to commercial formula which has < 5% nonprotein nitrogen.[15,16] There is debate as to how much of these nonprotein nitrogen-containing compounds contribute to nitrogen utilization.[17,18] The rate of absorption of nonprotein nitrogen, determined by stable isotope methods, has been estimated at 13%–43%.[17,18]

There are two fractions of protein defined by their solubility in acid: whey and casein. Approximately 70% of the proteins in human milk are in the soluble whey fraction and 30% in the insoluble casein fraction, which differs from that in commercial formula derived from bovine milk (18% whey, 82% casein).[16] It is speculated that because the whey proteins remain in solution after acid precipitation, they are more easily digested and are associated with more rapid gastric emptying.[19] The whey protein fraction provides lower concentrations of phenylalanine, tyrosine, and methionine and higher concentrations of taurine than the casein fraction of milk and these amino acid patterns are reflected in blood concentrations.[20–23] This pattern of amino acids in the plasma of breastfed infants is used as a reference in infant nutrition.[24] As such, potentially toxic imbalances in the levels of various amino acids are avoided.

The type of proteins contained in the whey fraction differs between human and bovine milks. The major human whey protein is α-lactalbumin, a protein involved in the mammary gland synthesis of lactose and a nutritional protein for the infant. Lactoferrin, lysozyme, and secretory immunoglobulin A (sIgA) are specific human whey proteins involved in host defense.[25–27] Because these host defense proteins resist proteolytic digestion, they are capable of a first line of defense by lining the gastrointestinal tract. The three host defense proteins essentially are absent in bovine milk. The major whey protein in bovine milk is β-lactoglobulin.[16]

Lipid

Human milk lipid represents approximately 50% of the calories in the milk, and is unique in that the lipid system is structured to facilitate superior fat digestion and absorption.[28] The lipid system is comprised of an organized milk fat globule, a pattern of fatty acids which are characteristically distributed on the triglyceride molecule, and bile salt-stimulated lipase.[29,30] As the lipase is heat-labile, it is important to recognize that the superior fat absorption from human milk is reported only when unprocessed milk is fed.[31] The fatty acid pattern consists of a high proportion of long-chain fatty acids: palmitic (16:0), oleic (18:1), and the essential fatty acids, linoleic (18:2ω6),

and linolenic (18:3ω3). The lipid is structured in the form of triglycerides which uniquely have the major fatty acid, palmitic (16:0), esterified at the 2-position of the molecule. Upon intestinal hydrolysis, 2-monoglycerides are formed which are better absorbed than the free palmitic acid. Not only is fat absorption enhanced, but because free palmitic acid is not available to bind minerals, mineral absorption also is enhanced. To match the overall fat absorption from human milk, commercial formula has a greater quantity of passively absorbed medium chain-length fatty acids than human milk.

Of the macronutrients in human milk, fat is the most variable in content.[32] The milk fat content rises slightly throughout lactation, changes over the course of one day, increases within-feed, and varies from mother to mother.[8] Some investigators comment that the variability in fat content is related to the degree of breast emptying.[33] The interindividual variation in milk fat content tracks through lactation. The total fat content of human milk is not affected by maternal diet; it may be affected by maternal body composition.[34,35]

The lipid system in human milk also is unique in its content of very long-chain fatty acid derivatives of linoleic and linolenic acids. Arachidonic acid (20:4ω6) and docosahexaenoic acid (22:6ω3), derivatives of the essential fatty acids are found in human but not bovine milk.[36] Arachidonic and docosahexaenoic acids functionally have been associated with cognition, growth, and vision.[37]

Carbohydrate

The carbohydrate composition of human milk is important as a nutritional source of lactose, the major carbohydrate in milk, and for the presence of oligosaccharides. Although studies in full-term infants demonstrate a small proportion of unabsorbed lactose in the feces, the presence of lactose is assumed to be a normal physiological effect of feeding human milk.[38,39] A softer stool consistency, non-pathogenic bacterial fecal flora, and improved absorption of minerals have been attributed to the lactose in human milk.[40] Oligosaccharides are carbohydrate polymers and glycoproteins that are important in the host defense of the infant because their structure mimics specific bacterial antigen receptors.[41] By preventing bacterial attachment to the host mucosa, oligosaccharides serve a protective role in the infant.[42]

Mineral and trace elements

The concentration of calcium and phosphorus in human milk is significantly lower than in commercial formula, and relatively constant through lactation. The macrominerals in human milk are more bioavailable than those in commercial formula because of the manner in which they are packaged. In human milk, the minerals are bound to digestible proteins and also present in complexed and ionized states which are readily bioavailable.[43] Thus, despite differences in mineral intake, bone mineral content of breastfed infants is similar to that of infants fed commercial formula.[44]

The concentrations of iron, zinc, and copper decline through lactation but appear adequate to meet the infant's nutritional needs through 6 months.[45,46] To prevent deficiencies, iron and micronutrient-containing complementary foods should be introduced beyond 6 months of breastfeeding.[47]

Vitamins

Maternal vitamin status may affect the content of vitamins in the milk. Maternal deficiency may result in low concentrations in milk that increase in response to dietary supplementation. This is more common for water-soluble than fat-soluble vitamins. Vegan mothers may be deficient in the water-soluble vitamin B_{12}. Infants of vegan mothers should receive a vitamin supplement. Vitamin K deficiency may be a concern in the breastfed infant. Bacterial flora are responsible for providing adequate vitamin K. The intestinal flora of the breastfed infant make less menaquinone and the content of vitamin K in human milk is low. Therefore, to meet vitamin K needs, a single dose of vitamin K is given at birth.[48] The content of vitamin D in human milk is low. Adequate sunlight exposure is needed to maintain vitamin D sufficiency. Life-style changes and concern about the risk of skin cancer have been associated with decreased unprotected sunlight exposure. Vitamin D deficiency has been reported in breastfed infants who have dark skin pigmentation and/or inadequate exposure to sunlight. Supplementation of all infants with vitamin D (200 IU day^{-1}) is indicated.

Non-nutritional factors

Nucleotides

Nucleotides represent 2%–5% of the nonprotein nitrogen in human milk.[49] Although they can be synthesized endogenously, it appears that exogenous nucleotides may have a role in a variety of metabolic functions, including effects on immune, gastrointestinal, and hepatic systems, and in lipid metabolism.[49,50] In addition, the growth of non-pathogenic bifidobacteria in stool is enhanced by exogenous nucleotides.[49]

Components affecting gastrointestinal function

Hormones (e.g., cortisol, somatomedin-C, insulin-like growth factors, insulin, thyroid hormone) and growth factors (e.g., epidermal growth factor, nerve growth factor) and gastrointestinal mediators (e.g., neurotensin, motilin) are present in human milk that may affect gastrointestinal function. Epidermal growth factor (EGF) is a polypeptide that stimulates DNA synthesis, protein synthesis, and cellular proliferation in intestinal cells.[51] EGF resists proteolytic digestion, is found in the intestinal lumen in suckling animals, and has been associated in experimental models with protection from necrotizing enterocolitis.[52] Nerve growth factor may play a role in the innervation of the intestinal tract. The hormonal components in milk may affect intestinal growth and mucosal function. Free amino acids such as taurine may be trophic for intestinal growth, and glutamine may be a fuel for the small intestine.[51] As a consequence of the total available human milk components, the gastrointestinal tract is protected against invasive disease.[53,54]

Components affecting host defense

A variety of heterogeneous agents that possess antimicrobial activity are found in human milk.[25,27,42,55] Many of these agents persist through lactation and are resistant to the digestive enzymes in the infant's gastrointestinal tract. The antimicrobial activities generally are found at mucosal surfaces, such as the gastrointestinal, respiratory, and urinary tracts.

Specific factors such as lactoferrin, lysozyme, and sIgA comprise the whey fraction of human milk protein, generally resist proteolytic degradation, and line mucosal surfaces preventing microbial attachment and inhibiting microbial activity.[25–27,56] Lactoferrin has antimicrobial activity when not conjugated to iron (apolactoferrin). It may function with other host defense proteins to effect microbial killing. Lysozyme is active against bacteria by cleaving cell walls. SIgA is synthesized by plasma cells against specific antigens. The enteromammary and bronchomammary immune systems summarize the important part of the protective nature of human milk.[57,58] In these systems the mother produces sIgA antibody when exposed either via her respiratory or gastrointestinal tract to foreign antigens. The plasma cells traverse the lymphatic system and are secreted at mucosal surfaces, including the mammary gland. Ingestion of milk, therefore, provides the infant with passive sIgA antibody against the offending antigen. The systems are active in infants against a variety of antigens.[25,57,58]

The products of lipid hydrolysis, free fatty acids, and monoglycerides, may exhibit antimicrobial activity against a variety of pathogens.[59] These lipid end products may prevent attachment and infection with viruses and protozoa, such as *Giardia*. The activity of human milk bile salt stimulated lipase also may affect host defense. Polyunsaturated fatty acids modulate inflammatory reactions and may protect the gastrointestinal tract.[60]

Oligosaccharides and glucoproteins affect intestinal bacterial flora to facilitate the growth of bifidobacteria and *Lactobacillus* species.[61] These agents also mimic bacterial epithelial receptors in the respiratory tract and in doing so, prevent attachment of pathogenic agents to epithelial lining of mucosal surfaces. There are a variety of oligosaccharides and glycoproteins that act as receptor analogs for multiple antimicrobial agents.[41,42]

There are specific enzymes in human milk, such as platelet activating factor (PAF)-acetylhydrolase. This enzyme degrades PAF, a potent mediator in the intestinal injury induced during necrotizing enterocolitis (NEC).[62] The cytokine, interleukin-10, also functions as an anti-inflammatory mediator and may have a role in protecting the infant from NEC.[63,64]

There are white cells (90% of which are neutrophils and macrophages) in human milk that contribute to the antimicrobial activity through phagocytosis and intracellular killing.[26] The lymphocytes in human milk may contribute to cytokine production (T-cells) or IgA production (B-cells).[26,55]

Benefits of breastfeeding for the infant

Body composition

Clinicians agree that the growth of the breastfed infant is the model on which infant growth is based. However, when plotted on standard US growth charts, the rates of weight gain of breastfed infants appear lower than those fed commercial formula.[65] More recent US growth charts, comprised of a heterogeneous population with limited exclusive breastfeeding, reflect a slight decline in rate of weight gain after 6 months. The divergence is viewed more as a concern with representation of the growth chart rather than a concern with nutrient adequacy.[66-68]

Although lower concentrations of calcium and phosphorus are observed in human milk compared with commercial formula, measures of bone mineralization are similar between human milk or commercial formula fed full-term infants during the first year of life.[43,69] Long-term bone mass also is affected by breastfeeding. Children at 8 y have

significantly greater bone mass if they breastfed compared with those not breastfed, and the effect is greater if they breastfed for more than 3 months.[73] Several studies have linked long-term obesity reduction with the duration of breastfeeding in infancy.[70-72] Children who were breastfed had nearly one-half the prevalence of obesity than children fed commercial formula, and the prevalence of obesity was related positively to the dose of human milk received by the infant.[74]

Gastrointestinal function

Gastric emptying is faster following the feeding of human milk than with commercial formula.[19,75] The clinical impression is that large gastric residual volumes are reported less frequently in premature infants fed human milk. Many factors in human milk may stimulate gastrointestinal growth and motility, and enhance maturity of the gastrointestinal tract. In studies of early trophic feeding in premature infants, those infants fed human milk had significantly greater intestinal lactase activity than infants fed preterm formula.[76] Further studies indicate that feeding of human milk favors a decrease in intestinal permeability early in life compared with preterm formula.[77]

Morbidity and mortality

There are numerous studies conducted in developing countries that delineate the protective effects of breastfeeding. In developing areas, the incidence of gastroenteritis and respiratory disease and overall morbidity and mortality are lower in breastfed infants than infants fed milk substitutes.[78 80] In developed countries, such as in the USA, breastfed infants have lower rates of diarrhea, lower respiratory tract illness, acute and recurrent otitis media, and urinary tract infection.[81-83] Not only is the attack rate lower, but the duration and severity of illness appear to be shortened in the breastfed infant.[84]

In developed countries, even in higher socioeconomic groups, a reduction is found in the incidence of gastroenteritis.[78,85] The incidence of diarrheal disease in infants breastfed for 12 months is one-half that of commercial formula-fed infants.[84] When adjusting for potential confounding variables, such as sibling number and day-care attendance, the differences remain significant. Infants who breastfed for at least 13 weeks have a significantly lower incidence of gastroenteritis (vomiting or diarrhea as a discrete illness lasting 48 hours or more) to 1 year of age than commercial formula-fed infants.[86] These observations remain significant after adjustment for social class, maternal age, and smoking.

The incidence of otitis media and recurrent otitis media are reduced in infants breastfed for 4 or more months.[87,88] This protective effect is observed after adjustment for confounding variables, such as family history of allergy, family size, use of day care, and smoking. Not only is otitis media reduced in infants breastfed for 1 year, but the duration of each episode is reduced significantly compared with infants fed commercial formula.[84] Respiratory illnesses are reduced in frequency and/or in duration in breastfed infants.[85,86,89,90] The incidence of wheezing is less and overall lower respiratory tract infection is decreased.[85,90] Studies of upper respiratory infections in former premature infants during their first year report a lower incidence of disease if, after discharge, they receive any human milk compared with commercial formula.[91]

A case-controlled study reported that the incidence of urinary tract infection was reduced in breastfed infants when compared with commercial formula-fed infants matched for hospitalization, age, gender, social class, birth order, and smoking status of the mother.[92] A mechanism for this protection has been suggested based on the known urinary excretion of oligosaccharides, lactoferrin, and sIgA in breastfed infants.[93] Urinary oligosaccharides reduce bacterial adhesion to urinary epithelial cells.[94]

The incidence of sepsis is reduced in premature infants receiving human milk.[95–98] Premature infants fed human milk have a lower incidence of NEC if they receive human milk compared with receiving commercial formula.[96,98–100] The lower incidence of NEC is observed even if the supply of mother's milk is low and commercial formula is used as a supplement. Thus, partial as well as exclusive feeding of mother's milk appears to protect the premature infant from NEC. Although the mechanism for the protection from NEC is unclear, one study observed that the feeding of an IgA–IgG preparation was associated with a decreased incidence of NEC.[101] Additional studies suggest that factors in human milk, such as PAF-acetylhydrolase, polyunsaturated fatty acids, and interleukin-10, also might explain the association between human milk feeding and protection from NEC.[62–64,102,103] These data suggest that by lining the gastrointestinal tract with human milk host defense factors, the infant may be protected.[53]

Chronic disease in pediatrics

Perhaps the most intriguing data are those suggesting that specific chronic pediatric disorders have a lower incidence in children who were breastfed as infants. There are associations between the duration of breastfeeding and a reduction in incidence of Crohn's disease, lymphoma, specific genotypes of type I juvenile diabetes mellitus,

and certain allergic conditions.[104–107] There are conflicting data regarding the protection against allergy afforded by breastfeeding.[108] In some reports, maternal diet may not have excluded potentially offending antigens. Breastfeeding appears to be protective against food allergies.[27,42] Atopic dermatitis may be lessened in infants whose mothers' follow a restricted diet. A lower incidence of atopic conditions is reported in breastfed infants with a family history of atopy.[109] Children from atopic as well as nonatopic families had a lower incidence of asthma if they breastfed exclusively for more than 3 months.[110]

There appears to be a relationship between breastfeeding and the development of type I insulin dependent diabetes mellitus (IDDM).[106] IDDM is more likely when breastfeeding duration is less than 3 months and bovine milk proteins are introduced before 4 months of age.[106] Elevated concentrations of specific IgG antibody to bovine serum albumin that cross reacts with β-cell-specific surface protein have been identified in children with IDDM.[111] It is estimated that up to 30% of type I IDDM could be prevented by removing bovine milk from the diet for the first 3 months.[106]

Blood cholesterol and lipoprotein concentrations appear to be strong risk factors for adult coronary artery disease. Breastfeeding is associated with increased cholesterol and low density lipoprotein concentrations in infancy, but lower blood concentrations in adolescence and adult life.[112]

Neurobehavioral aspects

Maternal–infant bonding is enhanced during breastfeeding. Several studies have linked improved cognitive and motor development later in childhood and adolescence to breastfeeding, and observed that the benefit to development is associated with the duration of breastfeeding.[113,114] Even when adjusted for socioeconomic status and parent education, at 3, 4, and 5 years there were significant increments in a limited set of cognitive test scores that paralleled the duration of breastfeeding.[115] Improved long-term cognitive development in premature infants also has been correlated with the receipt of human milk during their hospitalization.[116–119] An interesting observation in children with phenylketonuria is that those breastfed prior to the confirmed diagnosis had better intellectual outcomes than those who were fed commercial formula.[120]

A series of studies have indicated that human milk-fed full-term and premature infants have improved visual function related to the content of docosahexaenoic acid compared with infants not receiving this fatty acid.[121,122] Premature infants also have less severe retinopathy of prematurity if fed human milk than commercial formula.[123] This association may relate to the substantial antioxidant capacity of human milk compared with commercial formula.[124] Auditory-evoked responses also mature faster in breastfed premature infants.[125]

Thus, small but statistically significant, neurodevelopmental advantages in children who were formerly fed human milk have been demonstrated. Long-term advantage is more consistently demonstrated for cognitive than for motor skills. Although results of the studies cannot be assumed to be representative of all infants, there is some evidence of a dose-response.

Benefits of breastfeeding to the mother

Recovery from childbirth is accelerated by the oxytocin's action on uterine involution.[126] Maternal cardiovascular function is affected positively to protect breastfeeding.[127] Although breastfeeding should not be considered an entirely reliable means of contraception, breastfeeding prolongs the period of postpartum anovulation.[128] Frequency, intensity, and timing of feeds affect the endocrinologic responses that modulate ovulatory status.[129]

Prolonged breastfeeding may confer some advantage in terms of weight loss.[130] Bone demineralization occurs during lactation, with a compensatory remineralization after weaning.[131,132] Lactation has been shown to confer a protective effect against osteoporosis and bone fracture in later life,[133] but this has not been confirmed in all studies.[134]

A protective effect of breastfeeding against breast cancer has been found in a number of studies.[135–138] The effects were even greater in premenopausal women who had a cumulative total of 24 months of breastfeeding or who were 20 years or younger when they first lactated.

Contraindications to breastfeeding

A beneficial aspect of breastfeeding is that relatively few true contraindications exist.[139] Infants with galactosemia cannot ingest lactose-containing milk. Therefore, as the principal carbohydrate in human milk is lactose, infants with galactosemia should not breastfeed. Infants with other inborn errors of metabolism may ingest some human milk, but this recommendation would depend upon the desired protein intake and other factors. Women in the USA who are infected with human immunodeficiency virus (HIV) and those with human T-cell lymphotropic virus should not breastfeed. Women with HIV also should be counseled about the risks to the infant of breastfeeding. Globally, the health risks of not breastfeeding must be balanced with the risk of HIV acquisition. Indeed, some studies suggest that exclusive breastfeeding may decrease maternal to child transmission of HIV compared with mixed feedings. Women with miliary tuberculosis should not breastfeed until they are no longer contagious, approximately 2 weeks. When herpetic lesions are localized to the breast, women should not breastfeed. But women with vaginal herpes should be allowed to breastfeed. Women with varicella lesions on the breast should provide expressed milk to their infant until their lesions are crusted over, and the infant should receive varicella immune globulin. Women with breast cancer should not delay treatment so they can breastfeed. Depending upon the therapy, women receiving antimetabolite chemotherapy should not breastfeed. Most other medications are compatible with breastfeeding or a substitute medication may exist. Women ingesting drugs of abuse need counseling and should not breastfeed until they are free of the abused drugs.[140]

Economic impact of breastfeeding

The economic advantages of breastfeeding can be tangibly calculated at the personal and national levels.[141] The obvious personal advantage is in the savings accrued by not buying commercial formula, a figure conservatively estimated to be about $1000 per year. Thus, the increased rates of illness in non-breastfed infants translate into significantly increased costs to medical insurers, employers, government, and even to those uninsured.

From the perspective of the national economy, the expected savings for infants in the US' WIC Program who were breastfed exclusively for 6 months were estimated to be over $950 million annually in 1997 compared with not breastfeeding for 6 months.[142] These savings would come from a combined reduction in household expenditure on commercial formula, as well as reductions in expenditures for healthcare. In light of these data, the major gains in breastfeeding prevalence among WIC participants have contributed to the resurgence in breastfeeding in the USA in the last decade. The costs of not breastfeeding also have been computed from a health maintenance organization population. Compared with never breastfeeding, those infants who breastfed for 3 months or more had fewer medical office visits, medications, procedures, and hospitalizations, saving $331 per single infant in short-term acute medical care costs only. In the managed care setting, it has been estimated that full breastfeeding is associated with a 20% reduction in total medical expenses compared with never breastfeeding.[143] Not included in these cost estimates are the fewer absences from work of families who are breastfeeding their infants. Furthermore, the cost savings from reducing the incidence of chronic diseases in childhood and reducing the incidence of premenopausal breast cancer in women would be substantial. Thus, the economic incentives for a society to breastfeed are strong and should be promoted. Some corporations have recognized the significant cost savings from prolonging breastfeeding rates and have instituted vigorous promotion and support programs.

REFERENCES

1 Section on Breastfeeding, American Academy of Pediatrics. Breastfeeding and the use of human milk. *Pediatrics* 2005;**115**:496–506.

2 U.S. Department of Health and Human Services and Office on Women's Health. *Breastfeeding: HHS Blueprint for Action on Breastfeeding*. Washington, DC; 2000.

3 American College of Obstetricians and Gynecologists. Breastfeeding: maternal and infant aspects. Washington, DC: ACOG Educational Bulletin. 2000;**258**:1–16.

4 Freed, G. L., Landers, S., Schanler, R. J. A practical guide to successful breast-feeding management. *Am. J. Dis. Child.* 1991;**145**:917–21.

5 Ryan, A. S. The resurgence of breastfeeding in the United States. *Pediatrics* 1997;99.

6 Ryan, A. S., Wenjun, Z., Acosta, A. Breastfeeding continues to increase into the new millennium. *Pediatrics* 2002;**110**: 1103–9.

7 Schanler, R. J., O'Connor, K. G., Lawrence, R. A. Pediatricians' practices and attitudes regarding breastfeeding promotion. *Pediatrics* 1999a;**103**:e35.

8 Neville, M. C., Keller, R. P., Seacat, J. *et al.* Studies on human lactation. I. Within-feed and between-breast variation in selected components of human milk. *Am. J. Clin. Nutr.* 1984;**40**:635–46.

9 Mennella, J. A. Mother's milk: a medium for early flavor experiences. *J. Hum. Lact.* 1995;**11**:39–43.

10 Atkinson, S. A., Bryan, M. H., Anderson, G. H. Human milk: Difference in nitrogen concentration in milk from mothers of term and premature infants. *J. Pediatr.* 1978;**93**:67–9.

11 Butte, N. F., Garza, C., Johnson, C. A., Smith, E. O., Nichols, B. L. Longitudinal changes in milk composition of mothers delivering preterm and term infants. *Early Hum. Dev.* 1984a;**9**:153–62.

12 Schanler, R. J., Oh, W. Composition of breast milk obtained from mothers of premature infants as compared to breast milk obtained from donors. *J. Pediatr.* 1980;**96**:679–81.

13 Gross, S. J., David, R. J., Bauman, L., Tomarelli, R. M. Nutritional composition of milk produced by mothers delivering preterm. *J. Pediatr.* 1980;**96**:641–4.

14 Dewey, K. G., Cohen, R. J., Rivera, L. L., Canahuati, J., Brown, K. H. Do exclusively breast-fed infants require extra protein? *Pediatr. Res.* 1996;**39**:303–7.

15 Carlson, S. E. Human milk nonprotein nitrogen: occurrence and possible functions. In: Barness, L. A., ed. *Advances in Pediatrics*. Chicago, IL: Year Book Medical Publishers; 1985: 43–70.

16 Hambraeus, L. Proprietary milk versus human breast milk in infant feeding, a critical appraisal from the nutritional point of view. *Pediatr. Clin. N. Am.* 1977;**24**:17–35.

17 Heine, W., Tiess, M., Wutzke, K. D. 15N tracer investigations of the physiological availability of urea nitrogen in mother's milk. *Acta Paediatr. Scand.* 1986;**75**:439–43.

18 Fomon, S. J., Bier, D. M., Matthews, D. E. *et al.* Bioavailability of dietary urea nitrogen in the breast-fed infant. *J. Pediatr.* 1988;**113**:515–17.

19 Billeaud, C., Guillet, J., Sandler, B. Gastric emptying in infants with or without gastro-oesophageal reflux according to the type of milk. *Eur. J. Clin. Nutr.* 1990;**44**:577–83.

20 Rassin, D. K., Gaull, G. E., Raiha, N. C. R., Heinonen, K. Milk protein quantity and quality in low-birth-weight infants. IV. Effects on tyrosine and phenylalanine in plasma and urine. *J. Pediatr.* 1977;**90**:356–60.

21 Gaull, G. E., Rassin, D. K., Raiha, N. C. R., Heinonen, K. Milk protein quantity and quality in low-birthweight infants. III. Effects on sulfur amino acids in plasma and urine. *J. Pediatr.* 1977;**90**:348–55.

22 Jarvenpaa, A. L., Raiha, N. C., Rassin, D. K. Feeding the low-birth-weight infant: I. Taurine and cholesterol supplementation of formula does not affect growth and metabolism. *Pediatrics* 1983;**71**:171–8.

23 Jarvenpaa, A. L., Rassin, D. K., Raiha, N. C. R., Gaull, G. E. Milk protein quantity and quality in the term infant. II. Effects on acidic and neutral amino acids. *Pediatrics* 1982;**70**: 221–30.

24 Picone, T. A., Benson, J. D., Moro, G. *et al.* Growth, serum biochemistries, and amino acids of term infants fed formulas with amino acid and protein concentrations similar to human milk. *J. Pediatr. Gastroenterol. Nutr.* 1989;**9**:351–60.

25 Goldman, A. S., Chheda, S., Keeney, S. E., Schmalsteig, F. C., Schanler, R. J. Immunologic protection of the premature newborn by human milk. *Semin. Perinatol.* 1994;**18**:495–501.

26 Lonnerdal, B. Biochemistry and physiological function of human milk proteins. *Am. J. Clin. Nutr.* 1985;**42**:1299–317.

27 Hanson, L. A., Ahlstedt, S., Andersson, B. *et al.* Protective factors in milk and the development of the immune system. *Pediatrics* 1985;**75**:172–6.

28 Jensen, R. G. The lipids in human milk. *Prog. Lipid Res.* 1996;**35**:53–92.

29 Hernell, O., Blackberg, L. Human milk bile salt-stimulated lipase: functional and molecular aspects. *J. Pediatr.* 1994;**125**:S56–61.

30 Jensen, R. G., Jensen, G. L. Specialty lipids for infant nutrition. I. Milks and formulas. *J. Pediatr. Gastroenterol. Nutr.* 1992;**15**:232–45.

31 Jensen, R. G., Hagerty, M. M., McMahon, K. E. Lipids of human milk and infant formulas: a review. *Am. J. Clin. Nutr.* 1978;**31**:990–1016.

32 Butte, N. F., Garza, C., Smith, E. O. Variability of macronutrient concentrations in human milk. *Eur. J. Clin. Nutr.* 1988;**42**: 345–9.

33 Daly, S. E., Di, Rosso, A., Owens, R. A., Hartmann, P. E. Degree of breast emptying explains changes in the fat content, but not fatty acid composition, of human milk. *Exp. Physiol.* 1993;**78**:741–55.

34 Nommsen, L. A., Lovelady, C. A., Heinig, M. J., Lonnerdal, B., Dewey, K. G. Determinants of energy, protein, lipid, and lactose concentrations in human milk during the first 12 months of lactation: the DARLING study. *Am. J. Clin. Nutr.* 1991;**53**:457–65.

35 Butte, N. F., Garza, C., Stuff, J. E., Smith, E. O., Nichols, B. L. Effect of maternal diet and body composition on lactational performance. *Am. J. Clin. Nutr.* 1984b;**39**:296–306.

36 Sauerwald, T. U., Demmelmair, H., Koletzko, B. Polyunsaturated fatty acid supply with human milk. *Lipids* 2001;**36**: 991–6.

37 Uauy, R., Hoffman, D., Peirano, P., Birch, D., Birch, E. E. Essential fatty acids in visual and brain development. *Lipids* 2001;**36**:885–95.

38 Whyte, R. K., Homer, R., Pennock, C. A. Faecal excretion of oligosaccharides and other carbohydrates in normal neonates. *Arch. Dis. Child.* 1978;**53**:913–15.

39 MacLean, W. C., Fink, B. B. Lactose malabsorption by premature infants: magnitude and clinical significance. *J. Pediatr.* 1980;**97**:383–8.

40 Ziegler, E. E., Fomon, S. J. Lactose enhances mineral absorption in infancy. *J. Pediatr. Gastroenterol. Nutr.* 1983;**2**:288–94.

41 Kunz, C., Rudloff, S. Biological functions of oligosaccharides in human milk. *Acta Paediatr.* 1993;**82**:903–12.

42 Hanson, L. A., Adlerberth, I., Carlsson, B. *et al.* Host defense of the neonate and the intestinal flora. *Acta Paediatr. Scand.* 1989;**351**:122–5.

43 Neville, M. C., Watters, C. D. Secretion of calcium into milk: a review. *J. Dairy Sci.* 1983;**66**:371–80.

44 Venkataraman, P. S., Luhar, H., Neylan, M. J. Bone mineral metabolism in full-term infants fed human milk, cow milk-based, and soy-based formulas. *Am. J. Dis. Child.* 1992;**146**:1302–5.

45 Casey, C. E., Hambidge, K. M., Neville, M. C. Studies in human lactation: zinc, copper, manganese, and chromium in human milk in the first month of lactation. *Am. J. Clin. Nutr.* 1985;**41**:1193–200.

46 Dallman, P. R., Siimes, M. A., Stekel, A. Iron deficiency in infancy and childhood. *Am. J. Clin. Nutr.* 1980;**33**:86–118.

47 Lonnerdal, B., Hernell, O. Iron, zinc, copper and selenium status of breast-fed infants and infants fed trace element fortified milk-based infant formula. *Acta Paediatr.* 1994;**83**:367–73.

48 Greer, F. R., Suttie, J. W. Vitamin K and the newborn. In: Tsang, R. C., Nichols, B. L., eds. *Nutrition during Infancy.* Philadelphia, PA: Hanley & Belfus; 1988:289–97.

49 Uauy, R., Quan, R., Gil, A. Role of nucleotides in intestinal development and repair: implications for infant nutrition. *J. Nutr.* 1994;**124**:1436S–41S.

50 Carver, J. D., Walker, W. A. The role of nucleotides in human nutrition. *Nutr. Biochem.* 1995;**6**:58–72.

51 Sheard, N. F., Walker, W. A. The role of breast milk in the development of the gastrointestinal tract. *Nutr. Rev.* 1988;**46**:1–8.

52 Dvorak, B., Halpern, M. D., Holubec, H. *et al.* Epidermal growth factor reduces the development of necrotizing enterocolitis in a neonatal rat model. *Am. J. Physiol. Gastrointest. Liver Physiol.* 2001;**282**:G156–64.

53 Claud, E. C., Walker, W. A. Hypothesis: inappropriate colonization of the premature intestine can cause neonatal necrotizing enterocolitis. *FASEB J.* 2001;**15**:1398–403.

54 Steinwender, G., Schimpl, G., Sixl, B., Wenzl, H. H. Gut-derived bone infection in the neonatal rat. *Pediatr. Res.* 2001;**50**: 767–71.

55 Goldman, A. S., Sharpe, L. W., Goldblum, R. M. Anti-inflammatory properties of human milk. *Acta Paediatr. Scand.* 1986;**75**:689–95.

56 Goldman, A. S., Smith, C. W. Host resistance factors in human milk. *J. Pediatr.* 1973;**82**:1082–90.

57 Kleinman, R. E., Walker, W. A. The enteromammary immune system. *Dig. Dis. Sci.* 1979;**24**:876–82.

58 Fishaut, M., Murphy, D., Neifert, M., McIntosh, K., Ogra, P. L. Bronchomammary axis in the immune response to respiratory syncytial virus. *J. Pediatr.* 1981;**99**:186–91.

59 Isaacs, C. E., Kashyap, S., Heird, W. C., Thormar, H. Antiviral and antibacterial lipids in human milk and infant formula feeds. *Arch. Dis. Child.* 1990;**65**:861–4.

60 Caplan, M. S., Jilling, T. The role of polyunsaturated fatty acid supplementation in intestinal inflammation and neonatal necrotizing enterocolitis. *Lipids* 2001;**36**:1053–7.

61 Boehm, G., Lidestri, M., Casetta, P. *et al.* Supplementation of a bovine milk formula with an oligosaccharide mixture increases counts of faecal bifidobacteria in preterm infants. *Arch. Dis. Child. Fetal Neonatal.* 2002;**86**:F178–81.

62 Caplan, M. S., Lickerman, M., Adler, L., Dietsch, G. N., Yu, A. The role of recombinant platelet-activating factor acetylhydrolase in a neonatal rat model of necrotizing enterocolitis. *Pediatr. Res.* 1997;**42**:779–83.

63 Garofalo, R., Chheda, S., Mei, F. *et al.* Interleukin-10 in human milk. *Pediatr. Res.* 1995;**37**:444–9.

64 Fituch, C. C., Palkowetz, K. H., Hurst, N. M., Goldman, A. S., Schanler, R. J. Interleukin-10 concentrations in milk of mothers delivering extremely low birth weight infants. *Pediatr. Res.* 2001;**49**:398A.

65 Dewey, K. G., Peerson, J. M., Brown, K. H. *et al.* Growth of breast-fed infants deviates from current reference data: a pooled analysis of US, Canadian, and European data sets. *Pediatrics* 1995b;**96**:495–503.

66 Dewey, K. G. Nutrition, growth, and complementary feeding of the breastfed infant. *Pediatr. Clin. N. Am.* 2001;**48**:87–104.

67 Cohen, R. J., Brown, K. H., Canahuati, J., Rivera, L. L., Dewey, K. G. Effects of age of introduction of complementary foods on infant breast milk intake, total energy intake, and growth: a randomised intervention study in Honduras. *Lancet* 1994;**343**:288–93.

68 Stuff, J. E., Nichols, B. L. Nutrient intake and growth performance of older infants fed human milk. *J. Pediatr.* 1989;**115**:959–68.

69 Greer, F. R., Searcy, J. E., Levin, R. S. *et al.* Bone mineral content and serum 25-OH D concentrations in breast-fed infants with and without supplemental vitamin D: One year follow-up. *J. Pediatr.* 1982;**100**:919–22.

70 Armstrong, J., Reilly, J. J. Child Health Information Team. Breastfeeding and lowering the risk of childhood obesity. *Lancet* 2002;**360**:1249–50.

71 Gillman, M. W., Rifas-Shiman, S. L., Camargo Jr, C. A. *et al.* Risk of overweight among adolescents who were breastfed as infants. *J. Am. Med. Assoc.* 2001;**285**:2461–7.

72 Toschke, A. M., Vignerova, J., Lhotska, L. *et al.* Overweight and obesity in 6- to 14-year-old Czech children in 1991: protective effect of breastfeeding. *J. Pediatr.* 2002;**141**:764–9.

73 Jones, G., Riley, M., Dwyer, T. Breastfeeding in early life and bone mass in prepubertal children: a longitudinal study. *Osteoporosis Int.* 2000;**11**:146–52.

74 von Kries, R., Koletzko, B., Sauerwald, T. *et al.* Breast feeding and obesity: cross sectional study. *Br. Med. J.* 1999;**319**: 147–50.

75 Cavell, B. Gastric emptying in infants fed human milk or infant formula. *Acta Paediatr. Scand.* 1981;**70**:639–41.

76 Shulman, R. J., Schanler, R. J., Lau, C. *et al.* Early feeding, feeding tolerance, and lactase activity in preterm infants. *J. Pediatr.* 1998a;**133**:645–9.

77 Shulman, R. J., Schanler, R. J., Lau, C. *et al.* Early feeding, antenatal glucocorticoids, and human milk decrease intestinal permeability in preterm infants. *Pediatr. Res.* 1998b;**44**: 519–23.

78 Popkin, B. M., Adair, L., Akin, J. S. *et al.* Breast-feeding and diarrheal morbidity. *Pediatrics* 1990;**86**:874–82.

79 Glass, R. I., Stoll, B. J. The protective effect of human milk against diarrhea. *Acta Paediatr. Scand.* 1989;**351**:131–6.

80 Leon-Cava, N., Lutter, C., Ross, J., Martin, L. Quantifying the benefits of breastfeeding: a summary of the evidence. *Food and Nutrition Program, Pan American Health Organization.* 2002;1–168.

81 Cunningham, A. S. Morbidity in breast-fed and artificially fed infants. *J. Pediatr.* 1977;**90**:726–9.

82 Cunningham, A. S. Morbidity in breast-fed and artificially fed infants. II. *J. Pediatr.* 1979;**95**:685–9.

83 Cunningham, A. S., Jelliffe, D. B., Jelliffe, E. F. P. Breast-feeding and health in the 1980s: a global epidemiologic review. *J. Pediatr.* 1991;**118**:659–66.

84 Dewey, K. G., Heinig, M. J., Nommsen-Rivers, L. A. Differences in morbidity between breastfed and formula-fed infants. *J. Pediatr.* 1995a;**126**:696–702.

85 Kovar, M. G., Serdula, M. D., Marks, J. S., Fraser, D. W. Review of the epidemiologic evidence for an association between infant feeding and infant health. *Pediatrics* 1984;**74**:S615–38.

86 Howie, P. W., Forsyth, J. S., Ogston, S. A., Clark, A., Florey, C. V. Protective effect of breastfeeding against infection. *Br. Med. J.* 1990;**300**:11–16.

87 Rubin, D. H., Leventhal, J. M., Krasilnikoff, P. A. *et al.* Relationship between infant feeding and infectious illness: a prospective study of infants during the first year of life. *Pediatrics* 1990;**85**:464–71.

88 Duncan, B., Ey, J., Holberg, C. J. *et al.* Exclusive breast-feeding for at least 4 months protects against otitis media. *Pediatrics* 1993;**91**:867–72.

89 Frank, A. L., Taber, L. H., Glezen, W. P. *et al.* Breast-feeding and respiratory virus infection. *Pediatrics* 1982;**70**:239–45.

90 Wright, A. L., Holberg, C. J., Martinez, F. D., Morgan, W. J., Taussig, L. M., Group Health Medical Associates. Breast feeding and lower respiratory tract illness in the first year of life. *Br. Med. J.* 1989;**299**:945–8.

91 Blaymore-Bier, J., Oliver, T., Ferguson, A., Vohr, B. R. Human milk reduces outpatient upper respiratory symptoms in premature infants during their first year of life. *J. Perinatol.* 2002;**22**:354–9.

92 Pisacane, A., Graziano, L., Mazzarella, G., Scarpellino, B., Zona, G. Breast-feeding and urinary tract infection. *J. Pediatr.* 1992;**120**:87–9.

93 Goldblum, R. M., Schanler, R. J., Garza, C., Goldman, A. S. Human milk feeding enhances the urinary excretion of immunologic factors in low birth weight infants. *Pediatr. Res.* 1989;**25**:184–8.

94 Coppa, G. V., Gabrielli, O., Giorgi, P. *et al.* Preliminary study of breastfeeding and bacterial adhesion to uroepithelial cells. *Lancet* 1990;**335**:569–71.

95 Narayanan, I., Prakash, K., Gujral, V. V. The value of human milk in the prevention of infection in the high-risk low-birth-weight infant. *J. Pediatr.* 1981;**99**:496–8.

96 Schanler, R. J., Shulman, R. J., Lau, C. Feeding strategies for premature infants: Beneficial outcomes of feeding fortified human milk *vs* preterm formula. *Pediatrics* 1999b;**103**: 1150–7.

97 Hylander, M. A., Strobino, D. M., Pezzullo, J. C., Dhanireddy, R. Association of human milk feedings with a reduction in retinopathy of prematurity among very low birthweight infants. *J. Perinatol.* 2001;**21**:356–62.

98 Contreras-Lemus, J., Flores-Huerta, S., Cisneros-Silva, I. *et al.* Disminucion de la morbilidad en neonatos pretermino alimentados con leche de su propia madre. *Biol. Med. Hosp. Infant Mex.* 1992;**49**:671–7.

99 Yu, V. Y. H., Jamieson, J., Bajuk, B. Breast milk feeding in very low birthweight infants. *Aust. Paediatr. J.* 1981;**17**:186–90.

100 Lucas, A., Cole, T. J. Breast milk and neonatal necrotizing enterocolitis. *Lancet* 1990;**336**:1519–23.

101 Eibl, M. M., Wolf, H. M., Fürnkranz, H., Rosenkranz, A. Prevention of necrotizing enterocolitis in low-birth-weight infants by IgA-IgG feeding. *N. Engl. J. Med.* 1988;**319**:1–7.

102 Carlson, S. E., Montalto, M. B., Ponder, D. L., Werkman, S. H., Korones, S. B. Lower incidence of necrotizing enterocolitis in infants fed a preterm formula with egg phospholipids. *Pediatr. Res.* 1998;**44**:491–8.

103 Caplan, M. S., Russell, T., Xiao, Y. *et al.* Effect of polyunsaturated fatty acid (PUFA) supplementation on intestinal

inflammation and necrotizing enterocolitis (NEC) in a neonatal rat model. *Pediatr. Res.* 2001;**49**:647–52.

104 Davis, M. K., Savitz, D. A., Graubard, B. I. Infant feeding and childhood cancer. *Lancet* 1988;**1**:365–8.

105 Koletzko, S., Sherman, P., Corey, M., Griffiths, A., Smith, C. Role of infant feeding practices in development of Crohn's disease in childhood. *Br. Med. J.* 1998;**298**:1617–18.

106 Gerstein, H. C. Cow's milk exposure and type I diabetes mellitus. *Diabetes Care* 1994;**17**:13–19.

107 Beral, V., Fear, N. T., Alexander, F., Appleby, P. Breastfeeding and childhood cancer. *Br. J. Cancer* 2001;**85**:1685–94.

108 Kramer, M. S. Does breast feeding help protect against atopic disease? Biology, methodology, and a golden jubilee of controversy. *J. Pediatr.* 1988;**112**:181–90.

109 Saarinen, U. M., Backman, A., Kajosaari, M., Siimes, M. A. Prolonged breast-feeding as prophylaxis for atopic disease. *Lancet* 1979;**ii**:163–6.

110 Gdalevich, M., Mimouni, D., Mimouni, M. Breast-feeding and the risk of bronchial asthma in childhood: asystematic review with meta-analysis of prospective studies. *J. Pediatr.* 2001;**139**:261–6.

111 Karjalainen, J., Martin, J. M., Knip, M. *et al.* A bovine albumin peptide as a possible trigger of insulin-dependent diabetes mellitus. *N. Engl. J. Med.* 1992;**327**:302–7.

112 Owen, C. G., Whincup, P. H., Odoki, K., Gilg, J. A., Cook, D. G. Infant feeding and blood cholesterol: a study in adolescents and a systematic review. *Pediatrics* 2002;**110**:597–608.

113 Anderson, J. W., Johnstone, B. M., Remley, D. T. Breastfeeding and cognitive development: a meta-analysis. *Am. J. Clin. Nutr.* 1999;**70**:525–35.

114 Mortensen, E. L., Michaelsen, K. F., Sanders, S. A., Reinisch, J. M. The association between duration of breastfeeding and adult intelligence. *J. Am. Med. Assoc.* 2002;**287**:2365–71.

115 Rogan, W. J., Gladen, B. C. Breast-feeding and cognitive development. *Early Hum. Dev.* 1993;**31**:181–93.

116 Lucas, A., Morley, R., Cole, T. J., Lister, G., Leeson-Payne, C. Breast milk and subsequent intelligence quotient in children born preterm. *Lancet* 1992;**339**:261–4.

117 Horwood, L. J., Mogridge, N., Darlow, B. A. Cognitive, educational, and behavioral outcomes at 7 to 8 years in a national very low birthweight cohort. *Arch. Dis. Child. Fetal Neonatal* 1998;**79**:F12–20.

118 Horwood, L. J., Darlow, B. A., Mogridge, N. Breast milk feeding and cognitive ability at 7–8 years. *Arch. Dis. Child. Fetal Neonatal* 2001;**84**:F23–7.

119 McKinley, L. T., Thorp, J. W., Tucker, R. Outcomes at 18 months corrected age of very low birth weight (VLBW) infants who received human milk during hospitalization. *Pediatr. Res.* 2000;**47**:1720A.

120 Riva, E., Agostoni, C., Biasucci, G. *et al.* Early breastfeeding is linked to higher intelligence quotient scores in dietary treated phenylketonuric children. *Acta Paediatr.* 1996;**85**:56–8.

121 Anderson, G. J., Connor, W. E., Corliss, J. D. Docosahexaenoic acid is the preferred dietary n-3 fatty acid for the development of the brain and retina. *Pediatr. Res.* 1990;**27**:89–97.

122 Carlson, S. E., Werkman, S. H., Rhodes, P. G., Tolley, E. A. Visual-acuity development in healthy preterm infants: effect of marine-oil supplementation. *Am. J. Clin. Nutr.* 1993;**58**: 35–42.

123 Hylander, M. A., Strobino, D. M., Pezzullo, J. C., Dhanireddy, R. Association of human milk feedings with a reduction in retinopathy of prematurity among very low birthweight infants. *J. Perinatol.* 2001;**21**:356–62.

124 Friel, J. K., Martin, S. M., Langdon, M., Herzberg, G. R., Buettner, G. R. Milk from mothers of both premature and full-term infants provides better antioxidant protection than does infant formula. *Pediatr. Res.* 2002;**51**:612–18.

125 Amin, S. B., Merle, K. S., Orlando, M. S., Dalzell, L. E., Guillet, R. Brainstem maturation in premature infants as a function of enteral feeding type. *Pediatrics* 2000;**106**:318–22.

126 Riordan, J. Anatomy and psychophysiology of lactation. In: Riordan, J., Auerbach, K. G., eds. *Breastfeeding and Human Lactation.* Boston, MA: Jones and Bartlett; 1993:81–104.

127 Mezzacappa, E. S., Kelsey, R. M., Myers, M. M., Katkin, E. S. Breast-feeding and maternal cardiovascular function. *Psychophysiology* 2001;**38**:988–97.

128 Wang, I. Y., Fraser, I. S. Reproductive function and contraception in the postpartum period. *Obstet. Gynecol. Survey* 1994;**49**:56–63.

129 Campbell, O. M., Gray, R. H. Characteristics and determinants of postpartum ovarian function in women in the United States. *Am. J. Obstet. Gynecol.* 1993;**169**:55–60.

130 Dewey, K. G., Heinig, M. J., Nommsen, L. A. Maternal weight-loss patterns during prolonged lactation. *Am. J. Clin. Nutr.* 1993;**58**:162–6.

131 Specker, B. L., Tsang, R. C., Ho, M. L. Changes in calcium homeostasis over the first year postpartum: effect of lactation and weaning. *Obstet. Gynecol.* 1991;**78**:56–62.

132 Sowers, M. F., Corton, G., Shapiro, B. *et al.* Changes in bone density with lactation. *J. Am. Med. Assoc.* 1993;**269**:3130–5.

133 Cumming, R. G., Klineberg, R. J. Breastfeeding and other reproductive factors and the risk of hip fracture in elderly women. *Int. J. Epidemiol.* 1993;**2**:684–91.

134 Bauer, D. C., Browner, W. S., Cauley, J. A. *et al.* Factors associated with appendicular bone mass in older women. *Ann. Intern. Med.* 1993;**118**:657–65.

135 Yoo, K., Tajima, K., Kuroishi, T. *et al.* Independent protective effect of lactation against breast cancer: a case control study in Japan. *Am. J. Epidemiol.* 1992;**135**:726–33.

136 Newcomb, P. A., Storer, B. E., Longnecker, M. P. *et al.* Lactation and a reduced risk of premenopausal breast cancer. *N. Engl. J. Med.* 1994;**330**:81–7.

137 Furberg, H., Newman, B., Moorman, P., Millikan, R. Lactation and breast cancer risk. *Int. J. Epidemiol.* 1999;**28**:396–402.

138 Zheng, T., Holford, T. R., Mayne, S. T. *et al.* Lactation and breast cancer risk: a case-control study in Connecticut. *Br. J. Cancer* 2001;**84**:1472–6.

139 Lawrence, R. M., Lawrence, R. A. Given the benefits of breastfeeding, what contraindications exist? *Pediatr. Clin. N. Am.* 2001;**48**:235–52.

140 Committee on Drugs and American Academy of Pediatrics. The transfer of drugs and other chemicals into human milk. *Pediatrics* 2001;**108**:776–89.

141 Weimer, J. P. Economic benefits of breastfeeding: a review and analysis. Washington, DC: USDA Food Assistance and Nutrition Research Report. 2001;**13**:1–14.

142 Montgomery, D. L., Splett, P. L. Economic benefit of breast-feeding infants enrolled in WIC. *J. Am. Diet. Assoc.* 1997;**97**:379–85.

143 Ball, T. M., Bennett, D. M. The economic impact of breastfeeding. *Pediatr. Clin. N. Am.* 2001;**48**:253–62.

27

Fortified human milk for premature infants

Richard J. Schanler

Neonatal-Perinatal Medicine, Schneider Children's Hospital at North Shore, North Shore University Hospital, Manhasset, NY
and Pediatrics, Albert Einstein College of Medicine, Bronx, NY

Introduction

Nutrition support of the premature infant must be designed to compensate for metabolic and gastrointestinal immaturity, immunologic compromise, and associated medical conditions. Nutritional needs are determined based on intrauterine rates of growth and nutrient accretion.[1] The beneficial effects of human milk extend to the feeding of premature infants (Chapter 26). Human milk is capable of satisfying most of the needs of premature infants if careful attention is given to nutritional status. Nevertheless, because of their specialized needs the human milk-fed premature infant may require nutrient supplementation, or fortification, to maintain optimal nutritional status while deriving benefits from enhanced host defense, neurologic development, and gastrointestinal function. The nutritional adequacy of human milk for premature infants may be limited for several reasons. The nutrient content of the milk may be inadequate for their needs and the variability in nutrient content results in an unpredictable nutrient intake for an infant who cannot feed *ad libitum*. Infants often receive restricted milk intakes. Mothers often are unable to supply sufficient milk to meet the needs of the infant throughout the hospitalization. As a consequence, nutrient inadequacy may manifest in the premature infant fed unfortified human milk. This review will focus on the feeding of fortified human milk to the premature infant.

Composition of preterm milk

Milk from mothers who give birth prematurely (preterm milk) generally has greater concentrations of immune proteins, lipid, energy, vitamins, calcium, sodium, and trace elements than in corresponding term milk.[2–5] There is a trend for nutrient concentrations in preterm milk to decline as lactation progresses, a pattern of change also observed in term milk (Table 27.1). Thus, while the higher nutrient concentrations of "early" milk might meet the nutrient needs of the premature infant, exclusive feeding of mature preterm milk from 2 weeks postnatally and onward may lead to nutrient deficiencies in the rapidly growing premature infant.

Availability

Despite the desire to provide milk for their premature infants, mothers often do not sustain adequate milk production to meet their infants' needs. Several factors have been implicated: delayed initiation of milk expression, infrequent milk expression, stress, fatigue, return to work, poor maternal health, sudden changes in the infant's condition, and, possibly, biological immaturity of the mammary gland. Indeed, fatigue and pain result in stimulation of prolactin inhibitory factor, which serves to blunt milk synthesis induced by prolactin.

Fluid restriction is part of the management of many premature infants because of their clinical condition, their inability to feed on demand, and because of feeding intolerance. Usually premature infants, especially those of extremely low birth weight, do not easily tolerate volumes of intake above 180 ml kg^{-1} day^{-1}; many such infants are restricted to fluid intakes of 150–160 ml kg^{-1} day^{-1}. Although the intake of some nutrients would be adequate, most could not be met unless 200 ml kg^{-1} day^{-1} or more

Neonatal Nutrition and Metabolism. Second Edition, ed. P. Thureen and W. Hay. Published by Cambridge University Press.

Table 27.1. Nutrient composition of transitional and mature preterm human milk compared with mature term milk[49]

Component (unit L^{-1})	Source	Preterm transitional 6–10 days	Preterm mature 22–30 days	Term mature $\geq$ 30 days
Total protein, g	A	19 ± 0.5	15 ± 1	12 ± 1.5
IgA, mg per g protein	A	92 ± 63	64 ± 70	83 ± 25
Non-protein nitrogen, % total nitrogen	A	18 ± 4	17 ± 7	24
Fat, g	B	34 ± 6	36 ± 7	34 ± 4
Carbohydrate, g	B	63 ± 5	67 ± 4	67 ± 5
Energy, kcal	B	660 ± 60	690 ± 50	640 ± 80
Ca, mmol	A	8.0 ± 1.8	7.2 ± 1.3	6.5 ± 1.5
P, mmol	A	4.9 ± 1.4	3.0 ± 0.8	4.8 ± 0.8
Mg, mmol	A	1.1 ± 0.2	1.0 ± 0.3	1.3 ± 0.3
Iron, mmol (mg)	B	23 (0.4)	22 (0.4)	22 (0.4)
Zn, μmol	B	58 ± 13	33 ± 14	15–46
Cu, μmol	B	9.2 ± 2.1	8.0 ± 3.1	3.2–6.3
Mn, μg (median)	B	6 ± 8.9	7.3 ± 6.6	3–6
Na, mmol	A	11.6 ± 6.0	8.8 ± 2.0	9.0 ± 4.1
K, mmol	A	13.5 ± 2.2	12.5 ± 3.2	13.9 ± 2.0
Cl, mmol	B	21.3 ± 3.5	14.8 ± 2.1	12.8 ± 1.5

A = Average $\pm$ SD[1] of values.[2]

B = Average $\pm$ SD of published values derived from milk samples obtained from 24 hour collections and similar stages of lactation.

Table 27.2. Premature recommended nutrient intakes for stable-growing premature infants >1 kg birth weight and the volume of human milk needed to meet the nutrient intake for selected nutrients[6, 49]

Component (units)	Recommended nutrient intakes for premature infant (unit kg^{-1} day^{-1})	Volume of preterm human milk needed to meet recommended intake of nutrient (mL kg^{-1} day^{-1})
Energy, kcal	105–135	145–185
Protein, g	3.0–3.6	180–210
Potassium, mmol	2.5–3.5	155–220
Zinc, mmol	7.7–12.3	120–190
Copper, mmol	0.1–1.9	115–200
Vitamin E, mg	0.5–0.9	120–200

were tolerated by the infant (Table 27.2).[6] Even if human milk is available, many infants do not achieve full enteral feedings for several weeks after birth. Thus, adequacy of nutrient intake may be jeopardized by the unavailability of milk and limited fluid volume that can be tolerated by the infant in need for maintenance as well as catch-up nutrition support.[7]

Variability in milk composition

The adequacy of nutrient intake is further compromised by the variability in nutrient composition, both inherent to milk and imposed by circumstances of collection and distribution of the milk. A large variation in the energy and protein contents of human milk brought to the neonatal nursery by the mother is observed.[8] This variation may arise because of differences in methods of milk collection and storage, the feeding of "spot" samples (individual samples of expressed milk from one or both breasts, or milk partially expressed from one breast), and the use of feeding tubes.

The most variable nutrient in human milk is fat, the content of which differs during lactation, throughout the day, from mother to mother, and within a single milk expression.[9, 10] As human milk is not homogenized, upon standing, the fat content separates from the body of milk. Much of the variation in energy content of milk as used in the nursery is a result of differences in and/or losses of fat in the unfortified milk.[11–13] In one report, the range in fat contents of milk brought to the nursery was 2.2–4.7 g dL^{-1}.[8] Therefore, when collecting, mixing, and/or storing milk, efforts must be directed to avoid allowing the fat to separate from the milk and be discarded inadvertently.

The use of continuous tube-feeding methods also reduces fat delivery to the infant compared with intermittent-bolus feeding.[11] Should the clinical condition mandate continuous tube-feeding, the milk syringe should be oriented with tip upright, a short length of feeding tube should be used, and the syringe should be emptied completely into the infant at end of the infusion. This practice will ensure the least loss of fat because the fat will flow along with the remainder of the milk.

The within-feed change in fat content (from foremilk to hindmilk) also can be used to benefit the infant if the mother's milk production is in excess of the infant's need. Hindmilk may have 2- to 3-fold greater fat content than foremilk and can be utilized to provide significantly more fat and, therefore, energy for growth.[9] As fat is the most variable nutrient and many mothers do not produce sufficient volumes to allow fractionation into foremilk and hindmilk, the use of vegetable oil supplements has been recommended. Because exogenous fat does not mix with human milk, the fat should be given in divided doses directly into the feeding tube before a tube-feeding.

There is a significant decline in the content of protein from transitional to mature milk which contributes to the problem of nutrient variability. Although concentrations of protein and sodium decline through lactation, the nutrient needs of the premature infant remain higher than those of term infants until sometime after term postmenstrual age. Therefore, the decline in milk concentration precedes the reduction in nutrient needs and results in an inadequate nutrient supply from human milk for the premature infant. The content of other nutrients (e.g., calcium, phosphorus) have less variability through lactation but remain too low with respect to the needs of the premature infant. Technical reasons associated with collection, storage, and delivery of milk to the infant also result in a decreased quantity of available nutrients (e.g., vitamin C, vitamin A, riboflavin).

Consequences of feeding unfortified human milk

Growth

The exclusive feeding of unfortified human milk in premature infants, generally infants with birth weights less than 1500 g, has been associated with poorer rates of growth and nutritional deficits, during and beyond the period of hospital stay.[14–18] As growth rates in excess of 15 g kg^{-1} day^{-1} are desired, unfortified human milk would not meet this target.

Protein status

Indices of protein nutritional status, e.g., blood urea nitrogen, serum albumin, total protein, and transthyretin, are lower and continue to decline over time when premature infants are fed unfortified human milk.[14,17,19]

Mineral status

As a consequence of the low intakes of calcium and phosphorus, infants fed unfortified human milk have progressive decreases in serum phosphorus, increases in serum calcium, and increases in serum alkaline phosphatase activity compared with infants fed preterm formula.[15,20,21] Follow-up investigations of such infants at 18 months report that infants having the highest alkaline phosphatase in-hospital have as much as a 2-cm reduction in linear growth.[22] Evaluation of this cohort at 9–12 y of age found that attained height was inversely related to the neonatal serum alkaline phosphatase activity.[23] These data suggest that long-term mineralization might be affected by neonatal diet.

The low milk sodium intake, especially if diuretics are given to the infant, may be associated with late hyponatremia.[24]

Human milk fortification

The nutrient deficits that arise from feeding unfortified human milk can be corrected with nutrient supplementation.[7] Protein and energy supplementation are associated with improved rates of weight gain, nitrogen balance, and indices of protein nutritional status: blood urea nitrogen, serum albumin, total protein, and transthyretin.[17,25] The efficacy of protein fortification of human milk (~1.5 g protein kg^{-1} day^{-1} added to human milk) was of short-term benefit resulting in increases in weight gain, and increments in length and head circumference growth. Although the measured gains were small, the effects were cumulative.[26] The source of protein in the fortifier also has been studied. Similar responses to bovine compared with human milk protein sources have been reported.[27]

Supplementation with both calcium and phosphorus results in normalization of biochemical indices of mineral status: serum calcium, phosphorus, and alkaline phosphatase activity, and urinary excretion of calcium and phosphorus.[20,28] Mineral supplementation of unfortified human milk has been associated with improved linear growth and increased bone mineralization during and beyond the neonatal period.[29] A normalization of serum sodium has been reported following the supplementation of unfortified human milk with sodium.[30]

Table 27.3. Variability in nutrient composition of commercial human milk fortifiers (2002)[49]

Nutrient	Enfamil HMF	Similac HMF	SMA BMF	Milupa Eoprotin	Nutriprem Cow & Gate	Aptamil FMS Milupa	FM$_{85}$ Nestle
How supplied	4 packets	4 packets	2 sachets	3 scoops	2 sachets	powder	powder
Quantity	4 g	4 g	4 g	3 g	3 g	3.4 g	5 g
Energy, kcal	14	14	15	11	10	12	18
Protein, g	1.1	1	1	0.6	0.7	0.8	0.8
Fat, g	0.65	0.36	0.16	0.02	0	0	0.015
Carbohydrate, g	1.1	1.8	2.4	2.1	2	2.2	3.6
Calcium, mg	90	117	90	38	60	69	51
Phosphorus, mg	45	67	45	26	40	46	34
Magnesium, mg	1	7	3	2.1	6	6.8	2
Iron, mg	1.44	0.35	0	0	0	0	0
Manganese, μg	10	7.2	4.6	0	6	10	0
Zinc, μg	720	1000	260	0	300	350	0
Copper, μg	44	170	0	0	26	30	0
Sodium, mmol	0.5	0.7	0.8	0.9	0.3	0.3	1.2
Potassium, mmol	0.5	1.6	0.7	0.006	0.1	0.1	0.3
Chloride, mmol	0.3	1.1	0.5	0.4	0.2	0.2	0.5
Increment in osmolality, mOsm	63	90	137	70	60	57	105
Vitamin A, μg	285	186	270	30	130	150	0
Vitamin D, μg	4	3	7.6	0	5	5.7	0
Vitamin E, mg	4.6	3.2	3	0.3	2.6	2.9	0
Vitamin K$_1$, μg	4.4	8.3	11	0.2	6.3	7.1	0
Thiamin, μg	150	233	220	0	130	150	0
Riboflavin, μg	220	417	260	0	170	190	0
Vitamin B$_6$, μg	115	211	260	0	110	120	0
Vitamin B$_{12}$, μg	0.18	0.64	0.3	0	0.2	0.2	0
Niacin, mg	3	3.57	3.6	0	2.5	2.8	0
Folic acid, μg	25	23	0	0	50	57	0
Pantothenic acid, mg	0.73	1.5	0	0	0.75	0.85	0
Biotin, μg	2.7	26	0	0	2.5	2.8	0
Vitamin C, mg	12	25	40	15	12	14	0

Enfamil Human Milk Fortifier (Mead Johnson Nutritionals, Evansville, IN).
Similac Human Milk Fortifier (Ross Laboratories, Columbus, OH).
SMA Breast Milk Fortifier (Wyeth Nutritionals International, Philadelphia, PA).
Eoprotin (Milupa, Friedrichsdorf, Germany).
FM$_{85}$ (Nestle, Vevey, Switzerland).
Nutriprem (Cow & Gate).
Aptamil FMS (Milupa).

A systematic review that addressed multinutrient fortification of human milk included a meta-analysis of 10 controlled trials ($n > 600$ infants with birth weight generally <1850 g) of human milk fortification compared with the feeding of unfortified human milk.[29] The addition of multinutrient fortifiers to human milk resulted in short-term improvements in weight gain and increments in both length and head circumference growth during hospital stay.

Reformulations of human milk fortifiers

Comparison of human milk fortifiers (in 2002) indicate a wide range of nutrient compositions (Table 27.3). Few direct comparisons have been reported. The growth of premature infants fed fortified human milk has been reported to be lower than that of similar infants receiving preterm formula in most studies.[28,31–33] Several explanations have been advanced for this observation. The protein intake from fortified human milk is lower than preterm formula, especially if comparisons are made of fortified *mature* milk and formula. Studies of formulations of fortified human milk in the early 1990s reported lower fat absorption than infants fed preterm formula.[34] The variability in the fat content of human milk, the lack of fat in the human milk fortifiers used in the 1990s, and the soluble mineral preparations interacting with the fat globule, together, could result in lower rates of fat absorption. The addition of a large quantity of minerals to human milk may have created an unfavorable milieu for the human milk lipid system. The fat globule may be disrupted by osmotic forces generated by the high mineral content of the fortifier, and result in the liberation of free fatty acids. The free fatty acids may bind minerals and form soaps. In the intestinal tract soap formation may hinder fat absorption.[35,36]

Commercial human milk fortifiers in the USA have been reformulated to improve protein intake, fat absorption, and reduce the incidence of hypercalcemia.[31] Two randomized, multicenter trials of human milk fortifiers, comparing protein, fat, and mineral composition, found improved growth in infants fed the higher protein and fat formulations.[37,38] Beneficial effects on growth were observed in response to mean differences in protein intake of 0.3–0.4 g kg^{-1} day^{-1} fed over 20 to 29 days while in hospital. Indices of protein nutritional status tended to decline during one study.[38] This observation suggested that optimal protein intakes were not achieved. Although no major differences were reported in energy intake, it is argued that a more favorable milieu (less bioavailable mineral suspension prevented interaction with milk fat globule) and greater fat intake resulted in better fat absorption. Serum calcium and phosphorus were lower, in the normal range, in infants receiving the fortifier containing less soluble mineral sources.[38] Mildly elevated plasma alkaline phosphatase activity in the group receiving greater protein intake was considered a supportive of enhanced linear growth.[38] In addition, the fortifiers differed markedly in their contents of zinc and copper. Despite no added copper to one of the fortifiers, serum copper and ceruloplasmin concentrations were similar between groups with and without copper fortification.[37] These data suggest that the copper content of unfortified human milk is adequate for premature infants. Neither randomized trial reported any safety issues or differences in morbidity between study groups.

Non-nutritional outcomes of feeding fortified human milk

Feeding tolerance

Questions have been raised as to whether the addition of commercial formula-derived human milk fortifiers affects feeding tolerance in premature infants. Gastric residual volumes often are used to assess feeding tolerance. The residual volume may be affected by gastric emptying. The data on gastric emptying, however, are controversial. Novel ultrasound techniques to assess gastric cross-sectional areas have reported conflicting results.[39,40] In contrast, it clearly has been reported that use of fortified human milk is not associated with feeding intolerance, as manifest by abdominal distention, vomiting, changes in stool frequency, or volume of gastric aspirate.[33] An investigation of feeding tolerance indices 5 days before v. 5 days after addition of human milk fortifier (HMF) revealed that of the 10 indices assessed, only gastric residual volume ≥ 2 mL kg^{-1} and emesis were statistically greater after the addition of HMF. However, infants manifesting these feeding intolerance indices were no more likely to have delays in achieving full tube-feeding or full oral feeding than infants not experiencing increases in feeding intolerance indices. Furthermore, no differences in feeding tolerance were reported in a meta-analysis comparing premature infants fed fortified human milk or unfortified human milk.[29] Moreover, premature infants fed human milk fortified with a variety of commercial multinutrient fortifiers have not manifest any differences in feeding tolerance.[37,38] Lastly, in comparison with infants fed preterm formula, those fed fortified human milk had similar tolerance to feeding.[31] Thus, concerns about feeding tolerance should not dissuade clinicians from using HMF.

Host defense

A theoretical concern with human milk fortification is that the added nutrients may affect the intrinsic host defense system of the milk. The relationship between diet and the incidence of infection in premature infants has been examined. Human milk-fed infants had a 26% incidence of documented infection compared with 49% in formula-fed infants.[41] Results of a randomized trial of fortified human milk indicated no increases in the incidence of either confirmed infection or necrotizing enterocolitis compared with controls.[33] When the latter two events were combined, however, the group fed fortified human milk had more events than infants in the control group. The data, however, are difficult to interpret because study infants in both groups received more than 50% of their diet as preterm formula.[42] When compared with premature infants fed preterm formula, those infants fed exclusively fortified human milk had a significantly lower incidence of necrotizing enterocolitis and/or sepsis, fewer positive blood cultures, and less antibiotic usage.[31] Infants receiving the most human milk had the fewest positive blood cultures. Infants fed exclusively fortified human milk also had more episodes of skin-to-skin contact with their mothers and shorter hospital stays. From these data, it appears that by reducing infectious morbidity, feeding premature infants fortified human milk might have a marked effect on reducing the cost of medical care.

Extremely premature infants fed their mothers' milk supplemented with human milk fortifier had less episodes of sepsis and/a NEC but sepses and/or NEC was increased if the infants received preterm formula or fortified, pasteurized donor human milk. So as substitutes for mother's own milk no short-term advantages were noted for preterm formula or donor human milk.[50]

The effect of nutrient fortification on some of the general host defense properties of milk have been evaluated.[43,44] Fortification did not affect the concentration of IgA in milk.[43,44] When fortified human milk was evaluated under simulated nursery conditions, bacterial colony counts were not significantly different after 20 hours' storage at refrigerator temperature, but did increase from 20–24 hours when maintained at incubator temperature. The overall increase in bacterial colony counts at 24 hours, however, was no different from values at time 0.[43] Based on these data, changes are unlikely to be necessary in regard to the current practice of how fortifiers are used in the nursery.

Other outcomes

Unfortunately, there have been insufficient data to evaluate long-term outcomes of fortification of human milk on growth or neurodevelopment. One limited study found no differences in neurodevelopmental outcome at 18 months in premature infants fed fortified or minimally supplemented human milk in hospital.[33] Accordingly, several investigators have made a plea for further research that is designed to address both the short-term and long-term outcomes of protein and multinutrient fortification of human milk.[29]

Methods of human milk fortification

The fortification of human milk can be performed using a liquid commercial formula mixed with human milk or powdered commercial products. Most authorities recommend that the supplement provide multinutrient as opposed to single nutrient fortification. The powdered products have the obvious advantage of not diluting the human milk, are reported to be preferred by parents, and have a positive impact on duration of breastfeeding.[45] Few randomized comparisons among fortifiers have been reported. A casual comparison between a liquid preterm formula mixed with human milk (1:1, vol:vol) and a powdered human milk fortifier can be derived from the literature.[31,46] Protein intake and net retention were lower with the liquid preparation than the powder. Calcium, phosphorus, and zinc intakes also were lower with the liquid compared with the powdered preparation used in the early 1990s. Not only are the nutrient intakes lower with the liquid preparation, but the achieved net nutrient retentions are well below expected rates of intrauterine nutrient accretion. The use of a liquid fortifier should be reserved for situations when the mother is unable to provide sufficient milk to meet her infant's needs. However, when sufficient human milk is unavailable, an alternative approach is to feed fortified human milk (using powdered fortifier) for as many feedings as there is milk available, then alternating with preterm formula for the remaining feedings.

In-hospital feeding practices

The use of multinutrient fortification of human milk for premature infants is recommended.[31,34,47,48] A variety of protocols are used for feeding fortified human milk. In one such protocol, human milk is fortified when the infant achieves an enteral intake of 100 mL kg^{-1} day^{-1}.[31] The volume is maintained for approximately 2 days while the concentration is increased by the addition of fortifier. The intake of fortified human milk is then advanced daily to maintain a body weight gain of greater than 15 g kg^{-1} day^{-1}. No additional vitamin supplements are needed. To support the low iron stores of the premature infant, if the fortifier has insufficient iron content, an exogenous source of elemental iron is supplied after complete enteral feeding is achieved.

Fortified human milk is prepared daily and stored at refrigerator temperature in individual feeding syringes until used within 24 hours. However, recent data suggest that fortified human milk could be stored at refrigerator temperature for up to 72 hours.[51] Milk should be handled and checked carefully to ensure that the donor and recipient identities match. An aggressive approach toward lactation support is critical for successful milk production in mothers of premature infants.

REFERENCES

1 Ziegler, E. E., O'Donnell, A. M., Nelson, S. E., Fomon, S. J. Body composition of the reference fetus. *Growth* 1976;**40**:329–41.

2 Atkinson, S. A. The effects of gestational stage at delivery on human milk components. In: Jensen, R. G., ed. *Handbook of Milk Composition*. San Diego, CA: Academic Press; 1995:222–37.

3 Aquilio, E., Spagnoli, R., Seri, S., Bottone, G., Spennati, G., Trace element content in human milk during lactation of preterm newborns. *Biol. Trace Elem. Res.* 1996;**51**:63–70.

4 Friel, J. K., Andrews, W. L., Jackson, S. E. *et al.* Elemental composition of human milk from mothers of premature and full-term infants during the first 3 months of lactation. *Biol. Trace Elem. Res.* 1999;**67**:225–47.

5 Perrone, L., Di Palma, L., Di Toro, R., Gialanella, G., Moro, R. Interaction of trace elements in a longitudinal study of human milk from full-term and preterm mothers. *Biol. Trace Elem. Res.* 1994;**41**:321–30.

6 Nutrition Committee and Canadian Paediatric Society. Nutrient needs and feeding of premature infants. *Can. Med. Assoc. J.* 1995;**152**:1765–85.

7 Schanler, R. J. The use of human milk for premature infants. *Pediatr. Clin. N. Am.* 2001;**48**:207–20.

8 Polberger, S. Quality of growth in preterm neonates fed individually fortified human milk. In: Battaglia, F. C., Pedraz, C., Sawatzki, G. *et al.*, eds. *Maternal and Extrauterine Nutritional Factors. Their Influence on Fetal and Infant Growth*. Madrid: Ediciones Ergon SA; 1996: 395–403.

9 Neville, M. C., Keller, R. P., Seacat, J. *et al.* Studies on human lactation. I. Within-feed and between-breast variation in selected components of human milk. *Am. J. Clin. Nutr.* 1984;**40**:635–46.

10 Valentine, C. J., Hurst, N. M., Schanler, R. J. Hindmilk improves weight gain in low-birth-weight infants fed human milk. *J. Pediatr. Gastroenterol. Nutr.* 1994;**18**:474–7.

11 Greer, F. R., McCormick, A. Improved bone mineralization and growth in premature infants fed fortified own mother's milk. *J. Pediatr.* 1988;**112**:961–9.

12 Schanler, R. J. Special methods in feeding the preterm infant. In: Tsang, R. C., Nichols, B. L., eds. *Nutrition during Infancy*. Philadelphia, Pa: Hanley & Belfus; 1988:314 25.

13 Weber, A., Loui, A., Jochum, F., Bührer, C., Obladen, M. Breast milk from mothers of very low birthweight infants: variability in fat and protein content. *Acta Pædiatr.* 2001;**90**:772–5.

14 Atkinson, S. A., Bryan, M. H., Anderson, G. H. Human milk feeding in premature infants: protein, fat and carbohydrate balances in the first two weeks of life. *J. Pediatr.* 1981;**99**:617–24.

15 Atkinson, S. A., Radde, I. C., Anderson, G. H. Macromineral balances in premature infants fed their own mothers' milk or formula. *J. Pediatr.* 1983;**102**:99–106.

16 Cooper, P. A., Rothberg, A. D., Pettifor, J. M., Bolton, K. D., Devenhuis, S. Growth and biochemical response of premature infants fed pooled preterm milk or special formula. *J. Pediatr. Gastroenterol. Nutr.* 1984;**3**:749–54.

17 Kashyap, S., Schulze, K. F., Forsyth, M. *et al.* Growth, nutrient retention, and metabolic response of low-birth-weight infants fed supplemented and unsupplemented preterm human milk. *Am. J. Clin. Nutr.* 1990;**52**:254–62.

18 Gross, S. J. Growth and biochemical response of preterm infants fed human milk or modified infant formula. *N. Engl. J. Med.* 1983; **308**:237–41.

19 Polberger, S. K. T., Axelsson, I. A., Räihä, N. C. R. Urinary and serum urea as indicators of protein metabolism in very low birthweight infants fed varying human milk protein intakes. *Acta Paediatr. Scand.* 1990;**79**:737–42.

20 Rowe, J. C., Wood, D. H., Rowe, D. W., Raisz, L. G. Nutritional hypophosphatemic rickets in a premature infant fed breast milk. *N. Engl. J. Med.* 1979;**300**:293–6.

21 Pettifor, J. M., Rajah, R., Venter, A. Bone mineralization and mineral homeostasis in very low-birth-weight infants fed either human milk or fortified human milk. *J. Pediatr. Gastroenterol. Nutr.* 1989;**8**:217–24.

22 Lucas, A., Brooke, O. G., Baker, B. A., Bishop, N. Morley, R. High alkaline phosphatase activity and growth in preterm neonates. *Arch. Dis. Child.* 1989;**64**:902–9.

23 Fewtrell, M. S., Cole, T. J., Bishop, N. J., Lucas, A. Neonatal factors predicting childhood height in preterm infants: evidence for a persisting effect of early metabolic bone disease? *J. Pediatr.* 2000;**137**:668–73.

24 Roy, R. N., Chance, G. W., Radde, I. C. *et al.* Late hyponatremia in very low birthweight infants. *Pediatr. Res.* 1976; **10**:526–31.

25 Polberger, S. K. T., Axelsson, I. A., Räihä, N. C. R. Growth of very low birth weight infants on varying amounts of human milk protein. *Pediatr. Res.* 1989;**25**:414–19.

26 Kuschel, C. A., Harding, J. E. Protein supplementation of human milk for promoting growth in preterm infants (Cochrane Review). *The Cochrane Library*. 2005.

27 Polberger, S., Räihä, N. C., Juvonen, P. *et al.* Individualized protein fortification of human milk for preterm infants: comparison of ultrafiltrated human milk protein and a bovine whey fortifier. *J. Pediatr. Gastroenterol. Nutr.* 1999;**29**:332–8.

28 Schanler, R. J., Garza, C. Improved mineral balance in very low birth weight infants fed fortified human milk. *J. Pediatr.* 1987;**112**:452–6.

29 Kuschel, C. A., Harding, J. E. Multicomponent fortified human milk for promoting growth in preterm infants (Cochrane Review). *The Cochrane Library*. 2005.

30 Kumar, S. P., Sacks, L. M. Hyponatremia in very low-birth-weight infants and human milk feedings. *J. Pediatr.* 1978;**93**:1026–7.

31 Schanler, R. J., Shulman, R. J., Lau, C. Feeding strategies for premature infants: beneficial outcomes of feeding fortified human milk *vs* preterm formula. *Pediatrics* 1999;**103**:1150–7.

32 Wauben, I. P., Atkinson, S. A., Grad, T. L., Shah, J. K., Paes, B. Moderate nutrient supplementation of mother's milk for preterm infants support adequate bone mass and short-term growth: a randomized, controlled trial. *Am. J. Clin. Nutr.* 1998;**67**:465–72.

33 Lucas, A., Fewtrell, M. S., Morley, R. *et al.* Randomized outcome trial of human milk fortification and developmental outcome in preterm infants. *Am. J. Clin. Nutr.* 1996;**64**:142–51.

34 Schanler, R. J., Abrams, S. A. Postnatal attainment of intrauterine macromineral accretion rates in low birth weight infants fed fortified human milk. *J. Pediatr.* 1995;**126**:441–7.

35 Schanler, R. J., Henderson, T. R., Hamosh, M. Fatty acid soaps may be responsible for poor fat absorption in premature infants fed fortified human milk. *Pediatr. Res.* 1999; **45**:290A.

36 Chappell, J. E., Clandinin, M. T., Kearney-Volpe, C., Reichman, B., Swyer, P. W. Fatty acid balance studies in premature infants fed human milk or formula: effect of calcium supplementation. *J. Pediatr.* 1986;**108**:439–47.

37 Porcelli, P., Schanler, R., Greer, F. *et al.* Growth in human milk-fed very low birth weight infants receiving a new human milk fortifier. *Ann. Nutr. Metab.* 2000;**44**:2–10.

38 Barrett-Reis, B., Hall, R. T., Schanler, R. J. *et al.* Enhanced growth of preterm infants fed a new powdered human milk fortifier: a randomized controlled trial. *Pediatrics* 2000;**106**:581–8.

39 Ewer, A. K., Yu, V. Y. H. Gastric emptying in pre-term infants: the effect of breast milk fortifier. *Acta Paediatr.* 1996;**85**:1112–15.

40 McClure, R. J., Newell, S. J. Effect of fortifying breast milk on gastric emptying. *Arch. Dis. Child.* 1996;**74**:F60–2.

41 Hylander, M. A., Strobino, D. M., Pezzullo, J. C., Dhanireddy, R. Association of human milk feedings with a reduction in retinopathy of prematurity among very low birthweight infants. *J. Perinatol.* 2001;**21**:356–62.

42 Schanler, R. J. Human milk fortification for premature infants. *Am. J. Clin. Nutr.* 1996;**64**:249–50.

43 Jocson, M. A. L., Mason, E. O., Schanler, R. J. The effects of nutrient fortification and varying storage conditions on host defense properties of human milk. *Pediatrics* 1997;**100**:240–3.

44 Quan, R., Yang, C., Rubinstein, S. *et al.* The effect of nutritional additives on anti-infective factors in human milk. *Clin. Pediatr.* 1994;**33**:325–8.

45 Fenton, T. R., Tough, S. C., Belik, J. Breast milk supplementation for preterm infants: parental preferences and postdischarge lactation duration. *Am. J. Perinatol.* 2000;**17**:329–33.

46 Schanler, R. J., Abrams, S. A., Garza, C. Bioavailability of calcium and phosphorus in human milk fortifiers and formula for very low birth weight infants. *J. Pediatr.* 1988;**113**:95–100.

47 Greer, F. R., McCormick, A. Improved bone mineralization and growth in premature infants fed fortified own mother's milk. *J. Pediatr.* 1988;**112**:961–9.

48 Berseth, C. L., Van Aerde, J. E., Gross, S., Stolz, S. I., Haris, C. L., Honsen, J. W. Growth, efficacy, and safety of feeding an iron-fortified human milk fortifier. *Pediatrics* 2004;**114**:e699–e706.

49 Schanler, R. J., Atkinson, S. A., Human milk. In: Tsang, R. C., Koletzka, B., Uauy, R., Zlotkin, S. (eds.). *Nutrition of the Preterm Infant, Scientific Basis and Practical Guidelines*, 2nd edn. Digital Educational Publishing, Cincinnati: 2005.

50 Schanler, R. J., Lau, C., Hurst, N. M., Smith, E. O. Randomized trial of donor human milk versus preterm formula as substitutes for mothers' own milk in the feeding of extremely premature infants. *Pediatrics* 2005;**116**:400–6.

51 Santiago, M., Codipilly, C., Potak, D., Schanler, R. J. Effect of human milk fortifiers on bacterial growth in human milk. *J. Perinatol.* 2005;**25**(10):647–9.

28

Formulas for preterm and term infants

Deborah L. O'Connor and Joan Brennan

University of Toronto, The Hospital for Sick Children, Toronto, Ontario, Canada

Introduction

Breastfeeding is the gold standard and strongly preferred method of feeding healthy term infants.[1,2] The American Academy of Pediatrics recommends human milk as the exclusive nutrient source for feeding full-term infants for the first 6 months after birth and indicates that it should be continued with the addition of solid foods, until 12 months of life.[2] Likewise, the Canadian Pediatric Society recommends exclusive breastfeeding for a minimum of 4 months and suggests that it may continue for up to 2 years and beyond.[1] The duration of exclusive breastfeeding by the latter authoritative body is currently under review. Recently the World Health Organization made the recommendation that full-term infants be exclusively breastfed until the introduction of complementary foods at 6 months with continued breastfeeding thereafter.[3] The scientific rationale for recommending breastfeeding as the preferred feeding choice is extensively reviewed elsewhere in this book.

In the event that breastfeeding is contraindicated or a mother chooses not to breastfeed, a commercially prepared infant formula is the next best option. The American Academy of Pediatrics recommends that when breastfeeding is not initiated or is discontinued before an infant's first birthday, a standard cow's milk-based formula is the feeding of choice for term-born infants.[2] Canadian Health officials recommend use of cow's milk-based, iron-fortified formulas until 9–12 months of age.[1] Available data suggest that approximately 70% of North American women currently initiate breastfeeding.[4,5] At 6 months postpartum, however, only 32.5% of American women are still breastfeeding.[5] While these data suggest that additional efforts need to be undertaken to increase both the initiation and duration of breastfeeding, they also underscore the fact that a significant number of infants in North America continue to be fed by means other than breast milk. While the trend toward increased breastfeeding since its nadir in 1971 is associated with a decrease in early postnatal formula use, infants are also being introduced to unmodified cow's milk much later. Contrary to popular perception, the net result has been an increase in the percentage of infants being fed formulas after 4 months of age.[6] It is estimated that approximately 20% of 6-month-old infants were formula-fed in 1971 compared with greater than 50% in 1980. Together these data emphasize that a large proportion of infants rely on commercially prepared infant formula as a significant source of nutrition at some juncture during their first year of life. Educating healthcare professionals who care for infants about the formulas available and their indications for use could have a significant impact on the nutritional status of infants in North America and, indeed, anywhere that infant formula constitutes a significant portion of an infant's diet.

The purpose of this chapter, then, is to provide the clinician with a working knowledge of the major infant formulas available, their indications for use and to understand the basics of formula preparation. In addition, this chapter provides an overview of the models used to develop and make changes in the composition of commercially prepared infant formula, and the regulatory safeguards that provide assurance that these products are safe if used as intended. Finally, a number of current controversies surrounding the composition of infant formulas are presented.

Neonatal Nutrition and Metabolism. Second Edition, ed. P. Thureen and W. Hay. Published by Cambridge University Press.
© Cambridge University Press 2006.

Table 28.1. Composition of human milk, cow's milk and selected cow's milk-based formulas marketed for feeding term infants in North America

	Human milk (mature)[a]	Minimum required LSRO, 1998[b]	Minimum required, infant formula Act, 1985[c]	Whole cow's milk[d]	Evaporated cow's milk formula[e]	Milk-based infant formula[f,g]
Kcal dL^{-1}	70	63	Not stated	61	68.2	67–68
Protein g dL^{-1}	1.0	1.1	1.2	3.3	2.3	1.4–1.5
Protein g 100 kcal^{-1}	1.4	1.7	1.8	5.4	3.4	2.1–2.2
Fat g dL^{-1}	4.4	2.9	2.2	3.3	2.6	3.5–3.7
Fat g 100 kcal^{-1}	6.2	4.4	3.3	5.4	3.8	5.2–5.5
CHO g dL^{-1}	6.9	6.0	Not stated	4.7	8.1	7.1–7.5
CHO g 100 kcal^{-1}	9.9	9.0	Not stated	7.7	11.9	10.5–11.1
Na mmol dL^{-1}	0.74	0.73	0.58	2.1	1.5	0.7
Na mg dL^{-1}	17	16.8	13.4	49	35.3	16
K mmol dL^{-1}	1.3	1.03	1.4	3.9	2.6	1.7–1.9
K mg dL^{-1}	51	40.2	53.6	152	101	66.3–74
Cl mmol dL^{-1}	1.2	0.96	1.05	2.9	Not av.	1.1–1.2
Cl mg dL^{-1}	42	33.5	36.9	102	Not av.	38.5–42
Vit. A ug dL^{-1}	62	40.2	50.3	38	24	60.5
Vit. A IUdL^{-1}	241	134	167.5	126	80	200–203
Vit. D IUdL^{-1}	4	26.8	26.8	40	28.8	40–41
Vit. D μg dL^{-1}	0.1	0.67	0.67	1.06	0.72	1.0
Vit. E mg dL^{-1}	0.9	0.33	0.47	0.1	0.06	1.0–1.3
Vit. E IUdL^{-1}	0.9	0.33	0.47	0.1	0.06	1.0–1.3
Vit. K μg dL^{-1}	0.06	0.67	2.7	0.3	Not av.	5.4–5.5
Vit. C mg dL^{-1}	5	4.0	5.4	0.9	5.5	5.4–8.1
Ca mmol dL^{-1}	0.8	0.84	1.0	3.0	2.2	1.1–1.3
Ca mg dL^{-1}	32	33.5	40.2	119	87	44–52
P mmol dL^{-1}	0.45	0.43	0.65	3.0	2.2	0.8–1.2
P mg dL^{-1}	14	13.4	20.1	93	67.7	25–37
Fe mg dL^{-1}	0.03	0.13	0.1	0.05	0.06	1.0–1.2

[a] Energy and nutrient values obtained from:[177–180]

[b] Source [181]

[c] Source [14]

[d] Values obtained from:[178]

[e] Recipe from:[1,178]

[f] Composition of Enfamil, Similac Advance, and Good Start.

[g] See www.meadjohnson.com, www.verybestbaby.com (Carnation/Nestle) or www.ross.com for most recent product information.

History of formula feeding

Safe and acceptable human milk substitutes are a recent phenomenon of the twentieth century that are becoming more sophisticated as we better appreciate the impact of biological immaturity on nutrient requirements and, in turn, the impact of nutrients on biological maturation. Even at the beginning of the twentieth century, the major biochemical differences between human milk and cow's milk were understood.[6] Some of these differences are summarized in Table 28.1. It was understood that a human

milk substitute based on cow's milk required dilution with water and that carbohydrate needed to be added. A number of commercial infant formulas were, in fact, patented by this time; however, few infants were fed these products. In 1915 Gerstenberger developed the first complete infant formula of modern times.[7] De-fatted and diluted cow's milk formed the base of this product. Cod liver oil and beef tallow was added at a level of 4.6% to mimic the fat content of human milk. This product was called SMA for "synthetic milk adapted." This product and name remained on the market in North America until recently, but the formulation was modified extensively over time. The fat blend was replaced with vegetable oils, lactose was added, and the vitamin and mineral composition was modified.

From the 1920s until the 1950s most formulas fed to infants in North America were prepared in the home by mixing evaporated or fresh cow's milk with water and adding carbohydrate. Both options were inexpensive and evaporated milk did not require refrigeration. Evaporated milk assured sterility (at least until opened) at a time when the purity of fresh cow's milk was not always certain. Further, the process of sterilizing evaporated milk also modified casein such that it produced a finer curd and improved the digestibility of the product. While the current use of these formulations for infant feeding in the USA is virtually nonexistent, they are still used in some Northern Canadian communities due to cost, convenience, and tradition.[1] While Canadian Health authorities do not recommend homemade evaporated milk formulas as an alternative to breast milk or commercial infant formula, they do provide a suggested recipe to ensure proper dilution and that appropriate amounts of energy, protein, and carbohydrate are fed.[1] Due to their low iron content, iron deficiency is common among infants using these products.[6,8] Their high renal solute load puts young infants at risk of developing hypernatremic dehydration during illness.[6,9] Essential fatty acid intake is low and vitamin C deficiency, specifically scurvy, is observed, albeit less frequently since orange juice was recommended as a source of vitamin C for infants fed these preparations. Currently in North America, all evaporated milk is fortified with vitamin D. Vitamin C is also added as a fortificant in Canada.

The evaporated whole milk formula recipe recommended for the first 6 months of life is a 1:2 dilution of evaporated whole milk to water plus white table sugar. For example, 30 ml evaporated whole milk, 60 ml water and 1 teaspoon sugar will lower the protein and sodium content to an appropriate level for young infants. After 6 months of age, a 1:1 dilution of evaporated whole milk to water is recommended with no addition of sugar. The energy and select nutrient composition of the formulation for younger infants can be found in Table 28.1.

Since the 1950s, commercially prepared infant formulas have gradually replaced home-made preparations due to the introduction of liquid concentrates, iron-fortification, endorsement by physicians and infant formula industry marketing.[6] Years ago, formula concentrates were perceived as being more convenient than home formulations or commercially available powders which, at the time, were difficult to reconstitute.

Models used in formula development

Term infants

The composition of standard term starter formula, and research initiatives to make further improvements, are guided by our current understanding of the composition of human milk. The composition of human milk is extremely complex and it is unlikely that it will be duplicated. In addition to the presence of nutrients, human milk contains hormones, immunologic agents, enzymes, and live cells to name a few. It is also known that the bioavailability of nutrients and bioactive components is very much dependent on the presence or absence of other milk components. Because of this, it is flawed logic to assume that a nutrient or bioactive component ingested by exclusively human milk-fed infants will produce an identical response in formula-fed infants. So while the composition of human milk should serve as the starting point for modifications to infant formula, the ultimate goal should be to provide nutrients/bioactive components in a concentration and form that produces a metabolic response in the formula-fed infant that most closely resembles that of the breast-fed infant. In 1998 an Expert Panel made recommendations for revision of the Code of Federal Regulations as it applied to the nutrient content of infant formulas.[10] This recommended reference is a comprehensive review of the research literature regarding the nutrient requirements for infant formulas designed for term-born infants.

Preterm infants

Whilst the composition of human milk and performance of the exclusively breast-fed infant is the "gold standard" for the development of standard term formulas, this approach is not appropriate for developing and modifying formulas designed for the preterm infant. Under more ideal circumstances, premature infants during their early postnatal course would be receiving their nutrients via transplacental transfer and amniotic fluid. Despite the impressive list of advantages, human milk feeding alone during initial hospitalization will not meet the nutritional requirements of many premature infants, especially those born <1500 g (very low birth weight, VLBW).[2,11] As such, the nutrient composition of the first formulas designed for the premature infant were generally determined from estimates of the maximum intrauterine accretion rate for each nutrient accounting for endogenous losses, incomplete digestion, absorption, or retention by the premature infant. Daily accretion rates for nutrients such as nitrogen, calcium, and phosphorus were estimated from body composition data of fetuses at various weights and from intrauterine growth curves.[12,13] Subsequent modification of the nutrient levels in preterm formulas have occurred secondary to research that has more comprehensively examined the nutrient in question. To date, however, growth and tolerance are often used as the primary criteria for many compositional changes.

In 2002 an Expert Panel made recommendations for revision of the Code of Federal Regulations as it applies to the nutrient content of preterm infant formulas.[14] This recommended reference provides a comprehensive review of the research literature as it pertains to the nutrient requirements for infant formulas designed for prematurely born infants.[15] Readers are advised to refer to a document produced by the Nutrition Committee of the Canadian Pediatric Society for nutrient requirements for infant formulas designed for preterm infants after hospital discharge.[11]

Compositional differences between whole cow's milk and human milk

Protein

Whole (full-fat), 2%, 1% or skim cow's, goat's milk, and evaporated milk are not recommended for use during the first 9[1] or 12 months of life.[2] As illustrated in Table 28.1, the nutrient composition of whole cow's milk differs quite markedly from human milk.

The amount of protein in cow's milk is much higher than that of human milk and in comparison remains constant over time at approximately 3.5 g dL^{-1}.[16] In contrast mature human milk (1.0 g dL^{-1}) starts out with a higher protein concentration in early lactation and gradually decreases over time.[17] The protein in cow and human milk is composed of three major fractions: casein, whey, and nonprotein nitrogen. Human milk and cow's milk differ in their casein, whey, and nonprotein nitrogen ratios. The term casein and whey were developed by the dairy industry as a way to articulate physical properties of milk. Casein precipitates out into curds when acidified while the whey proteins remain in solution.[18] Cow's milk is casein predominant with a whey:casein ratio of 18:82. Conversely, human milk is whey predominant and the whey:casein ratio varies over time. The whey: casein ratio in early lactation is 90:10 and changes to 50:50 later on as the proportion of immunological proteins found in the whey fraction declines.[19] The protein and amino acid composition of the casein and whey fractions differs markedly between human and cow's milk. For example, the major constituents of the whey fraction of human milk are lactoferrin, alpha-lactalbumin and immunoglobulins whereas in cow's milk, it is beta-lactoglobulin.[16] The nonprotein nitrogen component of milk refers to the remainder of heterogeneous nitrogen-containing compounds left once the protein fraction has been removed. It consists of urea, peptides, free amino acids, creatine, creatinine, uric acid, ammonia, nucleotides, nitrogen-containing carbohydrates, and other nitrogenous substances.[20] It comprises about 5%–6%[21] and 20%–25%[22] of the total nitrogen content in cow's milk and human milk respectively. It appears that the peptides and free amino acids are nutritionally available but the contribution of urea to protein metabolism has yet to be clearly defined.[23]

Lipid

Next to water, the largest constituent of human or cow's milk is the lipid fraction. It also provides the greatest proportion of total energy. This fraction is composed of triglycerides (>98% of the lipid component) made up of some 167 and 437 identified fatty acids in human and cow's milk, respectively.[24] Seven and 12 of these fatty acids, respectively, are present at concentrations of >1% of total fatty acids.[25,26] In addition the lipid component consists of phospholipids, sphingolipids, and sterols. It is the most variable constituent of human milk with individual fatty acids varying in concentration over a feeding, from breast to breast, over a day's time, with parity and gestational age of offspring at birth and between individuals. Maternal diet has a major impact on the fatty acid profile of human milk.[25] For example, milk from lacto-ovo vegetarians contains a lower proportion of fatty acids derived from animal sources and a higher proportion of fatty acids from vegetable sources.[25] In contrast, the fatty acid composition of cow's milk is relatively unaffected by diet because of the biohydrogenation and production of short-chain fatty acids in the rumen of the cow.[26] In addition to differences between human milk and cow's milk in regard to the profile and concentration of individual fatty acids, the distribution of fatty acids on the glycerol backbone of triglyceride is unique to each species. These structural differences affect the bioavailability of individual fatty acids. In human milk most of the 16:0 (palmitic acid) is at the sn-2 position, 12:0 at the sn-3 position, and 18:0 (oleic acid) at sn-1, and 18:1 and 18:2 (linoleic acid) at sn-1 and sn-3.[25] In cow's milk, most 4:0–8:0 are at the sn-3 position and 12:0, 14:0, and 16:0 are at the sn-2 position.[26]

Carbohydrate

The predominant source of carbohydrate in human and cow milk is lactose. The concentration of lactose in human milk ($\sim$6.1 g dL^{-1}) is significantly higher than that of cow's milk ($\sim$4.8 g dL^{-1}).[27] Lactose is a disaccharide composed of the two monosaccharides, galactose and glucose. Other milk sugars in milk include glucose and galactose in low concentrations, neutral and acid oligosaccharides, and the peptide-bound and protein-bound carbohydrates. The concentration of oligosaccharides, the largest constituent of human milk after water, lipid, and lactose, is about ten times higher than that in cow's milk. More than 80 neutral and acidic oligosaccharides have been identified, several of which are known to play a role in promoting colonization of the gastrointestinal tract with bifidobacteria and inhibition of the binding of enteropathogens to epithelial surfaces.

Minerals

Human and cow's milk also differ with respect to the non-energy-containing nutrients.[28] For example, the mineral content of cow's milk is significantly higher than that of human milk and is thought to reflect the higher growth rate of calves compared with human infants. Calcium, phosphorus, magnesium, and sodium levels are reported to be 3–7 times higher in cow compared with human milk (Table 28.1).

The higher concentrations of protein, sodium, potassium, and chloride in unmodified cow's milk increases its renal solute load compared with human milk or commercially available formula.[29] Renal solute load by definition represents the solutes excreted per liter of milk or formula consumed. The higher solute load in cow's milk puts an unnecessarily high demand on the immature kidney relative to that of human milk and significantly increases urine osmolality.[30] Whilst the kidney of a healthy term infant can handle this increase, this might not be the case at times of increased water loss that occurs during a bout of acute febrile illness, diarrhea, and/or vomiting. Cow's milk, in these situations, may not supply sufficient free water.[31] Consumption of unmodified cow's milk has also been associated with blood loss in the stool of infants less than 6 months of age.[10,30] The mechanism for this loss is presumably mediated via an allergic-type reaction between some component of cow's milk protein and the enterocyte of the gastrointestinal tract. Further, the higher concentration of cow's milk proteins and calcium may negatively impact on the bioavailability of iron, increasing the infant's risk of iron-deficiency anemia.

Choosing the right Formula

There are numerous infant formulas available on the market in North America. What follows below are descriptions of the major categories of formulas available, their ingredient and nutrient composition, and indications for use. The text, in conjunction with the algorithm provided in Figure 28.1, will provide clinicians with direction on infant formula selection. As the ingredient and nutrient composition of formulas frequently change, the reader is strongly advised to refer to the most up-to-date product information provided by the manufacturer.

Cow's milk-based term formula

Cow's milk-based formulas for term-born infants currently on the market in North America provide approximately 67 kcal dL^{-1} energy (Table 28.1). Both brand name and generic varieties are available. To the best of our knowledge companies, or their global subsidiaries, that produce brand varieties manufacture all generics available in North America. However, brand varieties and generics produced by the same company may differ significantly in their ingredient composition and nutrient content.

Protein

The protein concentration of term cow's milk-based formulas is significantly lower than that of unmodified cow's milk and more similar to that of human milk (Table 28.1). Marketed formulas do differ in their whey:casein ratio (Table 28.2). For example, Carnation Good Start (Nestle Good Start in Canada) is made up of 100% partially hydrolyzed whey. In contrast, Enfamil (called Enfalac or Enfamil in Canada), Similac and one of the generics available in Canada (President's Choice) have whey:casein ratios of 60:40, 48:52 and 18:82, respectively. Historically, formula manufacturers increased the whey relative to casein content of formulas with the rationale that a greater proportion of human milk protein was in the whey versus casein fraction. As discussed above, however, proteins in the whey fraction of cow and human milk do differ and hence the logic for this is flawed. It has been shown that increasing the whey fraction of a protein mixture does not necessarily produce a plasma essential amino acid profile that better matches that of the breastfed infant. In one study, a formula containing approximately equal concentrations of whey and casein produced an amino acid profile in formula-fed infants most similar to the breastfed infant compared with infants fed either 100% whey or a whey-dominant formula.[32,33] The clinical significance of these observed differences is unknown. However,

Suggested Enteral Feeding for Infants**

Breastfeeding is the preferred feeding for preterm and term infants – if breastmilk is not available, or when weaning, choose:

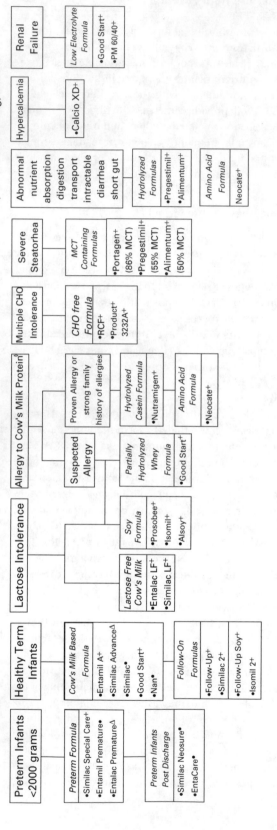

Preterm Infants <2000 grams

Preterm Formula
- Similac Special Care+
- Entamil Premature•
- Entalac Premature-Δ

Preterm Infants Post Discharge
- Similac Neosure•
- EntaCare•

Healthy Term Infants

Cow's Milk Based Formula
- Entamil A+
- Similac AdvanceΔ
- Similac•
- Good Start+
- Nan•

Follow-On Formulas
- Follow-Up+
- Similac 2+
- Follow-Up Soy+
- Isomil 2+

Lactose Intolerance

Lactose Free Cow's Milk
- Entalac LF+
- Similac LF+

Soy Formula
- Prosobee+
- Isomil+
- Alsoy+

Allergy to Cow's Milk Protein◊

Suspected Allergy

Partially Hydrolyzed Whey Formula
- Good Start+

Proven Allergy or strong family history of allergies

Hydrolyzed Casein Formula
- Nutramigen+

Amino Acid Formula
- Neocate+

Multiple CHO Intolerance

CHO free Formula
- RCF+
- Product+ 3232A+

Severe Steatorrhea

MCT Containing Formulas
- Portagen+ (86% MCT)
- Pregestimil+ (55% MCT)
- Alimentum+ (50% MCT)

Abnormal nutrient absorption digestion transport intractable diarrhea short gut

Hydrolyzed Formulas
- Pregestimil+
- Alimentum+

Amino Acid Formula
Neocate+

Hypercalcemia
- Calcio XD+

Renal Failure

Low Electrolyte Formula
- Good Start+
- PM 60/40+

+ Cdn and US
• US only
Δ Cdn only
◊ Infants with documented cow's milk protein enteropathy or enterocolitis may be as sensitive to soy protein and should not be given soy formula. They should be given an extensively hydrolyzed formula. Many infants with documented IgE-mediated allergy to cow's milk protein will tolerate a soy formula.
**This list is not exclusive. Additional products exist that may be equally suitable to an infant's needs.

Figure 28.1. A guide for clinicians on enteral feeding selection.

Table 28.2. Macronutrient and ingredient content of select cow's milk-based formula[a]

	Enfamil/Enfalac	Similac Advance	Good Start/NAN	Store brand
Protein (g 100 kcal^{-1})	2.1	2.1	2.2	2.2
Protein source	Reduced minerals whey nonfat milk	Nonfat milk, whey protein concentrate	Whey protein concentrate, nonfat dry milk	Nonfat milk
Carbohydrate (g 100 kcal^{-1})	10.9	10.8	11.2	10.6
Carbohydrate source	Lactose	Lactose	Lactose, corn syrup	Lactose
Fat (g 100 kcal^{-1})	5.3	5.4	5.1	5.3
Fat source	Palm olein oil, soy oil, coconut oil, high oleic sunflower, + or − single cell oils	High oleic sunflower oil, safflower oil, soy oil, coconut oil, + or − single cell oils	Palm olein oil, soy oil, coconut oil, high oleic safflower oil, + or − single cell oils	Proportions vary depending on brand manufacturer

[a] www.meadjohnson.com, www.verybestbaby.com (Carnation/Nestle) or www.ross.com for the most recent product information.

there are a number of examples in the adult and infant literature which illustrate that dietary amino acid composition can affect plasma amino acid patterns, which in turn may affect maturation and behavior.[32,34–38]

A number of studies, though not all, suggest that whey-based formulas accelerate gastric emptying relative to casein-based cow's milk formula and may be associated with fewer episodes of emesis and gastroesophageal reflux.[39–43] Indeed, bovine beta-casein produces a firmer curd in the stomach compared with either human milk kappa-casein or whey, serving to slow gastric emptying. It is not clear whether the level of hydrolysis of whey protein affects the rate of gastric emptying.[39,40] According to product literature, the 100% whey proteins in Carnation Good Start are "broken down into smaller pieces to be easy to digest in your baby's tummy." These proteins are called Comfort Proteins™ in advertising material. There is no scientific evidence that we are aware of which supports a tolerance advantage claim for healthy term infants in using this product.

Carbohydrate

The carbohydrate in cow's milk-based starter formulas is composed of lactose or a combination of lactose and maltodextrin (Table 28.2). Maltodextrins are oligosaccharides of 5–10 glucose units, produced from the hydrolysis of starch.

Lipids

Like human milk, fat provides 40%–50% of the energy in cow's milk-based formula. The butter-fat of whole cow's milk is removed and replaced with a combination of the following vegetable oils to mimic, in small part, the fatty acid profile of human milk: coconut, high oleic

sunflower, high oleic safflower, soybean, and palm olein oils (Table 28.2). Oleo oils (i.e., destearinated beef fat) are one of the oils used in many of the generics (formerly SMA, Wyeth Nutritionals) marketed in the USA. While formula manufacturers have done a good job of matching some of the most prevalent fatty acids found in human milk, oil blends do not approach mimicking the presence or concentration of all 167 fatty acids identified in human milk nor its triacylglycerol profile. Likewise the oil blend in infant formula differs from human milk with regard to the presence and concentration of a whole host of sterols (most prevalent is cholesterol), phospholipids, sphingomyelins, neutral glycosylceramides and acidic glycosphingolipids or gangliosides.

Coconut oil is an excellent source of saturated relatively short-chain fatty acids. Palm oil is a source of long-chain saturated fatty acids, and soy, corn, and safflower oils provide polyunsaturated fatty acids. Genetic variants of sunflower and safflower oil are used to increase the monounsaturate content of the fat blend. Available oil blends provide the essential fatty acids linoleic and linolenic acid in ample quantities. None provide a significant source of cholesterol, which is found in human milk. More recently, single cell oils have been added to formulas as a source of the long chain polyunsaturated fatty acids docosahexaenoic (DHA, 22:6n-3) and arachidonic acid (ARA, 20:4n-6).

There has been considerable discussion in the literature and research community about the relative efficacy of various base oil blends in promoting fat absorption and the benefit and safety of adding DHA and ARA to term formula. Human milk contains a significant quantity of palmitic acid (16:0, 20.5% of total fatty acids).[44] Many formulas contain substantially less palmitic acid than found in human milk. Palm olein, a lower-melting fraction of palm oil, has been added to some commercially available standard term formulas to increase its palmitic acid content. Palm oil is one of the few plant oils rich in palmitic acid; however, unlike human milk, palmitic acid in palm oil is esterified predominantly in the sn-1 and sn-3 positions as opposed to the sn-2 position.[45] When palmitic acid is in the sn-2 position, as is the case in human milk, it is better absorbed than in the sn-1 or sn-3 positions.[46–48] The fat absorption of infants consuming formulas containing palm olein is less than that of formulas devoid of this oil.[45,49,50] Likewise, calcium absorption is reduced presumably due to the formation of insoluble calcium soaps produced by the binding of dietary calcium with unabsorbed fatty acids. Despite this, Hansen et al.[51,52] report that infants consuming one brand of formula containing palm olein had calcium absorption and bone mineral content similar to that of breastfed infants. Koo et al.[53] report that feeding a formula containing palm olein for the first 6 months of life reduced the whole body bone mineral content and bone density of infants compared with that of infants fed a formula devoid of this oil. Together these data suggest that infants fed a standard cow's milk-based term formula containing palm olein have similar rates of bone mineralization compared with breastfed infants but lower rates compared with infants fed formula without palm olein. The clinical relevance of these observations is unknown, as is the impact on long-term bone health, osteoporosis, and bone fracture rates.

Docosahexaenoic (DHA) and arachidonic acid (ARA)

The recent addition of DHA and ARA to term infant formulas in the North American market has resulted in much discussion, confusion, and controversy. DHA and ARA are the major long chain polyunsaturated fatty acids found in the nonmyelin membranes of the brain, particularly the cortical synaptic terminals, and retina. These fatty acids are found in breast milk, the concentration of which is strongly influenced by maternal diet. For example, the DHA content of milk from women consuming large amounts of marine foods can be as high as 1.4% of fatty acids, though the DHA concentration in milk collected from women consuming a typical North American diet is generally in the range of 0.2%–0.4% of total fatty acids.[10,54,55]

While the polyunsaturated vegetable oils used to manufacture formulas do contain the precursors of DHA and ARA, alpha-linolenic acid and linoleic acid, they do not contain DHA and ARA. Neither linoleic acid nor alpha-linolenic acid can be synthesized by mammalian cells. As has been shown in studies using stable isotopes, infants have the enzymatic machinery to convert alpha-linolenic acid to DHA and linoleic acid to ARA.[10,56–59] These studies alone, however, provide insufficient data to assess whether

sufficient quantities of DHA and ARA are synthesized to meet the infants requirements. Infants fed formulas without DHA and ARA but containing adequate levels of alpha-linolenic and linoleic acid have lower levels of DHA and ARA in their blood compared with either breastfed infants or infants fed formulas supplemented with these fatty acids.[10] As with DHA and ARA in milk, the profile and concentration of these fatty acids in the blood will reflect dietary intake and do not provide sufficient data to assess whether endogenous biosynthesis of DHA and ARA is adequate to meet requirements. Analysis of postmortem samples of infant brain have shown lower concentrations of DHA, but not ARA, in the cerebral cortex of infants fed formula (devoid of added DHA and ARA) compared with breastfed infants.[60–62] The range of human cerebral DHA contents that is associated with normal function is not known; however, reduced brain DHA has been shown to decrease visual function and performance on learning tasks and altered serotonin and dopamine metabolism in animals.[55,63–66]

Unlike the situation for preterm infants, the results from clinical trials with term-born infants designed to evaluate the efficacy of DHA and ARA addition are mixed. For example, Birch et al.[67] evaluated the effects of feeding breast milk, term formula (1.5 and 14.6% of fatty acids as alpha-linolenic and linoleic, respectively) and term formula containing DHA alone or DHA and ARA (single cell microbial oil; 0.36% and 0.72% of fatty acids, respectively) on the visual acuity of full-term infants.[67] Infants fed term formula without DHA and ARA added had lower visual acuity (as measured by an electrophysiological Visual Evoked Potential VEP) procedure at 6, 17, and 52 weeks but not 26 weeks than infants fed breast milk, formula containing DHA alone or DHA plus ARA. Similarly, Birch et al.[68] evaluated the effects of feeding term formula (~1.5% and 15% of fatty acids as alpha-linolenic and linoleic, respectively) without added DHA and ARA and with DHA and ARA (0.36% and 0.72% of fatty acids, respectively) after weaning from breast milk after 6 weeks postpartum.[68] Despite a dietary source of DHA and ARA from breast milk during the first 6 weeks of life, infants weaned to term formula devoid of these fatty acids had poorer visual acuity at 17, 26 and 52 weeks of age. Finally, Birch et al. (2000) report that term-born infants fed formulas containing DHA and ARA (0.36% and 0.72% of fatty acids, respectively) had a 7-point higher score on the Mental Development Index of the Bayley Scales of Infant Development–II compared with formula-fed infants not fed these fatty acids.[69]

In contrast, Auestad et al.[70,71,73] did not find differences in visual acuity (as measured by VEP or Teller acuity card procedures), cognitive development, or motor development among infants fed formula without DHA and ARA compared with those fed formulas supplemented with either DHA or DHA and ARA. In the first study by Auestad *et al.*, term-born infants were randomly assigned to one of three formula regimens: control (no DHA or ARA), egg-yolk supplemented (0.12% and 0.43% of DHA and ARA, respectively) and fish-oil supplemented (0.23% and 0.07% of DHA and eicosapentaenoic acid (EPA), respectively).[70,72,73] Vocabulary comprehension scores were significantly lower in the fish oil (DHA alone) group compared with the breast-fed group. There was also a trend for vocabulary production scores to be lower for the fish oil (DHA alone) compared to the breastfed group. These infants were followed again at 3.25 years and no differences were found among formula groups with respect to infant IQ and measures of vocabulary.[73] In the second study, infants in the formula groups were randomized to a control formula with no DHA or ARA or one of two otherwise identical formulas containing ARA and DHA from either an egg-derived triglyceride or a fish and fungal oil source (0.14% and 0.46% DHA and ARA, respectively).[71] The alpha-linolenic and linoleic content of formulas in both studies was ~2% and 20% of fatty acids respectively. Reference groups of infants' breastfed and weaned to formulas with and without DHA and ARA were also included. No differences were found in the latter study between infants fed control formula without DHA and ARA and breastfed infants.

Other studies of term-born infants are similarly mixed with some showing at least a short-term benefit[74-77] on either visual or cognitive development of DHA and ARA supplementation of term formula and others showing no benefit at all.[78,79]

Iron

Standard term cow's milk-based formula can be purchased containing either a low (0.22–0.7 mg 100 kcal^{-1}) or a higher level of iron (1.5–1.8 mg 100 kcal^{-1}) though there is movement to phase out the latter. As iron is listed on the ingredient panel of both products, specific instructions should be provided to families on how to identify the higher iron-containing product. The higher iron-containing product is referred to as iron fortified; however, no standard term formula is available without added iron.

Infant formula providing iron at a level of 0.2 mg 100 kcal^{-1} would produce an estimated net rate of iron absorption similar to that of an exclusively human milk-fed infant.[10] Unless infants ingesting the low iron formula consume a medicinal iron supplement or foods rich in iron such as meats, they are at increased risk of iron deficiency in the latter half of their first year. The widespread decline in the prevalence of anemia among infants and preschool children in the USA during the 1960s and 1970s has been attributed to the widespread use of iron and ascorbic acid fortified formulas.[31] Results from a series of recent clinical studies suggest that an intermediate level of iron fortification between that currently available from low iron and higher iron-fortified formulas may be equally efficacious in the prevention of iron deficiency.[10] Presently in the USA approximately 9% of toddlers are iron-deficient (defined by increased free erythrocyte protoporphyrin and decreased transferrin saturation and serum ferritin).[80] There is no scientific support for claims that higher iron-containing formulas result in gastrointestinal intolerance, most notably constipation.[2,10,81] Higher iron-containing formulas, in particular, will produce green-colored stools that markedly differ from the yellow stools of exclusively breastfed infants.

Indications for use

The American Academy of Pediatrics recommends that when breastfeeding is not used or is stopped before 1 year of age, a standard cow's milk-based formula is the feeding of choice for full-term infants until 1 year of age.[2] Canadian Health officials recommend use of cow's milk-based, iron-fortified formulas until 9–12 months of age.[1]

Cow's milk-based preterm formula

Cow's milk-based formulas designed for preterm infants during their initial in-hospital course, commonly called premature formulas, provide either 68 or 81 kcal dL^{-1} (Similac Special Care Advance or Enfamil Premature LIPIL; Enfamil A+ Premature in Canada) (Tables 28.3 and 28.4). These products are available in either low or high iron varieties. Once full enteral feeding is established (e.g., intakes $\geq$100 kcal kg^{-1} day^{-1} and/or 150 ml kg^{-1} day^{-1}), the 81 kcal dL^{-1} variety is most often chosen as it provides the most logical compromise between the premature infants-limited ability to tolerate volume and their limited urinary excretory capacity.[15] Practices vary considerably from institution to institution on whether the 68 or 81 kcal dL^{-1} product is used, diluted or provided at full-strength, prior to establishment of full enteral feeding.

Protein

Premature formulas are higher in protein than standard term formulas in order to facilitate in utero rates of tissue growth and nitrogen accretion. Current premature formulas on the North American market contain either 2.7 or 3.0 g protein 100 kcal^{-1} which is well within the guidelines published by several authoritative bodies (2.5–3.0 g 100 kcal^{-1};[11] 2.9–3.3 g 100 kcal^{-1};[2] 2.5–3.6 kcal^{-1} 100 kcal^{-1}).[15] At intakes of 110–130 kcal kg^{-1} day^{-1}, current premature formulas provide at least 3.0 g kg^{-1} day^{-1}. The

Table 28.3. Composition of human milk and selected cow's milk-based formulas marketed for premature infants in North America

	Human milk (mature)[a]	Human milk (preterm)[b]	Minimum required for premature formulas[c] (LSRO, Klein 2002)	Milk-based premature formulas[c,d] 20 kcal per fld oz	Milk-based premature formulas[c,d] 24 kcal per fld oz	Milk-based post-discharge formulas[d,e] 22 kcal per fld oz
Kcal dL^{-1}	70	73.3	67	67.6	80.6	74.6–75.1
Protein g dL^{-1}	1.0	1.5	1.7	1.8–2.0	2.2–2.4	1.9–2.1
Protein g 100 kcal^{-1}	1.4	2.1	2.5	2.7–3.0	2.7–3.0	2.6–2.8
Fat g dL^{-1}	4.4	3.2	2.9	3.4–3.7	4.1–4.4	4.0–4.1
Fat g 100 kcal^{-1}	6.3	4.4	4.4	5.1–5.4	5.1–5.4	5.3–5.5
CHO g dL^{-1}	6.9	6.8	6.4	7.2–7.5	8.6–9.0	7.7–8.0
CHO g 100 kcal^{-1}	9.9	9.3	9.6	10.0–11.0	10.0–11.0	10.3–10.4
Na mmol dL^{-1}	0.74	1.1	1.4	1.1–1.3	1.4–1.5	1.1
Na mg dL^{-1}	17	25.3	31.4	26.4–29.1	31.5–34.7	24.6–26.3
K mmol dL^{-1}	1.3	1.5	1.2	1.8–2.2	2.1–4.5	2.0–2.7
K mg dL^{-1}	51	58.5	48.3	69.6–87.2	83.1–104.0	78.9–106.0
Cl mmol dL^{-1}	1.2	1.2	1.4	1.6	1.9–2.0	1.6–1.7
Cl mg dL^{-1}	42	42	48.3	54.7–57.4	65.3–68.5	56.0–58.6
Vit. A μg dL^{-1}	62	120	169	253	302	101–103
Vit. A IUdL^{-1}	241	400	564	845	1008	338–343
Vit. D μg dL^{-1}	0.1	0.3	1.5	2.5–4.6	3.0–5.4	1.3–1.5
Vit. D IU dL^{-1}	4	1.2	60.5	101.4–182.4	121.0–217.7	52.2–60.1
Vit. E mg dL^{-1}	0.9 (ATE)	0.75	1.6	2.7–4.3	3.2–5.1	2.7–3.0
Vit. E IUdL^{-1}	0.9	0.75	1.6	2.7–4.3	3.2–5.1	2.7–3.0
Vit. K μg dL^{-1}	0.3	0.3	3.2	5.4–8.1	6.5–9.7	6.0–8.2
Vit. C mg dL^{-1}	5	1.2–1.3	6.7	13.5–25.0	16.1–29.8	1.1–1.2
Ca mmol dL^{-1}	0.8	0.70	2.5	2.8–3.0	3.3–3.6	2.0–2.3
Ca mg dL^{-1}	32	28	99.1	111.5–121.6	133.1–145.2	78.4–90.2
P mmol dL^{-1}	0.45	0.48	2.1	1.8–2.2	2.2–2.6	1.5–1.6
P mg dL^{-1}	14	14.9	66.1	56.1–67.6	66.9–80.6	46.3–49.6
Fe mg dL^{-1}	0.03	0.09	1.4	1.2 (0.17–0.25)	1.5 (0.20–0.30)	13.4–13.5

[a] Values obtained from:[177–180]
[b] Values obtained from:[16,179,180,182–187]
[c] Assumes an infant is consuming a 24 kcal per fld oz formula.
[d] Enfamil Premature LIPIL and Similac Special Care Advance. Available at two levels of iron.
[e] See www.meadjohnson.com or www.ross.com for most recent product information.
[f] CHO, carbohydrate, EnfaCare LIPIL and Similac NeoSure Advance.

Expert Panel commissioned by the Life Sciences Research Office recently recommended a minimum intake of protein of 3.4 g kg^{-1} day^{-1} on the basis that this level promoted growth and improved plasma markers of protein nutritional status.[15] Infants provided with unmodified formulas containing 2.7 and 3.0 g protein 100 kcal^{-1} would need to consume 125 kcal kg^{-1} and 115 kcal kg^{-1}, respectively, in order to meet this recommendation. The American Academy of Pediatrics[2] currently recommends 3.5–4.0 g kg^{-1} day^{-1} of protein to mimic fetal accretion rates of protein. Health Canada recommends 3.5–4.0 g kg^{-1} day^{-1} of protein for stable growing infants born less than 1000 g

and 3.0–3.6 g kg^{-1} day^{-1} of protein for infants born 1000 g or greater.[23]

The protein component of currently available premature formulas is whey predominant (whey:casein ratio of 60:40) composed of nonfat milk and whey protein concentrate. It is believed that these whey-predominant infant formulas produce concentrations of plasma free amino acids that are more like those in infants fed pooled human milk than would a casein-predominant formula.[15] Whey-predominant formulas produce higher blood levels of the amino acids cyst(e)ine and threonine and lower levels of tyrosine and phenylalanine, which may be advantageous

Table 28.4. Macronutrient and ingredient content of formulas designed for premature infants[a]

	Enfamil Premature LIPIL[b]	Similac Special Care Advance[a]	EnfaCare LIPIL	NeoSure Advance
Protein (g 100 kcal^{-1})	3.0	2.7[d]	2.8	2.6
Protein source	Nonfat milk, whey protein concentrate	Nonfat milk, whey protein concentrate	Whey protein, concentrate, nonfat milk	Nonfat milk, whey protein concentrate
Carbohydrate (g 100 kcal^{-1})	11.0	10.6	10.4	10.3
Carbohydrate source	Corn syrup solids and lactose	Corn syrup solids and lactose	Lactose and corn syrup solids	Corn syrup solids and lactose
Fat (g 100 kcal^{-1})	5.1	5.4	5.3	5.5
Fat source[c]	40% MCT oil, soy oil, high oleic vegetable oil (sunflower and/or safflower), single cell oils	50% MCT oil, soy oil, coconut oils, single cell oils	High oleic vegetable oil, soy oil, 20% MCT oil, coconut oil, single cell oils	Soy oil, 25% MCT oil, coconut oil, single cell oils

[a] see www.meadjohnson.com or www.ross.com for most recent product information.

[b] Available as low-iron and higher iron 20 and 24 kcal per fld oz formula.

[c] Fat blends may differ depending on whether a concentrate, ready-to-feed or powder.

[d] In Canada contains 3.0 g 100 kcal^{-1} protein.

to the premature infant. Cysteine and threonine are conditionally and classically essential amino acids, respectively. Cysteine is thought to be essential in the diet of the premature infant due to inadequate enzymatic activity of cystathionase, a critical enzyme in its synthesis. High levels of tyrosine can be toxic. One of the most common human disorders of amino acid metabolism is transient neonatal tyrosinemia, a condition most often affecting premature infants and thought to be the result of a lag in the development of enzyme activity involved in tyrosine degradation.

Carbohydrate

The carbohydrate fraction of premature formulas is composed of lactose and glucose polymers (Table 28.4). Glucose polymers are oligosaccharides of 3–5 glucose units per molecule provided as corn syrup solids in infant formula. Glucose polymers are used to reduce the lactose content and osmolality of the formula. Glycosidase enzymes capable of breaking down glucose polymers are active in the intestine of premature infants. Premature infants may not be able to completely digest lactose because lactase activity is not fully active in fetal intestine until quite late in gestation (36–40 weeks). It is estimated that between 35% and 70% of ingested lactose might pass undigested into the colon where it is fermented and much of the constituent energy absorbed as short-chain fatty acids and lactate.[15] Excessive amounts of undigested carbohydrates

entering the large intestine could result in gas production and intestinal distension via the osmotic effect of lactose.

Many clinicians report that the enteral feeding tolerance of some VLBW infants is significantly improved with the introduction of a low lactose-containing formula. These anecdotal reports are supported by a study conducted by Griffin and Hansen.[82] These researchers report that effectively eliminating the lactose from premature formula improved feeding outcome as measured by a composite score consisting of weight gain, formula intake, gastric residuals and the number of days to reach full enteral feedings (115 kcal kg^{-1} day^{-1}). However, the relationship between prematurity and ability to tolerate lactose is complex. For example, most premature infants tolerate exclusive human milk very well despite a carbohydrate source that is predominantly composed of lactose. Arguably, there may be other components in human milk that facilitate the breakdown of lactose. There is some evidence to suggest that early feeding of lactose to premature infants increases intestinal lactase activity.

Lipids

Approximately half of the energy in premature formulas is provided as fat. The fat blend is made up of a combination of medium chain triglycerides (approximately half of the fat blend), soy oil, high oleic vegetable oils (sunflower and safflower), and coconut oil. As with term formulas, the fatty acids DHA and ARA have been added to the fat blend of premature formulas in North America using the single cell oils derived from *Mortierella alpina* and *Crypthecodinium*. Other sources of DHA and ARA include egg yolk lipid, phospholipid, and triglyceride and fish oil.

Docosahexaenoic and arachidonic acid

Unlike clinical trial results with term infants, results from studies with preterm infants consistently suggest at least a short-term developmental (visual, cognitive, and language) advantage of supplementing premature formulas with DHA and ARA. From a biological perspective there are several reasons why premature infants might be at increased risk of suboptimal DHA and ARA status and poor development compared with term-born infants. Premature infants have low stores of DHA and ARA. It is known, for example, that ~80% of intrauterine DHA and ARA accumulation occurs in the fetus during the third trimester of pregnancy.[83] As the physiologic maternal-to-fetal supply of these fatty acids is terminated as a result of premature delivery, fetal stores of DHA and ARA are greatly diminished. Second, supply may also be limited by immature de novo synthesis of DHA and ARA from the dietary essential precursor fatty acids, alpha-linolenic and linoleic acid, respectively.[84] Third, standard treatment modalities in neonatal intensive care units (e.g., drugs, oxygen therapy) and negative energy balance may impact on de novo synthesis of DHA and ARA. At a time when stores of ARA and DHA are low, the most rapid accumulation of DHA and ARA in the brain and retina occurs – during the last trimester of pregnancy and early months after birth.

The first clinical trials of premature infants consuming formulas with DHA alone (i.e., no ARA) suggest more rapid maturation of retinal function,[85] visual function[74,86,87] and neurodevelopment.[88,89] Infants in these three studies were fed premature formula (24 kcal per fld oz) with or without DHA beginning the first 2 weeks of life and until infants reached 1800 g or were 36–48 weeks postconceptional age. A standard term formula was fed thereafter. DHA, provided as marine oil, supplied between 0.2%–0.35% of total fatty acids as DHA and negligible to 0.65% of fatty acids as EPA in the premature formulas. Infants were fed DHA until they were 2–9 months-corrected age. Safety concerns were raised as growth in the Carlson studies and a third report by Ryan *et al.* (0.2% of total fatty acid as DHA and 0.06% of total fatty acids as EPA) was negatively affected by DHA-supplementation.[90–92] Presumably this occurred because incorporation of DHA into infant formulas, in the absence of ARA supplementation, resulted in an inhibition of the conversion of linoleic acid to ARA by n-3 fatty acids in the DHA supplemented formulas. The observed decrease in ARA status of premature infants with DHA-alone supplementation suggests that a balanced addition of ARA and DHA is necessary to achieve normal tissue accretion of both of these fatty acids.[93,94]

As expected, growth in most,[94–99] but not all,[100] subsequent studies was not negatively affected when DHA supplementation was accompanied by ARA. This latter set of much larger clinical trials incorporated DHA and ARA at levels of 0.17%–0.33% and 0.31%–0.60% of total fatty acids, respectively, from single cell, egg-derived triglyceride or marine oils. Duration of DHA and ARA-supplementation ranged from an average of 30 days to 16 months. The studies varied with respect to whether infants received a standard term formula after discharge or a specially designed nutrient-enriched feeding. O'Connor *et al.*[99] reported that ARA plus DHA supplementation resulted in improved visual development of preterm infants at 6 months corrected age. The improvement corresponded to approximately 1 line on a Snellen eye chart (e.g., 2/70 v. 20/50). In addition, there was evidence of improved motor development among infants <1250 g birth weight randomized to the ARA+DHA fish/fungal group compared with control infants. Finally a post-hoc analysis suggested that among a subset of infants (English-speaking singletons), those fed ARA + DHA had higher vocabulary comprehension scores at 14 months corrected age.[99] Similarly, Clandinin *et al.*[96] reported improved mental and cognitive development among VLBW infants at 18 months corrected age fed DHA + ARA. To date, researchers have not examined the benefit of feeding these oils to premature infants during the first year of life on developmental outcomes beyond 18 months corrected age. We do not know what impact early supplementation of ARA and DHA will have on school performance, for example.

Minerals

The calcium and phosphorus content of premature formulas currently available in North America range from 112–145 mg dL^{-1} (165–180 mg 100 kcal^{-1}) and 56–81 mg dL^{-1} (83–100 mg 100 kcal^{-1}), respectively. This value is significantly higher than that of standard term formula (44–52 mg dL^{-1} (64–78 mg 100 kcal^{-1}) and 25–37 mg dL^{-1} (36–53 mg 100 kcal^{-1}), respectively) and is necessary to facilitate the very rapid rate of bone mineralization which occurs during the third trimester of pregnancy. Mineral accretion rates are estimated to be nearly three times as high in the last trimester of pregnancy compared with the period immediately following a term birth.[15] It is estimated that the intrauterine accretion rate of calcium and phosphorus is in the order of 150 and 60–80 mg kg^{-1} day^{-1}, respectively;[101,102] levels that clearly can not be obtained from standard term formula.

In addition to the absolute quantity of calcium and phosphorus provided, the ratio between these two minerals is important in terms of optimal calcium retention. The calcium-to-phosphorus ratio of human milk is 2.0:1 (or 1.6:1 in terms of moles). Currently available preterm formulas provide this ratio.

Low birth weight infants, and in particular VLBW infants, have a high fractional rate of sodium excretion during the first 2 weeks of life. VLBW infants often experience difficulty with sodium regulation and have a high prevalence of hyponatremia. Infants born <1000 g typically need to have serum sodium levels regulated by adjusting their intake based on urinary losses. Late hyponatremia may also occur in this smaller group of infants between 2 and 6 weeks of age. The sodium content of premature formula (1.7–1.9 mmol 100 kcal^{-1} or 39–43 mg 100 kcal^{-1}) is higher than that of standard term formula (1.0–1.2 mmol 100 kcal^{-1} or 24–27 mg 100 kcal^{-1}). This higher sodium content reduces the risk of hyponatremia and promotes positive sodium balance and fetal accretion rates of sodium (1.6 mmol kg^{-1} day^{-1}).

Indications for use

Premature formulas are designed for use in-hospital as the sole source of nutrition for preterm infants who are not breastfed. Also, premature formulas may be used to supplement human milk feedings if the supply of the latter is inadequate. Some very small and/or fluid-restricted infants may benefit from the use of premature formulas after hospital discharge if nutrient intake goals cannot be accomplished using either a standard term or a post-discharge nutrient-enriched formula.

Cow's milk-based preterm post-discharge formula

Cow's milk-based formulas designed for prematurely born infants after hospital discharge are commonly called post-discharge nutrient-enriched formulas or simply post-discharge formulas. These products were developed in recognition of the fact that low birth weight infants, particularly those of VLBW, often have unique nutritional requirements after leaving hospital. These products provide approximately 75 kcal dL^{-1} (22 kcal per fld oz) and contain at least 13 mg dL^{-1} iron (Tables 28.3 and 28.4). The two products available on the market in North America are Neosure Advance by Ross and EnfaCare LIPIL by Mead Johnson. In addition to being more energy dense, they provide a more concentrated source of protein, vitamins, and minerals than term formulas but less than what is found in premature formulas. EnfaCare has a whey:casein ratio

of 60:40 and that of Neosure Advance is a ratio of 48:52. Both formulations contain a combination of lactose and glucose polymers and the fat blend is made up of vegetable and MCT oils (Table 28.4).

Today, many VLBW infants are discharged home at about half the weight of an infant born at term. They often have decreased nutrient stores, inadequately mineralized bones, and an accumulated energy deficit. Lemons et al.[103] studied ~4500 VLBW infants born at 14 US centers during 1995 and 1996. Twenty-two per cent were born <10th percentile for weight for gestational age, and by 36 weeks corrected 97% of the cohort were <10th percentile. As well, Merko et al. studied a cohort of Canadian infants born less than 28 weeks' gestation in 1998 and 1999 and found that 52% were below the 3rd centile for weight for gestational age at 36 weeks corrected.[104] These data are amazingly consistent with those published by Lucas[105] and Hack.[106]

Lucas et al. reported that by 9 months, premature infants fed a nutrient-enriched post-discharge formula were at the 25th centile for weight and the 50th centile for length; whereas those fed a term formula were between the 3rd and 10th centiles for weight and the 10th and 25th centiles for length. They also found a significant increase in bone mineral content in infants that received the enriched formula at 3 and 9 months corrected age.[107,108]

Consistent with these results, Cooke et al. found that male infants ≤1750 g at birth fed a standard term formula after hospital discharge tended to have poorer weight, length and head circumference gains compared with infants fed a nutrient-enriched formula.[109] Likewise, Wheeler reported that healthy preterm infants with birth weights <1800 g fed a 20 kcal fld oz nutrient-enriched formula after leaving hospital had better length and head circumference gains up to 12 weeks after hospital discharge compared with those fed term formula.[110] Brunton et al. demonstrated greater linear growth and lean and bone mass post-discharge among Canadian-born VLBW infants with bronchopulmonary dysplasia fed a nutrient-enriched 22 kcal per fld oz formula v. a comparable group fed a standard term formula with only energy enhancement.[111] Carver showed superior weight gains among infants born <1800 g fed nutrient-enriched 22 kcal per fld oz formula from discharge to 2 months corrected age. The infants in the cohort born <1250 g fed the enriched formula were larger at 6 months corrected and had larger head circumference at term, 1, 3, 6, and 12 months corrected age.[112] Together, data from the aforementioned studies suggest that nutrient-enrichment of formula designed for post-discharge feeding does not just make babies fatter but they promote a significant increase in lean body mass accretion and bone mineralization.

Table 28.5. Macronutrient and ingredient content of cow's milk-based lactose-free and soy formulas[a]

	Enfamil LactoFree	Similac Lactose Free	Nestle Alsoy	Similac Isomil	Enfamil Prosobee
Protein (g 100 kcal^{-1})	2.1	2.1	2.8	2.45	2.5
Protein source	Milk protein isolate	Milk protein isolate	Soy protein isolate, L-methionine and taurine	Soy protein isolate, L-methionine and taurine	Soy protein isolate, L-methionine and taurine
Carbohydrate (g 100 kcal^{-1})	10.9	10.7	11.0	10.3	10.6
Carbohydrate source	Corn syrup solids	Corn syrup solids, maltodextrin and sucrose	Sucrose and corn maltodextrin	Corn syrup and sucrose	Corn syrup
Fat (g 100 kcal^{-1})	5.3	5.4	4.9	5.46	5.3
Fat source[b]	Palm olein oil, soy oil, coconut oil, high oleic sunflower oils	High oleic safflower, soy oil, coconut oil	Palm olein oil, soy oil, coconut oil, high oleic safflower oil	High-oleic safflower oil, coconut oil, soy oil	Palm olein oil, soy oil, coconut oil, high oleic sunflower oil

[a] www.meadjohnson.com, www.verybestbaby.com (Carnation/Nestle) or www.ross.com for the most recent product information.
[b] Inclusion of single cell oils is being phased in at the time of writing. Fat blends may differ depending on whether a concentrate, ready-to-feed, or powder.

While feeding a nutrient-enriched formula to term-born small-for-gestational-age (SGA) babies may likewise improve their growth, there is preliminary evidence to suggest that this feeding regimen may produce a lower neurodevelopmental outcome in these same babies at 18 months corrected age.[113]

Indications for use

In its most recent communication the American Academy of Pediatrics acknowledged that the use of specially designed nutrient-enriched discharge formulas for LBW infants after hospital discharge and until 9 months corrected age may promote better linear growth, weight gain, and bone mineral content.[2]

Lactose-free cow's milk-based formulas

Lactose-free formulas currently on the retail market in North America (Enfamil LactoFree and Similac Lactose free) are free of lactose but contain cow's milk-based protein isolate as their protein source (Table 28.5). As summarized in Table 28.6, they provide 67 kcal dL^{-1} energy and are iron-fortified. Their carbohydrate fraction is composed of corn syrup solids (Enfamil LactoFree) or maltodextrin and sucrose (Similac Lactose free). Their fat blend is similar to their respective lactose-containing parent brands (Table 28.5).

Growth of infants fed lactose-free formulas appears to be comparable with that of infants consuming lactose-containing formulas.[114] While the data are mixed, it is generally accepted that lactose plays a role in mineral absorption, specifically with the minerals calcium, magnesium, manganese, zinc, and iron.[31] Clinical studies examining the effects of lactose on calcium absorption of infants have yielded conflicting results with some showing lower calcium absorption with lactose-free or lactose-reduced formulas and others showing no negative effect.[115–118] Most recently, Abrams et al.[119] measured the absorption of calcium and zinc from infant formulas by using a multitracer, stable-isotope technique and found that indeed the presence of lactose in a cow's milk-based formula did increase the absorption of calcium but not zinc. The authors point out, however, that the absorption of calcium from the lactose-free formula was adequate to meet the calcium needs of full-term infants when the formula's calcium content is similar to that of lactose-containing cow's milk-based infant formulas.

The unique linkage of the two monosaccharides in lactose (galactose beta[1–4]glucose) is thought to preclude its digestion by a large number of microbes commonly found in the environment and to promote growth of microorganisms in the colon that are able to split lactose.[27] Establishment of the latter group of microorganisms serves to exclude many potential pathogens from colonizing the gastrointestinal tract.

Table 28.6. Energy and nutrient composition of lactose-free, soy and protein hydrolysate formula marketed for term infants in North America[a]

	Lactose-free formulas[b]	Soy formulas[c]	Protein hydrolysate formulas[d]
Kcal dL^{-1}	67–68	67–68	67–68
Protein g dL^{-1}	1.4	1.6–1.9	1.8–1.9
Protein g 100 kcal^{-1}	2.1	2.5	2.8
Fat g dL^{-1}	3.6	3.3–3.7	3.6–3.7
Fat g 100 kcal^{-1}	5.3–5.4	4.4–5.5	5.3–5.6
CHO g dL^{-1}	7.2–7.3	6.9–7.4	6.8–6.9
CHO g 100 kcal^{-1}	10.7–10.9	9.8–10.6	10.2–10.3
Na mmol dL^{-1}	0.87	1.0–1.3	1.3–1.4
Na mg dL^{-1}	20.1	22–29.5	29.5–31.5
K mmol dL^{-1}	1.9–2.5	1.9–2.1	1.9–2.0
K mg dL^{-1}	71.7–73.7	72.4–80.4	73.7–79.1
Cl mmol dL^{-1}	1.2–1.3	1.2–1.5	1.5–1.6
Cl mg dL^{-1}	43.6–44.9	41.5–53.6	53.6–57.6
Vit. A ug dL^{-1}	60.4	60.4–62.5	60.4–76.6
Vit. A IUdL^{-1}	201	201–208	201–255
Vit. D IUdL^{-1}	40.2	40–40.2	30.1–33.5
Vit. D μg dL^{-1}	1.0	1.0	0.75–0.84
Vit. E mg dL^{-1}	1.3–2.0	1.0–2.0	1.3–2.7
Vit. E IUdL^{-1}	1.3–2.0	1.0–2.0	1.3–2.7
Vit. K μg dL^{-1}	5.4	5.4–7.4	5.4–10
Vit. C mg dL^{-1}	6.0–8.0	6.0–11.0	6.0–8.0
Ca mmol dL^{-1}	1.4	1.8	1.6–1.9
Ca mg dL^{-1}	54.9–56.3	70–70.4	63–77
P mmol dL^{-1}	1.2	1.3–1.8	1.4–1.6
P mg dL^{-1}	36.9–37.5	41–55.6	42.2–50.3
Fe mg dL^{-1}	1.2	1.2	1.2

[a] see www.meadjohnson.com, www.ross.com, and www.verybestbaby.com for most recent product information. At the time of writing inclusion of single cell oils were being phased into these formulas. Fat blends may differ depending on whether a concentrate, ready-to-feed, or powder.

[b] Similac Lactose Free and Enfamil Lactofree.

[c] Alsoy, Isomil and Prosobee.

[d] Pregestimil, Alimentum, Nutramigen.

Indications for use

As reviewed in the cow's milk-based premature formula section above, some preterm infants may require formulas with lower lactose. Thus premature formulas are lactose-reduced with corn syrup solids providing 50%–60% of the total carbohydrate. The lactose-free cow's milk-based formulas currently on the market in North America (Enfamil LactoFree and Similac Lactose Free) were developed to meet the nutrient needs of term infants and hence are not appropriate for feeding LBW infants

during their initial in-hospital course. Because these products are lactose-free, they are appropriate for use in term infants with congenital lactase deficiency, a relatively rare disorder. Though somewhat controversial, they may also be useful during periods of secondary disaccharidase deficiency due to acute enteritis or chronic conditions affecting the integrity of the small intestine such as diarrhea, enteropathies and Crohn's disease.[1,2] It is known that lactase activity declines dramatically with intestinal injury to mature epithelial cells. Generally, children recovering from a mild bout of diarrhea are able to tolerate breast milk or full-strength lactose-containing formula unless they demonstrated a prior history of lactose intolerance.[2] Careful clinical monitoring is always a must and children receiving a lactose-containing feeding that demonstrate a sudden increase in stool output should be re-assessed and a nonlactose-containing product considered, at least temporarily.

Many families self-prescribe a lactose-free formula in response to often nonspecific concerns that their baby is excessively fussy, gassy, and/or they suspect that their infant is sensitive to lactose. Likewise, healthcare professionals will often recommend a switch to a lactose-free product based on the aforementioned parental concerns as they view the change as relatively benign and that it might help and won't hurt. In fact, these products are sometimes marketed with these perceived indications in mind and without scientific evidence supporting either a need or efficacy. As discussed previously there are known benefits of consuming lactose for mineral absorption and colonic health. In addition, not all infants tolerate all brands of formula or forms of the same brand equally and some infants seem particularly sensitive to formula change especially if the switch is done abruptly. Regardless of whether a decision is made to switch formula or not, parents should be counseled on a range of gas, fussiness, spit-up etc. that is normal/expected in healthy term infants.

Neither of the currently available lactose-free products on the North American market are indicated for galactosemia as they contain low, but variable, levels of galactose.

Soy protein-based formulas

The isolated soy-based formulas currently on the market in North America are free of cow's milk-protein and lactose (Table 28.5). As summarized in Table 28.6, they provided 67 kcal dL^{-1} energy and are fortified with iron and zinc. The soy protein is a soy isolate supplemented with L-methionine, L-carnitine, and taurine. The first limiting amino acid in soy is methionine, hence the biological value of the protein is improved with the addition of methionine. Carnitine is deficient in foods of plant origin and is added to soy formula to the level found in breast milk. Carnitine is required for the optimal oxidation of long-chain fatty acids. Taurine is also added at levels found in breast milk. Taurine acts as an antioxidant and along with glycine functions as a major conjugate of bile acids in early infancy. Originally soy flour, and not soy protein isolate, was used as the protein source in these products. Because of the presence of indigestible carbohydrates (primarily stachyose and raffinose) in soy flour, infants frequently experienced diarrhea and excessive intestinal gas. The higher soy phytate content of the soy flour formulations is thought responsible for the often-cited unpredictable mineral absorption that has seemingly been rectified with the use of soy protein isolate (contains approximately 1.5% phytates) and improved product stability.

The fat content of soy-based formulas is made up primarily of vegetables oils (e.g., a combination of any of the following: high-oleic safflower oil, high oleic sunflower oil, coconut oil, soy oil, palm olein) and most recently a source of the long chain polyunsaturated fatty acids (DHA and ARA) have been added to some brands. Instead of lactose, carbohydrate is provided as starch, corn syrup solids, and sucrose.

It is estimated that approximately 18% of infants in the USA or 750 000 American infants are fed soy-based formulas annually.[120] Concern has been expressed about using these formulas without a clear clinical indication because of their phytoestrogen (specifically, isoflavone) content. Phytoestrogens, dietary estrogens, and plant estrogens are interchangeable terms used to describe heat-stable components found in many foods including soybeans that are similar to naturally occurring steroidal estrogens in structure but have weaker biologic activity.[121] Isoflavones, the major category of phytoestrogens found in legumes (e.g., soybeans), are 10 000–140 000 times less potent in animal and in vitro models than estradiol, the major endogenous estrogen found in humans. However, exposure of small laboratory animals (e.g., rodents and monkeys) to phytoestrogens have produced physiologic effects such as altered sexual development in some, but not all, studies.[121,122] Likewise, animals fed diets high in estrogenic substances are known to have reproductive disturbances. For example, a lower contraceptive rate has been observed in sheep after prolonged exposure to clover pastures rich in isoflavones.[121]

It is difficult to extrapolate data generated from these animal experiments to human infants because of the well-documented fact that the effects of isoflavones are very much species-specific. Nonetheless, concern has been expressed that the actual intake of isoflavones by human infants fed soy-based formulas and their blood levels exceed that shown to influence the menstrual cycle of humans.[123–125] These data do not consider the relative theoretical potency of these compounds (as determined in animal or in vitro models) compared with endogenous estrogen, nor do they confirm a biologic or clinical effect in infants. A recent retrospective cohort study based on telephone interviews reported no overt reproductive problems in young adults fed as infants soy-based formulas.[120] Also, it is argued that no major adverse effects of feeding soy-based formulas have come to light after decades of use.[121]

Indications for use

The indications for use of soy protein-based formulas have been reviewed by the American Academy of Pediatrics.[126] Briefly, because these products are lactose-free, they are appropriate for use in term infants with hereditary lactose deficiency or demonstrated temporary lactose intolerance secondary to acute gastroenteritis. While not significant from a nutritional perspective, the duration of diarrhea has been shown to be shorter among infants receiving soy-based infant formulas.[127,128] One soy-based infant formula (Similac Isomil DF), suitable for infants over 6 months of age, contains soy polysaccharide fiber which may help reduce the duration of diarrhea following acute gastroenteritis[129] or the duration of antibiotic-induced diarrhea in older infants and toddlers.[130]

Not all soy formulas are suitable for the management of infants with galactosemia because of low but variable levels of galactose. Likewise some soy protein-based formulas contain sucrose (Enfamil ProSobee does not) as the carbohydrate source and, as such, are contraindicated in sucrase-isomaltase deficiency and hereditary fructose intolerance.

Most (≥90%) infants with documented IgE-mediated allergy to cow's milk protein will do well on isolated soy-based formula.[2,131,132] Infants with documented cow's milk protein-induced enteropathy or enterocolitis, however, are frequently sensitive to soy protein as well; hence, they should be provided with formula derived from hydrolyzed protein or synthetic amino acids.[2,133–135]

Soy formulas would be suitable for term infants of families that wish to follow a vegetarian-based diet and request a supplement or replacement for breastfeeding. Soy-based formulas are not designed to meet the nutritional needs of the preterm infant.[126]

Table 28.7. Macronutrient content of protein hydrolysate-based formulas and amino acid formulation[a]

	Enfamil Pregestimil	Similac Alimentum	Enfamil Nutramigen	SHS Neocate
Protein (g 100 kcal^{-1})	2.8	2.75	2.8	3.7 amino acids, 3.1 g protein equivalent
Protein source	Hydrolyzed casein with added cystine, tyrosine, tryptophan, and taurine	Hydrolyzed casein with added cystine, tyrosine, tryptophan, and taurine	Hydrolyzed casein with added cysteine, tyrosine, tryptophan, and taurine	100% free amino acids including taurine and carnitine
Carbohydrate (g 100 kcal^{-1})	10.2	10.2	10.3	11.7
Carbohydrate source	Corn syrup solids, modified corn starch, + or − dextrose	Sucrose, + or − modified tapioca starch, + or − corn maltodextrin	Corn syrup solids and modified corn starch	Corn syrup solids
Fat (g 100 kcal^{-1})	5.6	5.5	5.3	4.5
Fat sources[b]	55% MCT oil, soy oil, corn oil, high oleic safflower, sunflower oil	33 % MCT oil, safflower oil, soy oil	Palm olein oil, soy oil, coconut oil, high oleic sunflower oil	High oleic safflower oil, coconut oil (5% as MCT), soy oil

[a] see www.meadjohnson.com, www.ross.com and www.shsna.com for the most recent product information.
[b] Inclusion of single cell oils is being phased in at the time of writing. Fat blends may differ depending on whether a concentrate, ready-to-feed, or powder.

Protein hydrolysate-based formulas

Protein hydrolysate-based formulas currently available on the market in North America can be loosely categorized according to the extent that the protein component is hydrolyzed: (1) 100% free amino acid-containing formula (SHS Neocate); (2) extensively hydrolyzed protein-containing formula (Enfamil Nutramigen, Enfamil Pregestimil, Similac Alimentum); and (3) partially hydrolyzed protein-containing formula (Carnation Good Start) (Table 28.7). All provide 67–68 kcal dL^{-1} energy and are iron-fortified (Table 28.6). The nitrogen in extensively hydrolyzed products is enzymatically hydrolyzed casein and is supplemented with three amino acids – L-cysteine, L-typtophan, and L-tyrosine. These products contain most nitrogen in the form of free amino acids and peptides <1500 kDa. As the name implies, less extensively hydrolyzed products have a greater proportion of the total nitrogen content comprised of larger peptides. The only partially hydrolyzed protein-containing product currently on the market in North America (Good Start/NAN) is derived from a whey source of cow's milk. In general, the level of hydrolysis dictates the cost of the formula with the 100% amino acid-containing formulas being the most expensive and partially hydrolyzed products the least expensive.

The fat content of protein hydrolysate-based formulas contains a combination of the following oils: corn oil, soy oil, high oleic safflower or sunflower oil, coconut oil, and palm olein (Table 28.7). Whereas both Alimentum and Pregestimil contain approximately one-third and one-half of total fatty acids, respectively, as medium-chain triglycerides, Neocate contains 5% of total fatty acids as MCT oil, and Nutramigen and Good Start are devoid of MCT oil.

The carbohydrate fraction of protein hydrolysate formulas is made up of a combination of the following: modified corn starch, modified tapioca starch, maltodextrins, corn syrup solids, lactose, and sucrose (Table 28.7). One hundred percent free amino acid and extensively hydrolyzed products are devoid of lactose.

Indications for use

Protein-hydrolysate formulas are currently used for: (1) infants with severe milk allergy; (2) infants at high risk of developing milk allergy; and (3) infants with significant malabsorption due to gastrointestinal or hepatobiliary disease. It is important to note that protein hydrolysate formulas cannot be used interchangeably for the aforementioned conditions. The American Academy of Pediatrics recently published a position statement clarifying what formula, if any, should be considered in response to protein hypersensitivity (protein allergy) in infants.[136] As breastfeeding is the optimal source of nutrition for infants, it is recommended that when breastfed infants develop symptoms of food allergy, mothers consider restricting their intake of cow's milk, egg, fish, peanuts, and tree nuts. If this approach is unsuccessful, an extensively protein-hydrolyzed formula or a 100% free amino acid-containing formula should be considered if allergic symptoms persist. In this context, extensively protein-hydrolyzed and 100% free amino-acid containing formulas are called hypoallergenic formulas. Formulas labeled hypoallergenic must demonstrate in randomized double-blind, placebo controlled trials that they do not provoke allergic reactions in 90% of infants or children with confirmed cow's milk allergy with 95% confidence. Breastfed infants with confirmed IgE-associated milk allergy not rectified with maternal restriction of cow's milk protein may benefit from the use of a soy-based formula. Soy formulas are considerably less expensive than the 100% free amino acid or extensively hydrolyzed formulas. Likewise, formula-fed infants may benefit from the use of protein hydrolysate or soy formulas as described for the breastfed infant. Formulas based on partially hydrolyzed cow's milk protein are not intended or recommended for the treatment of cow's milk allergy. The presence of significantly larger peptides and the presence of intact cow's milk protein will provoke allergic reactions in a significant number of infants with cow's milk allergy.

While they acknowledge that more studies are needed to produce a definitive recommendation regarding allergy prevention, The American Academy of Pediatrics[136] recommends that infants at high risk for developing allergy as identified by a strong family history should be breastfed for the first year of life or longer. Breastfeeding mothers should eliminate peanuts and tree nuts (e.g., almonds, walnuts, etc.) and consider eliminating eggs, cow's milk, fish and perhaps other foods from their diets. Solids should not be introduced to high-risk infants until 6 months of age, with dairy products delayed until 1 year, eggs until 2 years and peanuts, nuts, and fish until 3 years of age. During this time, if a supplement to breastfeeding is required, a hypoallergenic formula is recommended. In a recent Cochrane review[137] Ram et al. conclude that breast milk should remain the feeding of choice for all babies. In infants with at least one first-degree relative with atopy, extensively hydrolyzed formula for a minimum of 4 months combined with dietary restrictions and environmental measures (dust-mite reduction measures for example) may reduce the risk of developing asthma or wheeze in the first year of life. They found insufficient evidence to suggest that soy-based formula had any benefit.

More recent evidence suggests that partially hydrolyzed formulas may also be efficacious in allergy prevention among infants with a family history of allergy.[138,139–141] As partially hydrolyzed products are considerably cheaper than their extensively hydrolyzed counterparts, and are better tasting, they may be a suitable alternative for many families. These products should not be used where there is a risk of a severe allergic reaction to cow's milk protein. Again, partially hydrolyzed formulas should not be fed to infants that are already known to have an allergy to cow's milk.

Certain extensively hydrolyzed formulas (Pregestimil, Alimentum, Neocate) are also designed for the dietary management of infants with malabsorption disorders including intractable diarrhea, short gut syndrome, steatorrhea, cystic fibrosis, and severe protein-calorie malnutrition.

There has been considerable discussion in the research literature and popular press regarding the role that cow's milk-based formulas may play in the development of Type I diabetes.[142,143] The current understanding of the pathogenesis of Type I diabetes is that environmental factors (i.e., viral, dietary factors, toxins) either alone or in combination trigger in genetically susceptible individuals an autoimmune response in which T lymphocytes infiltrate the pancreatic islets and destroy the insulin-producing beta-cells. Epidemiological observations of infant feeding practices led to the theory that cow's milk consumption is somehow related to the development of Type I diabetes, though a number of observational studies do not find such a relationship. Serological studies examining the impact of cow's milk ingestion or ingestion of several cows' milk proteins on the immune response of humans (e.g., patients with newly diagnosed diabetes) are likewise suggestive. At present, a large multisite international prospective study (TRIGR study) is being conducted to determine whether the incidence of Type I diabetes can be reduced among high-risk infants when weaned from human milk to a protein hydrolysate versus a cow's milk-based formula. At present insufficient evidence is available to suggest that using a protein hydrolysate formula over a cow's milk-based formula will reduce the risk of developing Type I diabetes.

Follow-up formulas

Nutrient compositional guidelines for follow-up formulas designed for term-born infants were first developed by the European Society of Pediatric Gastroenteroloy and Nutrition (ESPGN) in 1981.[144] The rationale was to develop a formula that more closely met the nutritional needs of older infants receiving some solid food compared with infants receiving either a routine starter formula or whole cow's milk. These guidelines assume the ingestion of at least 500 ml of formula in addition to solid foods.[145] In addition to the ESPGN, international guidelines have been published by Codex[146] and the European Communities Directive.[147] Specific compositional criteria have not been established in Canada or the USA. In a double blind crossover design study, infants were fed either whole cow's milk, a milk-based starter formula, or a milk-based follow-up formula. Compared with whole cow's milk, infants fed either formula showed better fat absorption and a decreased renal solute load. Weight gain was similar in the three groups. The authors concluded that follow-up formulas had metabolic advantages compared with whole cow milk but not to starter formulas.[30] Follow-up formulas are available in milk-based and soy-based formulations in North America. There is some controversy surrounding the amount of protein, fat, calcium, and phosphorus in follow-up formulas.

Some follow-up formulas have a slightly higher protein concentration than routine starter formulas. In fact, the protein requirements are lower per unit body weight in the second 6 months of life; hence the need for, and safety of, higher protein-containing follow-up formulas has been questioned.[148,149] In a randomized double-blind controlled trial, infants between 4 and 7 months of age were randomized to receive one of three follow-up formulas with 1.5, 2.2, or 2.9 g dL^{-1} protein in addition to 25 g dL^{-1} cereal. Infants fed formulas with 2.2 or 2.9 g dL^{-1} had elevated urea and lower serum zinc levels when compared with the 1.5 g dL^{-1} protein intake group. The authors concluded that formulas with higher protein levels may be excessive.[148] No follow-up formulas marketed in North America contain more than 1.7 g protein dL^{-1}.

Whole cow's milk is low in essential fatty acids. Because many weaning foods are low in fat and intake of essential fatty acids may be suboptimal, Roy stated that follow-up formulas should not contain less fat than starter formulas.[149] Starter formulas contain 3.4–3.7 g dL^{-1}. Carnation Follow-up, Enfamil Next Step, and Similac Advance Step 2 contain 2.8 g dL^{-1}, 3.3 g dL^{-1} and 3.7 g dL^{-1} respectively.

Follow-up formulas contain more calcium and phosphorus than starter formulas. The National Institute of Health in 1994 stated that the calcium requirements were higher in the second 6 months of life, at 600 mg day^{-1}.[150] Adequacy of starter formulas to meet needs for bone mineralization have been questioned by Ernst and Fomon.[151,152] However, Hanning stated that there is no evidence that lower mineral intakes from starter formulas result in suboptimal bone growth.[153] In addition, the American Academy of Pediatrics published a statement on calcium requirements of infants, children, and adolescents. It stated that there is no evidence demonstrating sustained increases in bone mineralization in infants taking in more calcium than breastfed infants receiving solid food.[154] The most appropriate reference standard with which to determine optimal bone mineralization in formula-fed infants is unknown.

Indications for use

The Canadian Pediatric Society (CPS) and the American Academy of Pediatrics state that follow-up formulas have advantages as compared to whole cow milk but superiority to starter formulas has not been established.[1,2] One often-quoted benefit of follow-up formulas is that they are cheaper than starter formulas. However, this is not always the case.

Specialized formulations, modular formulations, and dietary supplements

Specialized formulations are enteral formulas designed commercially or by the addition of the dietary supplements, vitamins, and/or minerals to meet the unique nutritional needs of infants unable to tolerate one or more of the specific components found in human milk or human milk substitutes.[155] These preparations are designed to reduce the amount of or remove the offending nutrient and provide sufficient energy and other nutrients to meet the specific needs of the patient. Unique formulations exist for metabolic diseases including inborn errors of metabolism and disorders of carbohydrate, fat, and protein metabolism.

Dietary supplements or medical modules are nutrient(s) that are commercially available and can be added to standard or specialized products (Table 28.8). These formulations allow flexibility in providing nutrients in quantities that address individual tolerance issues and unique nutrient needs.

Carbohydrate

Carbohydrate modules are available as starch, polysaccharides plus oligosaccharides, disaccharides, glucose polymers, and monosaccharides, and are the least expensive of all nutrient modules. The choice of carbohydrate form is influenced by its ability to be digested and absorbed. Powder carbohydrate supplements are easily dissolved in liquid and some are also available in a liquid form. Carbohydrate modules impact the osmolality of the formulation with the longest chain glucose polymers, made from the partial hydrolysis of corn starch, contributing the least to the final osmolality.[156]

Fat

Fat modules are energy dense and contribute minimally to the final osmolality of the formulation. Depending on the purpose for using fat as the module of choice, either long-chain triglycerides (LCT) or medium-chain triglycerides (MCT) can be used. Because MCTs do not require bile salts for digestion and absorption and bypass the lymphatics, they are useful when diseases of fat malabsorption and/or maldigestion are present. MCT oil does not contain essential fatty acids and does not allow for transport

Table 28.8. Dietary supplements

Product	Manu-facturer	Composition/source	Form[a]	Kcal per ml or g	Protein g per 100 ml or g	Fat g per 100 ml or g	CHO g per 100 ml or g
Protein							
Casec	Mead Johnson	Calcium caseinate, soy lecithin	P	3.8	90	<2	
Promod	Ross	Whey protein, soy lecithin	P	4.2	76	<9	<10.2
Essential AA	SHS	Essential amino acids	P	3.2	79		
Complete AA	SHS	Essential and non-essential amino acids	P	3.3	82		
Polycose	Ross	Glucose polymers from hydrolyzed corn starch	P	3.8			94
			L	2			50
Caloreen	Nestle	Glucose polymers from hydrolyzed corn starch	P	3.8			96
Moducal	Mead Johnson	Maltodextrin	P	3.8			95
Dextrose		Corn syrup sugar/monosaccharide	P	4.0			99
Sucrose		Cane or beet sugar/disaccharide	P	4.0			99
Corn syrup		Light corn syrup/vanilla	L	4.0			100
Fructose		Fruit sugar/monosaccharide	P	4.0			100
Corn oil or safflower oil		Corn or safflower oil	L	8.4/ml 9.0/g		93	
MCT oil	Mead Johnson	Fractionated coconut oil 6%, >C10 <4%	L	7.7/ml 8.3/g		93	
Microlipid	Mead Johnson	Emulsified safflower oil	L	4.5/ml		50	

Sources: www.meadjohnson.ca, www.shsna.com, www.abbott.com,
Adapted from *Formulary of Infant and Enteral Formulas 2002*. The Hospital for Sick Children, Toronto, Canada. MCT, medium-chain triglycerides.

of vitamins out of the enterocyte. Careful calculations are necessary to ensure adequate amounts of essential fatty acids are present in the final formulation. Serum levels of fat-soluble vitamins should be monitored in infants on high MCT containing formulations to ensure adequate intake. Unlike MCT oil, over-the-counter LCT oils are an inexpensive energy supplement in situations where no malabsorption and/or maldigestion is present. Many contain both linoleic acid and linolenic acid (canola and soybean oil) which are considered essential nutrients and should be included in enteral feedings that are the sole source of nutrition.[157] Corn oil, which contains only linoleic acid, is not recommended for use as an energy supplement unless ratios of both linoleic and linolenic acid already exist within the formula. Both MCT and LCT modules are insoluble and will separate out if left to sit in the feeding tube or bottle, making it difficult for the patient to receive 100% of the desired amount.[158–160] An emulsified LCT formulation does exist (safflower oil) which ensures adequate delivery of the supplement with minimal adherence to the feeding apparatus.

Protein

Protein modules exist either as intact protein, hydrolyzed protein, or crystalline amino acids. Intact protein requires digestion to smaller peptides before absorption at the brush border. Proteins may be further broken down either by chemical or enzymatic means into peptides and free amino acids. As a supplement, intact protein tends to be more palatable and does not contribute as much to the osmolality as do free amino acids. Selecting the appropriate protein source, will be determined by the total amount of protein desired, the mineral content of the protein source, and the solubility of the protein source in the final formulation. Protein modules have a high renal solute load and will impact on the patient's fluid needs and limit the quantity of other solids added to the formulation.[161]

Diligent calculations of amounts and ratios of nutrients in any specialized feeding are necessary to ensure such problems as increased osmolality, increased renal solute load, or under or overdelivery of specific nutrients do not result in iatrogenic medical problems.

Choosing the right form of formula

Powders, ready-feed, and concentrates

Infant formulas are available in three forms: powder, concentrated liquid, and ready-to-feed. Powdered formula is the least expensive option.[162] It must be measured and mixed with clean water that has been boiled for infants under the age of 4 months. Recommended boiling times vary. The American Academy of Pediatrics and Health Canada recommend a rolling boil for at least 1 and 2 minutes, respectively.[1,2] Once the can is opened it can be stored for up to 1 month before discarding; hence, this form is the best option for mothers that are only using formula occasionally to supplement breastfeeding. It is important to note that powdered infant formulas are not commercially sterile products. Unlike liquid formulas, which are subjected to sufficient heat or are aseptically prepared to render them commercially sterile, powdered infant formulas are not processed at high enough temperatures for sufficient time to achieve commercial sterility. This is not usually an issue for healthy term infants, however, it could be for infants in the neonatal intensive care setting and for immunocompromised infants.

The fact that powders are not commercially sterile has been highlighted by health authorities in both the US and Canada in response to a number of outbreaks of *Enterobacter sakazakii* infection among neonates fed milk-based, powdered infant formulas.[163,164] *Enterobacter sakazakii* is a rare, but life-threatening cause of neonatal meningitis, sepsis, and necrotizing enterocolitis. In general, the reported case-fatality rate varies from 40%–80% among newborns diagnosed with this type of severe infection. When feeding immunocompromised infants or those in the neonatal care setting, an alternative to powdered formulas, such as ready-to-feed and concentrated liquid formulas aseptically prepared with sterile water, should be chosen if possible. If there is no alternative, reconstitution of powdered infant formulas in a laminar flow hood by trained personnel and using sterilized water will minimize contamination from the environment. Refer to the following document for detailed procedures of formula reconstitution in institutional settings: Preparation of Formula for Infants: Guidelines for Health-Care Facilities, American Dietetic Association (updated November, 2002, Website: www.eatright.org/formulaguide.html).

A liquid concentrate is easier to measure and mix than the powdered variety but is typically 30%–40% more expensive and must be used within 48 hours of opening and within 24 hours after being mixed with water. Again, water must be clean and brought to a rolling boil when feeding infants under 4 months of age, immunocompromised infants, and those infants in the neonatal intensive care unit setting.

Ready-to-feed formula is the most convenient since it requires no mixing and does not depend on a clean water supply; however, it is by far the most expensive way to buy formula, at up to four times the cost of the powdered option. While most types of formula are available in the powdered option, not all types of specialty formulas are available in liquid concentrate and in the ready-to-feed options.

Federal regulations regarding infant formula

The Food and Drug Administration (FDA) under the provisions of the federal Food, Drug and Cosmetic Act as amended, is responsible for ensuring the safety and nutritional quality of infant formulas sold in the United States (21 Code of Federal Regulations 107).[14] Known as the Infant Formula Act, this piece of legislation specifies the minimum concentration of 29 nutrients and maximum concentrations of nine of these nutrients (Table 28.1). Likewise in Canada, Health Canada, under the provision of the federal Food and Drug Regulations (Part B Division 25), has set out extensive nutritional requirements for infant formulas (www.hc-sc.gc.ca/food-aliment).[165] In the USA, formulas designed for LBW infants are considered exempt formulas under the Infant Formula Act and its 1986 amendment. Exempt formulas may have nutrients or nutrient levels that differ from those specified in the Act after the FDA approves the rationale for the deviation provided by the manufacturer. Health Canada has published guidelines for the Composition and Clinical Testing of Premature Formulas.[23]

In 1998 and again in 2002, Expert Panels assembled at the request of the FDA made recommendations for revision of the Infant Formula Act as it applied to the nutrient levels in standard term and premature formulas, respectively.[10,15] At the time of writing, legislation to change the Infant Formula Act to incorporate these suggested revisions has not occurred.

Increasing the nutrient density of formulas

Formulas may be altered in nutrient density for infants with specific requirements or with unique medical situations such as: (1) decreased formula intake (decreased stamina for oral feedings, transition from gavage to oral feedings or restricted fluids); (2) increased energy expenditure; and (3) increased energy/nutrient losses through malabsorption and/or maldigestion.

The use of energy dense formula has been shown to increase energy intake and weight gain in infants with nonorganic failure to thrive.[166] Concentrating a formula by reducing the amount of water added to either a liquid concentrate or powder formula increases levels of all macro and micronutrients and results in a more balanced formulation. Once the maximum levels of limiting nutrients are reached using the reduced water to concentrate method, energy modules, either carbohydrate or fat, are added to further increase energy alone. Specialized ready-to-feed infant formula (e.g., preterm formula) that is not manufactured as either powder or liquid concentrate can have levels of all nutrients increased by the addition of a commercial liquid concentrate (in-hospital use) or powder concentrate (home use). Similarly, once maximum levels of specific nutrients have been met, energy modules as either carbohydrate or fat are added to increase energy content alone. Determining which method to use to enhance nutrient composition will depend on the patient's medical condition as well as individual goals for weight, gain, composition of weight, and overall growth. Kashyap *et al.* showed that carbohydrate is more effective than fat in enhancing growth and protein accretion in enterally fed LBW infants suggesting that varying the source of nonprotein energy can impact on the quality of weight gain.[167] Van Goudo-

ever also showed that by reducing the energy content of formula and maintaining protein intake, VLBW infants fed lower energy formulas had a lower percentage of fat, suggesting that body composition can be altered by changing the ratio and amount of macronutrients.[168]

Increasing the nutrient composition of a formula also increases the osmolality. The American Academy of Pediatrics recommends that infant formulas have concentrations of less than 450 mOsm per kg water.[157] Osmolality and caloric density of liquid feedings are known to influence the rate of gastric emptying.[169,170] High osmolality feedings have been shown to empty from the stomach more slowly than isotonic solutions and are associated with an increased incidence of nausea, vomiting, diarrhea, and gastroesophageal reflux in infants.[170–173] Models are available to predict the osmolality of modified formulations quickly and accurately before feeding.[174] Calculation of the renal solute load is an important step in determining the suitability of a modified feeding for a patient.[29] The nitrogen and electrolyte content of the diet comprise the majority of the renal solute load. The Potential Renal Solute Load (PRSL) refers to the sum of dietary nitrogen, sodium, potassium, chloride, and phosphorus and will determine the osmolar concentration of the urine. Calculation of PRSL is important especially for infants who are consuming a nutrient-dense infant formula, are fluid restricted, have high sensible and/or insensible fluid losses, or poor renal concentrating ability. A formulation with a high renal solute load may lead to a negative fluid balance and subsequent dehydration. Recommended safe PRSL for infant formulas have been estimated to be 135–177 mOsmol L^{-1} or 20–26 mOsmol 100 $kcal^{-1}$ and maximum PRSL of approximately 221 mOsmol L^{-1} and 33 mOsmol 100 $kcal^{-1}$.[9,29]

Many excellent resources exist to aid the practitioner in calculating the most suitable "recipe" for nutrient-enriched formula for a particular patient.[175,176] Always refer to the most current product information available from the formula manufacturer for changes in ingredients, scoop size etc.

Calculations: potential renal solute load

Potential Renal Solute Load (mOsm L^{-1}) = (protein in g L^{-1} ÷ 0.175*) + (Na in mEq L^{-1} + K in mEq L^{-1} + Cl in mEq L^{-1}) + (Pa** in mg L^{-1} ÷ 31)

* This factor assumes that all dietary N from protein is converted to urea. The protein part of the equation can also be calculated as mg N/L ÷ 28 mg N/mOsm.

Pa** = available phosphorus; assumed to be total phosphorus of human milk and milk-based formulas, and two-thirds of the phosphorus of soy-based formulas.[9]

REFERENCES

1 Canadian Paediatric Society, Dietitians of Canada and Health Canada. *Nutrition for Healthy Term Infants*. Ottawa, ON: Minister of Public Works and Government Services; 1998.

2 American Academy of Pediatrics, Committee on Nutrition. Pediatric *Nutrition Handbook*. 4th edn. Elk Grove Village, IL; AAP 1998.

3 World Health Organization. *Global Strategies for Infant and Young Child Feeding*. Resolution Passes at: Fifty-fourth World Health Assembly; May 9, 2001.

4 Statistics Canada. *National Longitudinal Survey on Children and Youth, 1994/1995 and 1996/1997 Data*. Ottawa, ON: Statistics Canada; 2001.

5 Ryan, A. S., Wenjun, Z., Acosta, A. Breastfeeding continues to increase into the new millennium. *Pediatrics* 2002;**110**:1103–9.

6 Fomon, S. J. Infant formula feeding in the 20th century: formula and Beikost. *J. Nutr.* 2001;**131**:409S–20S.

7 Anderson, S. A., Chinn, H. I., Fisher, K. D. History and current status of infant formulas. *Am. J. Clin. Nutr.* 1982;**35**:381–97.

8 Friel, J. K., Andrews, W. L., Edgecombe, C. *et al.* Eighteen-month follow-up of infants fed evaporated milk formula. *Can. J. Public Health* 1999;**90**:240–3.

9 Fomon, S. J., Ziegler, E. E. Renal solute load and potential renal solute load in infancy. *J. Pediatr.* 1999;**134**:11–14.

10 Raiten, D. J., Talbot, J. M., Waters, J. H. Assessment of nutrient requirements for infant formulas. *J. Nutr.* 1998;**128**:2059S–293S.

11 Nutrition Committee of the Canadian Paediatric Society. Nutrient needs and feeding of preterm infants. *Can. Med. Assoc. J.* 1995;**152**:1765–85.

12 Widdowson, E. M., Spray, C. M. Chemical development in utero. *Arch. Dis. Child.* 1951;**26**:205–14.

13 Usher, R., McLean, F. Intrauterine growth of live-born Caucasian infants at sea level: standards obtained from measurements in 7 dimensions of infants born between 25 and 44 weeks of gestation. *J. Pediatr.* 1969;**74**:901–10.

14 Food and Drug Administration: Rules and regulations. *Nutrient requirements for infant formulas (21 CFR Part 107). Fed. Reg.* 1985;**50**:45106–8.

15 Klein, C. J. Nutrient requirements for preterm infant formulas. *J. Nutr.* 2002;**132**:1395S–577S.

16 George, D.E., DeFrancesca, B. A. Human milk comparison to cow milk. In: Lebenthal, E., ed. *Textbook of Gastroenterology and Nutrition in Infancy*. 2nd ed. New York, NY: Raven Press; 1989:239–61.

17 Lonnerdal, B, Atkinson, S. A. Human milk proteins. In: Jenson, R. G., ed. *Handbook of Milk Composition*. San Diego, CA: Academic Press; 1995:351–68.

18 Benson, J., Neylan, M., Masor, M., Paule, C., O'Connor, D. Approaches and considerations in determining the protein and amino acid composition of term and preterm infant formula. *Int. Dairy J.* 1998;**8**:405–12.

19 Kunz, C., Lonnerdal, B. Re-evaluation of the whey protein/casein ratio of human milk. *Acta Paediatr.* 1992;**81**:107–12.

20 Lonnerdal, B. Nutritional importance of non-protein nitrogen. In Raiha, N. C., ed. *Nestle Nutrition Workshop Series*. New York, NY: Raven Press; 1994:105–16.

21 Alston-Mills, B. Nonprotein nitrogen compounds in bovine milk. In Jenson, R. G., ed. *Handbook of Milk Composition*. San Diego, CA: Academic Press, 1995:468–72.

22 Atkinson, S. A, Lonnerdal, B. Nonprotein nitrogen fractions of human milk. In: Jenson, R. G., ed. *Handbook of Milk Composition*. San Diego, CA: Academic Press; 1995:369–87.

23 Health Canada Health Protection Branch. Guidelines for the composition and clinical testing of formulas for preterm infants. *Report of an Ad Hoc Expert Consultation to the Health Protection Branch, Health Canada*. Ottawa, ON: Canadian Government Publishing Center; 1995.

24 Lawrence, R. A., Lawrence, R. M. *Breast Feeding: A Guide for the Medical Profession*. 5th edn. St. Louis, MO: Mosby; 1999.

25 Jensen, R. G., Bitman, J., Carlson, S. E. *et al.* Human milk lipids. In Jensen, R. G., ed. *Handbook of Milk Composition*. San Diego, CA: Academic Press.; 1995:495–542.

26 Jensen, R. G., Newburg, D. S. Bovine milk lipids. In Jensen, R. G., ed. *Handbook of Milk Composition*. San Diego, CA: Academic Press Inc.; 1995:543–75.

27 Newburg, D. S, Neubauer, S. H. Carbohydrates in milks: analysis, quantities and significance. In: Jensen, R. G., ed. *Handbook of Milk Composition*. San Diego, CA: Academic Press; 1995:273–349.

28 Atkinson, S. A., Alston-Mills, B., Lonnerdal, B., Neville, M. C. Major minerals and ionic constituents of human and bovine milks. In Jensen, R. G., ed. *Handbook of Milk Composition*. San Diego, CA: Academic Press; 1995:593–622.

29 Ziegler, E. E., Fomon, S. J. Potential renal solute load of infant formulas. *J. Nutr.* 1989;**119**:1785–8.

30 Fuchs, G. J., Gastanaduy, A. S., Suskind, R. M. Comparative metabolic study of older infants fed infant formula, transition formula, or whole cow's milk. *Nutr. Res.* 1992;**12**:1467–78.

31 Fomon, S. J. *Nutrition of Normal Infants*. St. Louis, MO: Mosby; 1993.

32 O'Connor, D., Masor, M., Paule, C., Benson, J. Amino acid composition of cow's milk and human requirements. In Welch, R. A. S., ed. *Milk Composition, Production and Biotechnology*. Wallingford, UK: CAB International; 1997:203–13.

33 Paule, C., Wahrenberger, D., Jones, W., Kuchan, M., Masor, M. A novel method to evaluate the amino acid response to infant formulas. *FASEB J.* 1996;**10**:A554.

34 Yogman, M. W., Zeisel, S. H. Diet and sleep patterns in newborn infants. *N. Engl. J. Med.* 1983;**309**:1147–9.

35 Heine, W. E. The significance of tryptophan in infant nutrition. *Adv. Exp. Med. Biol.* 1999;**467**:705–10.

36 Oberlander, T. F., Barr, R. G., Young, S. N., Brian, J. A. Short-term effects of feed composition on sleeping and crying in newborns. *Pediatrics* 1992;**90**:733–40.

37 Steinberg, L. A., O'Connell, N. C., Hatch, T. F., Picciano, M. F., Birch, L. L. Tryptophan intake influences infants' sleep latency. *J. Nutr.* 1992;**122**:1781–91.

38 Rassin, D. K. Essential and non-essential amino acids in neonatal nutrition. In: Raiha, N. C. ed. *Protein Metabolism During Infancy.* New York, NY: Raven Press; 1994: 183–95.

39 Fried, M. D., Khoshoo, V., Secker, D. J. *et al.* Decrease in gastric emptying time and episodes of regurgitation in children with spastic quadriplegia fed a whey-based formula. *J. Pediatr.* 1992;**120**:569–72.

40 Khoshoo, V., Zembo, M., King, A. *et al.* Incidence of gastroesophageal reflux with whey- and casein-based formulas in infants and in children with severe neurological impairment. *J. Pediatr. Gastroenterol. Nutr.* 1996;**22**:48–55.

41 Billeaud, C., Guillet, J., Sandler, B. Gastric emptying in infants with or without gastro-oesophageal reflux according to the type of milk. *Eur. J. Clin. Nutr.* 1990;**44**:577–83.

42 Tolia, V., Lin, C. H., Kuhns, L. R. Gastric emptying using three different formulas in infants with gastroesophageal reflux. *J. Pediatr. Gastroenterol. Nutr.* 1992;**15**:297–301.

43 Thorkelsson, T., Mimouni, F., Namgung, R. *et al.* Similar gastric emptying rates for casein- and whey-predominant formulas in preterm infants. *Pediatr. Res.* 1994;**36**:329–33.

44 Lammi-Keefe, C. J., Jensen, R. G. Lipids in human milk: a review. 2: Composition and fat-soluble vitamins. *J. Pediatr. Gastroenterol. Nutr.* 1984;**3**:172–98.

45 Nelson, S. E., Frantz, J. A., Ziegler, E. E. Absorption of fat and calcium by infants fed a milk-based formula containing palm olein. *J. Am. Coll. Nutr.* 1998;**17**:327–32.

46 Lien, E. L., Boyle, F. G., Yuhas, R., Tomarelli, R. M., Quinlan, P. The effect of triglyceride positional distribution on fatty acid absorption in rats. *J. Pediatr. Gastroenterol. Nutr.* 1997;**25**: 167–74.

47 Filer, L. J., Jr., Mattson, F. H., Fomon, S. J. Triglyceride configuration and fat absorption by the human infant. *J. Nutr.* 1969;**99**:293–8.

48 Carnielli, V. P., Luijendijk, I. H., Goudoever Van, J. B. *et al.* Structural position and amount of palmitic acid in infant formulas: effects on fat, fatty acid, and mineral balance. *J. Pediatr. Gastroenterol. Nutr.* 1996;**23**:553–60.

49 Nelson, S. E., Rogers, R. R., Frantz, J. A., Ziegler, E. E. Palm olein in infant formula: absorption of fat and minerals by normal infants. *Am. J. Clin. Nutr.* 1996;**64**:291–6.

50 Ostrom, K. M., Borschel, M. W., Westcott, J. E., Richardson, K. S., Krebs, N. F. Lower calcium absorption in infants fed casein hydrolysate- and soy protein-based infant formulas containing palm olein versus formulas without palm olein. *J. Am. Coll. Nutr.* 2002;**21**:564–9.

51 Hansen, J. W., Huston, R., Ehreukranz, R., Bell, E. F. Impact of palm olein in infant feedings on fat and calcium absorption in growing premature infants. *J. Am. Coll. Nutr.* 1996;**15**:526.

52 Hansen, J. W., Diener, U. Challenges of matching human milk fatty acid patterns technically and functionally. *Eur. J. Med. Res.* 1997;**2**:74–8.

53 Koo, W. W., Hammami, M., Margeson, D. P., Montalto, M. B., Lasekan, J. B. Reduced bone mineralization in infants fed palm olein-containing formula: a randomized, double-blind, prospective trial. *Pediatrics* 2003;**111**:1017–23.

54 Innis, S. M., Kuhnlein, H. V. Long-chain n-3 fatty acids in breast milk of Inuit women consuming traditional foods. *Early Hum. Dev.* 1988;**18**:185–9.

55 Innis, S. M. Essential fatty acids in growth and development. *Prog. Lipid Res.* 1991;**30**:39–103.

56 Demmelmair, H., von Schenck, U., Behrendt, E., Sauerwald, T., Koletzko, B. Estimation of arachidonic acid synthesis in full term neonates using natural variation of 13C content. *J. Pediatr. Gastroenterol. Nutr.* 1995;**21**:31–6.

57 Pawlosky, R. J., Sprecher, H. W., Salem, N., Jr. High sensitivity negative ion GC-MS method for detection of desaturated and chain-elongated products of deuterated linoleic and linolenic acids. *J. Lipid Res.* 1992;**33**:1711–17.

58 Sauerwald, T. U., Hachey, D. L., Jensen, C. L. *et al.* Effect of dietary alpha-linolenic acid intake on incorporation of docosahexaenoic and arachidonic acids into plasma phospholipids of term infants. *Lipids* 1996;**31**:S131–5.

59 Salem, N., Jr., Wegher, B., Mena, P., Uauy, R. Arachidonic and docosahexaenoic acids are biosynthesized from their 18-carbon precursors in human infants. *Proc. Natl. Acad. Sci USA.* 1996;**93**:49–54.

60 Farquharson, J., Cockburn, F., Patrick, W. A., Jamieson, E. C., Logan, R. W. Infant cerebral cortex phospholipid fatty-acid composition and diet. *Lancet* 1992;**340**:810–13.

61 Jamieson, E. C., Abbasi, K. A., Cockburn, F. *et al.* Effect of diet on term infant cerebral cortex fatty acid composition. *World Rev. Nutr. Diet.* 1994;**75**:139–41.

62 Makrides, M., Neumann, M. A., Byard, R. W., Simmer, K., Gibson, R. A. Fatty acid composition of brain, retina, and erythrocytes in breast- and formula-fed infants. *Am. J. Clin. Nutr.* 1994;**60**:189–94.

63 Neuringer, M., Connor, W. E., Lin, D. S., Barstad, L., Luck, S. Biochemical and functional effects of prenatal and postnatal omega 3 fatty acid deficiency on retina and brain in rhesus monkeys. *Proc. Natl. Acad. Sci. USA.* 1986;**83**:4021–5.

64 de la Presa, Owens, S., Innis, S. M. Docosahexaenoic and arachidonic acid prevent a decrease in dopaminergic and serotoninergic neurotransmitters in frontal cortex caused by a linoleic and alpha-linolenic acid deficient diet in formula-fed piglets. *J. Nutr.* 1999;**129**:2088–93.

65 Neuringer, M., Connor, W. E., Petten Van C., Barstad, L. Dietary omega-3 fatty acid deficiency and visual loss in infant rhesus monkeys. *J. Clin. Invest.* 1984;**73**:272–76.

66 Neuringer, M., Connor, W. E., Lin, D. S., Anderson, G. J. Effects of n-3 fatty acid deficiency on retinal physiology and visual function. In: Sinclair, A., Gibson, R., eds. *Essential Fatty Acids and Eicosanoids. Invited Papers from the Third International Congress.* Adelaide, Australia: American Oil Chemists' Society; 1992:161–4.

67 Birch, E. E., Hoffman, D. R., Uauy, R., Birch, D. G., Prestidge, C. Visual acuity and the essentiality of docosahexaenoic acid

and arachidonic acid in the diet of term infants. *Pediatr. Res.* 1998;**44**:201–9.

68 Birch, E. E., Hoffman, D. R., Castaneda, Y. S. *et al.* A randomized controlled trial of long-chain polyunsaturated fatty acid supplementation of formula in term infants after weaning at 6 wk of age. *Am. J. Clin. Nutr.* 2002;**75**:570–80.

69 Birch, E. E., Garfield, S., Hoffman, D. R., Uauy, R., Birch, D. G. A randomized controlled trial of early dietary supply of long-chain polyunsaturated fatty acids and mental development in term infants. *Dev. Med. Child Neurol.* 2000;**42**:174–181.

70 Auestad, N., Montalto, M. B., Hall, R. T. *et al.* Visual acuity, erythrocyte fatty acid composition, and growth in term infants fed formulas with long chain polyunsaturated fatty acids for one year. Ross Pediatric Lipid Study. *Pediatr Res.* 1997;**41**:1–10.

71 Auestad, N., Halter, R., Hall, R. T. *et al.* Growth and development in term infants fed long-chain polyunsaturated fatty acids: a double-masked, randomized, parallel, prospective, multivariate study. *Pediatrics* 2001;**108**:372–81.

72 Scott, D. T., Janowsky, J. S., Carroll, R. E. *et al.* Formula supplementation with long-chain polyunsaturated fatty acids: are there developmental benefits? *Pediatrics.* 1998;**102**:E59.

73 Auestad, N., Scott, D. T., Janowsky, J. S. *et al.* Visual, cognitive, and language assessments at 39 months: a follow-up study of children fed formulas containing long-chain polyunsaturated fatty acids to 1 year of age. *Pediatric* 2003;**112**:177–83.

74 Carlson, S. E., Ford, A. J., Werkman, S. H., Peeples, J. M., Koo, W. W. Visual acuity and fatty acid status of term infants fed human milk and formulas with and without docosahexaenoate and arachidonate from egg yolk lecithin. *Pediatr. Res.* 1996;**39**:882–8.

75 Makrides, M., Neumann, M., Simmer, K., Pater, J., Gibson, R. Are long-chain polyunsaturated fatty acids essential nutrients in infancy? *Lancet* 1995;**345**:1463–8.

76 Agostoni, C., Trojan, S., Bellu, R. *et al.* Developmental quotient at 24 months and fatty acid composition of diet in early infancy: a follow up study. *Arch. Dis. Child.* 1997;**76**:421–4.

77 Willatts, P., Forsyth, J. S., DiModugno, M. K., Varma, S., Colvin, M. Effect of long-chain polyunsaturated fatty acids in infant formula on problem solving at 10 months of age. *Lancet* 1998;**352**:688–91.

78 Makrides, M., Neumann, M. A., Simmer, K., Gibson, R. A. A critical appraisal of the role of dietary long-chain polyunsaturated fatty acids on neural indices of term infants: a randomized, controlled trial. *Pediatrics* 2000;**105**:32–8.

79 Lucas, A., Stafford, M., Morley, R. *et al.* Efficacy and safety of long-chain polyunsaturated fatty acid supplementation of infant-formula milk: a randomised trial. *Lancet* 1999;**354**:1948–54.

80 Looker, A. C., Dallman, P. R., Carroll, M. D., Gunter, E. W., Johnson, C. L. Prevalence of iron deficiency in the United States. *J. Am. Med. Assoc.* 1997;**277**:973–6.

81 Oski, F. A. Iron-fortified formulas and gastrointestinal symptoms in infants: a controlled study with the cooperation of the Syracuse Consortium for Pediatric Clinical Studies. *Pediatrics* 1980;**66**:168–170.

82 Griffin, M. P., Hansen, J. W. Can the elimination of lactose from formula improve feeding tolerance in premature infants? *J Pediatr.* 1999;**135**:587–92.

83 Clandinin, M. T., Chappell, J. E., Leong, S. *et al.* Intrauterine fatty acid accretion rates in human brain: implications for fatty acid requirements. *Early Hum. Dev.* 1980;**4**:121–9.

84 Carlson, S. E. Long-chain polyunsaturated fatty acid supplementation of preterm infants. In Dobbing, J., ed. *Developing Brain and Behavior: The Role of Lipids in Infant Formula.* San Diego, CA: Academic Press; 1997:41–102.

85 Uauy, R. D., Birch, D. G., Birch, E. E., Tyson, J. E., Hoffman, D. R. Effect of dietary omega-3 fatty acids on retinal function of very-low-birth-weight neonates. *Pediatr. Res.* 1990;**28**:485–92.

86 Birch, E., Birch, D., Hoffman, D. *et al.* Breast-feeding and optimal visual development. *J. Pediatr. Ophthalmol. Strabismus* 1993;**30**:33–8.

87 Carlson, S. E., Werkman, S. H., Rhodes, P. G., Tolley, E. A. Visual-acuity development in healthy preterm infants: effect of marine-oil supplementation. *Am. J. Clin. Nutr.* 1993;**58**:35–42.

88 Werkman, S. H., Carlson, S. E. A randomized trial of visual attention of preterm infants fed docosahexaenoic acid until nine months. *Lipids* 1996;**31**:91–7.

89 Carlson, S. E., Werkman, S. H. A randomized trial of visual attention of preterm infants fed docosahexaenoic acid until two months. *Lipids* 1996;**31**:85–90.

90 Carlson, S. E., Werkman, S. H., Tolley, E. A. Effect of long-chain n-3 fatty acid supplementation on visual acuity and growth of preterm infants with and without bronchopulmonary dysplasia. *Am. J. Clin. Nutr.* 1996;**63**:687–97.

91 Carlson, S. E., Cooke, R. J., Werkman, S. H., Tolley, E. A. First year growth of preterm infants fed standard compared to marine oil n-3 supplemented formula. *Lipids* 1992;**27**:901–7.

92 Ryan, A. S., Montalto, M. B., Groh-Wargo, S. *et al.* Effect of DHA-containing formula on growth of preterm infants to 59 weeks postmenstrual age. *Am. J. Human. Biol.* 1999;**11**:457–67.

93 Carlson, S. E., Werkman, S. H., Peeples, J. M., Cooke, R. J., Tolley, E. A. Arachidonic acid status correlates with first year growth in preterm infants. *Proc. Natl. Acad. Sci. USA.* 1993;**90**:1073–7.

94 Innis, S. M., Adamkin, D. H., Hall, R. T. *et al.* Docosahexaenoic acid and arachidonic acid enhance growth with no adverse effects in preterm infants fed formula. *J. Pediatr.* 2002;**140**:547–54.

95 Lim, H., Antonson, D., Clandinin, M. T. *et al.* Formulas with docosahexaenoic acid (DHA) and arachidonic acid (ARA) for low-birth-weight infants (LBW) are safe. *Ped Res.* 2002;**51**:1854.

96 Clandinin, M. T., Aerde Van J., Antonson, D. *et al.* Formulas with docosahexaenoic acid (DHA) and arachidonic acid (ARA) promote better growth and development scores in very-low-weight infants (VLBW). *Ped. Res.* 2002;**51**:1092.

97 Vanderhoof, J., Gross, S., Hegyi, T. *et al.* Evaluation of a long-chain polyunsaturated fatty acid supplemented formula on growth, tolerance, and plasma lipids in preterm infants up to

48 weeks postconceptional age. *J. Pediatr. Gastroenterol. Nutr.* 1999;**29**:318–26.

98 Vanderhoof, J., Gross, S., Hegyi, T. A multicenter long-term safety and efficacy trial of preterm formula supplemented with long-chain polyunsaturated fatty acids. *J. Pediatr. Gastroenterol. Nutr.* 2000;**31**:121–7.

99 O'Connor, D. L., Hall, R., Adamkin, D. *et al.* Growth and development in preterm infants fed long-chain polyunsaturated fatty acids: a prospective, randomized controlled trial. *Pediatrics* 2001;**108**:359–71.

100 Fewtrell, M. S., Morley, R., Abbott, R. A. *et al.* Double-blind, randomized trial of long-chain polyunsaturated fatty acid supplementation in formula fed to preterm infants. *Pediatrics* 2002;**110**:73–82.

101 Ziegler, E. E., Biga, R. L., Fomon, S. J. Nutritional requirements of the preterm infant. In: Suskind, R. M., ed. *Textbook of Pediatric Nutrition.* New York, NY: Raven Press; 1981:29–39.

102 Widdowson, E. M. Trace elements in foetal and early postnatal development. *Proc. Nutr. Soc.* 1974;**33**:275–84.

103 Lemons, J. A., Bauer, C. R., Oh, W. *et al.* Very low birth weight outcomes of the National Institute of Child Health and Human Development Neonatal Research Network, January 1995 through December 1996. NICHD Neonatal Research Network. *Pediatrics* 2001;107:E1.

104 Merko, S., Shah, P. S., Wong, K. Y. *et al.* Nutrient intakes and growth of very preterm infants born <28 weeks gestation. *Can. J. Diet. Pract. Res.* 2002; **62**(2):S105.

105 Lucas, A. Nutrition, growth and development of postdischarge preterm infants. *Posthospital Nutrition in the Preterm Infant.* Columbus, OH: Ross Products Division, Abbott Laboratories, 1996:81–9.

106 Hack, M., Merkatz, I. R., McGrath, S. K., Jones, P. K., Fanaroff, A. A. Catch-up growth in very-low-birth-weight infants. Clinical correlates. *Am. J. Dis. Child.* 1984;**138**:370–375.

107 Lucas, A., Bishop, N. J., King, F. J., Cole, T. J. Randomised trial of nutrition for preterm infants after discharge. *Arch Dis Child.* 1992;**67**:324–27.

108 Bishop, N. J., King, F. J., Lucas, A. Increased bone mineral content of preterm infants fed with a nutrient enriched formula after discharge from hospital. *Arch. Dis. Child.* 1993;**68**:573–8.

109 Cooke, R. J., Griffin, I. J., McCormick, K. *et al.* Feeding preterm infants after hospital discharge: effect of dietary manipulation on nutrient intake and growth. *Pediatr Res.* 1998;**43**:355–60.

110 Wheeler, R. E., Hall, R. T. Feeding of premature infant formula after hospital discharge of infants weighing less than 1800 grams at birth. *J. Perinatol.* 1996;**16**:111–16.

111 Brunton, J. A., Saigal, S., Atkinson, S. A. Growth and body composition in infants with bronchopulmonary dysplasia up to 3 months corrected age: a randomized trial of a high-energy nutrient-enriched formula fed after hospital discharge. *J. Pediatr.* 1998;**133**:340–5.

112 Carver, J. D., Wu, P. Y., Hall, R. T. *et al.* Growth of preterm infants fed nutrient-enriched or term formula after hospital discharge. *Pediatrics* 2001;**107**:683–9.

113 Morley, R., Fewtrell, M. S., Abbott, R. A. *et al.* Neurodevelopment in children born small for gestational age: a randomized trial of nutrient-enriched versus standard formula and comparison with a reference breastfed group. *Pediatrics* 2004;**113**:515–21.

114 Heubi, J., Karasov, R., Reisinger, K. *et al.* Randomized multicenter trial documenting the efficacy and safety of a lactose-free and a lactose-containing formula for term infants. *J. Am. Diet Assoc.* 2000;**100**:212–17.

115 Moya, M., Cortes, E., Ballester, M. I., Vento, M., Juste, M. Short-term polycose substitution for lactose reduces calcium absorption in healthy term babies. *J. Pediatr. Gastroenterol. Nutr.* 1992;**14**:57–61.

116 Moya, M., Lifschitz, C., Ameen, V., Euler, A. R. A metabolic balance study in term infants fed lactose-containing or lactose-free formula. *Acta Paediatr.* 1999;**88**:1211–15.

117 Ziegler, E. E., Fomon, S. J. Lactose enhances mineral absorption in infancy. *J. Pediatr. Gastroenterol. Nutr.* 1983;**2**:288–94.

118 Kobayashi, A., Kawai, S., Obe, Y., Nagashima, Y. Effects of dietary lactose and lactase preparation on the intestinal absorption of calcium and magnesium in normal infants. *Am. J. Clin. Nutr.* 1975;**28**:681–3.

119 Abrams, S. A., Griffin, I. J., Davila, P. M. Calcium and zinc absorption from lactose-containing and lactose-free infant formulas. *Am. J. Clin. Nutr.* 2002;**76**:442–6.

120 Strom, B. L., Schinnar, R., Ziegler, E. E. *et al.* Exposure to soy-based formula in infancy and endocrinological and reproductive outcomes in young adulthood. *J. Am. Med. Assoc.* 2001;**286**:807–14.

121 Klein, K. O. Isoflavones, soy-based infant formulas, and relevance to endocrine function. *Nutr. Rev.* 1998;**56**:193–204.

122 Anthony, M. S., Clarkson, T. B., Hughes, C. L., Jr., Morgan, T. M., Burke, G. L. Soybean isoflavones improve cardiovascular risk factors without affecting the reproductive system of peripubertal rhesus monkeys. *J. Nutr.* 1996;**126**:43–50.

123 Sheehan, D. M. The case for expanded phytoestrogen research. *Proc. Soc. Exp. Biol. Med.* 1995;**208**:3–5.

124 Sharpe, R. M., Martin, B., Morris, K. *et al.* Infant feeding with soy formula milk: effects on the testis and on blood testosterone levels in marmoset monkeys during the period of neonatal testicular activity. *Hum. Reprod.* 2002;**17**:1692–703.

125 Setchell, K. D., Zimmer-Nechemias, L., Cai, J., Heubi, J. E. Exposure of infants to phyto-oestrogens from soy-based infant formula. *Lancet* 1997;**350**:23–27.

126 American Academy of Pediatrics. Committee on Nutrition. Soy protein-based formulas: recommendations for use in infant feeding. *Pediatrics* 1998;**101**:148–53.

127 Allen, U. D., McLeod, K., Wang, E. E. Cow's milk versus soy-based formula in mild and moderate diarrhea: a randomized, controlled trial. *Acta Paediatr.* 1994;**83**:183–7.

128 Santosham, M., Goepp, J., Burns, B. *et al.* Role of a soy-based lactose-free formula in the outpatient management of diarrhea. *Pediatrics* 1991;**87**:619–22.

129 Brown, K. H., Perez, F., Peerson, J. M. *et al.* Effect of dietary fiber (soy polysaccharide) on the severity, duration, and

nutritional outcome of acute, watery diarrhea in children. *Pediatrics* 1993;**92**:241–7.

130 Burks, A. W., Vanderhoof, J. A., Mehra, S., Ostrom, K. M., Baggs, G. Randomized clinical trial of soy formula with and without added fiber in antibiotic-induced diarrhea. *J. Pediatr.* 2001;**139**:578–82.

131 Bock, S. A., Atkins, F. M. Patterns of food hypersensitivity during sixteen years of double-blind, placebo-controlled food challenges. *J. Pediatr.* 1990;**117**:561–7.

132 Ladodo, K. S., Borovick, T. E. The use of an isolated soy protein formula for nourishing infants with food allergies. In Steinke, F. H., Waggle, D. H., Volgarev, M. N., eds. *New Protein Foods in Human Health: Nutrition, Prevention, and Therapy.* Boca Raton, FL: CRC Press; 1992:85–9.

133 Burks, A. W., Casteel, H. B., Fiedorek, S. C., Williams, L. W., Pumphrey, C. L. Prospective oral food challenge study of two soybean protein isolates in patients with possible milk or soy protein enterocolitis. *Pediatr. Allergy Immunol.* 1994;**5**:40–5.

134 Eastham, E. J. Soy protein allergy. In Hamburger, R. N., ed. *Food Intolerance in Infancy: Allergology, Immunology, and Gastroenterology. Carnation Nutrition Education Series.* New York, NY: Raven Press;1989:223–36.

135 Whitington, P. F., Gibson, R. Soy protein intolerance: four patients with concomitant cow's milk intolerance. *Pediatrics* 1977;**59**:730–2.

136 American Academy of Pediatrics Committee on Nutrition. Hypoallergenic infant formulas. *Pediatrics* 2000;**106**(2):346–9.

137 Ram, F. S., Ducharme, F. M., Scarlett, J. Cow's milk protein avoidance and development of childhood wheeze in children with a family history of atopy. *The Cochrane Database of Systematic Reviews.* 2003.

138 Marini, A., Agosti, M., Motta, G., Mosca, F. Effects of a dietary and environmental prevention programme on the incidence of allergic symptoms in high atopic risk infants: three years' follow-up. *Acta Paediatr. Suppl.* 1996;**414**:1–21.

139 Baumgartner, M., Brown, C. M., Secretin, M. C., Van't Hof, M., Haschke, F. Controlled trials investigating the use of one partially hydrolyzed whey formula for dietary prevention of atopic manifestations until 60 months of age: an overview using meta-analytical techniques. *Nutr. Res.* 1998;**18**:1425–42.

140 Chandra, R. K. Five-year follow-up of high-risk infants with family history of allergy who were exclusively breast-fed or fed partial whey hydrolysate, soy, and conventional cow's milk formulas. *J. Pediatr. Gastroenterol. Nutr.* 1997;**24**:380–8.

141 von Berg, A., Koletzko, S., Grubl, A. *et al.* The effect of hydrolyzed cow's milk formula for allergy prevention in the first year of life: the German Infant Nutritional Intervention Study, a randomized double-blind trial. *J. Allergy Clin. Immunol.* 2003;**111**:533–40.

142 Schrezenmeir, J., Jagla, A. Milk and diabetes. *J. Am. Coll. Nutr.* 2000;**19**:176S–90S.

143 Akerblom, H. K., Vaarala, O., Hyoty, H., Ilonen, J., Knip, M. Environmental factors in the etiology of type 1 diabetes. *Am. J. Med. Genet.* 2002;**115**:18–29.

144 ESPGN Committee on Nutrition. Guidelines on infant nutrition. Recommendations for the composition of follow-up formulas and beikost. *Acta Paediatr. Scand.* 1981;**70**:S287.

145 ESPGN Committee on Nutrition. Comment on the composition of cow's milk based follow-up formulas. *Acta Paediatr. Scand.* 1990;**79**:250–4.

146 Codex Alimentarius, 1994; **4**:42–51, Codex Standard for Follow-Up Formula, Codex Stan 156, 1987 (amended 1989).

147 Official Journal of the European Communities, **49**:12–16 Feb 28, 1996, Commission Directive 96/EC of Feb 16, 1996, amending Directive 91/321/EEC on infant formula and follow-up formula.

148 Lonnerdal, B., Chen, C. L. Effects of formula protein level and ratio on infant growth, plasma amino acids and serum trace elements. II. Follow-up formula. *Acta Paediatr. Scand.* 1990;**79**:266–73.

149 Roy, C. Do we need follow-on formulas? A Canadian symposium on optimal nutrition in the second six months of life. *Can. J. Paediatr.* 1993;**1**:61–3.

150 NIH Consensus Development Panel on Optimal calcium intake. *J. Am. Med. Assoc.* 1994;**272**(24):1942–8.

151 Ernst, J. A., Brady, M. S., Rickard, K. A. Food and nutrient intake of 6- to 12-month-old infants fed formula or cow milk: a summary of four national surveys. *J. Pediatr.* 1990;**117**:S86–100.

152 Fomon, S. J., Sanders, K. D., Ziegler, E. E. Formulas for older infants. *J. Pediatr.* 1990;**116**:690–6.

153 Hanning, R. Vitamins and minerals. A Canadian symposium on optimal nutrition in the second six months of life. *Can. J. Paediatr.* 1993;**1**:22–30.

154 American Academy of Pediatrics, Committee on Nutrition. Calcium requirements of infants, children and adolescents. *Pediatrics* 1999;**104**(5):1152–6.

155 Klish, W. J., Potts, E., Ferry, G. D., Nichols, B. L. Modular formula: an approach to management of infants with specific or complex food intolerances. *J. Pediatr.* 1976;**88**:948–52.

156 Davis, A., Baker, S. The use of modular nutrients in pediatrics. *J. Pareuter. Enterol. Nutr.* 1996;**20**:228–36.

157 American Academy of Pediatrics, Committee on Nutrition. Commentary on breast feeding and infant formulas, including proposed standards. *Pediatrics* 1976;**57**:278–85.

158 Mehta, N. R., Hamosh, M., Bitman, J., Wood, D. L. Adherence of medium-chain fatty acids to feeding tubes of premature infants fed formula fortified with medium-chain triglyceride. *J. Pediatr. Gastroenterol. Nutr.* 1991;**13**:267–9.

159 Mehta, N. R., Hamosh, M., Bitman, J., Wood, D. L. Adherence of medium-chain fatty acids to feeding tubes during gavage feeding of human milk fortified with medium-chain triglycerides. *J. Pediatr.* 1988;**112**:474–6.

160 Stocks, R. J., Davies, D. P., Allen, F., Sewell, D. Loss of breast milk nutrients during tube feeding. *Arch. Dis. Child.* 1985;**60**:164–6.

161 Smith, J. L., Heymsfield, S. B. Enteral nutrition support: formula preparation for modular ingredients. *J. Parenter. Enteral. Nutr.* 1983;**7**:280–8.

162 Kalnins, D., Saab, J. Better baby food. *Your Essential Guide to Nutrition, Feeding & Cooking for All Babies & Toddlers.* Toronto, Ontario: Robert Rose; 2001.

163 http://www.hc-sc.gc.ca/food-aliment/mh-dm/mhe-dme/e˙enterobacter˙sakazakii.html

164 http://vm.cfsan.fda.gov/~dms/inf-ltr3.html

165 *Food and Drug Directorate: Food and Drug Regulations.* Division 25, Canada Gazette; 1990;**124**:73E–H.

166 Khoshoo, V., Reifen, R. Use of energy-dense formula for treating infants with non-organic failure to thrive. *Eur. J. Clin. Nutr.* 2002;**56**:921–4.

167 Kashyap, S., Ohira-Kist, K., Abildskov, K. *et al.* Effects of quality of energy intake on growth and metabolic response of enterally fed low-birth-weight infants. *Pediatr. Res.* 2001;**50**:390–7.

168 van Goudoever, J. B., Sulkers, E. J., Lafeber, H. N., Sauer, P. J. Short-term growth and substrate use in very-low-birth-weight infants fed formulas with different energy contents. *Am. J. Clin. Nutr.* 2000;**71**:816–21.

169 Siegel, M., Lebenthal, E., Krantz, B. Effect of caloric density on gastric emptying in premature infants. *J. Pediatr.* 1984;**104**:118–22.

170 Minami, H., McCallum, R. W. Dietary caloric density and osmolality influence gastroesophageal reflux in infants. *Gastroenterology* 1984;**97**:601–4.

171 Carroll, A. E., Garrison, M. M., Christakis, D. A. A systematic review of nonpharmacological and nonsurgical therapies for gastroesophageal reflux in infants. *Arch. Pediatr. Adolesc. Med.* 2002;**156**:109–13.

172 Sutphen, J. L., Dillard, V. L. Dietary caloric density and osmolality influence gastroesophageal reflux in infants. *Gastroenterology* 1989;**97**:601–4.

173 Salvia, G., De Vizia B., Manguso, F. *et al.* Effect of intragastric volume and osmolality on mechanisms of gastroesophageal reflux in children with gastroesophageal reflux disease. *Am. J. Gastroenterol.* 2001;**96**:1725–32.

174 Anderson, K., Kennedy, B. A model for the prediction of osmolalities of modular formulas. *J. Parenter. Enteral Nutr.* 1986;**10**:646–9.

175 Brylinsky, C. M., Bastian, C. H. A step-wise approach to calculating modular feedings. *J. Am. Diet. Assoc.* 1989;**89**: 1489–91.

176 Groh-Wargo, S., Thompson, M., Hovasi Cox, J. *Nutritional Care for High-Risk Newborns.* Revised 3rd edn. Chicago, IL: Precept Press; 2000.

177 US Department of Agriculture (USDA), National Agricultural Library, The Food and Nutrition Information Centre website. Available at: www.nal.usda.gov/fnic/. Accessed 13, February, 2003.

178 The Canadian Nutrient File, Health Canada. Available at: http://www.hc-sc.gc.ca/food-aliment/ns-sc/nr-rn/surveillance/cnf-fcen/e˙index.html. Accessed 21, February, 2003.

179 Atkinson, S. A., Radde, I. C., Chance, G. W., Bryan, M. H., Anderson, G. H. Macro-mineral content of milk obtained during early lactation from mothers of premature infants. *Early Hum. Dev.* 1980;**4**:5–14.

180 Canfield, L. M., Hopkinson, J. M., Lima, A. F., Silva, B., Garza, C. Vitamin K in colostrum and mature human milk over the lactation period – a cross-sectional study. *Am. J. Clin. Nutr.* 1991;**53**:730–5.

181 American Society of Nutritional Sciences, Life Science Research Office. *Assessment of Nutrient Requirements for Infant Formula.* Bethesda, MD; 1998.

182 Mendelson, R. A., Anderson, G. H., Bryan, M. H. Zinc, copper and iron content of milk from mothers of preterm and full-term infants. *Early Hum. Dev.* 1982;**6**:145–51.

183 Bolisetty, S., Gupta, J. M., Graham, G. G., Salonikas, C., Naidoo, D. Vitamin K in preterm breastmilk with maternal supplementation. *Acta Paediatr.* 1998;**87**:960–2.

184 Lemons, J. A., Moye, L., Hall, D., Simmons, M. Differences in the composition of preterm and term human milk during early lactation. *Pediatr. Res.* 1982;**16**:113–17.

185 Chappell, J. E., Francis, T., Clandinin, M. T. Vitamin A and E content of human milk at early stages of lactation. *Early Hum. Dev.* 1985;**11**:157–67.

186 Lammi-Keefe, C.J. Vitamins D and E in human milk. In Jenson, R. G., ed. *Handbook of Milk Composition.* New York, NY: Academic Press; 1995:706–17.

187 Udipi, S. A., Kirksey, A., West, K., Giacoia, G. Vitamin B6, vitamin C and folacin levels in milk from mothers of term and preterm infants during the neonatal period. *Am. J. Clin. Nutr.* 1985;**42**:522–30.

29

Differences between metabolism and feeding of preterm and term infants

Scott C. Denne and Brenda B. Poindexter

Department of Pediatrics, Indiana University School of Medicine, Indianapolis, IN

Understanding differences in nutrient metabolism between premature and term neonates has important implications for the nutritional management of these infants in the neonatal intensive care unit. Prematurity and critical illness can impact the response to nutrient intake. Providing optimal nutritional support of both premature and critically ill neonates born at term remains an elusive challenge to neonatologists. Although less than 20% of extremely-low-birth-weight infants (ELBW) (<1000 g birth weight) are small for gestational age at the time of birth, growth failure is nearly universal by the time these infants approach discharge from the hospital.[1] The long-term impact that early nutritional deficiencies may have on growth and neurodevelopment is only beginning to be appreciated.

It would seem obvious that there are substantial differences in metabolism between preterm and term infants, yet precisely defining those differences is surprisingly challenging. Metabolic studies in preterm and term infants have often been carried out using different techniques and under varied clinical circumstances, making comparisons difficult. Furthermore, information in normal term infants is often limited. Nevertheless, understanding developmental differences is fundamental to providing appropriate nutritional and metabolic support to preterm and term infants. This chapter will focus on presenting the differences between preterm and term infants with regard to protein, glucose, and energy metabolism.

Protein metabolism

A first step in understanding protein requirements is to assess protein losses under basal conditions. In a series of studies, our laboratory has measured the rate of catabolism of the essential amino acid phenylalanine using stable isotopic techniques in preterm and term infants receiving 6 mg kg^{-1} min^{-1} of intravenous glucose.[2-4] Overall rates of protein loss can be calculated from these rates based on the phenylalanine content of protein (280 µmol per g protein). Extremely premature (26 weeks' gestation; ~850 g birth weight), clinically stable premature (32 weeks' gestation; 1600 g birth weight) and healthy term infants were studied in the first week of life.[2-4] As illustrated in Figure 29.1, protein losses are inversely related to gestational age, with losses in extremely premature infants 2-fold higher than in term infants. Other investigators have obtained similar results using nitrogen balance techniques.[5-7]

It is useful to understand the protein kinetic components of the higher protein losses in extremely preterm infants. Protein loss can be driven by high rates of proteolysis, low rates of protein synthesis, or a combination of both. Figure 29.2 shows rates of proteolysis and protein synthesis in extremely preterm and term infants during the 6 mg kg^{-1} min^{-1} glucose infusion.[3,4] Protein synthesis rates are not lower but in fact approximately 20% higher in extremely preterm infants compared to term infants. However, rates of proteolysis are even higher (~30%) in extremely preterm infants. Consequently, it is these high rates of proteolysis that result in the higher rates of protein losses in extremely premature compared with term infants. Rates of proteolysis, like rates of overall protein loss, vary inversely with gestational age. It has been speculated that high rates of proteolysis may be required to provide a continuous supply of amino acids needed for remodeling of tissue in rapid growth. It is useful to examine the regulators of proteolysis in neonates, and how they may differ between preterm and term newborns.

Neonatal Nutrition and Metabolism. Second Edition, ed. P. Thureen and W. Hay. Published by Cambridge University Press.

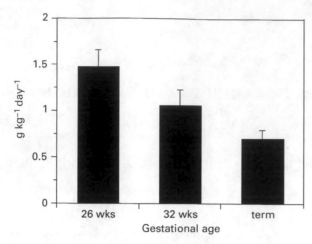

Figure 29.1. Rates of protein loss measured in preterm and term infants during an intravenous glucose infusion of 6 mg kg^{-1} min^{-1}. Protein losses calculated from phenylalanine kinetics.[2–4]

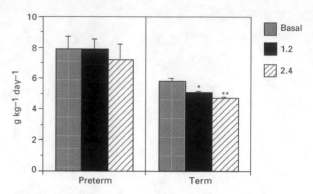

Figure 29.3. Rates of proteolysis in preterm and term infants during a basal glucose infusion of 6 mg kg^{-1} min^{-1}, and in response to a graded amino acid infusion of 1.2 g kg^{-1} day^{-1} and 2.4 g kg^{-1} day^{-1}. Proteolysis calculated from phenylalanine kinetics. Significant dose-dependent reductions in proteolysis were observed in term infants ($<$0.001) but not in preterm infants.[3,10]

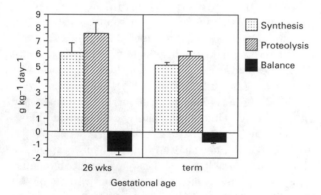

Figure 29.2. Protein synthesis, proteolysis, and protein balance in 26 weeks' gestation preterm infants and normal term neonates. Protein kinetics calculated from phenylalanine kinetics during intravenous glucose infusion of 6 mg kg^{-1} min.$^{-1}$ [2,4]

In both term and preterm infants, glucose infusions, which result in significant increases in insulin concentrations, do not result in reductions in overall proteolysis.[8,9] The ability of intravenous amino acids to reduce overall rates of proteolysis has also been evaluated in both preterm and term infants. In normal healthy term infants, a graded infusion of intravenous amino acids produces a dose dependent suppression of proteolysis (Figure 29.3).[3] At an amino acid intake of 1.2 g kg^{-1} day^{-1}, proteolysis is reduced by approximately 10%. In response to a doubling of amino acid intake to 2.4 g kg^{-1} day^{-1}, proteolysis is reduced by 20%. These changes in proteolysis are independent of any changes in glucose and insulin concentrations.

Premature neonates, on the other hand, demonstrate resistance to changes in proteolysis in response to intravenous amino acids. Clinically stable premature ($\sim$32 weeks' gestation) infants have been studied in the first week of life using a protocol identical to that used in the term infant study described above.[10] In contrast to their term counterparts, rates of proteolysis are unchanged in response to the graded infusion of intravenous amino acids. Figure 29.3 illustrates these differences between the two populations.

It must be noted that in both preterm and term infants, amino acid infusions increase overall rates of protein synthesis by approximately 13% in both populations.[3,10] In response to graded amino acid intake, protein balance improves in both groups, as illustrated in Figure 29.4. However, because preterm infants increase protein synthesis but do not suppress proteolysis in response to amino acids, overall protein balance is significantly less than that obtained in term infants at the same level of amino acid intake.

Developmental differences in the antiproteolytic response to full parenteral nutrition (containing glucose, lipid, and amino acids) have also been documented. Normal term infants and premature infants (ranging in gestation from 23–35 weeks) have been studied under an identical protocol, which determined overall rates of proteolysis in the basal state and in response to parenteral nutrition (90 kcal kg^{-1} day^{-1}, 2.5 g kg^{-1} day^{-1} of protein).[2,4] As shown in Figure 29.5, there is a direct relationship between gestational age and the ability of this

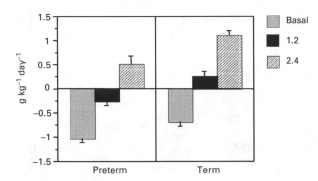

Figure 29.4. Protein balance calculated from phenylalanine kinetic data in preterm and term infants during a basal glucose infusion of 6 mg/kg/min and during amino acid infusions of 1.2 and 2.4 g/kg/day.[3,10]

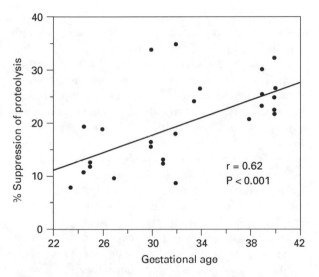

Figure 29.5. Relationship between the percent suppression of proteolysis in response to parenteral nutrition and gestational age. Results based on phenylalanine kinetics.[2,4]

parenteral nutrition solution to reduce overall proteolysis. Similar to the response to amino acids alone, full parenteral nutrition increased protein synthesis at all gestations by ~15%, so that overall protein balance was improved for all neonates. However, differences in the ability to reduce overall proteolysis resulted in smaller improvements at earlier gestational ages.[4]

These developmental differences in protein metabolism have important clinical implications. Based on higher basal protein losses and a reduced antiproteolytic response to amino acids, the overall protein requirements of preterm infants increases as gestational age decreases. Therefore, not only are there differences between the preterm infants

as a group and term infants, but there are also substantial differences between extremely preterm (23–27 weeks' gestation) infants compared with less premature (32–35 weeks' gestation) infants. These developmental differences must be taken into account when providing early amino acid nutritional support in the preterm infants. In addition, these findings raise significant questions about the protein adequacy of existing preterm formulas for extremely preterm infants; these formulas were designed over 20 years ago to support 30–35 week gestation preterm infants. Many clinicians use a variety of approaches to supplement existing preterm formulas, but none of these approaches have been systematically evaluated. Based on existing information about protein requirements in extremely preterm infants, studies evaluating nutritional strategies to better support these requirements are urgently needed.

Glucose metabolism

As glucose is the primary source of fuel for the brain, the use and regulation of glucose is a fundamental aspect of metabolism and one likely to show developmental differences. However, precisely defining the differences between premature and term infants across a range of gestational ages can be difficult, because proper comparison requires that study conditions be identical or at least similar for preterm and term infants. Existing data allow some assessment of the differences and similarities between preterm and term infants with regard to endogenous glucose production, the regulation of endogenous glucose production by exogenous glucose, and gluconeogenesis.

Endogenous glucose production

Endogenous glucose production is the rate of glucose released into the system from glycogenolysis or gluconeogenesis, and is often measured in the basal state (usually a short fast in neonates). The rate of endogenous glucose production provides important insight into basal glucose needs (in particular to support brain metabolism) and the ability of the neonate to maintain an adequate glucose supply. Endogenous glucose production has been measured between 3 and 5 mg kg^{-1} min^{-1} in studies of both preterm and term infants, so it may seem that there is little difference between preterm and term infants in this regard.[11,12] However, studies that have determined similar rates in preterm and term infants have studied more mature preterm infants (34–36 weeks' gestation).[11,12] When preterm infants are

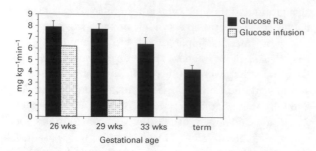

Figure 29.6. Total glucose rate of appearance measured by isotopic tracer dilution in preterm and term infants. Rate of exogenous glucose infusion (if any) is also shown.[8,9,13,14]

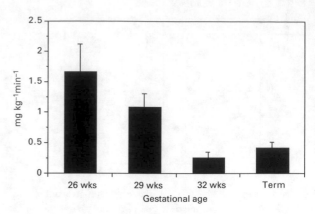

Figure 29.7. Endogenous glucose production rates during exogenous glucose infusions of ~6mg kg^{-1} min^{-1} in preterm and term infants.[8–10,15]

studied at earlier gestations, a different pattern emerges. Figure 29.6 shows glucose production rates measured in preterm and term infants within the first 3 days of life using the same technique (6, 6 d$_2$ glucose tracer dilution).[8,9,13,14] Term infants and 33 weeks' gestation preterm infants were studied after a brief fast; glucose production is approximately 50% greater in the 33-week preterm compared with the term infants.[9,14] Two studies have determined glucose production rates in clinically stable 26 weeks' gestation infants.[8,13] However, for ethical reasons, true fasting conditions cannot be obtained in this population. Some glucose was infused to these extremely preterm infants in the two studies reported, and nearly identical total glucose rates of appearance (~8 mg kg^{-1} min^{-1}) have been measured, despite the substantial differences in the exogenous glucose infusion rates between the two studies. Therefore, 8 mg kg^{-1} min^{-1} appears to be a reasonable approximation of basal glucose production in 26 weeks' gestation infants; this rate is 2-fold greater than that measured in term infants. These data strongly suggest significant differences in glucose production (and utilization) between preterm and term infants, at least when preterm infants ≤33 weeks' gestation are studied.

Regulation of endogenous glucose production by exogenous glucose

The normal adult response to an exogenous glucose infusion is effective suppression of endogenous glucose production (greater than 90%). Similar studies have been performed in both term newborns and premature infants of various gestational ages. Figure 29.7 shows endogenous glucose production (the difference between total measured glucose rate of appearance and exogenous glucose infusion) in preterm and term infants studied in the first week of life during an exogenous glucose infusion of approximately 6 mg kg^{-1} min.$^{-1}$ [8–10,15] This rate of glucose

infusion in all these studies resulted in similar glucose (80–110 mg dL^{-1}) and insulin (4–7 μg mL^{-1}) concentrations. These conditions effectively suppressed (greater than 90%) glucose production in term infants and 32 weeks' gestation preterm infants.[9,10] However, glucose production was less effectively suppressed in preterm infants of earlier gestations, with the highest residual glucose production rates in the most immature (26 weeks' gestation) infants.[8,15] It appears that very premature infants are more resistant to suppression of endogenous glucose production by exogenous glucose infusion. However, 26 weeks' gestation infants can suppress endogenous glucose production to levels similar to that obtained in term infants, but it requires a higher glucose infusion rate (9.5 mg kg^{-1} min^{-1}) resulting in higher glucose (136 mg dL^{-1}) and insulin (13 μg mL^{-1}) concentrations.[8] From a clinical perspective, glucose infusion rates of 8–9 mg kg^{-1} min^{-1} appear to be necessary in extremely preterm infants in order to best supply glucose needs and preserve endogenous stores. In more mature preterm infants (≥32 weeks gestation) and in term newborns, glucose infusion rates of ~6 mg kg^{-1} min^{-1} appear to adequately meet basal glucose requirements and preserve glucose stores.

Gluconeogenesis

The normal fetus is dependent upon the mother for a continuous supply of glucose, and endogenous glucose production and gluconeogenesis are inactive during fetal life.[16] After birth, the rapid ability to initiate gluconeogenesis is crucial to support endogenous glucose production, as both term and especially preterm infants have limited glycogen stores. Gluconeogenesis has been assessed in both preterm and term infants using a variety of approaches

Table 29.1. Resting energy expenditure measured by respiratory calorimetry in preterm and term infants in the first week of life

Gestation (wks)	BWT (g)	REE (kcal kg^{-1} day^{-1})	Total n	Source	Comments
27 wks	960	39	32	22,23	18 subjects ventilated, 5 subjects nasal CPAP
29 wks	1105	41	52	24,25	All subjects ventilated
32 wks	1450	47	85	23,26,27	Subjects in room air
40 wks	3275	44	34	28–30	Normal newborns in room air

BWT, body weight; REE, resting energy expenditure; CPAP, continuous positive airway pressure.

and under a number of different circumstances.[15,17–21] Gluconeogenesis is inherently difficult to quantify, and differing study conditions and approaches have been used in term and preterm infants. For these reasons, direct comparisons between these two groups are difficult. Nevertheless, qualitative if not quantitative comparisons are possible.

Perhaps the most significant qualitative finding is that both preterm and term infants have the capacity to initiate measurable and significant gluconeogenesis to support glucose production within the first 2 days after birth.[17,19,21] Although the exact quantitative relationship between gluconeogenesis and gestational age remains undefined, significant rates of gluconeogenesis have been measured in a variety of studies of extremely preterm infants with gestations as low as 24 weeks.[18,19] Studies in preterm and term infants have demonstrated that the gluconeogenesis substrates pyruvate and glycerol both contribute to glucose production. Gluconeogenesis accounts for ~30% of overall glucose production in term infants during fasting;[21] in preterm infants, gluconeogenesis contributes 30%–80% of residual glucose production during exogenous glucose or parenteral nutrition administration.[15,18,21] Glycerol appears to be the primary gluconeogenic substrate in extremely preterm infants during the administration of parenteral nutrition, which includes lipid.[18] Studies under similar conditions in term infants have not been performed. Available data regarding gluconeogenesis suggest many similarities between preterm and term infants. Developmental differences, if they exist, remain to be elucidated.

Energy expenditure

An accurate assessment of energy expenditure is necessary to appropriately provide for the energy needs of preterm and term infants. Similar to other aspects of metabolism, it would be logical to assume that there may be a developmental aspect to energy expenditure. Intuitively, higher rates (per kg) of energy expenditure might be anticipated in preterm infants, with their smaller body mass, susceptibility to thermal stresses, and their frequent requirement for ventilatory support.

However, the rather extensive data measuring resting energy expenditure in both preterm and term infants in the first week of life does not necessarily support this intuition. Table 29.1 shows rates of resting energy expenditure measured by respiratory calorimetry in term infants and in preterm infants of varying gestational ages.[22–30] Over 200 subjects from nine different studies are represented; different investigators have obtained remarkably similar results. Surprisingly, rates of resting energy expenditure are similar from 27 weeks' gestation through term, with no suggestion that more immature individuals have higher rates. Preterm infants requiring and not requiring mechanical ventilation have been included, and there is no indication that mechanical ventilation significantly influences measured energy expenditure in these studies. It also must be noted that although nutrient intake has an important influence on energy expenditure, both preterm and term infants were studied under similar conditions of nutrient intake (fasting or low caloric intakes). Therefore it seems unlikely that true differences between preterm and term infants were obscured by altered nutrient intakes.

Although the available data suggest similar energy expenditures in preterm and term infants, it is important to point out a number of caveats. First, these determinations were made by respiratory calorimetry, which can be technically challenging and perhaps less accurate when used in patients requiring supplemental oxygen and/or mechanical ventilation.[31] Technical difficulties may therefore contribute to the difficulty of demonstrating differences between preterm and term infants, but seem unlikely to play the primary role. Second, respiratory calorimetry is typically obtained over a relatively short period of time (2–4 hours) with close attention being paid to the thermal environment of the patients during the period of measurement. These short measurement intervals may underestimate inadvertent thermal stresses and other factors which contribute to total energy expenditure over longer periods. There is some preliminary evidence that when total energy expenditure is measured using the doubly labeled water

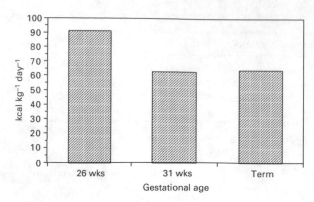

Figure 29.8. Total energy expenditure measured by either doubly labeled water technique or 24-hour respiratory calorimetry in preterm and term infants at ~3 weeks of age.[33–44]

technique, higher rates of energy expenditure are evident in extremely preterm infants in the first week of life.[32] Further studies determining energy expenditure over longer periods of time may ultimately be better able to demonstrate differences in energy expenditure between preterm and term infants. At present, the currently available data about resting energy expenditure in preterm and term infants remains difficult to reconcile with the higher rates of protein turnover and glucose production in preterm infants (both energy requiring processes), the higher rates of glucose utilization in preterm infants, and the poor growth outcomes of ELBW infants.[1]

A number of published studies have determined total energy expenditure in preterm and term infants slightly later in postnatal life, at approximately 3 weeks of age. Total energy expenditure was determined over 5–7 days using the doubly labeled water technique, or using 24-hour respiratory calorimetry. Figure 29.8 shows these rates of total energy expenditure in term infants (total n = 44 in three studies),[33–35] 31 weeks' gestation preterm infants (total n = 62 in eight studies),[36–43] and 26 weeks' gestation preterm infants (total n = 12 in one study).[44] Total energy expenditure is remarkably similar in 3-week-old 31 weeks' gestation preterm infants and term infants of a similar age. However, total energy expenditure in 3-week-old 26 weeks' gestation infants is approximately 50% higher. It must be noted that this only represents one study with a relatively limited number of subjects, and all subjects studied required mechanical ventilation. Nevertheless, the data do suggest that energy expenditure may be substantially higher in the most immature group of preterm infants. Clearly additional studies examining total energy expenditure in this group will be necessary to more precisely establish differences between this group and more mature preterm and term infants.

What are the clinical implications of these energy expenditure determinations? A minimum of 40 kcal kg^{-1} day^{-1} of energy intake is necessary for both preterm and term infants in the first week of life. It remains possible that higher energy intakes are necessary and desired, especially for the extremely preterm infant. As postnatal and nutrient intake advances, energy expenditure increases and intakes of approximately 65 kcal kg^{-1} day^{-1} are required for preterm infants ≥ 31 weeks' gestation and term infants to achieve a zero energy balance. Obviously higher intakes are required to achieve positive energy balance in normal growth. In extremely preterm infants (26 weeks' gestation) higher energy intakes of up to 90 kcal kg^{-1} day^{-1} may be necessary just to prevent negative energy balance, although the data remain limited. Currently available information on energy expenditure provides a minimum caloric target so that significant energy deficits might not accumulate. Nevertheless, additional information about energy requirements in both term and preterm infants need to be developed.

Summary

Although precise metabolic comparisons between preterm and term infants can be difficult, developmental differences in protein and glucose metabolism have been clearly established. Baseline protein losses increase with decreasing gestational age, and preterm infants have a more limited ability to reduce whole body rates of proteolysis in response to nutrients compared with term infants. Clinically, this information emphasizes the higher protein requirements of preterm infants and the necessity to minimize rapidly accumulating protein deficits. Developmental differences in glucose metabolism are also apparent, with high rates of glucose production and utilization, which decrease gradually to term gestation values. A glucose infusion rate of 6 mg kg^{-1} min^{-1} provides sufficient glucose to meet needs and preserve endogenous stores in term and moderately preterm (≥ 32 weeks' gestation) infants. Higher glucose infusion rates of 8–10 mg kg^{-1} min^{-1} appear to be necessary to produce the same result in more immature (26 weeks' gestation) infants. Similar rates of resting energy expenditure of ~40 kcal kg^{-1} day^{-1} have been measured in preterm and term infants in the first week of life, perhaps suggesting similar energy needs across gestational ages. However, some preliminary data would suggest that extremely preterm infants may have higher requirements in early postnatal life. At 3 weeks of age, ~64 kcal kg^{-1} day^{-1} appears to be necessary to meet energy expenditure requirements for both term and moderately preterm

(31 weeks' gestation) infants. The energy required to match energy expenditure in extremely preterm infants requiring mechanical ventilation at 3 weeks of age may be substantially higher (90 kcal kg^{-1} day^{-1}), although the data remain limited.

REFERENCES

1 Lemons, J. A., Bauer, C. R., Oh, W. *et al.* Very low birth weight outcomes of the National Institute of Child Health and Human Development Neonatal Research Network, January 1995 through December 1996. *Pediatrics* 2001;**107**:E1.

2 Clark, S. E., Karn, C. A., Ahlrichs, J. A. *et al.* Acute changes in leucine and phenylalanine kinetics produced by parenteral nutrition in premature infants. *Pediatr. Res.* 1997;**41**:568–74.

3 Poindexter, B. B., Karn, C. A., Ahlrichs, J. A. *et al.* Amino acids suppress proteolysis independent of insulin throughout the neonatal period. *Am. J. Physiol.* 1997;**272**:E592–9.

4 Denne, S. C., Karn, C. A., Ahlrichs, J. A. *et al.* Proteolysis and phenylalanine hydroxylation in response to parenteral nutrition in extremely premature and normal newborns. *J. Clin. Invest.* 1996;**97**:746–54.

5 Kashyap, S., Heird, W. C. *Protein Requirements of Low Birthweight, Very Low Birthweight, and Small for Gestational Age Infants.* New York, NY: Vevey/Raven Press; 1994.

6 Van Goudoever, J. B., Colen, T., Wattimena, J. L. D. *et al.* Immediate commencement of amino acid supplementation in preterm infants: effect on serum amino acid concentrations and protein kinetics on the first day of life. *J. Pediatr.* 1995;**127**:458–65.

7 Rivera, A., Bell, E. F., Bier, D. M. Effect of intravenous amino acids on protein metabolism of preterm infants during the first three days of life. *Pediatr. Res.* 1993;**33**:106–11.

8 Hertz, D. E., Karn, C. A., Liu, Y. M., Liechty, E. A., Denne, S. C. Intravenous glucose suppresses glucose production but not proteolysis in extremely premature newborns. *J. Clin. Invest.* 1993;**92**:1752–8.

9 Denne, S. C., Karn, C. A., Wang, J., Liechty, E. A. Effect of intravenous glucose and lipid on glucose production and proteolysis in normal newborns. *Am. J. Physiol.* 1995;**269**:E361–7.

10 Poindexter, B. B., Karn, C. A., Leitch, C. A., Liechty, E. A., Denne, S. C. Amino acids do not suppress proteolysis in premature neonates. *Am. J. Physiol. Endocrinol. Metab.* 2001;**281**:E472–8.

11 Kalhan, S., Oliven, A., King, K., Lucero, C. Role of glucose in the regulation of endogenous glucose production in the human newborn. *Pediatr. Res.* 1986;**20**:49–52.

12 Cowett, R. M., Wolfe, R. R. Glucose and lactate kinetics in the neonate. *J. Dev. Physiol.* 1991;**16**:341–7.

13 Sunehag, A., Ewald, U., Larsson, A., Gustafsson, J. Glucose production rate in extremely immature neonates (<28 weeks) studied by use of deuterated glucose. *Pediatr. Res.* 1993;**33**:97–100.

14 Farrag, H. M., Nawrath, L. M., Healey, J. E. *et al.* Persistent glucose production and greater peripheral sensitivity to insulin in the neonate vs the adult. *Am. J. Physiol.* 1997;**272**:E86–93.

15 Van Kempen, A., Romijn, J. A., Ackermans, M. T. *et al.* Adaptation of glucose production and gluconeogenesis to diminishing glucose infusion in preterm infants at varying gestational ages. *Pediatr. Res.* 2003;**53**:628–34.

16 Kalhan, S., Parimi, P. Gluconeogenesis in the fetus and neonate. *Semin. Perinatol.* 2000;**24**:94–106.

17 Sunehag, A., Gustafsson, J., Ewald, U. Glycerol carbon contributes to hepatic glucose production during the first eight hours in healthy term infants. *Acta Paediatr.* 1996;**85**:1339–43.

18 Sunehag, A. L., Haymond, M. W., Schanler, R. J., Reeds, P. J., Bier, D. M. Gluconeogenesis in very low birth weight infants receiving total parenteral nutrition. *Diabetes* 1999;**48**:791–800.

19 Sunehag, A., Ewald, U., Gustafsson, J. Extremely preterm infants (<28 weeks) are capable of gluconeogenesis from glycerol on their first day of life. *Pediatr. Res.* 1996;**40**:553–7.

20 Sunehag, A. L. Parenteral glycerol enhances gluconeogenesis in very premature infants. *Pediatr. Res.* 2003;**53**:635–41.

21 Kalhan, S. C., Parimi, P., Van Beek, R. *et al.* Estimation of gluconeogenesis in newborn infants. *Am. J. Physiol. Endocrinol. Metab.* 2001;**281**:E991–7.

22 Bauer, K., Laurenz, M., Ketteler, J., Versmold, H. Longitudinal study of energy expenditure in preterm neonates < 30 weeks' gestation during the first three postnatal weeks. *J. Pediatr.* 2003;**142**:390–6.

23 Mayfield, S. R. Technical and clinical testing of a computerized indirect calorimeter for use in mechanically ventilated neonates. *Am. J. Clin. Nutr.* 1991;**54**:30–4.

24 Forsyth, J. S., Crighton, A. Low birthweight infants and total parenteral nutrition immediately after birth. I. Energy expenditure and respiratory quotient of ventilated and nonventilated infants. *Arch. Dis. Child Fetal Neonatal Edn.* 1995;**73**:F4–7.

25 DeMarie, M. P., Hoffenberg, A., Biggerstaff, S. L. B. *et al.* Determinants of energy expenditure in ventilated preterm infants. *J. Perinat. Med.* 1999;**27**:465–72.

26 Denne, S., Karn, C., Liechty, E. Leucine kinetics after a brief fast and in response to feeding in premature infants. *Am. J. Clin. Nutr.* 1992;**56**:899–904.

27 Denne, S., Karn, C., Liu, Y., Leitch, C., Liechtyy, E. Effect of enteral *vs* parenteral feeding on leucine kinetics and fuel utilization in premature newborns. *Pediatr. Res.* 1994;**36**:429–35.

28 Steele, R. Influence of glucose loading and of injected insulin on hepatic glucose output. *Proc. N. Y. Acad. Sci.* 1959;**82**:420–30.

29 Denne, S., Kalhan, S. Glucose carbon recycling oxidation in human newborns. *Am. J. Physiol.* 1986;**251**:E71–7.

30 Denne, S., Rossi, E., Kalhan, S. Leucine kinetics during feeding in normal newborns. *Pediatr. Res.* 1991;**30**:23–7.

31 Kalhan, S. C., Denne, S. C. Energy consumption in infants with bronchopulmonary dysplasia. *J. Pediatr.* 1990;**116**:662–4.

32 Carr, B. J., Denne, S. C., Leitch, C. A. Total energy expenditure in extremely premature and term infants in early postnatal life. *Pediatr. Res.* 2000;**47**:284A.

33 Lucas, A., Ewing, G., Roberts, S., Coward, W. How much energy does the breast fed infant consume and expend? *Br. Med. J.* 1987;**295**:75–7.

34 Butte, N. F., Wong, W. W., Ferlic, L. *et al.* Energy expenditure and deposition of breast-fed and formula-fed infants during early infancy. *Pediatr. Res.* 1990;**28**:631–40.

35 Leitch, C. A., Karn, C. A., Peppard, R. J. *et al.* Increased energy expenditure in infants with cyanotic congenital heart disease. *J. Pediatr.* 1998;**133**:755–60.

36 Roberts, S., Coward, W., Schlingenseipen, K.-H., Nohria, V., Lucas, A. Comparison of the doubly labeled water (2H218O) method with indirect calorimetry and a nutrient-balance study for simultaneous determination of energy expenditure, water intake, and metabolizable energy intake in preterm infants. *Am. J. Clin. Nutr.* 1986;**44**:315–22.

37 Jensen, C. L., Butte, N. F., Wong, W. W., Moon, J. K. Determining energy expenditure in preterm infants: comparison of $^2H_2^{18}O$ method and indirect calorimetry. *Am. J. Physiol.* 1992;**263**: R685–92.

38 Bell, E., Rios, G., Wilmoth, P. Estimation of 24-hour energy expenditure from shorter measurement periods in premature infants. *Pediatr. Res.* 1986;**20**:646–9.

39 Roberts, S., Murgatroyd, P., Crisp, J. *et al.* Long-term variation in oxygen consumption rate in preterm infants. *Biol. Neonate* 1987;**52**:1–8.

40 Schulze, K., Stefanski, M., Masterson, J. *et al.* An analysis of the variability in estimates of bioenergetic variables in preterm infants. *Pediatr. Res.* 1986;**20**:422–7.

41 Freymond, D., Schutz, Y., Decombaz, J., Micheli, J.-L., Jequier, E. Energy balance, physical activity, and thermogenic effect of feeding in premature infants. *Pediatr. Res.* 1986;**20**:638–45.

42 Fjeld, C. R., Cole, F. S., Bier, D. M. Energy expenditure, lipolysis, and glucose production in preterm infants treated with theophylline. *Pediatr. Res.* 1992;**32**:693–8.

43 Westerterp, K., Lafeber, H., Sulkers, E., Sauer, P. Comparison of short term indirect calorimetry and doubly labeled water method for the assessment of energy expenditure in preterm infants. *Biol. Neonate* 1991;**60**:75–82.

44 Leitch, C. A., Ahlrichs, J. A., Karn, C. A., Denne, S. C. Energy expenditure and energy intake during dexamethasone therapy for chronic lung disease. *Pediatr. Res.* 1999;**46**:109–13.

30

Gastrointestinal reflux

Sudarshan Rao Jadcherla

Section of Neonatology, Columbus Children's Hospital, and Department of Pediatrics, The Ohio State University School of Medicine and Public Health, Columbus, OH

Gastrointestinal reflux (GIR) is a common problem in high-risk neonates and young infants, and is due to the retrograde flow of gastrointestinal contents from distal bowel into the more proximal region. This includes (1) duodeno-gastric reflux (DGR) when duodenal contents move into the stomach; (2) duodeno-gastroesophageal reflux (DGER) when duodenal and gastric contents move into the esophagus; and (3) the more common and well studied, gastroesophageal reflux (GER) when gastric contents reflux into the esophagus or supra-esophageal structures. The symptoms of the disease resulting from GIR in neonates and infants are protean. There are many excellent reviews on GER in adults and children.[1–8] There is considerable lack of information on GIR in neonates or high-risk infants. In this chapter we will discuss the three entities of GIR, specifically the applied physiology, pathology, clinical presentation, and available treatment options pertinent to young infants.

Significance of GIR

Gastric emptying, duodenal clearance and intestinal transit in healthy neonates are aboral, despite feeding frequently, suggesting that DGR and DGER are uncommon. However, both these conditions can occur in ill infants. On the other hand, GER is more common in neonates and young infants, and can be physiological if the infant is thriving well and has absence of symptoms inducible by gastric contents. Variable forms of GER, manifesting as regurgitation with movement of gastric contents into the mouth, can occur two or more times a day in nearly 50% of 2-month-old infants, but it occurs in only 1% of 1-year-old infants, thus indicating that regurgitation usually has spontaneous resolution and

that changes in dietary habits may alter its course.[9] In a recent study, GER with symptoms of disease was noted in 3–10% of infants who were born prematurely and weighed less than 1500 g.[10] In another study, over 90% of older children with gastroesophageal reflux disease were noted to have had emesis as one of their major symptoms before 6 weeks of age.[11] As the survival of premature and high-risk infants is increasing, so is the morbidity.[12] There are differences in incidence and prevalence of GIR among neonates from various studies, which may be related to an improvement in survival and therefore an increase in comorbidity factors.

Premature and stressed infants are at increased risk of GER, as are those that have chronic lung disease or congenital anomalies. The reasons for this increased association in neonates is unclear, but may be related to the tone of the abdominal wall muscles, diaphragmatic activity, esophageal dysmotility and tonicity of the lower esophageal sphincter (LES). Factors that create a common cavity between stomach and esophagus facilitate retrograde movement of refluxate. Similarly, an increase in intragastric pressure during relaxation of the LES favors the occurrence of GER.

Applied physiology related to GIR in the fetus, neonate, and young infant

Fetal swallowing of amniotic fluid begins by 11 weeks, sucking movements by 18–20 weeks, and by full-term gestation the fetus can swallow and circulate nearly 500 ml of amniotic fluid.[13,14] Thus, swallow-induced primary esophageal peristalsis occurs during fetal life.

Neonatal Nutrition and Metabolism. Second Edition, ed. P. Thureen and W. Hay. Published by Cambridge University Press.
© Cambridge University Press 2006.

Functional anatomy and physiology of swallowing and esophageal motility are well described.[15] Contrary to popular belief, anatomical LES does not exist, with gross and histological exam failing to identify a sphincter.[16] Electron microscopy studies show irregular muscle cell layers which have tonic activity. Electrophysiological studies show continuous electric spike activity and specialized calcium channel transport.[17] Endoscopically, in neonates the squamo-columnar junction differentiates boundaries at the Z-line.[18] Although LES is considered as an important functional segment in preventing GER, other neighboring structures including oblique sling fibers of the stomach, musculofacial diaphragmatic sling and intra-abdominal esophagus also contribute to prevention of GER.[16] Thus, it is conceivable that disorders of the foregut and abdominal wall defects may make GIR more apparent.

Similarly, congenital anomalies in the duodenum or jejunum, malrotation, acquired inflammatory conditions such as necrotizing enterocolitis, or functional or mechanical bowel obstruction can inhibit aboral peristalsis. In such conditions, DGER and gastric distension exist.

Pathophysiology of GIR

Variations in esophageal body and LES pressure characteristics are best determined by esophageal manometry. It was found that LES pressure rose from 3.8 mmHg in premature infants (<29 weeks' gestation) to 18.1 mmHg in term infants.[19,20] It was also found that premature infants (33–38 weeks', postconceptual age) have esophageal peristaltic motor patterns less frequently than nonperistaltic motor patterns in the esophagus.[21,22] In the latter study, GER mechanisms in premature infants were characterized, and swallow-unrelated transient lower esophageal sphincter relaxation (TLESR) lasted for a mean period of 15 seconds and had significantly low mean nadir pressures of 0.8 mm Hg in 82% of the episodes. Four possible mechanisms of GER were observed in neonates: (1) spontaneous transient LES relaxation; (2) transient LES relaxation after esophageal body contraction; (3) multiple swallows associated with LES relaxation; and (4) peristaltic failure associated with LES relaxation.

Other factors such as increased intra-abdominal pressure, excessive crying, delayed gastric emptying, and sluggish esophageal motility have been associated with GER.[7,19]

Although not systematically studied in neonates and young infants, the nature of the refluxed material may also contribute to pathogenesis. The refluxed material may be acidic from gastric acid, alkaline from biliary and pancreatic juices derived from DGER, neutral from milk feeds, or by gas reflux from simple air distension. Gastric pepsins and pancreatic trypsins may also disrupt mucosal integrity by virtue of their proteolytic nature, but their role in neonates is not completely understood.

Gastric acidity varies with feeding regimens, and may be a primary factor in inducing esophagitis, which may further aggravate reflux.[5] However, during regurgitation air from the stomach may distend the esophagus and cause symptoms reflexively. Although acid reflux has been considered the gold standard in the diagnosis and pathology of GER, non-acid or gas reflux episodes are underestimated in this thought process. Infantile reflux has been considered physiological to some extent.[10] The changes in reflux frequency per day and the proportion of time the distal esophageal pH is less than 4 vary during development.[5,23] Reflux frequency is high during the neonatal period and infancy, and the total reflux time, an indicator of acid clearance, is much greater in infants than adults. This suggests that acid clearance mechanisms are less in infants than adults, though little is known about defense mechanisms against GER in neonates and infants.

Esophageal and airway defense mechanisms against GIR in young infants are not completely understood. Thach and Menon have identified the presence of a laryngeal chemoreflex in infants with GER, in which there is an occurrence of reflexive apnea with reflux. This apnea may be protecting the airway against aspiration.[24] Recently Wenzl *et al.* found an association of apnea and nonacid gastroesophageal reflux in infants using the technique of intraluminal impedance measurement.[25] In this study, out of 49 apneic episodes that were associated with gastroesophageal reflux, only 22.4% showed acid reflux with pH < 4, while the rest were nonacid events that could be gas or alkaline or neutral pH materials.

With the use of upper esophageal sphincter (UES) sleeve manometry technique in neonates, we characterized the esophageal motor defense mechanisms against abruptly induced esophageal distension or acidification.[26] In this study, we observed one of the three responses to esophageal stimulation: (1) occurrence of esophageal peristalsis unrelated to a swallow (secondary esophageal peristalsis); (2) increase in UES pressure; (esophago-UES contractile reflex); and (3) occurrence of a swallow-induced primary esophageal peristalsis (esophago-deglutition response). These motor events may be considered as protecting the esophagus and the airway. Similarly, during spontaneous GER events, all three mechanisms are evident, as shown in Figures 30.1 and 30.2.

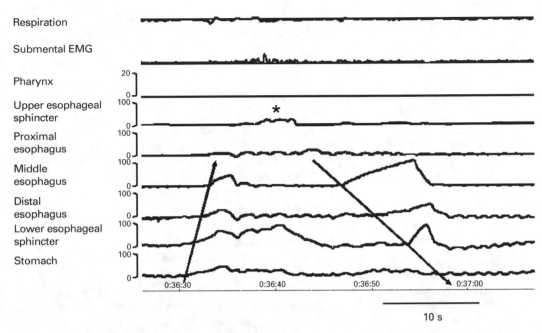

Figure 30.1. This figure illustrates an esophageal manometry recording identifying a reflux event depicted by the upward arrow. In response to this event, the upper esophageal sphincter pressure increased (*) and was followed by swallow independent secondary peristalsis (downward arrow). The latter two mechanisms may facilitate esophageal protection and clearance.

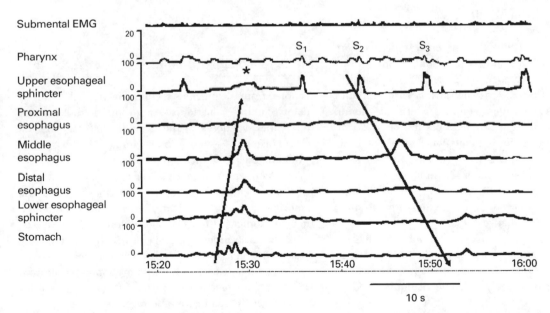

Figure 30.2. This figure illustrates an esophageal manometry recording identifying a reflux event depicted by the upward arrow. In response to this event, the upper esophageal sphincter pressure increased (*) transiently, which was followed by multiple swallows S1, S2, S3. Note that each pharyngeal swallow is associated with upper esophageal sphincter relaxation; however only the S2 propagated distally (downward arrow). This is a swallow-dependent primary peristalsis, which is another mechanism for esophageal clearance.

Table 30.1. *Differences in evaluation of physiological v. pathological gastroesophageal reflux (GER)*

Physiological reflux "Happy Spitters"	Pathological reflux "Scrawny Screamers"
Weight gain adequate	Failure to thrive
Effortless regurgitation	Painful regurgitation, with crying/discomfort
Feeding well on oral feeds	Poor feeding, often need gavage feeds
Strong sucking skills	Poor sucking skills
Good swallowing skills	Poor swallow coordination
Emesis is usually milk curds or acid	Emesis is milk, acid, blood tinged, or bile
Normal activity and behavior	Developmental delay or immaturity
Neurologically normal	Abnormal neurological exam may be present
No respiratory disease	Respiratory disease may be present
Absence of apneas or bradycardias	Apneas and/or bradycardias may be present
Absence of anemia	Iron-deficiency anemia
Gastric emptying of feeds normal	Delayed gastric emptying (residuals)

Clinical presentation of GIR

As noted from the previous sections, clinical presentation may be directly related to gastrointestinal reflux, to the associated complications, or to sequelae. Clinical features directly resulting from GIR in neonates may vary from simple regurgitation to frequent vomiting after feeds. About 20% of normal infants regurgitate, but less than 2% of these may require diagnostic evaluation.[5,10] Some of these infants may be considered "happy spitters" who are usually asymptomatic except for episodes of small emesis, but who may also ruminate and thereby re-swallow the refluxed material. These infants gain weight appropriately, despite causing social inconvenience (Table 30.1).

More frequent GIR episodes can injure esophageal mucosa and perpetuate esophagitis, whether the origin of reflux is from stomach (acidic medium and proteolytic enzymes) or duodenum (alkaline medium, bile salts and proteolytic enzymes). In the absence of appropriate esophageal clearance, prolonged contact time may be associated with esophageal dysmotility, poor oral feeding patterns, irritability from esophagitis, and excessive crying, particularly during feeds ("scrawny screamers," Table 30.1).[27,28] In these infants, problems due to frequent emesis lead to nutrient deprivation and failure to thrive. Sometimes, blood loss in the emesis can be a cause for iron-deficiency anemia. These unpleasant experiences to the neonate may result in feeding difficulties.[28]

Apneas and bradycardias can occur in the neonate independently of GIR. However, an apneic response to the presence of noxious stimulus in the pharynx (due to refluxate) may be protective to the airway, thus preventing aspiration.[29,30] Presence of refluxate in the pharynx stimulates a swallow, thus clearing the pharynx.[31] However, some pathologic apneic events can be life-threatening. The association of GER and apnea is still controversial. The apneic events associated with GIR appear to be of an obstructive type, commonly suggesting an inadequate clearance mechanism.

Respiratory manifestations of GER can present as the following: (1) central apnea due to chemoreceptor stimulation; (2) obstructive apnea due to laryngospasm; (3) airway hyper-reactivity and increased airway resistance due to bronchospasm; (4) stridor; (5) narrowing of airways from plugging or reflex-mediated (vagal) constriction; (6) parenchymal lung disease or pneumonia due to chronic microaspiration or macroaspiration of refluxed material into the lungs; and (7) chronic lung disease. Neonates rarely cough when refluxate is in the esophagus or pharynx, thus lacking efficient airway clearance, and they adapt by swallowing more frequently (Figure 30.2).

Differential diagnosis of GIR

As noted from the previous section, diagnosis of GIR is by history, clinical evaluation, and appropriate studies. Other differential diagnoses in the neonate that may present with a history of emesis, apneas and respiratory illness should be excluded, including sepsis, metabolic diseases (disorders of amino acid metabolism, urea cycle defects, galactosemia, congenital adrenal hyperplasia), structural abnormalities of brain and foregut (intestinal malrotation, tracheo-esophageal fistulas), and diaphragmatic defects. Infectious gastrointestinal etiologies such as necrotizing enterocolitis, ileus, or gastroenteritis can present with emesis or increased gastric residuals, often containing bile from DGER. Nongastrointestinal syndromes such as sepsis, urinary tract sepsis, meningitis, and respiratory viral illnesses should be excluded. Formula intolerance can also present with emesis and irritability. Acute abdominal conditions such as volvulus, adhesions, intestinal obstruction, meconium ileus and Meckel's diverticulum can present with emesis and respiratory distress.

Table 30.2. *Investigations in the diagnosis of gastroesophageal reflux (GER)*

Method	Advantages	Disadvantages
pH probe study	Sensitive for acid reflux only. Reproducible (18–24 h study) comparative data available. Bedside test	Discomfort of probe. Not specific for DGER.* Nearly 60–90% of GER episodes in infants are non-acid (milk or gas)
Upper gastrointestinal fluoroscopy	Defines structural anatomy. Readily available	Very short duration of study. Risk of aspiration. Unsafe in infants with swallowing problems
Esophageal manometry study	Defines pathophysiological mechanism of GER. Evaluation of esophageal clearance and peristalsis. Evaluation of sphincter dynamics. Measure of esophageal length. Can be done at bedside.	Limited availability. Skilled personnel required
Technetium[99] scan (scintigraphy)	Determines gastric emptying	Not portable. Poor sensitivity
Endoscopy	Documents esophagitis. Permits biopsy	Anesthesia needed. Specialized procedure

* DGER = duodeno-gastroesophageal reflux.

Evaluation of GIR

Careful history and clinical evaluation ruling out conditions listed in the previous section is important. Bilious emesis or aspirates, DGR or DGER should be considered pathologic until proven otherwise, and must be evaluated for etiologies that may need urgent intervention. Specifically, diagnosis of acute medical and surgical problems may be reversible when intervened upon early.

Evaluation for GER can be considered after determining whether it is physiological or pathological. In general, infants with physiological GER are "happy spitters" who continue to feed well and gain weight, usually outgrow symptoms with maturation and do not have any complications. Infants with pathological GER are "scrawny screamers" who usually fail to feed well and therefore have poor weight gain; these infants are usually unhappy, irritable, fussy, and have associated complications related to GER.[28,32] The differences between these two entities are summarized in Table 30.1.

Investigations may be necessary to confirm clinical evidence supporting pathological GER, to understand the mechanism of GER, to detect consequences of GER, or to monitor disease progress and treatment efficacy. There are no tests currently available to detect DGER in infants. Multi intraluminal impedance measurement can identify episodes of reflux irrespective of the nature of pH; however, these studies are for research use at present.[25] Some investigations suitable for application in the neonatal period and infancy are listed in Table 30.2, and are further summarized below.

Esophageal pH study indications are well defined.[33,34,35] Accurate probe placement in the distal esophagus (at the level of right atrium or third thoracic vertebra) is a necessary precondition for the reliability of data to be interpreted, in addition to documenting symptom index. Well performed esophageal pH studies can provide the following data: (1) reflux frequency per 24 hour period; (2) reflux index, or the percentage of the day with esophageal pH less than 4; (3) mean duration per reflux episode; (4) number of episodes longer than 5 min; and (5) duration of the longest episode. The latter two pieces of information reflect esophageal clearance abilities.[5,36,37] Postprandial states, feeding period duration, type of feeds, and use of medications such as antacids, antibiotics, or prokinetics may affect the gastric pH and therefore may under- or overestimate reflux episodes.

Fluoroscopy studies, including videoswallow studies, esophageal fluoroscopy, or upper gastrointestinal barium swallow studies have been used to identify sucking and swallowing problems, anatomical detail, and the presence of reflux.[5,38] These studies record very brief events, run the risk of radiation and aspiration, and are not generally suitable in tube fed infants, neurologically abnormal infants, and those with airway disease.[39] Upper gastrointestinal series are useful in identifying structural abnormalities of the foregut.

Esophageal manometry studies permit evaluation of motility events, and their correlation with feeding state may help identify the pathophysiological mechanism of GER or esophageal clearance. Such studies can be valuable in tube-fed neonates and young infants with feeding problems. These studies can identify the characteristics of esophageal peristalsis, the velocity of propagation, the sphincter responses to swallow and reflux events, and the mechanism of GER. Although these studies can be done at the bedside, the biggest limitation is lack of skilled personnel and availability of specialized equipment.

Gastroduodenal manometry studies may help identify the motor patterns during fasting and fed states, and motor patterns in asphyxiated infants and formula-fed infants, some of which may be associated with delayed gastric emptying or feeding intolerance.[40,41]

Gastroesophageal scintigraphy helps in evaluation of gastric emptying and determining the presence of reflux or pulmonary aspiration. The technique uses technetium[99] sulfur colloid to document the movement of the tracer isotope. However, the sensitivity of this test is poor.[38]

Endoscopy permits direct visualization of esophageal mucosa, documentation of inflammation, and ability to obtain biopsy for histopathological analysis. Normal limits of morphometric criteria for esophagitis in infants have been determined.[27,41] This technique requires skilled personnel, anesthesia, and is of limited use for identification of complications of GER.

It is important to note that the "gold standard" esophageal pH probe study underestimates reflux by not considering the nonacid events. Furthermore, no single test can predict infants at risk for gastroesophageal reflux disease.

Management of GIR

Management of DGR or DGER is done by identifying the cause and then instituting appropriate medical or surgical treatment. Management approaches include gastric decompression, correction of fluid and electrolyte imbalance, supportive parenteral nutrition, and appropriate antibiotics when sepsis is suspected.

Management of GER in neonatal life and young infancy has no consensus among practitioners. This may stem from the fact that many GER events are physiological and usually resolve with normal maturation and growth. However, infants with pathological gastroesophageal reflux, as stated in Table 30.1, may need treatment and follow-up. There is no specific drug suitable for GER in neonates. Approaches to the management of symptom reduction or modifying complications of GER include: (1) non-pharmacological approaches; (2) pharmacological therapy; and (3) surgical treatment. These are summarized below.

Nonpharmacological approaches, based on principles of applied physiology

Identify and avoid factors that aggravate reflux

In neonates and high-risk infants, factors such as suctioning, chest physical therapy, and supine positioning have been associated with increased reflux episodes.[5,43] Medications such as xanthines and betamimetic agents, used commonly in neonates as respiratory stimulants, have side-effects such as increased LES relaxation and therefore result in more frequent reflux episodes. Thus, the use of these agents should be reviewed based on their need.

Posture

Supine posture, right lateral position, and infant car seat position (upright position in a car seat) can make reflux worse, while prone position with a 30° elevation and left lateral position are associated with fewer episodes of reflux.[35,43–46] Symptomatic infants in the nursery or neonatal intensive care unit are usually monitored, and therefore prone or left-lateral positioning is a reasonable option. However, both prone and left-lateral positioning are recognized risk factors for sudden infant death syndrome.[44]

Dietary changes and feeding strategies

Heacock *et al.* demonstrated that breast-fed neonates had shorter GER episodes than formula-fed neonates (3.0 v. 8.3 min/hour) as gastric emptying is faster; however the lower median esophageal pH for breast-fed neonates was significantly less than in formula-fed newborns (2.0 v. 2.5).[47] Changing the type of feeding may not alter GER. Premature infant formulas usually contain medium-chain triglycerides, and these have been shown to accelerate gastric emptying when compared with long-chain triglycerides.[48]

In the neonatal period, feeding increments are usually regulated cautiously based on tolerance. GER worsens after feeds, particularly with increasing volumes per feed, indicating that gastric distension and delay in gastric emptying make GER worse.[49,50] GER is also influenced by the osmolality of the feeds. GER episodes may be minimized with certain feeding strategies such as feeding more frequently but with lower volumes per feed, or minimizing the use of oral medications that are hyperosmolar.

Thickening agents

Thickening feeds using rice cereal, carob flour, or sodium alginate have been used for infants with varied success.[1,51,52] Their beneficial role in the neonatal period is not well known, although addition of rice cereal is being practiced in symptomatic neonates. Thickening agents may decrease the frequency of postprandial reflux episodes, but the duration of reflux remains prolonged, suggesting that esophageal clearance may be further delayed. Potential side effects of adding rice cereal may include constipation and postprandial cough.

Pharmacological approaches

No ideal pharmacological agent exists for the treatment of symptomatic GER in neonates or infants.[1] Available drugs fall into three broad categories: (1) prokinetics; (2) acid-suppression agents; and (3) acid-neutralizing agents. Side effects and lack of response are the main problems with use of these agents.

Prokinetic agents

These agents increase gastrointestinal motility by various mechanisms, including: (1) increasing cholinergic drive (e.g., bethanechol); (2) inhibiting dopamine receptors (e.g., metoclopramide); (3) stimulating serotoninergic receptors of the myenteric neurons to increase acetylcholine release (e.g., cisapride, which is no longer approved for use); and (4) stimulating motilin receptors (e.g., erythromycin). It must be recognized that GER may be caused by different pathogenetic mechanisms even though the symptoms may be common. Therefore, a particular drug that is efficacious in one individual may not be useful in another.

Side effects of prokinetic agents are many and preclude their use. Bethanechol increases salivary and bronchial secretions, and may contribute to bronchospasm. Therefore, side effects of this agent are not acceptable in the high-risk neonate with respiratory illness. Metoclopramide can cause deleterious side effects such as extrapyramidal symptoms, irritability, sedation, and exacerbation of feeding problems, and some of these side effects may be dose-dependent. Cisapride is no longer used because it has been associated with serious side effects such as prolongation of the QTc interval and life-threatening ventricular arrhythmias. It is important to recognize that most macrolide antibiotics and H2 blockers have been known to elevate plasma cisapride levels. Erythromycin, a macrolide antibiotic, has gastroprokinetic effects by its ability to act on motilin receptors; however, such effects are not found in very premature infants.[53] Erythromycin does not affect esophageal or LES motility, but may improve gastric emptying in selective cases.

Acid-reduction strategies

The indications for using an acid-reducing medication in neonates and young infants are not clear. In general, these agents may be used to try to prevent complications from GER such as esophagitis, in infants with possible reflux who have poor respiratory reserve, following surgical repair of the esophagus (as in esophageal atresia or tracheo-esophageal fistula), or in tracheostomized infants. H2 blockers act by inhibiting the H2-receptors, thus limiting the interaction of histamine-released from the

histamine secreting mast cells.[42] Proton pump inhibitors have been used in resistant cases of esophagitis that have been unresponsive to H2-blockers.[54] These agents act by irreversible inhibition of H^+K^+-ATPase in the parietal cell. However, adverse effects have been reported with these medications. The side effects of using H2-blockers include elevation of cisapride levels, bronchospasm, sinus node dysfunction, and dystonic reactions. Proton pump inhibitors have caused drug-induced hepatitis.[23,35,54] Acid suppressing agents minimize the acid protective immunity, and favor the overgrowth of bacteria. Furthermore, by decreasing the gastric pH, they affect the function of acid-dependent gastric and lingual lipases and pepsin.

Acid-neutralizing agents such as antacids may facilitate healing in the presence of esophagitis in older infants. They are not routinely used in neonates because of constipation (calcium and aluminum-containing antacids) or diarrhea (magnesium-containing antacids).

Surgical treatment

Operative management of surgical etiologies of DGER or DGR should be carefully considered. Surgical treatment often relieves symptoms in cases of structural abnormalities such as intestinal malrotation, duodenal atresia or stenosis, annular pancreas, and with acute surgical conditions such as bowel obstruction. However, there is no consensus about the indications for the type or timing of surgery for pathological GER in neonates or young infants. Surgery in pathological GER in neonates and young infants is often considered when conservative and medical therapy fails, and sequelae and complications from GER are worsening. Certain neonates and young infants, such as infants with structural foregut anomalies (esophageal atresia, tracheo-esophageal fistula), infants with chronic respiratory disease and proven aspiration, and infants who are unable to protect their airway, may benefit from fundoplication and/or gastrostomy.[55] However, there is a considerable risk from anterograde aspiration when swallowing function or esophageal motility are abnormal. There are two types of fundoplication commonly performed in the surgical practice: the Nissen fundoplication in which 360° wrapping of the fundus around the LES may maintain resistance to backward reflux, and the Thal procedure in which 270° wrapping of the fundus around LES is done to avoid obstruction to forward peristalsis.[54]

In summary, DGER and DGR are usually pathologic conditions. GER may be physiologic in asymptomatic neonates, and many infants outgrow this condition over time. However, many aspects of gastroesophageal reflux disease in neonates and young infants remain to be explored. Diagnostic and therapeutic availability is necessary in infants with gastroesophageal reflux disease.

REFERENCES

1   NASPGHAN medical position statement: Pediatric GE reflux clinical practice guidelines. *J. Pediatr. Gastroenterol. Nutr.* 2001; **32**(Suppl. 2):S1–31.

2   Hrabovsky, E. E., Mullett, M. D. Gastroesophageal reflux and the premature infant. *J. Pediatr. Surg.* 1986; **21**:583–7.

3   Kumar, Y. and Sarvananthan, R. Gastroesophageal reflux in children. *Clinical Evidence (Br. Med. J.)* 2000;**4**:217–23.

4   Novak, D. A. Gastroesophageal reflux in the preterm infant. *Clin. Perinatol.* 1996;**23**:305–20.

5   Orenstein, S. R. Gastroesophageal reflux. *Curr. Probl. Pediatr.* 1991;**21**:193–241.

6   Orenstein, S. R. Controversies in pediatric gastroesophageal reflux. *J. Pediatr. Gastroenterol. Nutr.* 1992;**14**:338–48.

7   Sondheimer, J. M. Gastroesophageal reflux: update on pathogenesis and diagnosis. *Pediatr. Clin. N. Am.* 1988; **35**:103–18.

8   Jadcherla, S. R. Gastroesophageal reflux in the neonate. *Clin. Perinatol.* 20022; **29**:135–58.

9   Kibel, M.A. Gastroesophageal reflux. In Gellis, S., ed. *Report of the Seventy-Sixth Ross Conference on Pediatric Research.* Columbus, OH: Ross Laboratories, 1979:39–42.

10 Orenstein, S. R. Infantile reflux: different from adult reflux. *Am. J. Med.* 1997; **103**(3S):114S–19S.

11 Herbst, J. J. *Textbook of Gastroenterology and Nutrition in Infancy.* 2nd edn. New York, NY: Ravens Press; 1989:803–813.

12 Hack, M., Horbar, J. D., Malloy, M. *et al.* Very low birth weight infants: outcomes of the NICHD Neonatal Network. *Pediatrics* 1991;**87**:587–97.

13 Sadler, T. W. Special embryology, respiratory system. *Langman's Medical Embryology.* 7th edn. New York, NY: Williams and Wilkins; 1995: Part II, 232–41.

14 Sadler, T. W. Special embryology, digestive system. *Langman's Medical Embryology.* 7th edn. New York, NY: Williams and Wilkins; 1995: Part II, 241–71.

15 Goyal, R. K. and Sivarao, D. V. Functional anatomy and physiology of swallowing and esophageal motility. In Castell, D. O., Richter, J. E., eds. *The Esophagus.* 3rd edn. Philadelphia, PA: Lippincott Williams and Wilkins; 1999:1–31.

16 Kumar, D. Gross morphology of the gastrointestinal tract. In Kumar, D., Wingate, D., eds. *An Illustrated Guide to Gastrointestinal Motility.* Churchill Livingstone, 2nd edn. 1993:3–9.

17 Gabella, G. Structure of smooth muscle. In Kumar, D., Wingate, D., edn. *An Illustrated Guide to Gastrointestinal Motility.* 2nd edn. Churchill Livingstone 1993:32–48.

18 Biller, J. A., Winter, H. S., Grand, R. J., Allred, E. N. Are endoscopic changes predictive of histologic esophagitis in children? *J. Pediatr.* 1983;**103**:215–18.

19 Newell, S. J., Booth, I. W., Morgan, M. E. I. *et al.* Gastroesophageal reflux in preterm infants. *Arch. Dis. Child.* 1989;**64**:780–6.

20 Newell, S. J., Sarkar, P. K., Durbin, G. M., Booth, I. W., McNeish, A. S. Maturation of the lower oesophageal sphincter in the preterm baby. *Gut* 1988;**29**:67–172.

21 Omari, T. I., Miki, K., Fraser, R. *et al.* Esophageal body and lower esophageal sphincter function in healthy premature infants. *Gastroenterology* 1995;**109**:1757–64.

22 Omari, T. I., Benninga, M. A., Haslam, R. R. *et al.* Lower esophageal sphincter position in premature infants cannot be correctly estimated with current formulas. *J. Pediatr.* 1999;**135**:522–5.

23 Orenstein, S. R., Kocoshis, S. A., Orenstein, D. M., Proujansky, R. Stridor and gastroesophageal reflux: diagnostic use of intraluminal esophageal acid perfusion (Bernstein Test). *Pediatr. Pulmonol.* 1987;**3**:420–4.

24 Thach, B., Menon, A. Pulmonary protective mechanisms in human infants. *Am. Rev. Respir. Dis.* 1985;**131**:S55–8

25 Wenzl, T. G., Schenke, S., Peschgens, T. *et al.* Association of apnea and nonacid gastroesophageal reflux in infants: investigations with the intraluminal impedance technique. *Pediatr. Pulmonol.* 2001;**31**:144–9.

26 Jadcherla, S. R., Shaker, R. Esophageal and upper esophageal sphincter motor function in babies. *Am. J. Med.* 2001;**111**(8A):64–8S.

27 Black, D. D., Haggit, R. C., Orenstein, S. R. *et al.* Esophagitis in infants: morphometric histologic diagnosis and correlation with measures of gastroesophageal reflux. *Gastroenterology* 1990;**98**:1408–13.

28 Hyman, P. E. Gastroesophageal reflux: one reason why babies won't eat. *J. Pediatr.* 1994;**125**:S103–10.

29 Thach, B., Menon, A. Pulmonary protective mechanisms in human infants. *Am. Rev. Respir. Dis.* 1985;**131**:S55–8.

30 Thach, B. Reflux associated apnea in infants: evidence for a laryngeal chemoreflex. *Am. J. Med.* 1997;**103**:120S–4S.

31 Menon, P., Schefft, G. L., Thach, B. T. Apnea associated with regurgitation in infants. *J. Pediatr.* 1985;**106**:625–30.

32 Spitzer, A. R., Boyle, J. T., Tuchman, D. N. *et al.* Awake apnea associated with gastroesophageal reflux: A specific clinical syndrome. *J. Pediatr.* 1984;**104**:200–5.

33 Colletti, R. B., Christie, D. L., Orenstein, S. R. Indications for pediatric esophageal pH monitoring. Statement of the North American Society for Pediatric Gastroenterology and Nutrition. *J. Pediatr. Gastroenterol. Nutr.* 1995;**21**:253–62.

34 Sondheimer, J. M. Continuous monitoring of distal esophageal pH: a diagnostic test for gastroesophageal reflux in infants. *J. Pediatr.* 1980;**96**:804–7.

35 Vandenplas, Y., Belli, D., Benhamou, P. H. *et al.* Current concepts and issues in the management of regurgitation of infants: a reappraisal. Management guidelines from a working party. *Acta Paediatrica* 1996;**85**:531–4.

36 Vandenplas, Y., Goyvaerts, H., Helven, R., Sacre, L. Gastroesophageal reflux, as measured by 24-hour pH monitoring, in 509 healthy infants screened for risk of sudden infant death syndrome. *Pediatrics* 1991;**88**:834–40.

37 Vandenplas, Y., Sacre-Smits, L. Continuous 24-hour esophageal pH monitoring in 285 symptomatic infants 0–15 months old. *J. Pediatr. Gastroenterol. Nutr.* 1987;**6**:220–4.

38 Orenstein, S. R., Klein, H. A., Rosenthal, M. S. Scintigraphic images for quantifying pediatric gastroesophageal reflux: a study of simultaneous scintigraphy and pH probe using multiplexed data and acid feedings. *J. Nucl. Med.* 1993;**34**:1228–34.

39 Splaingard, M. L., Hutchins, B., Sulton, L. D., Chaudhuri, G. Aspiration in rehabilitation patients: videofluoroscopy vs bedside clinical assessment. *Arch. Phys. Med. Rehabil.* 1988;**69**:637–40.

40 Berseth, C. L., McCoy, H. H. Birth asphyxia alters neonatal intestinal motility in term neonates. *Pediatrics* 1992;**90**:669–73.

41 Jadcherla, S. R. and Berseth, C. L. Acute and chronic intestinal motor activity responses to two infant formulas. *Pediatrics* 1995;**96**:331–5.

42 Kuusela, A. L., Ruuska, T., Karikoski, R. *et al.* A randomized, controlled study of prophylactic ranitidine in preventing stress-induced gastric mucosal lesions in neonatal intensive care unit patients. *Crit. Care Med.* 1997;**25**:346–51.

43 Orenstein, S. R., Whitington, P. F. Positioning for prevention of infant gastroesophageal reflux. *J. Pediatr.* 1983;**103**:534–7.

44 Dwyer, T., Ponsonby, A. B., Newman, N. M. *et al.* Prospective cohort study of prone sleeping position and SIDS. *Lancet* 1991;**337**:1244–7.

45 Ewer, A. K., James, M. E., Tobin, J. M. Prone and left lateral positioning reduce gastroesophageal reflux in preterm infants. *Arch. Dis. Child Fetal Neonatal Edn.* 1999;**81**:F201–5.

46 Tobin, J. M., McCloud, P., Cameron, D. J. S. Posture and gastroesophageal reflux: a case for left lateral positioning. *Arch. Dis. Child.* 1997;**76**:254–8.

47 Heacock, H. J., Jefrey, H. E., Baker, J. L., and Page, M. Influence of breast versus formula milk on physiological gastroesophageal reflux in healthy, newborn infants. *J. Pediatr. Gastroenterol. Nutr.* 1992;**14**:41–6.

48 Sutphen, J. L., Dillard, V. L. Medium chain triglyceride in the therapy of gastroesophageal reflux. *J. Pediatr. Gastroenterol. Nutr.* 1992;**14**:38–40.

49 Sutphen, J. L., Dillard, V. L. Dietary caloric density and osmolality influence gastroesophageal reflux in infants. *Gastroenterology* 1989;**97**:601–4.

50 Sutphen, J. L., Dillard, V. L. Effect of feeding volume on gastroesophageal reflux in infants. *J. Pediatr. Gastroenterol. Nutr.* 1988;**7**:185–8.

51 Aggett, P. J., Agostoni, C., Goulet, O. *et al.* Medical Position Statement: Antireflux or antiregurgitation milk products for infants and young children: A commentary by the ESPGHAN committee on nutrition. *J. Pediatr. Gastroenterol. Nutr.* 2002;**34**:496–8.

52 Orenstein, S. R., Magill, H. L., Brooks, P. Thickening of infant feedings for therapy of gastroesophageal reflux. *J. Pediatr.* 1987;**110**:181–6.

53 Jadcherla, S. R., Berseth, C. L. Effect of erythromycin on gastroduodenal contractile activity in developing neonates. *J. Ped. Gastroenterol. Nutr.* 2002;**34**:16–22.

54 Gunasekharan, T. S., Hassall, E. G. Efficacy and safety of omeprazole for severe gastroesophageal reflux in children. *J. Pediatr.* 1993;**123**:148–54.

55 Nakayama, D.K. Esophageal atresia and tracheoesophageal fistula. In Nakayama, D. K., Bose, C. L., Chescheir, N. C., Valley, R. D., eds. *Critical Care of the Surgical Newborn.* Futura Publishing; 1996:227–49.

31

Hypo- and hyperglycemia and other carbohydrate metabolism disorders

Jane E. McGowan

Division of Neonatology, The Johns Hopkins Hospital, Baltimore, MD

Disorders of glucose homeostasis

The presence of neonatal hypoglycemia or hyperglycemia signals a failure of the normal transition from fetal to post-natal patterns of glucose homeostasis. Under normal conditions, glucose from maternal circulation is transported across the placenta via specific glucose transporters to be used by the fetus. The high fetal insulin : glucagon ratio suppresses glycogenolysis and gluconeogenesis and stimulates hepatic glycogen deposition during late gestation.

At delivery, glucose delivery to the infant stops abruptly. Until an exogenous supply of substrate is provided, the infant must rely on hepatic glucose production to meet metabolic needs. Both glycogenolysis and gluconeogenesis contribute to glucose homeostasis during the first few days of extrauterine life. However, hepatic glucose production via these two pathways requires availability of glycogen and gluconeogenic precursors, appropriate levels and activity of hepatic enzymes necessary for glycogenolysis and gluconeogenesis, and a normal endocrine response. The absence of any of these components may result in neonatal hypoglycemia or hyperglycemia.

Hypoglycemia

Incidence and clinical presentation

The reported incidence of neonatal hypoglycemia varies depending on the population studied, the method used for glucose measurement, and the definition of hypoglycemia used. In appropriate-for-gestational-age (AGA) term infants the incidence ranges from 5%–30%,[1–4] but may be as high as 50% in preterm infants,[5,6] and 70% in small-for-gestational-age (SGA) infants.[7–10] Clinical signs of hypoglycemia are nonspecific and may include lethargy, jitteriness, poor feeding, seizures, and temperature disturbances. The frequency of observation of the most common findings is listed in Table 31.1. However, most newborns with hypoglycemia are asymptomatic and are detected during routine screening.

Identifying infants with hypoglycemia

Many nurseries screen infants at risk for hypoglycemia by measuring blood glucose levels according to a pre-established protocol. Three important issues must be resolved in order for such a protocol to be successful. The first is identifying the high-risk newborn. In addition to preterm and SGA infants, other high-risk groups include infants of diabetic mothers (IDMs)[11–13] and other macrosomic infants.[8,14] Screening protocols should also take into account the time of initial presentation of hypoglycemia in various populations; for example, macrosomic infants rarely present with hypoglycemia beyond the first 8 hours of age, while the SGA infant or the IDM may not manifest hypoglycemia until the second or third postnatal day.[8,15].

The second issue is the choice of method for measuring glucose concentrations. Although laboratory enzymatic assays remain the "gold standard," these are not practical for use in screening protocols. Instead, rapid measurement methods using a quantitative analyzer in combination with a reagent test strip are commonly used. Results obtained using these methods are subject to technical inconsistencies that may significantly affect results. Screening with

Neonatal Nutrition and Metabolism. Second Edition, ed. P. Thureen and W. Hay. Published by Cambridge University Press.
© Cambridge University Press 2006.

Table 31.1. Frequency of occurrence of signs of neonatal hypoglycemia

Sign	Frequency
Seizures	47%
Apnea	27%
Hypotonia	27%
Tremors/jitteriness	26%
Cyanosis	18%
Irregular respirations	16%
Diaphoresis	11%
Poor feeding	11%
Irritability	5%

Adapted with permission.[65]

reagent strips is estimated to detect approximately 85% of cases of hypoglycemia; conversely, the false positive rate may be as high as 25%.[16–18]

Defining the blood glucose concentration that corresponds to neonatal hypoglycemia is the third, and still unresolved, issue. Early studies reported the presence of symptomatic hypoglycemia at a blood glucose concentration of <1 mmol L^{-1} (20 mg dL^{-1}) in preterm and <1.7 mmol L^{-1} (30 mg dL^{-1}) in term infants.[19] A review of the current literature suggests that 2.2–2.5 mmol L^{-1} (40–45 mg dL^{-1}) is commonly used as the lower limit of normal blood glucose concentrations during the first 72 hours of life. However, surveys in the UK demonstrated a continuing lack of consensus among practitioners as to the definition of hypoglycemia, with reported values ranging from <1 mmol L^{-1} (20 mg dL^{-1}) to <4 mmol L^{-1} (70 mg dL^{-1}).[20,21] A review of relevant publications confirms the results of these surveys, as the definitions of hypoglycemia used range from 1.1–2.6 mmol L^{-1} (20–48 mg dL^{-1}).[14,22,23]

Neither the minimum blood glucose concentration necessary for optimal brain function nor the concentration below which irreversible neuronal injury occurs has been established in the newborn. From a physiologic standpoint, hypoglycemia occurs when glucose supply is inadequate to meet energy demand. Unfortunately, there is no currently available method to establish this value in a given infant. Most often a statistical definition of hypoglycemia is used, meaning a blood glucose concentration >2 standard deviations below the mean value for a specific population. Such definitions have only limited physiologic significance, since such data reflect characteristics of the population, timing of first feeding, and adequacy of thermoregulation more than the presence of physiologic disturbances. Hypoglycemia may also be defined clinically, either as the glucose concentration associated with onset of clinical signs that resolve upon administration of glucose or, alternatively, the glucose concentration associated with longterm clinical consequences. However, it may be difficult to determine when symptoms first develop, and there is a general impression among clinicians that symptomatic hypoglycemia is associated with poor outcomes.

Evaluation of the overall metabolic and physiologic status of the infant in combination with the measured blood glucose concentration is essential in deciding when further investigation and/or intervention are required.[24,25] Using this premise, infants with increased demand or limited capability to alter glucose production rates may be considered at increased risk for impaired organ function at low blood glucose levels. In contrast, breast-fed infants may have normal energy metabolism even in the presence of "hypoglycemic" blood glucose values due to higher ketone levels. To date, there have been no systematic studies that establish the risks or benefits of using any one blood glucose value as the definition of "neonatal hypoglycemia" or an absolute indication for specific therapy in any newborn population.

Etiology of neonatal hypoglycemia

The etiologies of altered glucose metabolism in the newborn reflect the complex interactions between endocrine function, substrate availability, and metabolic activity. Neonatal hypoglycemia occurs via two basic mechanisms: normal metabolic demand for glucose in the presence of decreased substrate availability, or normal substrate availability in the presence of metabolic demand that exceeds the infant's capacity to compensate. Under some circumstances both of these mechanisms may contribute to hypoglycemia. The most common causes of neonatal hypoglycemia are listed in Table 31.2.

Preterm infants and infants with intrauterine growth retardation are the two largest populations of neonates at increased risk for hypoglycemia due to inadequate substrate availability. Preterm infants have not yet acquired the glycogen and fat stores that normally accumulate during the latter part of the third trimester in human pregnancy. Therefore, they have only a limited ability to release glucose from the liver via glycogenolysis or to produce gluconeogenic precursors via lipolysis. Activity of glucose-6 phosphatase, the enzyme required for the terminal steps of both glycogenolysis and gluconeogenesis (Figure 31.1), is also low in preterm infants. Hepatic glucose production may remain low for weeks to months after preterm birth, increasing the risk for episodes of hypoglycemia during periods of metabolic stress.[26]

Table 31.2. Common causes of neonatal hypoglycemia

Age at presentation	Differential diagnosis	Duration of hypoglycemia
Early (0–7 days)	IDM	Transient
	SGA	Transient
	Sepsis	Transient
	Endocrine disorders	Persistent
	Hypopituitarism	
	Adrenal insufficiency	
	Hyperinsulinism	Persistent
	Inborn errors of metabolism	Persistent
	Electron transport chain defects	
	Glycogen storage disease	
	Deficiencies of Krebs cycle enzymes	
Late (7–28 days)	Sepsis	Transient
	Malnutrition	Transient
	Endocrine disorders	Persistent
	Hyperinsulinism	Persistent
	Inborn errors of metabolism	Persistent
	Toxins	Transient
	Ethanol	
	Salicylates	
	Propranolol	

IDM, infant of diabetic mother; SGA, small-for-gestational-age.

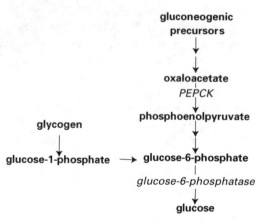

Figure 31.1. Metabolic pathways of glycogenolysis and gluconeogenesis, demonstrating the role of glucose-6-phosphatase in endogenous glucose production. PEPCK: phosphoenolpyruvate carboxykinase.

Infants with intrauterine growth retardation (IUGR) on the basis of placental insufficiency also have decreased glycogen and fat stores. IUGR infants may also have altered rates of glucose metabolism and/or insulin sensitivity.[27,28] As a result, hypoglycemia may persist beyond the first 72 h of life in up to 10% of IUGR infants in spite of adequate carbohydrate intake.[9] Inadequate substrate availability may also result from disorders that impair the infant's ability to use available substrate, such as glycogen storage disease Type I and other inborn errors of metabolism (see below and Table 31.2).

Hypoglycemia due to hyperinsulinemia

Hyperinsulinemia increases metabolic demand due to an insulin-induced increase in cellular glucose uptake and decreases endogenous glucose production by inhibiting glycogenolysis and gluconeogenesis.[29,30] Thus newborns with hyperinsulinemia are at high risk for severe hypoglycemia.

Transient hyperinsulinemia

Infants of diabetic mothers constitute the largest group of newborns at risk for hypoglycemia due to a transient increase in circulating insulin levels. During a diabetic pregnancy, the fetus may be exposed to episodes of maternal hyperglycemia with subsequent fetal hyperglycemia and increased fetal insulin production. Other diabetes-induced alterations in maternal metabolism, such as changes in serum amino acids, may also play a role. After delivery, hyperinsulinemia persists, inhibiting hepatic glucose production in the immediate postnatal period. IDMs also have an exaggerated pancreatic insulin response to a glucose load compared with non-IDMs.[31] Up to 50% of infants of diabetic mothers will have at least one low glucose value in the first 3 postnatal days,[11,32,33] with macrosomic infants at the highest risk. In most cases, the pancreatic insulin response normalizes over the first 24–72 hours of life.

Transient hyperinsulinemia may also result from non-metabolic causes. Infants with erythroblastosis fetalis have increased levels of insulin and an increase in pancreatic beta cell number.[34] Hyperinsulinemia may result from inactivation of circulating insulin by glutathione released from hemolyzed erythrocytes.[35] Exchange transfusions may exacerbate the problem because the high levels of dextrose used as a preservative in blood products stimulate more insulin release.[34,36] Use of beta-sympathomimetic tocolytic agents has been associated with hyperinsulinemia in the newborn, especially if the agent was used for more than 2 weeks and was discontinued less than 1 week prior to delivery.[37,38] Infants with Beckwith–Weidemann syndrome may also present with hypoglycemia due to increased pancreatic insulin production, but in most infants this resolves during the first week of life.[39] Mutations associated with Beckwith–Weidemann syndrome have been identified in the same region of chromosome 11p as those associated with idiopathic hyperinsulinemic hypoglycemia.[40,41]

Hyperinsulinemic hypoglycemia

Primary hyperinsulinemic hypoglycemia (HIHG, i.e., hyperinsulinemia not secondary to another disorder), is the most common cause of neonatal hypoglycemia persisting beyond the first week of life. These infants are often macrosomic and have frequent, severe episodes of symptomatic hypoglycemia. While 50% of infants present with neonatal seizures, 10%–25% of cases are diagnosed by routine neonatal screening.[42–44]

Normal insulin secretion is regulated by an ATP-sensitive potassium channel (K_{ATP} channel) that maintains the cell membrane potential (Figure 31.2). Closure of the K_{ATP} channel leads to insulin release, and abnormal function of the K_{ATP} channel may result in inappropriate release of insulin. Most cases of HIHG in infants and children are associated with one of several mutations that alter regulation of insulin secretion by the pancreatic β-cells.[45,46] Abnormal imprinting, with loss of maternal 11p gene expression and hemizygosity or uniparental disomy of a mutated paternal gene, may also result in neonatal hyperinsulinemia due to focal regions of abnormal beta cells with consequent hypoglycemia.[43,47] Two other metabolic abnormalities resulting from gene mutations, both with

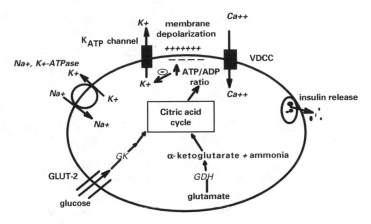

Figure 31.2. Schematic of mechanism of beta-cell insulin release. An increase in the ATP/ADP ratio leads to closure of the K_{ATP} channel, increase in intracellular calcium, and release of insulin via exocytosis. VDCC, voltage-dependent calcium channel; GK, glucokinase; GLUT-2: glucose transporter type 2; GDH: glutamate dehydrogenase.

autosomal dominant inheritance, are also associated with HIHG. Mutations in the gene for glucokinase, one of the enzymes in the pathway from glucose to pyruvate, result in levels of glucokinase activity that are inappropriately high for the intracellular glucose level, and also lead to excess release of insulin.[48] Mutations in the glutamate dehydrogenase gene are associated with leucine-sensitive hypoglycemia and mild to moderate hyperammonemia.[49,50]

Increased metabolic demand

Increased demand that exceeds the available substrate supply may occur in any neonate, including full-term AGA infants as well as preterm and SGA infants. The incidence of hypoglycemia is increased after perinatal asphyxia due to the rapid depletion of substrate supplies during the period of anaerobic metabolism. Hypoxic-ischemic damage to the liver may further impair hepatic glucose production. Transient hyperinsulinemia has also been reported after perinatal asphyxia.[51] Other conditions in the neonate that may lead to a shift from aerobic to anaerobic metabolism include hypotension, severe lung disease with hypoxemia and hypoventilation, and septic shock.

Hypothermia also leads to depletion of substrate due to rapid lipolysis of brown fat stores for thermogenesis and exhaustion of glycogen stores. It commonly occurs after out-of-hospital deliveries, but milder degrees may occur in the delivery room. Absence of adequate facilities for newborn care may contribute to the increased incidence of hypothermia and hypoglycemia observed in developing

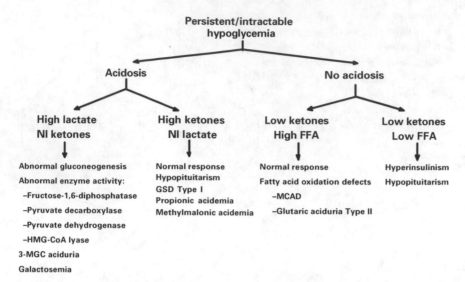

Figure 31.3. Decision tree for identifying causes of persistent or intractable hypoglycemia. FFA, free fatty acids; HMG, 3-hydroxy-3-methyglutaryl; MGC, methylglutaconic; GSD, glycogen storage disease; MCAD, medium-chain acyl-CoA dehydrogenase.

Table 31.3. Drugs associated with neonatal hypoglycemia

In utero exposure
Ritodrine
Valproate
Labetolol
Chlorpropamide
Neonatal exposure
Indomethacin
Gancyclovir

countries.[52] Hypoglycemia observed in infants with sepsis may be due to the presence of circulating endotoxins, which can increase the rate of glycolysis.[53]

Unusual causes of hypoglycemia

Although uncommon, several other etiologies must be considered in the differential diagnosis of the newborn with hypoglycemia, particularly when there is no previously identified cause. In addition to ritodrine, in utero or postnatal exposure to a number of drugs may be associated with neonatal hypoglycemia (Table 31.3). Global endocrine disturbances, including abnormalities of the hypothalamic-pituitary axis, adrenal failure, and primary hypothyroidism, are also associated with persistent neonatal hypoglycemia. Neonatal hypoglycemia may also be one of the early manifestations of an inborn error of metabolism, including defects of fatty acid oxidation, gluconeogenesis or mitochondrial function, disorders of amino acid metabolism, and some organic acidurias. Accompanying metabolic findings may be useful in identifying the specific metabolic disorder in infants presenting with persistent or intractable hypoglycemia (Figure 31.3).

Physiologic response to hypoglycemia and effects on the brain

In adults and older children, a decrease in blood glucose concentration triggers a counter-regulatory response characterized by release of catecholamines and increased cortisol, growth hormone, and glucagon levels that stimulate glycogenolysis and production of gluconeogenic substrates. However, newborns and young children have a diminished response to hypoglycemia. Increased cortisol levels have been reported in some hypoglycemic newborns.[54,55] However, growth hormone release in response to spontaneous hypoglycemia is less in children than in adults even in the absence of pituitary dysfunction or growth hormone deficiency.[56] The ability of the neonate to increase levels of ketones, free fatty acids, and lactate in response to hypoglycemia is also limited, particularly in preterm and SGA infants (Figure 31.4).[54,57,58] However, the extraction coefficient for ketones by brain tissue is highest in the newborn period.[59] Breast-feeding is associated with higher ketone levels; thus, breast-fed infants are able to meet energy requirements in spite of lower blood glucose values. In contrast, use of infant formulas may decrease ketogenesis, even in breast-fed infants.[58]

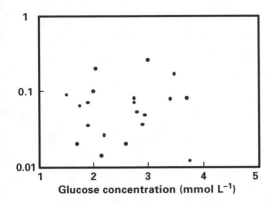

Figure 31.4. Lack of correlation between blood glucose concentration and levels of ketone bodies present in small-for-gestational-age infants. Adapted with permission.[43]

Cerebral glucose utilization accounts for as much as 90% of total glucose consumption in the newborn. In animal models, glucose deprivation induces widespread changes in brain function, including alterations in oxidative phosphorylation, amino acid metabolism, protein synthesis, neurotransmitter release, and transmembrane ion gradients.[60–64] Increases in cerebral blood flow have been reported in animal models as well as in human infants.[65–67] Hypoglycemic coma is associated with selective neuronal necrosis affecting the cortex, caudate/putamen, and hippocampus; however, in animal models, pathologic changes have not been reported with less severe hypoglycemia.[68,69] Limited postmortem studies in newborn infants with severe hypoglycemia in the absence of any other conditions associated with brain injury have shown a similar pattern of injury;[70] in addition, hypoglycemic newborns appear to have significant white matter injury.[59]

Imaging studies posthypoglycemia demonstrate a pattern of regional involvement similar to that seen histopathologically. Magnetic resonance imaging studies in newborns several weeks after onset of symptomatic hypoglycemia have shown signal abnormalities in the parietal and occipital cortex, as well as white matter changes.[71,72] Kinnala et al.[73] found that although 40% of term newborns with symptomatic hypoglycemia had abnormalities on initial MRI, these findings had resolved at 2 months of age. However, no neurologic follow-up was performed on these infants. In contrast, several investigators have reported that hypoglycemic newborns had evidence of cerebral atrophy and white matter injury on follow-up imaging studies several months after exposure to symptomatic hypoglycemia.[71,74,75]

Investigators and clinicians have attempted to determine the long-term effects of neonatal hypoglycemia on cognition and behavior for more than 40 years. However, the degree to which hypoglycemia can alter neurodevelopmental outcomes has yet to be determined, as a randomized, controlled trial is not practical, and hypoglycemic newborns often have other risk factors for adverse neurologic outcomes. Early studies in infants with symptomatic hypoglycemia suggested that the incidence of seizures and developmental delay was increased compared with normoglycemic infants,[76,77] but the number of infants examined was small and no standardized assessments were performed. Several follow-up studies of full-term infants with asymptomatic transient hypoglycemia have failed to identify any long-term adverse neurologic effects.[22,78] Although Koh et al. recorded an abnormal brainstem auditory evoked response (BAER) in five hypoglycemic neonates,[79] Cowett et al. found no correlation between blood glucose concentrations and BAER results.[80]

Results of follow-up studies in high-risk populations suggest that under some circumstances asymptomatic hypoglycemia may contribute to abnormal developmental outcomes. A retrospective analysis of outcome in over 600 preterm infants evaluated at 18–24 months of age found that those who had a recorded blood glucose concentration < 2.6 mmol L^{-1} on at least 5 days as neonates had lower mental and motor development scores and an increased risk of cerebral palsy compared with those who had fewer episodes or a single more severe episode.[23] In preterm infants with IUGR, a history of six or more episodes of blood glucose < 2.6 mmol L^{-1} was associated with a smaller head circumference during the first 5 years of life. Perceptive performance and motricity score were decreased at 2.5 years of age even if only one episode of hypoglycemia was recorded, suggestive of results in children with attention deficit–hyperactivity disorder (ADHD).[7] Similarly, IDMs with a history of neonatal hypoglycemia (glucose < 1.5 mmol L^{-1}) had more deficits in attention, motor control, and perception at 8 years of age than IDMs with no documented hypoglycemia or non-IDM controls.[13] These studies are limited by the fact that a standardized protocol for drawing blood glucose concentrations was not used, and the subjects were not followed to determine whether the differences observed initially persisted beyond early childhood and/or were associated with problems with behavior or learning at school age. However, the association with ADHD is supported by data from Rhesus monkeys exposed to neonatal hypoglycemia for up to 10 h. When tested in late childhood, these animals demonstrated problems with adaptability and motivation, with behaviors similar to those characteristic of human children with ADHD.

The long-term neurologic consequences of severe, symptomatic hypoglycemia associated with HIHG have

Table 31.4. Drugs used in the management of hypoglycemia

Drug	Mechanism of action	Side effects	Comments
Glucagon	Stimulates glycogenolysis and gluconeogenesis	↓ Secretion of gastric and pancreatic enzymes	Increased dose needed in presence of hyperinsulinemia
Hydrocortisone	↓ Peripheral glucose uptake ↓ insulin sensitivity ↑ lipolysis	Hypertension ↓ growth ↓ immune function	–
Diazoxide	K_{ATP} channel opener ↓ insulin release ↑ gluconeogenesis	Fluid retention Hypotension Hypertrichosis	–
Somatostatin/ octreotide	Activates G-protein-coupled K^+ channel ↓insulin release	↓ GH/TSH/ACTH ↓ growth steatorrhea	May cause sludging or stone formation in gallbladder
Nifedipine	Ca^{++} channel blocker ↓ insulin release	Hypotension	Experimental therapy only

K_{ATP}, ATP-dependent potassium channel; GH, growth hormone; TSH, thyroid-stimulating hormone; ACTH, adrenocorticotrophic hormone.

been more clearly defined. Children with HIHG are at significantly increased risk for neurologic abnormalities, including seizure disorders and mental retardation; only about 50% have normal development.[43,81,82] A critical deficit in our knowledge of the effect of hypoglycemia on the developing brain is the lack of animal or human data demonstrating whether there is a threshold glucose concentration below which brain injury occurs, or whether there is a continuous relationship between the degree of brain injury/dysfunction and the blood glucose concentration. Similarly, no data are available to establish the optimal blood glucose concentration to maintain in high-risk infants. Taken as a whole, available data suggest that asymptomatic hypoglycemia may lead to subtle changes in brain function that could affect long-term cognitive performance. However, more rigorous follow-up of large cohorts of at-risk infants, as well as additional studies in newborn animal models, are needed before the specific effects can be confirmed.

Management of hypoglycemia

Once the decision has been made that intervention is necessary in a hypoglycemic infant, the immediate goal is to normalize the blood glucose as quickly as possible. Infants in whom the presumed cause is expected to resolve quickly may be managed with frequent oral feedings of formula or breast milk. Dextrose/water solutions should be avoided as their use may be associated with rebound hypoglycemia due to stimulation of insulin secretion. In symptomatic infants as well as those with severe hypoglycemia (blood glucose < 1.3 mmol L^{-1} (24 mg dL^{-1}), those unable to feed, and those who have failed a trial of feeding, parenteral therapy with 10% dextrose/water is indicated. Once the etiology of the hypoglycemia is determined, specific therapy should be initiated when available (e.g., antibiotics, dietary management for metabolic disorders). Pharmacologic management of hypoglycemia is generally necessary only for stabilization while awaiting transport and for the treatment of HIHG (Table 31.4).

Distinguishing among the different types of HIHG is important to the successful management of these infants, as individuals with the autosomal dominant forms have normal K_{ATP} channels, and thus are likely to respond to medical management, while most cases with mutations of the K_{ATP} channel require surgical management. In the latter group, differentiating between diffuse and focal forms of pancreatic beta-cell dysfunction is critical. The diffuse form of the disorder often requires near-complete pancreatectomy to prevent recurrent hypoglycemia, increasing the subsequent risk for glucose intolerance and diabetes. In contrast, focal lesions can be successfully managed with more limited pancreatic resection in most cases, preserving normal glucose homeostasis postoperatively.[81,83,84]

Hyperglycemia

Hyperglycemia (blood glucose concentration > 8.3 mmol L^{-1} (150 mg dL^{-1})) most commonly occurs in very low birth weight (VLBW) infants receiving dextrose-containing IV infusions, with an incidence of $> 50\%$ in infants < 800 g.[85]

Mechanisms contributing to glucose intolerance in VLBW infants include decreased insulin release in response to glucose[5,85] and failure of suppression of endogenous glucose production during IV glucose infusion.[86,87] Proteolysis due to negative nitrogen balance may also be a stimulus for glucose production. Although intravenous lipid emulsions have been implicated as a cause of hyperglycemia, this is unlikely to occur at commonly used infusion rates.[88] Hyperglycemia in the VLBW infant is typically transient and resolves within the first 2 weeks of life, as the endocrine response to stress and exogenous glucose matures and nitrogen balance improves.

Hyperglycemia may also occur due to neonatal diabetes. The incidence is estimated at 1 per 400 000 live births, with approximately 50%–70% of cases due to transient neonatal diabetes (TNDM).[89,90] TNDM is a transient, self-limiting form that occurs primarily in full-term infants with IUGR,[91] and appears to be due to a relative deficiency in pancreatic insulin release. Mutations on chromosome 6 have been reported in 75% of infants with TNDM.[92] The majority of cases are identified during routine screening for hypoglycemia. Permanent neonatal diabetes (PNDM) has a significantly later onset than TNDM, and only 25% of infants with PNDM have IUGR compared with >70% of TNDM.[91] PNDM is more likely to present with ketoacidosis and dehydration than TNDM, and requirements for insulin are higher. No chromosomal abnormality has been identified in PNDM infants, although familial cases have been reported.[92] Infants with TNDM typically have resolution of glucose intolerance by 3 years of age, but longitudinal follow-up studies suggest these children are at increased risk of recurrence of glucose intolerance in adolescence.[89,90,91]

The differential diagnosis of neonatal hyperglycemia also includes gram-negative and fungal sepsis.[93] Methyl xanthine use has been shown to inhibit glucose transporter activity and may lead to hyperglycemia after administration of either therapeutic doses or an overdose.[94]

The physiologic consequences of neonatal hyperglycemia are not clear. Concerns include the possibility of dehydration due to osmotic diuresis and increased risk of intraventricular hemorrhage due to acute changes in intravascular volume caused by changes in intravascular osmolarity. Neonatal diabetes may present as dehydration and poor weight gain post-hospital discharge, particularly if there is a delay in making the diagnosis. However, no clinical studies have demonstrated any adverse effects due to hyperglycemia in the range usually encountered in the first 2 weeks of life. Nor has an association between IVH and hyperglycemia been established. Hyperglycemia is associated with higher mortality rates[95] and an increased incidence of severe retinopathy of prematurity[96] in VLBW infants, but high glucose concentrations may serve as an indicator of severity of illness rather than as a specific cause of morbidity and mortality. Thus, management of neonatal hyperglycemia remains controversial due to the relatively low associated morbidity.

When blood glucose concentrations exceed an arbitrarily chosen acceptable value (ranging from 160–250 mg dL^{-1}, depending on unit-specific policies), management options include decreasing the rate of glucose administration or treating with a continuous insulin infusion. Use of insulin has been reported to improve weight gain and nitrogen balance;[97,98] however, insulin infusions may result in iatrogenic hypoglycemia, and infants may become resistant to insulin effects with prolonged infusion.[99] Limiting glucose administration significantly reduces caloric intake in hyperglycemic infants and may have a long-term impact on rate of weight gain.[85] Given the lack of evidence that moderate hyperglycemia has deleterious effects, the impaired weight gain may be considered an iatrogenic problem.

Other carbohydrates

Although glucose is the most prominent carbohydrate in neonatal metabolism, both lactose and fructose also play a role in neonatal energy metabolism. Lactose is the major carbohydrate source in breast milk and is also found in most infant formulas, while fructose is present in sucrose-containing infant formulas. Although intestinal lactase activity is low in the fetus, and gradually increases to adult levels after birth,[100] clinical lactose intolerance, manifested by diarrhea, vomiting, and poor weight gain, is uncommon in newborns. In newborns lacking sufficient lactase to completely digest dietary lactose, the undigested sugar is metabolized by colonic flora and absorbed in the large bowel.[100] Early exposure of preterm infants to enteral feedings of any volume induces an increase in intestinal lactase activity and further facilitates lactose tolerance.[101] Conversely, administration of parenteral antibiotics may induce transient lactose intolerance in both full-term and preterm infants by altering colonic flora.[102]

Galactosemia is the most important disorder of non-glucose carbohydrates in the newborn, and results from inability of the newborn to metabolize galactose, one of the two sugars that comprise lactose. Galactosemia presents with hypoglycemia, unconjugated hyperbilirubinemia, cataracts, and hepatic failure; there is also an increased incidence of neonatal sepsis with gram-negative organisms.[33] The incidence is estimated at 2–10 per 100 000 live births. Three forms have been described: "classic," or Type 1, galactosemia results from a mutation in the gene coding for the enzyme galactose-1-phosphate uridyltransferase; Type 2 galactosemia is due to a defect in galactokinase activity, and Type 3 galactosemia results from a mutation in the gene coding for UDP-galactose-4-epimerase.[103] All three forms are inherited in an autosomal recessive pattern. Most cases of galactosemia are detected by newborn screening programs that are in place throughout the USA as well as internationally.

Disorders of fructose metabolism rarely present in the newborn period due to limited neonatal fructose intake. However, newborns with fructose-1,6-diphosphatase deficiency may present with hypoglycemic coma or even sudden, unexplained death in the newborn period. Two other defects in fructose metabolism, hereditary fructose intolerance (fructose-1-phosphate aldolase deficiency) and fructokinase deficiency, are usually asymptomatic in the newborn period but may present later in life.

REFERENCES

1 Anderson, S., Shakya, K. N., Shrestha, L. N., Costello, A. M. Hypoglycaemia: a common problem among uncomplicated newborn infants in Nepal. *J. Trop. Pediatr.* 1993;**39**:273–7.

2 Cole, M. D., Peevy, K. Hypoglycemia in normal neonates appropriate for gestational age. *J. Perinatol.* 1994;**14**:118–20.

3 Lubchenco, L. O., Bard, H. Incidence of hypoglycemia in newborn infants classified by birth weight and gestational age. *Pediatrics* 1971;**47**:831–4.

4 Srinivasan, G., Pildes, R. S., Caughy, M., Voora, S., Lilien, L. D. Plasma glucose values in normal neonates: a new look. *J. Pediatr.* 1986;**109**:114–17.

5 Farrag, H. M., Cowett, R. M. Glucose homeostasis in the micropremie. *Clin. Perinatol.* 2000;**27**:1–22.

6 Zanardo, V., Cagdas, S., Golin, R. *et al.* Risk factors of hypoglycemia in premature infants. *Fetal Diagn. Ther.* 1999;**14**:63–7.

7 Duvanel, C. B., Fawer, C. L., Cotting, J., Hohlfield, P., Matthieu, J. M. Long-term effects of neonatal hypoglycemia on brain growth and psychomotor development in small-for-gestational age infants. *J. Pediatr.* 1999;**134**:492–8.

8 Holtrop, P. C. The frequency of hypoglycemia in full-term large and small for gestational age newborns. *Am. J. Perinatol.* 1993;**10**:150–4.

9 Pallotto, E. K., Woelnerhannssen, B., Macones, G. A., Simmons, R. A. Hypoglycemia in small-for-gestational-age infants: how extensive is the problem and what are the risks? *Pediatr. Res.* 2003;**53**:499A.

10 Yamaguchi, K., Mishina, J. Mitsuishi, C., Nakabayashi, M., Nishida, H. Neonatal hypoglycemia in infants with intrauterine growth retardation due to pregnancy-induced hypertension. *Acta Paediatr Jpn.* 1997;**39**:S48–50.

11 Agrawal, R. K., Lui, K., Gupta, J. M. Neonatal hypoglycaemia in infants of diabetic mothers. *J. Paediatr. Child Health* 2000;**36**:354–6.

12 Curet, L. B., Izquierdo, L. A., Gilson, G. J. *et al.* Relative effects of antepartum and intrapartum maternal blood glucose levels on incidence of neonatal hypoglycemia. *J. Perinatol.* 1997;**17**:113–15.

13 Stenninger, E., Flink, R., Eriksson, B., Sahlen, C. Long-term neurological dysfunction and neonatal hypoglycaemia after diabetic pregnancy. *Arch. Dis. Child Fetal Neonatal Edn.* 1998;**79**:F174–9.

14 Schaefer-Graf, U. M., Rossi, R., Buhrer, C. *et al.* Rate and risk factors of hypoglycemia in large-for-gestational-age newborn infants of nondiabetic mothers. *Am. J. Obstet. Gynecol.* 2002;**187**:913–17.

15 Cowett, R. M., Schwartz, R. The infant of the diabetic mother. *Pediatr. Clin. N. Am.* 1982;**29**:1213–31.

16 Schlebusch, H., Niesen, M., Sorger, M., Paffenholz, I., Fahnenstich, H. Blood glucose determinations in newborns: four instruments compared. *Pediatr. Pathol. Lab. Med.* 1998;**18**:41–8.

17 Giep, T. N., Hall, R. T., Harris, K., Barrick, B., Smith, S. Evaluation of neonatal whole blood versus plasma glucose concentration by ion-selective electrode technology and comparison with two whole blood chromogen test strip methods. *J. Perinatol.* 1996;**16**:244–9.

18 Maisels, M. J., Lee, C. Chemstrip glucose test strips: correlation with true glucose values less than 80 mg/dL. *Crit. Care Med.* 1983;**71**:457–9.

19 Cornblath, M., Odell, G. B., Levin, E. Y. Symptomatic neonatal hypoglycemia associated with toxemia of pregnancy. *J. Pediatr.* 1959;**55**:545–62.

20 Koh, T. H., Eyre, J. A., Aynsley-Green, A. Neonatal hypoglycaemia – the controversy regarding definition. *Arch. Dis. Child.* 1988;**63**:1386–8.

21 Koh, T. H., Vong, S. K. Definition of neonatal hypoglycaemia: is there a change? *J. Paediatr. Child Health* 1996;**32**:302–5.

22 Griffiths, A. D., Bryant, G. M. Assessment of effects of neonatal hypoglycaemia. *Arch. Dis. Child.* 1971;**46**:819–27.

23 Lucas, A., Morley, R., Cole, T. J. Adverse neurodevelopmental outcome of moderate neonatal hypoglycaemia. *Br. Med. J.* 1988;**297**:1304–8.

24 Cornblath, M., Hawdon, J. M., Williams, A. *et al.* Controversies regarding definition of neonatal hypoglycemia: suggested operational thresholds. *Pediatrics* 2000;**105**:1141–5.

25 Kalhan, S., Peter-Wohl, S. Hypoglycemia: what is it for the neonate? *Am. J. Perinatol.* 2000;**17**:11–18.

26 Hume, R., McGeechan, A., Burchell, A. Developmental disorders of glucose metabolism in infants. *Child Care Health Dev.* 2002;**28**:S45–47.

27 Kliegman, R. M. Alterations of fasting glucose and fat metabolism in intrauterine growth-retarded newborn dogs. *Am. J. Physiol.* 1989;**256**:E380–5.

28 Marconi, A. M., Daviani, E., Baggiani, A. M. *et al.* An evaluation of fetal glucogenesis in intrauterine growth-retarded pregnancies. *Metabolism* 1993;**42**:860–4.

29 Hawdon, J. M., Aynsley-Green, A., Bartlett, K., Ward Platt, M. P. The role of pancreatic insulin secretion in neonatal glucoregulation. II. Infants with disordered blood glucose homoeostasis. *Arch. Dis. Child.* 1993;**68**:280–5.

30 Ktorza, A., Bihoreau, M., Nurjhan, N., Picon, L., Girard, J. Insulin and glucagon during the perinatal period: secretion and metabolic effects on the liver. *Biol. Neonate* 1985;**48**:204–20.

31 Pribylova, J., Kozlova, J. Glucose and galactose infusions in newborns of diabetic and healthy mothers. *Biol. Neonate* 1979;**36**:193–7.

32 Artal, R., Golde, S. H., Dorey, F. *et al.* The effect of plasma glucose variability on neonatal outcome in the pregnant diabetic patient. *Am. J. Obstetr. Gynecol.* 1983;**147**:537–41.

33 Chung, M. A. Galactosemia in infancy: diagnosis, management, and prognosis. *Pediatr. Nurs.* 1997;**23**:563–9.

34 Barrett, C. T., Oliver, T. K. Hypoglycemia and hyperinsulinism in infants with erythroblastosis fetalis. *N. Engl. J. Med.* 1968;**278**:1260–2.

35 Raivio, K. O., Osterlund, K. Hypoglycemia and hyperinsulinemia associated with erythroblastosis fetalis. *Pediatrics* 1969;**43**:217–25.

36 Schiff, D., Aranda, J. V., Colle, E., Stern, L. Metabolic effects of exchange transfusion. II. Delayed hypoglycemia following exchange transfusion with citrated blood. *J. Pediatr.* 1971;**79**:589–93.

37 Leake, R. D., Hobel, C. J., Okada, D. M., Ross, M. G., Williams, P. R. Neonatal metabolic effects of oral ritodrine hydrochloride administration. *Pediatr. Pharmacol.* 1983;**3**:101–6.

38 Procianoy, R. S., Pinheiro, C. E. A. Neonatal hyperinsulinism after short-term maternal beta sympathomimetic therapy. *J. Pediatr.* 1982;**101**:612–14.

39 DeBaun, M. R., King, A. A., White, N. Hypoglycemia in Beckwith–Weidemann syndrome. *Semin. Perinatol.* 2000;**24**:164–71.

40 Brown, K. W., Gardner, A., Williams, J. C. *et al.* Paternal origin of 11p15 duplications in the Beckwith–Wiedemann syndrome. A new case and review of the literature. *Cancer Genet Cytogenet.* 1992;**58**:66–70.

41 Waziri, M., Patil, S. R., Hanson, J. W., Bartley, J. A. Abnormality of chromosome 11 in patients with features of Beckwith–Wiedemann syndrome. *J. Pediatr.* 1983:**102**:873–6.

42 Cresto, J. C., Abdenur, J. P., Bergada, I., Martino, R. Long term follow up of persistent hyperinsulinaemic hypoglycaemia of infancy. *Arch. Dis. Child.* 1998;**79**:440–4.

43 De Lonlay, P., Fournet, J. C., Touati, G. *et al.* Heterogeneity of persistent hyperinsulinaemic hypoglycaemia. A series of 175 cases. *Eur. J. Pediatr.* 2002;**161**:37–48.

44 Glaser, B. Hyperinsulinism of the newborn. *Semin. Perinatol.* 2000;**24**:150–63.

45 Glaser, B., Ryan, F., Donath, M. *et al.* Hyperinsulinism caused by paternal-specific inheritance of a recessive mutation in the sulfonylurea-receptor gene. *Diabetes* 1999;**48**:1652–7.

46 Nestorowicz, A., Inagaki, N., Gonoi, T. *et al.* A nonsense mutation in the inward rectifier potassium channel gene, Kir6.2, is associated with familial hyperinsulinism. *Diabetes* 1997;**46**:1743–8.

47 Verkarre, V., Fournet, J. C., De Lonlay, P. *et al.* Paternal mutation of the sulfonylurea receptor (SUR1) gene and maternal loss of 11p15 imprinted genes lead to persistent hyperinsulinism in focal adenomatous hyperplasia. *J. Clin. Invest.* 1998;**102**:1286–91.

48 Glaser, B., Kesavan, P., Heyman, M. *et al.* Familial hyperinsulinism caused by an activating glucokinase mutation. *N. Engl. J. Med.* 1998;**338**:226–30.

49 Miki, Y., Taki, T., Ohura, T. *et al.* Novel missense mutations in the glutamate dehydrogenase gene in the congenital hyperinsulinism-hyperammonemia syndrome. *J. Pediatr.* 2000;**136**:69–72.

50 Stanley, C. A., Lieu, Y. K., Hsu, B. Y. *et al.* Hyperinsulinism and hyperammonemia in infants with regulatory mutations of the glutamate dehydrogenase gene. *N. Engl. J. Med.* 1998;**338**:1352–7.

51 Davis, D. J., Creery, W. D., Radziuk, J. Inappropriately high plasma insulin levels in suspected perinatal asphyxia. *Acta. Paediatrica Scand.* 2000;**88**:76–81.

52 Pal, D. K., Manandhar, D. S., Rajbhandari, S. *et al.* Neonatal hypoglycaemia in Nepal 1. Prevalence and risk factors. *Arch. Dis. Child. Fetal Neonatal Edn.* 2000;**82**:F46–51.

53 Leake, R. D., Fiser, R. H., Oh, W. Rapid glucose disappearance in infants with infection. *Clin. Pediatr.* 1981;**20**:397–401.

54 Hawdon, J. M., Weddell, A., Aynsley-Green, A., Ward Platt, M. P. Hormonal and metabolic response to hypoglycaemia in small for gestational age infants. *Arch. Dis. Child.* 1993;**68**:269–73.

55 Stanley, C. A., Anday, E. K., Baker, L., Delivoria-Papadopoulos, M. Metabolic fuel and hormone responses to fasting in newborn infants. *Pediatrics* 1979;**64**:613–19.

56 Hussain, K., Hindmarsh, P., Aynsley-Green, A. Spontaneous hypoglycemia in childhood is accompanied by paradoxically low serum growth hormone and appropriate cortisol counterregulatory hormonal responses. *J. Clin. Endocrinol. Metab.* 2003;**88**:3715–23.

57 Costello, A. M., Pal, D. K., Manandhar, D. S. *et al.* Neonatal hypoglycaemia in Nepal 2. Availability of alternative fuels. *Arch. Dis. Child. Fetal Neonatal Edn.* 2000;**82**:F52–8.

58 Hawdon, J. M., Ward Platt, M. P., Aynsley-Green, A. Patterns of metabolic adaptation for preterm and term infants in the first neonatal week. *Arch. Dis. Child.* 1992;**67**:357–65.

59 Vannucci, R. C., Vannucci, S. Hypoglycemic brain injury. *Semin. Neonatol.* 2001;**6**:147–55.

60 Belik, J., Wagerle, L. C., Stanley, C. A. *et al.* Cerebral metabolic response and mitochondrial activity following insulin-induced hypoglycemia in newborn lambs. *Biol. Neonate* 1989;**55**:281–9.

61 Katsura, K., Folbergrova, J., Bengtsson, F. *et al.* Recovery of mitochondrial and plasma membrane function following hypoglycemic coma: coupling of ATP synthesis, K^+ transport, and changes in extra- and intracellular pH. *J. Cerebr. Blood Flow Metabol.* 1993;**13**:820–6.

62 Kristian, T., Gido, G., Siesjö, B. K. Brain calcium metabolism in hypoglycemic coma. *J. Cereb. Blood Flow Metabol.* 1993;**13**:955–61.

63 Siesjö, B. K., Bengtsson, F. Calcium fluxes, calcium antagonists, and calcium-related pathology in brain ischemia, hypoglycemia, and spreading depression: a unifying hypothesis. *J. Cereb. Blood Flow Metabol.* 1989;**9**:127–40.

64 Wieloch, T., Harris, R. J., Symon, L., Siesjö, B. K. Influence of severe hypoglycemia on brain extracellular calcium and potassium activities, energy, and phospholipid metabolism. *J. Neurochem.* 1984;**43**:160–8.

65 Mujsce, D. J., Christensen, M. A., Vannucci, R. C. Regional cerebral blood flow and glucose utilization during hypoglycemia in newborn dogs. *Am. J. Physiol.* 1989;**256**:H1659–66.

66 Pryds, O., Christensen, N. J., Friis-Hansen, B. Increased cerebral blood flow and plasma epinephrine in hypoglycemic, preterm neonates. *Pediatrics* 1990;**85**:172–6.

67 Ruth, V. J., Park, T. S., Gonzales, E. R., Gidday, J. M. Adenosine and cerebrovascular hyperemia during insulin-induced hypoglycemia in newborn piglet. *Am. J. Physiol.* 1993;**265**:H1762–8.

68 Auer, R. N. Progress review: hypoglycemic brain damage. *Stroke* 1986;**17**:699–708.

69 Auer, R. N., Alimo, H., Olsson, Y., Siesjö, B. K. The temporal evolution of hypoglycemic brain damage. I. Light and electron microscopic findings in the rat cerebral cortex. *Acta Neuropathol.* 1985;**67**:13–24.

70 Bank, B. Q. The neuropathological effects of anoxia and hypoglycemia in the newborn. *Dev. Med. Child Neurol.* 1967;**9**:544–50.

71 Barkovich, A. J., Ali, F. A., Rowley, H. A., Bass, N. Imaging patterns of neonatal hypoglycemia. *Am. J. Neuroradiol.* 1998;**19**:523–8.

72 Chiu, N. T., Huang, C. C., Chang, Y. C. *et al.* Technetium-99m-HMPAO brain SPECT in neonates with hypoglycemic encephalopathy. *J. Nucl. Med.* 1998;**39**:1711–13.

73 Kinnala, A., Rikalainen, H., Lapinleimu, H. *et al.* Cerebral magnetic resonance imaging and ultrasonography findings after neonatal hypoglycemia. *Pediatrics* 1999;**103**:724–9.

74 Murakami, Y., Yamashita, Y., Matsuishi, T. *et al.* Cranial MRI of neurologically impaired children suffering from neonatal hypoglycaemia. *Pediatr. Radiol.* 1999;**29**:23–7.

75 Traill, Z., Squier, M., Anslow, P. Brain imaging in neonatal hypoglycaemia. *Arch. Dis. Child. Fetal Neonatal Edn.* 1998;**79**:F145–7.

76 Cornblath, M., Wybregt, S. H., Baens, G. S., Klein, R. I. Symptomatic neonatal hypoglycemia. Studies of carbohydrate metabolism in the newborn infant VIII. *Pediatrics* 1964;**33**:388–402.

77 Fluge, G. Neurological findings at follow-up in neonatal hypoglycaemia. *Acta. Paediatrica Scand.* 1975;**64**:629–34.

78 Yamaguchi, K., Mishina, J., Mitsuishi, C., Takamura, T., Nishida, H. Follow-up study of neonatal hypoglycemia. *Acta Paediatrica Jpn.* 1997;**39**:S51–3.

79 Koh, T. H., Aynsley-Green, A., Tarbit, M., Eyre, J. A. Neural dysfunction during hypoglycaemia. *Arch. Dis. Child.* 1988;**63**:1353–8.

80 Cowett, R. M., Howard, G. M., Johnson, J., Vohr, B. Brain stem auditory-evoked response in relation to neonatal glucose metabolism. *Biol. Neonate* 1997;**71**:31–6.

81 Meissner, T., Wendel, U., Burgard, P., Schaetzle, S., Mayatepek, E. Long-term follow-up of 114 patients with congenital hyperinsulinism. *Eur. J. Endocrinol.* 2003;**149**:43–51.

82 Menni, F., De Lonlay, P., Sevin, C. *et al.* Neurologic outcomes of 90 neonates and infants with persistent hyperinsulinemic hypoglycemia. *Pediatrics* 2001;**107**:476–9.

83 Aynsley-Green, A., Hussain, K., Hall, J. *et al.* Practical management of hyperinsulinism in infancy. *Arch. Dis. Child. Fetal Neonatal Edn.* 2000;**82**:F98–107.

84 Lovvorn, H. N. III, Nance, M. L., Ferry, R. Jr. *et al.* Congenital hyperinsulinism and the surgeon: lessons learned over 35 years. *J. Pediatr.* 1999;**34**:786–92.

85 Meetze, W., Bowsher, R., Compton, J., Moorehead, H. Hyperglycemia in extremely-low-birth-weight infants. *Biol. Neonate* 1998;**74**:214–21.

86 Cowett, R. M., Oh, W., Schwartz, R. Persistent glucose production during glucose infusion in the neonate. *J. Clin. Inv.* 1983;**71**:467–75.

87 Sunehag, A., Gustafsson, J., Ewald, U. Very immature infants (≤30 wk) respond to glucose infusion with incomplete suppression of glucose production. *Pediatr. Res.* 1994;**36**:550–5.

88 Vileisis, R. A., Cowett, R. M., Oh, W. Glycemic response to lipid infusion in the premature neonate. *J. Pediatr.* 1982;**100**:108–12.

89 Fosel, S. Transient and permanent neonatal diabetes. *Eur. J. Pediatr.* 1995;**154**:944–8.

90 Von Muhlendahl, K. E., Herkenhoff, H. Long-term course of neonatal diabetes. *N. Engl. J. Med.* 1995;**333**:704–8.

91 Marquis, E., Robert, J. J., Bouvattier, C. *et al.* Major difference in aetiology and phenotypic abnormalities between transient and permanent neonatal diabetes. *J. Med. Genet.* 2002;**39**:370–4.

92 Metz, C., Cave, H., Bertrand, A. M. *et al.* Neonatal diabetes mellitus: chromosomal analysis in transient and permanent cases. *J. Pediatr.* 2002;**141**:483–9.

93 James, T. III, Blessa, M., Boggs, T. R. Jr. Recurrent hyperglycemia associated with sepsis in a neonate. *Am. J. Dis. Child.* 1979;**133**:645–6.

94 Srinivasan, G., Singh, J., Cattamanchi, G., Yeh, T. F., Pildes, R. S. Plasma glucose changes in preterm infants during oral theophylline therapy. *J. Pediatr.* 1983;**103**:473–6.

95 Pildes, R. S., Pyati, S. P. Hypoglycemia and hyperglycemia in tiny infants. *Clin. Perinatol.* 1986;**13**:351–75.

96 Garg, R., Agthe, A. G., Donohue, P. K., Lehmann, C. U. Hyperglycemia and retinopathy of prematurity in very low birth weight infants. *J. Perinatol.* 2003;**23**:186–94.

97 Binder, N., Raschko, P. K., Benda, G. I., Reynolds, D. W. Insulin infusion with parenteral nutrition in extremely low birth weight infants with hyperglycemia. *J. Pediatr.* 1989;**114**: 273–80.

98 Ostertag, S. G., Jovanovic-Peterson, L., Lewis, B., Auld, P. Insulin pump therapy in the very low birth weight infant. *Pediatrics* 1986;**78**:625–30.

99 Goldman, S. L., Hirata, T. Attenuated response to insulin in very low birthweight infants. *Pediatr. Res.* 1980;**14**:50–3.

100 Murray, R. D., Boutton, T. W., Klein, P. D. *et al.* Comparative absorption of [13C]glucose and [13C]lactose by premature infants. *Am. J. Clin. Nutr.* 1990;**51**:59–66.

101 Shulman, R. J., Schanler, R. J., Lau, C. *et al.* Early feeding, feeding tolerance, and lactase activity in preterm infants. *J. Pediatr.* 1998;**133**:645–9.

102 Bhatia, J., Prihoda, A. R., Richardson, J. Parenteral antibiotics and carbohydrate intolerance in term neonates. *Am. J. Dis. Child.* 1986;**140**:111–13.

103 Novelli, G., Reichardt, J. K. Molecular basis of disorders of human galactose metabolism: past, present, and future. *Mol. Genet. Metab.* 2000;**71**:62–5.

32

The infant of the diabetic mother

Richard M. Cowett

CIGNA Insurance, Pittsburgh, PA

Introduction

The infant of the diabetic mother (IDM) is the premier example of the metabolic dysequilibrium that potentially exists in the neonate secondary to a maternal condition, i.e., diabetes.[1] Developmentally, the normal neonate is in a transitional state of glucose homeostasis.[2] The fetus is completely dependent on his/her mother for glucose delivery and the adult is considered to have precise control of glucose homeostasis.[3] However, maintenance of glucose homeostasis may be a major problem for the neonate born to the nondiabetic mother. The precarious nature of this equilibrium is emphasized by the numerous morbidities producing or associated with neonatal hypo- and hyperglycemia during the neonatal period. Although many IDMs have an uneventful perinatal course, there is still an increased risk of complications. Many can be minimized, but not currently eliminated, with appropriate obstetric and pediatric intervention. In fact, a recent analysis indicated that there is still much room for improvement due to the multiplicity of factors that impact on any specific pregnancy.[4] This discussion will enumerate many of the difficulties that the IDM may encounter, evaluate the pathophysiologic basis of their occurrence, and suggest treatment modalities.

Perinatal mortality and morbidity

Theoretically, the more metabolically controlled the diabetic pregnant patient is, the greater the potential for producing a normal neonate. Certainly the pregnancy of the diabetic mother should be considered to be of high risk.

Knowledge of the character of the maternal diabetic condition, prior pregnancy history, and complications occurring during pregnancy would allow the physician subsequently caring for the neonate to anticipate many of the potential fetal and neonatal complications (Table 32.1).

Studies of perinatal morbidity and mortality from diverse centers attest to the improving success of this principle of management. Pedersen et al. originally published a review of their experiences over a 26-year period with an analysis of 1332 diabetic pregnancies.[5] Perinatal mortality varied directly with severity of maternal diabetes as judged by two commonly used maternal classification schema: White's original classification of diabetes in pregnancy and Pedersen's Prognostically Bad Signs in Pregnancy (PBSP) classification. White's revised classification (Table 32.2) is based on duration of diabetes and the presence of late vascular complications,[6] while the PBSP classification (Table 32.3) includes abnormalities of the current pregnancy.

The relationship between PBSP and preeclampsia was studied by Diamond et al.[7] who evaluated 199 pregnancies. They noted that the presence of PBSP increased the perinatal mortality rate from 17.1% v. 7.3% in those insulin-dependent diabetic pregnancies without PBSB, and was predictive of pulmonary morbidity in general (31.6% v. 16.3%, respectively). The investigators concluded that the combination of the two were still as predictive as had originally been noted by Pedersen. While these investigators reported an improvement in nondiabetic pregnancy outcome during this same period, they emphasized that the improved classification schema combined with increased experience were the major reasons for the improved results in the diabetic pregnancy.

Neonatal Nutrition and Metabolism. Second Edition, ed. P. Thureen and W. Hay. Published by Cambridge University Press.
© Cambridge University Press 2006.

Table 32.1. Morbidities in the infant of the diabetic mother

Adrenal vein thrombosis
Asphyxia
Birth injury
Caudal regression
Congenital anomalies
Diaphragmatic hernia
Double outlet right ventricle
Heart failure
Hyperbilirubinemia
Hypertrophic obstructive cardiomyopathy
Hypocalcemia
Hypoglycemia
Hypomagnesemia
Increased blood volume
Macrosomia
Neurologic instability
Organomegaly
Polycythemia and hyperviscosity
Respiratory distress
Respiratory distress syndrome
Septal hypertrophy
Shoulder dystocia
Small left colon syndrome
Transient hematuria
Truncus arteriosus

Table 32.2. White's classification of diabetes in pregnancy (modified)

Gestational diabetes	Abnormal glucose tolerance test, but euglycemia maintained by diet alone or if diet alone insufficient, insulin required
Class A	Diet alone, any duration or onset age
Class B	Onset age 20 years or older and duration less than 10 years
Class C	Onset age 10–19 years or duration 10–19 years
Class D	Onset age under 10 years, duration over 20 years, background retinopathy, or hypertension (not preeclampsia)
Class R	Proliferative retinopathy or vitreous hemorrhage
Class F	Nephropathy with over 500 mg day^{-1} proteinuria
Class RF	Criteria for both R and F co-exist
Class H	Arteriosclerotic heart disease clinically evident
Class T	Prior renal transplantation

Table 32.3. Prognostically bad signs of pregnancy (PBSP)

Chemical pyelonephritis
Pre-coma or severe acidosis
Toxemia
"Neglecters"

Maternal glucose variability was studied in 154 pregnant diabetic patients who were hospitalized for a month prior to delivery.[8] An evaluation of the correlation for within-day plasma glucose variability showed that there is a significant association between maternal glucose variability and enhanced neonatal outcome (i.e., decreased incidence of complications) and that there was no correlation between maternal glucose variability and the neonate's birth weight. The investigators acknowledged that absence of glucose variability would not ensure prevention of neonatal complications. A variation of this theme was noted by Mello et al.[9] who reported that, overall, daily glucose concentrations ≤ 95 mg dL^{-1} were required in the second and third trimesters to avoid excess fetal growth.

Coustan and Imarah[10] first attempted to use prophylactic insulin treatment of the gestational diabetic to reduce the incidence of macrosomia, operative delivery, and birth trauma. The data indicated a partial decline of complications with tightened maternal metabolic control. This concept was reemphasized by Howorka et al.[11] who noted the normalization of pregnancy outcome by utilizing functional insulin treatment through individualization of insulin dosages during the day.

Finally, Hod et al.[12] reported data evaluating the effect of patient compliance, fasting plasma glucose, maternal body constitution, and method of treatment on perinatal outcome in the patient with gestational diabetes mellitus. Four hundred and seventy patients were compared with 250 control nondiabetics. Patient compliance reduced the rate of macrosomia (14.4%) and neonatal hypoglycemia (3.4%) but not to the level of the control population (5.2% and 1.2% respectively). Intensified insulin treatment was beneficial in terms of reducing the rate of perinatal complications in the obese parturient but, again, not to the level of the control group.

While most investigators have agreed on the importance of maintenance of euglycemia, the most optimal clinical method for achieving this has not been established. DeVeciana et al.[13] compared the efficacy of postprandial v. preprandial monitoring to achieve glycemic control in the gestational diabetic woman. The study involved 66 women at ≤ 30 weeks' gestation who were treated with insulin therapy following either preprandial monitoring or

Table 32.4. Components for the hypothesis of "hyperinsulinism" in the infant of the diabetic mother

Islet hyperplasia and b-cell hypertrophy
Obesity and macrosomia
Hypoglycemia with low free fatty acid concentration
Rapid glucose disappearance rate
  Higher plasma insulin-like activity after glucose
  Umbilical vein reactive immunoinsulin increase
C-peptide and proinsulin concentrations elevated

postprandial monitoring one hour after a meal. Adjusting insulin therapy in the mother according to postprandial blood glucose values decreased the risk of macrosomia, neonatal hypoglycemia, and lowered the delivery rate by cesarean section.

The maintenance of a normal metabolic state, including euglycemia, should diminish, but will not completely eradicate, the increased perinatal and neonatal mortalities and morbidities noted in the diabetic pregnancy.

Pathogenesis of the effects of maternal diabetes on the fetus

No single pathogenic mechanism has clearly defined the diverse problems observed in the IDM. Nevertheless, many of the effects can be attributed to maternal metabolic (i.e., originally primarily glucose) control. Pedersen originally emphasized the relationship between maternal glucose concentration and neonatal hypoglycemia (Table 32.4).[14] His hypothesis recognized that maternal hyperglycemia resulted in fetal hyperglycemia, which stimulated the fetal pancreas, resulting in islet cell hypertrophy and beta cell hyperplasia with increased insulin availability. Following delivery, the neonate was no longer supported by placental glucose transfer, and neonatal hypoglycemia occurred.

Hyperinsulinemia in utero affects diverse organ systems, including the placenta. Insulin acts as the primary anabolic hormone of fetal growth and development, resulting in visceromegaly, especially of heart and liver, and macrosomia. In the presence of excess substrate such as glucose, increased fat synthesis and deposition occur during the third trimester. Fetal macrosomia is reflected by increased body fat, muscle mass, and organomegaly but not an increased size of the brain or kidney.[15] After delivery there is a rapid fall in plasma glucose concentration with persistently low concentrations of plasma free fatty acids

(FFA), glycerol, and beta hydroxybutyrate. In response to an intravenous glucose stimulus, plasma insulin-like activity is increased, as is plasma immunoreactive insulin. This is determined in the absence of maternal insulin antibodies and plasma C-peptide concentration.[16]

MacFarlane et al.[17] suggested that the initial increase in fetal size due to fetal hyperinsulinemia produced developing hypoxemia. The limitation in fetal oxygen availability altered differential utilization of glucose. It also increased alpha glycerophosphate synthesis in the fetal adipocyte, which resulted in fetal adiposity.

Schwartz et al.[18] evaluated whether macrosomia in the fetus of the diabetic mother is related to fetal hyperinsulinemia and whether hyperinsulinemia and macrosomia are associated with maternal metabolic control. Ninety-five nondiabetic pregnant women were compared with 155 insulin treated pregnant women, subdivided according to the White classification, the presence of hypertension, the birth weight, and mode of delivery. Optimal care was provided and the neonate was evaluated. Macrosomia ($\geq$ 97.5%) was noted in 10%–27% of the diabetic groups and was correlated with umbilical total insulin, free insulin, and C peptide concentrations. Glycosylated hemoglobin was only a weak predictor of birth weight and fetal hyperinsulinemia. The investigators concluded that the etiology of macrosomia essentially remains unexplained, but that hyperinsulinemia remains the major stimulus for excessive fetal growth.

Finally, the cause of macrosomia in the IDM was further evaluated by the National Institute of Child Health and Human Development–Diabetes in Early Pregnancy Study, which recruited insulin-dependent diabetic and control women before conception. This study provided an opportunity to evaluate the relationship between maternal glycemia and percentile birth weight.[19] Data were analyzed from 323 diabetic and 361 control women. Fasting and nonfasting venous plasma glucose concentrations were measured on alternate weeks in the first trimester and monthly thereafter. Glycosylated hemoglobin was measured weekly in the first trimester and monthly thereafter. More infants of the diabetic women were at or above the 90th percentile for birth weight than infants of control women (28.5% v. 13.1%, $p < 0.001$). The third-trimester nonfasting glucose concentration, adjusted for data in prior trimesters, was the strongest predictor of percentile birth weight ($p = 0.001$). After adjusting for maternal hypertension, smoking, and ponderal index, the investigators concluded that monitoring of nonfasting glucose concentration rather than the fasting concentration, which is the more commonly monitored in clinical practice, is necessary to prevent macrosomia.

Metabolic analyses

Application of in vivo kinetic analysis has been utilized to evaluate the IDM metabolically. An early study using stable nonradioactive isotopes was reported by Kalhan *et al.* (using [1-^{13}C]glucose and the prime constant infusion technique).[20] They measured systemic glucose production rates in the infants of five normal (nondiabetic) women and five infants of insulin-dependent diabetics at 2 hours of age. As expected, the infant of the diabetic mother had a lower glucose concentration during the study compared with the infant of the nondiabetic mother. For the first time, they reported that the IDM had a lower systemic glucose production rate. They suggested that decreased glucose output was related to inhibited glycogenolysis. They speculated that increased insulin and decreased glucagon concentrations and catecholamine responses resulted in decreased systemic output. What was interesting about these data was that for the time studied, late 1970s, the diabetic women were considered to be in excellent control, with maternal blood glucose between 50–150 mg dL^{-1} (2.8–8.3 mmol L^{-1}).

A further evaluation of the IDM was reported by the same group 5 years later.[21] Again focusing on the neonate of the mother in "strict control," the investigators evaluated systemic glucose production in five infants of insulin-dependent mothers, one neonate of a gestational diabetic, and five neonates born to nondiabetic women. The blood glucose data were in a more restrictive range of 36–104 mg dL^{-1} (2.0–5.8 mmol L^{-1}) compared with that of the previous series. The systemic glucose production rate was similar in the infant of the diabetic compared with the control neonate. However, the investigators carried their analysis a step further. They infused exogenous glucose, which can diminish endogenous glucose production. The IDM did not evidence as great a suppression of endogenous glucose production as is seen in the adult.[3] The investigators concluded that altered regulation of glucose production may be secondary to intermittent maternal hyperglycemia, even in the strictly controlled woman.

These studies paralleled the work of Cowett *et al.*[22–25] Using 78% enriched D[U-^{13}C] glucose, 16 infants of diabetic women, of whom 10 were insulin-dependent and 6 were chemical-dependent, were compared with 5 infants of nondiabetic women. Four insulin-dependent mothers and five infants of chemical dependent diabetic mothers received 0.45% saline as the stable isotopic tracer diluent to determine basal endogenous glucose production. All of the mothers were evaluated relative to control mothers by utilization of hemoglobin A1c and maternal plasma glucose and/or cord vein glucose at delivery. There was a similarity in the basal glucose production rates in the neonates studied who had no exogenous glucose infusion. The investigators concluded that good metabolic control of the maternal diabetic state would help maintain euglycemia.[23] However, in a subsequent analysis in which the neonate of the nondiabetic mother received glucose exogenously to maintain euglycemia, a heterogeneity continued to exist in the ability of the neonate to depress endogenous glucose production.[24]

Baarsma *et al.*[26] followed 15 mother–infant pairs from the beginning of pregnancy until birth. Glucose kinetics were measured on the first day of life with stable isotopic dilution. In association with the above, plasma-free fatty acids and ketones were also measured. The neonates received 3.4 ± 0.7 mg kg^{-1} min^{-1} glucose during the study. No relationship existed between maternal control and glucose kinetics in the neonate. Total production was 5.2 ± 1.1 mg kg^{-1} min^{-1} and endogenous glucose production was 1.8 ± 1.1 mg kg^{-1} min^{-1} following subtraction of the glucose infusion. Endogenous glucose production was significantly lower in the neonates studied at the end of the first day of life. The lower production rate was associated with an increased concentration of ketone bodies. The investigators concluded that glucose kinetics in the infant of the tightly controlled diabetic mother are probably normal.

The realization that neonatal glucose homeostasis is in a transitional state and is not the only factor affecting neonatal birth weight is further supported by studies in which maternal control was evaluated in a group of gestationally diabetic women relative to the birth weight of the neonate.[27] If the Pedersen hypothesis were correct, birth weight of the neonate should correlate with the degree of control of the mother during the pregnancy. There was a lack of correlation between birth weight and mean maternal plasma glucose concentration during the third trimester of pregnancy in this group of gestational diabetics (Figure 32.1). This lack of correlation further supports the heterogeneity of the diabetic state and suggests that while control of glucose homeostasis is multifactorial, control of fetal growth is likewise. Similar conclusions led Freinkel and others to conclude that mixed nutrients (i.e., amino acids, free fatty acids, etc.) other than glucose are important in fetal–neonatal metabolic control as noted in the schematic (Figure 32.2).[28]

Support for this concept has been provided by Kalkhoff *et al.*[29] who studied the relationship between neonatal birth weight and maternal plasma amino acid profiles in lean and obese nondiabetic women and in Type I diabetic pregnant women. Hemoglobin A1c, plasma glucose concentration, and total amino acid profiles were elevated in the diabetic patient compared with controls. No differences were present between obese and lean control groups. Plasma

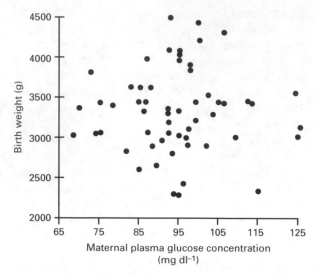

Figure 32.1. Lack of correlation between birth weight of the neonate and mean maternal plasma glucose concentration (mg dL^{-1}) during the last trimester of pregnancy in the glucose-intolerant group.[27]

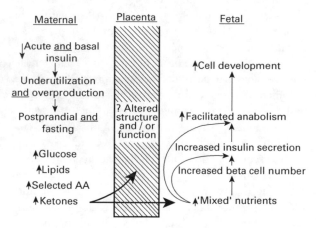

Figure 32.2. Fetal development in insulinogenic diabetic pregnancy utilizing maternal mixed nutrients as controlling factors.[28]

glucose concentrations and profiles of hemoglobin A1c did not correlate with relative weight of the neonate while average total plasma amino acid concentrations did. The investigators concluded that maternal plasma amino acid profiles may influence fetal weight generally and affect the development of neonatal macrosomia.

Further investigation relative to protein metabolism in pregnancy was performed by Whittaker *et al.*[30] They evaluated protein kinetics in six normal and five insulin-dependent diabetic women during and after pregnancy using stable isotopes and the hyperinsulinemic–

euglycemic clamp and amino acid infusions. Evaluation of protein breakdown measured using leucine kinetics was not higher than normal. Also, neither pregnancy nor Type I diabetes altered insulin sensitivity to amino acid turnover. The data were interpreted to suggest that alterations may support amino acid conservation for protein synthesis and accretion in late pregnancy.

Another data set, by Knopp *et al.*,[31] focused on the relationship between neonatal birth weight and substrate. It evaluated this relationship relative to plasma triglyceride concentration. They drew plasma samples for a number of metabolic parameters one hour after a 50-gram glucose load from 521 randomly selected negatively screened individuals, 264 positively screened individuals with a negative glucose tolerance test and 96 positively screened individuals with a positive glucose tolerance test at 24–28 weeks of gestation. Plasma triglyceride concentration was the only test elevated in the gestational diabetic subjects, but not in the negative glucose tolerance test group. Besides glucose concentration, only the plasma triglyceride concentration was significantly related to birth weight ratio (i.e., birth weight corrected for gestational age) and to glucose intolerance. The investigators concluded that plasma triglyceride may be a physiological contributor to neonatal birth weight (Figure 32.3).

This concept was further analyzed by Kitajima *et al.*[32] who evaluated plasma triglyceride concentrations between 24 and 32 weeks' gestation in women with positive diabetic screens but negative glucose tolerance tests. Hyper-triglyceridemia (defined as > the 75% value for these subjects, which was a plasma triglyceride concentration of >259 mg dL^{-1} [2.9 mmol L^{-1}]) was a significant factor in the development of macrosomia, independent of maternal obesity or maternal plasma glucose concentrations. Clearly metabolites rather than glucose contribute to the propensity of fetal/neonatal macrosomia and should be evaluated prospectively.

Congenital anomalies

While most of the morbidity and mortality data for the IDM has shown definite improvement with time, congenital anomalies remain a significant unresolved problem. In a population-based study of 7958 infants over a 12-year span, Becerra *et al.*[33] documented differences between the IDM and the non-IDM relative with congenital malformations. The relative risk for major malformations in the neonate born to the mother with insulin-dependent diabetes mellitus was 7.9 compared with the neonate of the nondiabetic mother. Likewise the relative risk for central nervous

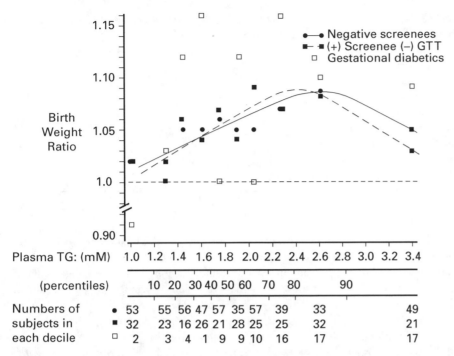

Figure 32.3. Relationship between birth weight ratio (neonatal birth weight adjusted for gestational age) and plasma triglyceride concentration.[31]

system and cardiovascular system defects was 15.5 and 18.0 respectively.

In a recent series a refinement of the above data was reported in a review of the relationship between specific birth weight and the presence of major congenital malformations. Waller et al.[34] reviewed the 8226 neonates in the Texas Birth Defects Monitoring files with a control group of neonates numbering almost 1 000 000 neonates without defects. Infants with 45 specific defects were more likely to have a birth weight > 4500 g than neonates who weigh less at birth. In contrast in another series Watkins et al.[35] reported that in the nondiabetic woman the odds ratio of delivering a neonate with congenital heart disease was higher if the prepregnancy weight of the woman indicated obesity.

The pathogenesis of the increase in congenital anomalies among IDMs has remained obscure, although several etiologies have been proposed to account for these, including: (1) hyperglycemia, either preconceptional or postconceptional; (2) hypoglycemia; (3) fetal hyperinsulinemia; (4) uteroplacental vascular disease; and/or (5) genetic predisposition. A review has cogently summarized the relevant data obtained from investigations during the 1980s.[36] While there are data to support each of these proposed mechanisms, currently the evidence seems best for the postconceptional hyperglycemia etiology.

In another study, 136 women with known prior gestational diabetes underwent preconceptional counseling at least 2 months before the onset of pregnancy and were compared to a group of 154 women who did not participate in this preconceptional counseling program. Evaluations included oral glucose tolerance testing, mean blood glucose concentration, and glycosylated hemoglobin level. Those that participated in the preconceptional counseling program delivered no neonates with congenital malformations compared with a 0.65% incidence rate among nonattenders.[37]

A number of studies have reported the strong association of preconceptional testing and control with a marked diminution in the incidence of congenital anomalies. These data parallel other reports suggesting that later control (after the first trimester) did not result in a fall in the incidence of congenital malformations although other morbidity did decrease. In fact, the neonatal malformation rate rose and was not influenced by maternal age or diabetic class.[38]

One rare congenital defect that is increased in frequency in the IDM is the small left colon syndrome.[39] The etiology is obscure. With conservative medical management, the condition usually resolves spontaneously.

A further evaluation of the association of congenital anomalies and the diabetic pregnancy, involving the association of maternal diabetes and cardiovascular malformations, was reported by Ferencz *et al.*[40] from the Baltimore–Washington Infant study, a population-based case-control study of cardiovascular malformations. The strongest associations with overt Type I diabetes were with double outlet right ventricle and truncus arteriosus. No association was noted with gestational diabetes.

Cardiomyopathy in the IDM can be congestive or hypertrophic. Hypertrophic cardiomyopathy in the neonate has been associated with poorly controlled diabetes in the parturient and neonatal hypoglycemia. Respiratory distress can be accompanied by septal hypertrophy,[41] with resolution of symptoms within 2–4 weeks and of the hypertrophy within 2–12 months.[42] Hypertrophy of the interventricular septum and walls of the right and left ventricles has also been reported.[43] Profound hypoglycemia after birth, consistent with the metabolic effects of neonatal hyperinsulinism, has been strongly associated with septal hypertrophy.[44] Fetal hyperinsulinism may contribute directly to septal hypertrophy.

Although cardiac hypertrophy apart from congenital heart disease has been recognized in autopsies of IDMs for the past three decades, only within the last decade has attention been directed to a peculiar form of subaortic stenosis similar to the idiopathic hypertrophic subaortic stenosis found in the adult.[45] This peculiar entity can be associated with symptomatic congestive heart failure. As with the adult variant in these neonates, therapy with digoxin is contraindicated because the resultant increased myocardial contractility has been reported to be deleterious. Propranolol appears to be the therapeutic drug of choice. Clinically this disorder resolves spontaneously over a period of weeks to months.

Macrosomia, birth injury, and asphyxia

At birth, the infant of the poorly controlled diabetic often will appear macrosomic in contrast to the infant born to either the well-controlled diabetic or the nondiabetic, nonobese mother. Also at birth, a consequence of undetected fetal macrosomia may be a difficult vaginal delivery due to shoulder dystocia with resultant birth injury and/or asphyxia. These potential birth injuries include cephalohematoma, subdural hemorrhage, facial palsy, ocular hemorrhage, brachial plexus injuries, and clavicular fracture. Injury to the brachial plexus may appear with a variety of presentations because the nerves of the brachial plexus may be variably damaged. In addition to the obvious injury to the nerves of the arm, diaphragmatic paralysis occurs when the phrenic nerve is injured. Because of the

Table 32.5. Potential birth injuries in the infant of the diabetic mother

Abdominal organ injury
Brachial plexus injury
Cephalohematoma
Clavicular fracture
Diaphragmatic paralysis
External genitalia hemorrhage
Facial palsy
Ocular hemorrhage
Subdural hemorrhage

associated organomegaly in the IDM, hemorrhage in the abdominal organs is possible, specifically the liver and the adrenal gland. Hemorrhage into the external genitalia of the large neonate has been reported. Other potential birth injuries are listed in Table 32.5.

Because the fetus is at high risk, intrapartum monitoring is essential to minimize potential complications. Clearly, early identification of macrosomia is critical. Mintz *et al.*[46] have suggested that shoulder soft tissue measurements and abdominal circumference may be the best individual predictors of the potential for macrosomia. The combination of abdominal circumference >90th percentile and shoulder soft tissue width >12 mm was the best predictor with a sensitivity of 96%, specificity of 89%, and accuracy of 93%.

While the specific etiology of asphyxia is unclear, it may be due to difficulty in the intrapartum period because of relative macrosomia. Asphyxia may have diverse consequences for the neonate. Acutely, asphyxia may affect respiratory, renal, and central nervous system function. Decreased fluid intake is usually recommended until the degree of injury to the renal and central nervous systems can be ascertained. An important complication of asphyxia in the neonate may be later respiratory difficulty. Mimouni *et al.*[47] studied the problem of asphyxia in the infant of the insulin-dependent diabetic woman. They suggested that poor glycemic control in the third trimester, diabetic vascular disease, preeclampsia, and smoking are significant risk factors for perinatal asphyxia. They prospectively studied 162 infants born to 149 diabetic mothers of White class B-R-T. Forty-four neonates (27.2%) had evidence of asphyxia. Its presence did not correlate with third trimester control, or the other factors listed, but did correlate with nephropathy occurring in pregnancy, maternal hyperglycemia before delivery, and prematurity. The investigators concluded that in the pregnant diabetic woman, maternal and subsequently fetal hyperglycemia before delivery leads to fetal hypoxemia.

Identification of maternal diabetes and maintenance of good metabolic control in the pregnant diabetic woman should diminish the frequency and magnitude of macrosomia and its attendant complications; careful obstetric management should prevent birth injury and asphyxia. Ogata et al.[48] reported data which seem to confirm this concept. Serial studies to estimate fetal biparietal diameter and abdominal circumference were used as differential indicators of intrauterine growth in fetuses of mothers who were White class A to C. Biparietal diameter was similar in fetuses of both groups. However, abdominal circumference was noted to be normal or enhanced. The latter group had an increased insulin concentration, weighed more at birth and had more subcutaneous fat. The investigators concluded that ultrasound was shown to be useful in the preliminary detection of macrosomia.

A recent study evaluated whether macrosomia is associated with increased perinatal morbidity and mortality. The question was whether the birth of a previous macrosomic neonate heralded the risk for a subsequent macrosomic neonate. A population-based cohort study utilizing birth data from Washington State between 1984 and 1990 identified a 7.0 times risk in this clinical situation. The overall prevalence was 22% and was interpreted to suggest that a mother with one macrosomic neonate is at markedly increased risk to deliver a second in a subsequent pregnancy.[49]

Respiratory distress syndrome

Respiratory distress, including respiratory distress syndrome (RDS), may be a relatively frequent and potentially severe complication in the IDM. While the increased susceptibility to RDS has been suspected in the IDM, a definitive retrospective analysis by Robert et al.[50] evaluated the relative risk of RDS in the IDM in a large series of diabetic pregnancies from the Joslin Clinic and the Boston Hospital for Women. The relative risk of RDS in the IDM was higher in comparison to the infant of the nondiabetic mother. If specific confounding variables are excluded, including gestational age, delivery by cesarean section, presence of labor, birth weight, sex, Apgar score at 5 minutes, hemorrhage, presence of hydramnios, maternal anemia, and maternal age, the relative risk is 5.6 times higher in the IDM. This effect is primarily confined to the neonate whose gestational age is ≤ 38 weeks. Present obstetric management has been noted to markedly reduce the frequency of RDS.

Other causes of respiratory distress in the IDM are depicted in Table 32.6. All of these conditions should be considered in the differential of the neonate with

Table 32.6. Causes of respiratory distress other than respiratory distress syndrome in the IDM

Cardiac disease
Diaphragmatic hernia
Meconium aspiration
Pneumomediastinum
Pneumothorax
Transient tachypnea

respiratory difficulty. Unfortunately, to date there have been no controlled trials of administration of any exogenous surfactant being delivered to the IDM specifically to determine if there is a different response to that of the neonate who is not an IDM.

Hypoglycemia

A decline in plasma glucose concentration following delivery is characteristic of the IDM especially in the neonate who is either large or small for gestational age and/or whose mother evidenced poor glycemic control during their pregnancy. Factors, besides hyperinsulinemia, that may contribute to the development of hypoglycemia include defective counter-regulation by catecholamines and/or glucagon.

The neonate exhibits transitional control of glucose metabolism, which suggests that a multiplicity of factors affect homeostasis. Many of the factors are similar to those which influence homeostasis in the adult. The difference in the neonate is the various stages of maturation that exist. Prior work, in conjunction with the previously mentioned glucose infusion studies, can be summarized to suggest that there is blunted splanchnic (hepatic) responsiveness to insulin in the neonate compared with the adult.[24] This is true for the IDM as well as preterm and term neonates of the nondiabetic mother. What has not been studied, but what is of particular interest, are the many contra-insulin hormones that influence metabolism. If insulin is the primary glucoregulatory hormone, then contra-insulin hormones assist in balancing the effect of insulin and other factors.

One should probably evaluate all of the contra-insulin hormones but those that have been of particular interest in the IDM have been those of the sympatho-adrenal neural axis. There are many publications that have evaluated epinephrine and norepinephrine concentrations in the IDM. The results are quite variable. A very early study involved 11 infants of diabetic mothers, only two of whom were gestational diabetics. Urinary excretion of catecholamines were measured and compared with 10 infants of normal mothers. Urinary norepinephrine and epinephrine concentrations did not increase in the IDMs who were severely hypoglycemic, but did increase in the neonate whose mother was mildly hypoglycemic.[51] Other studies have corroborated this report.[52–54]

Other factors related to sympatho-adrenal activity in the neonate may be of importance. In continuing evaluation of the transitional nature of neonatal glucose metabolism (both of insulin and contra-insulin factors) epinephrine was infused in two doses (50 mg or 500 mg kg^{-1} min^{-1} in a newborn lamb model and glucose kinetics (turnover) were measured with [6-^{3}H] glucose. The newborn lamb showed a blunted response to the lower dose of epinephrine infused. The investigators speculated that the newborn lamb evidenced decreased responsiveness to this important contra-insulin stimulus when compared with adult sheep.[55,56] This tendency was reaffirmed by recent data from the same laboratory.[57] It is possible that, if this occurs in the diabetic state, this would partially account for the presence of hypoglycemia noted clinically.

The infant of the diabetic mother is generally asymptomatic with a relatively low plasma glucose concentration. Signs and symptoms that may be observed in the symptomatic neonate are nonspecific and include tachypnea, apnea, tremulousness, sweating, irritability, and seizures. The asymptomatic neonate generally does not require parenteral treatment for maintenance of carbohydrate homeostasis.

Prompt recognition and treatment of the symptomatic neonate has minimized sequelae. To date, there is no uniformity of opinion about the potential of long-term sequelae secondary to hypoglycemia in the neonate.[58]

Blood for plasma glucose concentration should be obtained at delivery from the umbilical cord. The IDM may require parenteral treatment for maintenance of glucose homeostasis. Early administration of oral feeding at < 3–4 hours of age may be beneficial to maintain plasma glucose concentrations that are not in the hypoglycemic range.

The neonate who has a glucose concentration < 30 mg dL^{-1} (< 1.7 mmol L^{-1}) should be treated with glucose administered intravenously. As is generally well accepted, bolus injections without subsequent infusion will only exaggerate the hypoglycemia by a rebound mechanism and are contraindicated. Once the plasma glucose concentration stabilizes at > 45 mg dL^{-1} (> 2.5 mmol L^{-1}) the infusion rate should be slowly decreased while the oral feedings are initiated and/or advanced. If symptomatic hypoglycemia persists, higher glucose infusion rates of > 8–12 mg kg^{-1}min^{-1} may be indicated. Because most neonates are asymptomatic, glucagon administration to prevent hypoglycemia after delivery does not appear warranted. Furthermore, glucagon may stimulate insulin release that may exaggerate the tendency for hypoglycemia.

Ultimately, the neonate will require full supplementation per os. Although proprietary formula is available, there is no contraindication to breast-feeding by the mother who is metabolically stable. The treatment of hypoglycemia in the neonatal period has recently been reviewed in detail.[59] That discussion provides for an attempt at early introduction of oral or gavage feedings if the neonate is not symptomatic and/or has a glucose concentration > 30–45 mg dL^{-1}. Table 32.7 lists an algorithm for the treatment of symptomatic v. asymptomatic hypoglycemia depending on the plasma glucose concentration.

Hypocalcemia and hypomagnesemia

Hypocalcemia (< 7 mg dL^{-1} (0.39 mmol L^{-1})) ranks as one of the important metabolic derangements observed in the IDM.[60] Serum calcium concentration is elevated following an increase in parathyroid hormone (PTH) concentration by three mechanisms: mobilization of bone calcium, reabsorption of calcium in the kidney, and increased absorption of calcium in the intestine through action of vitamin D. In contrast, serum calcium concentration is decreased following an increase in calcitonin, which antagonizes the action of PTH. Serum calcium concentration may be increased by vitamin D (1,25(OH)2D), which improves both absorption of calcium in the intestine after feeding as well as reabsorption from bone.

During pregnancy, calcium is transferred from mother to fetus, concomitant with an increasing hyperparathyroid state in the mother. Calcium concentration is higher in the fetus than in the mother. This hyperparathyroid state functions as a homeostatic compensation to restore the maternal calcium that is diverted to the fetus. However, neither calcitonin nor the parathyroid hormone cross the placenta.

At birth, because of the concentration of calcitonin, and 1,25(OH)2D, serum calcium concentration declines following interruption of maternal–fetal calcium transfer. Increases in PTH and 1,25(OH)2D as early as 24 hours of age ensure correction of the low serum calcium concentration.

Tsang et al.[61–63] have shown that the neonate is prone to hypocalcemia, particularly the prematurely born neonate, the one who is asphyxiated, and the IDM. In an extension of the above studies, Noguchi et al.[64] evaluated parathyroid function in the hypocalcemic v. the normocalcemic IDM. In the hypocalcemic IDM serum PTH concentration did not increase in response to low serum calcium concentration, while in the normocalcemic IDM the PTH concentration

Table 32.7. Algorithm for treatment of neonatal hypoglycemia, following initial measurement of blood glucose at one hour after birth

---

Blood glucose (< 45 mg dL^{-1}(< 2.5 mmol L^{-1})) symptomatic

  If clinically **symptomatic** with one or more of the following: apnea, jitteriness, tremors, etc.

  Draw confirmatory laboratory specimen if initial measurement by meter or strip in clinical area unit

  Concurrently, give glucose bolus of 200 mg kg^{-1} (2 mL kg^{-1} of D$_{10}$W) and begin intravenous glucose administration at 6–8 mg kg^{-1}min^{-1}

  Check blood glucose after 30 minutes to 1 hour $\times$ 2; alter therapy until treatment produces euglycemia and confirm

  Begin breast-feeding or age-appropriate formula by gavage/orally when clinically appropriate

Blood glucose (<45 mg dL^{-1}(<2.5 mmol L^{-1}))asymptomatic

  If clinically **asymptomatic**, draw confirmatory laboratory specimen if initial measurement by meter or strip in clinical area unit

  Concurrently, if blood glucose is 30–45 mg dL^{-1} initiate breast-feeding or age-appropriate formula by gavage/ orally at appropriate intervals

  If blood glucose is < 30 mg dL^{-1}, give glucose bolus of 200 mg kg^{-1} (2 mL kg^{-1} of D$_{10}$W) and begin intravenous glucose administration at 6–8 mg kg^{-1}min^{-1}

  Check blood glucose 30 minutes to 1 hour after feeding and then before feeding to confirm euglycemia

  If blood glucose is < 45 mg dL^{-1} after feeding, begin intravenous glucose administration at 6–8 mg kg^{-1}min^{-1}

  Gradually increase feedings and decrease parenteral fluid administration while confirming maintenance of euglycemia

Blood glucose (> 45 mg dL^{-1}(<2.5 mmol L^{-1}))

  When clinically reasonable, begin breast-feeding or age-appropriate formula by gavage/orally at appropriate intervals

  Gradually increase feedings as tolerated while confirming maintenance of euglycemia before feeding

---

did increase in response to a slight decline in serum calcium concentration. These data in the IDM are interpreted to suggest that maternal diabetes may be an independent factor related to a suppressed neonatal parathyroid function.

More recently Namgung and Tsang[65] reported that several factors have been found to have a significant impact on newborn bone mineral content. Relative to the diabetic pregnancy, they reported that the infant of the diabetic mother whose mother had poor control of her glucose metabolism in the first trimester evidenced decreased bone mineral content at birth. They suggested that the poor bone mineral content related to decreased transplacental mineral transfer.

Hypomagnesemia (<1.5 mg dL^{-1} (0.62 mmol L^{-1})) has been found in as many as 33% of IDMs. As with hypocalcemia, the frequency and severity of clinical symptoms are correlated with the maternal status. Noguchi et al.[64] have correlated the neonatal magnesium concentration with that of the mother, as well as with the maternal insulin requirement and concentration of intravenous glucose administered to the neonate. They speculated that hypocalcemia in the IDM may be secondary to decreased hypoparathyroid function as a result of the hypomagnesemia. In a subsequent evaluation, these investigators correlated decreased material serum magnesium concentration with adverse fetal outcome in the insulin-dependent diabetic woman. They speculated that decreased magnesium concentration may contribute to the high spontaneous abortion and malformation rate in the insulin-dependent diabetic pregnancy.[66]

An algorithm for treatment of hypocalcemia and hypomagnesemia is listed in Table 32.8.

Table 32.8. Initial treatment of documented hypocalcemia, and hypomagnesemia in the infant of the diabetic mother

---

Symptomatic hypocalcemia

  Infusion of 1–2 mL kg^{-1} 10% calcium gluconate over 10–30 min

  Monitor heart rate and plasma concentration

  Maintenance therapy may be given intravenously or orally at 2–8 mL kg^{-1}day^{-1}

Symptomatic hypomagnesemia

  Intravenous or intramuscular injection of 0.1–0.2 mL kg^{-1} 50% solution

  Monitor heart rate and plasma concentration

  Repeat every 6–12 hours

Hyperbilirubinemia and polycythemia

Hyperbilirubinemia is observed more frequently in the IDM than in the normal neonate. Although a number of hypotheses have been suggested, the pathogenesis remains uncertain. Red cell life span, osmotic fragility, and deformability have not been found to be appreciably different in the IDM; neither has an increased umbilical cord bilirubin concentration nor has an increased postnatal rate of hemoglobin decline been demonstrated. Peevy *et al.*[67] suggested that only the macrosomic IDM was at risk for hyperbilirubinemia and that increased hemoglobin turnover was a significant factor in its pathogenesis. However, Stevenson *et al.*[68,69] suggested that delayed clearance of the bilirubin load was a factor, as measured by pulmonary excretion of carbon monoxide, an index of bilirubin production.

The fetal monkey, which is hyperinsulinemic in the last trimester of gestation in nondiabetic mothers, has been shown to have markedly elevated plasma erythropoietin concentrations as well as other evidence of increased fetal erythropoiesis such as an elevated reticulocyte count.[70] In addition, chronically catheterized fetal sheep who have been made hyperglycemic have been found to have increased oxygen consumption and decreased distal aortic arterial oxygen content.[71,72]

The polycythemia frequently observed in the IDM may well be the most important factor associated with hyperbilirubinemia. Mimouni *et al.*[73] found a 29.4% incidence of polycythemia in the IDM versus 5.9% in the control neonate. Indirect evidence for fetal hypoxia in the IDM may explain the neonatal preponderance for polycythemia and hyperbilirubinemia. In one-third of a group of 61 IDMs, umbilical cord erythropoietin concentration (which is stimulated by hypoxia), was found to be higher than the narrow range seen in control neonates.[70] There was also an association with relative hyperinsulinemia at birth.

Another consideration is the concept of ineffective erythropoiesis in the IDM. Further support for this concept comes from a study of gestational age-matched controls, and IDMs in whom increased carbon monoxide excretion, derived from heme metabolism, was observed.[68,69] Hemoglobin concentration was not significantly higher in the IDM. Hemolysis was not present as confirmed by the absence of Coombs positive blood group incompatibility. Increased ineffective erythropoiesis, defined as erythroid precursors harbored in body organs such as the liver and spleen and not released into the peripheral circulation, was postulated as an etiology for the observed increased bilirubin concentration in the IDM. In related data, Perrine *et al.*[74] reported delay in the fetal globin switch in the IDM. The mechanism of this delay is unknown.

In a study of 32 mother–infant pairs, Green *et al.*[75] published data indicating a correlation between maternal total glycosylated hemoglobin at delivery and neonatal hematocrit. The investigators concluded that improved maternal glycemic control during late gestation may decrease the incidence of neonatal polycythemia.

In a study of the mechanisms involving neonatal polycythemia in the IDM, a complete blood count, serum iron, transferrin and ferritin concentrations were evaluated in samples from the umbilical cord of neonates born to nine gestational diabetic mothers, 21 noninsulin-dependent diabetic mothers, and eight insulin-dependent diabetic mothers. While there were no differences in serum iron concentration, transferrin concentration was higher and ferritin concentration was significantly lower in the IDM compared with a control population. The investigators concluded that iron storage is reduced in the fetus of the diabetic mother.[76]

Renal vein thrombosis

Renal vein thrombosis is a severe, life-threatening, but rare occurrence in the perinatal period.[77] Its occurrence is more frequently associated with maternal diabetes mellitus compared with the normal nondiabetic population. Although Pedersen failed to mention this condition in his monograph,[14] in one postmortem survey of 16 cases of neonatal renal vein thrombosis, five were found in the IDM.[78] Seven other neonates were born to mothers without known diabetes but with fetal macrosomia and pancreatic b-cell hypertrophy and hyperplasia. Another center reported a case of an IDM who had nearly a totally occlusive thrombosis in the umbilical vein.[79]

The pathogenesis of this lesion remains obscure although most of the speculation has centered on the possible etiologic role of polycythemia. Sludging of the red cell, combined with a further reduction in cardiac output as a result of diabetic cardiomyopathy, may be a contributing factor. Stuart *et al.*[80] have suggested that because platelet endoperoxides are increased in the IDM, the normal balance between pro-aggregatory platelets and anti-aggregatory vascular prostaglandins is disrupted in the IDM, favoring the development of thrombosis. In a subsequent evaluation, Stuart *et al.*[81] evaluated abnormalities in vascular arachidonic acid metabolism in the IDM. They noted that decreased prostacyclin formation has been suggested as a cause of an atherothrombotic tendency in the adult. The investigators studied 6-ketoprostaglandin F_1 in the IDM, and found it was normal in umbilical cord blood if the mother was in good control. Inhibition of 6 ketoprostaglandin F_1 alpha was noted if the mother's hemoglobin A1c was elevated, indicating poor diabetic control. The investigators suggested that the correlation observed between plasma 6-keto F_1 alpha prostaglandin formation and endogenous vascular prostaglandin formation in the IDM indicated that an in vitro deficiency of prostacyclin formation reflected a concomitant in vivo abnormality. Why this lesion shows selectivity for the kidney is obscure. Birth trauma is an unlikely initiating factor, since this lesion has been observed in both the stillborn and the IDM delivered by cesarean section.

Long-term prognosis and follow-up

The previous discussion has focused on problems primarily encountered during the neonatal period. Of equal concern and perhaps of greater ultimate importance are the long-term effects on growth and development, on psychosocial intellectual capabilities, and finally on the risk to the neonate of subsequently developing diabetes. One of the most important factors influencing long-term prognosis is the improvement in management of the pregnant diabetic and her neonate. Assuming that many of the deleterious effects of the diabetic pregnancy are being modified by normalization of metabolic status in both the pregnant woman and her conceptus, the poor prognosis that has been reported in previous retrospective studies should be ameliorated in future prospective evaluations.

Silverman et al.[82] tested the hypothesis that long-term postnatal development may be modified by the in utero metabolic experience. They enrolled offspring of women with insulin-dependent diabetes mellitus, noninsulin-dependent diabetes mellitus, and gestational diabetes in a prospective study from 1977 through 1983. Fetal b-cell function was assessed by measurement of amniotic fluid insulin at 32–38 weeks' gestation. Postnatally, plasma glucose and insulin concentrations were measured yearly from 1.5 years of age after fasting and 2 hours after 1.75 g kg^{-1} oral glucose tolerance test. Control subjects had a single oral glucose challenge at 10–16 years of age. In the offspring of the diabetic mother, the prevalence of impaired glucose tolerance was 1.2% at < 5 years, 5.4% at 5–9 years, and 19.3% at 10–16 years. The 88 offspring of diabetic mothers (12.3 ± 1.7 years), when compared with 80 control subjects of the same age and pubertal stage, had higher 2-h glucose and insulin concentrations. Impaired glucose tolerance was not associated with the etiology of the mother's diabetes or macrosomia at birth. Impaired glucose tolerance was recorded in only 3.7% of adolescents whose amniotic fluid insulin was normal and 33.3% of those with elevated concentrations. The investigators concluded that impaired glucose tolerance in the offspring is a long-term complication of maternal diabetes. Excessive insulin secretion in utero, as assessed by amniotic fluid insulin concentration,

is a strong predictor of impaired glucose tolerance in childhood. These investigators subsequently restated the significance of these data.[83]

The outcome of children at 1, 3, and 5 years of age was evaluated by Stebhens et al.[84] Psychological evaluations suggested that at 3 and 5 years of age, the IDM was more vulnerable to intellectual impairment, especially if the neonate was born small for gestational age or if the pregnancy was complicated by acetonuria. This concept was reinforced by the work of Petersen et al.[85] They studied early growth delay in diabetic pregnancy in relation to psychomotor development at age 4 years. Their studies of 99 consecutive insulin-dependent and 101 nondiabetic pregnant women led them to conclude that the children with a history of growth delay in early diabetic pregnancy should be screened at 4–5 years of age by Denver Developmental Screening for possible developmental impairment.

The presence of hypoglycemia per se has not been related to later neuropsychological defects. Persson & Gentz[86] found no evidence that asymptomatic hypoglycemia leads to intellectual impairment by 5 years of age. No obvious relationship was found between maternal acetonuria during pregnancy, infant birth weight, blood glucose concentration during the first hours after birth, or neonatal complications and the IQ of these children. A correlation did exist between maternal and child IQ. Hadden et al.[87] studied 123 children of Type I insulin-dependent diabetic mothers and 124 children of nondiabetic mothers. No differences were found following pediatric assessment or by a psychologically based maternal and teacher questionnaire of the emotional state or academic achievement of the child.

Questioning to what extent maternal metabolism during pregnancy affects cognitive and behavioral function of the offspring by altering brain development, Rizzo et al.[88] correlated measures of metabolism in the pregnant diabetic and nondiabetic woman with intellectual development of their offspring. Of 223 pregnant women, 89 had pregestational diabetes mellitus, 99 had gestational diabetes, and 35 had normal carbohydrate metabolism. Carbohydrate and lipid metabolism were evaluated with respect to two measures of infant development: The Bayley Scale at age 2 years and the Stanford–Binet at 3, 4, and 5 years age. The Bayley Scale at 2 years of age was inversely correlated with the mother's third trimester plasma beta hydroxyl butyrate concentration and the Stanford–Binet correlated inversely with third trimester plasma beta hydroxybutyrate and free fatty acid concentrations. The investigators concluded that ketoacidosis and accelerated starvation should be avoided in pregnancy because of their potential long-term adverse consequences.

More recently, Ornoy et al.[89] studied the neurobehavioral effects that pregestational and gestational diabetes might have on offspring of mothers with the disease studied at school age compared with children of control mothers. Pregestational and gestational diabetes was reported to adversely affect attention span and motor functions of the offspring at school age. Their cognitive ability was not affected. The effects were negatively correlated with the degree of maternal glycemic control and were more pronounced when observed in the younger child.

An early prospective study of growth and development of the IDM suggested that excessive weight is almost 10 times more common in children of diabetic mothers than unusually low weight, which may represent a potential "return to obesity" noted at birth in this group of neonates.[14] Vohr et al.[90] suggested that macrosomia in the IDM may be a predisposing factor for later obesity, because at 7 years of age, 8/19 IDMs who had been large for gestational age at birth were obese, whereas only 1/14 who had been appropriate for gestational age was obese. When body weight and length and head circumference were evaluated from birth through 48 months of age, children of mothers with poor control during pregnancy showed higher values for weight and weight-height ratio in infancy compared with neonates of well-controlled mothers.[91]

Thus it is apparent that both immediate and potentially long-term effects are noted in the offspring born to the insulin-dependent Type I diabetic and gestational diabetic mother. Further research is clearly required to refine the operative pathophysiology so that enhanced treatment modalities can be developed and studied. Clearly the goal is to afford the pregnant woman, who is afflicted with diabetes either before or during her pregnancy, the opportunity to deliver as normal and unaffected a neonate as possible.

REFERENCES

1 Cowett, R. M. The infant of the diabetic mother. In Cowett, R. M., ed. *Principles of Perinatal-Neonatal Metabolism.* New York, NY: Springer-Verlag;1998:1105–30.

2 Cowett, R. M., Farrag, H. M. Neonatal glucose metabolism. In Cowett, R. M., ed. *Principles of Perinatal Neonatal Metabolism.* New York, NY: Springer Verlag;1998:686–722.

3 Wolfe, R. R., Allsop, J., Burke, J. F. Glucose metabolism in man: responses to intravenous glucose. *Metab. Clin. Exp.* 1979;**28**:210–20.

4 Carrapato, M. R., Marcelino, F. The infant of the diabetic mother: the critical developmental windows. *Early Pregnancy* 2001;**5**:57–8.

5 Pedersen, J., Molsted-Pedersen, L., Andersen, B. Assessors of fetal perinatal mortality in diabetic pregnancy. Analyses of 1,332 pregnancies in the Copenhagen series 1946–1972. *Diabetes* 1974;**23**:302–5.

6 Hare, J. W., White, P. Gestational diabetes and the White classification. *Diabetes Care* 1980;**3**:394.

7 Diamond, M. D., Salyer, S. L., Vaughn, W. K., Cotton, R., Boehm, F. H. Reassessment of White's clarification and Pedersen's prognostically bad signs of diabetic pregnancies in insulin dependent diabetic pregnancies. *Am. J. Obstet.* 1987;**156**:599–604.

8 Artal, R., Golde, S. H., Dorey, F. *et al.* The effect of plasma glucose variability on neonatal outcome in the pregnant diabetic patient. *Am. J. Obstet. Gynecol.* 1983;**147**:537–41.

9 Mello, G., Parretti, E., Mecacci, F. *et al.* What degree of maternal metabolic control in women with type 1 diabetes is associated with normal body size and proportions in full term infants? *Diabetes Care* 2000;**10**:1494–8.

10 Coustan, D. R., Imarah, J. Prophylactic insulin treatment of gestational diabetes reduces the incidence of macrosomia, operative delivery, and birth trauma. *Am. J. Obstet. Gynecol.* 1984;**150**:836–42.

11 Howorka, K., Pumpria, J., Gabriel, M. *et al.* Normalization of pregnancy outcome in pre-gestational diabetes through functional insulin treatment and modular outpatient education adapted for pregnancy. *Diab. Med.* 2001;**18**:965–72.

12 Hod, M., Rabinerson, D., Kaplan, B. *et al.* Perinatal complications following gestational diabetes: how sweet is it? *Acta Obstet. Gynecol. Scan.* 1996;**75**:809–15.

13 deVeciana, M., Major, A., Morgan, M. A. *et al.* Postprandial versus preprandial blood glucose monitoring in women with gestational diabetes mellitus requiring insulin therapy. *N. Eng. J. Med.* 1995;**333**:1237–41.

14 Pedersen, J. *The Pregnant Diabetic and her Newborn.* 2nd edn. Baltimore, MD: Williams & Wilkins, 1977.

15 Susa, J. B., McCormick, K. L., Widness, J. A. *et al.* Chronic hyperinsulinemia in the fetal rhesus monkey. Effects on fetal growth and composition. *Diabetes* 1979;**28**:1058–63.

16 Block, M. B., Pildes, R. S., Mossabhoy, N. A., Steiner, D. F., Rubinstein, A. H. C-peptide immunoreactivity (CRP): a new method for studying infants of insulin-treated diabetic mothers. *Pediatrics* 1974;**53**:923–8.

17 MacFarlane, C. M., Tsakalakos, N. The extended Pedersen hypothesis. *Clin. Physiol. Biochem.* 1988;**6**:68–73.

18 Schwartz, R., Gruppuso, P. A., Pelzold, K. *et al.* Hyperinsulinemia and macrosomia in the fetus of the diabetic mother. *Diabetes Care* 1994;**17**:640–8.

19 Jovanovic-Peterson, L., Peterson, C. M., Reed, G. F. *et al.* Maternal postprandial glucose levels and infant birth weight: The Diabetes in Early Pregnancy Study. *Am. J. Obstet. Gynecol.* 1991;**164**:103–11.

20 Kalhan, S. C., Savin, S. M., Adam, P. A. J. Attenuated glucose production rate in newborn infants of insulin-dependent diabetic mothers. *N. Engl. J. Med.* 1977;**296**:375–6.

21 King, K. C., Tserng, K. Y., Kalhan, S. C. Regulation of glucose production in newborn infants of diabetic mothers. *Pediatr. Res.* 1982;**16**:608–12.

22 Cowett, R. M., Susa, J. B., Giletti, B., Oh, W., Schwartz, R. Variability of endogenous glucose production in infants of insulin dependent diabetic mothers. *Pediatr. Res.* 1980;**14**: 570A.

23 Cowett, R. M., Susa, J. B., Giletti, B., Oh, W., Schwartz, R. Glucose kinetics in infants of diabetic mothers. *Am. J. Obstet. Gynecol.* 1983;**146**:781–6.

24 Cowett, R. M., Oh, W., Schwartz, R. *et al.* Persistent glucose production during glucose infusion in the neonate. *J. Clin. Invest.* 1983;**71**:467–73.

25 Cowett, R. M., Andersen, G. E., Maguire, C. A., Oh, W. Ontogeny of glucose kinetics in low birth weight infants. *J. Pediatr.* 1988;**112**:462–5.

26 Baarsma, R., Reijngoud, D. J., van Asselt, W. A. *et al.* Postnatal glucose kinetics in newborns of lightly controlled insulin dependent diabetic mothers. *Pediatr. Res.* 1993;**34**: 443–7.

27 Widness, J. A., Cowett, R. M., Coustan, D. R., Carpenter, M. W., Oh, W. Neonatal morbidities in infants of mothers with glucose intolerance in pregnancy. *Diabetes* 1985;**34**:61–5.

28 Freinkel, N. Of pregnancy and progeny. Banting Lecture. *Diabetes* 1980;**29**:1023–35.

29 Kalkhoff, R. K., Kandaraki, E., Morrow, P. G. *et al.* Relationship between neonatal birth weight and maternal plasma amino acid profiles in lean and obese non-diabetic women and in type I diabetic pregnant women. *Metabolism* 1988;**37**: 234–9.

30 Whittaker, P. G., Lee, C. H., Taylor, R. Whole body protein kinetics in women: effect of pregnancy and IDDM during anabolic stimulation. *Am. J. Physiol. Endocrinol. Met.* 2000;**279**: E978–88.

31 Knopp, R. H., Magee, M.S, Walden, C. E., Bonet, B., Benedetti, T. S. Prediction of infant birth weight by GDM screening tests: importance of plasma triglyceride. *Diabetes Care* 1992;**15**:1605–13.

32 Kitajima, M., Oka, S. Yasuchi, I. *et al.* Maternal serum triglyceride at 24–32 weeks' gestation and newborn weight in nondiabetic women with positive diabetic screens. *Obstet. Gynecol.* 2001;**97**;776–80.

33 Becerra, J. E., Koury, M. J., Cordero, J. F., Erickson, J. D. Diabetes mellitus during pregnancy and the risks for specific birth defects: a population based case control study. *Pediatrics* 1990;**85**:1–9.

34 Waller, D. K., Keddie, A. M., Canfield, M. A. Do infants with major congenital anomalies have an excess of macrosomia? *Teratology* 2001;**64**;311–17.

35 Watkins, M. L., Botto, L. D. Maternal prepregnancy weight and congenital heart defects in offspring. *Epidemiology* 2001;**12**;439–46.

36 Metzger, B. E., Buchanan, T. A. eds. Diabetes and birth defects: Insights from the 1980s, prevention in the 1990s. *Diabetes Spectrum* 1990;**3**:149–89.

37 Dicker, D., Feldberg, D., Yeshaya, A. *et al.* Pregnancy outcome in gestational diabetes with preconceptional diabetes counseling. *Aust. NZ. J. Obstet. Gynecol.* 1987;**27**:184–7.

38 Ballard, J. L., Holroyde, J., Tsang, R. C. *et al.* High malformation rates and decreased mortality in infants of diabetic mothers managed after the first trimester (1956–1978). *Am. J. Obstet. Gynecol.* 1984;**148**:111–18.

39 Davis, W. S., Allen, R. P., Favara, B. E., Sloves, T. L. Neonatal small left colon syndrome. *Am. J. Roent. Rad. Therap. Nucl. Med.* 1974;**120**:327–9.

40 Ferencz, C., Rubin, J. D., McCarter, R. J., Clark, E. B. Maternal diabetes and cardiovascular malformations: predominance of double outlet right ventricle and truncus arteriosus. *Teratology* 1990;**41**:319–26.

41 Way, G. L., Wolfe, R. R., Eshaghpour, H. D. *et al.* The natural history of hypertrophic cardiomyopathy in infants of diabetic mothers. *Pediatrics* 1979;**95**:1020–5.

42 Reeler, M. D., Kaplan, S. Hypertrophic cardiomyopathy in infants of diabetic mothers: an update. *Am. J. Perinatol.* 1988;**4**:353–8.

43 Mace, S., Hirshfield, S. S., Riggs, T., Fanaroff, A., Merkatz, I. R. Echocardiographic abnormalities in infants of diabetic mothers. *J. Pediatr.* 1979;**95**:1013–9.

44 Breitweser, J. A., Mayer, R. A., Sperling, M. A., Tsang, R. C., Kaplan, S. Cardiac septal hypertrophy in hyperinsulinemic infants. *J. Pediatr.* 1980;**96**:535–9.

45 Halliday, H. L. Hypertrophic cardiomyopathy in infants of poorly controlled diabetic mothers. *Arch. Dis. Child.* 1981;**56**:258–63.

46 Mintz, M. C., Landon, M. B., Gabbe, S. G. Shoulder soft tissue width as a predictor of macrosomia in diabetic pregnancies. *Am. J. Perinatol.* 1989;**6**:240–3.

47 Mimouni, F., Miodounik, M., Siddigi, T. A., Khoury, J., Tsang, R. C. Perinatal asphyxia in infants of insulin dependent diabetic mothers. *J. Pediatr.* 1988;**113**:345–53.

48 Ogata, E. S., Sabbagha, R., Metzger, B. E. *et al.* Serial ultrasonography to assess evolving fetal macrosomia. Studies in 23 pregnant women. *J. Am. Med. Assoc.* 1980;**243**:2405–8.

49 Davis, R., Woelk, G., Mueller, B. A., Daling, J. The role of previous birthweight on risk for macrosomia on a subsequent birth. *Epidemiology* 1995;**6**:607–11.

50 Robert, M. F., Neff, R. K., Hubbell, J. P., Taeusch, H. W., Avery, M. E. Association between maternal diabetes and the respiratory distress syndrome in the newborn. *N. Engl. J. Med.* 1976;**294**:357–60.

51 Light, I. J., Sutherland, J. M., Loggie, J. M., Gaffney, T. E. Impaired epinephrine release in hypoglycemic infants of diabetic mothers. *N. Engl. J. Med.* 1967;**277**:394–8.

52 Artal, R., Platt, L. D., Kummula, R. K. *et al.* Sympatho-adrenal activity in infants of diabetic mothers. *Am. J. Obstet. Gynecol.* 1982;**142**:436–9.

53 Artal, R., Doug, N., Wu, P., Sperling, M. Circulating catecholamines and glucagon in infants of strictly controlled diabetic mothers. *Biol. Neonate* 1988;**53**:121–5.

54 Broberger, U., Hansson, U., Lagercrantz, H., Persson, B. Sympatho-adrenal activity and metabolic adjustment during the first 12 hours after birth in infants of diabetic mothers. *Acta Pediatr. Scand.* 1984;**73**:620–5.

55 Cowett, R. M. Decreased response to catecholamines in the newborn: effect on glucose kinetics in the lamb. *Metabolism* 1988;**37**:736–40.

56 Cowett, R. M. Alpha adrenergic agonists stimulate neonatal glucose production less than beta adrenergic agonists in the lamb. *Metabolism* 1988;**37**:831–6.

57 Cowett, R. M., Rapoza, R. E., Gelardi, N. L. Insulin counter regulatory hormones are ineffective in neonatal hyperinsulinemic hypoglycemia. *Metabolism* 1999;**48**;568–74.

58 Cornblath, M., Schwartz, R., Aynsley-Green, A., Lloyd, J. K. Hypoglycemia in infancy: the need for a rational definition. *Pediatrics* 1990;**85**:834–7.

59 Cowett, R. M., Loughead, J. L. Neonatal glucose metabolism: differential diagnosis, evaluation and treatment of hypoglycemia. *Neonatal Netw.* 2002;**21**:9–19.

60 Tsang, R. C., Brown, D. R., Steichen, J. J. Diabetes and calcium disturbances in infants of diabetic mothers. In Merkatz, I. R., Adam, P. A. J., eds. *The Diabetic Pregnancy. A Perinatal Perspective.* New York, NY: Grune and Stratton; 1979:207–25.

61 Tsang, R. C., Kleinman, L. I., Sutherland, J. M. Hypocalcemia in infants of diabetic mothers: studies in Ca, P and Mg metabolism and in parathyroid hormone responsiveness. *J. Pediatr.* 1972;**80**:384–95.

62 Tsang, R. C., Light, I. J., Sutherland, J. M., Kleinman, L. I. Possible pathogenetic factors in neonatal hypocalcemia of prematurity. *J. Pediatr.* 1973;**82**:423–9.

63 Tsang, R. C., Chen, I., Atkinson, W. *et al.* Neonatal hypocalcemia in infants with birth asphyxia. *J. Pediatr.* 1974;**84**: 428–33.

64 Noguchi, A., Erin, M., Tsang, R. C. Parathyroid hormone in hypocalcemia and normocalcemic infants of diabetic mothers. *J. Pediatr.* 1980;**97**:112–14.

65 Namgung, R., Tsang, R. C. Factors affecting newborn bone mineral content: in utero effects on newborn bone mineralization. *Proc. Nutr. Soc.* 2000;**59**;55–63.

66 Mimouni, F., Miodovnik, M., Tsang, R. C. *et al.* Decreased maternal serum magnesium concentration and adverse fetal outcome in insulin-dependent diabetic women. *Obstet. Gynecol.* 1987;**70**:85–8.

67 Peevy, K. J., Landaw, S. A., Gross, S. A. Hyperbilirubinemia in infants of diabetic mothers. *Pediatrics* 1980;**66**:417–19.

68 Stevenson, D. K., Ostrander, C. R., Cohen, R. S., Johnson, J. D., Schwartz, H. C. Pulmonary excretion of carbon monoxide in the human infant as an index of bilirubin production. *Eur. J. Pediatr.* 1981;**137**:255–9.

69 Stevenson, D. K., Ostrander, C. R., Hopper, A. O., Cohen, R. S., Johnson, J. D. Pulmonary excretion of carbon monoxide as an index of bilirubin production. IIa. Evidence for possible delayed clearance of bilirubin in infants of diabetic mothers. *J. Pediatr.* 1981;**98**:822–4.

70 Widness, J. A., Susa, J., Garcia, J. F. *et al.* Increased erythropoiesis and elevated erythropoietin in infants born to diabetic mothers and in hyperinsulinemic rhesus fetuses. *J. Clin. Invest.* 1981;**67**:637–42.

71 Carson, B. S., Philipps, A. F., Simmons, M. A., Battaglia, F. C., Meschia, G. Effects of a sustained insulin infusion upon glucose uptake and oxygenation of the ovine fetus. *Pediatr. Res.* 1980;**14**:147–52.

72 Philipps, A. F., Widness, J. A., Garcia, J. F., Raye, J. R., Schwartz, R. Erythropoietin elevation in the chronically hyperglycemia fetal lamb. *Proc. Soc. Exp. Biol. Med.* 1982;**170**: 42–7.

73 Mimouni, F., Miodovnik, M., Siddiqi, T. A. *et al.* Neonatal polycythemia in infants of insulin-dependent diabetic mothers. *Obstet. Gynecol.* 1986;**68**:370–2.

74 Perrine, S. P., Greene, M. F., Faller, D. V. Delay in the fetal globin switch in infants of diabetic mothers. *N. Engl. J. Med.* 1985;**312**:334–8.

75 Green, D. W., Khoury, J., Mimouni, F. Neonatal hematocrit and maternal glycemic control in insulin dependent diabetes. *J. Pediatr.* 1992;**120**:302–5.

76 Murata, K., Toyoda, N., Ichio, T., Ida, M., Sugiyama, Y. Cord transferrin and ferritin values for erythropoiesis in newborn infants of diabetic mothers. *Endocrinol. Jpn.* 1989;**36**: 827–32.

77 Avery, M. E., Oppenheimer, E. H., Gordon, H. H. Renal vein thrombosis in newborn infants of diabetic mothers. *N. Eng. J. Med.* 1957;**265**:1134–8.

78 Takeuchi, A., Benirschke, K. Renal vein thrombosis of the newborn and its relation to maternal diabetes. *Biol. Neonate* 1961;**3**:237.

79 Fritz, M. A., Christopher, C. R. Umbilical vein thrombosis and maternal diabetes mellitus. *J. Reprod. Med.* 1981;**26**: 320–3.

80 Stuart, M. J., Sunderji-Shirazali, G., Allen, J. B. Decreased prostacyclin production in the infant of the diabetic mother. *J. Lab. Clin. Med.* 1981;**98**:412–16.

81 Stuart, M., Sunderje, S. C., Walenga, R. W. *et al.* Abnormalities in vascular arachidonic acid metabolism in the infant of the diabetic mother. *Br. Med. J.* 1983;**290**:1700–2.

82 Silverman, B. L., Metzger, B. E., Chon, H., Loeb, C. A. Impaired glucose tolerance in adolescent offspring of diabetic mothers. Relationship to fetal hyperinsulinemia. *Diabetes Care* 1995;**18**:611–17.

83 Silverman, B. L., Rizzo, T. A., Cho, N. H., Metzger, B. E. Long term effects of the intrauterine environment. The northwestern university diabetes in pregnancy center. *Diabetes Care* 1998;**21**:B142–9.

84 Stehbens, J. A., Baker, G. L., Kitchell, M. Outcome at ages 1, 3, and 5 years of children born to diabetic women. *Am. J. Obstet. Gynecol.* 1977;**127**:408–13.

85 Petersen, M. B., Pedersen, S. A., Greisen, G., Pedersen, J. F., Molsted-Pedersen, L. Early growth delay in diabetic pregnancy: relation to psychomotor development at age 4. *Br. Med. J.* 1988;**296**:598–600.

86 Persson, B., Gentz, J. Follow up of children of insulin dependent and gestational diabetic mothers. Neuropsychological outcome. *Acta Paediatr. Scand.* 1983;**73**:349–58.

87 Hadden, D. R., Bryne, E., Trotter, I. *et al.* Physical and psychological health of children of Type I (insulin dependent) diabetic mothers. *Diabetologia* 1983;**26**:250–4.

88 Rizzo, T., Metzger, R. E., Burns, W. J., Burn, K. Correlations between antepartum maternal metabolism and child intelligence. *N. Engl. J. Med.* 1991;**325**:911–6.

89 Ornoy, A., Ratson, N., Greeenbaum, C., Wolf, A., Dulitzky, M. School-age children born to diabetic mothers and to mothers with gestational diabetes exhibit a high rate of inattention and fine and gross motor impairment. *J. Pediatr. Endocrinol. Metab.* 2001;**14**:681–9.

90 Vohr, B. R., Lipsitt, L. P., Oh, W. Somatic growth of children of diabetic mothers with reference to birth size. *J. Pediatr.* 1980:**97**:196–9.

91 Gerlini, G., Arachi, S., Gori, M. G. *et al.* Developmental aspects of the offspring of diabetic mothers. *Acta Endocrinol. Suppl.* 1986;**277**:150–5.

33

Neonatal necrotizing enterocolitis: clinical observations and pathophysiology

Michael S. Caplan and Tamas Jilling

Department of Pediatrics, Evanston Northwestern Healthcare, Northwestern University, Feinberg School of Medicine, Evanston IL

Establishment of appropriate enteral feedings in the premature infant is a frequent cause of concern in the neonatal intensive care unit due to the dreaded complication of neonatal necrotizing enterocolitis (NEC), an ischemic and inflammatory necrosis of bowel that results in significant mortality, longer lengths of stay, increased costs, and possibly increased risk for abnormal neurodevelopmental outcomes.[1,2] The disease incidence varies between centers and across continents, but ranges between 3% and 28% with an average of approximately 8%–10% in infants born weighing less than 1500 g.[3] Despite significant advances in neonatal care, the morbidity and mortality resulting from NEC has not improved over the last three decades, with recent reports of NEC mortality ranging between 10%–30%.

Clinical presentation

The disease presents clinically in premature neonates with variable symptoms of intestinal bleeding, emesis, abdominal distension, lethargy, and apnea and bradycardia, and signs of abdominal tenderness, thrombocytopenia, metabolic acidosis, tachycardia, respiratory failure, and, if severe, shock.[4] The diagnosis is typically made by the identification of pneumatosis intestinalis (air in the bowel wall) on abdominal radiograph, although in some cases of NEC, commonly in un-fed patients, pneumatosis is not appreciated. In these situations, NEC may be diagnosed surgically or pathologically, or in some instances by ultrasound appreciation of portal venous air. Bell and colleagues suggested a classification scheme that differentiates feeding intolerance (stage I) from true NEC (stage II) and advanced NEC (stage III with peritonitis and/or perforation).[5] Clues to the etiology are suggested by the pathological changes observed in surgical specimens and autopsy material, including coagulation necrosis (suggesting some component of ischemic injury), inflammation (acute and/or chronic), and less commonly ulceration, hemorrhage, reparative change, bacterial overgrowth, edema, and pneumatosis intestinalis.[6]

Pathophysiology of NEC

Despite extensive investigation over the last 30 years, the etiology of NEC has remained elusive. Epidemiologic analyses of this disease have identified the important risk factors of feeding, prematurity, ischemia/asphyxia, and bacterial colonization. Furthermore, recent studies have begun to delineate the mechanisms that link the risk factors to the final common pathway of bowel necrosis, and it has been suggested that activation of the inflammatory cascade may play a vital role.

Enteral feeding

Enteral alimentation has long been considered an important risk factor on the initiation of NEC, with greater than 90% of cases presenting in premature infants after feedings were introduced. While the onset of disease used to occur several days following the first feed, in reports of extremely low birth weight (ELBW) infants from the 1990s, NEC is

Neonatal Nutrition and Metabolism. Second Edition, ed. P. Thureen and W. Hay. Published by Cambridge University Press.
© Cambridge University Press 2006.

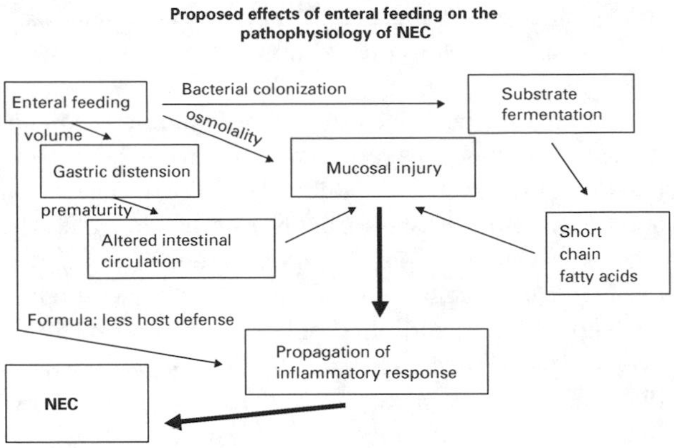

Figure 33.1. Effect of enteral feeding on the pathophysiology of NEC.

Table 33.1. Breast milk factors: molecules that may protect against NEC

Molecule	Effective in animal model	Effective in human trial
IgA, IgG	+	+/−
Leukocytes	+	
Oligosaccharides		
PUFA	+	+/−
Lactoferrin		
Glutamine	+	−
Arginine	+	+/−
PAF-AH	+	
EGF	+	
IL-10	+	

IgA, immunoglobulin A; IgG, immunoglobulin G; PUFA, polyunsaturated fatty acids; PAF-AH, PAF-acetylhydrolase; EGF, epidermal growth factor.

often diagnosed several weeks later.[3,7] Current neonatal practice initiates early trophic or hypocaloric feedings, but studies have failed to identify an increased risk of NEC in these patients.[8–10] While the precise relationship between enteral feedings and NEC remain poorly understood, studies have identified the importance of breast milk (v. formula), volume and rate of feeding advancement, osmolality, and substrate fermentation as important factors (Figure 33.1).[11–14]

Breast milk feeding appears to reduce the incidence of NEC in human studies and in carefully controlled animal models.[15,16] Breast milk contains multiple bioactive factors that influence host immunity, inflammation, and mucosal protection including secretory immunoglobulin A (IgA), leukocytes, lactoferrin, lysozyme, mucin, cytokines, growth factors, enzymes, oligosaccharides, and polyunsaturated fatty acids (PUFA), some of which are absent in neonatal formula preparations. Specific intestinal host defense factors acquired from breast milk such as epidermal growth factor (EGF), PUFA, PAF-acetylhydrolase, immunoglobulin A (IgA), and macrophages are effective in reducing the incidence of disease in animals,[17–20] and some have been effective in limited human trials (Table 33.1).[21,22] Nonetheless, breast milk is not completely protective against NEC in premature infants; the largest prospective trial identified a reduction by 50% in most birthweight-specific groups.[16,23] Nonetheless, there have been no randomized, controlled trials that have identified a statistically significant reduction in NEC from breast milk feeding, and due to ethical considerations, it seems unlikely that such an investigation will ever occur. Since most premature infants receive breast milk via the nasogastric route after artificial collection by mothers and subsequent freezing, it has been suggested that the lack of the normal maternal–infant physical inter-

action during feeding interferes with specific milk immunity thereby reducing the protection against the neonate's microbial flora. As discussed below, the unique microbial profile in the neonate's intestinal environment may contribute to initiation of NEC.

Specific components of milk feedings have been implicated to cause mucosal injury in the high-risk neonate and stimulate the subsequent development of NEC. Studies have shown that hyperosmolar formulae resulted in disease, and that addition of medication to feedings can markedly increase osmolality.[24,25] Animal studies have shown that short-chain fatty acids such as propionic or butyric acid can cause damage to developing intestine, and that colonic fermentation leading to production of these acids by the host microflora may occur in situations of carbohydrate malabsorption.[26–28] This pathway may be especially problematic in the premature infant, deficient in lactase activity and other brush border enzymes.

Different approaches to feeding have been associated with the initiation of NEC. Early studies suggested that rapid volume increases with full-strength formula increased the incidence of disease, and protocols were designed to limit feeding advancement. Several studies have shown that early, hypo-caloric or trophic feedings are safe and improve gastrointestinal function in very low birth weight (VLBW) infants.[8–10,29] Feeding advancement has been evaluated recently, and the results suggest that judicious volume increase may be safer.[12] It has been postulated that over-distention of the stomach with aggressive volumes may compromise splanchnic circulation leading to intestinal ischemia.

Prematurity

Greater than 90% of NEC cases occur in premature infants; there is clearly a higher risk with lower gestational age and birthweight.[3,16,30] While there are many differences between preterm and full-term neonates, the specific underlying mechanisms responsible for the predilection of NEC in the premature condition remain incompletely elucidated. Studies in humans and animals have identified alterations in multiple components of intestinal host defense,[31-33] motility,[34-37] bacterial colonization,[15,38-41] blood-flow regulation,[42-44] and inflammatory response[19,45,46] that may contribute to the development of intestinal injury in this unique population.

Host defense

Intestinal host defense involves a complex combination of factors that function to prevent intraluminal pathogens and toxins from resulting in disease while allowing for normal absorption of nutrients. This intricate system includes (1) physical barriers such as skin, mucus membranes, intestinal epithelia and microvilli, epithelial cell tight junctions, and mucin; (2) immune cells like polymorphonuclear leukocytes, macrophages, eosinophils, and lymphocytes; and (3) various biochemical factors.[33,47-55] Although not exhaustively studied, many of these important functions appear to be abnormal in the premature infant, and may therefore put this population at risk for NEC. Intestinal permeability to macromolecules including immunoglobulins, proteins, and carbohydrates is known to be greater in the neonate compared with older children and adults, and in premature infants this permeability may be more pronounced.[53,56] Although mucosal permeability is beneficial for developing animals to augment passive immunity and nutrient absorption, the precise mechanisms accounting for these differences are poorly understood. The microvilli and tight junctional barrier may be deficient in the premature infant, but the data are inconclusive.[57] It is known that intestinal mucus, a complex gel consisting of water, electrolytes, mucins, glycoprotein, immunoglobulins, and glycolipids, protects against bacterial and toxin invasion, and is abnormal in developing animals and perhaps premature infants.[49,58] Additionally, key bacteriostatic proteins are secreted from epithelium that bind to or inactivate the function of invading organisms. Intestinal trefoil factor is one such molecule that appears to be developmentally regulated and therefore deficient in the premature neonate.[59-61] Human defensins (or cryptidins) are bacteriostatic proteins synthesized and secreted from paneth cells that protect against bacterial translocation and are altered in premature infants and those with NEC.[62,63]

Immunologic host defense is abnormal in developing animals.[64-66] It is known that intestinal lymphocytes are decreased in neonates (B and T cells), and do not approach adult levels until 3–4 weeks of life. Newborns have markedly reduced secretory IgA in salivary samples, reflecting the decreased activity presumed in intestine.[22,67] Breast milk-feeding provides significant supplementation; formula-fed neonates have impaired intestinal humoral immunity, and this deficiency may predispose to the increased incidence of infectious diseases noted in this population.[68,69]

Several biochemical factors that are present in the intestinal milieu play an important role in the maintenance of gut health and integrity. Substances such as lactoferrin,[70] glutamine,[71,72] growth factors such as EGF,[19] TGF,[73] IGF,[74] and erythropoietin,[75,76] gastric acid, oligosaccharides,[77] PUFAs,[17,21] nucleotides,[78] and many others affect mucosal barrier function, intestinal inflammation, and the viability of intraluminal bacteria. Many of these factors are deficient or absent in the preterm neonate, especially in those patients not receiving breast milk-feedings. Intensive research is ongoing to define the specific role of each on gut integrity and the development of intestinal inflammation and necrosis.

Motility

Peristalsis in the premature infant is immature; normal patterns of intestinal motility (migratory motor complexes) appear around 34–35 weeks' gestation.[34,79] Abnormal peristaltic activity may allow for bacterial overgrowth that could increase endotoxin exposure and predispose the infant to NEC.

Bacterial colonization

Premature infants hospitalized in the neonatal intensive care unit have different patterns of gut bacterial colonization than healthy breast-fed term infants.[80] While there have been epidemics of NEC associated with specific bacteria (*Clostridia* sp., *Escherichia coli*, *Klebsiella* sp., *Staphylococcus epidermidis*, etc.), most cases occur endemically and demonstrate a variety of bacterial isolates from stool cultures.[41,81] Blood cultures are positive in only 20%–30% of affected cases, and this likely represents the degree of mucosal damage at presentation. At birth, the intestine is a sterile environment, and no cases of NEC have been described in utero, supporting the importance of bacterial colonization in the pathophysiology. Healthy breast-fed infants develop colonization by several species by 1 week of age that includes anaerobic species of Bifidobacteria and Lactobacilli, while the hospitalized, extremely premature infant intestine has less species diversity and fewer anaerobes.[69,82–84] This imbalance may allow for pathologic proliferation, binding, and invasiveness of otherwise nonpathogenic intestinal bacteria. Recent evidence suggests that contamination/colonization of nasogastric feeding tubes in formula-fed premature infants predisposes some infants to develop NEC.[85] It remains unclear whether bacterial translocation into submucosa is a prerequisite for disease, or rather the activation of the toll-like receptors from endotoxin is adequate to initiate the final common pathway of intestinal injury.[39,86–88] Nonetheless, certain bacteria such as adherent *E. coli* produce disease in a rabbit model of NEC, while nonpathogenic strains of Gram-positive organisms prevent disease.[89] Furthermore, preliminary work has suggested that early colonization by probiotics (facultative anaerobes, e.g., Bifidobacteria and Lactobacilli) reduces the risk of NEC in animal and human studies.[38,90] In summary, bacterial colonization is an important factor in the initiation of intestinal injury, but the specific events in the pathophysiology are not well delineated.

Intestinal blood flow regulation

Early observations on the pathophysiology of NEC suggested that profound intestinal ischemia was a critical predisposing factor.[91,92] Similar to the "diving reflex" observed in aquatic mammals, it was hypothesized that in periods of stress, blood flow was diverted away from the splanchnic circulation resulting in intestinal necrosis. While early epidemiologic observations identified asphyxia as an important risk factor, subsequent studies have shown that the majority of NEC cases are not associated with profound impairment in intestinal perfusion.[4] In animal models, studies have shown that the reperfusion following intestinal ischemia is required in the initiation of bowel necrosis,[93,94] and therefore, recent experimentation on the role of intestinal ischemia on the pathophysiology of NEC is focused on this construct.

Neonatal animals have been shown to have differences in the intestinal circulation that may predispose them to NEC. The basal intestinal vascular resistance is elevated in the fetus, and soon following birth decreases significantly, allowing for rapid increase in intestinal blood flow.[42] Intestinal and somatic growth is dramatic in developing animals, and therefore sufficient flow is mandatory. It has been shown that this change in the resting vascular resistance is dependent on the balance between the dilator (nitric oxide) and constrictor (endothelin) molecules, and the myogenic response.[95,96] Perhaps more relevant than basal vascular tone, studies have shown that the newborn has alterations in response to circulatory stress, resulting in compromised intestinal flow and/or vascular resistance. In response to hypotension, newborn animals (3-day-old but not 30-day-old swine) appear to have defective pressure-flow autoregulation, resulting in compromised intestinal oxygen delivery and tissue oxygenation.[43,44,97] In addition, in the face of arterial hypoxemia the newborn intestinal circulatory response differs from older animals. Although following modest hypoxemia, intestinal vasodilation and increased intestinal perfusion occurs; severe hypoxemia causes vasoconstriction, intestinal ischemia and/or hypoxia, mediated in part by loss of nitric oxide production. There are multiple chemical mediators (nitric oxide, endothelin, substance P, norepinephrine, and angiotensin) that impact on intestinal vasomotor tone, and in the stressed newborn abnormal regulation of these may result in compromised circulatory autoregulation, leading to perpetuation of intestinal ischemia and tissue necrosis.[98–100]

In summary, the premature neonate has several unique features that may increase their susceptibility to NEC, but the precise interrelationship of these factors in the final common pathway of intestinal necrosis remains unclear.

Final common pathway: the inflammatory cascade

Based on a growing body of evidence obtained from humans and animal/tissue experimentation, the final common pathway of intestinal injury appears to result from the activation of the inflammatory cascade.[55,101,102] This cascade involves a complex balance of pro and anti-inflammatory endogenous mediators, receptors, signaling pathways, second messengers, and a variety of downstream effects, that ultimately results in end-organ damage in certain circumstances. Inflammation can be initiated by a variety of factors, most notably the exposure to the bacterial cell wall product, endotoxin. Following endotoxin stimulation of the toll receptor family in animals, tissue, or cells, several mediators are rapidly produced including Platelet-activating factor (PAF), TNF, IL-1, and IL-8.[103–107] In intestine, subsequent events lead to chemotaxis, transmigration, and activation of leukocytes, and synthesis and release of many products from epithelial and

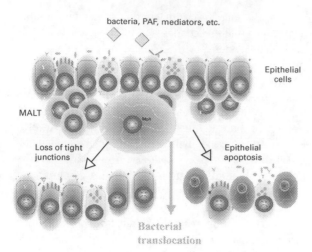

Figure 33.2. Hypothetical pathomechanism: effect of intraluminal ligands (bacteria, PAF, cytokine mediators, etc.) on intestinal epithelium leading to bacterial translocation.

inflammatory cells such as IL-6, IL-8, IL-10, IL-18, arachidonic acid metabolites, thromboxanes, leukotrienes, and prostaglandins, nitric oxide, endothelin-1, and oxygen-free radicals.[108–115] If counter-regulatory responses are insufficient (i.e., with decreased or absent IL-1 receptor antagonist, IL-11, IL-12, PAF-acetylhydrolase, etc.), pathologic changes to gut mucosa occur, and may include accentuated apoptosis of epithelial cells, perturbation of tight junctional proteins and complexes, increased mucosal permeability, bacterial translocation, alterations of vascular tone and microcirculation, and additional neutrophil infiltration and accumulation (Figure 33.2). The process may then be perpetuated by the activation of the secondary inflammatory response, and the final common pathway will result in intestinal necrosis. While these events remain localized in some cases, in others this activation results in the systemic inflammatory response syndrome, in which patients develop capillary leak, hypotension, metabolic acidosis, thrombocytopenia, renal failure, respiratory failure, and often, death.[116]

Although endotoxin is a well-characterized activator of inflammation, additional factors may play a role in stimulating the NEC cascade in premature infants. Asphyxia and/or ischemia-reperfusion activates the early mediators of inflammation in many tissues including intestine. Neonatal animal studies have shown that the stress of formula feeding stimulates phospholipase A$_2$ gene expression, intestinal PAF production, and stimulation of apoptosis and the inflammatory response with resulting NEC.[102,117] Therefore, many of the purported risk factors for NEC may

activate the inflammatory response that results in the final common pathway described above.

The evidence suggests that the premature neonate may have an abnormal balance between pro- and anti-inflammatory mediator production, thereby increasing their predisposition for diseases such as NEC. PAF is a potent phospholipid inflammatory mediator that is associated with NEC in several experimental models and human analyses.[118–122] PAF infusion causes intestinal necrosis in animals, and PAF receptor antagonists prevent injury following hypoxia, endotoxin challenge, TNF infusion, and ischemia-reperfusion.[123–125] It has been shown that neonates are markedly deficient in their ability to degrade PAF due to decreased activity of the PAF-specific enzyme PAF-acetylhydrolase.[45] PAF-acetylhydrolase is present in breast milk but absent in commercial formula, and this may in part explain the beneficial effects of breast milk-feeding. IL-10 is an anti-inflammatory cytokine thought to be important in reducing intestinal inflammation and possibly NEC in animals and humans.[126,127] In neonatal rats, maternal milk feedings increased IL-10 and reduced the incidence of NEC, while in human milk specimens, a significant percentage of NEC patient-pairs were deficient in this important cytokine. Studies have compared proinflammatory response to endotoxin and/or IL-1 in different cell lines, and have found that IL-8 response is significantly higher in fetal intestinal epithelium compared with mature, adult intestine.[46] These results suggest that

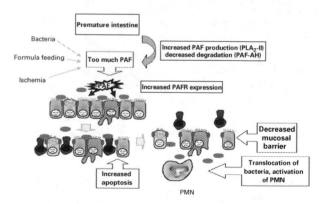

Figure 33.4. Model for NEC pathogenesis. In the premature animal (neonate) the risk factors of feeding, bacterial colonization, and altered intestinal blood flow increase platelet-activating factor (PAF) production via the PAF-synthesizing enzyme PLA$_2$-II. Since PAF degradation is deficient (low PAF-AH) in neonates, local PAF accumulates and activates PAF receptor on intestinal epithelium, leading to apoptosis, mucosal permeability, and bacterial translocation. PMN = Polymorphonuclear leucocyte.

the neonatal balance of the inflammatory response may be weighted towards the pro-inflammatory side and more likely to result in the pathologic outcome of NEC.

Although multiple mediators are implicated in the pathogenesis of NEC, the precise cellular mechanisms responsible for intestinal epithelial injury are less clear. Studies suggest that stimuli such as bacteria, PAF, and other mediators can bind to and activate intestinal epithelium, leading to signal transduction mechanisms that activate mucosal permeability, apoptosis, and pro-inflammatory gene transcription. In our neonatal rat model of asphyxia and formula stress, apoptosis is markedly accentuated following stress compared with control animals, and it appears that this event precedes necrosis (see color plate 33.3)*. Bacterial translocation occurs following loss of mucosal integrity, and the secondary inflammatory response is activated that ultimately leads to full-blown NEC accompanied by the systemic inflammatory response syndrome (Figure 33.4).

* Colour plates now on back cover.

Summary

In conclusion, NEC is a complex and poorly understood neonatal disease. Formula feeding, in the presence of prematurity, bacterial colonization, and intestinal ischemia/hypoxia stimulate a final common pathway that stimulates the inflammatory cascade and results in intestinal injury, and in some cases systemic disease and death. The premature infant differs from term infants and older patients in multiple ways, including the complex system of intestinal host defense, intestinal motility, bacterial colonization patterns, autoregulation of splanchnic blood flow, and the regulation of the inflammatory cascade. Since each case of NEC is different, and the importance of each of the complex factors may vary between cases, no single approach has been completely successful in preventing this dreaded disease. Although preventing prematurity would be the most successful approach to prevent NEC, several strategies have been tested in humans and animals. Nonetheless, no strategies have proven completely effective in reducing the incidence or severity of NEC. Future trials in high-risk premature infants will be needed to significantly reduce this morbidity and mortality that currently plagues neonatal intensive care units worldwide.

REFERENCES

1 Kliegman, R. M., Fanaroff, A. A. Necrotizing enterocolitis. *N. Engl. J. Med.* 1984;**310**:1093–103.

2 Vohr, B. R., Wright, L. L., Dusick, A. M. *et al.* Neurodevelopmental and functional outcomes of extremely low birth weight infants in the National Institute of Child Health and Human Development Neonatal Research Network, 1993–1994. *Pediatrics* 2000;**105**:1216–26.

3 Uauy, R. D., Fanaroff, A. A., Korones, S. B. *et al.* Necrotizing enterocolitis in very low birth weight infants: biodemographic and clinical correlates. National Institute of Child Health and Human Development Neonatal Research Network. *J. Pediatr.* 1991;**119**:630–8.

4 Walsh, M. C., Kliegman, R. M. Necrotizing enterocolitis: treatment based on staging criteria. *Pediatr. Clin. N. Am.* 1986;**33**:179–201.

5 Bell, M. J., Ternberg, J. L., Feigin, R. D. *et al.* Neonatal necrotizing enterocolitis. Therapeutic decisions based upon clinical staging. *Ann. Surg.* 1978;**187**:1–7.

6 Ballance, W. A., Dahms, B. B., Shenker, N., Kliegman, R. M. Pathology of neonatal necrotizing enterocolitis: a ten-year experience. *J. Pediatr.* 1990;**117**:S6–13.

7 Brown, E. G., Sweet, A. Y. Preventing necrotizing enterocolitis in neonates. *J. Am. Med. Assoc.* 1978;**240**:2452–4.

8 Dunn, L., Hulman, S., Weiner, J., Kliegman, R. Beneficial effects of early hypocaloric enteral feeding on neonatal gastrointestinal function: preliminary report of a randomized trial. *J. Pediatr.* 1988;**112**:622–9.

9 Troche, B., Harvey-Wilkes, K., Engle, W. D. *et al.* Early minimal feedings promote growth in critically ill premature infants. *Biol. Neonate* 1995;**67**:172–81.

10 Slagle, T. A., Gross, S. J. Effect of early low-volume enteral substrate on subsequent feeding tolerance in very low birth weight infants. *J. Pediatr.* 1988;**113**:526–31.

11 Stoll, B. J., Kanto, W. P. Jr, Glass, R. I., Nahmias, A. J., Brann, A. W. Jr. Epidemiology of necrotizing enterocolitis: a case control study. *J. Pediatr.* 1980;**96**:447–51.

12 Kamitsuka, M. D., Horton, M. K., Williams, M. A. The incidence of necrotizing enterocolitis after introducing standardized feeding schedules for infants between 1250 and 2500 grams and less than 35 weeks of gestation. *Pediatrics* 2000;**105**:379–84.

13 Tyson, J. E., Kennedy, K. A. Minimal enteral nutrition for promoting feeding tolerance and preventing morbidity in parenterally fed infants. *Cochrane Database Syst Rev.* 2000;CD001241.

14 Di Lorenzo, M., Bass, J., Krantis, A. An intraluminal model of necrotizing enterocolitis in the developing neonatal piglet. *J. Pediatr. Surg.* 1995;**30**:1138–42.

15 Caplan, M. S., Hedlund, E., Adler, L., Hsueh, W. Role of asphyxia and feeding in a neonatal rat model of necrotizing enterocolitis. *Pediatr. Pathol.* 1994;**14**:1017–28.

16 Lucas, A., Cole, T. J. Breast milk and neonatal necrotising enterocolitis [see comments]. *Lancet* 1990;**336**:1519–23.

17 Caplan, M. S., Russell, T., Xiao, Y. *et al.* Effect of polyunsaturated fatty acid (PUFA) supplementation on intestinal inflammation and necrotizing enterocolitis (NEC) in a neonatal rat model. *Pediatr. Res.* 2001;**49**:647–52.

18 Caplan, M. S., Lickerman, M., Adler, L., Dietsch, G. N., Yu, A. The role of recombinant platelet-activating factor

acetylhydrolase in a neonatal rat model of necrotizing enterocolitis. *Pediatr. Res.* 1997;**42**:779–83.

19 Dvorak, B., Halpern, M. D., Holubec, H. *et al.* Epidermal growth factor reduces the development of necrotizing enterocolitis in a neonatal rat model. *Am. J. Physiol. Gastrointest. Liver Physiol.* 2002;**282**:G156–64.

20 Pitt, J., Barlow, B., Heird, W. C. Protection against experimental necrotizing enterocolitis by maternal milk. I. Role of milk leukocytes. *Pediatr. Res.* 1977;**11**:906–9.

21 Carlson, S. E., Montalto, M. B., Ponder, D. L., Werkman, S. H., Korones, S. B. Lower incidence of necrotizing enterocolitis in infants fed a preterm formula with egg phospholipids. *Pediatr. Res.* 1998;**44**:491–8.

22 Eibl, M. M., Wolf, H. M., Furnkranz, H., Rosenkranz, A. Prevention of necrotizing enterocolitis in low-birth-weight infants by IgA–IgG feeding. *N. Engl. J. Med.* 1988;**319**:1–7.

23 Kliegman, R. M., Pittard, W. B., Fanaroff, A. A. Necrotizing enterocolitis in neonates fed human milk. *J. Pediatr.* 1979;**95**:450–3.

24 Willis, D. M., Chabot, J., Radde, I. C., Chance, G. W. Unsuspected hyperosmolality of oral solutions contributing to necrotizing enterocolitis in very-low-birth-weight infants. *Pediatrics* 1977;**60**:535–8.

25 White, K. C., Harkavy, K. L. Hypertonic formula resulting from added oral medications. *Am. J. Dis. Child.* 1982;**136**:931–3.

26 Butel, M. J., Roland, N., Hibert, A. *et al.* Clostridial pathogenicity in experimental necrotising enterocolitis in gnotobiotic quails and protective role of bifidobacteria. *J. Med. Microbiol.* 1998;**47**:391–9.

27 Clark, D. A., Thompson, J. E., Weiner, L. B. *et al.* Necrotizing enterocolitis: intraluminal biochemistry in human neonates and a rabbit model. *Pediatr. Res.* 1985;**19**:919–21.

28 Clark, D. A., Miller, M. J. Intraluminal pathogenesis of necrotizing enterocolitis. *J. Pediatr.* 1990;**117**:S64–7.

29 Schanler, R. J., Shulman, R. J., Lau, C., Smith, E. O., Heitkemper, M. M. Feeding strategies for premature infants: randomized trial of gastrointestinal priming and tube-feeding method [see comments]. *Pediatrics* 1999;**103**:434–9.

30 Ryder, R. W., Shelton, J. D., Guinan, M. E. Necrotizing enterocolitis: a prospective multicenter investigation. *Am. J. Epidemiol.* 1980;**112**:113–23.

31 Furlano, R. I., Walker, W. A. Immaturity of gastrointestinal host defense in newborns and gastrointestinal disease states. *Adv. Pediatr.* 1998;**45**:201–22.

32 Bines, J. E., Walker, W. A. Growth factors and the development of neonatal host defense. *Adv. Exp. Med. Biol.* 1991;**310**:31–9.

33 Walker, W. A. Role of nutrients and bacterial colonization in the development of intestinal host defense. *J. Pediatr. Gastroenterol. Nutr.* 2000;**30**:S2–7.

34 Berseth, C. L. Gestational evolution of small intestine motility in preterm and term infants. *J. Pediatr.* 1989;**115**:646–51.

35 Berseth, C. L. Neonatal small intestinal motility: motor responses to feeding in term and preterm infants. *J. Pediatr.* 1990;**117**:777–82.

36 Berseth, C. L. Gut motility and the pathogenesis of necrotizing enterocolitis. *Clin. Perinatol.* 1994;**21**:263–70.

37 Bueno, L., Ruckebusch, Y. Perinatal development of intestinal myoelectrical activity in dogs and sheep. *Am. J. Physiol.* 1979;**237**:E61–7.

38 Caplan, M. S., Miller-Catchpole, R., Kaup, S. *et al.* Bifidobacterial supplementation reduces the incidence of necrotizing enterocolitis in a neonatal rat model. *Gastroenterology* 1999;**117**:577–83.

39 Deitch, E. A. Role of bacterial translocation in necrotizing enterocolitis. *Acta Paediatr. Suppl.* 1994;**396**:33–6.

40 Duffy, L. C., Zielezny, M. A., Carrion, V. *et al.* Concordance of bacterial cultures with endotoxin and interleukin-6 in necrotizing enterocolitis. *Dig. Dis. Sci.* 1997;**42**:359–65.

41 Duffy, L. C., Zielezny, M. A., Carrion, V. *et al.* Bacterial toxins and enteral feeding of premature infants at risk for necrotizing enterocolitis. *Adv. Exp. Med. Biol.* 2001;**501**:519–27.

42 Nowicki, P. T., Miller, C. E. Autoregulation in the developing postnatal intestinal circulation. *Am. J. Physiol.* 1988;**254**:G189–93.

43 Nowicki, P. T., Nankervis, C. A., Miller, C. E. Effects of ischemia and reperfusion on intrinsic vascular regulation in the postnatal intestinal circulation. *Pediatr. Res.* 1993;**33**:400–4.

44 Nowicki, P. T. Effects of sustained flow reduction on postnatal intestinal circulation. *Am. J. Physiol.* 1998;**275**:G758–68.

45 Caplan, M., Hsueh, W., Kelly, A., Donovan, M. Serum PAF acetylhydrolase increases during neonatal maturation. *Prostaglandins* 1990;**39**:705–14.

46 Nanthakumar, N. N., Fusunyan, R. D., Sanderson, I., Walker, W. A. Inflammation in the developing human intestine: a possible pathophysiologic contribution to necrotizing enterocolitis. *Proc. Natl. Acad. Sci. USA.* 2000;**97**:6043–8.

47 Haller, D., Bode, C., Hammes, W. P. *et al.* Non-pathogenic bacteria elicit a differential cytokine response by intestinal epithelial cell/leucocyte co-cultures. *Gut* 2000;**47**:79–87.

48 Kagnoff, M. F. Immunology of the intestinal tract. *Gastroenterology* 1993;**105**:1275–80.

49 Laboisse, C. L. Structure of gastrointestinal mucins: searching for the Rosetta stone. *Biochimie* 1986;**68**:611–17.

50 Pang, K. Y., Bresson, J. L., Walker, W. A. Development of the gastrointestinal mucosal barrier V. Comparative effect of calcium binding on microvillus membrane structure in newborn and adult rats. *Pediatr. Res.* 1983;**17**:856–61.

51 Pang, K. Y., Bresson, J. L., Walker, W. A. Development of the gastrointestinal mucosal barrier. Evidence for structural differences in microvillus membranes from newborn and adult rabbits. *Biochim. Biophys. Acta.* 1983;**727**:201–8.

52 Pang, K. Y., Newman, A. P., Udall, J. N., Walker, W. A. Development of gastrointestinal mucosal barrier. VII. In utero maturation of microvillus surface by cortisone. *Am. J. Physiol.* 1985;**249**:G85–91.

53 Udall, J. N., Pang, K., Fritze, L., Kleinman, R., Walker, W. A. Development of gastrointestinal mucosal barrier. I. The effect of age on intestinal permeability to macromolecules. *Pediatr. Res.* 1981;**15**:241–4.

54 Udall, J. N. Jr. Gastrointestinal host defense and necrotizing enterocolitis. *J. Pediatr.* 1990;**117**:S33–43.

55 Hsueh, W., Caplan, M. S., Sun, X. *et al.* Platelet-activating factor, tumor necrosis factor, hypoxia and necrotizing enterocolitis. *Acta Paediatr. Suppl.* 1994;**396**:11–17.

56 Weaver, L. T., Laker, M. F., Nelson, R. Intestinal permeability in the newborn. *Arch. Dis. Child.* 1984;**59**:236–41.

57 Smith, S. D., Cardona, M. A., Wishnev, S. A., Kurkchubasche, A. G., Rowe, M. I. Unique characteristics of the neonatal intestinal mucosal barrier. *J. Pediatr. Surg.* 1992;**27**:333–8.

58 Snyder, J. D., Walker, W. A. Structure and function of intestinal mucin: developmental aspects. *Int. Arch. Allergy Appl. Immunol.* 1987;**82**:351–6.

59 Lin, J., Holzman, I. R., Jiang, P., Babyatsky, M. W. Expression of intestinal trefoil factor in developing rat intestine. *Biol. Neonate* 1999;**76**:92–7.

60 Sands, B. E., Podolsky, D. K. The trefoil peptide family. *Annu. Rev. Physiol.* 1996;**58**:253–73.

61 Tan, X. D., Hsueh, W., Chang, H., Wei, K. R., Gonzalez-Crussi, F. Characterization of a putative receptor for intestinal trefoil factor in rat small intestine: identification by in situ binding and ligand blotting. *Biochem. Biophys. Res. Commun.* 1997;**237**:673–7.

62 Salzman, N. H., Polin, R. A., Harris, M. C. *et al.* Enteric defensin expression in necrotizing enterocolitis. *Pediatr. Res.* 1998;**44**:20–6.

63 Ouellette, A. J. Paneth cells and innate immunity in the crypt microenvironment. *Gastroenterology* 1997;**113**:1779–84.

64 Guy-Grand, D., Griscelli, C., Vassalli, P. The mouse gut T lymphocyte, a novel type of T cell. Nature, origin, and traffic in mice in normal and graft-versus-host conditions. *J. Exp. Med.* 1978;**148**:1661–77.

65 Rieger, C. H., Rothberg, R. M. Development of the capacity to produce specific antibody to an ingested food antigen in the premature infant. *J. Pediatr.* 1975;**87**:515–18.

66 Perkkio, M., Savilahti, E. Time of appearance of immunoglobulin-containing cells in the mucosa of the neonatal intestine. *Pediatr. Res.* 1980;**14**:953–5.

67 Roberts, S. A., Freed, D. L. Neonatal IgA secretion enhanced by breast feeding. *Lancet* 1977;**2**:1131.

68 Villalpando, S., Hamosh, M. Early and late effects of breast-feeding: does breast-feeding really matter? *Biol. Neonate.* 1998;**74**:177–91.

69 Wold, A. E., Adlerberth, I. Breast feeding and the intestinal microflora of the infant – implications for protection against infectious diseases. *Adv. Exp. Med. Biol.* 2000;**478**:77–93.

70 Lee, W. J., Farmer, J. L., Hilty, M., Kim, Y. B. The protective effects of lactoferrin feeding against endotoxin lethal shock in germfree piglets. *Infect. Immun.* 1998;**66**:1421–6.

71 Neu, J., Roig, J. C., Meetze, W. H. *et al.* Enteral glutamine supplementation for very low birth weight infants decreases morbidity. *J. Pediatr.* 1997;**131**:691–9.

72 Neu, J., DeMarco, V., Li, N. Glutamine: clinical applications and mechanisms of action. *Curr. Opin. Clin. Nutr. Metab. Care* 2002;**5**:69–75.

73 Neurath, M. F., Fuss, I., Kelsall, B. L. *et al.* Experimental granulomatous colitis in mice is abrogated by induction of TGF-beta-mediated oral tolerance. *J. Exp. Med.* 1996;**183**:2605–16.

74 Riegler, M., Sedivy, R., Sogukoglu, T. *et al.* Effect of growth factors on epithelial restitution of human colonic mucosa in vitro. *Scand. J. Gastroenterol.* 1997;**32**:925–32.

75 Juul, S. E., Joyce, A. E., Zhao, Y., Ledbetter, D. J. Why is erythropoietin present in human milk? Studies of erythropoietin receptors on enterocytes of human and rat neonates. *Pediatr. Res.* 1999;**46**:263–8.

76 Ledbetter, D. J., Juul, S. E. Erythropoietin and the incidence of necrotizing enterocolitis in infants with very low birth weight. *J. Pediatr. Surg.* 2000;**35**:178–82.

77 Dai, D., Nanthkumar, N. N., Newburg, D. S., Walker, W. A. Role of oligosaccharides and glycoconjugates in intestinal host defense. *J. Pediatr. Gastroenterol. Nutr.* 2000;**30**:S23–33.

78 Tanaka, M., Lee, K., Martinez-Augustin, O. *et al.* Exogenous nucleotides alter the proliferation, differentiation and apoptosis of human small intestinal epithelium. *J. Nutr.* 1996;**126**:424–33.

79 Bisset, W. M., Watt, J. B., Rivers, R. P., Milla, P. J. Ontogeny of fasting small intestinal motor activity in the human infant. *Gut* 1988;**29**:483–8.

80 Lawrence, G., Bates, J., Gaul, A. Pathogenesis of neonatal necrotising enterocolitis. *Lancet* 1982;**1**:137–9.

81 Peter, C. S., Feuerhahn, M., Bohnhorst, B. *et al.* Necrotising enterocolitis: is there a relationship to specific pathogens? *Eur. J. Pediatr.* 1999;**158**:67–70.

82 Tomkins, A. M., Bradley, A. K., Oswald, S., Drasar, B. S. Diet and the faecal microflora of infants, children and adults in rural Nigeria and urban U.K. *J. Hyg. (Lond).* 1981;**86**:285–93.

83 Rubaltelli, F. F., Biadaioli, R., Pecile, P., Nicoletti, P. Intestinal flora in breast- and bottle-fed infants. *J. Perinat. Med.* 1998;**26**:186–91.

84 Gewolb, I. H., Schwalbe, R. S., Taciak, V. L., Harrison, T. S., Panigrahi, P. Stool microflora in extremely low birthweight infants. *Arch. Dis. Child. Fetal Neonatal Edn.* 1999;**80**:F167–73.

85 Mehall, J. R., Kite, C. A., Saltzman, D. A. *et al.* Prospective study of the incidence and complications of bacterial contamination of enteral feeding in neonates. *J. Pediatr. Surg.* 2002;**37**:1177-82.

86 Yoshimura, A., Lien, E., Ingalls, R. R. *et al.* Cutting edge: recognition of Gram-positive bacterial cell wall components by the innate immune system occurs via Toll-like receptor 2. *J. Immunol.* 1999;**163**:1–5.

87 Deitch, E. A., Specian, R. D., Berg, R. D. Endotoxin-induced bacterial translocation and mucosal permeability: role of xanthine oxidase, complement activation, and macrophage products. *Crit. Care Med.* 1991;**19**:785–91.

88 Birchler, T., Seibl, R., Buchner, K. *et al.* Human Toll-like receptor 2 mediates induction of the antimicrobial peptide human beta-defensin 2 in response to bacterial lipoprotein. *Eur. J. Immunol.* 2001;**31**:3131–7.

89 Panigrahi, P., Gupta, S., Gewolb, I. H., Morris, J. G. Jr. Occurrence of necrotizing enterocolitis may be dependent on patterns of bacterial adherence and intestinal colonization: studies in Caco-2 tissue culture and weanling rabbit models. *Pediatr. Res.* 1994;**36**:115–21.

90 Hoyos, A. B. Reduced incidence of necrotizing enterocolitis associated with enteral administration of *Lactobacillus acidophilus* and *Bifidobacterium infantis* to neonates in an intensive care unit. *Int. J. Infect. Dis.* 1999;**3**:197–202.

91 Alward, C. T., Hook, J. B., Helmrath, T. A., Mattson, J. C., Bailie, M. D. Effects of asphyxia on cardiac output and organ blood flow in the newborn piglet. *Pediatr. Res.* 1978;**12**:824–7.

92 Touloukian, R. J., Posch, J. N., Spencer, R. The pathogenesis of ischemic gastroenterocolitis of the neonate: selective gut mucosal ischemia in asphyxiated neonatal piglets. *J. Pediatr. Surg.* 1972;**7**:194–205.

93 Schoenberg, M. H., Beger, H. G. Reperfusion injury after intestinal ischemia. *Crit. Care. Med.* 1993;**21**:1376–86.

94 Crissinger, K. D. Animal models of necrotizing enterocolitis. *J. Pediatr. Gastroenterol. Nutr.* 1995;**20**:17–22.

95 Nankervis, C. A., Nowicki, P. T. Role of endothelin-1 in regulation of the postnatal intestinal circulation. *Am. J. Physiol. Gastrointest. Liver Physiol.* 2000;**278**:G367–75.

96 Nankervis, C. A., Nowicki, P. T. Role of nitric oxide in regulation of vascular resistance in postnatal intestine. *Am. J. Physiol.* 1995;**268**:G949–58.

97 Nowicki, P. T., Hansen, N. B., Hayes, J. R., Menke, J. A., Miller, R. R. Intestinal blood flow and O_2 uptake during hypoxemia in the newborn piglet. *Am. J. Physiol.* 1986;**251**:G19–24.

98 Nowicki, P. T., Minnich, L. A. Effects of systemic hypotension on postnatal intestinal circulation: role of angiotensin. *Am. J. Physiol.* 1999;**276**:G341–52.

99 Reber, K. M., Nankervis, C. A., Nowicki, P. T. Newborn intestinal circulation. Physiology and pathophysiology. *Clin. Perinatol.* 2002;**29**:23–39.

100 Nankervis, C. A., Reber, K. M., Nowicki, P. T. Age-dependent changes in the postnatal intestinal microcirculation. *Microcirculation* 2001;**8**:377–87.

101 Caplan, M. S., MacKendrick, W. Inflammatory mediators and intestinal injury. *Clin. Perinatol.* 1994;**21**:235–46.

102 Caplan, M. S., Jilling, T. New concepts in necrotizing enterocolitis. *Curr. Opin. Pediatr.* 2001;**13**:111–15.

103 O'Neill, L. A. The interleukin-1 receptor/Toll-like receptor superfamily: signal transduction during inflammation and host defense. *Sci. STKE.* 2000;**2000**:RE1.

104 Medzhitov, R. Toll-like receptors and innate immunity. *Nature Rev. Immunol.* 2001;**1**:135–45.

105 Read, R. C., Wyllie, D. H. Toll receptors and sepsis. *Curr. Opin. Crit. Care.* 2001;**7**:371–5.

106 Tracey, K. J., Beutler, B., Lowry, S. F. *et al.* Shock and tissue injury induced by recombinant human cachectin. *Science* 1986;**234**:470–4.

107 Benveniste, J. PAF-acether, an ether phospho-lipid with biological activity. *Prog. Clin. Biol. Res.* 1988;**282**:73–85.

108 Hsueh, W., Gonzalez-Crussi, F., Arroyave, J. L. Sequential release of leukotrienes and norepinephrine in rat bowel after platelet-activating factor. A mechanistic study of platelet-activating factor-induced bowel necrosis. *Gastroenterology* 1988;**94**:1412–18.

109 Hsueh, W., Gonzalez-Crussi, F., Arroyave, J. L. Release of leukotriene C4 by isolated, perfused rat small intestine in response to platelet-activating factor. *J. Clin. Invest.* 1986;**78**:108–14.

110 Cueva, J. P., Hsueh, W. Role of oxygen derived free radicals in platelet activating factor induced bowel necrosis. *Gut* 1988;**29**:1207–12.

111 Ford, H., Watkins, S., Reblock, K., Rowe, M. The role of inflammatory cytokines and nitric oxide in the pathogenesis of necrotizing enterocolitis. *J. Pediatr. Surg.* 1997;**32**:275–82.

112 Hammerman, C., Goldschmidt, D., Caplan, M. S. *et al.* Amelioration of ischemia-reperfusion injury in rat intestine by pentoxifylline-mediated inhibition of xanthine oxidase. *J. Pediatr. Gastroenterol. Nutr.* 1999;**29**:69–74.

113 Wallace, J. L., Cirino, G., McKnight, G. W., Elliott, S. N. Reduction of gastrointestinal injury in acute endotoxic shock by flurbiprofen nitroxybutylester. *Eur. J. Pharmacol.* 1995;**280**:63–8.

114 Tan, X., Sun, X., Gonzalez-Crussi, F. X., Gonzalez-Crussi, F., Hsueh, W. PAF and TNF increase the precursor of NF-kappa B p50 mRNA in mouse intestine: quantitative analysis by competitive PCR. *Biochim. Biophys. Acta.* 1994;**1215**:157–62.

115 Sun, X., Rozenfeld, R. A., Qu, X. *et al.* P-selectin-deficient mice are protected from PAF-induced shock, intestinal injury, and lethality. *Am. J. Physiol.* 1997;**273**:G56–61.

116 Takakuwa, T., Endo, S., Inada, K. *et al.* Assessment of inflammatory cytokines, nitrate/nitrite, type II phospholipase A2, and soluble adhesion molecules in systemic inflammatory response syndrome. *Res. Commun. Mol. Pathol. Pharmacol.* 1997;**98**:43–52.

117 Caplan, M. S., Hedlund, E., Adler, L., Lickerman, M., Hsueh, W. The platelet-activating factor receptor antagonist WEB 2170 prevents neonatal necrotizing enterocolitis in rats. *J. Pediatr. Gastroenterol. Nutr.* 1997;**24**:296–301.

118 Caplan, M. S., Sun, X. M., Hseuh, W., Hageman, J. R. Role of platelet activating factor and tumor necrosis factor-alpha in neonatal necrotizing enterocolitis. *J. Pediatr.* 1990;**116**:960–4.

119 Caplan, M. S., Sun, X. M., Hsueh, W. Hypoxia, PAF, and necrotizing enterocolitis. *Lipids* 1991;**26**:1340–3.

120 Hsueh, W., Gonzalez-Crussi, F., Arroyave, J. L. Platelet-activating factor-induced ischemic bowel necrosis. An investigation of secondary mediators in its pathogenesis. *Am. J. Pathol.* 1986;**122**:231–9.

121 Gonzalez-Crussi, F., Hsueh, W. Experimental model of ischemic bowel necrosis. The role of platelet-activating factor and endotoxin. *Am. J. Pathol.* 1983;**112**:127–35.

122 Rabinowitz, S. S., Dzakpasu, P., Piecuch, S. *et al.* Platelet-activating factor in infants at risk for necrotizing enterocolitis. *J. Pediatr* 2001;**138**:81–6.

123 Mozes, T., Braquet, P., Filep, J. Platelet-activating factor: an endogenous mediator of mesenteric ischemia-reperfusion-induced shock. *Am. J. Physiol.* 1989;**257**: R872–7.

124 Sun, X. M., Hsueh, W. Bowel necrosis induced by tumor necrosis factor in rats is mediated by platelet-activating factor. *J. Clin. Invest.* 1988;**81**:1328–31.

125 Caplan, M. S., Sun, X. M., Hsueh, W. Hypoxia causes ischemic bowel necrosis in rats: the role of platelet-activating factor (PAF-acether). *Gastroenterology* 1990;**99**:979–86.

126 Edelson, M. B., Bagwell, C. E., Rozycki, H. J. Circulating pro- and counterinflammatory cytokine levels and severity in necrotizing enterocolitis. *Pediatrics* 1999;**103**:766–71.

127 Lindsay, J. O., Ciesielski, C. J., Scheinin, T., Hodgson, H. J., Brennan, F. M. The prevention and treatment of murine colitis using gene therapy with adenoviral vectors encoding IL-10. *J. Immunol.* 2001;**166**:7625–33.

34

Neonatal short bowel syndrome

Judith Sondheimer

Division of Gastroenterology, The Children's Hospital, Denver, CO.

Neonatal short bowel syndrome (SBS) is a diagnosis with three major elements. The neonate has a shortened small intestine, either congenital or via surgical resection, has intestinal malabsorption to a degree that standard feeding practices cannot support normal growth, and requires intravenous nutrition (IVN) support for a "significant" period. Some authors state that the diagnostic criterion for neonatal short bowel syndrome is the loss of 50% of the small intestine.[1,2] Several factors make this definition inappropriate. Intestinal resection in the neonate is usually a surgical emergency. In this setting, measurements of the resected and remaining intestine may not be made or may be inaccurate because of bowel necrosis, edema, and adhesions. Factors other than the length of residual bowel also have an impact on the neonate's subsequent dependence on IVN. The anatomic area of bowel resected, the presence or absence of the ileocecal valve and colon, the viability of the remaining intestine and associated medical and surgical problems all have an impact on intestinal absorptive function that might produce intestinal insufficiency even after a modest resection.

The causes of neonatal short bowel syndrome are fairly predictable but the relative frequency depends upon the patient population of the individual center providing the statistics (Table 34.1). Most series of neonates and infants report four major causes – neonatal necrotizing enterocolitis (NEC), mid-gut volvulus, intestinal atresias, and gastroschisis. In most nurseries, NEC accounts for about 50% of all cases of neonatal SBS, with volvulus, atresia, and gastroschisis accounting together for about 40%. The remaining 10% is made up of more unusual causes such as meconium peritonitis, extensive intestinal angiomata or lymphangiomata, congenital short bowel, intussusception, severe motility disorders, trauma and vascular accidents.[3–8]

Pathophysiology

The basic problem of the infant with short bowel syndrome is the loss of intestinal absorbing surface. The length of the newborn intestine is not clearly established. Whether measurements taken during abdominal surgery or at autopsy reflect accurately the length of the healthy intestine in situ is debated. Autopsy measurements indicate that the small intestine length is 115 cm ± 21 cm (mean ± SD) in the fetus between 19 and 27 weeks' gestation and that the intestine doubles in length during the last trimester. Autopsy measurements estimate the normal newborn intestinal length at 248 cm ± 40.[13] The diameter of the newborn small intestine is estimated to be 1.5 cm. In adults by contrast, the small bowel length is estimated to be between 600–1500 cm with a diameter of 3–4 cm. There appears to be a direct relationship between crown heel length and intestinal length in normal infants from 32 weeks' gestation through 3–4 years of age. Beyond 3–4 years, the relationship between height and small bowel length has not been determined. However, the rate of intestinal lengthening clearly levels off at about 3–4 years of age (Figure 34.1).[14] Urban and Weser have shown a direct relationship between the mucosal surface area and the body weight and surface area.[15] The absorbing surface of 1 cm^2 of intestine is roughly 600 cm^2, as a result of the villi and microvilli of the mucosal surface. It has been estimated that the neonate must absorb 1 kcal through every 2 cm^2 of mucosal surface while the adult has 3.5 cm^2 of surface area available for the absorption of every kcal.[1]

Neonatal Nutrition and Metabolism. Second Edition, ed. P. Thureen and W. Hay. Published by Cambridge University Press.
© Cambridge University Press 2006.

Table 34.1. Causes of neonatal short bowel syndrome

Surgical resection
   Necrotizing enterocolitis
   Congenital small bowel atresias
     Multiple jejunal and/or ileal
     Christmas tree/apple peel deformity
   Midgut volvulus
     Congenital, secondary to intestinal malrotation
     Secondary to adhesive bands either congenital or acquired
   Gastroschisis
     Associated small bowel obstruction and necrosis
     Associated small bowel atresias
   Meconium ileus
   Vascular thrombosis of mesenteric arteries or veins
     Sepsis with coagulopathy
     Hypercoagulability syndromes
   Trauma
   Radiation enteritis with ischemia
Congenital
Congenital short bowel syndrome [9–11]
Absence of critical intestinal function resulting in resection
   Total intestinal aganglionosis [12]
   Intestinal dysmotility syndromes – intestinal pseudo-obstruction
   Microvillous inclusion disease

Digestive and absorptive functions are not evenly distributed along the intestinal length. The mucosal villi of the jejunum are longer with a greater absorbing surface than those of the ileum. The duodenum and jejunum are the main sites for digestion and/or absorption of carbohydrate, fat, protein, and fluid. Mucosal disaccharidases and peptidases are found in higher concentration in the jejunal enterocytes than they are distally. The majority of electrolytes, minerals, and vitamins are absorbed in the proximal small bowel. In the intact intestine, the ileum plays a lesser role in these same jejunal functions. The ileum is the primary site for active absorption of vitamin B_{12} and conjugated bile salts. The ileocecal valve controls the passage of small bowel contents into the colon. The release of ileal contents is in part hormonally mediated in response to the concentration of nutrients in the ileal lumen. Delayed release into the colon may be important in providing time for ileal mucosal absorption of nutrients malabsorbed proximally. The ileocecal valve is also a barrier against contamination of the small bowel by colon organisms. The colon is a key site for the retrieval of salt and water if their absorption has been inadequate in the small bowel. The colon is capable of absorbing free fatty acids, the end product of bacterial fermentation of unabsorbed carbohydrate, and thus may salvage carbohydrate calories lost through small intestinal malabsorption.[16–18]

Resection of the jejunum removes the site of maximum transport of hydrolyzed protein, fat, and carbohydrate as well as fluid, electrolytes, minerals and all vitamins but B_{12}. The major nutritional complication of loss of the jejunum is generalized malabsorption with calorie deficiency. Specific nutritional deficiencies may occur when the ileum fails to compensate adequately for one of the jejunal functions. The jejunum is the principal site of iron absorption. The ileum may not completely compensate for the absent jejunum in absorption of iron, possibly because the higher pH of its contents puts the iron into the poorly absorbed ferric state. Calcium and magnesium deficiency may be a secondary result of fat malabsorption associated with jejunal resection. Fat malabsorption increases the luminal concentration of fatty acids, which form insoluble soaps with dietary calcium and magnesium. These cannot be absorbed by the ileum and thus calcium and magnesium are lost in the stool.

Loss of the ileum leads to three major nutritional sequelae. The first is vitamin B_{12} deficiency. Active transport of intrinsic-factor-bound B_{12} occurs only in the ileum. The jejunum is unable to adapt to this function. Some passive transport of B_{12} does occur in the jejunum, but it may be insufficient to maintain hepatic stores. Although B_{12} deficiency is not generally a problem in neonates because of their large hepatic reserves, anemia and neurologic sequelae may be late, unanticipated complications of ileal resection, even when no other nutritional deficits are apparent.[19,20]

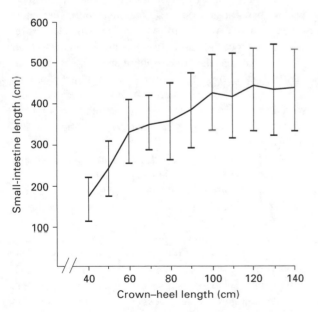

Figure 34.1. Small-intestine length v. crown-heel length (mean±SD). Autopsy study of children without bowel disease. Reproduced with permission.[14]

Second, active bile salt transport is a specific function of the ileum which cannot be performed by the jejunum whose cells lack bile salt receptors. When unabsorbed in the ileum, conjugated bile salts reach the colon where they undergo bacterial deconjugation and dehydroxylation, producing dihydroxy bile acids. These abnormal bile acids provoke fluid and electrolyte secretion by the colon. Fecal losses of malabsorbed conjugated bile salts deplete the bile acid pool, impairing fat absorption and increasing the potential for cholelithiasis by producing a lithogenic bile with low bile salt concentration. In some series of neonatal short bowel patients, 15%–25% of patients eventually develop cholelithiasis.[21,22] Steatorrhea from inadequate bile salt pool results in an increased concentration of unabsorbed long chain fatty acids in the colon. These fatty acids are hydroxylated by colon flora and can stimulate fluid secretion by the colon.

Finally, ileal resection is associated with hyperoxaluria and nephrolithiasis. Normally, dietary oxalate combines with calcium in the intestinal lumen forming insoluble calcium oxalate, which is then excreted in the stool. After terminal ileal resection, the reduced bile acid pool size impairs micellar solubilization and absorption of fatty acids. Fatty acids then complex with intraluminal calcium, increasing the concentration of free oxalate in the intestinal lumen and increasing its absorption. Hyperoxaluria results and promotes the formation of oxalate stones.[23,24]

Adaptation to small bowel resection

The key to survival after massive small intestinal resection is the ability of the small bowel to accommodate for the loss of absorbing surface area. It is convenient to view the process of adaptation in the neonate with short bowel syndrome as consisting of three stages – early, intermediate, and late.

The early phase of adaptation has been the most intensively studied probably because it lends itself to animal models. The changes in this phase, characterized by hypertrophy (increased in tissue or organ size) and hyperplasia (increase in cell number) of the residual intestine, are complete within 3–6 months of the resection. Whether these changes are the most critical factor in the neonate's eventual freedom from nutrition support is not established. Hypertrophy and hyperplasia of the residual intestine begin within 48 hours of partial intestinal resection. Anatomic changes include lengthening of the villi, deepening of the crypts, an increased number of enterocytes per villus and thickening of the entire wall of the intestine including the muscular layers.[25] Indicators such as mucosal dry weight, protein, and DNA per centimeter have been used to document the increases in mucosal mass per centimeter of intestine.[26] Glucose and fluid absorption per centimeter also increases. The ileum, which normally has fairly short villi, has a greater capacity for these adaptive changes than does the jejunum. Exposure of the intestinal mucosa to enteral nutrients, particularly glucose, provides fuel for the adaptive hyperplasia. Without enteral nutrition, the hyperplastic changes are blunted.[27–29] Immediately after intestinal resection in the rat, the amount of mRNA from the proapoptotic gene, *Bax*, increases and that of the prosurvival gene, *Bcl-w*, decreases suggesting that there is an immediate change in the balance between enterocyte apoptosis and survival in the intestinal mucosa which favors increased cell proliferation.[30] Biliary and pancreatic secretions also induce ileal mucosal hyperplasia, possibly via the epidermal growth factor they contain.[31] Intravenous administration of secretin and cholecystokinin, which increase pancreato-biliary secretions, also induces hyperplasia in residual intestine in part by increasing the contact of the bowel with these trophic secretions. Even when pancreatic and biliary secretions are diverted however, intravenous secretin and CCK induce mucosal hyperplastic changes.[32] The absorptive capacity and enzyme activity of each enterocyte are probably either unchanged or decreased in this process of rapid cell proliferation. However, the total absorptive capacity of the residual intestine increases because of the increase in cell number per centimeter.

In other experiments, it has been found that the blood of animals subjected to intestinal resection contains elements which when transfused into unoperated controls stimulate intestinal hypertrophy. If the animals undergoing resection do not receive enteral feedings postoperatively, their blood does not contain the trophic elements. These experiments suggest that enteral nutrition is not only a luminal stimulant for intestinal adaptation, but also that it induces secretion of hormones that stimulate the process.[33] Over the years, a large body of research has identified some of these hormones.[34]

Enteroglucagon and enteroglucagon-like substances were the first to be identified as hormonal stimulants to intestinal adaptation.[35,36] Released in large quantities from the ileal mucosa of animals with proximal small bowel resection, these hormones produce the typical hyperplastic changes of adaptation when administered intravenously to control animals. Antibodies to enteroglucagon do not prevent the adaptive changes, so the assumption is that enteroglucagon-like substances, not enteroglucagon itself, are the mediators of the process.[37,38] Proglucagon mRNA is found in large amounts in the residual bowel of animals after intestinal resection.[39] Peptide YY blood levels also increase after intestinal resection. This compound may promote hypertrophy but also slows intestinal transit in the ileum and may promote better absorption by increasing exposure time in the ileum.[40–42] Gastrin levels often increase after intestinal resection and in a small proportion of humans with proximal small bowel resection, hypergastrinemia may produce clinically significant hyperacidity.[43] Gastrin is a trophic hormone. However, the hypertrophic changes associated with gastrin are mainly in the stomach and upper small bowel. Pharmacologic doses are necessary to produce mucosal hypertrophy in the ileum, suggesting that hypergastrinemia is not an adaptive hormonal response to intestinal resection.[44,45]

Other hormones both of GI and extra GI origin induce mucosal hyperplasia and perhaps offer therapeutic options to maximize the residual intestine's adaptation to resection. It is unlikely that these substances are part of the natural adaptive process, however, as their blood and tissue levels do not increase after intestinal resection. Growth hormone binds to receptors in the intestinal mucosa, stimulating calcium absorption, crypt cell division and gastrin and IGF-1 secretion. Although these effects could possibly promote intestinal function, there is little support for the initial enthusiasm for growth hormone as a therapy for SBS, especially in neonates.[46–48] In adult short bowel patients, growth hormone has been associated with improved weight gain, but this may simply reflect edema.[49,50] Furthermore, it is unclear whether the beneficial effect of growth hormone reported in some patients persists after the course of growth hormone ends. Patients with massive small bowel resection have been found to have low serum IGF-1 and IGFBP-1 levels suggesting that these substances might be markers for intestinal failure.[51] Whether normalizing the serum levels promotes bowel adaptation is unclear. IGF-1 does stimulate proliferation of enterocytes in vitro. Receptors for IGF-1 are present in crypt cells. In rats with intestinal resection, exogenous IGF-1 causes duodenal and jejunal hyperplasia and increased ileal disaccharidase activity.[52,53] Glucagon-like peptide 2, which is released from the ileum in response to meals, is also reduced in the blood of animals with SBS.[39,54,55] There is no information about glucagon-like peptide use in inducing mucosal hyperplasia in humans. Epidermal growth factor is present in pancreato-biliary secretions and perhaps is the mediator for the trophic effects of these secretions. EGF is required for stimulating polyamine synthesis without which cell proliferation cannot occur.[56–58] Keratinocyte growth factor has also been used to stimulate mucosal hyperplasia in experimental animals.[59] The cytokine interleukin-11 has also been shown to stimulate intestinal cellular proliferation.[60]

There has been a search for specific enteral nutrients that promote mucosal hypertrophy. Research into the effects of diet in animal models of short bowel syndrome indicate that long-chain fats have a hyperplastic effect superior to short-chain fats, protein, and carbohydrate, possibly through a specific effect on the stimulation of peptide YY production.[61] Menhaden oil, a long-chain, polyunsaturated fish oil, is more trophic than the saturated long-chain fats.[62] Dietary glutamine functions as a direct small intestinal fuel and also prevents bacterial translocation to portal lymph nodes from the intestine. Its function as an agent for stimulating intestinal mucosal hypertrophy is not supported by experimental data.[63–66] Soluble plant fibers such as pectin are fermented to short-chain fatty acids – butyric, propionic, and acetic acid – in the colon. These compounds are important luminal fuel for colon enterocytes. Their presence may improve retrieval of water and electrolyte in the colon and may thus change the fluidity of the stool. However, fiber probably has little effect on stimulating mucosal hypertrophy.[67] Some experimental data support an effect of intravenously administered short-chain fatty acids on mucosal hypertrophy.[68,69]

The intense research into the immediate mucosal hyperplastic process after intestinal resection has resulted in an appreciation of the importance of luminal nutrition to the adaptive process. There is often a sense of urgency about introducing enteral "trophic" feedings to infants after intestinal resection. It should be stressed that although failure to establish enteral feedings directly after intestinal resection may delay mucosal hyperplasia, no permanent loss of adaptive potential occurs if feedings cannot be introduced immediately after surgery. Just as intestinal mucosal atrophy occurs any time feedings are withheld, mucosal hypertrophy can be induced at any time after resection by starting feedings.

The intermediate phase of intestinal adaptation commonly is said to involve two processes – gradual dilation of the residual intestine and a gradual increase in intestinal transit time.[26] This process can be seen on the radiographs of patients with neonatal short bowel syndrome and the changes are usually complete within the first 18 months after resection. The potential adaptive advantage of these changes is that dilation and delayed transit maximizes the contact of the intestinal mucosa with luminal contents and thus improves nutrient absorption.[70] There is some experimental evidence to support this supposition. However, there are many phenomena associated with dilation of the small bowel and delayed transit time that are probably counterproductive. Dilation and slow transit might promote small bowel bacterial overgrowth with subsequent adverse events such as bacterial translocation, deconjugation of bile acids, d-lactic acidemia, and hydroxylation of fatty acids. More research is needed to prove whether these two processes that characterize the gut in the first 18 months after resection are truly adaptive.

In contrast to adults who undergo massive small bowel loss, there is a late adaptation to intestinal resection in infants that dramatically improves their outlook. In a word, as infants grow in height, their bowel grows in length. Bowel length has been shown to increase pari passu with height, at least until the age of 3–4 years, and possibly beyond.[14] Residual bowel length does not increase in adults. Furthermore, as the child grows in height and weight, the calorie requirement per kg body weight or per cm^2 of body surface decreases. Thus, the requirement for calorie absorption per surface area of intestine decreases as the child grows. The key to this late adaptive process is the maintenance of normal growth and nutrition and the prevention of complications of therapy that hinder growth. It is not clear whether there is a time limit on late intestinal adaptation. Most studies report that the process of adaptation appears to decrease as the child reaches 3–5 years.[8] Clinicians will predict that if a child hasn't "gotten off TPN" by age 5, he/she never will. This observation does not always prove true, but is consistent with the observation that the velocity of bowel lengthening seems to plateau at about this age. Other studies have indicated that the premature infants may have a small advantage in late adaptation, presumably since they have a greater potential for bowel elongation than term infants. The intestine naturally doubles in length during the last trimester of gestation.[13] The implication is that a centimeter of residual bowel in a premature infant may have more potential for elongation than a centimeter of bowel in a term neonate.

Medical management

The initial medical care of the neonate with a short bowel centers on the careful assessment and replacement of fluids and electrolytes. Losses of sodium, potassium, calcium, phosphorus, magnesium, and zinc may be massive through diarrhea and particularly via stoma losses. Initiation of IV nutrition, which provides calorie, mineral, and vitamin needs and replaces losses, is critical. It is rare that peripheral intravenous alimentation is adequate for these neonates, and an immediate use of central alimentation is recommended.

Even in the absence of enteral feedings, the losses of fluid and electrolyte from stomas or per rectum may be great as a consequence of residual inflammation, post obstructive secretory diarrhea and the immediate failure of distal small bowel or colon to adapt to the increased demand for absorption of normal proximal small intestinal secretions.

It is estimated that the zinc losses from a jejunostomy may double an infant's daily requirements.

The sodium losses in stoma or stool may be as high as 140 mEq L^{-1}. Routine measurement of Na, K, Cl, and Zn in stool or stoma assists in the calculation of intravenous fluids. The large electrolyte and fluid losses from small bowel stomas are a major reason that continuity between the proximal portion of bowel and the distal portion should be re-established as soon as possible. The colon plays a critical role in the salvage of water and sodium in these patients.[71–73]

Although the ability to deliver adequate nutrition to neonates with SBS via central venous lines is the single most important factor in the improved survival of these infants since the 1970s, it is also the major source of the morbidity associated with their long-term care. A major consideration for personnel in neonatal units is the prevention of catheter-related sepsis. Any fever in a patient with SBS and a central venous line should be considered line sepsis until proven otherwise, and immediate broad-spectrum antibiotics instituted to prevent the devastating immediate and long-term effects of bacterial or fungal sepsis. Coverage for Gram-positive and Gram-negative bacteria should be routinely used until culture results are available. The central line must be kept infection-free by meticulous care of the IV tubing, connectors and skin dressings, and a medication regimen that minimizes entry into the line. The best way to treat sepsis related to a central venous line is to remove the line. However, in the patient with SBS who may be dependent upon central venous nutrition for many years, hasty removal of the central line should be avoided. Many episodes of bacterial sepsis can be treated without removal of the central line. Fungal sepsis almost always requires removal of the line.

Other sources of infection should be aggressively sought in the neonate with SBS who develops fever. Surgical and medical staff should remain aware of whether the original surgery was performed in the setting of bowel hypoperfusion or perforation. Late development of abdominal abscess or stricture may be the source of recurrent fever and infection without positive blood cultures. Abdominal wound cellulitis should be investigated and aggressively treated rather than observed and treated locally as it may be a manifestation of underlying abdominal sepsis. Early septic events seem to be linked to the gradual development of hepatic failure in neonates with SBS.[21] Prevention and rapid effective therapy of infection is critical in this early stage.

There is no firm guideline on how to introduce enteral feedings to an infant with short bowel syndrome. The first step is to assess the absorptive deficit of the patient. The child who has only lost 50 cm of mid small bowel and has an intact colon may be expected to tolerate enteral feedings given by mouth with fewer complications than the patient with 50 cm of jejunum ending in a jejunostomy. Feeding an infant with SBS requires daily assessment of the child's "tolerance." This loosely defined parameter includes the volume of stool output relative to enteral intake, the electrolyte losses in stool or stoma, abdominal distension, emesis, the presence of unabsorbed carbohydrate (reducing substances) in the stool, and the state of the perianal skin. Daily small increases in the amount of enteral feeding given to the neonate who appears to tolerate feedings will allow staff to gradually achieve the goal of maximal utilization of the infant's residual absorbing surface without creating fluid and electrolyte problems secondary to malabsorption. As long as intravenous nutrition can be administered in an uninterrupted fashion, a gradual approach to the advancement of feedings is safe and prevents complications.

Enteral feedings should be initiated as soon as postoperative ileus has resolved and the condition of the neonate is stable. Choice of delivery route (oral, nasogastric, gastrostomy) and the frequency of feeding (intermittent bolus or continuous drip) depend in part on the length of the remaining small bowel. In patients with greater than 75% loss of the small bowel, continuous enteral feedings by drip appear to be the most effective method to maximize the absorptive capacity of the intestine without unduly tiring the patient by frequent feedings.[74] Patients with more than 25% residual small bowel may do well with small bolus feedings by mouth. As the patient demonstrates tolerance of feedings, small boluses may be given to the patient with extensive resections.

The choice of formula depends on many considerations. Any enteral nutrition will stimulate the early mucosal adaptation, even simple glucose. Studies in rats indicate that a diet containing polyunsaturated long-chain fats is more trophic than diets containing short-chain or saturated fat. There are no clear guidelines as to the most trophic protein or carbohydrate formulation. Clearly other considerations must be taken into account in choosing a formula. Lactose is poorly tolerated in neonates with extensive small bowel loss because of the decrease in available mucosal lactase. An acid watery diarrhea may result in SBS patients after lactose ingestion. The intestinal reserves of sucrase and maltase are greater suggesting that these carbohydrates might be better hydrolyzed and absorbed. Glucose requires no hydrolysis, however, the osmotic load of glucose may in itself result in excessive fluid loss. Assessment of fecal reducing substances may help guide the choice of carbohydrate. The impact of glucose polymers in inducing a carbohydrate-driven diarrhea may

be underestimated by measurement of stool-reducing substances, since long-chain glucose polymers may only contain one reducing equivalent per chain. In fact, however, general experience indicates that glucose polymers are probably the best tolerated of the carbohydrate sources in formula.

Fat intake must often be limited in infants with SBS to prevent diarrhea, regardless of its potential trophic effects. Loss of absorptive area, rapid transit, bile acid depletion, reduced pancreatic enzyme release and bacterial overgrowth all contribute to fat malabsorption. Long-chain fats are the least efficiently absorbed nutrient in the small intestine. Medium-chain triglycerides (MCT) are better absorbed since micellar solubilization by bile acids is not required for their absorption. However, the trophic effects of long-chain fats must be considered and therefore, a formula that uses a combination of LCT and MCT, or one that at least contains a small amount of LCT, may be the appropriate choice. Essential fatty acid (EFA) deficiency is now rare in SBS patients because of the administration of intravenous lipid emulsions and enriched oral preparations (Microlipid). EFAs administered by the intravenous route do not produce the same serum levels as enterally absorbed EFAs. Thus, the intravenous dose of EFA may be higher than the recommended daily allowance (RDA) for enterally absorbed EFA.[75]

Protein is better tolerated than other nutrients, probably because the relative amount of protein in infant formulas is not enough to overload intestinal digestive capacity and produce osmotic diarrhea. In addition, unabsorbed protein and peptides are not fermented in the colon, as are fats and carbohydrates. Partially or completely hydrolyzed proteins are possibly better absorbed than whole proteins in the face of reduced absorptive surface area and decreased pancreatic enzyme output. Oligopeptides with 2–5 amino acids mimic the protein fragments encountered by the healthy small bowel during normal digestion and absorption and appear to be easily hydrolyzed by brush-border peptidases. Simple amino acids, such as those in elemental formulas, require no hydrolysis but do require specific carriers for absorption. Free amino acids increase the osmolality of a formula and may produce diarrhea. If an elemental formula is chosen, attention must be given to the composition of the amino acids. For example, glutamine appears to be the preferred fuel for enterocytes of the small bowel, and may be necessary for repair of damaged intestinal mucosa. Given enterally, it appears to decrease bacterial translocation and in some studies, the rate of bacterial sepsis. Most recent studies do not suggest that glutamine plays a major role in the adaptive process of mucosal hyperplasia however. It has been the observation of many pediatric gastroenterologists that infants with SBS seem to have an increased incidence of immediate allergic reactions to intact protein, especially cow's milk. Avoidance of cow's milk protein may be a judicious preventative measure, although there is little but observation to back up this measure.[76,77]

The best formula for feeding infants with SBS has not been identified. Breast milk is rich in growth factors such as epidermal growth factor and insulin-like growth factor, but its digestive complexity often results in significant malabsorption.[78] Elemental formulas induce early mucosal adaptation predominantly in the proximal intestine where they are almost completely absorbed. Less malabsorbed nutrient reaches the colon to stimulate salt and water secretion. These formulas are usually deficient in essential fatty acid content and the patient may require supplements if he/she is not simultaneously receiving intravenous lipids. In one clinical study, SBS patients with 30–150 cm of small bowel were fed a diet of polysaccharides, MCT oil, protein hydrolysates, and a high-viscosity tapioca starch by continuous slow enteral drip commencing 14 days postoperatively.[79] Because this diet was well tolerated, the authors concluded that completely elemental diets were not better than polymeric diets. The most commonly selected formulas contain protein hydrolysates, MCT oil, and glucose polymers. It is prudent to initiate feedings at one-half to one-quarter strength, using small amounts, either by bolus or drip, critically assessing the infant's tolerance within 24–48 hours. Strength and volume may then be increased. There is no agreement on whether the patient with SBS tolerates increased feedings in the form of increased volume or increased strength better. However, fluid overload is a concern in these small infants who require large intravenous fluid intakes in order to deliver required calories. Increased strength of formula is usually initiated first. Full strength elemental formulas may have very high osmolality and this factor alone may be sufficient reason to choose a more complex formula.

Infants with SBS routinely need both fat and water-soluble vitamin supplements after IV nutrition has been discontinued. Particular attention should be paid to the late onset of vitamin B_{12} deficiency, which is likely to become clinically significant within 1 year of discontinuing intravenous supplements. Routine measurements of vitamin B_{12}, methylmalonate and homocysteine should be made periodically in the infant who has lost a significant portion of the terminal ileum. A monthly dose of 100 μg is recommended. Some experts advocate the use of parenteral vitamin B_{12} for 4–5 years after the discontinuation of IV nutrition.[1] Patients with sufficient adaptation to grow on enteral feedings alone may still have enough fat malabsorption to cause deficiency of vitamins A, D, E, and K.

Similarly, mineral deficiencies may slowly develop in the child no longer on IV supplements.[80] Borderline sodium, potassium, calcium, magnesium, and zinc status is common. Routine stresses of childhood such as viral gastroenteritis may precipitate severe acidosis and electrolyte and mineral deficiencies. Latimer et al. reported two patients with SBS who developed severe zinc deficiency while on parenteral zinc doses of 40 mg kg^{-1} day^{-1}.[81] Replacement of the large losses of zinc in the stool corrected the clinical manifestations of acrodermatitis in these patients.

Normally, iron is absorbed in the proximal small bowel. Infants with proximal small bowel loss are at risk for iron-deficiency anemia, particularly as most IV nutrition mixtures do not contain iron. Generally, iron requirements can be met by enteral supplements after enteral feedings are successful. However, iron can be irritating to the gastrointestinal mucosa and supplements may not be well tolerated by young infants. Slow parenteral infusions of iron dextran can be given every 1–3 months in infants. However, consideration of possible impact of parenteral iron on white cell function and sepsis risk as well as the occasional shock-like reaction to parenteral iron should advise caution in giving parenteral iron. Other trace element deficiencies – selenium and chromium – may occur during IV nutrition administration. However, routine biochemical monitoring should avoid these complications.

Preservation of oral feeding function is a goal in the long-term feeding of infants with SBS. Like many infants who are unable to receive oral feedings directly after birth, oral aversion is a problem for infants and children with SBS. Unfortunately, pacifier sucking does not seem to preserve or promote normal feeding behavior in neonates. Thus, even in the neonate who is clearly unable to tolerate full enteral nutrition, some small oral feedings should be offered regularly if possible and continuous use of pacifiers avoided.[82]

As growth and late adaptation of the remaining intestine progress, intravenous nutrition support may be gradually withdrawn. Simultaneous monitoring of the child's growth rate and nutritional markers such as albumin, electrolytes, mineral, and vitamin levels will guide this gradual process of withdrawal of IV nutrition. When the child reaches 5–6 kg and has sufficient fat and hepatic glycogen stores to tolerate periods of fasting without hypoglycemia, IV nutrition may not be required around the clock. It is appropriate to allow the child some time free from intravenous tubing in order to promote normal development and parental bonding. Daily IV requirements can be consolidated into a reduced number of hours per day. If a significant fraction of the child's daily nutrition must be given intravenously, however, an acceptable intravenous infusion rate may limit the time the child can be free of the intravenous line. In older children, the use of lightweight portable pumps allows freedom of movement while receiving either enteral or parenteral feedings.

Medications may be useful in the management of infants with SBS. Cholestyramine and cholestipol are anion-binding resins that can bind luminal bile acids and improve bile acid-induced diarrhea. When used in a dose of 250 mg kg^{-1} day^{-1} in 3–4 divided doses, they may be of help in patients with ileal resection. In patients with more extensive resection, however, they can further deplete the bile acid pool and exacerbate steatorrhea. The exact length of ileal resection that correlates with a beneficial response to anion binding resin is not clear. Hyperchloremic acidosis has been reported during resin therapy and electrolytes should be monitored if these agents are used.[83] It should be remembered that anion binders may decrease the absorption of other anionic agents such as anticonvulsants and antibiotics. In patients with hyperacidity, H-2 receptor antagonists or proton pump inhibitors may raise the duodenal pH thereby improving pancreatic lipolytic activity and fat absorption. Unfortunately one clinical study has shown that water absorption but not sodium or macronutrient absorption improves with acid blocker therapy.[84] Potentially, very long-term use of acid blockers could promote small bowel bacterial overgrowth and impair intestinal absorption of vitamin B$_{12}$. The clinical importance of these long-term effects in SBS patients has not been assessed. Loperamide hydrochloride (Imodium), prolongs intestinal (mainly colon) transit time and may allow for better fluid, and possibly nutrient, absorption. A dose of 0.1 mg kg^{-1} given 2–3 times daily appears to be well tolerated. Use of nonabsorbed oral antibiotics such as colistin, gentamycin, neomycin, and the absorbed antibiotic flagyl has been proposed to reduce small bowel bacterial overgrowth and improve or prevent the complications of bile salt deconjugation, bacterial translocation steatorrhea, d-lactic acidosis, and possibly even cholelithiasis and liver disease.[85] Very little research has been done to validate these suggestions. Among untested therapies, the use of pancreatic supplements might improve fat and malabsorption in the hostile environment of the short intestine by improving the immediate contact of the luminal contents with larger amounts of lipase and proteases.[86] In infants with a depleted bile acid pool, exogenous conjugated bile acids might improve fat malabsorption. However, most available preparations also cause diarrhea. Recently, studies have shown that cholylsarcosine or ursodeoxycholic acid may increase fat absorption without causing diarrhea and may decrease the incidence of cholelithiasis by increasing bile flow.[87,88]

Ohlbaum reported using long-acting somatostatin to decrease the high volume ileal output of a 5-year-old child with SBS by prolonging the intestinal transit time and possibly by reducing the volume of pancreatic, biliary, and intestinal secretions.[89] Anti-inflammatory agents such as sulfasalazine and even prednisone have been used in older SBS patients who develop "short gut colitis," a condition that develops as enteral feedings are aggressively advanced.[90] This condition on biopsy appears both inflammatory and allergic, and the underlying cause is unknown but may be a nonspecific response of the colon to the abnormal amount of undigested material it encounters. A sulfasalazine dose of 25–50 mg kg^{-1} day^{-1} or prednisone dose of 1 mg kg^{-1} day^{-1} often results in prompt resolution of colitis. Neutropenia has been reported as a side effect of sulfasalazine and the child receiving it should be monitored.

Recently there has been enthusiasm for the use of probiotic and prebiotic agents in the treatment of SBS. Soluble fiber, a prebiotic, has several beneficial effects. It can be fermented in the colon and thus may increase the total calorie absorption through the production of short-chain fatty acids. Through its hygroscopic properties, it may also reduce the fluidity of the stool, improving perianal rashes and hygiene. It probably has little impact upon total water loss.[67] Commercially available products such as Certo™ or Sur-jel™ mix easily in enteral feedings and do not clog pumps. Probiotic agents have not been well enough studied to recommend them for routine use in SBS. Although some studies have shown a significant impact on diarrhea, presumably because of a reduction in Gram-negative aerobic overgrowth of the small intestine, others have not.[91,92] Administration of exogenous lactobacilli has been associated with the production of d-lactate, which causes acidosis and encephalopathy in SBS patients.[93]

It is often forgotten that short bowel reduces the absorption of medications prescribed for standard childhood conditions. The short gut must be considered especially when antipyretics, anticonvulsants and antibiotics are given by mouth. Intravenous, intrarectal, or intramuscular substitutes may have to be considered if the child fails to respond as expected.

Criteria for hospital discharge of an infant with SBS who is partly or completely dependent on intravenous nutrition are not clearly established. Factors that contribute to the decision include: (1) good weight gain on the in-hospital nutritional plan; (2) availability of adequate outpatient pharmacy and nursing services; (3) parental motivation, compliance, and reliability; (4) ability of the child to tolerate at least 6 hours without IV nutrition; (5) adequate financial resources to pay for home therapy; and (6) availability of skilled medical follow-up for GI and general pediatric needs. Many parents, who have become comfortable with the in-hospital care of their infants, are devastated by unexpected demands of outpatient care. Social service assistance is critical both before and after discharge as the parents cope directly with the care of their technologically dependent child at home.

Surgical management

At the time of the initial surgery, the surgeon's task is to assess the viability of the entire bowel and to preserve as much as possible. Distinguishing viable from nonviable bowel may be difficult. The use of intra-operative Doppler probe may aid in assessing blood flow in the major arteries when a pulse cannot be palpated. A second look laparotomy performed 24–48 hours after the initial emergency surgery allows the surgeon to reevaluate questionably viable intestinal segments and perhaps save centimeters that might have been resected at the first laparotomy. Performance of several diverting stomas along the length of the intestine allows for the removal of isolated segments of necrotic bowel. Reanastomosis of these segments can be performed electively later. If the viable mid-intestinal segments are too short to create stomas, blind segments of small bowel closed at either end may be constructed and left in the abdominal cavity for later reanastomosis. Other surgical reports have demonstrated that simply stenting these short intestinal segments may be sufficient as spontaneous anastomosis may occur.[94,95]

The surgeon contributes significantly to postoperative management and prognostication by providing subsequent caregivers an accurate idea of the length of bowel resected, the length of bowel remaining (generally measured along the antimesenteric border), the length of jejunum, the length of residual ileum, the relative diameters of the proximal and distal small bowel, and the presence or absence of the ileocecal valve and colon. A careful description of the intraoperative appearance and perfusion of the residual bowel helps alert postoperative caregivers to the potential for the later development of strictures. A careful drawing in the permanent patient record of the location and identity of any stomas on the abdominal wall will insure that postoperative caregivers have an accurate understanding of the child's anatomy. Inadvertent administration of fluid and medication through the wrong stoma is avoided.

Other decisions that are part of the initial operation include whether to place a central venous catheter and a gastrostomy. Postoperative dysmotility of the proximal small bowel is anticipated in infants with gastroschisis and mega duodenum. Placement of a gastrostomy helps in postoperative decompression of the stomach and upper small intestine. Both of these procedures may have to be delayed because of the unstable condition of the patient, however, their potential necessity should be made clear to parents.

When small bowel obstruction is present in utero, as in gastroschisis, meconium ileus, and intestinal atresias, there may be significant intestinal dilation proximal to the obstruction. Motility in the dilated segments may be poor, impeding the advancement of enteral feedings. End to end anastomosis of the dilated proximal bowel to the distal bowel may be difficult and functional obstruction after attempts at anastomosis may occur. A judicious tapering of the dilated proximal bowel may improve intestinal motility. When strictures occur postoperatively, a stricturoplasty, in which the strictured bowel is opened longitudinally and closed transversely, rather than simple resection of stricture, can save precious centimeters of intestine.[96–98]

Refeeding the effluent from a proximal stoma into the distal small bowel or colon is advocated by some surgeons as a means of saving fluid and electrolyte and of conditioning and dilating the distal unused bowel in preparation for anastomosis.[99] This is a somewhat messy procedure. Furthermore, it is not clear whether contamination of the stoma fluid might occur before it is collected and whether contamination makes the fluid harmful to the infant. As long as stoma losses are appropriately replaced intravenously, it is likely that 5% glucose and saline into the distal stoma is sufficient to start the process of dilating the distal segment in preparation for anastomosis.

Some authorities advocate prevention of proximal bowel dilation by early delivery of the fetus. The progress of proximal small bowel dilation is carefully followed by antenatal ultrasound. When duodenal diameter reaches 4 centimeters, early delivery should be considered if the fetus is mature enough.[100,101]

Surgical techniques to slow intestinal transit have for the most part been abandoned in neonates as complicated and ineffective. Reversed loops of small bowel, interposed colon segments, antiperistaltic electrical pacing, myenteric denervation, artificial valves in the small bowel to recreate the ileocecal valve, and recirculating loops of small bowel have been tried in an attempt to slow intestinal transit and improve absorption. These procedures generally cause obstructive symptoms and the improvement in absorption is rarely great enough to be of clinical significance.[98,102] Surgical techniques to increase mucosal surface area have also generally been abandoned. In these procedures, colon, abdominal wall muscle or prosthetic materials are fitted over a longitudinal small bowel enterotomy providing surface area over which regenerating mucosa can grow. The additional mucosal surface generated by these procedures is probably not of clinical significance.

Bowel lengthening procedures carry some therapeutic potential in neonatal short bowel syndrome. Bianchi designed the most commonly performed operation in which dilated bowel is divided longitudinally and the blood vessels of the two leaves of the mesentery are separated so that each segment has its own arterial supply. In this fashion, two separate intestinal tubes with half the diameter of the original are created and then anastomosed end to end in a pro peristaltic direction. Although the operation is a delicate one with complications such as bowel death, perforation, stricture and dysmotility, there have been excellent results in experienced hands. Generally, this operation is reserved for older infants who are no longer making any progress in their enteral feedings and who appear to be tied to IV nutrition indefinitely. The diameter of the bowel must be about 3–4 centimeters in order to create a reasonable diameter in the newly created segments.[103,104]

Small bowel transplantation is a final option for infants and children with massive small bowel resection or congenital short bowel syndrome. Every effort should be made treat the child medically in the hope that long-term adaptation will occur and the child will be free of intravenous alimentation and free of the chronic immunosuppression required after a small bowel transplant. In children with SBS and chronic liver disease, intestinal and liver transplant may be the only life-saving option. There is speculation and some experience to justify the idea that earlier intestinal transplant may halt the progression of liver disease in some SBS patients. A discussion of intestinal transplantation is beyond the scope of this chapter. Several excellent recent reviews of this topic are available.[105–110]

The onerous yet critical decision to withhold heroic surgical treatment may fall to the surgeon who takes the neonate to the operating room for the first exploratory laparotomy. Even in this emergency situation, honest preoperative consultation with the family and intraoperative consultation with the neonatologist is crucial for decision-making. A working knowledge of the established correlates of early and late mortality in SBS will assist in decision-making.

Complications and outcome

Wilmore published the first systematic assessment of the outcome of neonatal short bowel syndrome in 1972, before intravenous nutrition was commonly employed in neonates.[111] In this report of 50 infants with less than 75 cm of residual small bowel, mortality was 100% in those with

less than 15 cm. Mortality was also 100% in patients with less than 40 cm of remaining bowel if the ileocecal valve was resected. Mortality was 50% in patients with 15–38 cm of small bowel and an intact ileocecal valve. Only 18 of the 34 surviving patients had normal weight and height at long-term assessment. This study identified the ileocecal valve as being a critical determinant of survival in neonates with marginal length of remaining bowel (15–40 cm).

Most studies from the 1980s report 78–86% survival rate for neonates with resections of more than 50% of the small bowel.[2,4,7,112] In these reports, the ileocecal valve has not been generally found so critical to survival, probably because the routine use of IVN allows for adequate caloric intake and effective replacement of fluid and electrolyte losses. Most studies from the 1990s have reported similar 85–90% survival rates, suggesting that some limit has been reached for survival.[3,5,6,8,113] Although the absolute length of small bowel needed for survival has decreased since Wilmore's report, most recent reports suggest that a residual small bowel length less than 10 cm is incompatible with life. Although ultra-short bowel patients can be resuscitated and maintained briefly on IVN, the severity of their perioperative complications and the rapid onset of life-threatening liver disease almost always prevent long-term survival.[114] Since the routine use of IVN, the survival of neonates with SBS has improved from about 50% to about 85%. The mode of death has changed from inanition and surgical complications to the side effects of therapy – most commonly sepsis and liver failure.

Mortality as a measure of outcome may not be as important as the ability of the patient to achieve independence from IV nutrition. Several recent studies have evaluated the determinants of this endpoint with variable conclusions. All agree that the most important determinant of nutritional independence from IVN is the length of residual bowel. Sondheimer and colleagues, in a study of 44 neonates with SBS, found that two variables predicted whether a neonate would eventually develop intestinal sufficiency – the length of remaining intestine and the percent of total calories that were tolerated enterally at the adjusted age of 3 months.[8] A statistical model was created using intestinal length and percent daily calories given enterally at 3 months that can be used to roughly estimate the chances of independence from IV nutrition (Figure 34.2). Andorsky and colleagues found that the only independent predictor of duration of IVN dependence was residual intestinal length.[115] Other variables associated with reduced duration of IVN dependence were the use of either breast milk or an amino acid-based formula, and percent of daily calorie requirements taken enterally by 6 weeks postoperatively. Kaufman and colleagues also found that the

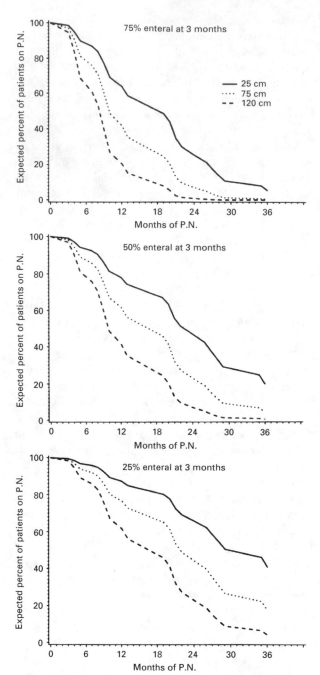

Figure 34.2. Plots derived from the Cox Proportional Hazard equation for three hypothetical patients with short bowel, all of whom receive 25% of their daily energy intake by the enteral route at 12 weeks adjusted age. Residual bowel lengths after initial surgery in these three patients are 25 cm, 75 cm and 120 cm. The range of potential dependence on parenteral nutrition in months can be estimated and the fiftieth percentile identified on the survivor function estimate on the vertical axis. Reproduced with permission.[8]

Table 34.2. Late complications of neonatal short bowel syndrome

Central venous catheter related
  Sepsis
  Thrombosis
  Mechanical obstruction
Nutritional
  Vitamin
  Mineral
  Caloric
Hepato-biliary
  Cholestasis
  Cholelithiasis
  Liver failure
Metabolic
  d-lactic acidosis[117]
  Osteopenia/osteoporosis
  Aluminum toxicity
Renal
  Oxalate stones
  Nephrotoxicity of drugs
Gastrointestinal
  Stricture
  Anastomotic ulcer with GI bleeding [118]
  Short bowel colitis
  Gastrointestinal allergy
  Hypergastrinemia and peptic ulcer
Behavioral
  Food refusal behavior
  Prolonged dependency
  Family emotional stress

length of remaining small bowel was the most important determinant of duration of IVN dependence.[116] However, they also found that intestinal inflammation, which they felt was secondary to bacterial overgrowth, was associated with longer IVN dependence. None of these three retrospective studies found that the presence of the ileo-cecal valve was an independent determinant of independence from IVN.

Even when nutritional management has been optimal, the child with neonatal SBS is at risk for many long-term complications. The complications come from three major sources – complications of associated genetic disorders, complications of the original intestinal crisis and its surgical therapy, and complications of therapy. A list of long-term complications is shown in Table 34.2.

The complication with the most impact on morbidity and mortality is cholestatic liver disease. A complete discussion of this very complex problem is beyond the scope of this chapter and the reader is referred to several recent reviews.[119,120] The incidence of cholestasis and liver failure in pediatric and adult patients on long-term IV nutrition who have not experienced intestinal resection is very low. The reasons for the high incidence of this complication in the neonate with SBS have not been determined. It is clear however, that the commonly used term "TPN cholestasis" is incomplete if not inaccurate. Other factors beside the use of intravenous nutrition play a critical part.

Most series report that direct hyperbilirubinemia occurs in about 67% of infants with neonatal short bowel syndrome. In the majority, the cholestasis occurs early in the nursery course and resolves spontaneously. However, about 10%–20% of short bowel patients, while still in the nursery, develop cholestatic jaundice, which progresses slowly and inexorably to liver failure. Predicting which patient will develop this life-threatening complication of SBS and IVN is not possible. Liver failure is associated with very short bowel, early bacterial infections, and, in some series, with the absence of the ileocecal valve and with intestinal dysmotility. Careful attention to reducing infections in the nursery, treating bacterial overgrowth vigorously, and promoting bowel motility are important.[121] Some investigators have found that increasing bile flow with intravenous cholecystokinin or oral choleretic bile acids reduces the severity of cholestasis.[122,123] It has been proposed that the intravenous amino acids, because they require active transport into the hepatocytes, may promote cholestasis by overwhelming the transport capacity of the cell. Others have proposed that photodegradation products of amino acids themselves are directly hepatotoxic. One intriguing study found that avoiding IV amino acids altogether, and giving all protein intake enterally was associated with normal nitrogen balance and a reduced incidence of cholestasis.[124] In many nurseries it is routine to "cycle" the amount of protein in the intravenous nutrition, giving $1\,\mathrm{g\,kg^{-1}day^{-1}}$ on one day and 2 or $3\,\mathrm{g\,kg^{-1}day^{-1}}$ the next in an attempt to avoid the continuous use of high concentrations of amino acids. There is no proof that this practice prevents cholestasis. Because of the perceived association between cholestasis and dysmotility, it is thought that small bowel bacterial overgrowth promotes liver disease by permitting the production and absorption of lipopolysaccharide enterotoxins into the portal circulation. There is some experimental support for this hypothesis.[125] The use of nonabsorbable antibiotics and probiotics may reduce bacterial overgrowth, but it has been impossible in these complex children to isolate the impact of this therapy on cholestasis. Enteral feedings stimulate bile flow and may improve the chances of avoiding cholestasis. Most retrospective reviews suggest that if cholestasis has not resolved by the age of 6–8 months, it is likely to progress to liver failure. Other factors promoting cholestasis in neonatal SBS include reduced antioxidant capacity of the infant liver and the toxic effects of medications.

Other long-term complications of patients with neonatal short bowel syndrome are listed in Table 34.2 and are discussed in the text. Infants with neonatal SBS require labor-intensive care during the perioperative period and meticulous outpatient management, sometimes for years. However, most are capable of eventually sustaining themselves by enteral feedings alone. Long-term morbidity and mortality depend on recognition of and prevention of complications. Nutritional status must be closely monitored for years after hospital discharge, inasmuch as deficiencies may occur insidiously. Height, weight, BMI, velocity of height, and weight gain must all be carefully assessed at regular intervals. A child whose growth has been satisfactory for years may experience a temporary deceleration of weight and height gain during adolescence when the absorption of nutrients may simply not be adequate for the increased demands of the pubertal growth spurt. A brief return to intravenous nutrition may sometimes be required to successfully complete the pubertal growth period. Regular biochemical monitoring for vitamin and mineral deficiency or excess are required. Long-term IV nutrition has been associated with aluminum toxicity and manganese deposition in the central nervous system even when these minerals are not added to the intravenous fluids. The possible development of d-lactic acidosis must be kept in mind as the child's diet begins to include more complex starches.

Improving the outcome of neonatal SBS will involve trials of new therapies to promote adaptation. A better understanding of the sources of cholestasis and its prevention in these patients is also critical to improved survival.

REFERENCES

1 Klish, W. K., Putnam, T. C. The short gut. *Am. J. Dis. Child.* 1981;**135**:1056–61.

2 Cooper, A., Floyd, T. F., Ross, A. J. *et al.* Morbidity and mortality of short-bowel syndrome acquired in infancy. *J. Pediatr. Surg.* 1984;**19**:711–18.

3 Georgeson, K. E., Breaux, C. W. Outcome and intestinal adaptation in neonatal short bowel syndrome. *J. Pediatr. Surg.* 1992;**27**:344.

4 Grosfeld, J. L., Rescorla, F. J., West, K. W. Short bowel syndrome in infancy and childhood. Analysis of survival in 60 patients. *J. Surg.* 1986;**151**:41.

5 Coran, A. G., Spivak, D., Teitelbaum, D. H. An analysis of morbidity and mortality of short bowel syndrome in the pediatric age group. *Eur. J. Ped. Surg.* 1999;**9**:228–30.

6 Kurkchubasche, A. G., Rowe, M. I., Smith, S. D. Adaptation in short bowel syndrome: reassessing old limits. *J. Pediatr. Surg.* 1993;**28**:1069.

7 Caniano, D. A., Starr, J., Ginn-Pease, M. E. Extensive short bowel syndrome in neonates: outcome in the 1980's. *Surgery* 1989;**105**:119.

8 Sondheimer, J. M., Cadnapaphornchai, M., Sontag, M. *et al.* Predicting the duration of dependence on parenteral nutrition after neonatal intestinal resection. *J. Pediatr.* 1997;**132**:80–4.

9 Schalamon, J., Schober, P. H., Gallippi, P. *et al.* Congenital short bowel: a case study and review of the literature. *Eur. J. Pediatr. Surg.* 1999;**9**:248–250.

10 Erez, I., Reish, O. *et al.* Congenital short bowel and malrotation: clinical presentation and outcome of 6 affected offspring in 3 related families. *Eur. J. Pediatr. Surg.* 2001;**11**:331–4.

11 Kern, I. B., Leece, A., Bohane, T. Congenital short gut, malrotation and dysmotility of the small bowel. *J. Pediatr. Gastroenterol. Nutr.* 1990;**11**:411–5.

12 Finaly, R., Cohen, Z., Mares, A. J. Near total intestinal aganglionosis with extreme short-bowel syndrome – a difficult surgical dilemma. *Eur. J. Ped. Surg.* 1999;**9**:253–5.

13 Touloukian, R. J., Walker-Smith, G. J. K. Normal intestinal length in preterm infants. *J. Pediatr. Surg.* 1983;**18**:720–3.

14 Siebert, J. R. Small intestinal length in infants and children. *Am. J. Dis. Child.* 1980;**134**:593–5.

15 Urban, E., Weser, E. Intestinal adaptation to bowel resection. In Stollerman, G. H., ed. *Advances in Internal Medicine, Vol 26.* Chicago, IL: Year Book Medical Publishers;1980:265–91.

16 Jeppessen, P. B., Mortensen, P. B. Colonic digestion and absorption of energy from carbohydrates and medium chain fat in small bowel failure. *J. Parenter. Enteral Nutr.* 1999;**23**:S101–5.

17 Nordgaard, I. What's new in the role of the colon as a digestive organ in patients with short bowel syndrome. *Nutrition* 1998;**14**:468–9.

18 Nordgaard, I. The colon as a digestive organ. The importance of colonic support for energy absorption as small bowel failure proceeds. *Dan. Med. Bull.* 1998;**45**:135–56.

19 Daview, B. W., Abel, G., Puntis, J. W. *et al.* Limited ileal resection in infancy: the long term consequences. *J. Ped. Surg.* 1999;**34**:583–7.

20 Valman, H. B., Roberts, P. D. Vitamin B12 absorption after resection of ileum in childhood. *Arch. Dis. Child.* 1974;**49**:171–3.

21 Sondheimer, J. M., Asturias, E., Cadnapapornchai, M. Infection and cholestasis in neonates with intestinal resection and long term parenteral nutrition. *J. Pediatr. Gastroenterol. Nutr.* 1998;**27**:131–7.

22 Nightengale, J. M. Management of patients with short bowel. *Nutrition* 1999;**15**:633–7.

23 Valman, H. B., Oberholzer, V. G., Palmer, T. Hyperoxaluria after resection of ileum in childhood. *Arch. Dis. Child.* 1974;**49**:171–3.

24 Nightengale, J. M., Lennard-Jones, J. E., Gertner, D. J. *et al.* Colon preservation reduces the need for parenteral therapy, increases the incidence of renal stones, but does not change the high prevelance of gall stones in patients with a short gut. *Gut* 1992;**33**:1493–7.

25 Jeppessen, P. B., Mortensen, P. B. Enhancing bowel adaptation in short bowel syndrome. *Curr. Gastroenterol. Rep.* 2002;**4**:338–47.

26 Vanderhoof, J. A. Invited review: Short bowel syndrome. *J. Pediatr. Gastroenterol. Nutr.* 1992;**14**:359.

27 Williamson, R. C. N. Intestinal adaptation: Part I. Structural function and cytokinetic changes. Part 2: Mechanisms of control. *N. Engl. J. Med.* 1978;**298**:1393–402, 1444–50.

28 Johnson, L. R., Copeland, E. M., Dudrick, S. J. *et al.* Structural and hormonal alterations in the gastrointestinal tract of parenterally fed rats. *Gastroenterology* 1975;**68**:1177–83.

29 Hughes, C. A., Dowling, R. H. Speed of onset of adaptive mucosal hypoplasia and hypofunction in the intestine of parenterally fed rats. *Clin. Sci.* 1980;**59**:317–27.

30 Stern, L. E., Falcone, R. A., Kemp, C. J. *et al.* Effect of massive small bowel resection on Bas/Bcl-w ratio and enterocyte apoptosis. *J. Gastroint. Surg.* 2000;**4**:93–100.

31 Altmann, G. G. Influence of bile acid and pancreatic secretion on the size of the intestinal villi in the rat. *Am. J. Anat.* 1971;**132**:167–78.

32 Hughes, C. A., Bates, T., Dowling, R. H. Cholecystokinin and secretin prevent the intestinal mucosal hypoplasia of total parenteral nutrition in the dog. *Gastroenterology* 1978;**75**:34–41.

33 Feldman, E. J., Dowling, R. H., McNaughton, R. J. Effects of oral vs intravenous nutrition on intestinal adaptation after small bowel resection in the dog. *Gastroenterology* 1976;**70**:712–9.

34 Adrian, T. E., Thompson, J. S., Quigley, E. M. Time course of adaptive regulatory peptide changes after massive small bowel resection in the dog. *Dig. Dis. Sci.* 1996;**41**:1194–203.

35 Bloom, S. R., Polak, J. M. The hormonal pattern of intestinal adaptation. A major role for enteroglucagon. *Scan. J. Gastroenterol.* 1982;**17**:91–103.

36 Sagor, G. R., Almukhtar, M. Y. T., Ghatei, M. A. *et al.* The effect of altered luminal nutrition on cellular proliferation and plasma concentrations of enteroglucagon and gastrin after small bowel resection in the rat. *Br. J. Surg.* 1982;**69**:14–18.

37 Holst, J. J., Sorensen, T. I. A., Andersen, A. N. *et al.* Plasma enteroglucagon after jejunoileal bypass with 3:1 or 1:3 jejunoileal ratio. *Scand. J. Gastroenterol.* 1979;**14**:205.

38 Fuller, P. J., Beveridge, D. J., Taylor, R. G. Ileal proglucagon gene expression in the rat: Characterization in intestinal adaptation using in situ hybridization. *Gastroenterology* 1993;**104**:459–64.

39 Gregor, M., Stallmach, A., Menge, H. *et al.* The role of gut glucagon-like immunoreactants in the control of gastrointestinal epithelial cell renewal. *Digestion* 1990;**46** (Suppl.):59–66.

40 Vanderhoof, J. A. Short bowel syndrome in children and small intestinal transplantation. *Ped. Clin. N. Am.* 1996;**43**:533.

41 Nightengale, J. M., Kamm, M. A., van der Sjip, J. R. *et al.* Gastrointestinal hormones in short bowel syndrome. Peptide

YY may be the colonic brake to gastric emptying. *Gut* 1996;**39**:267–72.

42 Litvak, D. A., Iseki, H., Evers, B. M. *et al.* Characterization of two novel proabsorptive peptide YY analogues, BIM-4373D and BIM-43004C. *Dig. Dis. Sci.* 1999;**44**:643–8.

43 Bohane, T. D., Haka-Iksa, K., Biggar, W. D. *et al.* A clinical study of young infants after small intestinal resection. *J. Pediatr.* 1979;**94**:522–8.

44 Morin, C. L., Ling, V. Effects of pentagastrin on the rat small intestine after resection. *Gastroenterology* 1978;**75**:224.

45 Thompson, J. S., Harty, R. F. Post resection hypergastrinemia correlates with malabsorption but not adaptation. *J. Invest. Surg.* 1994;**7**:469–76.

46 Shulman, D. I., Ju, C. S., Duckett, G. *et al.* Effects of short term growth hormone therapy in rats undergoing 75% small intestinal resection. *J. Pediatr. Gastroenterol. Nutr.* 1992;**14**:3–11.

47 Velasco, B., Lassaletta, L., Gracia, R. *et al.* Intestinal lengthening and growth hormone in extreme short-bowel syndrome: a case report. *J. Pediatr. Surg.* 1999;**34**:1423–4.

48 Waitzberg, D. L., Cukier, C., Mucerrino, D. R. *et al.* Small bowel adaptation with growth hormone and glutamine after massive resection of rat's small bowel. *Nutr. Hospitalaria* 1999;**14**:81–90.

49 Ling, L. I., Irving, M. The effectiveness of growth hormone, glutamine and low fat diet containing high carbohydrate on the enhancement of the function of remnant intestine among patients with short bowel syndrome: a review of published trials. *Clin. Nutr.* 2001;**20**:199–204.

50 Scolapio, J. S., Camillari, M., Fleming, C. R. *et al.* Effect of growth hormone, glutamine and diet on adaptation in short bowel syndrome: a randomized, controlled study. *Gastroenterology* 1997;**113**:1074–81.

51 Barksdale, E. M. Jr., Koehler, A. N., Yaworski, J. A. *et al.* IGF-1 and IGF-3 indices of intestinal failure in children. *J. Pediatr. Surg.* 1999;**34**:655–61.

52 Vanderhoof, J. A., McCusker, R. H., Clark, R. *et al.* Truncated and native insulin like growth factor-1 enhance mucosal adaptation after jejunoileal resection. *Gastroenterology* 1992;**102**:1949–56.

53 Lund, P. K. Molecular basis of intestinal adaptation: the role of the insulin like growth factor system. *Ann. N. Y. Acad. Sci.* 1998;**859**:18–36.

54 Jeppessen, P. B., Hartmann, B., Thulesen, J. *et al.* Glucagon-like peptide, released from ileum in response to meals is reduced in short bowel syndrome. *Gut* 1999;**45**:478–9.

55 Litvak, D., Hellmick, M. R., Evers, B. M. *et al.* Glucagon-like peptide 2 is a potent growth factor for small intestine and colon. *J. Gastrointest. Surg.* 1998;**2**:146–50.

56 Thompson, J. S. Epidermal growth factor and the short bowel syndrome. *J. Parenter. Enteral Nutr.* 1999;**23**:S113–16.

57 Feldman, E. J., Aures, D., Grossman, M. I. Epidermal growth factor stimulates ornithine decarboxylase activity in the digestive tract of the mouse. *Proc. Soc. Exp. Biol. Med.* 1978;**159**:400–2.

58 O'Loughlin, E. O., Winter, M., Shin, A. *et al.* Structural and functional adaptation following jejunal resection in rabbits: effect of epidermal growth factor. *Gastroenterology* 1994;**107**:87–93.

59 Johnson, W. F., DiPalma, C. R., Ziegler, T. R. *et al.* Keratinocyte growth factor enhances early gut adaptation in a rat model of short bowel syndrome. *Vet. Surg.* 2000;**29**:17–27.

60 Liu, Q., Su, X. X., Shindel, Z. X. The trophic effects of IL-11 in rats with experimental short bowel syndrome. *J. Pediatr. Surg.* 1996;**31**:1047–51.

61 Kollman, K. A., Lien, E. L., Vanderhoof, J. A. Dietary lipids influence intestinal adaptation after massive small bowel resection. *J. Pediatr. Gastroenterol. Nutr.* 1999;**28**:41–5.

62 Vanderhoof, J. A., Park, J. H. Y., Herrington, M. K. The effects of dietary menhaden oil on mucosal adaptation after small bowel resection in rats. *Gastroenterology* 1994;**106**:94–9.

63 Alavi, K., Kato, Y., Yu, D. *et al.* Enteral glutamine does not enhance the effects of hepatocyte growth factor in short bowel syndrome. *J. Pediatr. Surg.* 1998;**33**:1666–9.

64 Wiren, M. E., Permert, J., Skullman, S. P. *et al.* No difference in mucosal adaptive growth one week after intestinal resection in rats given enteral glutamine or deprived of glutamine. *Eur. J. Surg.* 1996;**162**:489–98.

65 Wiren, M., Adrian, T. E., Amelo, U. *et al.* Early gastrointestinal regulatory peptide response to intestinal resection in the rat is stimulated by enteral glutamine supplementation. *Dig. Surg.* 1999;**16**:197–203.

66 Yang, H., Larsson, J., Permert, J. *et al.* No effect of bolus glutamine supplementation on the post resectional adaptation of small bowel mucosa in rats receiving chow ad libitum. *Dig. Surg.* 2000;**17**:256–60.

67 Roth, J. A., Frankel, W. L., Zhang, W. *et al.* Pectin improves colonic function in rat short bowel syndrome. *J. Surg. Res.* 1995;**58**:240–6.

68 Tappenden, K. A., Thompson, A. B., Wild, G. E. *et al.* Short chain fatty acid supplemented total parenteral nutrition enhances functional adaptation to intestinal resection in rats. *Gastroenterology* 1997;**112**:792–802.

69 Tappenden, K. A., Thompson, A. B., Wild, G. E. *et al.* Short chain fatty acids increase proglucagon and ornithine decarboxylase mRNA after intestinal resection in the rat. *J. Parenter. Enteral Nutr.* 1996;**20**:357–62.

70 Kawaguchi, A. L., Dunn, J. C., Lam, M. *et al.* Glucose uptake in dilated small intestine. *J. Pediatr. Surg.* 1998;**33**:1670–3.

71 Ovesen, L., Chu, R., Howard, L. The influence of dietary fat on jejunostomy output in patients with severe short bowel syndrome. *Am. J. Clin. Nutr.* 1983;**38**:270–7.

72 Sandstrom, B., Davidsson, L., Bosaeus, I., *et al.* Selenium status and absorption of zinc (65Zn), selenium (75 Se) and manganese (54Mn) in patients with short bowel syndrome. *Eur. J. Clin. Nutr.* 1990;**44**:697–703.

73 Ladefoged, K. Intestinal and renal loss of infused minerals in patients with severe short bowel syndrome. *Am. J. Clin Nutr.* 1982;**36**:59–67.

74 Parker, P., Stroop, S., Greene, H. A controlled comparison of continuous versus intermittent feeding in the treatment of infants with intestinal disease. *J. Pediatr.* 1981;**99**:360–4.

75 Jeppessen, P. B., Hay, C. E., Mortensen, P. B. Differences in essential fatty acid requirements by enteral and parenteral routes of administration in patients with fat malabsorption. *Am. J. Clin. Nutr.* 1999;**70**:78–84.

76 Heyman, M., Grasset, E., Ducroc, R. *et al.* Antigen absorption by the jejunal epithelium of children with cows milk allergy. *Ped. Res.* 1988;**24**:197–202.

77 D'Antiga, L., Dhawan, A., Davenport, M. *et al.* Intestinal absorption and permeability in paediatric short bowel syndrome: a pilot study. *J. Pediatr. Gastroenterol. Nutr.* 1999;**29**:588–93.

78 Burrin, D. G., Stoll, B. Key nutrients and growth factors for the neonatal gastrointestinal tract. *Clin. Perinatol.* 2002;**29**:65–96.

79 Levy, E., Firleux, P., Sandrucci, S. *et al.* Continuous enteral nutrition during the early adaptive stage of the short bowel syndrome. *Br. J. Surg.* 1988;**75**:549–53.

80 Engles, L. G. J., van den Hamer, C. J. A., van Tongeren, J. H. M. Iron, zinc and copper balance in short bowel patients on oral nutrition. *Am. J. Clin. Nutr.* 1984;**40**:1038–41.

81 Latimer, J. S., McClain, C. J., Sharp, H. L. Clinical zinc deficiency during zinc-supplemented parenteral nutrition. *J. Pediatr.* 1980;**97**:434–7.

82 Linscheid, T. R., Tarnowski, K. J., Rasnake, L. K. *et al.* Behavioral therapy for food refusal in a child with short bowel syndrome. *J. Pediatr. Psychol.* 1987;**12**:451–9.

83 Scheel, P. J. Jr, Whelton, A., Rossiter, K. *et al.* Cholestyramine induced hyperchloremic metabolic acidosis. *J. Clin. Pharm.* 1992;**32**:536–8.

84 Jeppessen, P. B., Staun, M., Tjellesen, L. *et al.* Effect of intravenous ranitidine and omeprazole on intestinal absorption of water, sodium and macronutrients in patients with intestinal resection. *Gut* 1998;**43**:763–9.

85 Lichtman, S. N., Keku, J., Clark, R. L. *et al.* Biliary tract disease in rats with experimental small bowel bacterial overgrowth. *Hepatology* 1991;**13**:766–72.

86 Hardt, P. D., Helfrich, C., Klauke, T. *et al.* Liquid pancreatic enzyme therapy for a patient with short bowel syndrome and chronic pancreatitis in a complicated case of Crohn's disease. *Eur. J. Med. Res.* 1999;**4**:345–6.

87 Gruy-Kapral, C., Little, K. H., Fordtran, J. S., *et al.* Conjugated bile acid replacement therapy for short bowel syndrome. *Gastroenterology* 1999;**116**:15–21.

88 Heydorn, S., Jeppessen, P. B., Mortensen, P. B. Bile acid replacement therapy with cholylsarcosine for short bowel syndrome. *Scand. J. Gastroenterol.* 1999;**34**:818–23.

89 Ohlbaum, P., Galperine, R. I., Demarquez, J. *et al.* Use of a long acting somatostatin analogue (SMS201–995) in controlling a significant ileal output in a 5 year old child. *J. Pediatr. Gastroenterol. Nutr.* 1987;**6**:466–70.

90 Taylor, S. F., Sondheimer, J. M., Sokol, R. J. *et al.* Noninfectious colitis associated with short gut syndrome in infants. *J. Pediatr.* 1991;**119**:24–8.

91 Vanderhoof, J. A., Young, R. J., Murray, N. *et al.* Treatment strategies for small bowel bacterial overgrowth in short bowel syndrome. *J. Pediatr. Gastroenterol. Nutr.* 1998;**27**:155–60.

92 Sondheimer, J. M., Fidanza, S., Setchell, K. D. R. Intestinal function in short bowel syndrome (SBS): effect of *Lactobacillus casei* GG. *J. Pediatr. Gastroenterol. Nutr.* 1999;**29**:495. (Abstr.).

93 Bongaerts, G., Bakkeren, J., Severijnen, R. Lacobacilli and acidosis in children with short small bowel. *J. Pediatr. Gastroenterol. Nutr.* 2000;**30**:288–93.

94 Lessin, M. S., Schwartz, D. L., Wesselhoeft, C. W., Jr. Multiple spontaneous small bowel anastomoses in premature infants with multi segmental necrotizing enterocolitis. *J. Pediatr. Surg.* 2000;**35**:170–2.

95 Sapin, E., Carricaburu, E., De Boissieu, D. *et al.* Conservative intestinal surgery to avoid short bowel syndrome in multiple intestinal atresias and necrotizing enterocolitis: 6 cases treated by multiple anastomoses and Santulli type enterostomy. *Eur. J. Ped. Surg.* 1999;**9**:24–8.

96 Waang, K. L., Heller, K. Surgical techniques in short bowel syndrome. *Prog. Ped. Surg.* 1990;**25**:81.

97 Warner, B., Chaet, M. S. Nontransplant surgical options for management of the short bowel syndrome. *J. Pediatr. Gastroenterol. Nutr.* 1993;**17**:1.

98 Thompson, J. S., Langnas, A. N., Pinch, L. W. *et al.* Surgical approach to short bowel syndrome. Experience in a population of 160 patients. *Ann. Surg.* 1995;**222**:600–5.

99 Al-Harbi, K., Walton, J. M., Gardner, V. *et al.* Mucous fistula refeeding in neonates with short-bowel syndrome. *J. Pediatr. Surg.* 1999;**34**:1100–3.

100 Simmons, M., Georgeson, K. E. The effect of gestational age at birth on morbidity in patients with gastroschisis. *J. Pediatr. Surg.* 1996;**31**:1060–2.

101 Dykes, E. H. Prenatal diagnosis and management of abdominal wall defects. *Semin. Ped. Surg.* 1996;**5**:90–4.

102 Garcia, S. B., Kawasaky, M. C., Silva, J. C. *et al.* Intrinsic myenteric denervation: a new model to increase the intestinal absorptive surface in short-bowel syndrome. *J. Surg. Res.* 1999;**85**:200–3.

103 Bianchi, A. Experience with longitudinal intestinal lengthening and tailoring. *Eur. J. Surg.* 1999;**9**:256–9.

104 Waag, K. L., Hosie, S., Wersel, L. What do children look like after longitudinal intestinal lengthening? *Eur. J. Surg.* 1999;**9**:260–2.

105 Jan, D., Michel, J. L., Goulet, O. *et al.* Up-to-date evaluation of small bowel transplantation in children with intestinal failure. *J. Pediatr. Surg.* 1999;**34**:841–3.

106 Vanderhoof, J. A. Short bowel syndrome in children and small intestinal transplantation. *Ped. Clin. N. Am.* 1996;**43**:533.

107 Gotrand, F., Michaud, L., Bonnevalle, M. *et al.* Favorable nutritional outcome after isolated liver transplant for liver failure in a child with short bowel syndrome. *Transplant* 1999;**67**:632–4.

108 Kelly, D. Transplantation: new beginnings, new horizons. *J. Pediatr. Gastroenterol. Nutr.* 2002;**34**:S51–3.

109 Park, B. K. Intestinal transplantation in pediatric patients. *Prog. Trans.* 2002;**12**:97–113.

110 Sokal, E. M., Cleghorn, G., Goulet, O. *et al.* Liver and intestinal transplantation in children: working group report of the First World Congress of Pediatric Gastroenterology, Hepatology and Nutrition. *J. Pediatr. Gastroenterol. Nutr.* 2002;**35**:S159–72.

111 Wilmore, D. W. Factors correlating with a successful outcome following extensive intestinal resection in newborn infants. *J. Pediatr.* 1972;**80**:88.

112 Galea, M. H., Holliday, H., Carachi, R. *et al.* Short bowel syndrome; a collective review. *J. Pediatr. Surg.* 1992;**27**:592.

113 Mayr, J. M., Schober, P. G. H., Werssensteiner, U. *et al.* Morbidity and mortality of the short bowel syndrome. *Eur. J. Ped. Surg.* 1999;**9**:231–3.

114 Iacono, G., Carroccio, A., Montalto, G. *et al.* Extreme short bowel syndrome: a case for reviewing the guidelines for predicting survival. *J. Pediatr. Gastroenterol. Nutr.* 1993;**16**:216.

115 Andorsky, D. J., Lund, D. P., Lillehei, C. W. *et al.* Nutritional and other postoperative management of neonates with short bowel syndrome correlates with clinical outcomes. *J. Pediatr.* 2001;**139**:5–7.

116 Kaufman, S. S., Loseke, C. A., Lupo, J. V. *et al.* Influence of bacterial overgrowth and intestinal inflammation on duration of parenteral nutrition in children with short bowel syndrome. *J. Pediatr.* 1997;**131**:356–61.

117 Day, A. S., Abbot, G. D. D-lactic acidosis in short bowel syndrome. *N. Zealand Med. J.* 1999;**112**:277–8.

118 Sondheimer, J. M., Sokol, R. J., Narkewicz, M. R. *et al.* Anastomotic ulceration: a late complication of ileocolonic anastomosis. *J. Pediatr.* 1995;**127**:225–30.

119 Suita, S., Masumoto, K., Yamanouchi, T. *et al.* Complications in neonates with short bowel syndrome and long term parenteral nutrition. *J. Parenter. Enteral Nutr.* 1999;**23**:S106–9.

120 Sokol, R. J. Total parenteral nutrition related liver disease. *Acta Paed. Sin.* 1997;**328**:418–28.

121 Meehan, J. J., Georgeson, K. E. Prevention of liver failure in parenteral nutrition-dependent children with short bowel syndrome. *J. Pediatr. Surg.* 1997;**32**:473–5.

122 Teitelbaum, D. H., Han-Markey, T., Drongowski, R. A. *et al.* Use of cholecystokinin to prevent the development of parenteral nutrition associated cholestasis. *J. Parenter. Enteral Nutr.* 1997;**21**:100–3.

123 Rintala, R. J., Lindahl, H. G., Pohjavuori, M. Total parenteral nutrition associated cholestasis in surgical neonates may be reversed by intravenous cholecystokinin: a preliminary report. *J. Pediatr. Surg.* 1995;**31**:827–30.

124 Brown, M. R., Thunberg, B. J., Golub, L. *et al.* Decreased cholestasis with enteral instead of intravenous protein in the very low birth weight infant. *J. Pediatr. Gastroenterol. Nutr.* 1989;**9**:21–7.

125 Lichtman, S. L., Wang, J., Schwab, J. *et al.* Comparison of peptidoglycan polysaccharide and lipopolysaccharide stimulation of Kupffer cells to produce TNF and IL-1. *Hepatology* 1994;**19**:1013–22.

35

Acute respiratory failure

John E. E. Van Aerde and Michael Narvey

Stollery Children's Hospital, Edmonton, Alberta Canada

Feeding a patient with respiratory failure is more complicated in a neonatal than in an adult intensive care setting. For adults the goal is to maintain an acceptable energy balance without imposing extra metabolic and respiratory stress on the organism. In newborn infants, the caloric cost for growth has to be added to the energy balance which means that additional respiratory demands will be imposed on the neonate, because the growth process itself produces carbon dioxide and consumes oxygen.

Nutritional status affects the respiratory system directly by providing energy for the respiratory muscles and development of lung structure and function; indirectly, the level of energy intake (EI) and the dietary macronutrient composition modify the metabolic demands and affect the respiratory system by modifying central ventilatory drive and the respiratory gaseous exchange.

This chapter describes the effect of nutrition on the development and function of the respiratory system in newborns. The first portion describes the interactions between nutrition and structural, biochemical, and functional changes in the lung. The second part addresses metabolic needs of infants with acute respiratory distress and describes the effects of EI and/or diet composition on respiratory gas exchange and energy metabolism in intravenously fed neonates.

Nutrition, metabolism, and the respiratory system

Lung development and morphology

The preterm infant with a birth weight of 1000 g has an expendable nonprotein energy reserve of less than 200 kcal,

with 1%–2% of the body weight as fat and less than 1% as glycogen. Because accretion of expendable energy stores occurs in late gestation, energy and protein reserves in the preterm infant quickly deplete after short periods of insufficient nutritional intake. Critical illness and severe respiratory distress increase the infant's protein and energy demands.

Interference with somatic growth may affect lung structure, as lung size, alveolar number, and alveolar surface area are stature-dependent. A 50% reduction in energy intake in newborn rats during the first 21 days of life, results in lower lung weight than in the control group. There seems to be a permanent reduction in the number of lung cells during subsequent developmental stages.[1,2] When food restriction of equal duration is imposed later in the course of lung development, there is less of an effect on lung growth. Whereas early malnutrition impedes cell division with no recovery when feeding is re-instituted, malnutrition at a later stage of growth results in a reduction of cell size rather than absolute cell number allowing recovery when refeeding occurs.[2] In adult rats receiving 20%–33% of the control EI for periods of 1–6 weeks, the alveolar diameter increases, with a decrease in alveolar surface area and dissolution of connective tissue elements from within alveolar septa,[3,4] resulting in morphological lung changes similar to those seen in emphysema. The reduced alveolar surface area is further accompanied by limited in vivo pulmonary diffusing capacity.[5] In the starved human, emphysematous lesions have also been found in all age groups from childhood to geriatrics.[6]

In the newborn guinea pig, a 50% reduction in EI in the prenatal and weanling period results in reduced lung tissue volumes, reduced alveolar and capillary surface areas,

Neonatal Nutrition and Metabolism. Second Edition, ed. P. Thureen and W. Hay. Published by Cambridge University Press.
© Cambridge University Press 2006.

and diminished pulmonary diffusion capacity. As guinea pigs have more mature lungs than other rodents at birth, the postnatal lung is more resistant to alveolar hypoplasia than the prenatal lung. This is confirmed by complete recovery when the starved weanlings are re-fed, whereas animals starved prenatally show residual starvation effects as adult animals, demonstrating reduced tissue volumes, reduced alveolar and capillary surface areas, and diminished pulmonary diffusing capacity.[7] The development of lungs of prenatally starved guinea pigs is arrested in the saccular phase. Furthermore, the newborn guinea pig is born with considerable adipose tissue reserves, and pulmonary growth retardation seems minimized during starvation; lung growth might be protected by these energy reserves. In infants with a gestational age < 27 weeks, alveolarization has not occurred yet and energy reserves are minimal; alveolar development might therefore be delayed in preterm infants when fed inappropriately, as suggested by one report of an infant with bronchopulmonary dysplasia.[8]

Even short-term starvation or malnutrition (50% of energy of control group given as glucose for 60 hours) leads to failure of lung growth in terms of weight, protein content, and cell size in 21-day-old rats.[9]

Changes in connective tissue composition of the lung are also known to occur during malnutrition. In adult rats receiving one fifth of the calories of control animals, body and lung weight as well as lung content of crude connective tissue, elastin, hydroxyproline, and protein drop significantly.[10] After refeeding, elastin and protein content do not return to control values, indicating that the emphysema-like changes in the lungs of malnourished rats are at least partly related to the loss of connective tissue elements. The diet-induced loss of elastic recoil forces persists and resembles mechanical and morphological changes of experimental, elastase-induced emphysema.[3,4] Besides energy deprivation, protein deficiency also seems to be a major dietary factor contributing to nutrition-induced emphysema in rats.[11,12]

In summary, food restriction during early life impacts on lung growth, alveolar development and various connective tissue components. In rats, the severity and reversibility of the changes appear to depend on the stage of the lung growth during which food deprivation occurs. These are interesting findings in view of the fact that undernutrition early on in life has been mentioned to be a major contributing factor in the pathogenesis of bronchopulmonary dysplasia (BPD).[13]

Nutrition and surfactant synthesis

Phosphatidylcholine (PC), particularly desaturated phosphatidylcholine (DSPC) and phosphatidylglycerol (PG), are the main phospholipids of lung surfactant.[14] Food deprivation in adult rats for 2–3 days results in a decrease of total phospholipids and PC in total lung tissue expressed per DNA content,[15] but the ratio of saturated over unsaturated fatty acids in PC is maintained.[16] In adult rats, reduced surfactant synthesis and diminished release into the alveoli seems to occur after short-term food deprivation.[9,17] Brown et al. confirmed that fasting or calorie deprivation for 24–72 hours in adult rats results in diminished pools of total phospholipids, PC, DSPC, and PG in the intracellular fractions of the lung, however after 96 hours of complete fasting or 192 hours of calorie deprivation, the pool sizes return to control levels.[18] The activity of choline-phosphate cytidylyl transferase, the main regulatory enzyme in the synthesis of PC, increases markedly with the duration of fasting with maximum activity after 72 hours.[18,19] Sahebjami and Macgee[10] studied effects of more prolonged partial food deprivation on lung surfactant. Adult rats receiving one fifth of their normal measured daily food consumption for 3 weeks show a significant reduction in DSPC content both in lung tissue and lavage fluid compared with the age-matched control-fed group. After 7–10 days of refeeding, the DSPC content of both tissue and lavage fluid returns to normal.[10]

Gail et al. have shown that alveolar stability is maintained despite decreased surfactant phospholipids, probably by maintaining the ratio of saturated to unsaturated phosphatidylcholine in the extracellular surfactant fraction.[16] Whereas the status of pulmonary surfactant appears to be sufficient in the energy-deprived animal, it remains speculative whether the same is true for the infant with respiratory distress syndrome, who often has a surfactant deficient lung.

It is interesting to speculate whether diet composition, without energy deprivation, can also alter the quality of surfactant. Feeding a diet deficient in essential fatty acids to weanling rats for 12–14 weeks does not change the content of total PC in lung tissue and lavage material, but the content of DSPC is reduced significantly.[20,21] Within 24 hours of refeeding essential fatty acids, the return towards control fatty acid composition is evident and gradually completed in 7–14 days. Several recent studies have attempted to modify the saturation of lung phospholipids through dietary long-chain polyunsaturated fatty acids (LCPUFA).[22–25] The LCPUFA content of the lung tissue phospholipids increases when the diets provided to rats are supplemented with arachidonic acid (ARA) and docosahexaenoic acid (DHA). Given the recent interest in ARA and DHA with respect to the development of the brain and retina, it is important to determine if such modification would have a deleterious effect on surfactant composition. Recently, lung tissue and surfactant phospholipid composition were studied in newborn rat pups supplemented with DHA and ARA.[26] As found in the previous studies, the ratio of unsaturated to saturated fatty acids in lung tissue phospholipids increased but the ratio within surfactant resisted such change. Oxidative stress in piglets fed diets high in linoleic acid (61% of fat) or fish oil (38% of fat) is less well tolerated than in animals receiving a saturated fatty acid diet. In the groups receiving the unsaturated fatty acids the lungs demonstrated greater wet:dry weight, pulmonary edema, and vascular congestion.[27] The results may be explained by the change in unsaturated:saturated phosphatidylcholine observed in surfactant obtained from the piglets, suggesting an alteration of surfactant function as a possible explanation. Despite the fact that the dietary study LCPUFA level was abnormally high as compared with what is present in infant nutrition, it would be prudent to further study the effect of adding LCPUFA to intravenous lipid emulsions on the lung function of the ill neonate.

Finally, choline and inositol have been considered to have potential nutritional value for surfactant synthesis. After birth, neither glycogen nor exogenous choline seems to have a regulatory influence on lung lipid synthesis, but glucose continues to be an important precursor. As in energy deprivation, the surfactant PC pool size in lungs shows very little change with established choline deficiency, and the maximal choline incorporation into PC is unchanged by dietary choline deficiency.[28] Prior to the introduction of surfactant it seemed that there might be a place for inositol. Inositol administered by the intragastric or intravenous route had been shown to decrease the severity of respiratory distress syndrome (RDS),[29] probably secondary to an increased ratio of saturated phosphatidylcholine to sphingomyelin.[30] However, when inositol supplementation was studied in a group receiving surfactant as well, no additional benefit could be demonstrated. While originally promising, inositol does not likely have a role in neonatal lung function now that surfactant is widely available.[31]

In summary, even for short periods, food and calorie deprivation alters surfactant metabolism, leading to inadequate tissue stores and intra-alveolar levels; the quality of the surfactant on the alveolar surface is not altered considerably. It appears that the lung is capable of shifting its metabolic activity during short-term food deprivation toward maintaining essential lipid components in order to preserve the stability of lung mechanics.[32] Although the surfactant phospholipid production by the type II cells of the lungs eventually returns to normal, the initial marked reduction in surfactant production during experimental malnutrition might be important during the first few days of life in the ELBW and VLBW infant who is in a catabolic state. Conflicting animal data exist with regards to the effect of LCPUFA supplementation on surfactant composition.

Lung defense mechanisms

Nutritional interventions affect lung defense mechanisms and hence may reduce oxygen toxicity, barotrauma, and lung infection. The lung's repair capability, adaptive capacity and defense mechanisms might be compromised unless early nutritional support is instituted. The ultimate consequence of these damaging factors is the development of BPD which is beyond the scope of this chapter.

Nutrition and respiratory muscles

Nutritional studies in animals and human adults suggest that energy utilization and protein synthesis in viscera during undernutrition are maintained by degradation of skeletal muscle protein.[33] Despite their continuous use, the respiratory muscles are not spared from atrophy during nutritional deprivation. Two to three days of starvation cause the rate of protein synthesis in isolated rat diaphragm strips to fall by half and to more than double the rate of protein degradation.[34,35] In adults, undernutrition is associated with diaphragmatic muscle atrophy and a decrease in muscle force output.[36-38] The minority of the preterm diaphragmatic muscle fibers are of the fast-oxidative fatigue-resistant type,[39] indicating that the ventilatory muscles of the newborn infant are very susceptible to fatigue, particularly if there is superimposed lung disease.[40] There is controversy in this area, particularly as other investigators have found a high oxidative capacity and, in contrast to the findings of Keens et al.,[39] they found fatigue resistance in newborn monkeys[41,42] and piglets.[43] Because of the highly compliant rib cage, a substantial fraction of the force of the diaphragm is dissipated in distorting the rib cage rather than affecting gas volume exchange. Tachypnea is characteristic of lung disease in infancy, and the faster the repetition rate of muscle contraction, the shorter the time of its endurance. As in other skeletal muscles,[44] when the available chemical energy becomes limited, force generation will fail. The ability to sustain contractions has been found to depend on intramuscular glycogen stores.[45,46] Diaphragmatic glycogen depletion resulting in loss of force has been demonstrated.[47] It is interesting that the diaphragm at birth is rich in glycogen,[48] but it is unknown for how long these reserves are sufficient to cover the respiratory needs of the newborn infant. Apnea of prematurity has at least in part been attributed to respiratory muscle fatigue. Apart from the increased work of breathing due to the high chest wall compliance and paucity of high oxidative type fibers in the diaphragm of the preterm infant,[40] relative substrate deficiency has also been hypothesized to play a role.[49,50] A reduction in frequency of apneas has been observed in preterm infants receiving amino acids and glucose intravenously compared with those receiving only glucose.[51] This might have resulted from either the higher EI or an increase in ventilatory drive caused by amino acids, as is discussed in the next section.

Nutrition, metabolism, and ventilatory drive

Nutrition can affect the ventilatory drive directly by stimulating the central nervous ventilatory stimuli, and indirectly by modifying metabolism, and consequently the metabolic rate and respiratory gaseous exchange. In adults and infants, cardiac output and heart rate closely parallel changes in oxygen consumption,[52,53] while carbon dioxide production affects minute ventilation.[53] When adults are weaning from mandatory ventilation, the ability to breathe spontaneously is dependent on an appropriate level of EI;[54] in contrast, overfeeding might result in hypercapnea in the patient with borderline lung function.[53] In the latter situation, the ventilatory response to carbon dioxide may be diminished, either secondary to decreased chemosensitivity or because changes in ventilatory mechanics limit the response.[53] It may well be that the same rules apply to the preterm infant. On the one hand, the intensivist has the difficult task of minimizing the oxygen demands and the carbon dioxide burden in patients with borderline lung function; on the other hand, enough energy has to be provided to allow weaning from the ventilator. In newborn infants, there is the additional necessity of giving sufficient energy to allow structural lung maturation and growth of the body. This brittle balance might be particularly difficult to achieve in the very small premature infant.

A high carbohydrate load seems to increase minute ventilation by increasing carbon dioxide production in adults.[55–58] A similar correlation between glucose intake and carbon dioxide production has been reported in newborn infants receiving fat-free intravenous nutrition.[59–63] In adults, increasing protein intakes have been associated with increased oxygen consumption and ventilatory drive. A recent study in neonates, however, demonstrated that oxygen consumption and carbon dioxide production were correlated with EI but not with protein intake.[64]

The rise in carbon dioxide production may cause an increase in ventilation requirements. Wahlig et al.[65] found that as an infant's level of respiratory illness becomes more severe the oxygen consumption increases as well. One may thus extrapolate that infants with greater degrees of respiratory illness require a higher EI to prevent catabolism.

Without the ability of the chest wall and lung system to adequately respond, increasing the ventilatory drive in infants with limited lung function might cause problems. In those infants who cannot respond adequately, this may precipitate respiratory failure; in the infants who do respond, the increase in workload may lead to an excessively high level of work of breathing and induce respiratory muscle fatigue. In infants with BPD, energy expenditure increases by 0.7 kcal kg^{-1} day^{-1} per breath.[66] Clearly, one is dealing with a difficult dilemma: on one hand EI has to be sufficient to maintain bodily functions and support adequate growth; on the other hand, too much EI and unbalanced dietary composition might induce or accelerate respiratory failure in the infant with borderline lung function.

Acute respiratory disease and total parenteral nutrition

The majority of infants with acute respiratory distress cannot be fed enterally initially and, therefore, total parenteral nutrition (TPN) will be the main focus of this section. Many VLBW infants with birth weight under 1000 g are in a catabolic state during the most acute phase of their respiratory illness.[13,67] Although their energy stores are limited, providing too much energy might overload the already compromised lung function, while providing too little energy will lead to the development of a catabolic state.

Energy

Total parenteral nutrition is the main source of nutrition during the first week of life in 80% of the infants weighing less than 1000 g.[68] In the last decade, a shift to more aggressive introduction of parenteral and enteral nutrition during the first 24 hours of life has taken place.[69]

A caloric intake of 60 kcal kg^{-1} day^{-1} should provide enough energy to account for the resting metabolic state of the infant as well as to compensate for energy losses through temperature regulation and physical activity.[69] As enteral nutrition does not contribute significantly to EI in this population in the first few days of life, caloric losses through the gastrointestinal tract are insignificant. Caloric expenditure may be minimized in this population of ventilated newborns by maintaining a thermoneutral environment and providing adequate sedation and analgesia.

Energy expenditure (EE) in the first few days of life in ventilated ELBW and VLBW infants has been the subject of several recent studies.[64,70,71] More recent estimates of 40–50 kcal kg^{-1} day^{-1} to prevent catabolism are slightly lower than previous estimates of 60 kcal kg^{-1} day^{-1}. In ventilated

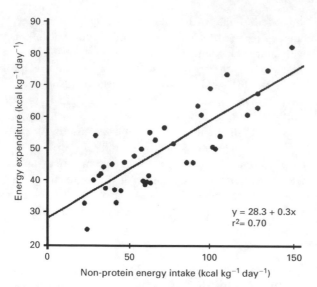

Figure 35.1. Energy expenditure increases by 30% for each additional kilocalorie of non-protein energy intake.[64]

newborns there is a strong correlation between EI and EE, but not with severity of illness (Figure 35.1).[64] Furthermore, in healthy, spontaneously breathing term infants, a correlation between EI and oxygen consumption and carbon dioxide production has been seen.[72]

The increase in EE cannot be necessarily accounted for by increased work of breathing to eliminate the increased carbon dioxide. Reduced EE in sick ventilated neonates as compared with nonventilated controls has been demonstrated.[70] Similarly no increase in EE following PDA ligation was found in a group of ventilated newborns.[71] These results are biologically plausible if one considers that any potential increase in EE by work of breathing is compensated for by increased support from the ventilators. Therefore, while these neonates might consume more energy if spontaneously breathing, ventilator support may offset this potential cost.

One must be cautious when interpreting results from EE studies. Errors may be derived from the use of indirect calorimetry to estimate energy requirements in intubated newborns. High oxygen concentrations and small variations in the flow by leaks around the endotracheal tube translate into large errors in the final result which may explain some of the variation seen across studies. Furthermore, while the estimated and measured EEs for a group may be similar, individual comparisons may be quite discordant.[73]

In summary, safe estimates of energy maintenance requirements are in the range of 60–70 kcal kg^{-1} day^{-1}. Growth will not be accomplished at this level of intake.

Protein and amino acids

The initial goal is not to attain weight gain but to provide adequate calories and nitrogen to prevent catabolism and promote positive nitrogen balance. It has been generally accepted that the provision of 60 kcal kg^{-1} day^{-1} and 2–2.5 g kg^{-1} day^{-1} of amino acids results in a positive nitrogen balance.[74,75] However, two recent studies suggest an amino acid intake as low as 1–1.5 g kg^{-1} day^{-1} may be sufficient to maintain positive nitrogen balance and prevent catabolism.[76,77] In the study by Thureen and coworkers, only 1/19 infants with a minimal intake of 1 g kg^{-1} day^{-1} of amino acids was found to be catabolic at the above EI. However, a group of infants receiving 3 g kg^{-1} day^{-1} of protein was safe and efficacious, causing 50% of the protein to be retained.

What does seem to be consistent is that nitrogen retention is dependent on total energy supply rather than the amounts of fat or glucose provided.[76,78] Despite previous findings in which 50 kcal kg^{-1} day^{-1} provided as glucose, led to an excretion of nitrogen at a rate of approximately 130 mg kg^{-1} day^{-1},[74] current evidence suggests that ventilated newborns may achieve positive nitrogen balance at intakes below 60 kcal kg^{-1} day^{-1}.[77,79] It is important to note however that this does not imply that intakes below 60 kcal kg^{-1} day^{-1} can achieve weight and length gain.

For those infants requiring parenteral nutrition for longer periods of time, the second goal, weight gain, must be achieved. Energy intakes above 70 kcal kg^{-1} day^{-1} (including 2.7–3.5 g of protein kg^{-1} day^{-1}) result in nitrogen accretion rates similar to in utero values,[80] indicating that basal and muscular activity caloric needs have been met. The combined effect of energy and nitrogen intake seems to be such that, at any level of EI, increasing nitrogen intake increases nitrogen retention; similarly, at any level of nitrogen intake, increasing EI up to 120 kcal kg^{-1} day^{-1} increases nitrogen retention. Metabolic acidosis as a result of a large range of protein intake is no longer seen in preterm infants.[76,81] Serum levels of amino acids did not increase at intakes of 1–1.5 g kg^{-1} day^{-1}, suggesting intact capabilities to utilize amino acids.[77] The ideal amino acid composition of the intravenous solutions is still being investigated.

There is some controversy to what extent increasing intake of amino acids contributes to rise in EE. In the preterm neonate, Weinstein *et al.*[82] have demonstrated that a moderate amount of intravenous amino acids (2 g kg^{-1} day^{-1}) does not affect EE compared with when glucose is given alone. In contrast, in adults, intravenous amino acids cause a rise in both oxygen consumption and EE, which is related to an increase in respiratory drive and circulating norepinephrine.[83] In preterm infants, there is also evidence of increasing EE with rising protein gain.[84,85]

Plasma levels or supplementation of specific amino acids in infants with respiratory disease have also been studied. Nitric oxide has become an established treatment for the term newborn with pulmonary hypertension and is derived endogenously from arginine. Studies in newborns have demonstrated a reduction in serum arginine levels in infants with persistent pulmonary hypertension of the newborn,[86,87] but have not shown a correlation between arginine levels and response to inhaled nitric oxide.[86] While there are no controlled trials using arginine as a nutritional supplement for persistent pulmonary hypertension (PPHN), McCaffrey[88] and colleagues have described a series of five patients treated with L-arginine. Their findings included increased oxygenation and a reduction in the oxygenation index of 33%–50% in four of five infants over a 5-hour trial. While the evidence is not conclusive for a respiratory benefit, preliminary evidence has shown reduced arginine levels in neonates with established necrotizing enterocolitis (NEC)[89,90] and a potential therapeutic role for arginine in reducing the incidence of NEC.[91] There may be an additional benefit by cosupplementation of inhaled NO with arginine to increase endogenous NO production but further trials are needed.

Cysteine, another amino acid used as a supplement in TPN, is the rate-limiting precursor for glutathione production, an antioxidant. Neonates in a hyperoxic environment produce greater amounts of oxygen-free radicals. Reduced cysteine levels have been demonstrated in a group of neonates with PPHN, which recovered after resolution of the pulmonary disease.[92] The reduced levels were presumably secondary to consumption of cysteine through increased conversion to glutathione. Further studies on the effect of cysteine on pulmonary morbidity need to be performed before widespread use can be recommended.

Glucose

Glucose is the main energy source in total parenteral nutrition. When giving human milk the glucose intake of the newborn infant is around 1.75 g kg^{-1} day^{-1} during the first 2 days, increasing to 2.75 g kg^{-1} day^{-1} on days 3 and 4, and to 6.3 g kg^{-1} day^{-1} 1 week after birth.[93] It has been demonstrated that low EI provided by glucose (38 kcal kg^{-1} day^{-1}) results in diminished activity of the sympathetic nervous system.[82] Increasing glucose intake from 38 to 64 kcal kg^{-1} day^{-1} induces a rise in EE, which is related to a surge in catecholamines. This indicates that the sympathetic nervous system in the preterm infant responds to

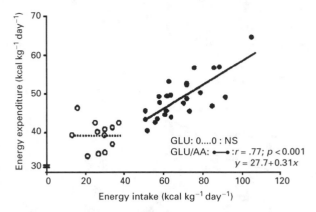

Figure 35.2. Energy expenditure increases with increasing energy intake for the glucose/amino acid group by 0.31 kcal per kcal administered. No effect can be demonstrated in the glucose group with energy intakes below maintenance energy requirements.[63]

varying levels of EI similarly to adults. We have investigated energy metabolism and respiratory gaseous exchange in full-term nonventilated infants receiving fat-free intravenous nutrition.[61,63] Twelve infants (group 1) received glucose between 3.5 and 10 g kg^{-1} day^{-1} (2.4 to 7.0 mg kg^{-1} min^{-1}), equivalent to an EI ranging from 13.1 to 37.5 kcal kg^{-1} day^{-1}. Twenty-six infants (group 2) received increasing amounts of a glucose/amino acid solution totalling between 10.9 and 24.1 g kg^{-1} day^{-1} for glucose, 2.06 to 3.90 g kg^{-1} day^{-1} for amino acids, and 51 to 105 kcal kg^{-1} day^{-1} for EI. There was no increase in EE with increasing glucose intake in group 1. For group 2, diet-induced-thermogenesis caused by the glucose-amino acid infusion resulted in an increment in resting EE of 0.31 kcal per extra kilocalorie supplied (Figure 35.2).

The major portion of this rise was due to increasing lipogenesis from glucose with increasing glucose intake.[60,63] Increasing EI using fat-free parenteral nutrition has also been shown to increase carbon dioxide production, EE and oxygen consumption.[60,63] Whereas increasing EI by increasing IV glucose results in a rise in EE and respiratory gas exchange, increasing an isonitrogenous caloric intake from 60 kcal kg^{-1} day^{-1} as glucose only to 85 kcal kg^{-1} day^{-1} by adding 2 g kg^{-1} day^{-1} of IV lipid does not result in an increase in metabolic rate, oxygen consumption, or carbon dioxide production.[94]

In adults, high glucose loads increase resting EE[56,95,96] and can induce temperature instability.[97] High glucose loads have also been demonstrated to increase carbon dioxide production,[56,98–101] resulting in a higher minute ventilation.[56,97,101–103] This can exacerbate respiratory failure in the patient on ventilatory support and with

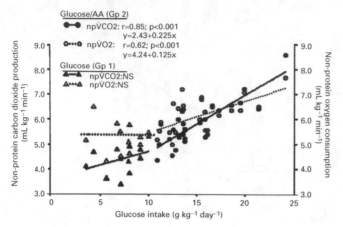

Figure 35.3. Effect of glucose intake on nonprotein respiratory gas exchange in full-term infants receiving fat-free intravenous nutrition. Nonprotein carbon dioxide production (npVCO2, closed circles), rose 0.225 ml kg^{-1} min^{-1} for each additional gram of glucose administered and nonprotein oxygen consumption (npVO2, open circles) rose 0.125 ml kg^{-1} min^{-1} in 26 full-term infants receiving a fat-free diet of glucose and amino acids (glucose/AA). Nonprotein respiratory quotient = 1.0 at a glucose intake of approximately 18 g kg^{-1} day^{-1}. Below an energy intake sufficient to cover maintenance energy requirements (triangles), there was no effect of glucose intake on respiratory gas exchange.[63]

borderline lung function.[56,57,104] We did not demonstrate a rise in carbon dioxide production or oxygen consumption below glucose intakes equivalent to 40 kcal kg^{-1} day^{-1} in full-term infants on fat-free parenteral nutrition (Figure 35.3). Nonprotein carbon dioxide production almost doubled from 4.7 to 7.9 mL kg^{-1} min^{-1} when the glucose intake increased from 10 to 24 g kg^{-1} day^{-1} (Figure 35.3). Nonprotein oxygen consumption increased slower and equaled nonprotein carbon dioxide production at a glucose intake of approximately 18 g kg^{-1} day^{-1}.[61,63] This is similar to findings in preterm infants on fat-free parenteral nutrition.[59] The difference between the slopes of nonprotein carbon dioxide production and nonprotein oxygen consumption in Figure 35.3 is the result of increasing lipogenesis with increasing glucose intake, as confirmed by Sauer *et al.*[60] Lipogenesis from glucose produces more carbon dioxide than it consumes oxygen[105] and will cause an increase in EE, because up to 24% of the glucose energy is required to cover the energy requirements for fatty acid synthesis from glucose.[106] This accounts at least partially for the rise in metabolic rate from 43 to 60 kcal kg^{-1} day^{-1} (group 2; glu/aa) observed in Figure 35.2.

A large carbohydrate load given to healthy adults increases carbon dioxide production by 43% and oxygen consumption by 13%, which results in a 47% increase in alveolar ventilation.[103] In adults with airway disease without carbon dioxide retention, a large oral carbohydrate load causes an increase in minute ventilation from 10.3 to 12.8 L min^{-1}.[102] Assuming that the basic caloric requirement for a full-term 3-kg neonate is equal to the average hepatic endogenous glucose production of 6 mg kg^{-1} min^{-1} [107,108] and assuming that the respiratory frequency averages 40 breaths min^{-1}, the nonprotein carbon dioxide production will total 13.1 mL min^{-1} or 0.33 mL per breath. Raising the glucose intake to 15 mg kg^{-1}min^{-1} will increase the nonprotein carbon dioxide production to 21.9 mL min^{-1}, an increase of 8.8 mL min^{-1} or approximately 67%. To eliminate this extra carbon dioxide, the minute ventilation will increase either by augmenting respiratory rate or volume. Assuming constant tidal volume, the respiratory rate would rise to approximately 65 breaths per minute. The workload of additional ventilation imposed by the increased carbon dioxide production occasioned by a high load of intravenous glucose could precipitate respiratory failure when respiratory function is compromised, and weaning from ventilatory support could be impeded. Assuming a caloric need of 0.7 kcal kg^{-1} day^{-1} per breath,[66] this would mean an increased energy expenditure of 17.5 kcal kg^{-1} day^{-1}.

In summary, increasing the energy supply progressively by only increasing glucose and amino acid intake would impose an additional workload on the respiratory system.

Effect of intravenous lipid emulsions on energy metabolism and respiratory gas exchange

In adults, a combination of intravenous glucose and lipid as the nonprotein energy source appears to be more physiologic than infusion of glucose alone.[109–111] Nose *et al.* found a substantial increase in basal metabolic rate in infants and children on TPN with glucose and amino acids alone compared with lipid-supplemented patients.[112] On the other hand, when intravenous fat alone is given as the nonprotein energy source, an increase in oxygen consumption has been reported.[113]

We compared two groups of nonintubated full-term infants on TPN with similar energy and protein intakes, but with a nonprotein energy supply of either only glucose or a combination of glucose and lipid with a caloric ratio of 3 : 1. At a caloric intake of approximately 85 kcal kg^{-1} day^{-1}, EE decreased significantly when an isocaloric amount of fat was substituted for glucose, leaving more energy for storage and growth. Both nonprotein carbon dioxide production

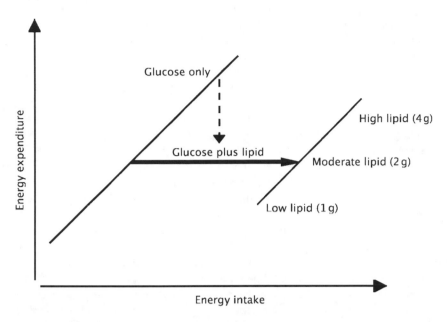

Figure 35.4. Energy expenditure increases with increasing energy intake when diet composition is constant (glucose only + AA). When glucose calories are isocalorically replaced by lipid, energy expenditure decreases. When energy intake is increased by adding lipid and changing the diet composition, there is no effect on energy expenditure. Different glucose : lipid ratios with different energy intake may result in different effects on energy expenditure.

and nonprotein oxygen consumption decreased.[62,63,114] The significant differences in carbon dioxide production, oxygen consumption, and metabolic rate between the two groups were due to suppression of lipogenesis from glucose in the lipid-supplemented group. This has been confirmed by studies combining indirect calorimetry and U-^{13}C-glucose.[114]

Piedboeuf and colleagues studied nonventilated newborns receiving isocaloric, isonitrogenous IV nutrition with either 1 g kg^{-1} day^{-1} or 3 g kg^{-1} day^{-1} of intralipid. Their findings of 11% higher carbon dioxide production and 11% lower pO$_2$ agree with previous reports of increased CO$_2$ and decreased oxygenation when receiving higher amounts of lipid infusions.[115] A subsequent study in ventilated infants with early BPD corroborated the observation that lipid intakes of 2–2.5 g kg^{-1} day^{-1} were not associated with elevated CO$_2$ production compared with isocaloric glucose-based intravenous nutrition.[116] It seems that the problem of increasing metabolic rate with increasing EI only applies when the diet composition is left constant. These data and the earlier work of Heim *et al.*[113] indicate that administering either glucose or fat as the only nonprotein energy source results in "metabolic stress," with an increase in oxygen consumption, carbon dioxide production, and EE. From the point of view of energy balance and respiratory gaseous exchange, intravenous nonprotein calories should be given

as a combination of glucose and lipid, but the ideal ratio still has to be determined (Figure 35.4).

Effect of intravenous lipid emulsions on lung function

Lipid emulsions have been blamed for causing pulmonary dysfunction. There is a lot of controversy reflecting differences in dose, duration, and rate of lipid infusion, fatty acid composition, type of animal models, and type of patients. The lung dysfunction had initially been attributed to the associated hyperlipidemia;[117] this might in fact only be correct with fat overload syndrome. Other studies have indicated that the decrease in PaO$_2$ is a result of ventilation/perfusion inequalities due to changes in prostanoid metabolism causing alterations in the pulmonary vascular tone.[118–123] Whereas a bolus of prostaglandin precursors has resulted in higher pulmonary pressure responses, continuous infusion has yielded net vasodilator responses in some studies[118,124,125] or no effect in other studies.[126] There is a much larger volume of studies in animals[121,127–129] demonstrating a vasoconstrictor response in the pulmonary circulation after either a bolus or low-dose continuous infusion. In human neonates, after 90 minutes of intravenous lipid infusion, the ratio of right ventricular pre-ejection period to ejection time rises significantly, suggesting increased pulmonary vascular resistance.[130] Using right ventricular pre-ejection period to ejection time as a measure of pulmonary artery blood pressure, we have demonstrated a dose–response relationship between dose of lipid infusion between 0 and 3 g kg^{-1} day^{-1} and elevation of pulmonary vascular resistance.[131] Interestingly this response is not seen until after 24 hours of exposure.

Infusion of soybean oil-based intravenous lipid emulsions might increase the incidence of BPD, and it is postulated that this effect is related to thromboxane A2[132,133] and leukotrienes.[134] A recent study in piglets receiving soybean-based emulsions failed to demonstrate a rise in thromboxane A2 during hypoxia-induced pulmonary vasoconstriction.[135] In the same study the hypoxia-induced pulmonary hypertension was much higher in the animals receiving an intravenous soybean oil emulsion as compared with controls or animals given an intravenous fish oil emulsion. It may be that the vasoconstriction is mediated by leukotrienes rather than thromboxane.

Despite higher levels of pulmonary vascular resistance, there are some data indicating a decrease in oxygen toxicity when feeding diets high in linoleic acid.[136] The explanation for the contradictory results might be due to differences in duration and in rate of infusion of the lipid emulsions in the respective studies and the resulting differences in the ratio of vasodilating over vasoconstricting eicosanoids. During a bolus or a rapid infusion, an excessive amount of substrate may overwhelm the enzymatic pathways for PGI$_2$ and PGE$_2$ metabolism, resulting in an increased production of potent vasoconstrictive thromboxanes.[122] Curiously, administration of indomethacin, an inhibitor of vasodilating prostaglandin production helps maintain stable pO$_2$s during intralipid infusions as has been shown in a rabbit model.[118] Pulmonary venous admixture is known to increase during intralipid infusion in adults.[137] This may arise due to local increases in pulmonary vasodilating prostaglandins causing shunting past poorly ventilated lung units. By inhibiting the release of these prostaglandins, indomethacin may decrease the extent of shunt during intravenous lipid infusion. Although some data from animal studies are available, there is presently insufficient clinical evidence to withhold intravenous lipid emulsions for pulmonary reasons, except perhaps in infants with persistent pulmonary hypertension. Expansion of this research into the neonatal area is warranted.

More recently, the use of MCT based parenteral lipid sources has been explored for their potential benefits. They undergo faster hydrolysis and oxidization and are oxidized more completely than long chain fatty acids. Despite these advantages, they must be combined with an LCT preparation containing essential fatty acids. An energy source that is metabolized more efficiently might be expected to prevent catabolism in an already stressed, ventilated neonate. Ball *et al.*[138] found that adults receiving an MCT preparation had higher glucose, insulin, nonesterified fatty acids, and ketone levels than a group receiving an LCT lipid source. These findings support the improved efficiency of MCTs as an energy source with the higher glucose and insulin levels being explained by the availability of ketones and nonesterified fatty acids as an alternative energy source. Furthermore, an adult study has shown a reduction in nitrogen loss when a combined MCT/LCT preparation is used versus an LCT preparation used alone.[139] Several investigators have measured eicosanoid levels and changes in pulmonary functions in patients receiving MCT lipids. There was no difference between prostanoid levels of ventilated adults receiving either an MCT or LCT emulsion. A decrease in levels occurred on withdrawal of the LCT but not the MCT preparation.[140]

In a study examining physiologic parameters, minute ventilation increased by 21% in the MCT/LCT group v. to 1% increase in the group receiving LCTs compared with baseline.[141] Furthermore, oxygen consumption increased 27% compared with 11% in the same groups reflecting the increase in oxidation. Interestingly though, in a group of critically ill adults, no difference in oxidation rates between a group receiving an LCT preparation v. those on a mixed preparation with MCT/LCT was shown.[142] The difference in the results may be explained by the presence of hyperglycemia in the latter study which may have been preferentially utilized as the primary energy source. Similarly, in stable, postsurgical, nonventilated infants receiving a low carbohydrate intake with an MCT/LCT lipid emulsion, lipid oxidation increased as compared with another group receiving a high carbohydrate intake.[143] Additionally, infants receiving LCT preparations regardless of carbohydrate intake have lower rates of lipid oxidation.

As Pediatric or Neonatal MCT-emulsions are not available in North America, many clinical questions remain unanswered.

Summary

In summary, during the acute stage of respiratory disease, catabolism should be avoided and a positive nitrogen balance achieved, to support lung repair and development, and to safeguard that appropriate amounts of nutrients are given during the "critical epochs" of growth and development. During the first 36–48 hours of the infant's life, the nutritional management should provide approximately 60 kcal kg^{-1} day^{-1} comprising 10 to 12 g kg^{-1} day^{-1} as glucose, 0.5–1.0 g kg^{-1} day^{-1} of intravenous lipid (which is enough to prevent essential fatty acid deficiency), and amino acid intake of 2 g kg^{-1} day^{-1}. Whereas fluid overload and the risk for lung edema[144] can be limited with this regimen, hyperglycemia is often a serious problem in the smallest preterm infants. Continuous infusion of low-dose insulin improves glucose tolerance in extremely low-birth-weight infants,[145,146] but there are no data regarding the effect on metabolic rate, respiratory gaseous exchange, or metabolic rate of glucose.

After a few days, one should aim for a more positive energy balance by progressively increasing the intravenous lipid intake to 3–4 g kg^{-1} day^{-1}, while monitoring the triglyceride levels.[126] A glucose : lipid ratio of 3 : 1 to 2 : 1 on a caloric basis minimizes the carbon dioxide stress, which is particularly important during the acute stage of impaired lung function. A progressive increase of protein intake to 3.0–3.5 g kg^{-1} day^{-1} should also be aimed for. This should result in an IV energy intake of 80–100 kcal kg^{-1} day^{-1} by the end of the first week of life.

Whereas data are available on energy requirements for the stable growing infant nourished either orally or intravenously, very limited data are available on the critically ill, ventilated, preterm infant. While calculations are available for predicting energy requirements for the sick preterm neonate, ideally they should be determined for each infant individually. However, indirect calorimetry in the intubated infant receiving high concentrations of oxygen is prone to errors. On a long-term basis, limited intake of energy and nutrients affects the development of the fast-growing nervous system, but it also affects lung growth and might contribute to the development of bronchopulmonary dysplasia. On one hand, a negative energy balance in infants with limited energy stores affects mortality and morbidity of the smallest preterm infants. On the other hand, feeding "too much" or "an inappropriate mix" results in high carbon dioxide production, with a potential for respiratory acidosis and an increase in EE. Finding the brittle equilibrium is a key part in the nutritional management of these infants.

Based on the studies reviewed in this chapter, early appropriate nutrition should be part of the total management of the prematurely born infant; this is important not only on a short-term basis for the acutely ill infant with limited energy reserves, but also in the long term, as it might limit lung damage leading to broncho-pulmonary dysplasia.

In managing the preterm infant, failing organs and body systems cannot be treated separately but have to be seen as part of a complex interaction in which energy balance and metabolism take a central position from the very beginning. The energy efficiency of any type of burning furnace or engine depends largely on the fuel administered.

REFERENCES

1 Goswami, T., Vu, M., Srivastava, U. Quantitative changes in the DNA, RNA and protein content of various organs of the young of undernourished female rats. *J. Nutr.* 1974;**104**: 1257–64.

2 Winick, M., Noble, A. Cellular response in rats during malnutrition at various ages. *J. Nutr.* 1966;**89**:300–6.

3 Sahebjami, H., Vassalo, C. Effects of starvation and refeeding on lung mechanics and morphometry. *Am. Rev. Respir. Dis.* 1979;**119**:443–51.

4 Sahebjami, H., Wirman, J. Emphysema-like changes in the lungs of starved rats. *Am. Rev. Respir. Dis.* 1981;**124**: 619–24.

5 Harkema, J., Mauderly, J., Gregory, R. *et al.* A comparison of starvation and elastase models of emphysema in the rat. *Am. Rev. Respir. Dis.* 1984;**129**:584–91.

6 Stein, J., Fenigstein, H. Anatomie pathologique de la maladie de famine. In Apfelbaum, E., ed. *Maladie de Famine.* American Joint Distribution Committee; 1946:21–7.

7 Lechner, A. Perinatal age determines the severity of retarded lung development induced by starvation. *Am. Rev. Resp. Dis.* 1985;**131**:638–43.

8 Sobonya, R., Logvinoff, M., Faussig, L. *et al.* Morphometric analysis of the lung in prolonged bronchopulmonary dysplasia. *Pediatr. Res.* 1983;**16**:969–72.

9 Gross, I., Ilic, I., Wilson, C. *et al.* The influence of postnatal nutritional deprivation on the phospholipid content of developing rat lung. *Biochim. Biophys. Acta* 1976;**441**:412–22.

10 Sahebjami, H., Macgee, J. Changes in connective tissue composition of the lung in starvation and refeeding. *Am. Rev. Respir. Dis.* 1983;**128**:644–7.

11 Kerr, J., Riley, D., Lanza-Jacoby, S. *et al.* Nutritional emphysema in the rat. *Am. Rev. Respir. Dis.* 1985;**131**:644–50.

12 Meyers, B., Dubick, M., Gerreits, J. *et al.* Protein deficiency: effects on lung mechanics and the accumulation of collagen and elastin in rat lung. *J. Nutr.* 1983;**113**:2308–15.

13 Frank, L., Sosenko, I. Undernutrition as a major contributing factor in the pathogenesis of bronchopulmonary dysplasia. *Am. Rev. Respir. Dis.* 1988;**138**:725–9.

14 Van Golde, L., Batenburg, J., Robertson, B. The pulmonary surfactant system: biochemical aspects and functional significance. *Physiol. Rev.* 1988;**68**:374–455.

15 Fariday, E. Effect of food and water deprivation on surface elasticity of lungs of rats. *J. Appl. Physiol.* 1970;**29**:493–8.

16 Gail, D., Hassaro, G., Hassaro, D. Influence of fasting on the lung. *J. Appl. Physiol.* 1977;**42**:88–92.

17 Rubin, J., Clowes, G., Macnicol, M. Impaired pulmonary surfactant synthesis in starvation and severe nonthoracic sepsis. *Am. J. Surg.* 1972;**123**:461–7.

18 Brown, L., Bliss, A., Longshore, W. Effect of nutritional status on the lung surfactant system. Food deprivation and caloric restriction. *Exp. Lung Res.* 1984;**6**:133–47.

19 Bruno, J., McMahon, K., Farrell, P. Lung surfactant phospholipids as related to hydration and choline status of fasted rats. *J. Nutr.* 1985;**115**:85–9.

20 Frank, L., Sosenko, I. Development of lung antioxidant enzyme system in late gestation: possible implications for the prematurely-born infant. *J. Pediatr.* 1987;**110**:9–14.

21 Kyriakides, E., Beeler, D., Edmonds, R. *et al.* Alterations in phosphatidyl choline species and their reversal in pulmonary surfactant during essential fatty acid deficiency. *Biochim. Biophys. Acta* 1976;**431**:399–407.

22 Huang, J., Craig-Schmidt, M. C. Arachidonate and docosahexaenoate added to infant formula influence fatty acid composition and subsequent eicosanoid production in neonatal pigs. *J. Nutr.* 1996;**126**:2199–208.

23 Suarez, A., del Carmen Ramirez, M., Faus, M. J., Gil, A. Dietary long-chain polyunsaturated fatty acids influence tissue fatty acid composition in rats at weaning. *J. Nutr.* 1996;**126**:887–97.

24 Baybutt, R. C., Smith, J. E., Gillespie, M. N., Newcomb, T. G., Yeh, Y. Y. Arachidonic acid and eicosapentaenoic acid stimulate type II pneumocyte surfactant secretion. *Lipids* 1994;**29**:535–9.

25 Palombo, J. D., DeMichele, S. J., Lydon, E. E., Gregory, T. J. *et al.* Rapid modulation of lung and liver macrophage phospholipid fatty acids in endotoxemic rats by continuous enteral feeding with n-3 and gamma-linolenic fatty acids. *Am. J. Clin. Nutr.* 1996;**63**:208–19.

26 Yeh, Y. Y., Whitelock, K. A., Yeh, S. M., Lien, E. L. Dietary supplementation with arachidonic and docosahexaenoic acids has no effect on pulmonary surfactant in artificially reared infant rats. *Lipids* 1999;**34**:483–8.

27 Wolfe, R. R., Martini, W. Z., Irtun, O., Hawkins, H. K. *et al.* Dietary fat composition alters pulmonary function in pigs. *Nutrition* 2002;**18**:647–53.

28 Farrell, P. Nutrition and infant lung functions. *Pediatr. Pulmonol.* 1986;**2**:44–59.

29 Hallman, M., Jarvenpaa, A. I., Pohjavuori, M. Respiratory distress syndrome and inositol supplementation in preterm infants. *Arch. Dis. Child.* 1986;**61**:1076–83.

30 Hallman, M., Arjornaa, P., Hoppu, K. Inositol supplementation in respiratory distress syndrome. Relationship between serum concentration, renal excretion, and lung effluent phospholipids. *J. Pediatr.* 1987;**110**:604–10.

31 Hallman, M., Bry, K., Hoppu, K., Lappi, M. *et al.* Inositol supplementation in premature infants with respiratory distress syndrome. *N. Engl. J. Med.* 1992;**326**:1233–9.

32 Rhoades, R. Influence of starvation on the lung: effect of glucose and palmitate utilization. *J. Appl. Physiol.* 1975;**38**:513–16.

33 Goldberg, A., Chane, T. Regulation and significance of amino acid metabolism in skeletal muscle. *Fed. Proc.* 1978;**37**:2301–7.

34 Fulks, R., Li, J., Goldberg, A. Effects of insulin, glucose and amino acids on protein turnover in rat diaphragm. *J. Biol. Chem.* 1975;**250**:290–8.

35 Goldberg, A., Odessey, R. Oxidation of amino acids by diaphragm from fed and fasted rats. *Am. J. Physiol.* 1972;**223**:1384–91.

36 Arora, N., Rochester, D. Respiratory muscle strength and maximal voluntary ventilation in undernourished patients. *Am. Rev. Respir. Dis.* 1982;**126**:6–8.

37 Arora, N., Rochester, D. Effect of body weight and muscularity on human diaphragm muscle mass, thickness and area. *J. Appl. Physiol.* 1982;**52**:64–70.

38 Kelly, S., Rosa, A., Field, S. Inspiratory muscle strength and body composition in patients receiving total parenteral nutrition therapy. *Am. Rev. Respir. Dis.* 1984;**130**:33–7.

39 Keens, T., Bryan, A., Levison, H. *et al.* Developmental pattern of muscle fiber types in human ventilatory muscles. *J. Appl. Physiol.* 1978;**44**:909–13.

40 Muller, N., Gulston, G., Cade, D. *et al.* Diaphragmatic muscle fatigue in the newborn. *J. Appl. Physiol.* 1979;**46**:688–95.

41 Maxwell, L., Kuehl, Y., Robotham, J. *et al.* Temporal changes after death in primate diaphragm muscle oxidative enzyme activity. *Am. Rev. Respir. Dis.* 1984;**130**:1147–51.

42 Maxwell, L., McCarter, R., Kuehl, T. *et al.* Development of histochemical and functional properties of baboon respiratory muscles. *J. Appl. Physiol.* 1983;**54**:551–61.

43 Maycock, D., Hall, J., Watchko, J. *et al.* Diaphragmatic muscle fiber type development in swine. *Pediatr. Res.* 1987;**22**:449–54.

44 Fraser, I., Jeejeebhoy, K., Atwood, H. Hypocaloric diet impairs force-length adaptation in the rat soleus. *Fed. Proc.* 1984;**43**:533.

45 Costill, D., Gollnick, P., Jansson, E. *et al.* Glycogen depletion pattern in human muscle fibers during distance running. *Acta Physiol. Scand.* 1973;**9**:374–89.

46 Gollnick, P., Pieml, K., Saubert, C. *et al.* Diet, exercise and glycogen changes in human muscle fibers. *J. Appl. Physiol.* 1972;**33**:421–5.

47 Aubier, M., Trippenbach, T., Foussos, C. Respiratory muscle fatigue during cardiogenic shock. *J. Appl. Physiol.* 1981;**51**:499–508.

48 Haddad, G., Akabas, S. Adaptation of respiratory muscles to acute and chronic stress. Considerations on energy and fuels. *Clin. Chest Med.* 1986;**7**:79–89.

49 Swyer, P. Nutrition, growth and metabolism in the newborn. In Prakash, O., ed. *Critical Care of the Child.* Boston, MA: Martinus Nijhoff; 1984:1–27.

50 Swyer, P., Hein, T. Nutrition in the high-risk newborn. In Fanaroff, A., Martin, R., eds. *Neonatal-Perinatal Medicine.* St. Louis, MO: CV Mosby Co; 1987:445–59.

51 Bryan, M., Wei, P., Hamilton, J. *et al.* Supplemental intravenous alimentation in low-birthweight infants. *J. Pediatr.* 1973;**82**:940–4.

52 Chessex, P., Reichman, B., Verellen, G. *et al.* Relation between heart rate and energy expenditure in the newborn. *Pediatr. Res.* 1981;**15**:1077–82.

53 Heymsfield, S., Erbland, M., Casper, K. *et al.* Enteral nutritional support: metabolic, cardiovascular, and pulmonary interrelations. *Clin. Chest Med.* 1986;**7**:41–67.

54 Laaban, J., Lemaire, F., Baron, J. *et al.* Influence of caloric intake on the respiratory mode during mandatory minute volume ventilation. *Chest* 1985;**87**:67–78.

55 Tappy, L., Schwarz, J. M., Schneiter, P., Cayeux, C. *et al.* Effects of isoenergetic glucose-based or lipid-based parenteral nutrition on glucose metabolism de novo lipogenesis, and respiratory gas exchanges in critically ill patients. *Crit. Care Med.* 1998;**26**:860–7.

56 Askanazi, J., Elwyn, D., Silverberg, P. *et al.* Respiratory distress secondary to a high carbohydrate load. *Surgery* 1980;**80**:596–8.

57 Covelli, H., Black, J., Olsen, M. *et al.* Respiratory failure precipitated by high carbohydrate loads. *Ann. Intern. Med.* 1981;**95**:579–81.

58 Zwillich, C., Sahn, S., Weil, J. Effects of hypermetabolism on ventilation and chemosensitivity. *J. Clin. Invest.* 1977;**60**:900–6.

59 Chessex, P., Putet, G., Verellen, G. *et al.* Influence of glucose load on the energy metabolism of preterm infants on fat-free parenteral nutrition. *Pediatr. Res.* 1984;**18**:192A.

60 Sauer, P., Van Aerde, J., Pencharz, P. *et al.* Glucose oxidation rates in newborn infants measured with indirect calorimetry and U-13 C-glucose. *Clin. Sci.* 1986;**70**:587–93.

61 Van Aerde, J., Sauer, P., Heim, T. *et al.* Effect of increasing glucose loads on respiratory gaseous exchange in the newborn infant. *Pediatr. Res.* 1986;**20**:420A.

62 Van Aerde, J., Sauer, P., Pencharz, P. *et al.* Glucose and fat requirements in the intravenously fed newborn infant. In Stern, L., Friis-Hansen, B., Orzalesi, M., eds. *Physiologic Foundations of Perinatal Care, Vol 3*. New York, NY: Elsevier Scientific Publishing; 1989;60–74.

63 Van Aerde, J. Intravenous nutritional energy support and macronutrient utilization in the neonate. PhD Thesis. *Acta Biomedica Lovaniensis* 1990;**22**.

64 DeMarie, M. P., Hoffenberg, A., Biggerstaff, S. L. *et al.* Determinants of energy expenditure in ventilated preterm infants. *J. Perinat. Med.* 1999;**27**:465–72.

65 Wahlig, T. M., Gatto, C. W., Boros, S. J. *et al.* Metabolic response of preterm infants to variable degrees of respiratory illness. *J. Pediatr.* 1994;**124**:283–8.

66 Meer, D. E. K, Westerterp, X. R., Houwen, R. H. J *et al.* Total energy expenditure in infants with bronchopulmonary dysplasia is associated with respiratory status. *Eur. J. Pediatr.* 1997;**56**:299–304.

67 Georgieff, M., Hoffman, J., Pereira, G. *et al.* Effect of neonatal caloric deprivation on head growth and 1-year developmental status in preterm infants. *J. Pediatr.* 1985;**107**:581–7.

68 Churella, H., Bachuber, B., MacLean, W. Survey: methods of feeding low-birthweight infants. *Pediatrics* 1985;**76**:243–9.

69 Ziegler, E. E., Thureen, P. J., Carlson, S. J. Aggressive nutrition of the very low birthweight infant. *Clin. Perinatol.* 2002;**29**:225–44.

70 Forsyth, J. S., Crighton, A. Low birthweight infants and total parenteral nutrition immediately after birth. I. Energy expenditure and respiratory quotient of ventilated and non-ventilated infants. *Arch. Dis. Child Fetal Neonatal Edn.* 1995;**73**:F4–7.

71 Garza, J. J., Shew, S. B., Keshen, T. H. *et al.* Energy expenditure in ill premature neonates. *J. Pediatr. Surg.* 2002;**37**:289–93.

72 Van Aerde, J. Acute respiratory failure and bronchopulmonary dysplasia. In Hay, W. W. Jr., ed. *Neonatal Nutrition and Metabolism*. New York, NY: Mosby Year Book Publishers; 1991:476–506.

73 Verhoeven, J. J., Hazelzet, J. A., van der Voort, E., Joosten, K. F. Comparison of measured and predicted energy expenditure in mechanically ventilated children. *Intens. Care Med.* 1998;**24**:464–8.

74 Anderson, T., Muttart, C., Bieber, M. *et al.* A controlled trial of glucose versus glucose and amino acids in preterm infants. *J. Pediatr.* 1979;**94**:947–51.

75 Joosten, K. F., Verhoeven, J. J., Hazelzet, J. A. Energy expenditure and substrate utilization in mechanically ventilated children. *Nutrition.* 1999;**15**:444–8.

76 Thureen, P. J., Anderson, A. H., Baron, K. A. *et al.* Protein balance in the first week of life in ventilated neonates receiving parenteral nutrition. *Am. J. Clin. Nutr.* 1998;**68**:1128–35.

77 Rivera, A. Jr, Bell, E. F., Bier, D. M. Effect of intravenous amino acids on protein metabolism of preterm infants during the first three days of life. *Pediatr. Res.* 1993;**33**:106–11.

78 Rubecz, I., Mestyan, J., Varga, P. *et al.* Energy metabolism, substrate utilization, and nitrogen balance in parenterally fed postoperative neonates and infants. *J. Pediatr.* 1981;**98**: 4246.

79 Van Goudoever, J. B., Colen, T., Wattimena, J. L. *et al.* Immediate commencement of amino acid supplementation in preterm infants: effect on serum amino acid concentrations and protein kinetics on the first day of life. *J. Pediatr.* 1995;**127**:458–65.

80 Zlotkin, S., Bryan, M., Anderson, G. Intravenous nitrogen and EIs required to duplicate in utero nitrogen accretion in prematurely born human infants. *J. Pediatr.* 1981;**99**:115–20.

81 Porcelli, P. J. Jr, Sisk, P. M. Increased parenteral amino acid administration to extremely low-birth-weight infants during early postnatal life. *J. Pediatr. Gastro. Nutr.* 2002;**34**:174–9.

82 Weinstein, M., Haugen, K., Bauer, J. *et al.* Intravenous energy and amino acids in the preterm newborn infant: effects on metabolic rate and potential mechanisms of action. *J. Pediatr.* 1987;**111**:119–23.

83 Takala, J., Askanazi, J., Weissman, C. *et al.* Changes in respiratory control induced by amino acid infusions. *Crit. Care Med.* 1988;**16**:465–9.

84 Catzeflis, C., Schutz, Y., Micheli, J. *et al.* Whole body protein synthesis and energy expenditure. *Pediatr. Res.* 1985;**19**:679–87.

85 Sauer, P., Van Aerde, J., Beesley, J. *et al.* Energy partition of protein synthesis in resting energy expenditure of neonates on TPN. *Pediatr. Res.* 1984;**18**:339A.

86 Kavvadia, V., Greenough, A., Lilley, J. *et al.* Plasma arginine levels and the response to inhaled nitric oxide in neonates. *Biol. Neonate* 1999;**76**:340–7.

87 Vosatka, R. J., Kashyap, S., Trifiletti, R. R. Arginine deficiency accompanies persistent pulmonary hypertension of the newborn. *Biol. Neonate* 1994;**67**:240–3.

88 McCaffrey, M. J., Bose, C. L., Reiter, P. D., Stiles, A. D. Effect of L-arginine infusion on infants with persistent pulmonary hypertension of the newborn. *Biol. Neonate* 1995;**67**:240–3.

89 Becker, R. M., Wu, G., Galanko, J. A. *et al.* Reduced serum amino acid concentrations in infants with necrotizing enterocolitis. *J. Peds.* 2000;**137**:785–93.

90 Zamora, S. A., Amin, H. J., McMillan, D. D. *et al.* Plasma L-arginine concentrations in premature infants with necrotizing enterocolitis. *J. Peds.* 1997;**131**:226–32.

91 Amin, H. J., Zamora, S. A., McMillan, D. D. *et al.* Arginine supplementation prevents necrotizing enterocolitis in the premature infant. *J. Peds.* 2002;**140**:425–31.

92 White, C. W., Stabler, S. P., Allen, R. H. *et al.* Plasma cysteine concentrations in infants with respiratory distress. *J. Peds.* 1994;**125**:769–77.

93 Aynsley-Green, A., Soltesz, G. The regulation of carbohydrate metabolism. In Aynsley-Green, A., Soltesz, G., eds. *Hypoglycemia in Infancy and Childhood.* Edinburgh: Churchill Livingstone; 1985:1–27.

94 Van Aerde, J. E., Sauer, P. J., Pencharz, P. B. *et al.* Metabolic consequences of increasing energy intake by adding lipid to parenteral nutrition in full-term infants. *Am. J. Clin. Nutr.* 1994;**59**:659–62.

95 Askanazi, J., Rosenbaum, S., Hyman, A. *et al.* Respiratory changes induced by the large glucose loads of total parenteral nutrition. *J. Am. Med. Assoc.* 1980;**14**:1444–7.

96 Nordenstrom, J., Jeevanandarn, M., Elwyn, D. *et al.* Increasing glucose intake during total parenteral nutrition increases norepinephrine excretion in trauma and sepsis. *Clin. Physiol.* 1981;**1**:525–34.

97 Askanazi, J., Rosenbaum, S., Michelsen, C. *et al.* Increased body temperature secondary to total parenteral nutrition. *Crit. Care Med.* 1980;**8**:736–7.

98 Askanazi, J., Carpentier, Y., Elwyn, D. *et al.* Influence of total parenteral nutrition on fuel utilization in injury and sepsis. *Am. Surg.* 1979;**191**:40–6.

99 Elwyn, D., Kinney, J., Gump, F. *et al.* Some metabolic effects of fat infusions in depleted patients. *Metabolism* 1980;**29**:125–32.

100 Hunker, F., Burton, C., Hunker, E. *et al.* Metabolic and nutritional evaluation of patients supported with mechanical ventilation. *Crit. Care Med.* 1980;**8**:628–32.

101 Rodriguez, J., Weissman, C., Askanazi, J. *et al.* Metabolic and respiratory effects of glucose infusion. *Anesthesiology* 1982;**57**:AI99.

102 Gieseke, T., Gurushanthaiah, G., Glauser, F. Effects of carbohydrate on carbon dioxide excretion in patients with airway disease. *Chest* 1977;**71**:55–8.

103 Saltzman, H., Salzano, J. Effects of carbohydrate metabolism upon respiratory gas exchange in normal men. *J. Appl. Physiol.* 1971;**30**:228–31.

104 Herve, P., Simonneau, G., Girard, P. *et al.* Enteral nutritional support: metabolic, cardiovascular, and pulmonary interrelations. *Clin. Chest Med.* 1986;**7**:41–67.

105 Frayn, K. Calculation of substrate oxidation rate in vivo from gaseous exchange. *J. Appl. Physiol.* 1983;**55**:628–34.

106 Flatt, J. The biochemistry of energy expenditure. In Bray, G., ed. *Recent Advances in Obesity Research.* Washington, DC: Newman Publishers; 1977:211–28.

107 Bier, D., Leake, R., Haymond, M. *et al.* Measurement of "true" glucose production rates in infancy and childhood with 6,6-dideutero-glucose. *Diabetes* 1977;**26**:1016–23.

108 Kalhan, S., Savin, S., Adam, P. *et al.* Estimation of glucose turnover with stable tracer glucose-1–13C. *J. Lab. Clin. Med.* 1977;**80**:285–94.

109 Heymsfield, S. B., Head, C. A., McManus, C. B. 3rd. *et al.* Respiratory, cardiovascular and metabolic effects of enteral hyperalimentation: influence of formula dose and composition. *Am. Clin. Nutr.* 1984;**40**:116–30.

110 Nordenstrom, J., Carpentier, Y., Askanazi, J. *et al.* Metabolic utilization of intravenous fat emulsion during total parenteral nutrition. *Ann. Surg.* 1982;**196**:221–31.

111 Thiebaud, D., Acheson, K., Schutz, Y. *et al.* Stimulation of thermogenesis in man after combined glucose-long-chain-triglyceride infusion. *Am. J. Clin. Nutr.* 1983;**37**:603–11.

112 Nose, O., Tipton, J., Ament, M. *et al.* Effect of the energy source on changes in energy expenditure, respiratory quotient and nitrogen balance during total parenteral nutrition in children. *Pediatr. Res.* 1987;**21**:538–41.

113 Heim, T., Putet, G., Verellen, G. *et al.* Energy cost of intravenous alimentation in the newborn infant. In Stem, L., Salle, B., Friis-Hansen, B., eds. *Intensive Care in the Newborn III.* New York, NY: Masson Publishing; 1981:219–38.

114 Van Aerde, J., Sauer, P., Pencharz, P. *et al.* The effect of replacing glucose with lipid on the energy metabolism of newborn infants. *Clin. Sci.* 1989;**76**:581–8.

115 Piedboeuf, B., Chessex, P., Hazan, J. *et al.* Total parenteral nutrition in the newborn infant: energy substrates and respiratory gas exchange. *J. Pediatr.* 1991;**118**:97–102.

116 Chessex, P., Belanger, S., Piedboeuf, B., Pineault, M. Influence of energy substrates on respiratory gas exchange during conventional mechanical ventilation of preterm infants. *J. Pediatr.* 1995;**126**:619–24.

117 Greene, H., Hazlett, D., Demaree, R. Relationship between intralipid-induced hyperlipemia and pulmonary function. *Am. J. Clin. Nutr.* 1976;**29**:127–35.

118 Hageman, J. R., McCulloch, K., Gora, P. *et al.* Intralipid alterations in pulmonary prostaglandin metabolism and gas exchange. *Crit. Care Med.* 1983;**11**:794–8.

119 Hageman, J., Hunt, C. Fat emulsions and lung function. *Clin. Chest Med.* 1986;**7**:69–77.

120 Inwood, R., Gora, P., Hunt, C. Indomethacin inhibition of intralipid induced lung dysfunction. *Prostaglandins Med.* 1981;**6**:503–14.

121 McKeen, C., Brigham, K., Bowers, R. Pulmonary vascular effects of fat emulsion infusion in unanesthetized sheep. *J. Clin. Invest.* 1978;**61**:1291–7.

122 Skeie, B., Askanazi, J., Rothkopf, M. *et al.* Intravenous fat emulsions and lung emulsions: a review. *Crit. Care Med.* 1988;**16**:183–94.

123 Mathru, M., Dries, D. J., Zecca, A. *et al.* Effect of fast vs. slow intralipid infusion on gas exchange, pulmonary hemodynamics, and prostaglandin metabolism. *Chest* 1991;**126**:619–24.

124 Hunt, C., Pachman, L., Hageman, J. *et al.* Liposyn infusion increases plasma prostaglandin concentrations. *Pediatr. Pulmonol.* 1986;**2**:154–8.

125 Kadowitz, P., Spannhake, E., Levin, J. Differential actions of the prostaglandins on the pulmonary vascular bed. *Adv. Prostaglandin Thromboxane Res.* 1980;**7**:731–43.

126 Brans, Y., Dutton, E., Andrew, D. *et al.* Fat emulsion tolerance in very low birth weight neonates. Effect on diffusion of oxygen in the lungs and on blood pH. *Pediatrics* 1986;**78**:79–84.

127 Coe, J., Van Aerde, J., Kolatat, T. *et al.* Intralipid induced pulmonary vasoconstrictions in newborn piglets. *Clin. Invest. Med.* 1988;**11**:1334.

128 Gurtner, G., Knoblauch, A., Smith, P. *et al.* Oxidant- and lipid-induced pulmonary vasoconstriction mediated by arachidonic acid metabolites. *J. Appl. Physiol.* 1983;**55**:949–54.

129 Tague, W., Ray, U., Braun, D. *et al.* Lung vascular effects of lipid infusion in awake lambs. *Pediatr. Res.* 1987;**22**:714–19.

130 Lloyd, T., Boucek, M. Effect of intralipid on the neonatal pulmonary bed: an echographic study. *J. Pediatr.* 1986;**108**:130–3.

131 Prasertsom, W., Phillipos, E. Z., Van Aerde, J. E., Robertson, M. Pulmonary vascular resistance during lipid infusion in neonates. *Arch. Dis. Child.* 1996;**74**:F95–8.

132 Hammerman, C., Aramburo, M. Decreased lipid intake reduces morbidity in sick premature neonates. *J. Pediatr.* 1988;**113**:1083–8.

133 Hammerman, C., Valaitis, S., Aramburo, M. Thromboxanes: The link between intralipid and pulmonary vasoconstriction in the newborn. *Pediatr. Res.* 1987;**21**:236A.

134 Broderick, K., Tyrala, E. Leukotrienes and their role in the development of bronchopulmonary dysplasia in the newborn. *Pediatr. Res.* 1987;**21**:445A.

135 Barrington, K. J., Chan, G., Van Aerde, J. E. Intravenous lipid composition affects hypoxic pulmonary vasoconstriction in the newborn piglet. *Can. J. Physiol. Pharmacol.* 2001;**79**:594–600.

136 Sosenko, I., Innis, S., Frank, L. Polyunsaturated fatty acids and protection of newborn rats from oxygen toxicity. *J. Pediatr.* 1988;**112**:630–7.

137 Venus, B., Smith, R. A., Patel, C., Sandoval, E. Hemodynamic and gas exchange alterations during intralipid infusion in patients with adult respiratory distress syndrome. *Chest* 1989;**95**:1278–81.

138 Ball, M. J., White, K. Metabolic effects of intravenous medium- and long-chain triacylglycerols in critically ill patients. *Clin. Sci. (Lond).* 1989;**76**:165–70.

139 Lindgren, B. F., Ruokonen, E., Magnusson-Borg, K., Takala, J. Nitrogen sparing effect of structured triglycerides containing both medium- and long-chain fatty acids in critically ill patients: a double blind randomized controlled trial. *Clin. Nutr.* 2001;**20**:43–8.

140 Planas, M., Masclans, J. R., Iglesia, R. *et al.* Eicosanoids and fat emulsions in acute respiratory distress syndrome patients. *Nutrition* 1997;**13**:202–5.

141 Chassard, D., Guiraud, M., Gauthier, J. *et al.* Effects of intravenous medium-chain triglycerides on pulmonary gas exchanges in mechanically ventilated patients. *Crit. Care Med.* 1994;**22**:248–51.

142 Delafosse, B., Viale, J. P., Pachiaudi, C. *et al.* Long- and medium-chain triglycerides during parenteral nutrition in critically ill patients. *Am. J. Physiol. Endocrinol. Metab.* 1997;**272**:E550–5.

143 Donnell, S. C., Lloyd, D. A., Eaton, S., Pierro, A. The metabolic response to intravenous medium-chain triglycerides in infants after surgery. *J. Pediatr.* 2002;**141**:689–94.

144 Brown, E., Stark, A., Sosenko, I. *et al.* Bronchopulmonary dysplasia. Possible relationship to pulmonary edema. *J. Pediatr.* 1978;**92**:982–4.

145 Binder, N., Raschko, P., Benda, G. *et al.* Insulin infusion with parenteral nutrition in extremely low birth weight infants with hyperglycemia. *J. Pediatr.* 1989;**114**:273–80.

146 Ostertag, G., Jovanovic, L., Lewis, B. *et al.* Insulin pump therapy in the very low birth weight infant. *Pediatrics.* 1986;**78**:625–30.

36

Nutrition for premature infants with bronchopulmonary dysplasia

Stephanie A. Atkinson

Department of Pediatrics, McMaster University, Hamilton, Ontario, Canada

Nutrition for extremely low birth weight infants (ELBW) at risk of developing bronchopulmonary dysplasia (BPD) is critical to the prevention, amelioration, and recovery from this severe lung disorder. A "new" form of BPD has emerged owing to increased survival of ELBW immature infants who have benefited from improved ventilatory regimens, use of prenatal and postnatal steroids and postnatal surfactant. The histopathologic picture of alveolar and capillary hypoplasia of the "new" BPD differs from the "old" BPD, such that the new BPD is less fibrotic than its earlier counterpart, and there is a significant component of delayed alveolar development and perhaps permanent alveolar underdevelopment.[1] Unfortunately, targeted treatment strategies to optimize normal lung development and prevent BPD remain elusive.

Bronchopulmonary dysplasia has been referred to as an "oxygen radical disease of prematurity."[2] A state of oxidative stress is a hallmark of BPD owing to a combination of exposure to high oxygen concentrations starting shortly after birth and increased production of reactive oxygen species as a result of cytokine activation during infections and inflammations.[3] The antioxidant availability to counter such oxidative stress is likely to be inadequate in ELBW infants due to extreme immaturity and meager nutritional stores. Administration of antioxidant nutrients such as vitamin E and N-acetylcysteine have been proposed as a means of prevention or attenuation of the severity of BPD. Vitamin A, which may stimulate re-epithelialization of lung tissues, and inositol, which promotes maturation of surfactant phospholipids, have been investigated as preventive measures against BPD.

Postnatal growth failure is common in infants with BPD, and usually extends beyond early neonatal life for several years. Such growth failure is multi-factorial including extreme prematurity at birth, exposure to corticosteroids drugs both antenatally and in early postnatal life, inadequate nutrition due to prolonged dependence on parenteral nutrition, fluid restriction or feeding intolerance, and possibly excess energy expenditure due to work of breathing. To date, no evidence-based nutrition recommendations exist for the nutritional management of infants with BPD. This chapter will examine the available evidence for a role of specific nutrients in the prevention and treatment of BPD and for nutritional rehabilitation and catch-up growth.

Antioxidants for the prevention of BPD

As recently reviewed,[1,3–5] oxidative stress leading to pulmonary oxygen injury results from the combined effect of antioxidant deficiency (e.g., deficiency of endogenous enzymatic antioxidants and/or antioxidant nutrients such as selenium or vitamin E) and an increased generation of reactive oxygen species (ROS). Neonatal oxidative stress resulting from high oxygen inspiration and exposure to infections and inflammatory processes that yield ROS may also contribute to risk for BPD. Studies in animal and human infants demonstrated that oxidative processes, particularly of lipids and proteins, in early life contribute to the development of BPD. Nutrient-based interventions (Table 36.1) for the prevention of, or reduction in, the severity of chronic lung disease have been investigated primarily for vitamin E and N-acetylcysteine.

Neonatal Nutrition and Metabolism. Second Edition, ed. P. Thureen and W. Hay. Published by Cambridge University Press.
© Cambridge University Press 2006.

Vitamin E

Vitamin E as adjunctive antioxidant therapy in ventilated infants was postulated to serve as a scavenger of excessive oxygen radicals produced during exposure to high oxygen delivery, thereby diminishing the risk of pulmonary oxygen toxicity that presents as BPD or retrolental fibroplasia. Intervention with supplemental vitamin E failed to prevent BPD in human infants,[8] an observation substantiated in premature baboons exposed to prolonged hyperoxia.[9] A meta-analysis of available studies found no evidence for a clinical benefit of vitamin E at intakes above that which maintains a normal serum alpha-tocopherol concentration (10–30 mg L^{-1}).[10] An adequate intake of vitamin E is available from full enteral feedings with mother's milk or preterm formula, or if necessary, from the standard prescribed dose of parenteral or enteral multivitamin preparations.

Selenium

Low antioxidant status in very early life measured as plasma selenium concentration was not associated with later development of BPD in one study.[11] In contrast, low plasma selenium at 28 days was associated with increased respiratory morbidity in preterm infants <1500 g birth weight in New Zealand, an area of selenium-deficient soils.[12] Additionally, both low plasma selenium and alpha-tocopherol (vitamin E) were significantly associated with severe respiratory disease and BPD in premature infants of ≤ 30 weeks gestation compared with healthy premature infants.[13] As a required constituent of the endogenous antioxidant glutathione peroxidase, selenium supplements were proposed to reduce oxidative stress and thus BPD. To date, no clinical trials have been conducted to prove the effectiveness of selenium as antioxidant therapy in improving respiratory morbidity.

N-acetylcysteine

Exogenous provision of N-acetylcysteine (NAC), the precursor to glutathione (GSH) in tissues, was proposed to enhance the availability of one of the natural antioxidant defenses in the tissues. Specifically, GSH functions to neutralize hydrogen peroxide, thereby reducing the amount of ROS. One randomized placebo-controlled multi-center trial tested whether intravenously administered NAC for 6 days starting at less than 36 hours of life would reduce oxidative stress and hence the occurrence of BPD.[14] The study, conducted in 391 infants in Nordic countries, found that NAC delivery was not associated with a reduction in BPD or deaths, the number of BPD survivors at 36 weeks of gestational age, or mean oxygen needs.[14] The authors suggested that perhaps the infants were cysteine-replete owing to delivery of this amino acid in parenteral amino acid solutions infused prior to the study or that lung injury had occurred either in utero or in the hours postbirth but prior to initiation of the NAC. Further clinical trials are required to fully explore the role of NAC as an antioxidant in the prevention of BPD.

Antioxidant enzymes

Administration of antioxidant enzymes normally produced endogenously was tested in animal studies where the antioxidant was given intratracheally or intravenously with some positive benefit demonstrated.[3] In human preterm infants, bovine superoxide dismutase (SOD) injected intramuscularly resulted in a reduction in need for positive airway pressure and a lower frequency of respiratory problems after hospital discharge.[15] More recently, in a multicenter study in 302 premature infants (<1220 g birth weight) recombinant human SOD given intratracheally did not reduce BPD or deaths compared with controls.[16] Remarkably, at follow-up at 1 year the SOD-treated infants had a 44% reduction in wheezing and a significantly lower incidence of respiratory illnesses that required pulmonary medication. While the antioxidant enzymes do not appear to prevent BPD, when given in early life they may provide some long-term benefits to respiratory health. Clearly, more clinical studies are required to validate the clinical effectiveness of antioxidant enzymes.

In summary, despite evidence that excessive oxidative processes contribute to the lung injury in early postnatal life that predisposes to BPD, administration of antioxidant nutrients and enzymes has been unsuccessful in ameliorating the progression of the disease. As noted by Welty,[6] it may be that the antioxidants have not been delivered sufficiently early postbirth or to the target area of the lung exposed to oxidative stress to be effective clinically.

Nutrients to improve lung function

Inositol

Myo-inositol is a six-carbon sugar alcohol naturally present as phosphatidylinositol in tissues and in cell membranes. It is proposed that an adequate supply of inositol enhances the synthesis and secretion of pulmonary surfactant, which could influence pulmonary mechanics and reduce severity of lung disease. Preterm human milk is known to

Table 36.1. Nutrient interventions targeted to prevent or ameliorate bronchopulmonary dysplasia (summary)

Nutrient	Amount/route/ duration	Review of evidence – reference
Antioxidant		
Nutrients	No proven effect	
n-acetylcysteine		3,5,6,7
Vitamin E		
Vitamin C		
Selenium		
Inositol	Intravenously or in formula from 48 hours of life for 5–10 days	21
Vitamin A	5000 IU by intramuscular ×3/week for 4 weeks	24–26

have a high concentration of inositol, and higher serum concentrations of inositol were observed in human milk-fed newborns compared with those fed parenteral nutrition solutions or infant formula.[17,18] Inositol supplementation in newborn infants resulted in an increase in the saturated phosphatidylcholine/sphingomyelin ratio in surfactant.[19,20]

To investigate a possible role for inositol in the prevention of BPD, a few randomized trials were conducted in which inositol was supplemented parenterally or in formula. A Cochrane review of available trials[21] summarized five reports of three trials (one report was a duplicate publication, and in a second report subjects who were randomized to treatment could not be separated from a nonrandomized group). In the two trials that measured similar outcomes, positive benefits of inositol supplementation for duration of 5–10 days included significant reductions in death or BPD combined, intraventricular hemorrhage (IVH) grade III/IV, and retinopathy of prematurity (ROP) stage 4 or ROP needing treatment. However, for a diagnosis of BPD alone at 28 days there was only a trend. No adverse effects such as necrotizing enterocolitis (NEC) or sepsis were observed in the studies summarized.[21] The authors of this systematic review concluded that despite the small number of studies and cumulative sample population, inositol supplementation did have a significant impact on reducing rates of death, death or BPD, IVH grades III and IV, and ROP stage 4 or needing treatment. However, further studies designed as large multi-centered trials are needed to confirm the role of

routine inositol supplementation in infants with respiratory disease and to clarify the dose, schedule, and route of administration.

Vitamin A

Infants of ELBW are at risk of vitamin A deficiency (defined as plasma retinol < 200 μgL^{-1}) because of low stores at birth.[22] Further, vitamin A accrual may be low in early neonatal life owing to meager dietary intakes or lack of delivery owing to loss through intravenous or oral plastic tubing or photo inactivation[23] unless intravenous and oral feedings are fortified with extra vitamin A. Vitamin A is proposed to have a role in the prevention of BPD by virtue of its action as a stimulant for the re-epithelialization of lung tissue after acute injury induced by barotrauma or oxygen toxicity.

A systematic review with meta analysis was conducted to determine if vitamin A supplementation prevented mortality and morbidity (defined as chronic lung disease, BPD, ROP) or had an effect on circulating vitamin A concentrations in infants of <1500 g birth weight.[24] Five of the 10 published studies met the eligibility criteria for this Cochrane review, although not all studies reported the same outcomes. All studies included in the review were randomized or quasi-randomized trials comparing high dose vitamin A (given intramuscularly or orally) to a placebo or no treatment. In total, the five studies reported measures in 149 infants treated with vitamin A and in 141 nontreated infants. Four of the studies gave intramuscular injections of water-soluble retinyl palmitate (2000–4000 IU vitamin A given alternate days or three times per week) for about 28 days, and one study gave an oral dose of 5000 IU daily. It is important to note that at the time these studies were conducted there was minimal or no use of antenatal or postnatal steroids, and no use of surfactant. The overall results of the meta-analysis found that high doses of vitamin A did not influence rate of death by 1 month of age, but there was a trend to reduction of dependence on oxygen therapy. If death and oxygen dependence were combined as outcomes, then a significant effect of high-dose vitamin A was found. There was only a trend for retinopathy of prematurity to be reduced by treatment with high dose vitamin A. For the studies that measured plasma retinol, supplemental vitamin A did support significantly higher concentrations, and the level attained was above 200 μg L^{-1}, a value below which is suggestive of marginal deficiency status. Since the Cochrane review in 1999,[24] two further randomized trials have been reported that support the use of a high-dose vitamin A of 5000 IU given intramuscularly 3 times per week.[25,26] Both were randomized trials in infants <1 kg birth weight. The intervention of high-dose vitamin A of 5000 IU per day intramuscularly resulted in reduced death (55% v. 62%) or BPD at 36 weeks compared with low-dose vitamin A, although there was no difference in ROP.[25] Since 22% of infants treated with high-dose vitamin A had low or absent vitamin A stores in the study from the National Institute of Child Health and Development (NICHD) Neonatal Research Network,[25] a subsequent study investigated higher doses given intramuscularly of 10 000 IU three times or 15 000 IU once per week compared to the 5000 IU three times per week.[26] In the latter study, the overall rate of death/BPD in the group receiving 5000 IU per dose three times per week was 48%, even lower than that observed in the previous study at the same dose (55%).[25] No benefits in clinical outcomes of BPD/death by 36 weeks, death by 36 weeks, or ROP were observed in groups who received the higher doses of vitamin A, although the study may have been underpowered to reach statistically significant differences in clinical outcomes. Notably, both of the higher vitamin A doses failed to reduce the incidence of vitamin A deficiency, and infants in the highest dose (10 000 IU once per week) actually had lower serum retinol concentrations on study day 28 compared with the other dosing groups.[26]

Taken together, the clinical trials on vitamin A interventions to prevent morbidity and mortality in infants at high risk of severe respiratory disease provide evidence that a dose of 5000 IU per dose three times per week for 4 weeks is effective in reducing BPD and death, even when vitamin A biochemical status is less than normal. Further study is required to optimize dosing regimens (oral or intravenous versus intramuscular delivery) and to evaluate both immediate and long-term clinical outcomes in relation to vitamin A nutrition in vulnerable very low birth weight (VLBW) infants.

Growth failure in BPD infants in early life

Since ELBW infants, especially those with BPD, have a multitude of feeding problems such as fluid restriction, reliance on long-term parenteral feeding, oral feeding intolerance and gastroesophageal reflux, it follows that the observed growth failure in this infant population may be attributed to the cumulative effects of inadequate nutrient delivery.

An example of early growth failure in BPD infants is shown in Table 36.2. At about 34 weeks postmenstrual age, a group of ELBW infants (n = 27) diagnosed with BPD by 28 days postnatally, had achieved a body weight of only 1500 g despite being fed a commercially available nutrient-enriched premature formula with energy density

Table 36.2. Growth and nutrient accretion in infants with bronchopulmonary dysplasia (n = 27) fed standard premature infant formula (Preemie SMA, Wyeth) in hospital at about 34 weeks postmenstrual age[29]

Weight at balance: 1.5 ± 0.2 kg (50th percentile = 2550 g)[27]
Weight gain during balance period = 15.5 ± 12.4 g kg^{-1} day^{-1}
Formula intake
Fluid volume = 144 ± 9 mL kg^{-1} day^{-1}
Energy = 112 ± 7 kcal kg^{-1} day^{-1}
Nutrient accretion measured in 72-hour metabolic balance study
Nitrogen retention = 316 mg kg^{-1} day^{-1}
(71% nitrogen retention)
Net protein accretion = 1.97 ± 0.49^a g kg^{-1} day^{-1}
Calcium retention = 2.1 mmol^b(84 mg) kg^{-1} day^{-1}
(75% calcium retention)
Phosphorus retention = 1.5 mmol ^{c}(46 mg) kg^{-1} day^{-1}
(89% phosphorus retention)
Zinc retention = 1.7 μmol (110 μg)^d kg^{-1} day^{-1}
(10% zinc retention)

$^{a, b, c, d}$ Reference intrauterine accretion: ^{a} Protein: 2–4 g kg^{-1} day^{-1}; ^{b} Calcium: 2.5–3 mmol kg^{-1} day^{-1}; ^{c} Phosphorus: 1.9 – 2.5 mmol kg^{-1} day^{-1}; ^{d} Zinc = 5.4 μmol kg^{-1} day^{-1}. [29]

of 810 kcal L^{-1}.[29] The average attained weight of these BPD infants at 8 weeks postnatal was 1500 g, considerably lower than a weight of 2550 g that represents the 50th percentile of growth at a similar postmenstrual age based on recent growth standards.[27] Metabolic balance studies completed on these infants showed that protein, calcium, and phosphorus accretion fell below predicted intrauterine accretion rates (Table 36.2). Fluid restriction and administration of dexamethasone to improve pulmonary compliance are additional factors that may have contributed to delayed growth performance in these infants. As the infants were born in the early 1990s, dexamethasone was prescribed rather liberally, and the measured cumulative dose of dexamethasone administered during hospitalization was 6.2 mg kg^{-1} body weight.[29] This amount of steroid drug most definitely contributed to the growth restriction during the first 2 postnatal months (see discussion later in chapter).

Energy needs

Higher energy need has been proposed as a cause of growth failure in BPD infants, linking this to an elevated basal metabolic rate or increased energy expenditure due to work of breathing. In a review of studies on energy expenditure measured using the classical method of indirect calorimetry, Denne[30] concluded that increased expenditure due to work of breathing was inconsistently observed in infants with chronic respiratory disease. It was proposed that measurement of energy expenditure in small infants would be improved by use of the doubly labeled water (DLW) technique with oral dosing and serial collections of urine for analysis of the stable isotopes of deuterium and oxygen 18-labeled water by mass spectrometry.[30]

Longitudinal measures of energy expenditure by DLW were obtained in my laboratory in infants with BPD (birth weight $= 867 \pm 194$ g, gestational age $= 26 \pm 1.4$ weeks) after discharge from hospital.[31] At 1 and 3 months corrected age, energy expenditure was 72 ± 21 and 76 ± 29 kcal kg^{-1} day^{-1}, respectively, which represented $63 \pm 22\%$ and $73 \pm 33\%$ of energy intake that was carefully measured using pre/postweighing of formula consumed. Although we did not measure energy expenditure in term-born infants at similar ages, it was possible to compare our observations in preterm BPD infants to published values for energy expenditure in term infants using the DLW method.[32] Term infants expended 64 ± 17 kcal kg^{-1} day^{-1} at 1.5 months ($n = 39$) and 67 ± 14 kcal kg^{-1} day^{-1} at 3 months ($n = 40$).[32] Thus, energy expenditure in BPD infants compared with term-born infants at similar corrected ages appears to be elevated for an extended period of early life during recovery from BPD. This observation is supported by doubly labeled water measurements in a small number of infants with BPD who demonstrated higher rates of energy expenditure compared to non-BPD infants.[33] From the data available it appears that infants with BPD may have higher energy needs than term-born infants, and indeed those of stable growing VLBW infants,[33] although the duration of excess energy expenditure in relation to recovery from lung disease needs to be defined.

Dexamethasone therapy

Another impediment to achieving optimal growth in ELBW infants is the use of exogenous glucocorticoids such as dexamethasone to improve pulmonary compliance. From the early to late 1990s,[34] the steroid dexamethasone was commonly used as therapy to induce lung maturation, thus allowing earlier weaning from the ventilator and possibly prevention of BPD. Unfortunately, negative effects of the potent steroid on growth and mineral and bone metabolism accompany any immediate clinical benefit of steroid therapy. In studies from my laboratory, tapered dosing regimens of dexamethasone administered to ELBW infants were associated with restriction in weight, length, and head circumference growth and abnormalities in biomarkers of bone turnover.[35,36] Inadequate nutrition was not the limiting factor to growth in the latter studies since nutrient intakes of the ELBW infants with and without treatment with dexamethasone met current guidelines for low birth weight infants.[35,36] Thus, the catabolic effects of dexamethasone on protein metabolism[37] and its interference with the growth hormone-insulin-like growth factor-I pathway,[36] are the more likely explanations for the immediate influence of the drug on normal development rather than inadequate nutrient intake. Using the doubly labeled water method to measure energy expenditure, no differences were observed between ELBW infants gaining 6.5 v. 20 g kg^{-1} day^{-1}, the former being infants who were receiving dexamethasone therapy.[38] Again, the slower growth is attributed to the alterations on nutrient metabolism induced by the steroid drug and not excessive energy expenditure.

Using the early weaned piglet model, we have reproduced the dexamethasone-induced abnormalities observed in ELBW infants, thus proving that the restrictions in growth and bone mineralization are a result of the steroid drug and not a result of the lung disease or extreme prematurity per se.[39,40] Furthermore, potential adjunctive therapies such as supplemental calcium, phosphorus, and calcitriol,[41] or recombinant growth hormone with or without insulin-like growth factor-1[40] given with dexamethasone failed to induce complete recovery of dexamethasone-induced reductions in bone mass and linear growth. Such observations in the animal model warrant long-term follow-up of ELBW infants who have been exposed to dexamethasone in early life.

In current neonatal practice in most centers, dexamethasone is prescribed much more conservatively than in the early 1990s, due in large part to the reported observation of adverse effects on growth and bone status, as well as a lack of evidence of long-term benefits to respiratory health.[42]

Nutrition intervention to promote growth in infants with chronic lung disease

While undernutrition and delayed growth are commonly observed in ELBW infants with BPD in early life, few studies have investigated possible avenues of nutritional management to optimize growth and development in this special preterm infant population. No benefit to growth from intervention with nutrient-enriched formula during neonatal hospitalization was observed in one study.[43] In infants with chronic lung disease (requiring oxygen at 28 days postnatal age), this randomized study tested a dietary intervention of a high-density (1000 kcal L^{-1} (30 kcal per oz)) formula that provided significantly higher energy

(143 v. 134 kcal kg^{-1} day^{-1}) and protein (3.9 v. 3.6 g kg^{-1} day^{-1}) intakes. No benefit to growth or respiratory status was observed. However, the calculated sample size (n = 35 infants per group) was not attained (27 infants in the low-density group and 33 infants in the high-density group) and use of antenatal steroids was greater in the low nutrient density group. Administration of antenatal steroids is known to result in lower birth weight and reduced fetal organ size in VLBW infants.[44]

To determine if aggressive nutritional support in the recovery period after hospital discharge would enhance growth in BPD infants, we conducted an intervention trial of high-energy formula with or without greater amounts of protein and minerals in which the intervention was implemented from about 35 weeks gestational age until 3 months corrected age.[29] This study was the first randomized, double-blinded, intervention trial to determine if nutrient-enriched formula with a higher protein : energy ratio than in term formula would improve rate and composition of growth (lean, fat, and bone mineral mass) when fed to 3 months corrected age. Infants of average birth weight of 870 g and gestational age of 26 weeks (appropriate for gestational age) were randomized to nutrient-enriched formula (energy density of 910 kcal L^{-1}, protein : energy ratio of 2.5 g 100 $kcal^{-1}$) or an iso-energetic formula but with a protein and mineral composition similar to term infant formula (protein : energy ratio of 1.6 g 100 $kcal^{-1}$). Feeding of the nutrient-enriched formula provided for retentions (based on 72-hour metabolic balance studies) of protein, calcium, phosphorus, and zinc that were significantly greater than the infants fed the standard formula, despite the moderate fluid restriction (142 mg kg^{-1} day^{-1}) during the balance study (Table 36.3). Net retention for all nutrients was in the range reported for intrauterine accretion for the infants fed the enriched formula only (Table 36.3). After 4 months on the experimental formulas, the infants on the enriched formula demonstrated a benefit in length and lean mass growth and had a lower percent body fat than infants randomized to the lower protein : energy ratio formula. Head circumference growth was similar between diet groups at all measurement times. Z-scores for length at 3 months were less negative in the high protein : energy formula group albeit still below reference standards age (Table 36.4).[40] At the end of the experimental intervention (3 months corrected age), the infants fed the formula with the lower protein : energy ratio had developed significantly greater adiposity than those on the high protein : energy formula despite similar total energy intakes. Percent body fat (measured by dual energy x-ray absorptiometry (DEXA)) was significantly higher in infants fed the low v. high protein : energy ratio formulas at 3 months

Table 36.3. Nutrient balance, weight gain and calculated protein accretion in BPD infants at about 38 weeks postmenstrual age after 3 weeks of being randomized to high energy formula with protein and minerals as in standard term formula (SF, birth weight = 836 ± 260 g, gestational age = 26.2 ± 1.6 weeks) or isoenergetic protein-mineral enriched formula (EF, birth weight = 841 ± 168 g, gestational age 25.7 ± 1.2 weeks) as their sole source of intake[29]

	SF	EF
	N = 17	N = 19
Weight gain (g kg^{-1} day^{-1})	11.9 ± 2.9	10.8 ± 3.0
Formula volume (mL kg^{-1} day^{-1})	145 ± 12	142 ± 22
Nutrient balance		
Calcium (mmol kg^{-1} day^{-1})		
Intake	1.53 ± 0.14	3.87 ± 0.70[b]
Retention	0.95 ± 0.25	2.52 ± 0.78[b]
Phosphorus (mmol kg^{-1} day^{-1})		
Intake	1.52 ± 0.12	3.11 ± 0.56[b]
Retention	1.20 ± 0.18	2.39 ± 0.54[b]
Nitrogen (mg kg^{-1} day^{-1})		
Intake	366 ± 28	490 ± 51[b]
Retention	262 ± 48	365 ± 34[b]
Net protein accretion (g kg^{-1} day^{-1})	1.51 ± 0.41	2.21 ± 0.17[b]

[a] Values are mean ± SD.
[b] EF v. SF, p < 0.01.

CA (30% v. 26% for males and 29% v. 22% for females, p < 0.025 for females). Intakes of protein and energy, which were carefully measured using pre-/postweighing method, for both diet groups met or exceeded the recommended intakes for preterm infants in the postdischarge period.[29,46]

No specialized infant formulas or fortifiers for human milk targeted for infants with BPD are currently marketed. In practice, this infant population is maintained on preterm infant formula (energy content up to 810 kcal L^{-1}) sometimes further enriched with modular products of carbohydrate, lipid, or addition of powdered or concentrated liquid infant formula. Such "recipes" usually provide an energy density of up to 1000 kcal L^{-1}, but may be hyperosmolar or sufficiently thickened to limit delivery flow through feeding tubes or nipples. One option for feeding older BPD infants (past term CA) is commercial pediatric enteral formulas. In a retrospective study, infants (n = 27) with fluid restriction (116 ml kg^{-1} day^{-1}) who were past term age and fed an enteral formula (PediaSure, Ross Products Division, Abbott Laboratories) had similar growth and feeding tolerance compared with preterm formula supplemented with modular units of carbohydrate, lipid, and protein.[47]

Table 36.4. Longitudinal growth as Z-scores for age in BPD infants (as described in Table 36.3) fed high-energy formula with protein and minerals as in standard term formula (SF) or protein-mineral enriched formula (EF) from about 35 weeks postmenstrual age to 3 months corrected age, then standard term formula after 3 months with weaning to whole cow milk after 9 months of age at parental discretion[29,45]

Age, mo corrected age	Weight Z-score		Length Z-score	
	SF	EF	SF	EF
1	-1.49 ± 0.8^a	-1.14 ± 0.8	-2.60 ± 1.1	-2.36 ± 1.1
3	-1.42 ± 0.9	-1.05 ± 1.1	-2.36 ± 0.9^b	-1.80 ± 1.2^c
6	-1.80 ± 0.7	-1.47 ± 1.1	-1.93 ± 0.9	-1.53 ± 1.1
12	-1.85 ± 1.0	-1.76 ± 1.1	-1.54 ± 1.0	-1.36 ± 1.1

[a] Values are mean $\pm$ SD.

[b,c] b v. c, SF group significantly different from EF group, $p < 0.05$.

Protein status was actually improved in the infants fed the ready-to-feed enteral formula. More research is needed to define optimal nutrient intakes for ELBW infants with BPD to achieve catch-up growth with special consideration for the protein to energy ratio in order to cover any extra need for energy expenditure but not in amounts that result in abnormal deposition of body fat. Ideally, safe and efficacious specially designed nutritional products that allow for fluid restriction but support optimal growth in infants recovering from BPD will be developed and marketed.

Growth and nutrition after hospital discharge in BPD infants

Growth of infants recovering from neonatal BPD is usually observed to be slower and body composition different than that of infants of similar birth weight who do not develop chronic lung disease or other major neonatal morbidities. Weight and length growth and body composition of infants with BPD over the first year of life are reported in two recent studies.[45,48]

Weight and length growth

The extent of growth recovery in BPD infants over the first year of life is demonstrated by the data on z-scores for weight and length in Table 36.4. At 3 months corrected age, BPD infants were disproportionately heavy for length, but by 12 months corrected age body proportions had reversed with infants being lean for length (Table 36.4). Similar observations of low Z-(SD) scores compared with term-born infants were reported in a prospective descriptive

study of Dutch infants (n = 29) followed through neonatal follow-up clinic from 6 weeks to 12 months corrected age.[48] Protein and energy intakes at 3 and 6 months were similar in infants in the two studies.[45,48] Of note, "catch-up" growth had not been achieved by 12 months of age in infants in either study, as the mean Z-scores were ≤ -1 for both weight and height.

Body composition

The proportions of fat and lean mass observed in VLBW–BPD infants appear to vary from that of term infants and may be related to the protein : energy ratio of the diet, total energy intake, or exposure to exogenous steroid drugs. It is impossible to compare values for lean and fat mass reported for BPD infants between available published studies since the methodologies employed – DLW, DEXA, or total body electric conductivity (TOBEC) – do not yield comparative values.[49] When the DLW method was used to estimate body fat, percent whole body fat rose from 9% $\pm$ 7% at 34.5 weeks of gestation to 13% $\pm$ 9% at 38 weeks, and 16% $\pm$ 9% and 20% $\pm$ 9% at 1 and 3 months corrected age, respectively.[31] Using TOBEC, a similar increase in percent body fat was observed between 6 weeks (15.3% $\pm$ 1.6% for boys and 17.0% $\pm$ 1.7% for girls) and 3 months (19% $\pm$ 1.5% for boys and 20.0% $\pm$ 1.6% for girls) corrected age.[48] Beyond 3 months, percent body fat in BPD infants rose in both studies to a maximum of 24% in boys at 9 months by TOBEC[48] and 27% by DEXA at 6 months in a mixed gender group.[45] In both studies, mean percent body fat declined at 12 months corrected age to 21.7% in boys and 18.2% $\pm$ 1.7% in girls,[48] and 23% $\pm$ 5% in the mixed gender group.[45] In both studies,[45,48] values for body fat were below that for term-born infants (31% $\pm$ 5%) at the corrected age of

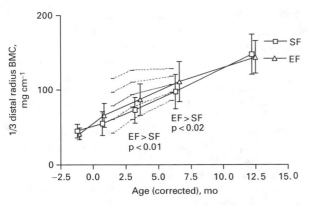

Figure 36.1. Bone mineral content (BMC) of the one-third distal radius in prematurely born infants of extremely low birth weight (n = 56, birth weight = 866 ± 16 g, gestational age = 24 ± 1.5 weeks) randomized to high energy formula with protein and minerals as in standard term formula (SF) or nutrient-enriched formula (EF) to 3 months corrected age [29] and then followed to 12 months corrected age while receiving standard infant formula and foods as selected by parents (Brunton and Atkinson, unpublished data). The infants fed EF had significantly higher radial BMC at 3 months (p = 0.01) and 6 months (p = 0.02) but by 12 months corrected age the BMC was similar between groups. Radial BMC in the EF preterm infants reached the mean value for term infants by 6 months corrected age. The data from term infants fed standard formula[52] are shown as mean (in solid line) ± 2 SD (in hatched lines) as a reference population.

1 year.[50] The cause of the observed growth deceleration and lower fat and lean mass observed in BPD compared with term-born infants after 6 months corrected age has not been investigated. Feeding problems and frequent infections, often requiring repeated hospitalizations, may be contributory factors.

Bone mass

In most infants born prematurely, bone mass at term CA is lower than for infants born at term.[51] Provision of a protein/mineral-enriched formula fed to 3 months CA in BPD infants supported greater accretion of radial bone mineral content (BMC) (measured by single photon absorptiometry (SPA)) (Figure 36.1) and whole body BMC (measured by DEXA) (Figure 36.2) than a formula with protein and mineral similar to term formula.[29] However, a sustained benefit to either measure of BMC was not apparent at 12 months corrected age. For radial BMC, the BPD infants had similar values to term infants[52] by 6 months corrected age (Figure 36.1). For whole body BMC, at 12 months CA BPD infants had mean values of about −1 SD that of term infants fed formula to 1 year of age (Figure 36.2). Dietary

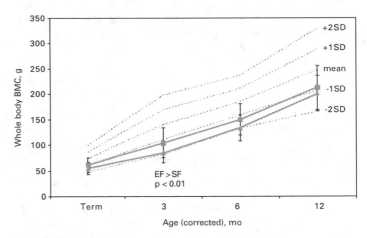

Figure 36.2. Whole body bone mineral content (BMC) for the same infants described in Figure 36.1 was significantly higher (87 ± 21 v. 74 ± 17 g, p < 0.01) in the EF group at 3 months only.[29,45] Whole body BMC increased about 3.5-fold in both diet groups from term to 12 months corrected age but remained about −1 SD below values for term reference infants. The data from term infants fed standard formula[50] are shown as mean (in solid line) ± 2 SD (in hatched lines) as a reference population.

intake of minerals after the diet intervention period should not have been limiting to bone accretion as intakes after 6 months CA were in excess of recommended intakes for preterm infants.[53] Calcium intake ranged from 13–18 mmol (520–720 mg) day^{-1}, phosphorus from 13–21 mmol (403–651 mg) day^{-1} and protein from 2.4–3.1 g kg^{-1} day^{-1}.[45] By 12 months CA most infants were weaned from formula to whole cow milk resulting in high intakes of calcium (about 22 mmol (880 mg) day^{-1} and of phosphorus (about 26 mmol (806 mg) day^{-1}),[45] well above the recommended intakes for age.[54] Vitamin D intake averaged 8 μg (800 IU) per day that is also in excess of recommendations.

Long-term growth outcomes in former VLBW–BPD infants

Suboptimal growth performance of former preterm infants with BPD that tracked into childhood has been reported out to 12 years of age[55–58] and at adolescence.[59] The studies reported in the 1990s preceded improvements in respiratory support and pharmacotherapy, and the survivors of BPD during these earlier times tended to be larger than the survivors of BPD since the late 1990s. In a study conducted after the introduction of surfactant and pre- and postnatal steroid therapy, follow-up growth measures were made at 7 years of age in three groups of infants: (1) VLBW infants diagnosed with BPD in neonatal life (need for oxygen and chest radiology findings consistent with BPD at 28 postnatal days) (birth weight $= 954 \pm 201$ g, gestational age $= 27 \pm 2$ weeks, n $= 31$); (2) VLBW infants not treated with steroids (birth weight $= 1127 \pm 236$ g, gestational age $= 29 \pm 2$ weeks, n $= 33$); and (3) term infants (n $= 33$).[58] The former VLBW–BPD infants were shorter and lighter with a significantly lower body mass index (BMI) (14.8 ± 1.7 kg m^{-2}) than term-born infants (16.1 ± 2.1 kg m^{-2}).[58] The BMI was below the 10th percentile in 58% of former VLBW–BPD children compared with 9% in the term infants.[58] However, none of the growth outcomes of the former VLBW–BPD infants were significantly different from former VLBW infants who did not develop BPD but who were of significantly greater birth weight and gestational age. Of note, while prenatal steroid exposure was similar between VLBW infant groups (32% compared with 39%), in the former VLBW–BPD infants 55% had received postnatal corticosteriods compared to only 12% in the non-BPD group, suggesting no sustained effect of steroid-induced growth failure in early neonatal life. However, there was no indication of dose or duration of postnatal dexamethasone therapy and the study was not powered on this outcome.

Summary

The clinical population of premature infants with BPD in the post-year 2000 era represents what has been termed the "new BPD."[1] A comparison of incidence and outcomes of infants with respiratory distress syndrome between the early (1990–1995) and late 1990s revealed that the incidence of respiratory disease did not change significantly but that smaller infants of lower gestation were increasingly surviving.[60] Moreover, the rate of chronic lung disease at 36 weeks postmenstrual age (about 16.5%) and at 1 year (about 8.6%) remained similar between the two time intervals. This pattern of survival in infants with respiratory disease impacts on nutritional management in at least two ways. First, the surviving infants are of more extreme low birth weight and thus will require intensive nutritional support until medically stable. Second, given that respiratory problems persist even up to the first year of life, continuing nutritional intervention and monitoring after hospital discharge will be key to ensuring normal nutritional status and sufficient nutrients to support catch-up growth.

Consensus of the studies summarized in this chapter is that growth of ELBW infants diagnosed with BPD is compromised in early neonatal life owing to a combination of factors including extreme low birth weight, restricted feeding due to fluid intolerance, exposure to exogenous

Table 36.5. Guidelines for nutritional management of infants with bronchopulmonary dysplasia or in the recovery phase as informed by the literature reviewed in this chapter

Early neonatal life (in hospital)

Vitamin A: given intramuscularly at 5000 IU 3 times per week for 4 weeks; given orally at 5000 IU once enteral feeds are established

Vitamin E: up to 4–5 mg day^{-1} will maintain normal serum alpha-tocopherol (available from ≥ 150 mL of mother's milk or premature infant formula or the standard dose of parenteral or enteral multivitamin preparations)

No evidence for effectiveness of other antioxidant vitamins or nutrients on outcomes of BPD

Fluid restriction: if fluid intake is restricted to less than 150 mL kg^{-1} day^{-1} then provide high nutrient density feedings as tolerated

Stable and growing period (pre/posthospital discharge to at least 3 months CA or longer)[a] Target intakes of nutrients in the following amounts

Protein: ≥ 3.0 g kg^{-1} day^{-1}

Energy: 120–130 kcal kg^{-1} day^{-1}

Calcium: 4 mmol kg^{-1} day^{-1}

Phosphorus: 3 mmol kg^{-1} day^{-1}

Zinc: 20 μmol kg^{-1} day^{-1}

Vitamin D: 400–800 IU day^{-1}

[a] If fluid intake is restricted, modular nutrient sources (lipid, carbohydrate, and protein) may need to be added to breast milk or preterm formulas or other nutrient-enriched enteral nutrition products used (see text for further discussion).

pre- and postnatal steroid drugs, and possibly elevated energy expenditure. Aggressive nutritional intervention from hospital discharge to 3 months corrected age provided short-term benefits to growth and bone mass accretion,[29] but such growth advantage was not sustained after the intervention was completed.[45] Accelerated growth to attain catch-up to normal growth percentiles does not occur by 1 year corrected age,[45,48] and indeed, even at 7 years of age short stature (height <10th percentile) and low BMI compared with term-born infants were observed in over half of VLBW–BPD infants.[58]

To date, there are insufficient data to develop evidence-based practice guidelines for the nutritional management of ELBW infants at risk for or with developed BPD. Guidance in key management issues can at least be informed by the literature reviewed in this chapter. Until further research provides more rigorously derived evidence, interim recommendations for nutritional support of BPD infants as provided in Table 36.5 may help to guide clinical practice.

REFERENCES

1 Welty, S. E. Antioxidants and oxidations in bronchopulmonary dysplasia: there are no easy answers. *J. Pediatr.* 2003;**43**:697–8.

2 Sullivan, J. L. Iron, plasma antioxidants, and the 'oxygen radical disease of prematurity'. *Am. J. Dis. Child.* 1988;**142**:1341–44.

3 Saugstad, O. D. Bronchopulmonary dysplasia – oxidative stress and antioxidants. *Semin. Neonatol.* 2003;**8**:39–49.

4 Pitkanen, O. M., Hallman, M. Evidence for increased oxidative stress in preterm infants eventually developing chronic lung disease. *Semin. Neonatol.* 1998;**3**:199–205.

5 Jankov, R. P., Negus, A., Tanswell, A. K. Antioxidants as therapy in the newborn: Some words of caution. *Pediatr. Res.* 2001;**50**:681–7.

6 Welty, S. E. Is there a role for antioxidant therapy in bronchopulmonary dysplasia? *J. Nutr.* 2001:**131**;947S–50S.

7 Welty, S. E., Smith, C. V. Rationale for antioxidant therapy in premature infants to prevent bronchopulmonary dysplasia. *Nutr. Rev.* 2001;**59**:10–17.

8 Watts, J. L., Milner, R., Zipursky, A. *et al.* Failure of supplementation with vitamin E to prevent bronchopulmonary dysplasia in infants less than 1,500 g birth weight. *Eur. Respir. J.* 1991;**4**:188–90.

9 Berger, T. M., Frei, B., Rifai, N. *et al.* Early high dose antioxidant vitamins do not prevent bonchopulmonary dysplasia in premature baboons exposed to prolonged hyperoxia: a pilot study. *Pediatr. Res.* 1998;**43**:719–26.

10 Specker, B. L., deMarini, S., Tsang, R. C. Vitamin and mineral supplementation. In Sinclair, J. C., Bracken, M. B., eds. *Effective Care of the Newborn*. New York: Oxford University Press; 1992:161–77.

11 Merz, U., Peschgens, T., Dott, W., Hornchen, H. Selenium status and bronchopulmonary dysplasia in premature infants <1,500 g. *Z. Geburtshilfe Neonatol.* 1998;**202**:203–6.

12 Darlow, B. A., Inder, T. E., Graham, P. J. *et al.* The relationship of selenium status to respiratory outcome in the very low birth weight infant. *Pediatrics* 1995;**96**:314–19.

13 Falciglia, H. S., Johnson, R. J., Sullivan, J. *et al.* Role of antioxidant nutrients and lipid peroxidation in premature infants with respiratory distress syndrome and bronchopulmonary dysplasia. *Am. J. Perinatol.* 2003;**20**:97–108.

14 Ahola, T., Lapatto, R., Raivo, K. O. *et al.* N-acetylcysteine does not prevent bronchopumonary dysplasia in immature infants: a randomized controlled trial. *J. Pediatr.* 2003;**143**:713–19.

15 Rosenfeld, W., Evans, H., Concepcion, L. *et al.* Prevention of bronchopulmonary dysplasia by administration of bovine superoxide dismutase in preterm infants with respiratory distress syndrome. *J. Pediatr.* 1984;**105**:781–5.

16 Davis, J. M., Richter, S. E., Biswas, S. *et al.* Long-term follow-up of premature infants treated with prophylactic intratracheal recombinant human CuZn superoxide dismutase. *J. Perinatol.* 2000;**20**:213–16.

17 Bromberger, P., Hallman, M. Myoinositol in small preterm infants: Relationship between intake and serum concentration. *J. Pediatr. Gastroenterol. Nutr.* 1986;**5**:455–8.

18 Pereira, G. R., Baker, L., Egler, J., Corcoran, L., Chiavacci, R. Serum myoinositol concentrations in premature infants fed human milk, formula for infants, and parenteral nutrition. *Am. J. Clin. Nutr.* 1990;**51**:589–93.

19 Hallman, M., Arjomaa, P., Hoppu, K. Inositol supplementation in respiratory distress syndrome: relationship between serum concentration, renal excretion, and lung effluent phospholipids. *J. Pediatr.* 1987;**110**:604–10.

20 Hallman, M., Bry, K., Hoppu Lappi, M., Pohjavuori, M. Inositol supplementation in premature infants with respiratory distress syndrome. *N. Engl. J. Med.* 1992;**326**:1233–9.

21 Howlett, A., Ohlsson, A. Inositol for respiratory distress syndrome in preterm infants. *Cochrane Database Syst Rev.* 2003;**4**:CD000366.

22 Koo, W. W. K., Krug-Wispe, S., Succop, P., Tsang, R. C., Neylan, M. Effects of different vitamin A intakes in very low birth weight infants. *Am. J. Clin. Nutr.* 1995;**62**;1216–20.

23 Green, H., Phillips, B. L., Franck, L. *et al.* Persistently low blood retinal levels during and after parenteral feeding of very low birth weight infants: examination of losses into intravenous administration sets and a method of prevention by addition to a lipid emulsion. *Pediatrics* 1987:**79**:894–900.

24 Darlow, B. A., Graham, P. J. Vitamin A supplementation for preventing morbidity and mortality in very low birth weight infants. *Cochrane Database Syst Rev.* 2000;**2**:CD000501.

25 Tyson, J. E., Wright, L. L., Oh, W. *et al.* Vitamin A supplementation for extremely-low-birth-weight infants. National Institute of Child Health and Human Development Neonatal Research Network. *N. Eng. J. Med.* 1999;**340**:1962–8.

26 Ambalavanan, N., Wu, T.-J., Tyson, J. E. A comparison of three vitamin A dosing regimens in extremely-low-birth-weight infants. *J. Pediatr.* 2003;**142**:656–61.

27 Kramer, M. S., Platt, R. W., Shi, W. W. *et al.* A new and improved population-based Canadian reference for birth weight for gestational age. *Pediatrics* 2001;**108**:1–7.

28 Ziegler, E. E., Biga, R. L., Fomon, S. J. Nutritional requirements of the premature infant. In Suskind, R. M., ed. *Textbook of Pediatric Nutrition*. New York: Raven Press; 1981:29.

29 Brunton, J. A., Saigal, S., Atkinson, S. A. Growth and body composition in infants with bronchopulmonary dysplasia up to 3 months corrected age: a randomized trial of a high-energy nutrient-enriched formula fed after hospital discharge. *J. Pediatr.* 1998;**133**:340–5.

30 Denne, S. C. Energy expenditure in infants with pulmonary insufficiency: is there evidence for increased energy needs. *J. Nutr.* 2001;**131**:935S–7S.

31 Brunton, J. A., Atkinson, S. A., Winthrop, A., Saigal, S. Measures of energy intake and expenditure by doubly labeled water in infants recovering from bronchopulmonary dysplasia up to 3 months corrected age. *Pediatr. Res.* 1996;**39**:305A.

32 Davies, P. S. W., Irving, G., Lucas, A. Energy expenditure in early infancy. *Br. J. Nutr.* 1989;**62**:621–9.

33 Leitch, C. A., Denne, S. C. Increased energy expenditure in premature infants with chronic lung disease. *Pediatr. Res.* 2000;**47**:291.

34 St. John, E. B., Carlo, W. A. Respiratory distress syndrome in VLBW infants: changes in management and outcomes observed by the NICHD Neonatal Research Network. *Semin. Perinatol.* 2003;**27**:288–92.

35 Weiler, H. A., Paes, B., Shah, J. K., Atkinson, S. A. Longitudinal assessment of growth and bone mineral accretion in prematurely born infants treated for chronic lung disease with dexamethasone. *Early Hum. Dev.* 1997;**47**:271–86.

36 Ward, W. E., Atkinson, S. A., Donovan, S., Paes, B. Bone metabolism and circulating IGF-I and IGFBPs in dexamethasone-treated preterm infants. *Early Hum. Dev.* 1999;**56**:127–41.

37 Weiler, H. A., Wang, Z., Atkinson, S. A. Whole body lean mass is altered by dexamethasone treatment through reductions in protein and energy utilization in piglets. *Biol. Neonate* 1997b;**71**:53–9.

38 Leitch, C. A., Ahlrichs, J., Karn, C., Denne, S. C. Energy expenditure and energy intake during dexamethasone therapy for chronic lung disease. *Pediatr. Res.* 1999;**46**:109–13.

39 Weiler, H., Wang, Z., Atkinson, S. A. Dexamethasone alters calcium metabolism and bone mineralization during early development in the piglet model. *Am. J. Clin. Nutr.* 1995;**61**:805–11.

40 Ward, W. E., Donovan, S. M., Atkinson, S. A. Dexamethasone-induced abnormalities in bone metabolism in piglets are partially attenuated by growth hormone with no synergistic effect of insulin-like growth factor-1. *Pediatr. Res.* 1998;**44**:215–21.

41 Weiler, H. A., Atkinson, S. A. Dietary intervention following dexamethasone (DEX) treatment is effective in ameliorating dexamethasone-induced growth delay and osteoporosis in infant pigs. *Am. J. Clin. Nutr.* 1995;**61**:910.

42 Shinwell, E. S., Karplus, M., Bader, D. *et al.* Neonatologists are using much less dexamethasone. *Arch. Dis. Child Fetal Neonatal Edn.* 2003;**88**:F432–3.

43 Fewtrell, M. S., Adams, C., Wilson, D. C. *et al.* Randomized trial of high nutrient density formulas versus standard formula in chronic lung disease. *Acta Pediatr.* 1197;**86**:577–82.

44 Kay, H. H., Bird, I. M., Coe, C. L., Dudley, D. J. Antenatal steroid treatment and adverse fetal effects: what is the evidence? *J. Soc. Gynecol. Investig.* 2000;**7**:269–78.

45 Brunton, J. A., Saigal, S., Atkinson, S. A. Nutrient intake similar to recommended values does not result in catch-up growth by 12 mo of age in very low birth weight infants (VLBW) with bronchopulmonary dysplasia (BPD). *Am. Soc. Clin. Nutr.* 1997;**102**.

46 Atkinson, S. A. Special nutritional needs of infants for prevention of and recovery from bronchopulmonary dysplasia. *J. Nutr.* 2001;**131**:942S–6S.

47 Puangco, M. A., Schanler, R. J. Clinical experience in enteral nutrition support for premature infants with bronchopulmonary dysplasia. *J. Perinatol.* 2000;**20**:87–91.

48 Huysman, W. A., de Ridder, M., de Bruin, N. C. *et al.* Growth and body composition in preterm infants with bronchopulmonary dysplasia. *Arch. Dis. Child Fetal Neonatal Edn.* 2003;**88**:F46–51.

49 Butte, N., Heinz, C., Hopkinson, J. *et al.* Fat mass in infants and toddlers: comparability of total body water, total body potassium, total body electrical conductivity and dual energy X-ray absorptiometry. *J. Pediatr. Gastroenterol. Nutr.* 1999;**29**:184–9.

50 Randall Simpson, J., Paes, B., Thompson, P., Atkinson, S. A. Body composition analysis by dual energy x-ray absorptiometery (DXA) of term infants from birth to 12 months. *Am. J. Clin. Nutr.* 1995;**61**:500.

51 Atkinson, S. A., Randall-Simpson, J. Factors influencing body composition of premature infants at term-adjusted age. In Yasumura, S., ed. *Annals New York Academy of Sciences. 5th International Symposium on In Vivo Body Composition Studies, New York.* 2000;**904**:393–400.

52 Mimouni, F., Campaigne, B., Neylan, M., Tsang, R. C. Bone mineralization in the first year of life in infants fed human milk, cow-milk formula or soy-based formula. *J. Pediatr.* 1993;**122**:348–54.

53 Nutrition Committee, Canadian Pediatric Society. Nutrient needs and feeding of premature infants. *Can. Med. Assoc. J.* 1995;**152**:1765–85.

54 Institute of Medicine. *Dietary Reference Intake for Calcium, Phosphorus, Magnesium, Vitamin D and Fluoride. Food and Nutrition Board.* Washington, DC: National Academy Press; 1997.

55 Vrlenich, L. A., Bozynski, M. E. A., Shyr, Y. *et al.* The effect of bronchopulmonary dysplasia on growth at school age. *Pediatrics* 1995;**95**:855–9.

56 Robertson, C. M. T., Etches, P. C., Goldson, E., Kyle, J. M. Eight year school performance, neurodevelopmental and growth outcome of neonates with bronchopulmonary dysplasia: a comparative study. *Pediatrics* 1992;**89**:365–72.

57 Giacoia, P. G., Venkataraman, S. P., Kerstin, I., West, W., Faulkner, M. J. Follow-up of school age children with bronchopulmonary dysplasia. *J. Pediatr.* 1997;**130**:400–8.

58 Korhonen, P., Hyodynmaa, E., Lenko, H.-L., Tammela, O. Growth and adrenal androgen status at 7 years in very low birth weight survivors with and without bronchopulmonary dysplasia. *Arch. Dis. Child.* 2004;**89**:320–4.

59 Northway, W. H., Moss, R. B., Carlisle, K. B. *et al.* Late pulmonary sequelae of bronchopulmonary dysplasia. *N. Engl. J. Med.* 1990;**323**:1793–9.

60 Koivisto, M., Marttila, R., Kurkinen-Raty, M. *et al.* Changing incidence and outcome of infants with respiratory distress syndrome in the 1990s: a population-based survey. *Acta Pediatr.* 2004;**93**:177–84.

37

Nutrition in infants with congenital heart disease

James S. Barry and Patti J. Thureen

University of Colorado Health Sciences Center, Denver, CO

Introduction

Congenital heart disease (CHD) occurs in 1% of newborns each year.[1] It is the most common major congenital defect, comprising 13% of all major congenital defects.[2] It is well known that infants with hemodynamically significant CHD have an increased rate of malnutrition and growth failure compared with healthy infants. In the early 1900s, William Osler described children with CHD as "rarely thriving and often displaying lethargy of body and mind." Unfortunately, in the modern era, this description may still be accurate for some infants and children with CHD.

The neonatal period is a critical time for organ growth and development that is adversely affected by malnutrition associated with CHD.[3] Many infants and children with CHD will need surgical correction of their congenital defect, with more than half requiring surgery during infancy.[4] Although no data are available in infants undergoing cardiac surgery, data in adults indicate that improved preoperative nutritional status results in decreased postoperative morbidity.[5] Therefore, it is imperative that early nutritional intervention is begun in infants with CHD, both to avoid long-term consequences of malnutrition during this period of rapid growth and development and to improve the metabolic response to surgery in those infants who require early surgical intervention.

There are few data regarding nutritional metabolism and growth in the neonatal period in infants with CHD. This chapter focuses on the physiology and pathophysiology of CHD, the descriptive studies of growth patterns in infants and children with CHD, and on the few investigations that have been done regarding the pathogenesis of the abnormal growth rates in these infants.

Growth in infants with CHD

It has generally been thought that infants with CHD usually have normal weight and length at birth, unless affected by other "in utero" conditions known to be associated with poor fetal growth, and that CHD-associated growth problems develop postnatally.[3,6,7] However, studies have reported prenatal growth failure in infants with CHD. Levy et al. found an 80% incidence of subnormal birth weights among neonates with major cardiac lesions.[8] In the Baltimore–Washington Infant Study, a population-based, case-control study of infants with CHD conducted from 1981 to 1987, Rosenthal et al. reported significant weight deficits at birth in infants with tetrology of Fallot (TOF), endocardial cushion defect, pulmonary stenosis (PS), hypoplastic left heart syndrome (HLHS), coarctation of the aorta (CoA), ventricular septal defect (VSD), and atrial septal defect (ASD). The only diagnostic group for which birth weight was normal occurred in infants with transposition of the great arteries (TGA).[9]

In other early studies it was often difficult for investigators to separate the relative contribution of CHD from other co-existing prenatal conditions that could potentially cause poor fetal growth (e.g., genetic disorders, metabolic disease, infections, environmental factors). Fortunately, there are increasingly more refined methodologies available to diagnose these disorders, enabling better understanding of the effect of specific heart defects on growth.

A number of studies have looked at postnatal growth rates in infants and children with CHD. However, it has been difficult to draw firm conclusions from these studies because of the significant differences in study design. Various reports have included only hospitalized patients, thus

Neonatal Nutrition and Metabolism. Second Edition, ed. P. Thureen and W. Hay. Published by Cambridge University Press.

selecting the "sickest" infants. Other studies have investigated growth rates in infants and children over wide age ranges when growth velocities are different, in subjects with a large spectrum of cardiac anomalies that were not always grouped based upon specific heart lesions, in study populations comprised of both pre-operative and postoperative patients, and in infants with other disorders known to intrinsically affect growth such as Trisomy 21. Additionally, many studies that assessed growth included patients with CHD diagnosed by a mixture of clinical and cardiac catheterization-based diagnosis, or were done prior to the use of echocardiographic surveys to define anatomy. Most of the studies focusing on growth and nutrition in this population are descriptive in nature and few are hypothesis-driven, prospective studies.

The largest study of growth in infants with CHD was by Mehrizi and Drash.[10] This study, albeit older and retrospective, described growth failure tendencies for specific heart lesions in 890 infants and children 35 years ago. They reported that 55% of children with CHD were below the 16th percentile for weight, 52% were below the 16th percentile for height, and 27% were below the 3rd percentile for both. In general, they found that the cyanotic heart lesions TOF and TGA caused growth stunting of weight and height. In their acyanotic group, lesions with large left to right shunts and elevated pulmonary artery pressures (e.g., VSD, ASD, or patent ductus arteriosus (PDA) had a more pronounced effect on weight than height or head circumference.

A more recent study by Varan et al. investigated malnutrition in infants and children grouped as cyanotic or acyanotic heart lesions with and without pulmonary hypertension measured by heart catheterization.[11] Overall, they found a higher incidence of poor growth compared to the Mehrizi and Drash study. Sixty-five percent of 89 patients studied were below the 5th percentile for weight, and 41% were below the 5th percentile for height. They found that their patients with cyanotic CHD and pulmonary hypertension had the highest rate of failure to thrive, defined as less than 5th percentile for weight and height. These studies illustrate that growth impairment is a major morbidity for infants and children with CHD, especially those with pulmonary overcirculation, cyanosis, or pulmonary hypertension.

Data from the Baltimore–Washington Infant Study suggests that fetal growth patterns may be specific to certain cardiac defects.[12] This retrospective, case-control study characterized fetal growth differences among control newborns (n = 276) and neonates with TGA (n = 69), TOF (n = 66), HLHS (n = 51), and CoA (n = 65). Newborns with HLHS were found to be smaller in relation to height, weight, and head circumference when compared with controls,

with head circumference disproportionately smaller than weight. Infants with CoA had proportionately reduced lengths and weights as compared with head circumference. Infants with TOF were symmetrically undergrown, while those with TGA were of normal weight, but relatively smaller head volume. It was suggested that alterations in fetal hemodynamics caused the abnormal fetal growth pattern. This study excluded infants with known genetic syndromes, fetal infections and exposures that may have confounded the growth pattern findings. However, it is still not known if the fetal hemodynamics directly caused the abnormal growth patterns or if it is a more global process that is an "intrinsic growth disturbance" during embryogenesis and cardiogenesis.

Normal cardiac physiology

To better understand the impact that CHD has upon nutrition and metabolism, one should fully understand the physiologic adaptations that occur in the transition from fetal to neonatal life. Serious structural heart disease, for the most part, is completely compatible with fetal life and it is not until after birth that the postnatal alterations in cardiopulmonary hemodynamics result in physiologic instability.

The fetal lamb has been the most commonly used model to investigate fetal circulatory patterns and applied to human physiology. In the present era of sensitive ultrasonography, human fetal hemodynamics are becoming better understood and, in general, it has been found that major blood flow patterns are the same between species.[13] Since fetal blood flow is dependent on a "parallel" circulation with unequal left and right ventricular outputs, fetal cardiac output is described as bi-ventricular.[14,15] The majority of fetal cardiac output is provided to the placenta (45%) with little directed towards the lungs (<10%). At birth, a rapid transition occurs as the low resistance placenta is replaced by the lungs as the organ for gas exchange. Alveolar distension with breathing and alveolar fluid resorption causes a dramatic decrease in pulmonary vascular resistance so that pulmonary blood flow greatly increases and returns normally to the left atrium. This increase in left atrial blood flow and pressure functionally closes the foramen ovale. As the arterial oxygen level is increased and the placental source of prostaglandin is removed, the ductus arteriosus functionally closes during the first day of life. Thus, the pulmonary and systemic circulations change from a "parallel" circuit to one that functions in "series" with equal right and left ventricular cardiac outputs.

In the fetus, the intestine is a relatively dormant organ that requires a small amount of blood flow and oxygen delivery (less than 5% of cardiac output).[16] After birth, the intestine has an increase in metabolic activity as it becomes the sole organ for nutrient exchange. Intestinal growth dramatically increases in the first weeks of life to enable effective gastrointestinal absorption, secretion, and motility. In the normal neonate, there is a large increase in mesenteric blood flow (20% of cardiac output) and doubling of oxygen delivery in the first weeks of life.[17,18] With certain cardiac defects intestinal blood flow and oxygen delivery may be compromised because of diastolic "run off" (e.g., patent ductus arteriosus, aortic-pulmonic window, aorto-pulmonary collaterals, aortic insufficiency), decreased systemic perfusion secondary to a left-sided heart obstruction (e.g., coarctation of aorta, aortic stenosis, interrupted aortic arch), or peripheral and mesenteric vasoconstriction resulting from hypoxemia.

Pathophysiology of CHD

There have been many classifications for CHD. In this chapter, focus will be directed toward two main groups: cyanotic and acyanotic cardiac defects. These two groups have differing pathophysiology, but both may result in growth failure and poor nutrition.

Two main classifications of malformations cause cyanotic CHD: (1) lesions that result in decreased pulmonary blood flow secondary to obstruction, and (2) defects that fail to create "in series" pulmonary and systemic circulations, resulting in a separation of the pulmonary and systemic circulations. Decreased pulmonary blood flow occurs with TOF, critical pulmonic stenosis (PS), tricuspid valve anomalies (e.g., Ebstein's anomaly) and hypoplastic right heart syndromes. In complete TGA and total anomalous pulmonary venous return there is admixing of oxygenated and deoxygenated blood with the poorly oxygenated blood entering the systemic circulation. With cyanotic lesions, systemic blood is poorly oxygenated and the degree is related to the severity of the heart lesion. Interestingly, the degree of cyanosis has not been found to correlate with growth failure, but the duration of cyanosis is directly correlated with growth impairment.[19,20]

Acyanotic heart lesions result in an "effective" increase in the pulmonary circulation. These infants and children have increased pulmonary blood flow, either secondary to an increased systemic-to-pulmonary blood flow ratio or to a left-sided obstructive lesion. These include defects such as PDA, VSD, atrioventricular septal defect (AVSD), CoA, aortic stenosis (AS), interrupted aortic arch and HLHS (note

that HLHS is often characterized as being both a cyanotic and an acyanotic lesion, and represents a spectrum of left heart hypoplasia). With PDA, VSD, AVSD, and HLHS pulmonary blood flow may be greater than systemic blood flow as pulmonary arterial pressures decrease to subsystemic levels in the first months of life. Blood is shunted down the pressure gradient from the higher pressure in the systemic circulation to the lower pressure in the pulmonary circulation. In left-sided obstructive lesions such as CoA and AS, there is an increase in pressure of the left heart (left ventricle and left atrium) secondary to a decrease in antegrade systemic blood flow. This results in elevation of the pulmonary venous pressure that is transmitted to the pulmonary capillary bed. With the elevated capillary hydrostatic pressure, fluid is forced into the pulmonary interstitium resulting in "effective" pulmonary overcirculation and a decreased pulmonary compliance. Thus, symptomatic acyanotic heart lesions tend to cause congestive heart failure (CHF) with symptoms of tachypnea, dyspnea, tachycardia, hepatomegaly and cardiomegaly that undoubtedly contribute to the growth failure in these infants.

With both cyanotic and acyanotic heart lesions, the most prominent hemodynamic alterations that adversely affect nutritional state are volume overload of the left or right ventricle, pulmonary arterial hypertension, congestive heart failure, chronic hypoxia, and myocardial dysfunction.[4]

Cardiac and extra-cardiac etiologies of growth failure

There are a variety of etiologies for growth failure in infants with CHD that can be divided into "cardiac" and "extra-cardiac" factors. Extra-cardiovascular etiologies for growth failure in infants and children with CHD have been well described and include, but are not limited to, the following: chromosomal abnormalities (e.g., Trisomy 21, Turner's syndrome), genetic abnormalities (e.g., DiGeorge syndrome, William's syndrome), intrauterine infections (e.g., rubella), and environmental factors (e.g., gestational hyperthermia, placental insufficiency, fetal toxins). Each of these may lead to a reduction in future growth potential. As noted above, these prenatal factors may produce both fetal and postnatal growth failure, and may be difficult to separate from "cardiac" etiologies as the source of failure to thrive.

Four main "cardiac" factors have been found to contribute to poor growth in a number of infants and children with CHD: (1) increased metabolic rate, (2) feeding difficulties resulting in inadequate intake, (3) malabsorption of macro- and micro-nutrients, and (4) poor growth originating from alterations at the cellular or molecular level.

These are described in detail below. Additionally, other etiologies for poor growth such as chronic respiratory infections have been described, but are not clearly substantiated by clinical studies.

Metabolic alterations with CHD

In infants with CHD, the main etiology of failure to thrive has long been thought to be an increase in energy expenditure. Several studies have demonstrated an increase in metabolic rate in infants with CHD, especially in those infants and children with congestive heart failure.[21–23] Although an exact metabolic mechanism of poor growth with CHD has not been defined, it is likely because of a discrepancy between energy expenditure and energy intake. Total energy expenditure (TEE) is comprised of three main elements: (1) resting energy expenditure (REE), (2) physical activity, and (3) thermal energy for nutrient processing and new tissue formation. In the early neonatal period, REE is the major component of TEE, with physical activity being a major contributor to TEE only as the infant becomes more active after the first weeks to months of life.

Energy expenditure has been assessed using both indirect calorimetry (measures both REE and TEE) and doubly-labeled water techniques (measures TEE). As with the difficulty of assessing growth in infants with CHD because of the numerous confounding variables present in most studies, the same problem exists in many investigations of energy expenditure in infants and children. Studies have evaluated energy expenditure over large age ranges, included study subjects with vastly differing cardiac lesions, and have often lacked control groups. As a result, conflicting TEE and REE results have been reported in infants and children with CHD. Nevertheless, on balance, they suggest an increase in energy expenditure with CHD.

Older studies tested the hypothesis that infants with CHD have an increased oxygen requirement and increased oxygen consumption because of an elevated metabolic rate. Several early studies[21,24] demonstrated that oxygen consumption rates correlate with the severity of congestive heart failure. Krauss et al.[22] reported that infants with CHD and CHF had increased oxygen consumption compared with infants that had CHD but no evidence of CHF. Kennaird[25] measured oxygen consumption in infants with cyanotic v. acyanotic CHD and found that oxygen consumption was low in the cyanotic group and significantly higher in the acyanotic group, particularly those infants with evidence of CHF. Therefore, with energy expenditure indirectly determined using oxygen consumption measurements, infants with CHF as a result of acyanotic CHD (specifically those with large systemic to pulmonary

shunting lesions), have a relative hypermetabolism compared with infants with cyanotic CHD.

REE in infants with CHD has been reported to be normal[7,26] and elevated[22,27,28] in various studies. In a study controlled for type of heart lesion (uncorrected cyanotic heart disease) and age at study (investigated twice, at 2 weeks and again at 3 months of age), REE was not elevated at either age when compared with control infants without CHD.[29] From a methodological standpoint this is perhaps the best study on REE in infants with CHD, and it suggests that, at least in cyanotic CHD, REE is not a major cause of growth failure in early infancy.

More recent studies have used the doubly-labeled water method to determine TEE by measuring the relative urinary elimination rates of ^{18}O and ^{2}H, a reflection of the rate of CO_2 production. In infants with severe CHD (including both cyanotic and acyanotic lesions, with and without CHF) at 3–6 months of age, TEE was significantly elevated when compared with control infants from the literature.[30] As noted above, Leitch et al.[29] studied 10 infants with cyanotic CHD without CHF and 12 age-matched, healthy control infants at 2 weeks of age and again at 3 months of age. At 2 weeks of age there were no significant differences between groups in REE and TEE, but at 3 months of age, there was a significant increase in TEE (30%) in the patients with cyanotic CHD when compared with TEE in control infants. Ackerman et al.[31] measured both TEE and REE in infants 3–5 months old with moderate to large VSDs compared with that in healthy, age-matched controls and demonstrated no difference in REE between groups. However, TEE was 40% higher in the VSD group. Farrell and colleagues[23] evaluated energy expenditure in infants with VSD at 3–5 months of age compared with age-matched healthy controls and found TEE to be increased by 51% in patients with symptoms of CHF and by 26% in patients with a VSD but without symptoms of CHF.

In both the Ackerman[31] and Farrell[23] studies, the difference between TEE and REE was found to be much greater in infants with CHD as compared with age-matched healthy controls. Neither of these studies found a significant difference in REE when compared with healthy control infants. The authors hypothesize that in infants with VSDs, this indicates an increase in the energy cost of physical activity (which tends to increase at 3–4 months of age) compared with control infants.

Feeding difficulties as cause of growth failure with CHD

Poor nutrition is a likely cause of failure to thrive in many infants with CHD. In infants with CHD there is often a fine balance between fluid restriction and adequate caloric intake. At times, fluid restriction prevents effective caloric intake and results in growth failure.

Insufficient nutrient intake has long been thought to be the main etiology for growth failure in infants with CHD[7,24,26,27,32–35] with a common finding of a direct correlation between caloric intake and body weight. However, other studies have reported no significant differences compared with healthy age-matched controls in caloric intake when calculated as kcal kg^{-1} day^{-1}.[29,31,36] Generally, caloric intake for weight is normal or "near-normal." However, when intake is expressed per expected weight for age (50th percentile), less than adequate intake is often found.[29,31,36]

The cause of poor intake in infants with CHD is multifactorial in origin. Infants with CHD commonly have fatigue with feeding that results in inadequate intake.[32] This is especially true for infants with CHF that already have increased baseline respiratory rates.[21] Infants with CHF may begin feeding vigorously but often tire quickly. Anorexia may also be a component of poor oral intake that is caused by hypoxia, medications, and a delayed gastric emptying. It is well known in adults that digoxin toxicity causes loss of appetite,[37] but it is unknown if this effect is significant in the therapeutic range in infants and children with CHD. Fluid restriction and diuretics are commonly utilized and can cause electrolyte abnormalities such as hyponatremia that may lead to anorexia. Early satiety and a depressed appetite may be related to the delayed gastric emptying that has been reported in infants with cyanotic CHD[38] and adults with CHF,[39] as well as to the decreased gastric capacity that can occur secondary to compression of the stomach from an enlarged liver or ascites.[40]

Inherent changes in gastro-intestinal function may limit the infant or child with CHD from taking adequate enteral feedings. Patients receiving chronic prostaglandin administration (e.g., infants with HLHS) may have altered gastric antral mucosal hyperplasia that can functionally create a gastric outlet obstruction.[41,42] Potentially, CHF and hepatomegaly can increase intra-abdominal pressure and lead to emesis. Ineffective caloric intake may also be related to the high incidence of gastroesophageal reflux that occurs with CHD.[43]

Thus, there are a multitude of reasons for an infant with CHD to feed poorly, necessitating an individualized approach to ensure proper nutrient intake.

Losses of macro- and micro-nutrients

Some patients with CHD have failure to thrive despite consuming adequate calories based upon weight and/or age. This has led some investigators to believe that nutrient losses may cause poor weight and height gain. This is presumed to occur primarily via gastrointestinal malabsorption of nutrients, but there can also be significant protein and energy loss in the urine.

The pathophysiological processes underlying malabsorption have not been defined clearly. Elevated right atrial pressures, CHF, low cardiac output states, and chronic hypoxemia may all result in intestinal venous or lymphatic congestion causing mesenteric hypoxia and functional abnormalities of the intestine leading to nutrient malabsorption. Sondheimer et al.[44] investigated the malabsorption profile of fat, protein, and carbohydrate in hospitalized infants less than 20 weeks of age with either chronic CHF or cyanotic CHD. They found that 24% of infants studied had increased stool fat loss and 60% of infants had an increase in stool protein (4 of 6 in the CHF group and 4 of 8 in cyanotic CHD group). Despite these findings, the infants were all in a positive nitrogen balance and had normal levels of serum albumin. The stool fat equated to a caloric loss of up to 20 kcal kg^{-1} day^{-1}. However, indirect measurements of body lipid markers such as serum levels of carotene, cholesterol, and vitamin A were normal. Several other studies of intestinal function in infants with CHD suggested an absence of significant malabsorption in these patients. Vaisman et al.[45] found that there was an increase in stool fat excretion in children with congestive heart failure requiring chronic diuretic usage. When stool fat was expressed as a percentage of daily caloric intake no significant difference was found when compared with controls. However, infants with increased total body water despite diuretic therapy had increased malabsorption when compared with euvolemic patients. Yahav et al.[46] studied 14 infants with CHD and growth failure during three differing nutrient regimens each lasting 3–7 days: (1) normal feeding, (2) increased enteric calories delivered orally, and (3) increased enteric calories delivered via nasogastric tube. They concluded that there were no abnormalities of intestinal function in infants with CHD when compared with controls. Of interest, in this study proximal intestinal biopsies were performed and there was edema noted in the lamina propria but it did not correlate with malabsorption.

Conflicting results from the above studies may be related to the differences in study populations. Sondheimer et al.[44] included ill hospitalized patients, all less than 20 weeks of age, with specific cardiac lesions: TGA for the cyanotic group and an acyanotic group consisting of infants with severe CHF. The other studies contained heterogeneous study populations.[45,46] Overall, it does not consistently appear that nutrient malabsorption is the main etiology of growth failure in infants and children with CHD, but it should be considered if a patient has a prominent stooling pattern and poor growth despite an adequate medical and nutritional regimen.

Alterations at the cellular and molecular level

Most investigations regarding intake and growth in infants and children with CHD have focused on macronutrient consumption. However, there may be abnormalities in micro-nutrient intake and/or systemic concentrations that may result in impaired growth secondary to altered cellular and molecular functions.

With CHF, clinical management usually includes fluid restriction and use of diuretics, a practice that commonly results in electrolyte abnormalities. In adults on diuretics, the level of potassium and magnesium in skeletal muscle has been found to be significantly decreased in half of the patients.[47] In animal studies reduced potassium, magnesium, and zinc cause a decrease in growth and protein synthesis that is proportional to insulin-like growth factor-1 (IGF-1) concentrations.[48,49] In adults with CHF, cachexia may occur secondary to increased levels of cytokines.[50]

Newborn lambs who were made hypoxemic for 2 weeks (oxygen saturation 60–74%) demonstrated that serum IGF-1 levels were decreased by 43% compared with control animals.[51] Recently, Barton et al.[52] studied 62 infants at 1 year of age who had been diagnosed with symptomatic CHD. They found that serum concentrations of IGF-1 and insulin-like growth factor binding protein-3 (IGFBP-3) were significantly reduced when compared with age-matched healthy controls. These are interesting findings that will need proper clinical trials to determine if deficiencies in electrolytes or micro-nutrients specifically lead to a decrease in serum IGF-1 levels in infants and children with CHD or if they are merely correlated with growth impairment.

Sasaki et al.[53] investigated the growth of children with surgically corrected CHD and continued growth impairment. Children in this study continued to have poor growth despite surgical correction of their CHD and were given recombinant growth hormone therapy over a 2-year period. They found an increase in growth rate (height) of 45% during the first year of treatment and an increase of 32% over the second year of study. Interestingly, these patients were not growth hormone deficient, but they did respond to recombinant growth hormone therapy.

Necrotizing enterocolitis and CHD

Necrotizing enterocolitis (NEC) is a life-threatening intestinal disease most often associated with premature infants,

however it is estimated that 7–25% of NEC cases occur in full-term infants.[54–56] Multiple studies have found that premature and full-term infants with CHD are at an increased risk for developing NEC.[54–61] The proposed etiology in this population is intestinal mucous membrane injury initiated by mesenteric ischemia. In 1969 Lloyd studied diving mammals and found that there was a neurogenic redistribution of blood flow away from the gastro-intestinal circulation toward more critical organs such as the heart and brain.[62] It was proposed that this "diving reflex" caused intestinal hypoxia and was the antecedent insult causing NEC. It has been found that a neurogenic redistribution of blood flow does occur in the neonate, but there is quickly an "autoregulatory escape" phenomenon that improves oxygen delivery to the newborn intestine if the neonate is hemodynamically stable. However, this protective "autoregulatory escape" mechanism does not sustain intestinal blood flow and adequate oxygen delivery in the face of added insults such as moderate to severe arterial hypotension or hypoxia.[63]

It is likely that ischemia of the intestinal tract may occur with specific CHD lesions in newborns and infants that result in a decreased intestinal blood flow. CHD lesions that create a decreased systemic cardiac output, a large left to right shunt with an increase in the Qp/Qs ratio, or a diastolic "run-off" may predispose the infant to intestinal ischemia. Patent ductus arteriosus in preterm neonates, a lesion of "diastolic steal" with decreased intestinal blood flow has been clearly associated with an increased incidence of NEC.[64,65] Feeding may also increase the risk of intestinal tissue hypoxia by increasing the metabolic demand on already "at risk" tissues.[66] These may be the antecedent insults that cause NEC in some patients with CHD.

The role of CHD in NEC has been studied in two specific manners: (1) determining the incidence of NEC in neonates with CHD, and (2) evaluating the incidence of CHD in neonates with NEC. The incidence of NEC in patients with CHD varies from 3.3–7% (Table 37.1).[59–61] In these studies, significant contributing factors to the increased incidence of NEC were prostaglandin E_2 administration that led to apnea and/or hypotension[60] and having at least one non-cardiac risk factor for NEC such as episodes of poor cardiac output and relative prematurity.[59] In studies by Leung et al.[60] and Cheng et al.,[61] no specific cardiac lesions were found to be significantly associated with NEC. However, McElhinney et al.[59] found that the cardiac lesions significantly associated with NEC were HLHS, AP window, and truncus arteriosus.

Several retrospective studies have been performed to investigate the role of CHD as a risk factor for NEC in newborns (Table 37.2).[56–58,67] These studies reported the incidence of CHD in patients with proven NEC to range from

Table 37.1. Incidence of necrotizing enterocolitis (NEC) in neonates with congenital heart disease (CHD)

Primary Author	Number of subjects	Gestational age (weeks)	Percent with NEC	Type of CHD	Comments
Leung et al.[60]	133	NI	7%	44% – Pulmonary outflow obstruction 33% – Left heart obstruction 23% – NI	All patients had symptomatic CHD Identified PGE$_2$ infusion as significant risk factor for NEC
Cheng et al.[61]	850	mean: 37 weeks 25% preterm	3.5%	47% – Pulmonary outflow obstruction 27% – VSD, ASD, PDA, or AV canal 17% – AS, CoA, IAA 10% – TGA	Institutional review from 1981–1997 PDA found in 80% of neonates with NEC and CHD Mortality 57% with NEC and CHD, compared with 20% in newborns without CHD
McElhinney et al.[59]	643	range: 31–42 weeks 62%<36 weeks	3.3%	48% – HLHS 10% for each of the following: TA, TOF, PA with IVS, CoA 5% for each of the following: AS, AP window, DORV	All 21 patients with NEC and CHD had at least one non-cardiac risk factor for NEC Significant lesions for NEC: HLHS, TA, AP window

Abbreviations: NI, not indicated; PGE$_2$, prostaglandin F$_2$; VSD, ventricular septal defect; ASD, atrial septal defect; PDA, patent ductus arteriosus; AV canal, atrio-ventricular canal; AS, aortic stenosis; CoA, coarctation of the aorta; IAA, interrupted aortic arch; TGA, transposition of the great arteries; HLHS, hypoplastic left heart; TA, tricuspid atresia; TOF, tetrology of Fallot; PA with IVS, pulmonary atresia with intact ventricular septum; AS, aortic stenosis; AP window, aorto-pulmonary window; DORV, double outlet right ventricle.

Table 37.2. Incidence of congenital heart disease (CHD) in patients with necrotizing enterocolitis (NEC)

Primary author	Number of subjects	Gestational age (weeks)	Percent with CHD	Type of CHD	Comments
Polin et al.[56]	13	39.5 weeks	39%	60% – HLHS 40% – NI	Institutional study HLHS associated with low cardiac output or CHF
Andrews et al.[57]	10	≥38 weeks	20%	10% – VSD (trisomy 21) 10% – VSD/ASD (trisomy 21)	No infants in this study had cyanotic CHD
Martinez-Tallo et al.[58]	24	100% > 2 kg, 66% > 36 weeks	12%	Specific heart lesions – NI	Significant risk factors: PROM, low Apgar score, CHD, hypoglycemia, respiratory distress, exchange transfusion
Bolisetty et al[67]	29	>37 weeks	35%	40% – TGA 20% – CoA 20% – PA 10% – TA 10% – VSD	Regional review of tertiary centers All but two infants had noncardiac risk factors for NEC

Abbreviations: NI, not indicated; HLHS, hypoplastic left heart; CHF, congestive heart failure; VSD, ventricular septal defect; ASD, atrial septal defect; PROM, premature rupture of the membranes; TGA, transposition of the great arteries; CoA, coarctation of the aorta; PA, pulmonary atresia; TA, tricuspid atresia.

12%–39%. However, some of these studies included premature infants. As prematurity is the most substantiated risk factor for NEC, it may confound the results associating CHD with NEC. When the studies included only full-term infants (>37 weeks) with CHD, the incidence of NEC ranged from 20%–30%. Overall, CHD is a significant risk factor for NEC. Specific heart lesions such as HLHS, truncus arteriosus, interrupted aortic arch and any other cardiac defects causing decrease in intestinal perfusion put a newborn at a much higher risk for NEC than the standard newborn population.

Nutritional assessment

Often, in the complex medical management of CHD, nutrition may be an afterthought as the clinical management of critical heart lesions takes the forefront. Nutritional assessment is of critical importance in both determining the need for nutritional intervention and in assessing the efficacy of the nutritional regimen in infants with CHD. For a detailed review of nutritional assessment techniques, see the chapter "Nutritional Assessment of the Neonate."

A detailed, standardized nutritional assessment format should be used for all infants with CHD who demonstrate, or are at risk for, growth failure. Historical information should include questions regarding types and volume of feeding with an estimate of calorie and protein intake, duration of feeds and work of feeding (is the infant tiring?), irritability, lethargy, vomiting, constipation, diarrhea.

Anthropometric measurements are critical to assessing growth. Weight, length and head circumference should be measured by trained personnel, preferably by the same person on each visit. Appropriate growth charts for age, gender, altitude, and racial/ethnic background should be used. Weight for length and growth velocities should be determined. Skinfold thickness and arm circumference can be used to estimate energy and protein loss and accretion. Laboratory assessment depends on the individual child, especially if unanticipated growth faltering is occurring (see chapter "Nutritional Assessment of the Neonate" for details).

Nutritional regimen

As noted above, infants and children with CHD are often noted to be "poor feeders," especially those with CHF and/or cyanosis. In many instances, alternative nutritional regimens and techniques are necessary to support adequate nutritional intake.

No studies have been performed to determine the most effective nutritional regimen for infants and children with CHD. It has been found that infants and children with CHD and poor growth improve with increased caloric delivery. Jackson et al.[27] studied the short-term effects of increasing caloric density in 14 infants, 1–5 months of age, that had failure to thrive and CHD. They studied infants on normal formula, and then on the same formula but fortified with glucose polymers to increase mean energy intakes by 32%. They found over the short study period of 2–3 days that the mean weight gain improved significantly from 1.3 g kg^{-1} day^{-1} to 5.8 g kg^{-1} day^{-1}. Unger et al.[68] investigated caloric intake and weight improvement after instituting a protocol for nutritional assessment and counseling in 35 patients aged 1 month to 2 years of age with CHD. They found that initially only 89% of RDA were being consumed. However, with intervention intake increased to 108% of RDA and resulted in improved weight for length measurements over the study period.

Studies have shown infants and children with poor growth secondary to CHD may benefit from nasogastric feeding. Vanderhoof et al.[68] studied the use of nasogastric feedings in 11 infants with complex CHD and poor growth despite receiving hypercaloric formulas and nutritional supplementation. By switching from oral to nasogastric feedings, the caloric intakes increased by 32% secondary to decreased emesis. A study by Schwarz et al.[34] investigated 19 infants with CHF receiving one of three different feeding regimens: (1) ad lib demand oral feedings, (2) 12 hours of nasogastric continuous feedings with 12 hour ad lib demand oral feedings, and (3) 24 hours of continuous nasogastric feedings. Only the patients in the group receiving 24 hours of continuous nasogastric feedings gained weight and height over the 5-month study period. The poorest growth rate was in the infants on ad lib demand feedings. Therefore, consideration should be given to implementing nasogastric feeds in select patients with continued poor growth. Recently, several studies have suggested that gastrostomy tube placement is a low risk procedure that may be preferable to nasogastric tube feedings because it does not interfere with oral feeding and dislocations requiring replacement.[70,71]

Nutritional intervention needs to be individualized. As noted above, simply an increase in caloric intake may improve growth. What is "optimal growth" in these patients is not well-defined; the gold standard for growth of the preterm infant is that of the reference fetus, or 15–18 g kg^{-1} day^{-1}.[72] For post-term infants over the first several months of life a common weight gain goal is 20–30 g day^{-1}.[73] In many patients, this has to be accomplished in the face of fluid restriction. Weight gain alone is probably not the optimal nutritional endpoint in these patients since this does not address the quality of the weight that is gained. The goal should be to avoid catabolism and to provide sufficient protein and energy to achieve a body composition that, at least in the first several months of life, reflects that of the breast-fed infant at the same gestational age. On a practical level, this is often difficult to achieve since body composition assessment methods are often not routinely available.

In many neonatal or cardiac intensive care units, nutritional management is to increase nutrient intake until weight gain occurs. In neonates and infants weight gain is often achieved by adding modular supplements (glucose, lipid, and protein) to formula. These supplements are increased in the same relative proportion until growth is improved or intolerance develops. Frequently this results in a caloric density of 28–30 kcal per ounce formula intake. In 1972 Fomon et al.[74] suggested a 1 kcal mL^{-1} formula preparation with a content of 9% protein, 31% fat, and 60% carbohydrate for infants with CHD and poor growth, a recommendation that is still appropriate for use in this population today. Carbohydrate intake above this level should be avoided in that it may result in a hypermetabolic state with increased energy expenditure.

Whenever concentrated formulas are used, attention must be given to the osmolality of the formula since such preparations may result in delivery of an excessive renal solute load to the kidney. The AAP recommends that enteral feedings have an osmolarity < 400 mOsm L^{-1}, which is an osmolality of approximately 450 mOsm kg^{-1} of liquid.[75] Osmolarity of medications are often overlooked in these patients, but they also need to be taken into consideration.[76] Additionally, the potential renal solute load needs to be considered, particularly in infants who are fluid restricted or on diuretic therapy.[77]

Efforts should be made to normalize serum electrolyte concentrations and micronutrient concentrations since deficiencies can be growth-limiting. Based on clinical history (medication use, dietary intake, etc.), it can be anticipated who is at risk for electrolyte and micronutrient deficiencies. If growth is still suboptimal, evaluate for possible malabsorption. Consider partial or full NG feedings if feeds are given enterally. If none of the enteral feeding approaches are successful, parenteral partial or full nutrition may be required for a period of time.

Conclusion

Growth problems are common in infants and children with CHD. An individualized nutritional approach is warranted

for the most "at risk" patients, particularly those with chronic hypoxemia, pulmonary hypertension, and CHF. The most common causes of growth failure in infants with CHD (i.e., poor intake, malabsorption, increased energy expenditure, and altered cellular metabolism) should be considered in each patient so that an individualized nutritional regimen and assessment strategy can be developed to aid in attaining maximal growth.

REFERENCES

1 Hoffman, J. I. Incidence of congenital heart disease: I. Postnatal incidence. *Pediatr. Cardiol.* 1995;**16**:103–13.

2 Holmes, L. B. Current concepts in genetics. Congenital malformations. *N. Engl. J. Med.* 1976;**295**:204–7.

3 Naeye, R. L. Anatomic features of growth failure in congenital heart disease. *Pediatrics* 1967;**39**:433.

4 Rosenthal, A. Nutritional considerations in the prognosis and treatment of children with congenital heart disease. In Suskind, R. M., Lewinter-Suskind, L., eds. *Textbook of Pediatric Nutrition.* 2nd Edn. New York, NY: Raven Press; 1993: 383–93.

5 Blackburn, G. L., Gibbons, G. W., Bothe, A. *et al.* Nutritional support in cardiac cachexia. *J. Thorac. Cardiovasc. Surg.* 1977;**73**:489–95.

6 Bayer, L. M., Robinson, S. J. Growth history of children with congenital heart disease. Size according to sex, age decade, surgical status, and diagnostic category. *Am. J. Dis. Child.* 1969;**117**:564–72.

7 Huse, D. M., Feldt, R. H., Nelson, R. A., Novak, L. P. Infants with congenital heart disease. Food intake, body weight, and energy metabolism. *Am. J. Dis. Child.* 1975;**129**:65–9.

8 Levy, R. J., Rosenthal, A., Fyler, D. C., Nadas, A. S. Birthweight of infants with congenital heart disease. *Am. J. Dis. Child.* 1978;**132**:249–54.

9 Rosenthal, G. L., Wilson, P. D., Permutt, T., Boughman, J. A., Ferencz, C. Birth weight and cardiovascular malformations: a population-based study. The Baltimore–Washington Infant Study. *Am. J. Epidemiol.* 1991;**133**:1273–81.

10 Mehrizi, A., Drash, A. Growth disturbance in congenital heart disease. *J. Pediatr.* 1962;**61**:418–29.

11 Varan, B., Tokel, K., Yilmaz, G. Malnutrition and growth failure in cyanotic and acyanotic congenital heart disease with and without pulmonary hypertension. *Arch. Dis. Child.* 1999;**81**:49–52.

12 Rosenthal, G. L. Patterns of prenatal growth among infants with cardiovascular malformations: possible fetal hemodynamic effects. *Am. J. Epidemiol.* 1996;**143**:505–13.

13 Rasanen, J., Wood, D. C., Weiner, S. *et al.* Role of the pulmonary circulation in the distribution of human fetal cardiac output during the second half of pregnancy. *Circulation* 1996;**9**:1068–73.

14 Rudolph, A. M. Distribution and regulation of blood flow in the fetal and neonatal lamb. *Circ. Res.* 1985;**57**:811–21.

15 Friedman, A. H. Fahey, J. T. The transition from fetal to neonatal circulation: normal responses and implications for infants with heart disease. *Semin. Perinatol.* 1993;**17**:106–21.

16 Reber, K. M., Nankervis, C. A., Nowicki, P. T. Newborn intestinal circulation: physiology and pathophysiology. *Clin. Perinatol.* 2002;**29**:23–39.

17 Stoddart, R. W., Widdowson, E. M. Changes in the organs of pigs in response to feeding for the first 24 h after birth. III. Fluorescence histochemistry of the carbohydrates of the intestine. *Biol. Neonate.* 1976;**29**:18–27.

18 Edelstone, D. I., Holzman, I. R. Fetal intestinal oxygen consumption at various levels of oxygenation. *Am. J. Physiol.* 1982;**242**:H50–4.

19 Feldt, R. H., Strickler, G. B., Weidman, W. H. Growth of children with congenital heart disease. *Am. J. Dis. Child.* 1969;**117**:573–9.

20 Linde, L. M., Dunn, O. J., Schireson, R., Rasof, B. Growth in children with congenital heart disease. *J. Pediatr.* 1967;**70**:413–19.

21 Stocker, F. P., Wilkoff, W., Miettinen, O. S., Nadas, A. S. Oxygen consumption in infants with heart disease. Relationship to severity of congestive heart failure, relative weight, and caloric intake. *J. Pediatr.* 1972;**80**:43–51.

22 Krauss, A. N., Auld, P. A. Metabolic rate of neonates with congenital heart disease. *Arch. Dis. Child.* 1975;**50**:539–41.

23 Farrell, A. G., Schamberger, M. S., Olson, I. L., Leitch, C. A. Large left to right shunts and congestive failure increase total energy expenditure in infants with ventricular septal defects. *Am. J. Cardiol.* 2001;**87**:1128–31.

24 Lees, M., Bristow, J. D., Griswold, H. E., Olmstead, R. W. Relative hypermetabolism in infants with congenital heart disease and undernutrition. *Pediatrics* 1965;**36**:183–91.

25 Kennaird, D. L. Oxygen consumption and evaporative water loss in infants with congenital heart disease. *Arch. Dis. Child.* 1976;**51**:34–41.

26 Menon, G. K., Poskitt, E. M. Why does congenital heart disease cause failure to thrive? *Arch. Dis. Child.* 1985;**60**:1134–9.

27 Jackson, M., Poskitt, E. M. The effects of high-energy feeding on energy balance and growth in infants with congenital heart disease and failure to thrive. *Br. J. Nutr.* 1991;**65**:131–43.

28 Lees, M., Bristow, J. D., Griswold, H. E., Olmstead, R. W. Relative hypermetabolism in infants with congenital heart disease and undernutrition. *Pediatrics* 1965;**36**:183–91.

29 Leitch, C. A., Karn, C. A., Peppard, R. J., *et al.* Increased energy expenditure in infants with cyanotic congenital heart disease. *J. Pediatr.* 1998;**133**:755–60.

30 Barton, J., Hindmarsh, P., Scrimgeour, C., Rennie, M., Preece, M. Energy expenditure in congenital heart disease. *Arch. Dis. Child.* 1994;**70**:5–9.

31 Ackerman, I. L., Karn, C. A., Denne, S. C., Ensing, G. J., Leitch, C. A. Total but not resting energy expenditure is increased in infants with ventricular septal defects. *Pediatrics* 1998;**102**:1172–7.

32 Hansen, S. R., Dorup, I. Energy and nutrient intakes in congenital heart disease. *Acta. Paediatr. Scand.* 1993;**82**:166–72.

33 Krieger, I. Growth failure and congenital heart disease. Energy balance in infants. *Am. J. Dis. Child.* 1970;**120**:497–502.

34 Schwarz, S. M., Gewitz, M. H., See, C. C., *et al.* Enteral nutrition in infants with congenital heart disease and growth failure. *Pediatrics* 1990;**86**:368–73.

35 Salzer, H. R., Haschke, F., Wimmer, M., Heil, M., Schilling, R. Growth and nutritional intake of infants with congenital heart disease. *Pediatr. Cardiol.* 1989;**10**:17–23.

36 Strangeway, A., Fowler, R., Cunningham, K., Hamilton, J. R. Diet and growth in congenital heart disease. *Pediatrics* 1976;**57**:75–86.

37 Holt, D. W., Volans, G. N. Gastrointestinal symptoms of digoxin toxicity. *Br. Med. J.* 1977;**2**:704.

38 Cavell, B. Gastric emptying in infants with congenital heart disease. *Acta. Paediatr. Scand.* 1981;**70**:517–20.

39 Pittman, J. G., Cohen, P. The pathogenesis of cardiac cachexia. *N. Engl. J. Med.* 1964;**271**:403–9.

40 Gervasio, M. R., Buchanan, C. N. Malnutrition in the pediatric cardiology patient. *CCQ.* 1985;**8**:49–56.

41 Babyn, P., Peled, N., Manson, D. *et al.* Radiologic features of gastric outlet obstruction in infants after long-term prostaglandin administration. *Pediatr. Radiol.* 1995;**25**:41–3.

42 Peled, N., Dagan, O., Babyn, P. *et al.* Gastric-outlet obstruction induced by prostaglandin therapy in neonates. *N. Engl. J. Med.* 1992;**327**:505–10.

43 Forchielli, M. L., McColl, R., Walker, W. A., Lo, C. Children with congenital heart disease; a nutrition challenge. *Nutr. Rev.* 1994;**52**:348–53.

44 Sondheimer, J. M., Hamilton, J. R. Intestinal function in infants with severe congenital heart disease. *J. Pediatr.* 1978;**92**:572–8.

45 Vaisman, N., Leigh, T., Voet, H. *et al.* Malabsorption in infants with congenital heart disease under diuretic treatment. *Pediatr. Res.* 1994;**36**:545–9.

46 Yahav, J., Avigad, S., Frand, M. Assessment of intestinal and cardiorespiratory function in children with congenital heart disease on high-caloric formulas. *J. Pediatr. Gastroenterol. Nutr.* 1985;**4**:778–85.

47 Dyckner, T., Wester, P. O. Plasma and skeletal muscle electrolytes in patients on long-term diuretic therapy for arterial hypertension and/or congestive heart failure. *Acta Med. Scand.* 1987;**222**:231–6.

48 Dorup, I., Clausen, T. Effects of potassium deficiency on growth and protein synthesis in skeletal muscle and the heart of rats. *Br. J. Nutr.* 1989;**62**:269–84.

49 Dorup, I., Flyvberg, A., Everts, M. E., Clausen, T. Role of insulin-like growth factor-1 and growth inhibition induced by magnesium and zinc deficiencies. *Br. J. Nutr.* 1991;**66**:505–21.

50 Feldman, A. M., Combes, A., Wagner, D., *et al.* The role of tumor necrosis factor in the pathophysiology of heart failure. *J. Am. Coll. Cardiol.* 2000;**35**:537–44.

51 Bernstein, D., Jasper, J. R., Rosenfeld, R. G., Hintz, R. L. Decreased serum insulin-like growth factor-1 associated with growth failure in newborn lambs with experimental cyanotic heart disease. *J. Clin. Invest.* 1992;**89**:1128–32.

52 Barton, J. S., Hindmarsh, P. C., Preece, M. A. Serum insulin-like growth factor 1 in congenital heart disease. *Archiv. Dis. Child.* 1996; **75**:162–3.

53 Sasaki, H., Baba, K., Nishida, Y., *et al.* Treatment of children with congenital heart disease and growth retardation with recombinant human growth hormone. *Acta. Paediatr. Scand.* 1996;**85**:251–3.

54 Kliegman, R. M., Fanaroff, A. A. Neonatal necrotizing enterocolitis: a nine-year experience. *Am. J. Dis. Child.* 1981;**135**:603–7.

55 Wiswell, T. E., Robertson, C. F., Jones, T. A., Tuttle, D. J. Necrotizing enterocolitis in full-term infants. A case control study. *Am. J. Dis. Child.* 1988;**142**:532–5.

56 Polin, R. A., Pollack, P. F., Barlow, B. Necrotizing enterocolitis in term infants. *J. Pediatr.* 1976;**89**:460–2.

57 Andrews, D. A., Sawin, R. S., Ledbetter, D. J., Schaller, R. T., Hatch, E. I. Necrotizing enterocolitis in term infants. *Am. J. Surg.* 1990;**159**:507–9.

58 Martinez-Tallo, E., Claure, N., Bancalari, E. Necrotizing enterocolitis in full-term or near-term infants: risk factors. *Biol. Neonate* 1997;**71**:292–8.

59 McElhinney, D. B., Hedrick, H. L., Bush, D. M., *et al.* Necrotizing enterocolitis in neonates with congenital heart disease: risk factors and outcomes. *Pediatrics* 2000;**106**:1080–7.

60 Leung, M. P., Chau, K., Hui, P., *et al.* Necrotizing enterocolitis in neonates with symptomatic congenital heart disease. *J. Pediatr.* 1988;**113**:1044–6.

61 Cheng, W., Leung, M. P., Tam, P. K. H. Surgical intervention in necrotizing enterocolitis with symptomatic congenital heart disease. *Pediatr. Surg. Int.* 1999;**15**:492–5.

62 Lloyd, J. The etiology of gastrointestinal perforations in the newborn. *J. Pediatr. Surg.* 1969;**4**:77–84.

63 Nowicki, P. T., Nankervis, C. A. The role of the circulation in the pathogenesis of necrotizing enterocolitis. *Clin. Perinatol.* 1994;**21**:219–34.

64 Cooke, R. W., Meradji, M., de Villenevue, V. H. Necrotising enterocolitis after cardiac catheterisation in infants. *Arch. Dis. Child.* 1980;**55**:66–8.

65 Wong, S. N., Lo, R. N., Hui, P. W. Abnormal renal and splanchnic arterial Doppler pattern in premature babies with symptomatic patent ductus arteriosus. *J. Ultrasound Med.* 1990;**9**:125–30.

66 Crissinger, K. D., Burney, D. L. Post-prandial hemodynamics and oxygenation in developing piglet intestine. *Am. J. Physiol.* 1991;**260**:G651–7.

67 Bolisetty, S., Lui, K., Oei, J., Wojtulewicz, J. A regional study of underlying congenital diseases in term infants with necrotizing enterocolitis. *Acta. Paediatr. Scand.* 2000; **89**:1226–30.

68 Unger, R., DeKleermaeker, M., Gidding, S. S., Christoffel, K. K. Abstract Calories count. Improved weight gain with dietary intervention in congenital heart disease. *Am. J. Dis. Child.* 1992;**146**:1078–84.

69 Vanderhoof, J. A., Hofschire, P. J., Baluff, M. A., *et al.* Continuous enteral feedings. *Am. J. Dis. Child.* 1982;**136**:825–7.

70 Hofner, G., Behrens, R., Koch, A., Singer, H., Hofbeck, M. Enteral nutritional support by percutaneous endoscopic gastrostomy in children with congenital heart disease. *Pediatr. Cardiol.* 2000;**21**:341–6.

71 Ciotti, G., Holzer, R., Pozzi, M., Dalzell, M. Nutritional support via percutaneous endoscopic gastrostomy in children with cardiac disease experiencing difficulties with feeding. *Cardiol. Young.* 2002;**12**:537–41.

72 American Academy of Pediatrics, Committee on Nutrition. Nutritional needs of preterm infants. In Kleinman, R., ed. *Pediatric Nutrition Handbook.* Elk Grove Village, IL: American Academy of Pediatrics; 1998: 55–87.

73 Fomon, S. J., Haschke, F., Ziegler, E. E., Nelson, S. E. Body composition of reference children from birth to 10 years. *Am. J. Clin. Nutr.* 1982;**35**:1169–75.

74 Fomon, S. J., Ziegler, E. E. Nutritional management of infants with congenital heart disease. *Am. Heart J.* 1972;**83**;581–8.

75 Committee on Nutrition, American Academy of Pediatrics. Commentary on breast-feeding and infant formulas, including proposed standard for formulas. *Pediatrics* 1976;**57**:278–85.

76 Jew, R., Oven, D., Kaufman, D. Osmolality of commonly used medications and formulas in the neonatal intensive care unit. *Nutr. Clin. Pract.* 1997;**12**:158–63.

77 Fomon, S. J., Ziegler, E. E. Renal solute load and *potential* renal solute load in infancy. *J. Pediatr.* 1999;**134**:11–14.

38

Nutrition therapies for inborn errors of metabolism

Janet A. Thomas, Anne Tsai, and Laurie Bernstein

Department of Pediatrics, The Children's Hospital, Denver, CO

Inborn errors of metabolism are rare, but important causes of disease in the neonate. They cause significant morbidity and mortality that can in some cases be ameliorated or prevented by nutritional treatment. An increasingly large number of inborn errors of metabolism are being described many of which present or can be identified in the newborn period.

Premature infants have no less risk of inborn errors of metabolism than full-term neonates. However, inborn errors may be less frequently suspected in the premature infant because symptoms may resemble more common problems expected in those patients. In addition, diagnostic tests in the premature infant may be altered by common treatments. For example, whole blood transfusions can give false negative results on newborn screening for galactosemia. Premature infants are actually at higher risk for transient forms of some inborn errors for which a critical enzyme shows maturation in the perinatal period. In addition, advances in technology have led to the description of an increasing number of inborn errors of metabolism.

For each disorder, identification of specific abnormal metabolites leads to understanding the unique biochemistry of the disorder and is the key to developing approaches to management. Nutrition plays an important role in the management of inborn errors of metabolism. The benefit of a phenylalanine-restricted diet for PKU was described by Bickel and associates in 1953 after it was shown that modification of dietary intake could alter the biochemical imbalances of the patient.[1] Since that time compliance with dietary therapy has been shown to result in normal intellectual development in patients with classic PKU.

The nutrition management of inborn errors has contributed to our knowledge of the requirements for various essential amino acids, fats, carbohydrates, vitamins, and minerals in healthy infants as well as infants with metabolic disorders. The first special dietary formulations for inborn errors of metabolism (e.g., PKU) were made from casein hydrolysates or free amino acids. It was not until several years later that commercially prepared special metabolic formulas were available for widespread use. Currently, a wide variety of commercial metabolic formulas are available for treatment of various inborn errors, and are used in combination with other nutritional and medical therapies to treat patients with these disorders.

The focus of this chapter is limited solely to inborn errors of metabolism that can be diagnosed in the newborn period, and for which efficacy of nutritional management in that period has been demonstrated. A variety of inherited enzymatic defects that may respond to specific nutritional therapies are shown in Table 38.1. It is not in the scope of this chapter to discuss diagnostic approaches or criteria for these disorders. It should be pointed out that treatment of these disorders (which may present with nonspecific symptoms) can be successful only if an inborn error of metabolism is suspected and identified by appropriate biochemical studies. With identification and appropriate treatment, neonates with the inborn errors of metabolism considered in this chapter can be expected to show improved, and sometimes normal, mental and physical development.

Physiology, pathophysiology, development, and disease

General principles of metabolism are illustrated in Figure 38.1. All metabolism is mediated by enzymes coded

Neonatal Nutrition and Metabolism. Second Edition, ed. P. Thureen and W. Hay. Published by Cambridge University Press.
© Cambridge University Press 2006.

Table 38.1. Nutrition therapies in selected metabolic disorders

Disorder	Nutrition therapy
Aminoacidopathies	
Phenylketonuria (classic)	Phenylalanine restriction, tyrosine
Hyperphenylalaninemia	Phenylalanine restriction may be required for some
Biopterin deficiency	Phenylalanine restriction, tetrahydrobiopterin, dopaminergic drugs
Tyrosinemia, type I	Phenylalanine and tyrosine restriction, cysteine, NTBC[a]
Neonatal tyrosinemia	Low protein diet, ascorbic acid
Tyrosinemia, type II	Phenylalanine and tyrosine restriction
Maple syrup urine disease	Branched chain amino acid restriction, valine and isoleucine
Homocystinuria	Methionine restriction, cysteine, betaine, folate, pyridoxine
Organic Acidemias	
Isovaleric acidemia	Lysine restriction, carnitine and/or glycine
Methylmalonic acidemia	Propiogenic amino acid restriction, carnitine
Propionic acidemia	Propiogenic amino acid restriction, carnitine, biotin
Cobalamin defects	Propiogenic amino acid restriction, hydroxycobalamin, carnitine, betaine, folate, pyridoxine
Pyruvate carboxylase deficiency	High fat, low carbohydrate or modified ketogenic diet, biotin
Pyruvate dehydrogenase deficiency	Ketogenic diet, thiamine, biotin, lipoic acid
Glutaric acidemia, type 1	Lysine and tryptophan restriction, carnitine
Urea cycle disorders	Low protein diet with nonessential amino acid restriction, citrulline or arginine, sodium benzoate, sodium phenylbutyrate, carnitine
Carbohydrate disorders	
Galactosemia (classic)	Galactose/lactose restriction, calcium
Galactosemia (Duarte)	Some centers support galactose restriction for first year of life
Galactokinase deficiency	Galactose/lactose restriction
Hereditary fructose intolerance	Fructose and sorbitol restriction
Glycogen storage diseases	
Type I (glucose-6-phosphate deficiency)	Galactose/fructose restriction, modified fat and moderate protein, frequent feedings, nocturnal drip, cornstarch
Type III (amylo-1,6-glucosidase deficiency)	Same as type I except high protein
Type IV (phosphorylase deficiency)	Frequent feedings
Type VIII (phosphorylase kinase deficiency)	High protein, frequent feedings
Fatty acid oxidation disorders	
Medium-chain acyl-CoA dehydrogenase deficiency	Frequent feeding, carnitine, some centers support medium chain fat restriction
Long-chain hydroxy-acyl-CoA dehydrogenase deficiency	Long chain fat restriction, frequent feedings, carnitine, docohexanoic acid, medium chain triglyerides
Peroxisomal disorders	
Adrenoleukodystrophy	Low fat diet supplemented with monosaturated fatty acids (erucic and oleic)
Infantile refsum disease	Phytanic restriction
Others	
Smith-Lemli-Opitz syndrome	Cholesterol, bile acids
Congenital disorder of glycosylation, type 1b	Mannose

[a] NTBC = 2-(2-nitro-4-trifluoro-methylbenzoyl)-1,3-cyclohexanedione.

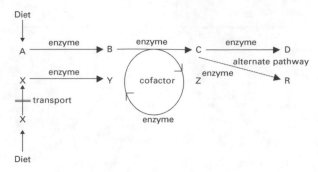

Figure 38.1. General principles of metabolism. Virtually all reactions are controlled by enzymes coded for by genes. Any compound can have more than one metabolic fate or origin, and some reactions may proceed in either direction depending on biochemical conditions. A transport system, enzyme, or cofactor may serve a single metabolic pathway or may be important for several. Any step that requires mediation of an enzyme is at risk for genetic error. A metabolic block may cause a decrease in levels of compounds after the block unless there is an alternative mechanism by which to produce the compound. Similarly, there is accumulation of compounds before a block depending on availability of other pathways of disposal or alternative metabolism of the compound.

for by genes. Some enzymes function independently, while some require a cofactor or a coenzyme, which may itself be synthesized or recycled by enzyme-mediated steps. Some biochemical pathways are necessary for every cell and are therefore present in all tissues, while some reactions are organ or tissue-specific. These variations of enzyme activity in tissues of the healthy individual must be the result of timed tissue-specific development. Only a few maturational defects of metabolic pathways have been suspected or demonstrated to cause human disease (e.g., transient hyperammonemia of the neonate, neonatal tyrosinemia). Most inborn errors of metabolism are single gene defects, usually autosomal recessive, but occasionally X-linked, dominant, or mitochondrially inherited.

There is a wide range of expression of each inborn error of metabolism. Phenotypic variation is most marked between families, but there may be significant variation between siblings and within a single patient over time. Variation of the defective enzyme activity between families and variation within families in the activity of other relevant pathways of metabolism alter the tolerance of and requirements for nutrients. Clinical variation is also due to different requirements for energy and for cell growth between individuals and over time. These variations, along with differences in feeding practices govern timing and severity of presentation of each disorder. There is little information

for each disorder about the special issues in the premature infant.

The clinical symptoms of each inborn error of metabolism must result from the abnormal metabolism. Usually, clinical expression can be related to elevated or depressed concentrations of some measurable metabolite. For most disorders there are short-term reversible effects and long-term irreversible damage in the untreated patient. Either deficiency or excess of a specific metabolite may directly or indirectly have an effect on the infant. "Direct effects" are usually well understood, but may be only a part of the pathophysiology of a disorder. An example of direct action is the formation of cataracts by galactitol accumulation in the lens of patients with galactosemia. In some diseases, secondary biochemical alterations occur. An example of this is in methylmalonic acidemia, in which some patients have hyperammonemia presumably due to interference with the urea cycle resulting from metabolites of methylmalonic acid. Secondary deficiencies can also be found in some inborn errors. For example, secondary carnitine deficiencies have been identified in patients with organic acidemias, possibly resulting from the increased excretion of acylcarnitine esters. Unfortunately, in many cases the exact pathophysiology remains a mystery. The interdependence and interconnectedness of the biochemical pathways makes it unlikely that simple explanations such as the effect of one biochemical pathway on one physiologic or developmental system will account for the expression of an inborn error of metabolism.

Principles of nutrition support

The basic principle in the management of inborn errors of metabolism is to manipulate the biochemistry so that the metabolite(s) is as normal as possible in the tissue where the defect has its pathophysiologic effect(s). The goals for nutrition support are:

(1) To provide all essential nutrients in quantities adequate to promote optimal physical and mental development.
(2) To supply the optimal amount of any nutrient that is restricted or supplemented in order to promote growth while preventing or correcting metabolic imbalances.

For each disease, management depends on the specific biochemistry and pathophysiology of the disease. The main strategies of nutrition support are:

(1) Dietary restriction of any compound or precursors of metabolites that accumulate as a result of the enzyme block.
(2) Replenishing any deficient end product distal to the enzyme block.

Table 38.2. Recommended nutrient intakes for inborn errors of amino acid metabolism which require specific amino acid restrictions[61]

Nutrient	Unit	Age range			
		0–3 mos	3–6 mos	6–9 mos	9–12 mos
Energy	kcal kg^{-1}	95–145	95–145	80–135	80–135
Fluid	mL kg^{-1}	125–200	130–160	124–145	120–135
Protein (total)[a]	g kg^{-1}	2.5–3.5	2.5–3.5	2.5–3.0	2.5–3.0
Carbohydrate	% total energy	←------	----35–50---	--------	------→
Fat	% total energy	←------	----40–50---	--------	------→
Isoleucine[b]	mg kg^{-1}	75–120	65–100	50–90	40–80
Valine[b]	mg kg^{-1}	75–105	65–90	35–75	30–60
Threonine[b]	mg kg^{-1}	75–135	60–100	40–75	20–40
Methione[b]	mg kg^{-1}	30–50	20–45	10–40	10–30
Isoleucine[c]	mg kg^{-1}	36–60	30–50	25–40	18–33
Leucine[c]	mg kg^{-1}	60–100	50–85	40–70	30–55
Valine[c]	mg kg^{-1}	42–70	35–60	28–50	21–38
Leucine[d]	mg kg^{-1}	80–150	70–140	60–130	50–120
Phenylalanine[e]	mg kg^{-1}	25–70	20–45	15–35	10–35
Methionine[f]	mg kg^{-1}	15–30	10–25	10–25	10–20
Lysine[g]	mg kg^{-1}	80–100	70–90	60–80	50–70
Tryptophan[g]	mg kg^{-1}	10–20	10–15	10–12	10–12
Tyrosine[h]	mg kg^{-1} Phe plus Tyr	65–155	55–135	50–120	40–105

[a] Protein amounts are total amounts and do not reflect amounts of natural or whole protein as a percentage of the total protein. In addition, the values for protein do not apply to disorders where total protein must be restricted, i.e., urea cycle disorders. Further information on protein restrictions are mentioned in the text for each disorder.

[b] Methylmalonic and propionic acidemia.[62]

[c] Maple syrup urine disease.

[d] Isovaleric acidemia.

[e] Phenylketonuria.

[f] Homocystinuria.

[g] Glutaric acidemia Type 1.

[h] Tyrosinemia.

Phe = phenylalanine; Tyr = tyrosine.

(3) Supplementing compounds that may combine with a toxic metabolite to promote its excretion or its safe metabolism.

(4) Providing cofactor in therapeutic doses, if a cofactor is deficient or if the enzyme can be activated by cofactor excess.

The use of nutrition support to treat inborn errors of metabolism has helped to clarify specific nutrient requirements in the healthy infant. When a specific nutrient (e.g., phenylalanine in PKU) has been over restricted, failure to thrive and protein malnutrition have resulted.

Substrate restriction in the treatment of inborn errors of metabolism can be very specific (a single amino acid, sugar, or fatty acid) or general (total protein, total carbohydrate, or total fat). When one specific nutrient is being restricted, it may be difficult to insure adequate intake of other related nutrients. It is the challenge to the metabolic nutritionist to insure optimal nutrition despite the restrictions of one or many nutrients.

Nutritional management of amino acid disorders requires the use of synthetic formulas (medical foods) that have been developed based on a knowledge of nutrition requirements in the healthy infant. Diets for amino acid disorders are designed individually using combinations of metabolic formulas and natural protein sources from standard infant formulas, breast milk, or foods.

Each diet prescription is calculated to provide required amounts of protein, energy, fluid, and the specific nutrients that must be restricted and/or supplemented. In some instances, the diet regimen may also specify avoidance of fasting, as many metabolic disorders worsen acutely with catabolism. Guidelines for calculating specific nutrient needs for amino acid disorders are found in Table 38.2. Strong caution is advised in attempting to utilize these guidelines in calculating dietary prescriptions for individual patients without consultation with a metabolic nutritionist.

Diet prescriptions should be evaluated for vitamin and mineral adequacy. Research has shown that trace mineral status of children treated with special metabolic formulas may be compromised.[2] The reliance on chemically defined metabolic formulas used in amino acid disorders can affect the bioavailability of several trace elements, including copper, zinc, and iron. Historically, special metabolic formulas did not contain certain recognized essential nutrients, such as selenium, molybdenum, chromium, taurine, and carnitine. Presently, most, if not all, formulas are adequate in trace elements. Periodic assessment of trace mineral status, however, still needs to be considered.

The special metabolic formulas are specific for each disorder and provide essential and nonessential amino acids, vitamins, minerals, and energy. Some formulas provide no fat or linoleic acid, and therefore less energy than others. Metabolic formulas are usually necessary to meet long-term protein requirements whenever specific amino acid(s) must be restricted. A "low-protein" diet alone using only standard infant formula to adequately restrict one or more specific amino acids will usually over restrict other essential amino acids and result in protein malnutrition. The total protein recommendations for many amino acid disorders are higher than the recommended dietary allowances (RDA) when the majority of protein is supplied by synthetic amino acids.

If the special metabolic formula chosen has a low energy: protein ratio, supplementation with a protein-free energy module is indicated to provide additional calories. These modules, which contain needed vitamins and minerals in addition to fats and carbohydrates, are preferable to using separate fat and carbohydrate sources for energy.

Many of the special metabolic formulas used to treat amino acid disorders are potentially hyperosmolar. Presence or absence of a fat source and the nature of the carbohydrates in the formula will affect osmolality. Hyperosmolar feedings may result in vomiting, diarrhea, and dehydration, which can trigger a catabolic crisis. Osmolality of formula should be analyzed when calculations suggest hyperosmolality.

Because of the variability found in most inborn errors of metabolism, the nutrition support must be individualized and constantly reevaluated according to the patient's clinical assessment and biochemical parameters. The dietary prescription must allow for age-related biochemical parameters, growth acceleration, and level of stress in acute situations. The metabolic status of the infant will also determine the energy, protein, and fluid requirements.

Frequent dietary changes in infancy are usually necessary to meet the demands of the rapidly developing infant. Management for all disorders includes anthropometrics and visceral protein status. Other biochemical parameters measured are specific to each disorder. For a number of disorders, assessment of plasma concentrations of carnitine should be performed, and levels of any cofactor that is supplemented should be monitored. Providing optimal nutrients during infancy may set precedents for future potential in regard to both mental and physical development and growth. Infants with inborn errors of metabolism require lifelong nutrition therapy.

Counseling and education of the family are a part of the dietary management of inborn errors. The success of the diet regimen requires cooperation between the clinicians and family. The clinicians must provide accurate instructions on all aspects of the diet including formula preparation and diet record keeping, as well as anticipatory guidance to help integrate the complicated diets into the family's lifestyle. Continued support, education, and encouragement increase compliance with the diet.

In this chapter, discussion of management for each disorder is generally restricted to the newborn period, but principles of chronic management are described, as these are important issues for the counseling of the family. Also, we restrict discussion to nutritional management generally, assuming that basic principles of medical management of vascular access, fluids, resuscitation, and so forth are applied. These issues are addressed only for disorders in which special problems related to the nutritional management of the disorder are expected.

Aminoacidopathies

Phenylketonuria (PKU)

Classic PKU, an autosomal recessive disease, was first described by Fölling in 1934.[3] It occurs in one of every 12 000 Caucasians and if untreated causes severe mental retardation, seizures, mousy odor, light pigmentation of eyes, hair, and skin, eczema, and behavior difficulties in most affected individuals. The defect in PKU is a deficiency of the enzyme, phenylalanine hydroxylase, a tetrahydrobiopterin dependent enzyme (Figure 38.2). The deficiency causes failure to metabolize phenylalanine, an essential amino acid, to tyrosine. This enzymatic pathway is the major fate of phenylalanine and defects cause significant elevation of phenylalanine and metabolites of phenylalanine, such as phenylpyruvic acid, phenyllactic acid, and phenylacetylglutamine.

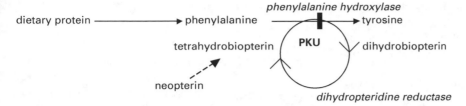

Figure 38.2. Phenylalanine metabolism. Tetrahydrobiopterin, synthesized from neopterin by a series of reactions, is the cofactor for phenylalanine hydroxylase. The tetrahydrobiopterin is oxidized to dihydrobiopterin in the reaction and is recycled by dihydropteridine reductase. Phenylketonuria (PKU) results from a deficiency of the enzyme phenylalanine hydroxylase. Solid bar indicates enzymatic block.

Tyrosine becomes an essential amino acid in infants with PKU. The biochemical mechanisms that lead to impaired brain development and function in PKU are still the subject of research. Elevated levels of phenylalanine appear to interfere with brain growth and nerve myelination. Phenylalanine is a large neutral amino acid (LNAA), which studies have suggested competes with other LNAAs for access across the blood–brain barrier.[4] Also, alteration of levels of biogenic amines, for which tyrosine is a precursor, are demonstrable in patients with hyperphenylalaninemia.[4]

The percentage of dietary phenylalanine that is hydroxylated to tyrosine is dependent on a person's age and rate of growth. In the rapidly growing infant approximately 50%–60% of the phenylalanine is used for protein synthesis, compared with 10% in the normal adult.

Classic PKU is generally diagnosed by newborn screening programs. Milder forms of phenylalanine hydroxylase deficiency are also detected with frequency similar to classic PKU, and there is apparently a transient form of enzyme deficiency probably due to a maturational defect. Hyperphenylalaninemia may also be due to defects in the synthesis of tetrahydrobiopterin, a coenzyme in the phenylalanine hydroxylase enzyme system. These disorders must be rapidly distinguished from classic PKU in the newborn period by determination of blood pterin and dihydropteridine reductase (DHPR) activity, as their management and outcome are quite different. Patients with cofactor defects will show a response of blood phenylalanine levels to dietary phenylalanine restriction, but retardation will not be prevented. Mild and transient hyperphenylalaninemia usually does not require treatment, and dietary restriction of phenylalanine in these individuals may be harmful to growth and development. Finally, offspring of mothers with PKU may present with a high phenylalanine on newborn screening if the screen is done earlier than recommended. These babies do not require dietary treatment. If the mother has had poor control of her PKU during the

pregnancy, the baby may also suffer from maternal PKU syndrome with resulting pre and postnatal growth deficiency, microcephaly, congenital defects of the heart and esophagus, and mental retardation. Overall, the most common error in nutritional management of PKU is probably the inappropriate institution of diet in a baby who does not require restriction.

Therapy

Nutritional therapy began in the first month of life, and ideally within the first 2 weeks of life, with blood phenylalanine levels maintained between 120 and 360 μmol L^{-1} (2–6 mg dL^{-1}), has resulted in normal mental and physical development for the majority of patients. It was previously believed that the phenylalanine-restricted diet could be discontinued in childhood, but results from the National PKU Collaborative Study and the problems associated with maternal PKU syndrome now support lifelong continuation of diet.[5–7]

The components of a phenylalanine-restricted diet prescription include phenylalanine, tyrosine, protein, and energy. The phenylalanine requirement must be individualized and is determined by age, growth acceleration, and the presence of any residual enzyme activity. Tyrosine supplementation may be necessary if blood tyrosine concentrations remain less than 44 μmol L^{-1}.

The basis for nutrition support of PKU is the use of low-phenylalanine or phenylalanine-free special metabolic formulas. Throughout infancy these special formulas supply approximately 80% of the total protein requirement and are used in conjunction with standard infant formulas or breast milk, to meet the infant's requirements for phenylalanine and tyrosine. Because the majority of the protein consumed by the infant with PKU comes from either a casein hydrolysate or free amino acid source, the diet prescription is calculated to supply a total protein intake greater than the recommended intakes for healthy infants. As the infant grows, natural foods are introduced into the dietary regimen. With time, the entire phenylalanine requirement will be supplied by natural foods, but metabolic formula consumption remains the mainstay of therapy lifelong.

Alternative methods for treating PKU have been attempted with limited success. Supplementation of branched-chain amino acids in patients with PKU resulted in decreased concentrations of phenylalanine in cerebrospinal fluid. The branched-chain amino acids may compete with phenylalanine at the blood–brain barrier since they follow similar transport systems. This approach has had limited success and should not replace the phenylalanine-restricted diet. More recently, PreKUnil tablets have been introduced. PreKUnil tablets contain large amounts of large neutral amino acids, such as tyrosine, tryptophan, leucine, isoleucine, arginine, valine, histidine, methionine, and threonine, which compete against phenylalanine at the blood–brain barrier. The idea is that the LNAAs will prevent excess phenylalanine from crossing the blood–brain barrier and therefore, reduce the concentration of phenylalanine in the central nervous system. Blood phenylalanine levels remain elevated. Use of PreKUnil tablets allows liberalization of the diet with an increased consumption of natural protein intake in order to meet protein needs. PreKUnil tablets are not recommended for children or women of childbearing age as the long-term consequence of elevated blood phenylalanine levels on brain development or on other body tissues is not known and a developing fetus must be protected against high blood phenylalanine levels. The role of PreKUnil tablets in the treatment of PKU may be limited to noncompliant adolescents and late diagnosed patients. Finally, some phenylalanine hydroxylase deficient patients may respond to supplementation with tetrahydrobiopterin as determined by tetrahydrobiopterin loading tests.[8,9]

Blood phenylalanine concentrations should be obtained at least weekly in infancy, and tyrosine concentrations are required periodically. The frequency of requested monitoring levels decreases with age, but generally not less than monthly. Trace mineral status, including iron indices, should be monitored.

Causes of hyperphenylalaninemia in the treated infant with PKU include illness leading to catabolism, improper dietary prescription, a change in growth velocity, inaccurate measurement of formula or food components, or decreased formula or food consumption. The clinician must be aware of hidden sources of phenylalanine, such as aspartame, which may be found in cough medicines.

Hereditary tyrosinemias

Tyrosinemia type I

Type I tyrosinemia, an autosomal recessive disorder, is a defect in the metabolism of tyrosine, due to a deficiency of the enzyme, fumarylacetoacetase (fumarylacetoacetase hydrolase [FAH]) (Figure 38.3). The enzyme block results in accumulation of fumarylacetoacetate and possibly maleylacetoacetate, which are alkylating toxic agents that are felt to cause the hepatorenal symptoms associated with this disease. Tyrosine, 4-OH-phenylpyruvate and its derivatives, and methionine are elevated in blood. The clinical presentation is heterogeneous, from acute to chronic. The acute form of the disease expresses itself in the neonatal period with findings of failure to thrive, vomiting, renal tubular dysfunction, jaundice, and hepatosplenomegaly. Death usually occurs before 8 months of age. Chronic cases usually become symptomatic after one year of age or in early childhood and are characterized by mild hepatomegaly, growth retardation, renal tubular dysfunction, and history of easy bruising. Other clinical findings include rickets, porphyria-like symptoms (because of ALA-dehydratase inhibition from the formation of succinylacetone), and hepatocellular carcinoma.

Therapy

Dietary treatment with restriction of phenylalanine and tyrosine has been employed for more than 30 years with variable clinical benefit. In 1992, a new drug, 2-(2-nitro-4-trifluoro-methylbenzoyl)-1,3-cyclohexanedione (NTBC), was introduced. It is a potent inhibitor of 4-hydroxyphenylpyruvate dioxygenase, therefore, decreasing the major toxic metabolites, fumarylacetoacetate and malylacetoacetate. The recommended dose is 1 mg kg^{-1}day.[10] While traditional diet therapy may relieve the acute symptoms and slow down the progression of renal dysfunction, the overall prognosis remains poor. NTBC is now considered an effective treatment. NTBC also helps to relieve porphyria-like symptoms and, at least in some cases, decreases the risk of early hepatocellular carcinoma.[10] Therefore, dietary treatment is now used in conjunction with NTBC.

A restricted phenylalanine and tyrosine diet may decrease the formation of toxic metabolites and may better prepare the infant for liver transplantation. Since elevations of plasma methionine apparently reflect the extent of liver insult rather than dietary intake of methionine, plasma methionine should not be aggressively regulated by dietary restriction. Methionine levels usually normalize as the liver function improves. Plasma phenylalanine and tyrosine concentrations are well correlated with dietary

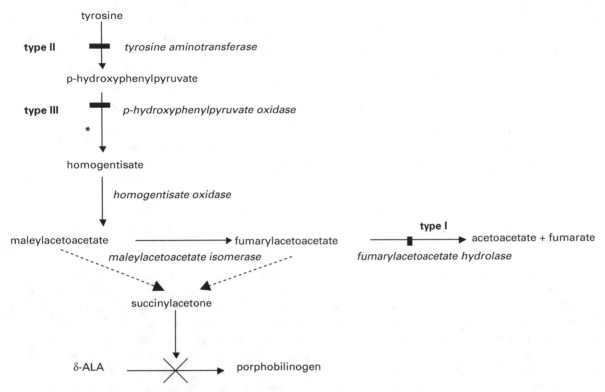

Figure 38.3. Tyrosine metabolism. The enzymes illustrated lead to primary disorders of tyrosine metabolism (tyrosinemia types I–III). Succinylacetone (broken lines) is a result of an alternative pathway of metabolism in the neonatal form of tyrosinemia with liver disease. Succinylacetone is a potent inhibitor of the heme biosynthetic enzyme, δ-aminolevulinic acid dehydratase, resulting clinically in porphyria-like symptoms. * = site of action of NTBC. Solid bar indicates enzymatic block.

intake. Over restriction of phenylalanine and tyrosine will lead to a phenylalanine-tyrosine deficiency syndrome, which has been found in the management of this disease. A combined dose at 90 mg kg^{-1} day^{-1} of phenylalanine plus tyrosine is sufficient for normal growth in infants and up to 700–900 mg day^{-1} is sufficient for older children.[11] Slightly more than half of the amount should be phenyl-alanine. Requirements for phenylalanine may be higher than that in patients with PKU. The amounts of nutrients required are determined by the patient's tolerance of these amino acids as monitored by plasma amino acid profiles. In NTBC-treated patients, the goal is to keep plasma tyrosine levels below 500 μmol L^{-1}.

Energy intakes should be high to prevent failure to thrive. Where growth delay has already occurred, catch-up growth can be achieved only by provision of the maximum calories tolerated by the infant. A standard rule of thumb is to provide up to 150% of calories based on ideal body weight for height, when height is calculated as being at the 50th percentile for chronological age.

Special metabolic formulas free of phenylalanine and tyrosine, and in some formulas methionine, are an essential component to nutrition support. Standard infant formulas supply the prescribed amounts of amino acids and additional nutrients necessary for growth. Additional protein-free energy supplements may be needed. Some researchers have recommended that high-carbohydrate feedings – up to 75% of total energy – should be given.[12]

Neonatal tyrosinemia

Neonatal tyrosinemia, also called transient tyrosinemia of the newborn, is caused by delayed maturation of p-hydroxyphenylpyruvate oxidase, and is more frequent in premature infants receiving high-protein diets. Some can present with poor feeding and lethargy, but most patients are asymptomatic and are usually identified through state newborn screening programs. The outcome of neonatal tyrosinemia is variable. Although it is considered a benign disorder, mild intellectual deficit has been associated with persistent hypertyrosinemia in some patients.

Incidence of transient tyrosinemia varies in neonates of various population groups, apparently according to infant feeding practices. The decreased incidence of this disease in infants weighing over 2500 g in Scandinavian countries has been attributed to the increase in breast-feeding and use of lower protein cow's-milk infant formula.[13]

Protein restriction to 1.5–2.0 g kg^{-1} day^{-1} can reduce plasma tyrosine levels. This can be achieved, in part, by changing from higher protein infant formulas, such as soy-protein-based infant formulas, to standard cow's-milk formula or breast milk. Therapeutic dosages of ascorbic acid, 400 mg day^{-1}, may accelerate maturation of the enzyme p-hydroxyphenylpyruvate oxidase and warrants a therapeutic trial.

Tyrosinemia type II

Unlike other tyrosinemias, type II tyrosinemia (Richner – Hanhart syndrome) is a chronic disorder. It results from a defect in hepatic cytosol tyrosine aminotransferase, the rate-limiting enzyme in tyrosine metabolism (Figure 38.3). The clinical findings are highly correlated with plasma tyrosine levels and include hyperkeratotic skin lesions on the palms and soles and ocular lesions. While more than 50% of patients are severely retarded, mental status varies from normal to severe retardation and is not strongly correlated with age of diagnosis. The age of presentation may vary from infancy up to adulthood. This disease is particularly frequent in persons of Italian origin.

Therapy
The goal of nutrition therapy is the amelioration of hyperkeratotic skin lesions through reduction of dietary tyrosine and phenylalanine. Information on early treatment in infants is limited, but patients treated early with a tyrosine and phenylalanine-restricted diet have shown normal psychomotor development.[14,15] The degree of tyrosine and phenylalanine restriction will vary depending on individual tolerance as demonstrated by monitoring of plasma levels. In the infant it is beneficial to monitor tyrosine and phenylalanine concentrations at least weekly throughout the first year of life. Plasma tyrosine concentrations ranging from 607–994 μmol L^{-1} can reduce the clinical signs and symptoms associated with this disorder. Untreated levels may be greater than 3313 μmol L^{-1}; a normal level is less than 221 μmol L^{-1}.

Tyrosinemia type III

A few cases of tyrosinemia type III have been reported in the literature. The first case was described as tyrosinemia without liver dysfunction due apparently to the deficiency of the enzyme, p-hydroxyphenylpyruvate oxidase, the same enzyme involved in neonatal tyrosinemia.[16] The patient also had acute intermittent ataxia and drowsiness, but rather normal psychomotor development.[16] Protein restriction and vitamin C therapy failed to correct the biochemical abnormality. Liver biopsy was histologically

normal. There is no evidence that diet restriction is actually needed for this condition, however, since high tyrosine levels can be associated with mental retardation, keeping the tyrosine level below 500 μmol L^{-1} is recommended.[17]

Maple syrup urine disease (branched-chain ketoaciduria)

Maple syrup urine disease (MSUD) is an autosomal recessive disorder of the metabolism of the branched-chain amino acids leucine, isoleucine, and valine (Figure 38.4). It is caused by a deficiency in the branched chain 2-keto acid dehydrogenase complex. Elevations in plasma and branched-chain ketoacids, and the presence of alloisoleucine, correlate with clinical symptoms.

Classic MSUD presents in neonates who at first appear normal, but within several days develop lethargy, failure to thrive, poor suck and feeding, vomiting, and ketoacidosis. The urine may smell like maple syrup. Variant forms of the disease exist, with milder clinical features (mild or intermediate). Some mild variants have symptoms only after febrile illness, infections, or a protein load (intermittent). Early diagnosis and treatment can prevent death, severe mental retardation, and neurologic deficits. Despite early treatment and diagnosis, some patients still present with compromised mental status.[18]

Another variant of MSUD is the thiamine-responsive type, first described by Scriver *et al.* in 1971 in an infant with MSUD who responded to therapeutic dosages of thiamine (10 mg day^{-1}).[19] Other researchers have since identified similar patients who have improved biochemical parameters with varying dosages of thiamine, up to 1000 mg day^{-1}. The effects of pharmacologic dosages of thiamine may not be expressed for several weeks.[20]

The most rare type of MSUD is due to deficiency of the E3 subunit of the enzyme complex. Patients usually develop lactic acidosis in addition to MSUD. No effective treatment to date is known, although diet therapy combined with high-dose thiamine, biotin, and lipoic acid supplementation is generally recommended.

Therapy
The neonate with classic MSUD must be treated aggressively. The acutely ill infant frequently requires withdrawal from formula and may require dialysis if the acidosis is severe. Prevention or inhibition of catabolism is essential. If the oral route is not possible, then parenteral nutrition utilizing glucose and lipids is indicated. Amino acid solutions free of branched-chain amino acids are now available for use in total parenteral nutrition.

Once formula is tolerated, a total restriction of branched-chain amino acids may still be necessary for a rapid

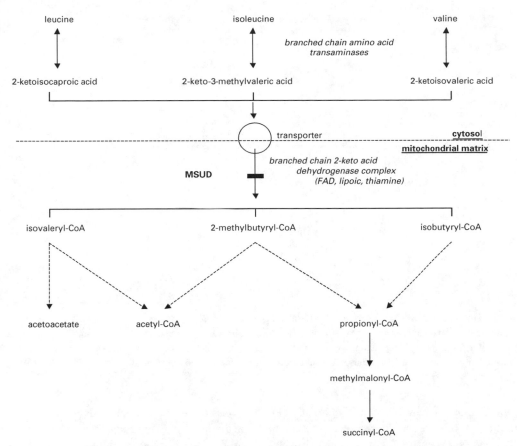

Figure 38.4. Branched chain amino acid metabolism. The branched chain amino acids share a common enzyme for decarboxylation and defects of that dehydrogenase complex cause maple syrup urine disease (MSUD). Other steps not discussed here are specific to the pathways of one or two branched chain amino acids or their metabolites. CoA = coenyzme A. FAD = flavin adenine dinucleotide. Solid bar indicates enzymatic block.

reduction of their levels in plasma. This can be accomplished by the use of branched-chain amino acid-free special metabolic formulas alone to provide the recommended amounts of protein. Higher total protein intakes may be required because of the source of protein from these special formulas. Intakes of 2.5–3.0 g kg^{-1} day^{-1} of protein supplied by special metabolic formulas may be needed to inhibit catabolism in the infant recovering from an acute episode. Extra energy is also needed during recovery, and protein-free energy modules may be used to provide these calories.

The total restriction of branched-chain amino acids will require daily monitoring of plasma amino acid concentrations to prevent a prolonged over-restriction of these essential amino acids. After several days of treatment, blood concentrations of valine and isoleucine may be reduced to therapeutic range while leucine is still elevated. Supplemental L-isoleucine (Ile) and L-valine (val) may be required. It has been suggested that supplementation of L-Ile and L-Val at 40–45 mg kg^{-1} without the addition of

leucine will help normalize all three branched-chain amino acids within a few days.[21] Once the patient has been stabilized and the plasma concentrations of branched-chain amino acids are within the therapeutic range, natural protein sources such as breast milk and infant formulas can be incorporated into the nutrition therapy.

Requirements for the branched-chain amino acids depend on age, growth velocity, state of health, and residual enzyme activity. Because most infants with classic MSUD have 0%–2% of the enzyme activity, the restriction of branched-chain amino acids is usually significant. The presently available metabolic formulas used in infants with MSUD have a more balanced energy to protein ratio (36:1) and may be used alone without the risk of being hyperosmolar which was the concern with older formula preparations.

In nature, leucine makes up a larger portion of all natural protein (8.5%) than valine and isoleucine. Tolerance to dietary leucine may significantly drop within the first 6 months of life. The dietary restriction of leucine necessary

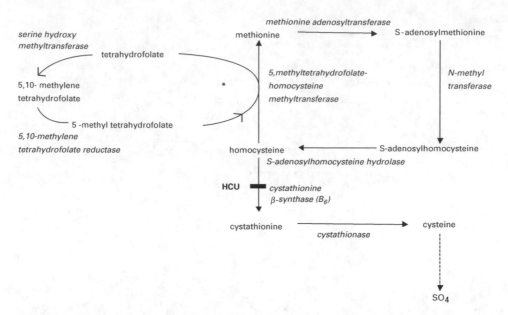

Figure 38.5. Sulphur amino acid metabolism. Diagram of metabolic origin and fate of methionine from exogenous and endogenous protein. Folate is required for metabolism of homocysteine to methionine, and pyridoxine is a required cofactor for action of cystathionine synthase. * = Betaine favors conversion of homocysteine to methionine through remethylation. Homocystinuria (HCU) is caused by a deficiency of the enzyme cystathionine β-synthase. Solid bar indicates enzymatic block.

to obtain a therapeutic range may over-restrict valine and isoleucine. Supplementation of these two amino acids as a solution (10 mg mL^{-1}) may be necessary. An excess or deficiency of any of these amino acids will have clinical consequences.

Nutrition therapy in thiamine-nonresponsive classic MSUD is lifelong. During episodes of illness, additional nutrients and energy to inhibit or prevent catabolism and acidosis may be needed. With time, these patients may develop increased tolerance to episodes of illness, but any ketosis or illness that causes decreased nutrient and fluid intake must be treated aggressively. Families are instructed on home monitoring of urine for presence of ketoacids using either 2,4-dinitrophenylhydrazine or ketone test strips to assess impending illness. Analysis of plasma branched chain amino acids should be performed at least weekly for the first year of life and, if stable, less frequently thereafter.

Homocystinuria

Homocystinuria (HCU) may result from a variety of enzyme defects. The most common cause is a deficiency of cystathionine β-synthase that results in the accumulation of methionine and homocystine with a concurrent depletion of cystine (Figure 38.5). Homocystine is also found in the urine of these patients. Because animals with high methionine levels are healthy, it is believed that homocysteine and not methionine is the major toxic compound in the pathophysiology of homocystinuria.[22] The presence of homocysteine and low blood levels of methionine is also found in the disorder of methylmalonic acidemia/homocystinuria complex due to cobalamin synthesis defects.

Screening tests which measure methionine in the blood of newborns leads to the diagnosis of homocystinuria in 1 in 200 000 live births. The mode of inheritance is autosomal recessive. Untreated patients may clinically present with dislocated optic lenses, osteoporosis, and thromboembolic events, and a limited life expectancy. Mentation is variable, with treated patients having less severe manifestations of the disorder.

Pyridoxine responsiveness is found in up to 40% of patients with homocystinuria.[23] Those responsive to pyridoxine are clinically healthier and tolerate more methionine than nonresponders.[24] Some completely responsive patients require no special diet. The majority of patients diagnosed by newborn screening are pyridoxine nonresponders.[23,24]

Therapy

Once diagnosed with homocystinuria, the patient should be tried on therapeutic doses of pyridoxine. Oral doses of pyridoxine ranging from 200–1200 mg day^{-1} have resulted

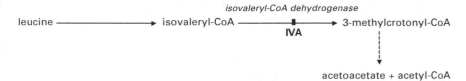

Figure 38.6. Leucine metabolism. Part of leucine metabolism, shared with other branched chain amino acids, is shown in Figure 38.4. Isovaleric acidemia (IVA) is a defect of an enzyme specific to leucine metabolism. CoA = coenzyme A. Solid bar indicates enzymatic block.

in decreases in plasma methionine concentrations and a significant reduction in plasma and urine homocysteine. It may take from days to several weeks of pharmacologic doses before a biochemical response is noted. Some patients do not respond because of folic acid depletion, therefore, concurrent folic acid supplementation at 1–5 mg day^{-1} is recommended. If the patient does not respond to a trial of pyridoxine, the pyridoxine dose should be decreased because prolonged periods of high doses of pyridoxine may cause peripheral neuropathy.[25] Those who do not respond to pyridoxine should receive dietary therapy with a methionine-restricted diet. Trimethylglycine (Betaine), a medication that increases the remethylation of homocysteine to methionine therefore decreasing plasma homocystine levels, should be used if diet alone is insufficient to offer good control. Ideal treatment range is to keep plasma total homocysteine levels below 50 μmol dL^{-1} and plasma methionine concentrations less than 150 μmol dL^{-1}.[26]

In patients not responsive to pyridoxine, supplementation of L-cysteine is necessary because cysteine becomes an essential amino acid. The amount of supplementation is variable. Total cysteine intake should range from 200 to 300 mg kg^{-1} day^{-1} in infants up to 12 months of age. Actual cysteine supplementation will need to be adjusted to maintain normal plasma concentrations.

The dietary prescription for the infant with homocystinuria includes a methionine-free special metabolic formula and a prescribed amount of natural protein from either standard infant formulas or breast milk to supply the requirements for methionine. Although breast-feeding of an infant being treated for homocystinuria has not been reported, it seems physiologically appropriate because breast milk is low in methionine and has a unique 1:1 ratio of methionine to cysteine. In contrast to breast milk, some soy and hypoallergenic infant formulas contain more methionine than found even in standard cow's-milk infant formulas. A change from soy formulas to other natural protein sources may assist in reducing plasma methionine.

Some special metabolic formulas used in the treatment of homocystinuria have a low ratio of energy to protein. Therefore, a protein-free energy module such as Protein-

Free Diet Powder or Protein Free Diet Powder 2, is indicated. Methionine requirements in nature are small in comparison to other essential amino acids. This limits the amounts of foods available for consumption.

Weekly analysis of plasma concentrations is recommended for the infant up to 6 months of age. Bimonthly assessment is recommended from 6 months to 1 year of age. Assessment of nutrition support should include protein, iron, and folate status. Because a large percentage of the protein is from synthetic amino acids, protein needs may be greater than the RDA.[27] Folic acid is utilized in the remethylation of homocysteine to methionine, and has been used with limited success in the treatment of this disorder. Therefore, supplementation of folic acid may be helpful to some patients. As with other special formulas, trace minerals may be suboptimal and periodic assessment of intake is warranted.

Organic acidemias

Isovaleric acidemia

Isovaleric acidemia, an autosomal recessive disorder, was the first organic acidemia to be described in humans, in 1966.[28] A defect in the metabolism of leucine secondary to a deficiency of the enzyme, isovaleryl-CoA hydrogenase, results in the accumulation of isovaleric acid (IVA), N-isovalerylglycine and 3-hydroxyvaleric acid (Figure 38.6). The presence of excess toxic IVA is responsible for the clinical features and distinctive "sweaty-feet odor" associated with this disease.

Isovaleric acidemia may be acute or chronic. Patients with acute isovaleric acidemia appear normal at birth, but within several days develop vomiting, lethargy, and coma. If not aggressively treated, death occurs, either from severe infection, ketoacidosis, or hyperammonemia. Seizures and hematologic abnormalities such as leukopenia, thrombocytopenia, and anemia may also be present in the infant. If the patient survives this severe neonatal episode, the subsequent course is similar to that of patients with chronic intermittent isovaleric acidemia and is characterized by recurrent episodes of vomiting, acidosis, lethargy, and coma. Symptoms are usually triggered by infections or protein loads. Metabolic acidosis may occur frequently in early infancy and childhood, but subsides with maturity likely directly related to a decrease in the frequency of infections. Mental development is variable and depends on early diagnosis and treatment and long-term therapeutic compliance.

Therapy

Limiting the production of IVA by utilizing a low leucine diet, and enhancing IVA excretion, via glycine and carnitine supplementation, are the backbones of therapeutic intervention. Such an approach can reduce the frequency and severity of acute ketotic episodes. The goal of therapy is to keep the urine free of IVA and 3-hydroxyvaleric acid.

During acute episodes of metabolic acidosis it is advisable to provide a leucine-free or drastically reduced leucine dietary regimen. In acute crisis, adequate protein and energy can be supplied by leucine-free metabolic formulas alone or in conjunction with protein-free energy modules. Parenteral nutrition using glucose and lipids has been used in treating acute episodes.

Glycine and isovaleryl-coenzyme A (CoA), the toxic acyl-CoA compound of this disorder, form isovalerylglycine, which is easily excreted in the urine, thus reducing accumulation of IVA.[29] During acute crisis, glycine supplementation, ranging from 250–600 mg kg^{-1} day^{-1}, has been used. Carnitine also conjugates with isovaleryl-CoA forming isovalerylcarnitine. This compound is then excreted in the urine thereby reducing the accumulation of free IVA.[30] The use of L-carnitine supplementation has been suggested to also replenish depleted tissue carnitine stores. Recommended intake of carnitine in this disorder during an acute crisis ranges from 100–400 mg kg^{-1} day^{-1}. Carnitine is generally tolerated orally, but intravenous preparations of L-carnitine are available for use in the acutely ill patient. The amount of glycine needed for chronic therapy varies, but 150–300 mg kg^{-1} day^{-1} may be optimal. The amount of carnitine for chronic therapy is generally in the range of 50–100 mg kg^{-1} day^{-1}. In the steady state, the need for both supplements is controversial, but both can be useful during acute crisis.

In the infant, dietary prescription is based on a leucine-free special metabolic formula. The necessary leucine requirements are provided by natural protein sources from standard infant formulas. Patients supplemented with glycine and/or carnitine have a relatively high leucine tolerance. Infants may tolerate up to 120 mg leucine kg^{-1} because of the efficiency of the glycine conjugating system.

In 3–5-year-old children, as much as 1300 mg day^{-1} of leucine could be handled by this system.[31] However, for infants, the use of protein restriction alone is not recommended, as without supplemental leucine-free protein from special metabolic formulas, their protein intake may not be sufficient for optimal growth. After the first year of life, though, strict low-leucine diets can be replaced by low-protein diets. Most children can tolerate 20–30 g of protein per day, which is sufficient to assure normal growth and development without supplementation with a special metabolic formula.[32] Therapy should be monitored by quantification of the urinary excretion of isovalerylglycine. Plasma amino acids should also be checked periodically to ensure appropriate nutritional status.

Methylmalonic/propionic acidemia (ketotic hyperglycinemia)

Propionic acidemia

Propionic acidemia is an autosomal recessive disorder of propionate metabolism. Propionic acid is normally metabolized to methylmalonic acid, and the metabolic block results in the accumulation of propionic acid (Figure 38.7). Elevated propionic acid in blood and urine, however, is not always observed. Rather, other organic acid byproducts, including propionylcarnitine, 3-hydroxypropionate, and methylcitrate are the major diagnostic metabolites. Plasma amino acids may reveal a striking elevation of glycine and glutamine. The disease can result from deficiency of the holoenzyme, propionyl-CoA carboxylase, or deficiency of the biotin cofactor. The propiogenic amino acids isoleucine, valine, threonine, and methionine are the major precursors of propionyl-CoA. Only a few patients with the carboxylase defect are clinically responsive to biotin therapy, although their cells often show a response to biotin, with increased enzyme activity.[33] A trial period of therapeutic dosages of 5–10 mg biotin per day should be attempted.

Methylmalonic acidemia

Methylmalonic acidemia results from decreased activity of the enzyme, methylmalonyl-CoA mutase, which converts L-methylmalony1-CoA to succinyl-CoA (Figure 38.7). The enzymatic block results in greatly increased amounts of methylmalonic acid in blood and urine. Also, owing to the secondary inhibition of propionyl-CoA carboxylase, propionic acid and other propionyl-CoA metabolites are also found in the urine. Plasma glycine and glutamine levels are again elevated. Several autosomal recessive mutations of this enzyme system have been identified. Defects in

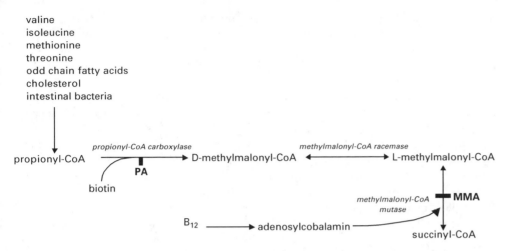

Figure 38.7. Propionic and methylmalonic acid metabolism. Propionic acid is formed from propiogenic amino acids, fatty acids, and cholesterol. Defects in propionyl-CoA carboxylase may be primary or may result from deficiency of the biotin cofactor resulting in propionic acidemia (PA). Similarly, defects in methylmalonyl-CoA mutase may be primary or result from abnormal B_{12} metabolism or deficiency of B_{12} resulting in methylmalonic acidemia (MMA). No inborn errors of metabolism of D- to L-methylmalonyl CoA have been described. CoA = coenzyme A. Solid bar indicates enzymatic block.

the mutase enzyme are most common. When the defect is in biosynthesis of adenosylcobalamin, a cofactor in the mutase enzyme system, the patient may be responsive to pharmacologic doses of cobalamin (vitamin B_{12}). Since cobalamin is also needed in the metabolism of homocystine, some of these patients excrete homocystine as well. All patients with methylmalonic acidemia should be initially treated with vitamin B_{12} until the specific defect can be determined. Patients responsive to pharmacologic doses of vitamin B_{12} may not require nutritional therapy. Prenatal vitamin B_{12} therapy in a diagnosed fetus has been utilized.[34]

There have been cases of methylmalonic aciduria due to B_{12} deficiency in infants who were breast-fed from vegan B_{12} deficient mothers.[35,36] Thus, vitamin B_{12} deficiency must be excluded when excessive urinary methylmalonic acid is found.

Diagnosis/clinical presentation
Both methylmalonic and propionic acidemias usually present in the neonatal period with vomiting, poor feeding, failure to thrive, profound metabolic acidosis, ketonuria, and lethargy often progressing to coma and death. Hyperammonemia may be present and contribute to clinical symptoms. These patients may also present with clinically significant neutropenia or thrombocytopenia and may be unusually prone to infections. Hypotonia may be impressive. If the patient survives this severe neonatal episode, the clinical course is characterized by recurrent episodes of ketoacidosis generally associated with an intercurrent illness, fasting, or a protein load. Survivors have many nutritional problems with poor growth and neurologic sequelae and the long-term clinical course may be complicated by anorexia, pancreatitis, cardiomyopathy, and chronic renal disease. Individuals with cobalamin defects and late-onset forms may have a better outcome.

Therapy
During acute presentation, correction of acidosis and provision of calories to reverse catabolism are essential. As management progresses to oral or nasogastric feedings, electrolyte solutions with a mixture of glucose polymers to make a 20 kcal per fluid ounce solution can assist in providing fluids and energy.

The cornerstone of dietary therapy is the restriction of those amino acids whose metabolism directly requires the utilization of the affected pathways. The so-called "propiogenic amino acids" include valine, methionine, isoleucine, and threonine. The propiogenic amino acids are restricted, but total protein is not restricted unless hyperammonemia is present. Natural protein sources, from either standard infant formulas or foods, supply the requirements for the essential propiogenic acids, while the additional protein requirements are supplied by synthetic amino acids from metabolic formulas. Metabolic formulas, free of, or markedly reduced in, propiogenic amino acids, can provide additional nitrogen for protein synthesis and assist in promoting anabolism. Since valine is one of the direct precursors of propionyl-CoA, the diet can be based on valine intake and the other amino acids provided in proportion. The restriction of the propiogenic amino acids sufficient to maintain normal plasma concentrations of methionine and threonine may over-restrict isoleucine and valine, and supplementation is recommended to balance the plasma profiles. The exact nutrients provided are determined by the child's age, biochemical data, growth parameters, and tolerance of propiogenic amino acids. Most B_{12} responsive patients need only mild protein restriction or none at all. Monitoring of treatment should include quantitative assay of relevant urinary metabolites and concentrations of amino acids in the blood. Blood or urinary methylmalonic acid levels should also be monitored in patients with methylmalonic acidemia.

The protein requirements of children with methylmalonic and propionic acidemia are not well established. Reports of protein intake in an infant with methylmalonic acidemia show an intake of 1.25 g kg^{-1} of natural protein was necessary for maximal nitrogen retention, with slight retention at 0.75 g kg^{-1} in the same infant.[37] Total protein intakes equaling 70%–85% of the RDA for protein for infants can provide adequate visceral and somatic protein stores and help reduce acidotic episodes. Optimal energy from carbohydrates and fat must be supplied to protect the infant's protein stores. Although researchers have shown that biotin and vitamin B_{12}-deficient animals process linoleic acid into the propionate pathway, a restriction of lipids in patients with methylmalonic acidemia has not been warranted.[38]

Many infants with methylmalonic acidemia or propionic acidemia develop anorexia and a poor suck early in infancy, and may require nasogastric feedings. Gastrostomy tubes are recommended if long-term tube feedings are expected. Some children also experience dysphagia and hyperactive gag reflex, both of which interfere with the provision of nutrients. The anorexia and food refusal may be both physiologic and behavioral. The physiologic component may be the result of an altered serotonin metabolism.[39] Fasting should be avoided.

Frequent infections and vomiting make it difficult to provide optimal nutrients for any extended period of time. Children are prone to recurrent infections and illness. During times of illness, the special formula mixture may need to be temporarily stopped. Parenteral nutrition calculated to provide the prescribed amounts of amino acids in conjunction with carbohydrate and fat can limit catabolism.

Adjunct therapies to the treatment of these disorders include supplementations of L-alanine and carnitine. Secondary carnitine deficiency has been identified in organic acidemias.[40,41] Carnitine increases propionyl-CoA

excretion and promotes detoxification. It also appears to reduce the propensity for ketogenesis.[42] Prophylactic treatment of 100 mg kg^{-1} day^{-1} of oral carnitine should be initiated. During acute crisis, intravenous carnitine up to 300 mg kg^{-1} day^{-1} has been utilized in patients with these disorders. The supplementation of exogenous L-alanine into the dietary regimen may spare the catabolism of branched-chain amino acids, but this is less widely utilized now than previously. Supplementation of 250 mg alanine kg^{-1} day^{-1} enhances nitrogen balance and may promote growth at lower intakes of protein. Also, the anabolic properties of human growth hormone have decreased the propensity for catabolism in some patients.[42]

Propionic acid is synthesized by the intestinal bacteria and this may be an important source of propionate and methylmalonate production in these patients.[42] Microbial propionate production can be suppressed by antibiotics, such as metronidazole and neomyocin. Therapy with these antibiotics has been found to be specifically effective in reducing urinary excretion of propionate metabolites by 40% in patients with methylmalonic or propionic acidemia.[42] Long-term metronidazole or neomyocin therapy (10–20 mg kg^{-1} day^{-1} and 50 mg kg^{-1} day^{-1}, respectively, given for 10 consecutive days each month) may have significant clinical benefit.[32]

Glutaric acidemia type I

Glutaric acidemia type 1 (GA1) is an autosomal recessive condition caused by a deficiency of the enzyme, glutaryl-CoA dehydrogenase, a mitochondrial flavin-adenine-dinucleotide (FAD) requiring enzyme within the catabolic pathway of lysine, hydroxylysine, and tryptophan (Figure 38.8). The enzymatic block results in the accumulation of glutaric acid and 3-hydroxyglutaric acid in blood and urine. Glutaryl-CoA is also esterified with carnitine leading to increased ratios of acylcarnitines to free carnitine in plasma and urine.[43] Glutarylcarnitine is excreted which contributes to secondary carnitine deficiency. Patients may also excrete metabolites indicative of mitochondrial dysfunction such as dicarboxylic acid, 2-oxoglutarate, and succinate.

The clinical presentation of GA1 is often in the first year of life, but not typically in the neonatal period. It is being included in this chapter because expanded newborn screening will make the diagnosis possible within the first weeks of life before the onset of symptoms. Generally, patients have a "presymptomatic" period characterized by "soft" neurological signs including hypotonia, head lag, irritability, jitteriness, and feeding difficulties. Macrocephaly is noted at or shortly after birth in the majority of patients. During this time, neuroimaging may

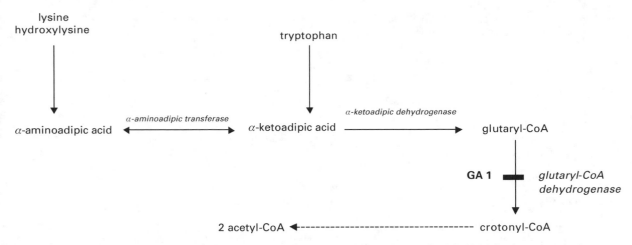

Figure 38.8. Lysine and tryptophan metabolism. Lysine, hydroxylysine, and tryptophan are degraded initially via separate pathways which converge in a common pathway starting with α-aminoadipic acid and α-ketoadipic acid. Glutaryl-CoA is oxidized and decarboxylated to crotonyl-CoA by glutaryl-CoA dehydrogenase which is deficient in glutaric acidemia type I (GAI). CoA = coenzyme A. Solid bar indicates enzymatic block.

reveal frontotemporal atrophy, enlarged sylvian fissures, or delayed myelination.[43] Infants are prone to suffer acute subdural hemorrhages after minor trauma, commonly around 1 year of age, due to the presence of enlarged subdural fluid spaces with associated bridging veins. Child abuse is often suspected. On average, at the age of 14 months, 75% of patients suffer an acute brain injury, mostly associated with an upper respiratory infection or gastrointestinal infection, a period of fasting (such as for surgery), following routine immunizations, or following minor head trauma.[43] Infants then present with an acute loss of skills, such as the ability to sit, pull to stand, and cruise, as well as loss of head control and suck and swallow reflexes. They appear alert with profound truncal hypotonia and extremity hypertonia with choreoathetotic movements of hands and feet. Over time, seizures and a severe dystonic movement disorder develop. At this time, neuroimaging reveals progressive frontotemporal atrophy and involvement of the basal ganglion. Although the majority of patients present with the characteristic symptoms and disease course, intrafamilial variability, and asymptomatic individuals have been reported. Death usually occurs before the end of the first decade of life.

Therapy

Early diagnosis and treatment is essential, as current therapy has little effect on the brain-injured child. Therapy prevents brain degeneration in more than 90% of affected infants who are treated prospectively.[43] Without treatment, more than 90% of affected children will develop severe neurological disabilities.[43] Fasting should be avoided and intercurrent illnesses should be treated aggressively with

frequent feedings, high carbohydrate and zero protein intake, followed by high-dose intravenous glucose and carnitine supplementation (100–300 g kg^{-1} day^{-1}).[43] Long-term carnitine supplementation is recommended to help prevent metabolic crises. An extremely rare patient may be riboflavin responsive, thus, a therapeutic trial of riboflavin is indicated.

Dietary therapy consists of either a low-protein diet or a lysine-restricted diet supplemented with a lysine-free amino acid mixture. Natural protein sources, from either standard infant formulas or foods, supply the lysine requirements, while the additional protein requirements are supplied by synthetic amino acids from special metabolic formulas. The intake of tryptophan should not be equally reduced as tryptophan contributes only 20% or less to total body glutarate production, and concentrations of tryptophan directly modulate the production of serotonin in the central nervous system.[43] In patients with neurologic symptoms, dietary therapy results in no major clinical improvement, but appears to halt the progression of the disease. Pharmacologic treatment of neurologic symptoms is also important. Monitoring of dietary intervention via plasma amino acids and quantitative plasma glutaric and 3-hydroxyglutaric acid levels is necessary.

Urea cycle disorders

Urea cycle disorders compromise a variety of enzymatic defects in the production of urea, the end product of nitrogen metabolism (Figure 38.9). The enzyme defects include:

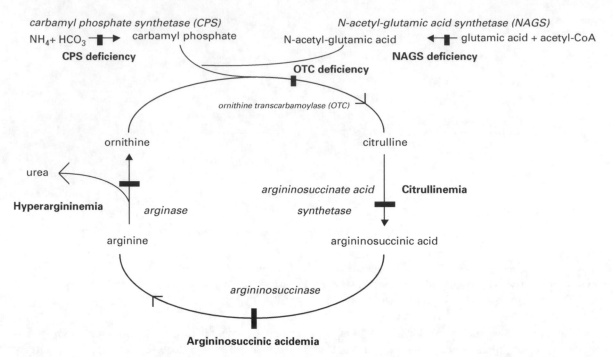

Figure 38.9. The urea cycle. Amino groups from exogenous and endogenous protein are the source of ammonia. The cycle converts the toxic ammonia molecule into the non-toxic product, urea, which is excreted in the urine. Disorders resulting from known enzyme deficiencies are noted. CoA = coenzyme A. Solid bar indicates enzymatic block.

(1) Carbamoyl-phosphate synthetase (CPS) deficiency

(2) Ornithine transcarbamoylase (OTC) deficiency

(3) Argininosuccinic acid synthetase deficiency (citrullinemia)

(4) Argininosuccinic acid lyase deficiency

(5) Arginase deficiency (arginemia)

(6) N-acetylglutamate synthetase (NAGS) deficiency.

Except for OTC deficiency, whose inheritance is X-linked, the enzyme defects in the urea cycle are transmitted as autosomal recessive traits.

The degradation of amino acids releases ammonia (primarily from glutamine and glutamate), which enters the urea cycle by way of carbamoyl phosphate. Hyperammonemia is the major biochemical abnormality of all the urea cycle defects and the accumulating ammonia itself is apparently an important neurotoxin. Ammonia increases the transport of tryptophan through the blood–brain barrier which leads to increased production of serotonin. Recently, magnetic resonance spectroscopy has demonstrated that increased glutamine in the central nervous system increases the osmolarity, hence, is responsible for the cellular swelling and brain edema which may complicate these diseases.[44,45]

With the exception of argininemia, the neonatal clinical features usually include vomiting, poor feeding, lethargy, respiratory distress, seizures, and coma. The prognosis relates to the age of onset and the severity and duration of hyperammonemic coma. Although rapid resolution of hyperammonemia may preserve mental development, those who present in the newborn period are likely to sustain neurological complications regardless of aggressive treatment. Mental retardation is common in infants surviving the neonatal course. The survival rate in infancy depends on the location of the enzymatic defect in the cycle, level of enzyme activity, and recognition and treatment of the disorder. In general, defects early in the cycle and patients with lower enzyme activity have the highest mortality. Mortality is highest for CPS deficiency and boys with classic OTC deficiency, and these respond poorly to therapy. Heterozygote girls with OTC deficiency may present neonatally or may be symptomatic only after a protein load or with an infection in childhood.[46] Family histories from female heterozygotes for OTC may reveal an intolerance and avoidance of high-protein foods.

Therapy

The components of the treatment regimen of urea cycle disorders include: (1) removal of waste nitrogen by promoting urinary excretion using sodium benzoate, sodium phenylacetate, and sodium phenylbutyrate; (2) limitation of production of waste nitrogen through restriction of intake of amino acids and protein; and (3) removal of waste

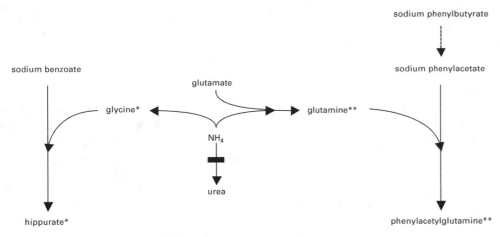

Figure 38.10. Ammonia diversion. The equilibrium of glutamine and glycine with ammonia may be used for disposal of ammonia by use of drugs such as sodium benzoate and sodium phenylacetate, which form complexes with glycine and glutamine that are excreted in the urine. * = moles of nitrogen excreted. Solid bar indicates enzymatic block.

nitrogen by supplementation of urea cycle intermediates distal to the enzymatic block.

Acute therapy

During acute hyperammonemic episodes, the major goal is to reduce plasma ammonia levels immediately. Fluid volume should be restricted if there is concern regarding brain edema. During acute crisis all exogenous protein sources are stopped. However, non-protein energy sources by intravenous or gastric feedings are necessary to inhibit or prevent catabolism. Reintroduction of protein should be performed slowly, starting at 0.5 g kg^{-1} day^{-1} and titrating to a tolerated intake approximately 1.0–1.5 g kg^{-1} day^{-1}. Sodium benzoate and sodium phenylacetate are standard drugs for reducing ammonia concentrations. They act by forming compounds with ammonia which are excreted in the urine[47] (Figure 38.10). Ammonul (Ucyclyd Pharma, Inc.), an intravenous 10% solution of these compounds, has now been used for many years in the acute therapy of these conditions at a standard dose of 250 mg kg^{-1} day^{-1}. Intravenous L-arginine at doses ranging from 210–660 mg kg^{-1}, with standard starting dose of 210 mg kg^{-1} day^{-1}, should be added, except for patients diagnosed with arginase deficiency. This will allow the rest of the cycle to continue to form urea and supplements arginine, which becomes an essential amino acid in patients affected by these disorders.

Aggressive measures using hemodialysis, or suboptimally peritoneal dialysis, may be required if hyperammonemia is not controlled. Hemodialysis, hemodiafiltration, or continuous venous-venous hemodialysis (CVVH) are the most effective. Exchange transfusions are not particularly beneficial.

Chronic therapy

To promote anabolism, a dietary prescription providing 145 kcal kg^{-1} day^{-1} and 1.0–1.5 g protein kg^{-1} day^{-1} is recommended as a baseline once the patient is ready for chronic therapy. Restricting protein intake to a minimum daily requirement may be sufficient to support protein synthesis and growth. It is essential that optimal calories from fat and carbohydrates be provided to inhibit gluconeogenesis. No less than 100 kcal kg^{-1} day^{-1} should be given to the infant up to 12 months of age.

The use of a mixture of essential L-amino acids prescribed as a percentage of the total protein may improve nitrogen retention and reduce waste nitrogen. However, use of the essential amino acids alone as the total protein intake may be limiting. Natural protein, in the form of standard infant formulas or food sources of protein, and essential amino acids in a 50:50 ratio is recommended to supply the total protein required. This regimen has been successful in promoting optimal visceral and somatic protein status and growth. Because protein intake is a small percentage of the total caloric intake per day (7%–10%), carbohydrates and fat must balance out the required energy.

Cyclinex 1 (Ross Laboratories) is an essential amino acid formulation available for use in infants. In addition to essential amino acids, it contains L-tyrosine, L-cystine, L-carnitine, vitamins, minerals, carbohydrates, and fat. Cyclinex 1 should be used in conjunction with natural protein and protein-free energy supplements to provide the required nutrients for the infant.

Dietary restriction of protein alone has had limited success.[46] The use of oral sodium benzoate therapy in conjunction with nutrition therapy can improve metabolic control. Sodium benzoate at doses of 250–500 mg kg^{-1} day^{-1} has resulted in reduced ammonia levels without significant toxicity. A newer compound, sodium phenylbutyrate (Buphenyl, Ucyclyd Pharma, Inc.), oxidizes to phenylacetate in the liver and subsequently binds glutamine and is rapidly excreted in the urine in the form of phenylacetylglutamine (Figure 38.10). Sodium phenylbutyrate is only available in an oral preparation and is more favorable as it does not have the peculiar mousy odor noted with sodium phenylacetate and more effectively binds and excretes nitrogen when compared with sodium benzoate. It is usually given at a dose of 250 mg kg^{-1} day^{-1}, but has been used in doses up to 650 mg kg^{-1} day^{-1}.[48] Oral supplementation of arginine must be continued for all patients except those with arginase deficiency. The aim should be to maintain plasma arginine concentrations between 50–200 μmol L^{-1}. A dose of 100–150 mg kg^{-1} day^{-1} appears to be sufficient for most patients.[48] In OTC and CPS, citrulline may be substituted for arginine in doses up to 170 mg kg^{-1} day^{-1}, as this will utilize an additional nitrogen molecule. Patients with citrullinemia and argininosuccinic aciduria have a higher requirement and may require doses up to 700 mg kg^{-1} day^{-1}.

Secondary carnitine deficiency may occur in patients with urea cycle disorders.[49–51] The deficiency may be more pronounced during hyperammonemic episodes. Prophylactic supplementation of oral L-carnitine (100 mg kg^{-1} day^{-1}) may be considered. Dietary restriction of tryptophan has reversed associated anorexia in some patients.[39]

Infants on restricted protein diets should be monitored at least monthly for the first year. Analysis of plasma amino acid profiles, ammonia, visceral protein status, anthropometrics, and growth assessment are recommended. Patients should be educated not to fast and to seek medical attention during illness to ensure adequate glucose intake and hydration to minimize catabolism. Intermittent episodes of hyperammonemia associated with intercurrent illnesses are felt to directly contribute to the poor neurologic outcome of these conditions. Families should be given the option of liver transplantation, which may offer a better long-term prognosis.

Disorders of carbohydrate metabolism

Galactosemia

Galactosemia is a biochemical defect in the metabolism of galactose, a monosaccharide milk sugar. The defect in classic galactosemia is a deficiency of the enzyme, galactose-1-phosphate uridyl transferase (gal-1-PUT), an enzyme necessary for the conversion of galactose to glucose (Figures 38.11). The biochemical block results in the accumulation of galactose-1-phosphate and galactose, and the formation of galactitol. The pathogenesis of the hepatic, renal, and cerebral disturbance is unclear, but is probably related to the accumulation of galactose-1-phosphate and galactose.[42] Cataract formation is explained by the accumulation of galactitol. Galactosemia can also occur due to enzymatic defects of galactokinase, and UDP-galactose-4-epimerase. All forms are autosomal recessive.

The neonatal presentation in patients with classic transferase deficiency can be catastrophic and includes vomiting, failure to thrive, liver disease, jaundice, hepatomegaly, edema, ascites, lethargy, *Escherichia coli* sepsis, and cataracts. Symptoms occur within a few days after birth, once the infant is exposed to lactose-containing formulas or breast milk. If undiagnosed, the infant may die of liver or renal failure or sepsis, or follow a course of recurring symptoms with failure to thrive and mental retardation. When a galactose restricted diet is instituted early, symptoms disappear promptly; jaundice resolves within days, cataracts may clear, liver and kidney function return to normal, and liver cirrhosis can be prevented. Various genotypes of transferase deficiency have been identified and have implications for the severity of illness.[52] Galactokinase deficiency presents with only cataracts. Many states perform newborn screening for galactosemia by assay of transferase activity and/or galactose level in blood.

Despite newborn screening and early intervention, patients with classic galactosemia may still have significant problems. Longitudinal studies have shown that infants diagnosed early and well managed have improved mental status and intellectual function, but are still below the intellectual quotients measured in their unaffected siblings.[53] Other findings in this same population include speech and language deficits, ovarian failure, and neurologic defects.

Therapy

A galactose-restricted diet regimen is used for patients with both classic transferase and galactokinase deficiency. Patients with some variants of transferase deficiency may also benefit from a galactose-restricted diet.[54]

Infants suspected of having galactosemia should immediately be removed from lactose-containing formulas. Although false positive newborn screening tests are common when the screen tests enzyme activity, treatment should be started while diagnosis is excluded or confirmed. Acceptable formula alternatives are Nutramigen, a casein

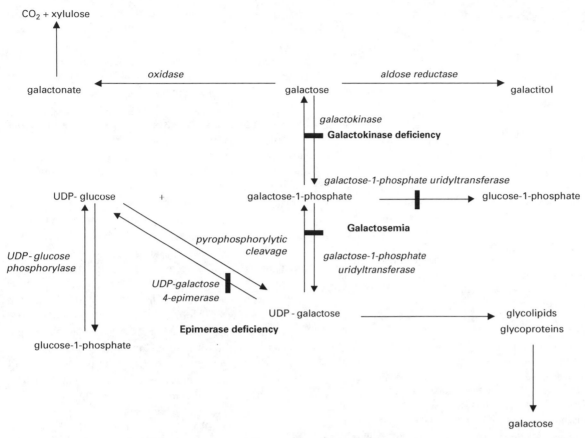

Figure 38.11. Selected pathways of carbohydrate metabolism. Galactose must be converted to glucose for use in energy metabolism. Any defect in galactose metabolism results in accumulation of galactitol as a result of an alternate pathway. Known disorders resulting from enzymatic blocks within the galactose metabolic pathway are noted. UDP = uridine diphosphate. Solid bar indicates enzymatic block.

hydrolysate (Mead Johnson Nutritionals), or soy protein formulas, such as ProSobee (Mead Johnson Nutritionals), and Isomil (Ross Laboratories). At one time the use of soy-protein formulas was questioned because of raffinose and stachyose, two galactose-containing oligosaccharides found in soybeans. Researchers now have shown that these sugars are not absorbed by human gut mucosa.[55] Soy-based formulas have since been used successfully in patients with galactosemia.

Free galactose sugars are not commonly found in natural foods. Lactose, a common disaccharide, comprising galactose and glucose, yields 50% galactose on hydrolysis. Therefore, all lactose-containing foods, such as milk and milk products, must be totally excluded from the diet. It is difficult to provide a diet regimen that is entirely free of exogenous galactose. Lactose is used in many processed foods including bread, cereals, dry mixes, and candies. Hidden sources of lactose are found in many "pill-form" medications and vitamin supplements, and as extenders

in artificial sweeteners. The steady increase in the use of processed foods has challenged many families. Food label reading is an absolute necessity for anyone managing a galactose-restricted diet. Table 38.3 lists foods and ingredients found on food labels that are considered unacceptable; they all contain lactose or galactose. Some investigators have suggested that the diet can be relaxed in school-age children,[56] but the consensus is now to continue the dietary regimen indefinitely.

There are major discrepancies in food lists for galactose-restricted diets. Some "questionable" foods that may contain either galactose or sugars that may be metabolized to galactose include some legumes, molasses, monosodium glutamate, sugar beets, soy sauce, and canned tuna fish. The lack of consensus regarding these foods has caused frustration for both families and practitioners. Determination of galactose-1-phosphate levels is helpful in monitoring adherence to the diet. Measurement of urinary galactitol for monitoring of treatment has not been

Table 38.3. Restricted ingredients for a galactosemic diet

Butter	Margarine[d]
Buttermilk	Milk
Buttermilk solids	Milk Chocolate
Calcium caseinate	Milk Solids
Casein	Nonfat dry milk
Cheese[a]	Nonfat dry milk solids
Cream	Nonfat milk
Dry milk	Organ meats[e]
Dry beans and peas[b]	
Hydrolyzed protein[c]	Sherbet[f]
Ice cream	Sodium caseinate
Lactalbumin (milk albuminate)	Sour Cream
Lactose	Whey and whey solids
Lactoglobulin	Yogurt

[a] Swiss cheeses of the Emmentaler, Gruyeres and Tilsiter types are galactose and lactose free.[57]

[b] Garbanzo beans, kidney beans, lima beans, lentils, split peas (this is only a partial list).

[c] Hydrolyzed protein is unacceptable if it is made from casein or whey.

[d] A few diet margarines do not contain any milk products and are acceptable. Check labels before using any brand. If "margarine" is listed as an ingredient in any processed food, check with the company to make sure it contains no milk products.

[e] Liver, heart, kidney, sweetbreads, and pancreas. Organ meats are often listed as "meat-by-products" on labels.

[f] Sherbet contains nonfat dry milk; however, many brands of sorbet do not and are acceptable.

Reprinted with permission.[63]

successful as only large amounts of ingested galactose are reflected and these are only detected after some delay.[57]

The nutritional requirements for the patient with galactosemia are similar to those of healthy infants and children. The need for supplementation of calcium or vitamin D is dependent on the quantity and quality of milk-substitute, infant formulas and natural foods supplied. If calcium or other vitamin-mineral supplements are indicated, care must be taken to ascertain whether they contain lactose fillers. Liquid preparations do not contain lactose. All medications should first be checked by a physician or pharmacist.

Type I glycogen storage disease

Type I glycogen storage disease (GSD; von Gierke's disease) is an inherited disorder of carbohydrate metabolism. GSD-1a results from an enzymatic deficiency of glucose-6-phosphatase, significantly impairing glycogenolysis and gluconeogenesis (Figure 38.12). Glucose-6-phosphate translocase deficiency, GSD-1b, results from insufficient translocase that transports the glucose-6-phosphate enzyme across the membrane. Historically, there is GSD-1c, due to defective transport of phosphate, and GSD-1d, due to defective transport of glucose. Because of the similar clinical presentations and because the enzymes that cause types 1b, 1c, and 1d all belong to a family of plasma membrane facilitative glucose transporters, these three types are currently categorized under GSD-1b.[58,59] The clinical findings and metabolic derangements are not discernible except for neutropenia and the susceptibility to infections seen in type 1b.

The young infant with GSD type I presents with failure to thrive, severe hypoglycemia, hepatomegaly, and lactic acidosis. Biochemical abnormalities include elevation of blood lactate, pyruvate, triglycerides, cholesterol, and uric acid. Blood ketone concentrations are surprisingly not elevated. This could be explained by the increased synthesis of fatty acids and cholesterol from the conversion of excess lactate and pyruvate into acetyl-CoA and subsequent conversion to malonyl-CoA, a potent activator of liponeogenesis and inhibitor of fatty acid oxidation.[60] Also, elevated malonyl-CoA will inhibit carnitine palmitoyl transferase 1 (CPT-1) and subsequently prevent entry of long chain fatty acyl-CoA into the mitochondria decreasing the oxidation and conversion to ketone bodies.[60]

Therapy

The goals of nutrition support for GSD type I include (1) steady supply of exogenous glucose to prevent hypoglycemia and reduce the biochemical derangements, while (2) avoiding excess glucose or energy to inhibit hepatic glycogen storage. The dietary prescription is a fructose-restricted, galactose-restricted diet with limited fat intake and moderate protein. Fructose (sucrose) and galactose (lactose) should be avoided because they cannot metabolize to glucose by the gluconeogenic pathway and may contribute to elevated blood lactate. Carbohydrate should be in the form of glucose and glucose polymers. Total fat ingestion should be restricted to prevent over accumulation of triglycerides, but hypertriglyceridemia may be a consequence of hypoglycemia rather than exogenous fat. The use of medium-chain triglycerides as a substitute for other fat sources may reduce blood triglycerides. Excess protein in the diet is not useful because amino acids cannot be readily converted to free glucose. An energy distribution of 60%–75% of calories as carbohydrate, 10%–15% as protein, and 20%–30% as fat is recommended.

Daytime formula feedings providing 1.5–2.5 g kg^{-1} per feed of predominantly complex carbohydrate every 3 hours have been beneficial in maintaining normoglycemia. The actual amount of prescribed carbohydrate per feed will

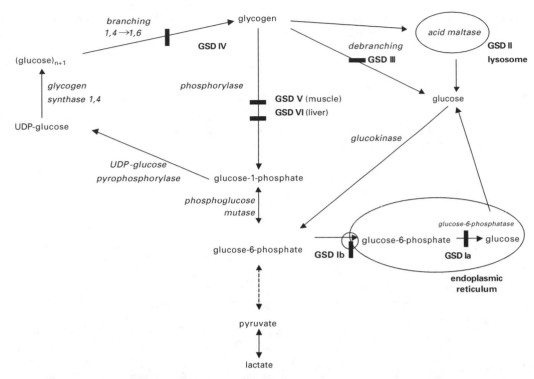

Figure 38.12. Glycogen metabolism. Glycogen synthase and branching enzyme are the enzymes for glycogen synthesis. The phosphorylase system, debranching enzyme, and glucose-6-phosphatase are the enzymes for glycogen degradation and glucose liberation. Some, but not all, forms of glycogen storage disorders (GSD) are noted. GSD II, Pompe disease, is generally considered a lysosomal storage disorder. GSD, Ib results from a defect in a membrane transporter. UDP = uridine diphosphate. Solid bar indicates enzymatic block.

depend on the individual infant and the source and physical nature of the carbohydrate. Adjustments of exogenous glucose may be necessary based on ascertainment of blood glucose levels before, after, and between feedings. Infants less than 6 months of age can use soy-based formulas without sucrose or carbohydrate-free formulations as the major nutrient source. These formulas must be used with either glucose polymers or uncooked cornstarch. Glucose polymers are necessary to allow for a slow absorption of glucose between feedings. Chemically defined formulas with glucose polymers as the carbohydrate source, have been used for daytime feedings. The high carbohydrate and low fat ratio in these formulas appears beneficial in preventing childhood obesity and promoting an acceptable blood glucose response. Ultimately, raw cornstarch provides a better blood glucose response than either dextrose or a carbohydrate module, but the decreased pancreatic amylase activity of young infants limits its use in neonates. However, pancreatic amylase activity can be stimulated with ingestion of oral starch, and partial digestion by salivary amylase if the oral route is utilized. Because of the variability of each infant's amylase enzyme activity, tolerance to cornstarch ingestion should be attempted in gradual dosages at

later infancy. Cornstarch is generally introduced at 1 year of age. Side effects of bowel distension, flatulence, and loose stools are usually transient and can be mitigated by slowly increasing the dose.[60]

Nocturnal continuous drip feedings of chemically defined formulas or dextrose have been beneficial in preventing hypoglycemia, reducing biochemical aberrations, and potentiating optimal growth. Infusion rates providing 7–9 mg glucose kg^{-1} minute^{-1} can prevent hypoglycemia. Intragastric feedings using dextrose alone instead of chemically defined formulas in these patients has also been used, however the latter is preferred.

Gastrostomy tube placement is indicated at the time of diagnosis in young infants and children because of the long-term dependence on nocturnal feedings. The gastrostomy tubes also provide an entry for feedings during times of illness or anorexia when the oral route is not sufficient for the provision of nutrients.

The recommended dietary needs for the infant with GSD type I are similar to those of healthy infants. Special attention should be given to insuring adequate intake of calcium, vitamin D, and ascorbic acid, as foods that supply these nutrients are restricted. GSD type 1b, which is commonly associated with neutropenia, requires appropriate antibiotic therapy as needed. In serious cases, granulocyte colony stimulating factor (GCSF) at a dose of 3–10 $\mu g\,kg^{-1}$ 2–4 times per week is recommended. The dose can be tapered as the patient improves clinically.

The use of frequent daytime high-carbohydrate feedings in conjunction with nocturnal infusion of carbohydrate results in optimal growth in these patients. Appropriate glucose infusion is necessary during acute illnesses to avoid complications from hypoglycemia or hyperglycemia. Careful monitoring of blood glucose concentrations and prevention of hyperglycemia and hypoglycemia can minimize the biochemical abnormalities associated with this disorder and ensure good life quality. Parents need to be taught to monitor for hypoglycemia at home.

Primary lactic acidosis

Lactic acidosis will not be discussed at length, but does deserve mention in a discussion of nutritional therapy of inborn errors of metabolism presenting in the neonate. One of the many causes of primary lactic acidosis, severe pyruvate dehydrogenase deficiency, presenting with overwhelming acidosis in the neonate, has the distinction of being the only inborn error of metabolism to worsen acutely with intravenous glucose. Generally, clinical intervention makes little difference to the outcome in neonates with severe pyruvate dehydrogenase deficiency. Treatment has been attempted in these and in more mildly affected patients with a modified ketogenic diet and various drugs and vitamins or other cofactor supplements. Response to treatment has been reported in a limited number of patients.

Another group of patients with primary lactic acidosis have gluconeogenic disorders and present with hypoglycemia and acidosis. These patients require treatment with provision of a steady glucose source. One important subset of this group are patients with disorders of fructose metabolism. Although there may be some lactic acidosis in the absence of fructose ingestion, significant symptoms usually occur only after fructose exposure. Some neonates are exposed to fructose by certain feeding practices and medications. A few patients with lactic acidosis due to disorders of the respiratory chain present as neonates. These patients usually do not respond to dietary manipulation. Infrequently, patients with primary lactic acidosis of various or unknown causes will present with hyperammonemia and protein intolerance. Understanding of the various presentations of and strategies for therapy of primary lactic acidosis is rapidly changing, and it is likely that any attempt to discuss more extensively the place of nutrition in the

management of neonates with these disorders would be out of date at publication.

Acknowledgment

The authors gratefully acknowledge Dr. Carol Greene and Dr. Steven Yannicelli, whose original version of this chapter provided the content backbone for this updated version.

REFERENCES

1 Bickel, H., Gerrard, J., Hickmans, E. M. Influence of phenylalanine intake on phenylketonuria. *Lancet* 1953;**265**:812–13.
2 Acosta, P. B., Fernhoff, P. M., Warshaw, H. *et al.* Zinc and copper status of treated children with phenylketonuria. *J. Parenter. Enteral Nutr.* 1981;**5**:406–9.
3 Folling, A. Uber Ausscheidung von Phenylbrenztrauben saure in den Harn als Stoffwechsel anomalie in Verbindemgmit Imbezillitat. *Hoppe-Seylers Z. Physiol Chem.* 1934;**277**:169–76.
4 Scriver, C. R., Kaufman, S. Hyperphenylalaninemia: phenylalanine hydroxylase deficiency. In Scriver, C. R., Beaudet, A. L., Sly, W. S., Valle, D., eds. *The Metabolic and Molecular Bases of Inherited Disease*. 8th edn. New York, NY: McGraw Hill; 2001:1667–724.
5 Koch, R., Friedman, E. G., Azen, C. G. *et al.* Report from the United States Collaborative Study of Children Treated for Phenylketonuria (PKU). In Bickel, H., Wachtel, U., eds. *Inherited Diseases of Amino Acid Metabolism*. Stuttgart, Federal Republic of Germany: George Thieme; 1985:134–50.
6 Lenke, R. R., Levy, H. L. Maternal phenylketonuria and hyperphenylalaninemia: an international survey of the outcome of untreated and treated pregnancies. *N. Engl. J. Med.* 1980;**303**:1202–8.
7 Phenylketonuria (PKU): Screening and Management. NIH Consensus Statement. 2000;**17**(3):1–33.
8 Kure, S., Hou, D.-C., Ohura, T. *et al.* Tetrahydrobiopterin-responsive phenylalanine hydroxylase deficiency. *J. Pediatr.* 1999;**135**:375–8.
9 Bernegger, C., Blau, N. High frequency of tetrahydrobiopterin-responsiveness among hyperphenylalaninemias: a study of 1919 patients observed from 1988 to 2002. *Mol. Genet. Metab.* 2002;**77**:304–13.
10 Holme, E., Lindstedt, S. Tyrosinemia type I and NTBC. *J. Inherit. Metab. Dis.* 1998;**21**:507–17.
11 Gilbert-Barness, E., Barness, L. *Metabolic Diseases: Fundamentals of Clinical Management, Genetics, and Pathology*. Natick, MA: Eaton Publishing; 2000:36–37.
12 Bonkowsky, H. L., Magnussen, C. R., Collins, A. R. *et al.* Comparative effects of glycerol and dextrose on porphyrin, precursor excretion in acute intermittent porphyria. *Metabolism* 1976;**25**:405–14.
13 Halvorsen, S. Screening for disorders of tyrosine metabolism. In Bickel, H., Guthrie, R., Hammersen, G., eds. *Neonatal

Screening for Inborn Errors of Metabolism. New York, NY: Springer-Verlag; 1980:45.

14 Buist, N. R. M., Kennaway, N. G., Fellman, J. H. Tyrosinemia Type II: Hepatic cytosol tyrosine aminotransferase deficiency. In Bickel, H., Wachtel, U., eds. *Inherited Diseases of Amino Acid Metabolism.* Stuttgart, Federal Republic of Germany: George Thieme; 1985:203–35.

15 Halvorsen, S., Skjelkvale, L. Tyrosine aminotransferase deficiency (TATD): First case diagnosed on newborn screening and successfully treated with Phe-Tyr restricted diet from early age. *Pediatr. Res.* 1977;**11**:1017.

16 Giardini, O., Cantani, A., Kennaway, N. G., D'Eufemia, P. Chronic tyrosinemia associated with 4-hydroxyphenyl-pyruvate dioxygenase deficiency with acute intermittent ataxia and without visceral and bone involvement. *Pediatr. Res.* 1983;**17**:25–9.

17 Kvittingen, E. A., Holme, E. Disorders of tyrosine metabolism. In Fernandes, J., Saudubray, J.-M., van den Berghe, G., eds. *Inborn Metabolic Diseases: Treatment and Diagnosis.* 3rd edn. Berlin: Springer; 2000:191.

18 Rousson, R., Guilbaud, P. Long term outcome of organic acidurias: survey of 105 French cases (1967–1983). *J. Inherit. Metab. Dis.* 1984;**7**(suppl. 1):10–12.

19 Scriver, C. R., Mackenzie, S., Clow, C. L. *et al.* Thiamine-responsive maple syrup urine disease. *Lancet* 1971;**1**:310–2.

20 Elsas, L., Danner, D., Lubitz, D. *et al.* Metabolic consequence in inherited defects in branched-chain alpha ketoacid dehydrogenase: mechanism of thiamine action. In Walser, M., Williamsen, J. R., eds. *Metabolism and Clinical Implications of Branched Chain Amino and Ketoacids.* New York, NY: Elsevier/North-Holland; 1981:369.

21 Naglak, M., Elsas, L. J. Nutrition support of maple syrup urine disease. *Metabolic Currents* 1989;**1**(3):15–20.

22 McCully, K. S. Vascular pathology of homocysteinemia: implications for the pathogenesis of arteriosclerosis. *Am. J. Pathol.* 1969;**56**:111–28.

23 Mudd, S. H., Skovby, F., Levy, H. L. *et al.* The natural history of homocystinuria due to cystathionine beta-synthase deficiency. *Am. J. Hum. Genet.* 1985;**37**:1–31.

24 Fowler, B. Recent advances in the mechanism of pyridoxine-responsive disorders. *J. Inherit. Metab. Dis.* 1985;**8**(Suppl. 1):76–83.

25 Andria, G., Fowler, B., Sebastio, G. Disorders of sulfur amino acid metabolism. In Fernandes, J., Saudubray, J.-M., van den Berghe, G., eds. *Inborn Metabolic Diseases: Treatment and Diagnosis.* 3rd edn. Berlin: Springer; 2000:228.

26 Yaghmai, R., Kashani, A. H., Geraghty, M. T. *et al.* Progressive cerebral edema associated with high methionine levels and betaine therapy in a patient with cystathionine beta-synthase (CBS) deficiency. *Am. J. Med. Genet.* 2002;**108**(1):57–63.

27 Gropper, S., Acosta, P. B. Effect of simultaneous ingestion of L-amino acids and whole protein on plasma amino acid concentrations and urea nitrogen in humans. *J. Parenter. Enteral Nutr.* 1991;**15**:48–53.

28 Tanaka, K., Budd, M. A., Efron, M. L. *et al.* Isovaleric acidemia: a new genetic defect of leucine metabolism. *Proc. Natl. Acad. Sci. USA* 1966;**56**:236–42.

29 Kreiger, I., Tanaka, K. Therapeutic effects of glycine in isovaleric acidemia. *Pediatr. Res.* 1976;**10**:25–9.

30 de Sousa, C., Chalmers, R. A., Stacey, T. E. *et al.* The response to L-carnitine and glycine therapy in isovaleric acidaemia. *Eur. J. Pediatr.* 1986;**144**:451–6.

31 Tanaka, K., Ikeda, Y. Isovaleric acidemia: clinical manifestations on biochemistry and genetics. In Bickel, H., Wachtel, U., eds. *Inherited Diseases of Amino Acid Metabolism.* Stuttgart, Federal Republic of Germany: George Thieme; 1985.

32 Ogier de Baulny, H., Saudubray, J.-M. Branched-chain organic acidurias. In Fernandes, J., Saudubray J.-M., van den Berghe, G., eds. *Inborn Metabolic Diseases: Treatment and Diagnosis.* 3rd edn. Berlin: Springer; 2000:197–207.

33 Wolf, B. Reassessment of biotin-responsiveness in "unresponsive" propionyl-CoA carboxylase deficiency. *J. Pediatr.* 1980;**97**:964–6.

34 Ampola, M. G., Mahoncy, M. J., Nakamura, E. *et al.* Prenatal therapy of a patient with vitamin B12-responsive methylmalonic acidemia. *N. Engl. J. Med.* 1975;**293**:313–17.

35 Specker, B. L., Miller, D., Norman, E. J. *et al.* Increased urinary methylmalonic acid excretion in breast-fed infants of vegetarian mothers and identification of an acceptable dietary source of vitamin B12. *Am. J. Clin. Nutr.* 1988;**47**:89–92.

36 Higginbottom, M. C., Sweetman, L., Nyhan, W. L. A syndrome of methylmalonic aciduria, homocystinuria, megaloblastic anemia and neurologic abnormalities in a vitamin B12 deficient breast-fed infant of a strict vegetarian. *N. Engl. J. Med.* 1978;**299**:317–23.

37 Ney, D., Bay, C., Saudubray, J. M. *et al.* An evaluation of protein requirements in methyl-malonic acidemia. *J. Inherit. Metab. Dis.* 1985;**8**:132–42.

38 Wolff, J. A., Sweetman, L., Nyhan, W. D. The role of lipid in the management of methylmalonic acidaemia: administration of linoleic acid does not increase excretion of methylmalonic acid. *J. Inherit. Metab. Dis.* 1985;**8**:100.

39 Hyman, S. L., Porter, C. A., Page, T. J. *et al.* Behavior management of feeding disturbances in urea cycle and organic acid disorders. *J. Pediatr.* 1987;**111**(4):558–62.

40 DiDonato, S., Rimoldi, M., Garavaglia, B. *et al.* Propionyl-carnitine excretion in propionic and methylmalonic acidurias: a cause of carnitine deficiency. *Clin. Chim. Acta.* 1984;**139**:13–21.

41 Chalmers, R. A., Stacy, T. E., Tracey, B. M. *et al.* L-carnitine insufficiency in disorders of organic acid metabolism: response to L-carnitine by patients with methylmalonic acidemia and 3-hydroxy-3-methyl-glutaric acidemia. *J. Inherit. Metab. Dis.* 1984;**7**(Suppl. 2):108–10.

42 Nyhan, W. L., Ozand, P. T. *Atlas of Metabolic Diseases.* London: Chapman and Hall Medical; 1998.

43 Hoffmann, G. F. Disorders of lysine catabolism and related cerebral organic-acid disorders. In Fernandes, J., Saudubray, J.-M., van den Berghe, G., eds. *Inborn Metabolic Diseases:*

Treatment and Diagnosis. 3rd edn. Berlin: Springer; 2000:245–50.

44 Bachmann, C. Mechanisms of hyperammonemia. *Clin. Chem. Lab. Med.* 2002;**40**(7):653–62.

45 Colombo, J. P. Urea cycle disorders, hyperammonemia and neurotransmitter changes. *Enzyme* 1987;**38**(1–4):214–19.

46 Batshaw, M. L., Thomas, G. H., Brusilow, S. W. New approaches to the diagnosis and treatment of inborn errors of urea synthesis. *Pediatrics* 1981;**68**:290–7.

47 Brusilow, S., Tinker, J., Batshaw, M. L. Amino acid acylation: a mechanism of nitrogen excretion in inborn errors of urea synthesis. *Science* 1980;**207**:659–61.

48 Leonard, J. V. Disorders of the urea cycle. In Fernandes, J., Saudubray, J.-M., van den Berghe, G., eds. *Inborn Metabolic Diseases: Treatment and Diagnosis.* 3rd edn. Berlin: Springer; 2000:219.

49 Matsuda, I., Ohtani, Y., Ohyanagi, K. *et al.* Hyperammonemia related to carnitine metabolism with particular emphasis on ornithine transcarbamylase deficiency. Recent advances in inborn errors of metabolism. Proc. 4th Int. Congr., Sendai. *Enzyme* 1987;**38**:251–5.

50 Ohtani, Y., Ohyanagi, K., Yamamoto, S. *et al.* Secondary carnitine deficiency in hyperammonemic attacks of ornithine transcarbamylase deficiency. *J. Pediatr.* 1988;**112**:404–14.

51 Mori, T., Tsuchiyama, A., Nagai, K. *et al.* A case of carbamylphosphate synthetase-I deficiency associated with secondary carnitine deficiency – L-carnitine treatment of CPS-I deficiency. *Eur. J. Pediatr.* 1990;**149**(4):272–4.

52 Holton, J. B., Walter, J. H., Tyfield, L. A. Galactosemia. In Scriver, C. R., Beaudet, A. L., Sly, W. S., Valle, D., eds. *The Metabolic and Molecular Bases of Inherited Disease.* 8th edn. New York, NY: McGraw Hill; 2001:1553–87.

53 Fishler, K., Donnell, G. N., Bergren, W. R. *et al.* Intellectual and personality development in children with galactosemia. *Pediatrics* 1972;**50**:412–19.

54 Schwarz, H. P., Zuppinger, K. A., Zimmerman, A. *et al.* Galactose intolerance with double heterozygosity for duarte variant and galactosemia. *J. Pediatr.* 1982;**100**:704–9.

55 Wiesmann, U. N., Rose-Beutler, B., Schluchter, R. Leguminosae in the diet: the raffinose-stachyose question. *Eur. J. Pediatr.* 1995;**154**:S93.

56 Kowrower, G. M. Galactosemia: thirty years on: the experience of a generation. *J. Inherit. Metab. Dis.* 1982;**5**(Suppl. 2):96–104.

57 Gitzelmann, R. Disorders of galactose metabolism. In Fernandes, J., Saudubray, J.-M., van den Berghe, G., eds. *Inborn Metabolic Diseases: Treatment and Diagnosis.* 3rd edn. Berlin: Springer; 2000:105.

58 Veiga-da-Cunha, M., Gerin, I., Van Schaftingen, E. How many forms of glycogen storage disease type I? *Eur. J. Pediatr.* 2000;**159**(5):314–18.

59 Veiga-da-Cunha, M., Gerin, I., Chen, Y. T. *et al.* The putative glucose 6-phosphate translocase gene is mutated in essentially all cases of glycogen storage disease type I non-a. *Eur. J. Hum. Genet.* 1999;**7**(6):717–23.

60 Fernandes, J., Smit, G. P. A. The glycogen-storage diseases. In Fernandes, J., Saudubray, J.-M., van den Berghe, G., eds. *Inborn Metabolic Diseases: Treatment and Diagnosis.* 3rd edn. Berlin: Springer; 2000:87–101.

61 Acosta, P. B., Yannicelli, S. *The Ross Metabolic Formula System Nutrition Support Protocols.* 4th edn. Columbus, Ohio: Abbott Laboratories; 2001.

62 Thomas, J. A., Bernstein, L. E., Greene, C. L., Koeller, D. M. Apparent decreased energy requirements in children with organic acidemias: preliminary observations. *J. Am. Diet Assoc.* 2000;**100**(9):1074–6.

63 Hartz, L., Pettis, K., van Calcar, S. *Understanding Galactosemia: A Diet Guide.* 2nd edn. Madison, WI: Biochemical Genetics Program, University of Wisconsin; 2000.

39

Nutrition in the neonatal surgical patient

Agostino Pierro and Simon Eaton

Department of Paediatric Surgery, The Institute of Child Health and Great Ormond Street Hospital for Children NHS Trust, University College London, London, UK

Introduction

The newborn infant is in a "critical epoch" of development not only for the organism as a whole but also for the individual organs and most significantly for the brain.[1] Adequate nutrition in the neonatal period is necessary to avoid the adverse effects of malnutrition on morbidity and mortality[2] and to minimise the future menace of stunted mental and physical development.[1]

The survival rate of newborn infants affected by isolated congenital gastrointestinal abnormalities has improved considerably over the past 20 years and is now in excess of 90% in most pediatric surgical centers. The introduction of parenteral nutrition and advancement in nutritional management are certainly among the main factors responsible for this improvement.

Historical background

Parenteral nutrition stepped forward from numerous historical anecdotes in the 1930s with the first successful infusion of protein hydrolysates in humans,[3] followed by the first report of successful total parenteral nutrition in an infant in 1944,[4] and given a huge boost by the first placement of a catheter in the superior vena cava to deliver nutrients for prolonged periods.[5] Using this system, Dudrick and Wilmore showed that adequate growth and development could be achieved in beagle puppies and in a surgical infant.[5] Following these initial reports Filler and co-authors reported the first series of surgical neonates with gastrointestinal abnormalities treated with long-term total parenteral nutrition.[6] During the 1970s and 1980s significant improvements were made in the technique itself and in reduction of complications, and the last 10 years have seen considerable changes in the nutritional management of surgical neonates. Various investigators have highlighted the importance of introducing enteral nutrition as soon as possible in surgical neonates. The beneficial effects of minimal enteral feeding on the immune system, infection rate and liver function have been elucidated.

Body composition

Newborn infants grow very rapidly, have lower caloric reserves than adults and therefore do not tolerate prolonged periods of starvation. The body composition of newborn infants is markedly different from that of adults. The total body water varies from 86% of body weight at 28 weeks of gestation to 69% at 40 weeks of gestation and 60% in adulthood. This decline in body water reflects also an increase in energy content of the body. The ratio between minimal metabolic rate to nonprotein energy reserve is only 1:2 at 28 weeks gestation, it decreases to 1:29 for term infants and 1:100 for the adult,[1] hence the urgent need for adequate caloric intake in very-low-birth-weight infants after birth. Full-term neonates have higher content of endogenous fat (approximately 600 g) and therefore can tolerate a few days of undernutrition.

Energy metabolism

Newborn infants have a significantly higher metabolic rate and energy requirement per unit body weight than children

Neonatal Nutrition and Metabolism. Second Edition, ed. P. Thureen and W. Hay. Published by Cambridge University Press.
© Cambridge University Press 2006.

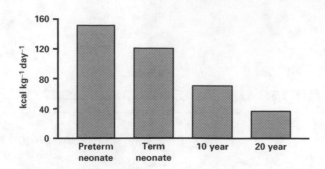

Figure 39.1. Total energy requirement according to age.

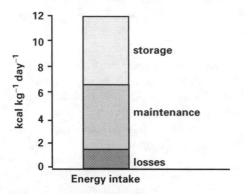

Figure 39.2. Partition of energy metabolism in surgical newborn infants.[8]

and adults (Figure 39.1).[7] They require approximately 40–70 kcal kg^{-1} day^{-1} for maintenance metabolism, 50–70 kcal kg^{-1} day^{-1} for growth (tissue synthesis and energy stored), and up to 20 kcal kg^{-1} day^{-1} to cover energy losses in excreta (Figure 39.2).[8,9] The total energy requirement for a newborn infant fed enterally is 100–120 kcal kg^{-1}day^{-1}, compared with 60–80 kcal kg^{-1} day^{-1} for a 10-year-old and 30–40 kcal kg^{-1} day^{-1} for a 20-year-old individual. Newborn infants receiving total parenteral nutrition (TPN) require fewer calories (80–100 kcal kg^{-1} day^{-1}). This is due to the absence of energy losses in excreta and to the fact that energy is not required for thermoregulation when the infant is nursed in a thermoneutral environment using a double-insulated incubator. Although energy expenditure may double during periods of activity, including crying, most surgical infants are at rest 80–90% of the time.[8] Significant differences in resting energy expenditure (REE) have been reported among full-term surgical newborn infants (range 33.3–50.8 kcal kg^{-1} day^{-1}),[8] and between premature and full-term babies. A full term infant requires 100–120 kcal kg^{-1} day^{-1}, and a premature infant 110–160 kcal kg^{-1} day^{-1} (Figure 39.1).[8,10] These variations in maintenance metabolism explain the different growth rates frequently

observed in surgical neonates receiving similar caloric intakes, and probably represent differences in metabolically active tissue mass i.e., organ and muscle size. Several equations have been published to predict energy expenditure in adults[11] and equations have been developed to predict REE in stable surgical neonates, to which the major contributing predictors are body weight, heart rate (providing an indirect measure of hemodynamic and metabolic status) and postnatal age.[12]

Operative trauma

In contrast with adults, the energy requirement of infants and children undergoing major operations seems to be modified minimally by the operative trauma per se. In adults, trauma or surgery causes a brief "ebb" period of a depressed metabolic rate followed by a "flow phase" characterised by an increase in oxygen consumption to support the massive exchanges of substrate between organs.[13] In newborn infants major abdominal surgery causes a moderate (15%) and immediate (peak at 4 hours) elevation of oxygen consumption and resting energy expenditure and a rapid return to baseline 12–24 hours postoperatively.[14] There is no further increase in energy expenditure in the first 5–7 days following an operation.[14,15] The timing of these changes corresponds with the postoperative changes in catecholamine levels and other biochemical and endocrine parameters.[16] It has been demonstrated that the postoperative increase in energy expenditure can, at least partially, result from severe underlying acute illness, which frequently necessitates surgery (i.e., sepsis or intense inflammation, see below).[17] Interestingly, infants having a major operation after the second day of life have a significantly greater increase in resting energy expenditure than infants undergoing surgery within the first 48 hours of life. A possible explanation for this may be greater secretion of endogenous opioids in the perinatal period blunting the endocrine and metabolic responses.[16,18,19]

Resting energy expenditure is directly proportional to growth rate in healthy infants, and growth is retarded during acute metabolic stress. Studies in adult surgical patients have shown that operative stress causes marked changes in protein metabolism characterised by a postoperative increase in protein degradation, negative nitrogen balance,[20,21] and a decrease in muscle protein synthesis.[22] However, changes in whole body protein flux, protein synthesis, amino acid oxidation or protein degradation do not seem to occur in infants and young children undergoing major operations,[23] which led us to speculate that infants and children divert protein and energy from growth to tissue repair, thereby avoiding the overall increase in energy expenditure and catabolism seen in the adult.[23–25]

Critical illness and sepsis

Nutritional problems in infants and children requiring surgery are not unusual. The real nutritional challenge is not represented by the operation per se but by the clinical condition of the patient. Examples include intrauterine growth retardation in small for gestational age preterm infants, infants who have suffered massive intestinal resection for necrotizing enterocolitis, and infants with motility disorders of the intestine following surgery for atresia, malrotation and midgut volvulus, meconium ileus or gastroschisis.

Nutritional integrity particularly in the neonatal period should be maintained regardless of the severity of the illness or organ failure due to the limited energy and protein stores in neonates. Infants and children require nutrition for maintenance of protein status as well as for growth and wound healing. One considerable challenge in pediatrics is represented by nutrition support during critical illness and sepsis. Keshen *et al.* [26] have shown that parenterally fed neonates on extracorporeal life support are in hypermetabolic and protein catabolic states. These authors recommend the provision of additional protein and nonprotein calories to attenuate the net protein losses.

Sepsis is an intriguing pathological condition associated with many complex metabolic and physiological alterations.[27] Studies in adults have shown that the metabolic response to sepsis is characterized by hypermetabolism,[28] increased tissue catabolism,[28] gluconeogenesis and hepatic release of glucose.[29] Energy is largely derived from fat, and increased protein catabolism provides precursors for enhanced hepatic gluconeogenesis.[29] However, fat mobilization is far greater than fat oxidation, implying considerable cycling[30] and in later stages of sepsis, oxidative metabolism[31] and fat utilization may become impaired.[32]

The existing knowledge on the metabolic response to sepsis in infants is limited. There are conflicting reports on whether critically ill infants are hypermetabolic.[33–39] However, recent studies suggest that infants with sepsis do not become hypermetabolic (Figure 39.3)[40,41] and that septic neonates with necrotizing enterocolitis do not show any increase in whole body protein turnover, synthesis and catabolism.[24]

From these studies, it is clear that the metabolic rate and hormonal response to surgery, stress and sepsis in infants may well be different from that of adults and therefore it is not possible to adapt nutritional recommendations

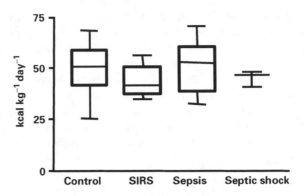

Figure 39.3. Resting energy expenditure in critically ill infants and controls. Indirect calorimetry was performed on infants and children with systemic inflammatory response syndrome (SIRS), sepsis, septic shock, and controls. Results are expressed as median, range, and interquartile range. There were no significant differences between the groups.[40]

made for adults to the neonatal population. It is possible that neonates divert the products of protein synthesis and breakdown from growth into tissue repair.

This may explain the lack of growth commonly observed in infants with critical illness or sepsis. Further studies are needed in this field to delineate the metabolic response of neonates and children to trauma and sepsis, explore the relationship between nutrition and immunity and to design the most appropriate diet.

Parenteral nutrition

Indications

Parenteral nutrition should be utilized when enteral feeding is impossible, inadequate, or hazardous for more than 4–5 days. The most frequent indications in neonatal surgery are intestinal obstruction due to congenital anomalies. Frequently after an operation on the gastrointestinal tract, adequate enteral feeding cannot be achieved for more than one week and parenteral nutrition becomes necessary. This modality of therapy has improved significantly the survival rate of newborns with gastroschisis, a condition which requires intravenous administration of nutrients for 2–3 weeks. Parenteral nutrition is also used in cases of necrotizing enterocolitis, short-bowel syndrome, and respiratory distress.

Components of parenteral nutrition

The parenteral nutrition formulation includes carbohydrate, fat, protein, electrolytes, vitamins, trace elements, and water. The caloric needs for total parenteral nutrition are provided by carbohydrate and lipid. Protein is not used as a source of calories, since the catabolism of protein to produce energy is an uneconomic metabolic process compared with the oxidation of carbohydrate and fat which produces more energy at a lower metabolic cost. The ideal total parenteral nutrition regimen therefore should provide enough amino acids for protein turnover and tissue growth, and sufficient calories to minimize protein oxidation for energy.

Fluid requirements

Any newborn infant deprived of oral fluids will lose body fluids and electrolytes in urine, stools, sweat and evaporative losses from the lungs and the skin. The insensible water losses from the skin are particularly high (up to 80–100 ml kg^{-1} day^{-1}) in low-birth-weight infants.[42] This is due to the very large surface area relative to body weight, to the very thin and permeable epidermis, to reduced subcutaneous fat, and to the large proportion of total body water and extracellular water.[42] The pre-term infant requires larger amounts of fluid to replace the high obligatory renal water excretion due to the limited ability to concentrate urine. In surgical newborns it is not unusual to have significant water losses from gastric drainage and gastrointestinal stoma. In order to reduce the water losses it is important to use double-walled incubators, to place the infant in relatively high humidity, to use warm humidified air via the endotracheal tube, and in premature babies to cover the body surface with an impermeable sheet. However, overhydration is potentially a problem, leading to complications such as pulmonary edema.

Energy sources

Carbohydrates and fat provide the main energy sources in the diet, and this is reflected by their importance as a source of calories in parenteral nutrition.

Glucose is a main energy source for body cells and is the primary energy substrate in parenteral nutrition. The amount of glucose that can be infused safely depends on the clinical condition and maturity of the infant. The ability of neonates to metabolize glucose may be impaired by prematurity and low birth weight. Carbohydrate conversion to fat (lipogenesis) occurs when glucose intake exceeds metabolic needs. The risks associated with this process are 2-fold: accumulation of the newly synthesized fat in the liver,[43] and aggravation of respiratory acidosis resulting from increased CO$_2$ production, particularly in patients with compromised pulmonary function.[44]

Since the 1960s, safe commercial intravenous fat emulsions have become widely used. These preparations have

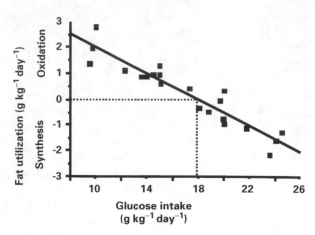

Figure 39.4.   Linear relationship between glucose intake and fat utilization (r = −0.9; p < 0.0001). Lipogenesis is significant when glucose intake exceeds 18 g kg^{-1} day^{-1}.[51]

a high caloric value (9 kcal g^{-1} of fat), prevent essential fatty acid deficiency,[45,46] and are isotonic, allowing adequate calories to be given via a peripheral vein.[47] A number of studies in both adults and infants have shown that combined infusion of glucose and lipids confers metabolic advantages over glucose, because it lowers the metabolic rate and increases the efficiency of energy utilisation.[48–50]

Jones et al.[51] have shown that in surgical infants receiving parenteral nutrition there is a negative linear relationship between glucose intake and fat utilization (oxidation and conversion to fat). Net fat synthesis from glucose exceeds net fat oxidation when the glucose intake is greater than 18 g kg^{-1} day^{-1} (i.e., in excess of energy expenditure) (Figure 39.4). Jones et al.[14] also found a significant relationship between glucose intake and CO$_2$ production. The slope of this relationship (i.e., increased CO$_2$ production) was steeper when glucose intake exceeded 18 g kg^{-1} day^{-1} than when glucose intake was less than 18 g kg^{-1} day^{-1}, indicating that lipogenesis results in a significantly increased CO$_2$ production. More recent studies on stable surgical newborn infants receiving fixed amounts of carbohydrate and amino acids and variable amounts of intravenous long-chain fat emulsion have shown that at a carbohydrate intake of 15 g kg^{-1} day^{-1}, the proportion of energy metabolism derived from fat oxidation does not exceed 20% even with a fat intake as high as 6 g kg^{-1} day^{-1}. At a carbohydrate intake of 10 g kg^{-1} day^{-1} this proportion can be as high as 50%.[52] This study seems to indicate that during parenteral nutrition in surgical infants the majority of the intravenous fat infused is not oxidized but deposited.

Fat tolerance has been extensively studied by monitoring fat clearance from plasma. However, clearance from plasma does not imply that the fat is being utilized to

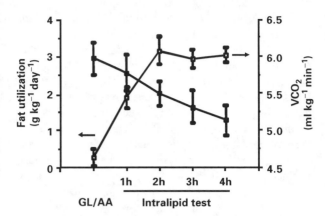

Figure 39.5. Intralipid utilization test: surgical newborn infants adapt very rapidly to the infusion of intravenous fat. The oxidation of exogenous fat is associated with a significant reduction in CO_2 production. Fat utilization open symbols; CO_2 production (VCO_2 closed symbols).[53]

meet energy requirements, since it may be being stored instead.[53,54] Pierro et al. have studied intravenous fat utilization by performing a "lipid utilisation test".[53] This consisted of infusing lipid for 4 hours in isocaloric and isovolemic amounts to the previously given mixture of glucose and amino acids. Gas exchange was measured by indirect calorimetry to calculate the patient's O_2 consumption and CO_2 production, and net fat utilization (Figure 39.5). The study showed that within 2 hours, more than 80% of the exogenous fat can be oxidized and that CO_2 production is reduced during fat infusion as a consequence of the cessation of carbohydrate conversion to fat (lipogenesis).[53]

Net fat oxidation seems to be significantly influenced by the carbohydrate intake and by the resting energy expenditure of the neonate. When the intake of glucose calories exceeds the resting energy expenditure of the infant, net fat oxidation is minimal regardless of fat intake.[52] In order to use intravenous fat as an energy source (i.e., oxidation to CO_2 and H_2O), it is therefore necessary to maintain carbohydrate intake below basal energy requirements. Glucose intake exceeding 18 g kg^{-1} day^{-1} is also associated with a significant increase in respiratory rate and plasma triglyceride levels. It is advisable therefore in stable surgical newborn infants requiring parenteral nutrition to not exceed 18 g kg^{-1} day^{-1} of intravenous glucose intake.[51,53]

Commonly used fat emulsions for parenteral nutrition in pediatrics are based on long-chain triglycerides (LCT). The rate of intravenous fat oxidation during total parenteral nutrition could potentially be enhanced by the addition of L-carnitine and/or medium-chain triglycerides (MCT) to the intravenous diet. L-carnitine is required for the oxidation of long-chain triglycerides, and although it is present in breast milk and infant formula, is not present in parenteral feeds. Although some authors have found decreased carnitine levels in parenterally fed neonates and/or reported enhanced fat oxidation upon carnitine supplementation,[55,56] carnitine levels have to fall extremely low before fatty acid oxidation is impaired[57,58] and although supplementation has been recommended by some groups, a systematic review found no evidence to support the routine supplementation of parenterally fed neonates with carnitine.[59] MCT are both cleared from the bloodstream and oxidized at a faster rate than LCT, and various studies have suggested that MCT/LCT mixtures in pediatric parenteral nutrition provide benefits over LCT alone.[60–62] However, randomized controlled trials are necessary before MCT/LCT mixtures find routine use in parenteral nutrition of neonates. We have recently investigated the metabolic response to intravenous medium-chain triglycerides in surgical infants and found that, providing that carbohydrate calories do not exceed energy expenditure, partial replacement of LCT by MCT can increase net fat oxidation without increasing metabolic rate.[63]

Amino acids

In contrast to healthy adults who exist in a state of neutral nitrogen balance, infants need to be in positive nitrogen balance in order to achieve satisfactory growth and development. Infants are efficient at retaining nitrogen, and can retain up to 80% of the metabolizable protein intake on both oral and intravenous diets.[64–66] Protein metabolism is dependent upon both protein and energy intake. The influence of dietary protein is well established. An increased protein intake has been shown to enhance protein synthesis,[67,68] reduce endogenous protein breakdown,[69] and thus enhance net protein retention.[65,69] The protein requirements of newborn infants are between 2.5 and 3.0 g kg^{-1} day^{-1}. The nitrogen source of TPN is usually provided as a mixture of amino acids. The solutions commercially available contain the eight known essential amino acids plus histidine, which is known to be essential in children.[70] Complications like azotemia, hyperammonemia, and metabolic acidosis have been described in patients receiving high levels of intravenous amino acids[42] but rarely seen with amino acid intake of 2–3 g kg^{-1} day^{-1}.[71] In patients with severe malnutrition or with additional losses (i.e., jejunostomy, ileostomy), protein requirements are higher.[70]

The influence of nonprotein energy intake on protein metabolism is more controversial. Protein retention can be enhanced by giving carbohydrate or fat,[72–77] which are thus said to be protein-sparing. Although some studies have suggested that the protein-sparing effect of carbohydrate is greater than that of fat,[72–74] others have suggested that the protein-sparing effect of fat may be either equivalent to, or greater than, that of carbohydrate.[75–77] The addition of fat calories to the intravenous diet of surgical newborn infants reduces protein oxidation, protein contribution to the energy expenditure, and increases protein retention.[77] In a further study, we compared protein metabolism in two groups of neonates receiving isonitrogenous and isocaloric total parenteral nutrition: one group received a high fat diet and the other, a high carbohydrate diet. There was no significant difference between the two groups with regard to any of the components of whole body protein metabolism: protein synthesis, protein breakdown, protein oxidation/excretion, and total protein flux, thus supporting the use of fat in the intravenous diet of surgical newborn infants.[78,79]

The ideal quantitative composition of amino acid solutions is still controversial. In newborn infants cysteine, taurine, and tyrosine seem to be essential amino acids. However, the addition of cysteine in the parenteral nutrition of neonates does not cause any difference in the growth rate and nitrogen retention.[65]

Glutamine

Nutrients can modulate immune, metabolic, and inflammatory responses. Of these nutrients, glutamine is of particular interest. Glutamine is the most abundant free amino acid in the body where it plays fundamental physiological roles. It is the predominant amino acid supplied to the fetus through the placenta[80] and is normally present in the enteral diet. Glutamine can be synthesized in the human body in substantial amounts and therefore is usually considered to be nonessential. However, in patients with acute and long-term sepsis and/or trauma, glutamine stores decline. This may be due to a combination of reduced glutamine production, possibly reflecting low muscle glycogen levels, glucose intolerance, and increased glutamine utilization. During sepsis, the liver and the immune system become major glutamine consumers such that net glutamine utilization exceeds production and glutamine becomes 'conditionally essential'.[81,82] In rats, glutamine oxidation supplies a third of the total energy requirement of the gut.[83] In humans who have sustained multisystem trauma or sepsis, glutamine concentration is 15% higher in arterial blood than in portal blood, confirming the selective uptake of glutamine in the gut.[84]

Until recently glutamine has been excluded from parenteral nutrition because of low solubility and instability in solution. However glutamine dipeptides with improved stability and solubility are now available ma-

king it possible to add glutamine to parenteral nutrition formulation.[85] There are several reasons why glutamine may be beneficial for critically ill patients receiving parenteral nutrition. Firstly, glutamine supplementation has been shown to be beneficial, both in vitro and in vivo, for the immune system.[86–88] The effect of glutamine supplementation on the prevention of infectious complications has been examined in randomized trials in adult patients receiving either glutamine-supplemented parenteral nutrition or isonitrogenous isocaloric parenteral nutrition. These trials included patients undergoing elective operation for colorectal cancer, patients with multiple trauma,[89] critically ill patients[90] and patients undergoing bone marrow transplantation.[86] All these studies showed that parenteral glutamine administration does reduce infectious complications. Secondly, glutamine has multiple effects on gastrointestinal function. Glutamine deficiency leads to gut atrophy and bacterial translocation[81,91,92] and supplemental glutamine may preserve the gut mucosal barrier during stress.[81,92–94] Glutamine prevents deterioration of gut permeability, prevents intestinal mucosal atrophy[95] and preserves mucosal structure in patients receiving parenteral nutrition.[96,97] Reduced nitrogen loss has been demonstrated in adult patients receiving glutamine-supplemented parenteral nutrition after major abdominal operations.[98]

Recent studies have shown that in a neonatal animal model, glutamine reverses the liver dysfunction caused by sepsis due to an increase in the production of glutathione, a major intracellular antioxidant, for which glutamine is an important precursor.[99,100]

There have been several trials of glutamine parenteral nutrition supplementation in adults. However, a recent Cochrane systematic review[101] has identified only two published randomized controlled trials of glutamine in neonates[102,103] including one on parenteral nutrition supplementation.[102] This trial did not identify any adverse effects attributable to glutamine.[102]

Glutamine administration was associated with a reduced duration of artificial ventilation, hospital admission, and parenteral nutrition[102] but effects on immunity or infection and its generalizability to other settings or patient groups remain unclear.[101] The Cochrane Review highlighted the requirement for a large randomized controlled trial of glutamine supplementation in neonates requiring parenteral nutrition.

Vitamins and trace elements

Vitamins and trace elements are important cofactors or components of enzymes, and provision of adequate supplies is important for the growing neonate. Vitamins and trace elements are particularly important in maintenance of the body's antioxidant defenses: vitamins C and E, selenium (for glutathione peroxidase), copper, zinc, and manganese (all for superoxide dismutases) are all added to parenteral nutrition. However, vitamins and trace elements are particularly vulnerable to photo-oxidation and loss, or to increased lipid peroxide production and various studies have suggested photoprotection of parenteral nutrition bags in order to minimize losses and peroxide generation.[104–107] Free radical production and lipid peroxidation will be considered in more detail below.

Complications of parenteral nutrition

Infectious complications

In spite of significant improvement in the management of parenteral nutrition including the introduction of nutrition support teams, recently published infection rates from large children's hospitals indicate that between 5% and 37% of infants may develop sepsis while receiving parenteral nutrition.[108–111] This may lead to impaired liver function,[111,112] critical illness and removal of central venous catheters. It has always been assumed that the central venous catheter is the major portal of entry for micro-organisms causing septicemia in patients on parenteral nutrition.[109] However, studies in animals[113] and surgical neonates[111] have reported microbial translocation (migration of micro-organisms from the intestinal lumen to the systemic circulation) during parenteral feeding. In a study on surgical neonates on parenteral nutrition [111] all but one episode of microbial translocation occurred in patients with elevated serum bilirubin (cholestasis). Pierro *et al.* have reported that almost half the surgical infants on parenteral nutrition develop abnormal flora and that all cases of septicemia were preceded by gut colonization with abnormal flora.[112] Furthermore, it has been reported[114,115] that parenteral nutrition itself impairs host defence mechanisms and contributes to the occurrence of infection in neonates.[116] This may be due to individual components of the parenteral nutrition solution, such as lipid emulsion,[117–120] or due to lack of nutrients, such as glutamine, normally present in the enteral diet.

Important factors in reducing the incidence of septic complications are placing intravenous catheters under strict aseptic conditions, preparing the parenteral nutrition solutions in pharmacy in aseptic conditions and using meticulous care when the catheters are used. Sepsis should be suspected when infants on parenteral nutrition present clinical features of generalized inflammation including one or more of the following features: temperature instability, poor perfusion, hypotension, lethargy, tachycardia,

Table 39.1. Metabolic complications of total parenteral nutrition

Carbohydrate administration
Hyperglycemia
Hypoglycemia
Fatty infiltration of the liver
Hyperosmolarity and osmotic diuresis
Increased CO_2 production
Protein administration
Hyperammonemia, azotemia
Abnormal plasma amino acid profiles
Hepatic dysfunction
Cholestatic jaundice
Fat administration
Hyperlipidemia
Fat overload syndrome
Displacement of albumin-bound bilirubin by free fatty acids
Peroxidation and generation of free radicals
Fluid administration
Patent ductus arteriosus
Pulmonary edema
Electrolyte imbalance
Sodium, potassium, chloride,
Calcium, phosphate
Trace element and vitamin deficiency

respiratory distress, and fever. In these neonates, blood culture should be performed from the central venous line and/or from a peripheral vein.

Metabolic complications

The metabolic complications most frequently observed in newborn infants receiving parenteral nutrition are listed in Table 39.1. These complications are related to inappropriate administration of nutrients, fluid, electrolytes, and trace elements or to the inability of the individual patient to metabolize the intravenous diet.

Hyperglycemia occurs frequently during the course of parenteral nutrition, particularly while the glucose concentration of the infusate is being increased, but most patients will produce adequate endogenous insulin to metabolize the carbohydrate load within hours. The treatment of symptomatic hyperglycemia is usually reduction of the infusion rate. Hypoglycemia usually results from sudden interruption of an infusion containing a high glucose concentration.

High doses of fat or an accidental rapid infusion of fat may lead to fat overload syndrome, characterized by an acute febrile illness with jaundice and abnormal

Table 39.2. Mechanical complications of parenteral nutrition

Extravasation of parenteral nutrition solution
Blockage of the central venous line
Migration of the central venous line
Breakage of the infusion line
Right atrium thrombosis
Cardiac tamponade (perforation of right atrium or vena cava)

Table 39.3. Patient risk factors for the development of parenteral nutrition-related cholestasis

Age
Prematurity
Immaturity of biliary secretory system
Absence of oral/enteral intake
Septicemia
Bacterial overgrowth in the small bowel
Short bowel length
Necrotizing enterocolitis
Hypoxia
Major abdominal operations
General anesthesia

coagulation.[121,122] The intravenous administration of fat emulsion in premature infants seems to increase the incidence of bronchopulmonary dysplasia and retinopathy.[123] Peroxidation in stored fat emulsions, occlusion-stored fat emulsions, and the generation of free radicals during intravenous infusion of fat in premature infants have been reported.[124] The release of free radicals may overwhelm the endogenous protective mechanisms, resulting in cellular damage (see below).[125]

Mechanical complications
Mechanical complications related to the intravenous infusion of nutrients are not uncommon. Table 39.2 lists the mechanical complications reported in the literature. Extravasation of parenteral nutrition solution is a common complication of peripheral parenteral nutrition. Unfortunately, even a low osmolarity solution is detrimental for peripheral veins leading to inflammation and extravasation of the solution, which can cause tissue necrosis and infection. Intravenous lines may become clogged from thrombus formation, calcium precipitates, or lipid deposition. There is disagreement on the ideal position of central venous lines (CVL) for parenteral nutrition in infants. Some authors advocate the atrium as the ideal position because this would give less chance of catheter dysfunction.[126,127] Others believe that placement in the superior vena cava would reduce the risk of perforation.[128,129] In a survey of 587 CVL inserted in neonates,[130] cardiac tamponade was the cause of death in two neonates (0.3%). In most of the cases reported in literature of cardiac tamponade following CVL insertion the perforation was thought to be in the right atrium.[128,129,131]

Hepatic complications
The hepatobiliary complications related to parenteral nutrition remain serious and often life threatening. The commonest hepatobiliary complication of parenteral nutrition in surgical neonates is cholestasis. The incidence of parenteral nutrition-related cholestasis varies widely from as low as 7.4%[132] to as high as 84%.[133] Although the frequency of this complication seems to be diminishing,[134,135]

this is probably related to the early initiation of oral feeding rather than to an improvement in the intravenous diet. The etiology of cholestatic jaundice in infants requiring parenteral nutrition is still unclear. However, infants requiring long-term parenteral nutrition still develop progressive jaundice, commonly preceded by elevation of biochemical nonspecific tests of hepatic damage, function, and excretion.

Various clinical factors are thought to contribute to the development of parenteral nutrition-related cholestasis (Table 39.3). These include prematurity, low birth weight, duration of parenteral nutrition, immature enterohepatic circulation, intestinal microflora, septicemia, failure to implement enteral nutrition, and number of operations.[136–140] Parenteral nutrition-related cholestasis has a higher incidence in premature infants than in children and adults. This may be due to the immaturity of the biliary secretory system since bile salt pool size, synthesis, and intestinal concentration are low in premature infants in comparison with full-term infants.[141] Parenteral nutrition-related cholestasis is a diagnosis of exclusion without any specific marker yet available. Therefore, infants with cholestasis who are receiving or have received parenteral nutrition must have an appropriate diagnostic evaluation to exclude other causes of cholestasis. These include bacterial and viral infections, metabolic diseases, and congenital anomalies.[142] Gallbladder sludge, which can progress to "sludge balls" and gallstones, appeared in 18 neonates (44%) after a mean period of 10 days of parenteral nutrition.[143] The cholestasis is progressive unless parenteral nutrition is ceased and enteral feeding introduced. Hepatosplenomegaly and severe jaundice are characteristic features of the advanced disease, and portal hypertension may develop. Although parenteral nutrition-related cholestasis resolves with time after discontinuation of parenteral nutrition, in a small percentage of cases it remains intractable and progresses to severe hepatic dysfunction and death.[144]

The etiology of parenteral nutrition-related cholestasis remains unclear. Possible causes include the toxicity of components of parenteral nutrition, lack of enteral feeding, continuous nonpulsatile delivery of nutrients and host factors.[138,145] Most of the components of parenteral nutrition have been implicated in the pathogenesis of cholestasis. Hepatic damage from the components of intravenous diet may result from excessive nutrient administration, deficient nutrient administration, toxicity of byproducts,[146,147] and abnormal metabolism in the neonate.

The clinical care of infants and children who require parenteral nutrition and develop progressive jaundice represents a real challenge, compounded by this lack of knowledge. Prevention of parenteral nutrition-related cholestasis is based on the early usage of enteral feeding and on the administration of intravenous feeding only when appropriate and necessary. In most patients the cholestasis resolves gradually as enteral feedings are initiated and parenteral nutrition is discontinued. It has been recently shown that minimal bolus enteral feeding (1 ml kg^{-1}) during parenteral nutrition in premature infants induces significant gallbladder contraction and after 3 days of starting minimal enteral feeds, the gallbladder volume returns to normal.[148] Unfortunately, as a consequence of gut dysfunction, enteral feeding is often not feasible. Maini et al.[149] suggested that cycling the parenteral nutrition may diminish cholestatic hepatic changes in adults. This may explain the less frequent liver disease in children receiving their parenteral nutrition cyclically at home. Experience with this technique in premature infants is extremely limited but encouraging.[150,151] Rebound hypoglycaemia is a common complication of this approach. Modification of the parenteral nutrition constituents has been proposed but no prospective trial has demonstrated any benefit in reducing or changing the intake of nutrients.

Several reports have described the attempts to use drug therapy to treat or prevent parenteral nutrition-related cholestasis. Cholecystokinin has been administered to diminish the gallbladder stasis and promote bile flow. Sitzmann et al.[152] have demonstrated in a randomized, double-blind controlled study in adults receiving parenteral nutrition that cholecystokinin given intravenously daily prevents stasis and sludge in the gallbladder. Rintala et al.[153] reported the reversal of parenteral nutrition-related cholestasis in seven infants by intravenous administration of cholecystokinin; however all the patients except one were completely weaned from parenteral nutrition before

the treatment with cholecystokinin. Teitelbaum et al. conducted a prospective trial of cholecystokinin in the prevention of parenteral nutrition-related cholestasis;[154] however, the patients were consecutive rather than randomized and there is a need for a randomized controlled trial of cholecystokinin in administration to neonates on parenteral nutrition.

Ursodeoxycholic acid can be used in infants and children on parenteral nutrition to correct the decreased secretion of endogenous bile acids.[134] Ursodeoxycholic acid is nontoxic and acts as a natural bile acid after conjugation. Although there have been limited trials of the use of ursodeoxycholic acid in preterm neonates on TPN,[155] results were inconclusive.

Cholecystectomy is the treatment of choice for patients with acute and symptomatic cholelithiasis and cholecystitis. Rintala et al.[156] have proposed laparotomy and operative cholangiography followed by biliary tract irrigation in patients with progressive cholestatic jaundice not responding to medical treatment. In some patients the hepatic disease may progress to cirrhosis, portal hypertension, and hepatic failure. In selected cases small bowel and liver transplantation have been used. The introduction of tacrolimus has allowed clinical intestinal transplantation to become feasible. However, infectious and immunological problems still cause significant morbidity and mortality, even 1–3 years after transplantation.[157]

Free radicals and parenteral nutrition

Free radicals are highly reactive short-lived species in possession of an unpaired electron, and are produced during many physiological processes. When neutrophils and macrophages engulf foreign particles, the particle is exposed to superoxide and hydroxyl radicals and a variety of other reactive compounds during the so-called "respiratory burst," which occurs as the white cell destroys the bacteria. Intracellular and extracellular antioxidants protect against uncontrolled free radical activity. These include enzymes (e.g., superoxide dismutase, catalase, glutathione peroxidase) and chemical antioxidants such as vitamins E and C. A pathologic increase in free radical activity may occur when the normal balance between free radical formation and protective antioxidant activity becomes disrupted, and free radicals can then attack and damage cells and tissues. TPN may exacerbate free radical activity in newborn infants by providing (1) the substrates for free radical production (polyunsaturated fatty acids), (2) the initiators of free radical reactions (carbon-centered radicals derived from fatty acids), and (3) the catalysts (transition metal ions) for chain reactions. However, TPN also provides (1) vitamins C and E (antioxidants), (2) metal ions

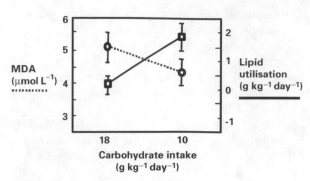

Figure 39.6. Free radical production (assessed as plasma malondialdehyde, MDA, concentration) in response to different carbohydrate contents of parenteral nutrition.[162]

that are important components of antioxidant enzymes (Cu, Zn, Mn, Se), (3) amino acids that are components of glutathione, and important intracellular antioxidants. An increased generation of free radicals during total parenteral nutrition (TPN) in premature infants was first reported by Wispe [158] and confirmed by other studies.[124,159,160] Bronchopulmonary dysplasia and retinopathy in premature infants are associated with fat infusions,[123,161] and these conditions have been linked to free radical-mediated cell damage. Reducing the exposure of premature infants to any unnecessary source of oxidative stress would be desirable. To this end it has been suggested that the use of intravenous fat infusion should be restricted;[123] however, we have shown that a reduction in the carbohydrate to fat ratio in PN diet will result in increased oxidation of administered fat and a decrease in free radical-mediated lipid peroxide formation (Figure 39.6).[162] It is interesting to note that the decrease in MDA accompanying increased fat utilization was of a similar magnitude to that observed when the fat infusion was discontinued. Therefore, it is not necessary to discontinue the infusion of fat to reduce the production of oxygen-derived free radicals. Manipulation of the carbohydrate to fat ratio therefore may be a powerful tool in changing the metabolism of fat infusions to mitigate their toxic effects while allowing continued administration.

Enteral nutrition

The energy requirement of an infant fed enterally is greater than the intravenous requirement because of the energetic cost of absorption from the gastrointestinal tract and energy lost in the stools. Even small amounts of enteral feeding allow the preservation of normal intestinal villi and the maintenance of the epithelial barrier function. Clinical[163,164] and labora-

tory [113,165–169] studies have shown that enteral feeding is associated with less infectious and immunological complications than parenteral nutrition. Moore et al.[164] demonstrated that patients receiving total enteral feeding experienced significantly fewer septic complications than patients on parenteral plus enteral nutrition. Kudsk et al. [165,166] showed that enteral feeding improved survival after hemoglobin-*Escherichia coli* peritonitis in both malnourished and well-nourished rats, compared with rats receiving total PN. The reason for these findings remains poorly understood. However, enteral feeding may act by stimulating a more effective immune response. Alverdy et al.[113] documented in a rodent model that enteral feeding maintains normal biliary concentrations of secretory IgA (S-IgA), which is an important component of mucosal immunity. In contrast, total parenteral nutrition decreases the biliary levels of this immunoglobulin. Furthermore, Lin et al.[169] demonstrated that the level of TNF-α in peritoneal lavage fluid was higher in enterally fed rats than in rats receiving total PN after 2 hours peritoneal bacterial challenge. TNF-α, which is mainly produced by macrophages, and lymphocytes, is an important factor in the activation of neutrophils, macrophages, and lymphocytes and may therefore be required for effective eradication of bacterial infections.

In surgical infants, enteral feeding often results in vomiting, interruption of feeding, inadequate calorie intake and rarely in necrotizing enterocolitis. In infants with congenital gastrointestinal anomalies, exclusive enteral feeding is commonly precluded for some time after surgery due to large gastric aspirate and intestinal dysmotility. Therefore, appropriate calorie intake is established initially by total parenteral nutrition. Supplementary enteral feeding is introduced when intestinal motility and absorption improves. The percentage of calories given enterally is gradually increased at the expense of intravenous calorie intake. This transition time from total parenteral nutrition to total enteral feeding could be quite long. The presence of significant gastric aspirate often induces clinicians and surgeons not to use the gut for nutrition. However, minimal enteral feeding can be implemented early in these patients even if its nutritional value is questionable. Minimal enteral feeding may be all that is required to enhance some immunological function. This is supported by studies in animals[170] and infants.[116] Shou et al.[170] reported that supplementation of parenteral nutrition with just 10% enteral calories as cow diet improved rat macrophage and splenocyte function. Okada et al.[116] have shown that the introduction of small volumes of enteral feed improved the impaired host bactericidal activity against coagulase negative staphylococci and the abnormal cytokine response observed during total parenteral nutrition. The increase in bactericidal activity against coagulase negative staphylococci after the addition of small enteral feeds in patients on parenteral nutrition was significantly correlated with the duration of enteral feeding. This implies that stimulation of the gastrointestinal tract may modulate immune function in neonates and prevent bacterial infection.

Feeding routes

Oral feeding is the preferred modality of feeding, with breast-feeding being the best physiological method up to 6 months of age. Surgical infants do not always tolerate oral feeding due to prematurity, critical illness, abnormalities of the swallowing mechanism, esophageal dysmotility, gastro-esophageal reflux or gastric outlet obstruction. Alternative feeding routes in these clinical situations include naso-gastric or oro-gastric tubes, naso-jejunal tubes, gastrostomy tubes, or jejunostomy tubes.

Gastric feeding is preferable to intestinal feeding because it allows for a more natural digestive process. In addition gastric feeding is associated with a larger osmotic and volume tolerance and a lower frequency of diarrhoea and dumping syndrome. Neonates are obligatory nose breathers and therefore oro-gastric feeding is preferable over naso-gastric feeding in preterm infants to avoid upper airway obstruction.

In surgical infants requiring gastric tube feeding for more than 6–8 weeks it is advisable to insert a gastrostomy tube. The tube can be inserted using an open, endoscopic or laparoscopic approach. In infants with significant gastro-esophageal reflux, fundoplication with gastrostomy tube or enterostomy tube placement is indicated. In preterm infants with gastro-esophageal reflux, enteral feeding can be established via a naso-jejunal tube inserted under fluoroscopy. Naso-jejunal feeding usually minimizes the episodes of gastro-oesophageal reflux and their consequences. However, it is common for these tubes to dislocate back in the stomach. Regular analysis of the pH in the aspirate is essential to monitor the correct position of the tube. Feeding jejunostomy tubes can be inserted through an existing gastrostomy or directly into the jejunum via laparotomy or laparoscopy.

Selection of enteral feeds

Breast milk is the ideal feed for infants because it has specific anti-infectious activities,[171] which protect them from gastrointestinal and respiratory diseases. In addition breast milk has high content of nonprotein metabolizable nitrogen notably urea.[172] When breast milk is not available chemically defined formulae can be used. If malabsorption persists, an appropriate specific formula should be introduced. A soy-based disaccharide-free feed is used when there is disaccharide intolerance resulting in loose stools containing disaccharides. For fat malabsorption, a formula containing medium-chain triglycerides (MCT) should be used. An elemental formula may be indicated when there is severe malabsorption due to short bowel syndrome or severe mucosal damage as in necrotizing enterocolitis. Infants recovering from neonatal necrotizing enterocolitis pose a particular problem, as malabsorption may be severe and prolonged. These infants may have had small bowel resected, in addition to which the remaining bowel may not have healed completely by the time feeds are begun. Feeding may provoke a relapse of the necrotising enterocolitis and feeding should therefore be introduced cautiously. Elemental formula preparations contain amino acids, glucose, and fats, including MCTs. Dipeptide preparations which include dipeptides as well as amino acids have the advantage of a lower osmolality, are well absorbed and have a more palatable taste.[173]

For persistent severe malabsorption, a modular diet may be necessary.[174,175] Glucose, amino acid, and MCT preparations are provided separately, beginning with the amino acid solution and adding the glucose and then the fats as tolerated. Minerals, trace elements, and vitamins are also added. These solutions have a high osmolality and if given too quickly may precipitate dumping syndrome, with diarrhoea, abdominal cramps, and hypoglycemia. It is important therefore to start with a dilute solution and increase slowly the concentration and volume of each component. This may take several weeks and infants will need parenteral nutritional support during this period.

Administration of enteral feeds

Enteral feeds can be administered as boluses, continuous feeds or combination of the two. Bolus feeds are more physiological and are known to stimulate intestinal motility, enterohepatic circulation of bile acids, and gallbladder contraction.[176] They mimic or supplement meals and are easier to administer than continuous feeds since a feeding pump is not required. Bolus feeds are usually given over 15–20 minutes and usually every 3 hours. In preterm neonates or in neonates soon after surgery 2-hourly feeds are occasionally given.

Continuous feeds should be administered via an infusion pump. This modality of feeding is used in infants with gastro-esophageal reflux, delayed gastric emptying, or intestinal malabsorption. Infants with a jejunal tube should receive continuous feeds and not bolus feeds. Continuous feedings are usually given over 24 hours. Term infants can tolerate a period of 4 hours without feeds before hypoglycemia occurs. This modality of tube feeding can be very advantageous, however, there is evidence to suggest that normal physiology may be altered when this approach is adopted. Jawaheer et al.[177] have shown that continuous enteral feeding leads to an enlarged, noncontractile gallbladder in infants. Contraction is observed immediately after resuming bolus enteral feeds and gallbladder volume returns to baseline after 4 days. Therefore the mode of feeding has important bearings on the motility of the extrahepatic biliary tree. Studies in adults[178–180] have reported biliary sludging in patients receiving continuous enteral nutrition, implying gallbladder stasis. In one study[180] the sludge cleared within 2 weeks of starting bolus oral feeds. This complication has not been reported in infants or children undergoing continuous enteral feeding. In preterm infants, continuous enteral feedings are associated with lower energy expenditure and better growth compared with bolus feedings.

Complications of enteral tube feeding

Enteral tube feeding is associated with fewer complications than parenteral feeding. The complications can be mechanical including tube blockage, tube displacement or migration and intestinal perforation. Other complications involve the gastrointestinal tract. These include: gastroesophageal reflux with aspiration pneumonia, dumping syndrome, and diarrhoea. Jejunostomy tubes inserted at laparotomy can be also associated with intestinal obstruction. The use of hyperosmolar feeds has been associated with development of necrotizing enterocolitis, dehydration, and rarely intestinal obstruction due to milk curds.

REFERENCES

1 Swyer, P. R., Heim, T. F. Nutrition, body fluids, and acid-base homeostasis. In Fanaroff, A. A., Martin, R. J., eds. *Neonatal–perinatal Medicine*. St. Louis, MO; 1987:445–60.

2 Coran, A. G. Nutrition of the surgical patient. In Welch, K. J., Randolph, J. G., Reed, D. J., eds. *Pediatric Surgery*. Chicago, IL; 1986:96–108.

3 Elman, R. Amino acid content of blood following intravenous injection of hydrolyzed casein. *Proc. Soc. Exp. Biol. Med.* 2937;**37**:437.

4 Helfrick, F. W., Abelson, N. M. Intravenous feeding of a complete diet in a child: report of a case. *J. Parenter. Enteral Nutr.* 1978;**2**:688–9.

5 Dudrick, S. J., Wilmore, D. W., Vars, H. M., Rhoads, J. E. Long-term total parenteral nutrition with growth, development, and positive nitrogen balance. *Surgery* 1968;**64**:134–42.

6 Filler, R. M., Eraklis, A. J., Rubin, V. G., Das, J. B. Long-term total parenteral nutrition in infants. *New Engl. J. Med.* 1969;**281**:589–94.

7 Teitelbaum, D. H., Coran, A. G. Perioperative nutritional support in pediatrics. *Nutrition* 1998;**14**:130–42.

8 Pierro, A., Carnielli, V., Filler, R. M. *et al.*. Partition of energy metabolism in the surgical newborn. *J. Pediatr. Surg.* 1991;**26**:581–6.

9 Freymond, D., Schutz, Y., Decombaz, J., Micheli, J. L., Jequier, E. Energy-balance, physical-activity, and thermogenic effect of feeding in premature-infants. *Pediatr. Res.* 1986;**20**:638–45.

10 ESPGAN Committee on Nutrition. Nutrition and feeding of preterm infants. *Acta Paediatr. Scand.* 1987;Suppl. 386.

11 Cunningham, J. J. Body composition as a determinant of energy expenditure: a synthetic review and a proposed general prediction equation. *Am. J. Clin. Nutr.* 1991;**54**:963–9.

12 Pierro, A., Jones, M. O., Hammond, P., Donnell, S. C., Lloyd, D. A. A new equation to predict the resting energy expenditure of surgical infants. *J. Pediatr. Surg.* 1994;**29**:1103–8.

13 Hill, A. G., Hill, G. L. Metabolic response to severe injury. *Br. J. Surg.* 1998;**85**:884–90.

14 Jones, M. O., Pierro, A., Hammond, P., Lloyd, D. A. The metabolic response to operative stress in infants. *J. Pediatr. Surg.* 1993a;**28**:1258–62.

15 Shanbhogue, R. L. K., Lloyd, D. A. Absence of hypermetabolism after operation in the newborn-infant. *J. Parenter. Enteral Nutr.* 1992;**16**:333–6.

16 Anand, K. J., Sippell, W. G., Aynsley-Green, A. Randomised trial of fentanyl anaesthesia in preterm babies undergoing surgery: effects on the stress response. *Lancet* 1987;**1**:62–6.

17 Chwals, W. J., Letton, R. W., Jamie, A., Charles, B. Stratification of injury severity using energy-expenditure response in surgical infants. *J. Pediatr. Surg.* 1995;**30**:1161–4.

18 Anand, K. J., Hickey, P. R. Halothane-morphine compared with high-dose sufentanil for anesthesia and postoperative analgesia in neonatal cardiac surgery. *New Engl. J. Med.* 1992;**326**:1–9.

19 Facchinetti, F., Bagnoli, F., Bracci, R., Genazzani, A. R. Plasma opioids in the first hours of life. *Pediatr. Res.* 1982;**16**:95–8.

20 Harrison, R. A., Lewin, M. R., Halliday, D., Clark, C. G. Leucine kinetics in surgical patients. II: A study of the effect of malignant disease and tumour burden. *Br. J. Surg.* 1989;**76**:509–11.

21 Carli, F., Webster, J., Pearson, M. *et al.* Postoperative protein metabolism: effect of nursing elderly patients for 24 h after abdominal surgery in a thermoneutral environment. *Br. J. Anaesth.* 1991;**66**:292–9.

22 Essen, P., McNurlan, M. A., Wernerman, J., Vinnars, E., Garlick, P. J. Uncomplicated surgery, but not general anesthesia, decreases muscle protein synthesis. *Am. J. Physiol.* 1992;**262**:E253–60.

23 Powis, M. R., Smith, K., Rennie, M., Halliday, D., Pierro, A. Effect of major abdominal operations on energy and

protein metabolism in infants and children. *J. Pediatr. Surg.* 1998;**33**:49–53.

24 Powis, M. R., Smith, K., Rennie, M., Halliday, D., Pierro, A. Characteristics of protein and energy metabolism in neonates with necrotizing enterocolitis – a pilot study. *J. Pediatr. Surg.* 1999;**34**:5–10.

25 Groner, J. I., Brown, M. F., Stallings, V. A., Ziegler, M. M., O'Neill-Ja, J. Resting energy expenditure in children following major operative procedures. *J. Pediatr. Surg.* 1989;**24**:825–7.

26 Keshen, T. H., Miller, R. G., Jahoor, F., Jaksic, T. Stable isotopic quantitation of protein metabolism and energy expenditure in neonates on- and post-extracorporeal life support. *J. Pediatr. Surg.* 1997;**32**:958–62.

27 Vlessis, A., Goldman, R., Trunkey, D. New concepts in the pathophysiology of oxygen-metabolism during sepsis. *Br. J. Surg.* 1995;**82**:870–6.

28 Plank, L. D., Connolly, A. B., Hill, G. L. Sequential changes in the metabolic response in severely septic patients during the first 23 days after the onset of peritonitis. *Ann. Surg.* 1998;**228**: 146–58.

29 Takala, J., Pitkanen, O. Nutrition support in trauma and sepsis. In Payne-James, J., Grimble, G., Silk, D., eds. *Artificial Nutrition in Support in Clinical Practice*. London: Edward Arnold; 1995:403–13.

30 Wolfe, R. R., Herndon, D. N., Jahoor, F., Miyoshi, H., Wolfe, M. Effect of severe burn injury on substrate cycling by glucose and fatty-acids. *New Engl. J. Med.* 1987;**317**:403–8.

31 Giovannini, I., Boldrini, G., Castagneto, M. *et al*. Respiratory quotient and patterns of substrate utilization in human sepsis and trauma. *J. Parenter. Enteral Nutr.* 1983;**7**:226–30.

32 Samra, J. S., Summers, L. K. M., Frayn, K. N. Sepsis and fat metabolism. *Br. J. Surg.* 1996;**83**:1186–96.

33 Tilden, S. J., Watkins, S., Tong, T. K., Jeevanandam, M. Measured energy-expenditure in pediatric intensive-care patients. *Am. J. Dis. Child.* 1989;**143**:490–2.

34 Phillips, R., Ott, L., Young, B., Walsh, J. Nutritional support and measured energy expenditure of the child and adolescent with head injury. *J. Neurosurg.* 1987;**67**:846–51.

35 White, M. S., Shepherd, R. W., McEniery, J. A. Energy expenditure in 100 ventilated, critically ill children: improving the accuracy of predictive equations. *Crit. Care Med.* 2000;**28**:2307–12.

36 Briassoulis, G., Venkataraman, S., Thompson, A. E. Energy expenditure in critically ill children. *Crit. Care Med.* 2000;**28**:1166–72.

37 Chwals, W. J., Lally, K. P., Woolley, M. M., Mahour, G. H. Measured energy expenditure in critically ill infants and young children. *J. Surg. Res.* 1988;**44**:467–72.

38 Jaksic, T., Shew, S. B., Keshen, T. H., Dzakovic, A., Jahoor, F. Do critically ill surgical neonates have increased energy expenditure? *J. Pediatr. Surg.* 2001;**36**:63–7.

39 Coss-Bu, J. A., Klish, W. J., Walding, D. *et al.*. Energy metabolism, nitrogen balance, and substrate utilization in critically ill children. *Am. J. Clin. Nutr.* 2001;**74**:664–9.

40 Turi, R. A., Petros, A., Eaton, S. *et al*. Energy metabolism of infants and children with systemic inflammatory response syndrome and sepsis. *Ann. Surg.* 2001;**233**:581–7.

41 Taylor, R. M., Cheeseman, P., Preedy, V. R., Baker, A. J., Grimble, G. K. Can energy expenditure be predicted in critically ill children? *Pediatr. Crit. Care Med.* 2003;**4**:176–80.

42 Kerner, J. A. Carbohydrate requirements. In Kerner, J. A., ed. *Manual of Pediatric Parenteral Nutrition*. New York, NY: John Wiley & Sons; 1983:79–88.

43 Stein, T. P. Why measure the respiratory quotient of patients on total parenteral nutrition? *J. Am. Coll. Nutr.* 1985;**4**:501–13.

44 Askanazi, J., Nordenstrom, J., Rosenbaum, S. H. *et al*. Nutrition for the patient with respiratory failure: glucose vs. fat. *Anesthesiology* 1981;**54**:373–7.

45 Cooke, R. J., Yeh, Y. Y., Gibson, D., Debo, D., Bell, G. L. Soybean oil emulsion administration during parenteral nutrition in the preterm infant: effect on essential fatty acid, lipid, and glucose metabolism. *J. Pediatr.* 1987;**111**:767–73.

46 Gutcher, G. R., Farrell, P. M. Intravenous infusion of lipid for the prevention of essential fatty acid deficiency in premature infants. *Am. J. Clin. Nutr.* 1991;**54**:1024–8.

47 Borresen, H. C., Coran, A. G., Knutrud, O. Metabolic results of parenteral feeding in neonatal surgery: a balanced parenteral feeding program based on a synthetic l-amino acid solution and a commercial fat emulsion. *Ann. Surg.* 1970;**172**:291–301.

48 Nordenstrom, J., Carpentier, Y. A., Askanazi, J. *et al*. Metabolic utilization of intravenous fat emulsion during total parenteral nutrition. *Ann. Surg.* 1982;**196**:221–31.

49 Nose, O., Tipton, J. R., Ament, M. E., Yabuuchi, H. Effect of the energy source on changes in energy expenditure, respiratory quotient, and nitrogen balance during total parenteral nutrition in children. *Pediatr. Res.* 1987;**21**:538–41.

50 van Aerde, J. E., Sauer, P. J., Pencharz, P. B., Smith, J. M., Swyer, P. R. Effect of replacing glucose with lipid on the energy metabolism of newborn infants. *Clin. Sci.* 1989;**76**:581–8.

51 Jones, M. O., Pierro, A., Hammond, P., Nunn, A., Lloyd, D. A. Glucose utilization in the surgical newborn infant receiving total parenteral nutrition. *J. Pediatr. Surg.* 1993b;**28**:1121–5.

52 Pierro, A., Jones, M. O., Hammond, P., Nunn, A., Lloyd, D. A. *Utilization of intravenous fat in the surgical newborn infant*. Proceedings of the Nutrition Society; 1993;**52**:237A.

53 Pierro, A., Carnielli, V., Filler, R. M., Smith, J., Heim, T. Metabolism of intravenous fat emulsion in the surgical newborn. *J. Pediatr. Surg.* 1989;**24**:95–101.

54 Heim, T., Putet, G., Verellen, G. *et al*. Energy cost of intravenous alimentation in the newborn infant. In Stern, L., Salle, B., Friis-Hansen, B., eds. *Intensive Care in the Newborn Vol. 3*. New York, NY: Masson; 1981:219–37.

55 Helms, R. A., Whitington, P. F., Mauer, E. C. *et al*. Enhanced lipid utilization in infants receiving oral L-carnitine during long-term parenteral nutrition. *J. Pediatr.* 1986;**109**:984–8.

56 Tibboel, D., Delemarre, F. M., Przyrembel, H. Carnitine deficiency in surgical neonates receiving total parenteral nutrition. *J. Pediatr. Surg.* 1990;**25**:418–21.

57 Eaton, S. Control of mitochondrial β-oxidation flux. *Prog. Lipid Res.* 2002;**41**:197–239.

58 Heinonen, O. J., Takala, J. Moderate carnitine depletion and long-chain fatty-acid oxidation, exercise capacity, and nitrogen-balance in the rat. *Pediatr. Res.* 1994;**36**:288–92.

59 Cairns, P. A., Stalker, D. J. Carnitine supplementation of parenterally fed neonates (Cochrane Review). *The Cochrane Library Issue* **4**, 2002.

60 Ulrich, H., Pastores, S. M., Katz, D. P., Kvetan, V. Parenteral use of medium-chain triglycerides: a reappraisal. *Nutrition* 1996;**12**:231–8.

61 Lai, H. S., Chen, W. J. Effects of medium-chain and long-chain triacylglycerols in pediatric surgical patients. *Nutrition* 2000;**16**:401–6.

62 Papavassilis, C. Use of medium-chain triacylglycerols in parenteral nutrition of children. *Nutrition* 2000;**16**:460–1.

63 Donnell, S. C., Lloyd, D. A., Eaton, S., Pierro, A. The metabolic response to intravenous medium-chain triglycerides in infants after surgery. *J. Pediatr.* 2002;**141**:689–94.

64 Snyderman, S. E., Boyer, A., Kogut, M. D., Holt, L. E. J. The protein requirement of the premature infant. I. The effect of protein intake on the retention of nitrogen. *J. Pedia.* 1969;**74**:872–80.

65 Zlotkin, S. H., Bryan, M. H., Anderson, G. H. Intravenous nitrogen and energy intakes required to duplicate in utero nitrogen accretion in prematurely born human infants. *J. Pediatri.* 1981;**99**:115–20.

66 Catzeflis, C., Schutz, Y., Micheli, J. L. *et al.* Whole-body protein-synthesis and energy-expenditure in very low birth-weight infants. *Pediatr. Res.* 1985;**19**:679–87.

67 Garlick, P. J., Clugston, G. A., Swick, R. W., Waterlow, J. C. Diurnal pattern of protein and energy metabolism in man. *Am. J. Clin. Nutr.* 1980;**33**:1983–6.

68 Golden, M., Waterlow, J. C., Picou, D. The relationship between dietary intake, weight change, nitrogen balance, and protein turnover in man. *Am. J. Clin. Nutr.* 1977;**30**:1345–8.

69 Pencharz, P. B., Masson, M., Desgranges, F., Papageorgiou, A. Total-body protein-turnover in human premature neonates – effects of birth-weight, intrauterine nutritional-status and diet. *Clin. Sci.* 1981;**61**:207–15.

70 Zlotkin, S. H., Stallings, V. A., Pencharz, P. B. Total parenteral nutrition in children. *Pediatr. Clin. N. Am.* 1985;**32**:381–400.

71 American Academy of Pediatrics Committee on Nutrition. Commentary on parenteral nutrition. *Pediatrics* 1983;**71**:547–52.

72 Chessex, P., Gagne, G., Pineault, M. *et al.* Metabolic and clinical consequences of changing from high-glucose to high-fat regimens in parenterally fed newborn-infants. *J. Pediatr.* 1989;**115**:992–7.

73 Long, J. M., Wilmore, D. W., Mason, J., Pruitt, J. Effect of carbohydrate and fat intake on nitrogen excretion during total intravenous feeding. *Ann. Surg.* 1977;**185**:417–22.

74 Tulikoura, I., Huikuri, K. Changes in nitrogen metabolism in catabolic patients given three different parenteral nutrition regimens. *Acta Chir. Scand.* 1981;**147**:519–24.

75 Rubecz, I., Mestyan, J., Varga, P., Klujber, L. Energy metabolism, substrate utilization, and nitrogen balance in parenterally fed postoperative neonates and infants. The effect of glucose, glucose + amino acids, lipid + amino acids infused in isocaloric amounts. *J. Pediatr.* 1981;**98**:42–6.

76 Bark, S., Holm, I., Hakansson, I., Wretlind, A. Nitrogen-sparing effect of fat emulsion compared with glucose in the postoperative period. *Acta Chir. Scand.* 1976;**142**:423–7.

77 Pierro, A., Carnielli, V., Filler, R. M., Smith, J., Heim, T. Characteristics of protein sparing effect of total parenteral nutrition in the surgical infant. *J. Pediatr. Surg.* 1988;**23**:538–42.

78 Jones, M. O., Pierro, A., Garlick, P. J. *et al.* Protein metabolism kinetics in neonates: effect of intravenous carbohydrate and fat. *J. Pediatr. Surg.* 1995;**30**:458–62.

79 Pierro, A., Jones, M., Garlick, P. *et al.* Nonprotein energy-intake during total parenteral-nutrition – effect on protein-turnover and energy-metabolism. *Clin. Nutr.* 1995;**14**:47–9.

80 Marconi, A. M., Battaglia, F. C., Meschia, G., Sparks, J. W. A comparison of amino acid arteriovenous differences across the liver and placenta of the fetal lamb. *Am. J. Physiol.* 1989;**257**:E909–15.

81 Souba, W. W., Austgen, T. R. Interorgan glutamine flow following surgery and infection. *J. Parenter. Enteral Nutr.* 1990;**14**:90S–3S.

82 Lacey, J. M., Wilmore, D. W. Is glutamine a conditionally essential amino acid? *Nutr. Rev.* 1990;**48**:297–309.

83 Windmueller, H. G., Spaeth, A. E. Uptake and metabolism of plasma glutamine by the small intestine. *J. Biol. Chem.* 1974;**249**:5070–9.

84 McAnena, O. J., Moore, F. A., Moore, E. E., Jones, T. N., Parsons, P. Selective uptake of glutamine in the gastrointestinal tract: confirmation in a human study. *Br. J. Surg.* 1991;**78**:480–2.

85 Furst, P., Pogan, K., Stehle, P. Glutamine dipeptides in clinical nutrition. *Nutrition* 1997;**13**:731–7.

86 Ziegler, T. R., Young, L. S., Benfell, K. *et al.* Clinical and metabolic efficacy of glutamine-supplemented parenteral nutrition after bone marrow transplantation. A randomized, double-blind, controlled study. *Ann. Intern. Med.* 1992;**116**:821–8.

87 Chang, W. K., Yang, K. D., Shaio, M. F. Effect of glutamine on Th1 and Th2 cytokine responses of human peripheral blood mononuclear cells. *Clin. Immunol.* 1999;**93**:294–301.

88 Dewitt, R. C., Wu, Y., Renegar, K. B., Kudsk, K. A. Glutamine-enriched total parenteral nutrition preserves respiratory immunity and improves survival to a *Pseudomonas* pneumonia. *J. Surg. Res.* 1999;**84**:13–18.

89 Houdijk, A. P. J., Rijnsburger, E. R., Jansen, J. *et al.* Randomised trial of glutamine-enriched enteral nutrition on infectious morbidity in patients with multiple trauma. *Lancet* 1998;**352**:772–6

90 Griffiths, R. D., Jones, C., Palmer, T. E. A. Six-month outcome of critically ill patients given glutamine-supplemented parenteral nutrition. *Nutrition* 1997;**13**:295–302.

91 Wilmore, D. W., Smith, R. J., O'Dwyer, S. T. *et al.* The gut: a central organ after surgical stress. *Surgery* 1988;**104**:917–23.

92 Burke, D. J., Alverdy, J. C., Aoys, E., Moss, G. S. Glutamine-supplemented total parenteral nutrition improves gut immune function. *Arch. Surg.* 1989;**124**:1396–9.

93 Inoue, Y., Grant, J. P., Snyder, P. J. Effect of glutamine-supplemented intravenous nutrition on survival after *Escherichia coli*-induced peritonitis. *J. Parenter. Enteral Nutr.* 1993;**17**:41–6.

94 Jiang, Z. M., Wang, L. J., Qi, Y. *et al.* Comparison of parenteral nutrition supplemented with L-glutamine or glutamine dipeptides. *J. Parenter. Enteral Nutr.* 1993;**17**:134–41.

95 Tremel, H., Kienle, B., Weilemann, L. S., Stehle, P., Furst, P. Glutamine dipeptide-supplemented parenteral-nutrition maintains intestinal function in the critically ill. *Gastroenterology* 1994;**107**:1595–601.

96 Allen, S. J., Pierro, A., Cope, L. *et al.* Glutamine-supplemented parenteral-nutrition in a child with short- bowel syndrome. *J. Pediatr. Gastroenterol. Nutr.* 1993;**17**:329–32.

97 van der Hulst, R. R., van Kreel, B. K., von Meyenfeldt, M. F. *et al.* Glutamine and the preservation of gut integrity. *Lancet* 1993;**341**:1363–5.

98 Stehle, P., Zander, J., Mertes, N. *et al.* Effect of parenteral glutamine peptide supplements on muscle glutamine loss and nitrogen balance after major surgery. *Lancet* 1989;**1**:231–3.

99 Markley, M. A., Pierro, A., Eaton, S. Hepatocyte mitochondrial metabolism is inhibited in neonatal rat endotoxaemia: effects of glutamine. *Clin. Sci.* 2002;**102**:337–44.

100 Babu, R., Eaton, S., Drake, D. P., Spitz, L., Pierro, A. Glutamine and glutathione counteract the inhibitory effects of mediators of sepsis in neonatal hepatocytes. *J. Pediatr. Surg.* 2001;**36**:282–6.

101 Tubman, T. R. J., Thompson, S. W. *Glutamine supplementation for preventing morbidity in preterm infants (Cochrane Review)*. Oxford, England: The Cochrane Library Update Software; 2001:1.

102 Lacey, J. M., Crouch, J. B., Benfell, K. *et al.* The effects of glutamine-supplemented parenteral nutrition in premature infants. *J. Parenter. Enteral Nutr.* 1996;**20**:74–80.

103 Neu, J., Roig, J. C., Meetze, W. H. *et al.* Enteral glutamine supplementation for very low birth weight infants decreases morbidity. *J. Pediatr.* 1997;**131**:691–9.

104 Laborie, S., Lavoie, J. C., Chessex, P. Increased urinary peroxides in newborn infants receiving parenteral nutrition exposed to light. *J. Pediatr.* 2000;**136**:628–32.

105 Laborie, S., Lavoie, J. C., Pineault, M., Chessex, P. Contribution of multivitamins, air, and light in the generation of peroxides in adult and neonatal parenteral nutrition solutions. *Ann. Pharmacother.* 2000;**34**:440–5.

106 Lavoie, J. C., Belanger, S., Spalinger, M., Chessex, P. Admixture of a multivitamin preparation to parenteral nutrition: The major contributor to in vitro generation of peroxides. *Pediatrics* 1997;**99**:E61–5.

107 Silvers, K. M., Sluis, K. B., Darlow, B. A. *et al.*. Limiting light-induced lipid peroxidation and vitamin loss in infant par-

enteral nutrition by adding multivitamin preparations to Intralipid. *Acta Paediatr.* 2001;**90**:242–9.

108 Bos, A. P., Tibboel, D., Hazebroek, F. W. *et al.* Total parenteral nutrition associated cholestasis: a predisposing factor for sepsis in surgical neonates? *Eur. J. Pediatr.* 1990;**149**:351–3.

109 Wesley, J. R., Coran, A. G. Intravenous nutrition for the pediatric patient. *Semin. Pediatr. Surg.* 1992;**1**:212–30.

110 Seashore, J. H. Central venous access devices in children: trends over 543 patient years. *Clin. Nutr.* 1994;**13**:27–A079.

111 Pierro, A., van Saene, H. K. F., Donnell, S. C. *et al.* Microbial translocation in neonates and infants receiving long-term parenteral-nutrition. *Arch. Surg.* 1996;**131**:176–9.

112 Pierro, A., van Saene, H. K. F., Jones, M. O. *et al.* Clinical impact of abnormal gut flora in infants receiving parenteral nutrition. *Ann. Surg.* 1998;**227**:547–52.

113 Alverdy, J. C., Aoys, E., Moss, G. S. Total parenteral nutrition promotes bacterial translocation from the gut. *Surgery* 1988;**104**:185–90.

114 Okada, Y., Klein, N. J., Pierro, A. Peter Paul Rickham Prize – 1998. Neutrophil dysfunction: the cellular mechanism of impaired immunity during total parenteral nutrition in infancy. *J. Pediatr. Surg.* 1999;**34**:242–5.

115 Okada, Y., Klein, N. J., van Saene, H. K. *et al.*. Bactericidal activity against coagulase-negative staphylococci is impaired in infants receiving long-term parenteral nutrition. *Ann. Surg.* 2000;**231**:276–81.

116 Okada, Y., Klein, N., van Saene, H. K., Pierro, A. Small volumes of enteral feedings normalise immune function in infants receiving parenteral nutrition. *J. Pediatr. Surg.* 1998;**33**:16–19.

117 Monson, J. R., Ramsden, C. W., MacFie, J., Brennan, T. G., Guillou, P. J. Immunorestorative effect of lipid emulsions during total parenteral nutrition. *Br. J. Surg.* 1986;**73**:843–6.

118 Sedman, P. C., Somers, S. S., Ramsden, C. W., Brennan, T. G., Guillou, P. J. Effects of different lipid emulsions on lymphocyte function during total parenteral nutrition. *Br. J. Surg.* 1991;**78**:1396–9.

119 Palmblad, J., Brostrom, O., Lahnborg, G., Uden, A. M., Venizelos, N. Neutrophil functions during total parenteral nutrition and intralipid infusion. *Am. J. Clin. Nutr.* 1982;**35**:1430–6.

120 Fisher, G. W., Hunter, K. W., Wilson, S. R., Mease, A. D. Diminished bacterial defences with intralipid. *Lancet* 1980;**2**:819–20.

121 Heyman, M. B., Storch, S., Ament, M. E. The fat overload syndrome. Report of a case and literature review. *Am. J. Dis. Child.* 1981;**135**:628–30.

122 Wesson, D. E., Hampton Rich, R., Zlotkin, S. H., Pencharz, P. B. Fat overload syndrome causing respiratory insufficiency. *J. Pediatr. Surg.* 1984;**19**:777–8.

123 Hammerman, C., Aramburo, M. J. Decreased lipid intake reduces morbidity in sick premature neonates. *J. Pediatr.* 1988;**113**:1083–8.

124 Pitkanen, O., Hallman, M., Andersson, S. Generation of free-radicals in lipid emulsion used in parenteral-nutrition. *Pediatr. Res.* 1991;**29**:56–9.

125 Hinder, R. A., Stein, H. J. Oxygen-derived free radicals. *Arch. Surg.* 1991;**126**:104–5.

126 Brandt, R. L., Foley, W. J., Fink, G. H., Regan, W. J. Mechanism of perforation of the heart with production of hydropericdium by a venous catheter and its prevention. *Am. J. Surg.* 1970;**119**:311–6.

127 Lucas, H., Attard-Montalto, S. P., Saha, V. Central venous catheter tip position and malfunction in a paediatric oncology unit. *Pediatr. Surg. Int.* 1996;**11**:159–63.

128 Bar, J. G., Galvis, A. G. Perforation of the heart by central venous catheters in infants: guidelines to diagnosis and management. *J. Pediatr. Surg.* 1983;**18**:284–7.

129 van Engelenburg, K. C., Festen, C. Cardiac tamponade: a rare but life-threatening complication of central venous catheters in children. *J. Pediatr. Surg.* 1998;**33**:1822–4.

130 Goutail-Flaud, M. F., Sfez, M., Berg, A. *et al.* Central venous catheter-related complications in newborns and infants: a 587-case survey. *J. Pediatr. Surg.* 1991;**26**:645–50.

131 Bagwell, C. E., Salzberg, A. M., Sonnino, R. E., Haynes, J. H. Potentially lethal complications of central venous catheter placement. *J. Pediatr. Surg.* 2000;**35**:709–13.

132 Bell, R. L., Ferry, G. D., Smith, E. O. Total parenteral nutrition-related cholestasis in infants. *J. Parenter. Enteral Nutr.* 1986;**10**:356–9.

133 Cohen, D., Olsen, M. Pediatric total parenteral nutrition. Liver histopathology. *Arch. Pathol. Lab. Med.* 1981;**105**:152–6.

134 Hofmann, A. F. Defective biliary secretion during total parenteral nutrition: probable mechanisms and possible solutions. *J. Pediatr. Gastroenterol. Nutr.* 1995;**20**:376–90.

135 Kubota, A., Yonekura, T., Hoki, M. *et al.* Total parenteral nutrition-associated intrahepatic cholestasis in infants: 25 years' experience. *J. Pediatr. Surg.* 2000;**35**:1049–51.

136 Drongowski, R. A., Coran, A. G. An analysis of factors contributing to the development of total parenteral nutrition-induced cholestasis. *J. Parenter. Enteral Nutr.* 1989;**13**:586–9.

137 Quigley, E. M. M., Marsh, M. N., Shaffer, J. L. *et al.* Hepatobiliary complications of total parenteral nutrition. *Gastroenterology* 1993;**104**:286–301.

138 Teitelbaum, D. H., Tracy, T. Parenteral nutrition-associated cholestasis. *Semin. Pediatr. Surg.* 2001;**10**:72–80.

139 Beath, S. V., Davies, P., Papadopoulou, A. *et al.* Parenteral nutrition-related cholestasis in postsurgical neonates: multivariate analysis of risk factors. *J. Pediatr. Surg.* 1996;**31**:604–6.

140 Moss, R. L., Das, J. B., Raffensperger, J. G. Necrotizing enterocolitis and total parenteral nutrition-associated cholestasis. *Nutrition* 1996;**12**:340–3.

141 Watkins, J. B., Szczepanik, P., Gould, J. B., Klein, P., Lester, R. Bile salt metabolism in the human premature infant. Preliminary observations of pool size and synthesis rate following prenatal administration of dexamethasone and phenobarbital. *Gastroenterology* 1975;**69**:706–13.

142 Pereira, G. R., Piccoli, D. A. Cholestasis and other hepatic complications. In Yu, V. Y. H., MacMahon, R. A., eds. *Intravenous Feeding of the Neonate.* London: Edward Arnold;1992s:153–65.

143 Matos, C., Avni, E. F., Van Gansbeke, D., Pardou, A., Struyven, J. Total parenteral nutrition (TPN) and gallbladder diseases in neonates. Sonographic assessment. *J. Ultrasound Med.* 1987;**6**:243–8.

144 Hodes, J. E., Grosfeld, J. L., Weber, T. R. *et al.* Hepatic failure in infants on total parenteral nutrition (TPN): clinical and histopathologic observations. *J. Pediatr. Surg.* 1982;**17**:463–8.

145 Moss, R. L., Amii, L. A. New approaches to understanding the etiology and treatment of total parenteral nutrition-associated cholestasis. *Semin. Pediatr. Surg.* 1999;**8**:140–7.

146 Iyer, K. R., Spitz, L., Clayton, P. BAPS prize lecture: new insight into mechanisms of parenteral nutrition-associated cholestasis: role of plant sterols. *J. Pediatr. Surg.* 1998;**33**:1–6.

147 Clayton, P. T., Bowron, A., Mills, K. A. *et al.* Phytosterolemia in children with parenteral nutrition-associated cholestatic liver disease. *Gastroenterology* 1993;**105**:1806–13.

148 Jawaheer, G., Lloyd, D. A., Shaw, N. J., Pierro, A. *Minimal enteral feeding promotes gallbadder contractility in neonates.* Proceedings of the Nutrition Society 1996;**183A**:55.

149 Maini, B., Blackburn, G. L., Bistrian, B. R. *et al.* Cyclic hyperalimentation: an optimal technique for preservation of visceral protein. *J. Surg. Res.* 1976;**20**:515–25.

150 Merritt, R. J. Cholestasis associated with total parenteral nutrition. *J. Pediatr. Gastroenterol. Nutr.* 1986;**5**:9–22.

151 Ternullo, S. R., Burkart, G. J. Experience with cyclic hyperalimentation in infants. *J. Parenter. Enteral Nutr.* 1979;**3**:516.

152 Sitzmann, J. V., Pitt, H. A., Steinborn, P. A., Pasha, Z. R., Sanders, R. C. Cholecystokinin prevents parenteral nutrition induced biliary sludge in humans. *Surg. Gynecol. Obstet.* 1990;**170**:25–31.

153 Rintala, R. J., Lindahl, H., Pohjavuori, M. Total parenteral nutrition-associated cholestasis in surgical neonates may be reversed by intravenous cholecystokinin: a preliminary report. *J. Pediatr. Surg.* 1995;**30**:827–30.

154 Teitelbaum, D. H., Han-Markey, T., Drongowski, R. A. *et al.* Use of cholecystokinin to prevent the development of parenteral nutrition-associated cholestasis. *J. Parenter. Enteral Nutr.* 1997;**21**:100–3.

155 Levine, A., Maayan, A., Shamir, R. *et al.* Parenteral nutrition-associated cholestasis in preterm neonates: evaluation of ursodeoxycholic acid treatment. *J. Pediatr. Endocrinol. Metab.* 1999;**12**:549–53.

156 Rintala, R., Lindahl, H., Pohjavuori, M., Saxen, H., Sariola, H. Surgical treatment of intractable cholestasis associated with total parenteral nutrition in premature infants. *J. Pediatr. Surg.* 1993;**28**:716–9.

157 Furukawa, H., Reyes, J., Abu-Elmagd, K. Clinical intestinal transplantation. *Clin. Nutr.* 1996;**15**:45–52.

158 Wispe, J. R., Bell, E. F., Roberts, R. J. Assessment of lipid peroxidation in newborn infants and rabbits by measurements of expired ethane and pentane: influence of parenteral lipid infusion. *Pediatr. Res.* 1985;**19**:374–9.

159 Basu, R., Muller, D. P. R., Papp, E. *et al.* Free radical formation in infants: the effect of critical illness, parenteral nutrition, and enteral feeding. *J. Pediatr. Surg.* 1999;**34**:1091–5.

160 Helbock, H. J., Motchnik, P. A., Ames, B. N. Toxic hydroperoxides in intravenous lipid emulsions used in preterm infants. *Pediatrics* 1993;**91**:83–7.

161 Cooke, R. W. Factors associated with chronic lung disease in preterm infants. *Arch. Dis. Child.* 1991;**66**:776–9.

162 Basu, R., Muller, D. P. R., Eaton, S., Merryweather, I., Pierro, A. Lipid peroxidation can be reduced in infants on total parenteral nutrition by promoting fat utilization. *J. Pediatr. Surg.* 1999;**34**:255–9.

163 Moore, F. A., Moore, E. E., Jones, T. N., McCroskey, B. L., Peterson, V. M. TEN versus TPN following major abdominal trauma – reduced septic morbidity. *J. Trauma* 1989;**29**: 916–22.

164 Moore, F. A., Feliciano, D. V., Andrassy, R. J. *et al.* Early enteral feeding, compared with parenteral, reduces postoperative septic complications. The results of a meta-analysis. *Ann. Surg.* 1992;**216**:172–83.

165 Kudsk, K. A., Carpenter, G., Petersen, S., Sheldon, G. F. Effect of enteral and parenteral feeding in malnourished rats with *E. coli*-hemoglobin adjuvant peritonitis. *J. Surg. Res.* 1981;**31**:105–10.

166 Kudsk, K. A., Stone, J. M., Carpenter, G., Sheldon, G. F. Enteral and parenteral feeding influences mortality after hemoglobin-*E. coli* peritonitis in normal rats. *J. Trauma* 1983;**23**: 605–9.

167 Deitch, E. A., Winterton, J., Li, M., Berg, R. The gut as a portal of entry for bacteremia. Role of protein malnutrition. *Ann. Surg.* 1987;**205**:681–92.

168 Alverdy, J., Chi, H. S., Sheldon, G. F. The effect of parenteral nutrition on gastrointestinal immunity. The importance of enteral stimulation. *Ann. Surg.* 1985;**202**:681–4.

169 Lin, M. T., Saito, H., Fukushima, R. *et al.* Route of nutritional supply influences local, systemic, and remote organ responses to intraperitoneal bacterial challenge. *Ann. Surg.* 1996;**223**: 84–93.

170 Shou, J., Lappin, J., Minnard, E. A., Daly, J. M. Total parenteral nutrition, bacterial translocation, and host immune function. *Am. J. Surg.* 1994;**167**:145–50.

171 Lucas, A. Human milk and infant feeding. In Boyd, R., Battaglia, F. C., eds. *Perinatal Medicine.* London: Butterworths; 1983:172–200.

172 Hambreus, L., Forsum, E., Lonnerdal, B. Nutritional aspects of breast milk versus cow's milk formula. In McFarlane, H., Hambreus, L., Hanson, L. A., eds. *Food and Immunology Symposia of the Swedish Nutrition Foundation XIII.* Stockholm, Sweden: Almquist and Wiksell; 1976:

173 Taylor, C. J., Jenkins, P., Manning, D. Evaluation of a peptide formula (milk) in the management of infants with multiple GIT intolerance. *Clin. Nutr.* 1988;**7**:183–90.

174 Francis, D. E. Treatment of multiple-malabsorption syndrome of infancy. *J. Hum. Nutr.* 1978;**32**:270–8.

175 Larcher, V. F., Shepherd, R., Francis, D. E., Harries, J. T. Protracted diarrhoea in infancy. Analysis of 82 cases with particular reference to diagnosis and management. *Arch. Dis. Child.* 1977;**52**:597–605.

176 Jawaheer, G., Pierro, A., Lloyd, D., Shaw, N. Gall-bladder contractility in neonates – effects of parenteral and enteral feeding. *Arch. Dis. Child.* 1995;**72**:F 200–2.

177 Jawaheer, G., Shaw, N. J., Pierro, A. Continuous enteral feeding impairs gallbladder emptying in infants. *J. Pediatr.* 2001;**38**:822–5.

178 Catnach, S., Hinds, C., Fairclough, P. Enteral nutrition does not protect against biliary sludge in critically ill patients. *Gut* 1993;**34**:S51.

179 Toursarkissian, B., Kearney, P. A., Holley, D. T. *et al.* Biliary sludging in critically ill trauma patients. *S. Med. J.* 1995;**88**: 420–4.

180 Schwesinger, W. H., Page, C. P., Strodel, W. E. *et al.* Biliary sludge formation during enteral nutrition: prevalence and natural history. *Surgery* 1998;**124**:768–71.

40

Nutritional assessment of the neonate

Robert Erick Ridout[1] and Michael K. Georgieff[2]

[1] University of Colorado Health Sciences Center, The Children's Hospital, Denver, CO
[2] Department of Pediatrics, University of Minnesota School of Medicine, Minneapolis, MN

Nutritional management decisions, as with most interventions in medicine, are meant to maximize benefit (growth and development) and minimize harm (toxicity). In order to achieve this goal, clinicians require tools that will allow careful monitoring of their patients' short- and longer-term responses to their nutritional management plan. Past and current research efforts have advanced the science of neonatal nutrition and helped guide present day nutrition strategies. This chapter will provide the clinician a review of those nutritional assessment tools that are currently readily available and also discuss future techniques. Given that the smallest preterm infants (those with birthweights < 1250 g) pose the greatest challenge to clinicians from nutritional management and assessment standpoints, the bulk of this chapter will address their specific needs. While this chapter will be divided into medical record review (maternal and neonatal), nutritional intake, laboratory measurements, and anthropometrics, in practice one should consider these concepts concomitantly when assessing the infant.

Medical record review

The foundation of a sound nutritional assessment plan starts with a comprehensive review of the patient's medical history. In the case of a neonate, the mother's medical history must also be considered. Figure 40.1 depicts the various maternal, nutritional, environmental, endocrinological, and fetal factors one must consider when reviewing the medical and nutritional history. Additional neonatal factors, not included in Figure 40.1, must also be taken into account. For example, neonates undergoing major surgery may have caloric needs 20%–30% higher than baseline, while neonates with severe sepsis may have caloric needs upwards of 40%–50% higher than baseline.

Nutritional intake

A key part of nutritional assessment is making certain the prescribed nutrient intake is actually provided. As the typical neonate undergoing a comprehensive nutritional assessment will be an inpatient in a nursery setting, the nutritional intake will likely be well documented in the patient record and bedside flow sheets. Although the focus of nutritional assessment typically is on the current nutritional management plan, it is critical to review all dietary intake since birth given the profound impact early nutritional management decisions can have on long-term growth and nutrient needs. The nutritional intake in neonates is divided into parenteral and enteral routes.

Parenteral intake

Most neonates requiring neonatal intensive care will receive parenteral nutrition. The smallest preterm neonate may be managed exclusively via the parenteral route over the first days to weeks of life pending a successful transition to the enteral route. A number of studies in preterm infants have demonstrated that infusion of amino acids as early as the first day of life decreases protein catabolism.[1–12] Many of these studies have shown an amino acid intake of as little as 1.5–$2.0\,\mathrm{g\,kg^{-1}\,day^{-1}}$, when given with $\geq 30\,\mathrm{kcal\,kg^{-1}\,day^{-1}}$

Neonatal Nutrition and Metabolism. Second Edition, ed. P. Thureen and W. Hay. Published by Cambridge University Press.
© Cambridge University Press 2006.

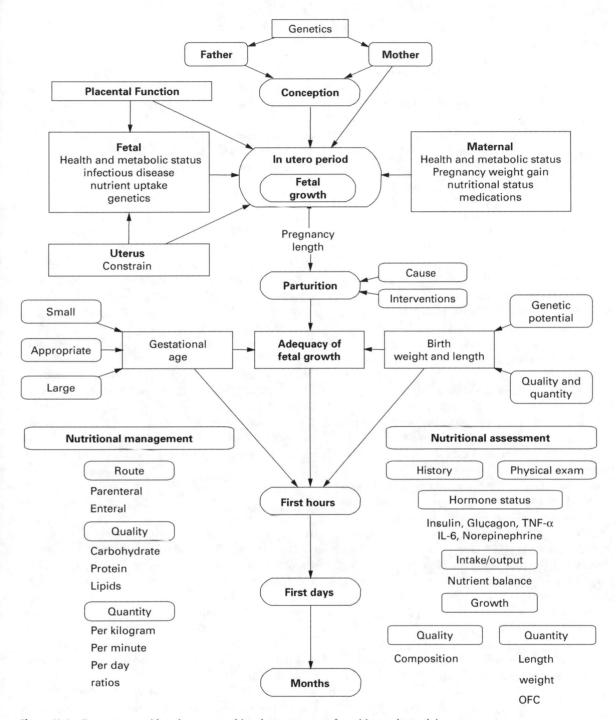

Figure 40.1. Factors to consider when approaching the assessment of nutrition and growth in any neonate.

of nonprotein calories, is sufficient to avoid catabolism in neonates.[13] Higher amino acid and energy intakes result in net anabolism.[14] With the goal of replicating intrauterine protein accretion rates, amino acid intakes of 3.5–

4.0 g kg^{-1} day^{-1} have been shown to be required, particularly for those infants with birthweights <1000 g.[15,16]

Given these data, a typical parenteral nutritional regimen, in a preterm low birth weight (LBW) infant, will likely include between 1.5–$4 \, g \, kg^{-1} \, day^{-1}$ of balanced crystalline amino acids, up to $12.5 \, mg^{-1} \, kg^{-1} \, minute^{-1}$ of dextrose delivery, and up to $4 \, g \, kg^{-1} \, day^{-1}$ of a balanced intravenous lipid emulsion, and an appropriate complement of vitamins and minerals. The caloric intake with such a regimen will usually lie between 80–$100 \, kcal \, kg^{-1} \, day^{-1}$. In addition to the above, parenteral solutions are occasionally supplemented with one or all of the following: albumin, erythropoietin, and carnitine.[17–20] When recording parenteral intake for an individual infant, it is important to record what was ordered and what was given as patient factors may dictate changes throughout the infusion period.

Enteral intake

Most infants will ultimately transition from full or partial parenteral nutrition to full enteral nutrition. With few exceptions, the American Academy of Pediatrics recommends the use of human milk in all infants, including the premature infant.[21] Human milk, therefore, has long been considered the gold standard against which all commercially available formulas are compared. Many commercial formulas exist, each with its own set of unique qualities. All formulas, however, should provide for balanced nutrition. When compared with the parenteral route, use of the enteral route has many potential benefits. Studies have shown early introduction of enteral feeds, and shorter duration of parenteral nutrition, may lead to faster weight gain.[22] As there is a higher energy cost associated with assimilating enteral nutrients, and the bioavailability of these nutrients may be less when compared with the parenteral route, the required enteral intake may be significantly higher. Caloric and fluid intakes will typically fall between 120–$140 \, kcal \, kg^{-1} \, day^{-1}$ and 120–$180 \, cc \, kg^{-1} \, day^{-1}$, respectively. Preterm infants often require higher caloric intakes via supplemented human milk or formula, and higher volume intakes to achieve the targeted reference intrauterine rate of growth. There exists a significant variety of commercially available formulas, modular and complete supplements which may be used as supplements. One must remember that any modification of human milk or commercial formula may affect its osmolality and renal solute load.

Laboratory assessment

Laboratory measurements serve a key role in the assessment of nutritional adequacy and toxicity. As with the other assessment tools discussed here, there is a trade-off between the information derived from the measurement and the impact it has on the infant. When ordering a test, consider other tests that may be required and could be run on the same aliquot of blood thereby minimizing the burden on the patient. Prior to checking laboratory parameters one must consider the following issues: availability of normal values, timeliness of results, pre-test plan, cost, and initial versus follow-up test. Additionally, one must be aware of the local laboratory's capabilities and reliability. When ordering a laboratory test, it will also be important to indicate time of day and frequency of the assessment.

Electrolytes

Electrolyte panels are among the most common routinely ordered labs in most nurseries. These panels provide information on fluid status and renal function, and help guide nutritional management decisions. It is important, however, to not base management decisions solely on a single set of electrolytes. When evaluating electrolytes, one must make an accurate determination of intake (fluid and electrolytes), output (measured and insensible), and progression of each individual patient's disease process. Electrolyte panels (sodium, potassium, chloride, bicarbonate) should be checked daily on all infants receiving total parenteral nutrition over the first week of life, as well as following any changes to the total parenteral nutrition prescription. Additionally, infants on enteral feeds should have electrolytes obtained twice weekly while receiving diuretic therapy.

Blood urea nitrogen

Urea is produced in the liver as a byproduct of amino acid metabolism (oxidation) and when excreted represents an irreversible loss of nitrogen from the body. In the human fetus, the capability of urea synthesis has been demonstrated as early as week 13 of gestation with the overall enzymatic activity increasing to approximately 90% of adult levels near term.[23,24] While the metabolism of dietary and endogenous urea has been well described in adults and older children, a similar "full" understanding in neonates does not exist.

Until recently, urea was felt to be metabolically unavailable to the human neonate. Ongoing research, the majority of it on term neonates, demonstrates that the minority (20%) of urea produced is excreted and is thereby metabolically "lost." In contrast, the remaining 80% has been shown to enter the gut, undergo hydrolysis, and return the nitrogen to the metabolically active (available) nitrogen pool.[25,26] Considering these findings along with data obtained from ovine studies where amino acids are transported from maternal to fetal compartments in excess of accretion requirements and the excess amino acids ultimately oxidized leading to high levels of urea synthesis, blood urea nitrogen (BUN) values in neonates can prove to be difficult to interpret.[27] An elevated BUN value may represent appropriate amino acid delivery, utilization, and subsequent appropriate oxidation (a robust BUN value) or it may represent amino acid intolerance (BUN as an indicator of a pathologic process).

In the smallest preterm infants a significant body of literature suggests that the early provision of amino acids leads to improved postnatal growth, nitrogen balance, and potentially long-term neurodevelopmental outcomes. Recent studies evaluating higher amino acid intakes in these preterm infants have not shown the increased BUN concentrations and metabolic acidosis found in prior studies,[28] complications which are currently felt to be related to the use of protein hydrolysate preparations in the prior studies. Indeed, a recent review of amino acid intake data and BUN concentrations in our institution has failed to show a clinically significant correlation between these two variables (Figure 40.3).

Given the increasing support of early and more aggressive amino acid delivery to preterm neonates, particularly those with birth weights <1000 g, and the multiple confounding traits of BUN concentration in this population and neonates in general, modification of amino acid intake should not be based on BUN concentration alone. Infants receiving parenteral nutrition typically have BUN and creatinine concentrations measured once per week. While no absolute levels exist at which amino acid intake should be altered, a continuously rising BUN value may indicate a mismatch between production and excretion.

Calcium, magnesium, phosphorus, and alkaline phosphatase

Calcium, phosphorus, and alkaline phosphatase levels are often followed in the management and surveillance of metabolic bone disease. Together with serum osteocalcin, and C-terminal procollagen peptide levels one can evaluate bone formation (osteoblastic activity) as it relates to metabolic bone disease.[29] Despite the long-standing use of serum laboratory values in the evaluation of metabolic bone disease, a relatively new modality available to assess neonates is dual energy x-ray absorptiometry (DEXA). DEXA provides a quantitative assessment of bone mass, is relatively noninvasive, and has been validated to work in neonates.[30,31] A more extensive discussion on the use of DEXA is provided elsewhere in this text.

Calcium, phosphorus, and magnesium levels are also utilized to assess acute excess or deficiency states as suggested by clinical presentation or history. Neonatal calcium homeostasis, as in adults, involves a complex interaction between bone stores, acid-base status, serum magnesium and phosphorus levels, parathyroid function, Vitamin D status, and dietary intake. Fetal and subsequently neonatal calcium homeostasis is critically dependent on an adequate calcium supply from a normo-calcemic maternal compartment. Presence of maternal hyper- or hypocalcemia may have an impact on fetal accretion and manifest as neonatal parathyroid dysfunction.

Magnesium levels can aid in the investigation of poor gut motility in a neonate born to a mother following magnesium sulphate tocolysis. Additionally, given that magnesium is required for normal parathyroid function, these levels are often included in an evaluation of refractory hypocalcemia. Approximately one-third of infants of diabetic mothers have been found to have hypomagnesemia (defined by a serum magnesium level $<1.5\,\mathrm{mg\,dL^{-1}}$), a finding which explains the associated parathyroid dysfunction and hypocalcemia.

The solubility of calcium and phosphorus limits the amounts of these ions that can be put in solution; thus, it is nearly impossible to provide enough to mimic intrauterine accretion rates while a patient remains on sole parenteral nutrition.[32]

Due to the effect of neonatal illness and the transition of the infant to its own parathyroid regulation, hypocalcemia and hypomagnesemia are a distinct possibility in the first week of life. Thus, serum calcium, magnesium, and phosphorus levels should be measured daily over the first 3 days of life and every other day thereafter until medically stable. In those infants less than 32 weeks gestation, serum phosphorus and alkaline phosphatase levels should be assessed weekly to monitor for osteopenia of prematurity. Serum calcium in this disease is frequently within the normal range (albeit in the low range of normal) since it is preserved at the expense of the calcium stores in the bone. Thus, a more direct way to assess the increased bone turnover that supplies calcium to the serum is to measure the serum alkaline phosphatase concentration. In assessing the causes and severity of osteopenia, one must also consider the negative impact medications may have on the infant's calcium, phosphorus, and magnesium balance (e.g., furosemide, caffeine citrate, glucocorticosteroids).

Lipids

Lipids provide a very concentrated source of nonprotein energy and have many critical biological functions. Lipids

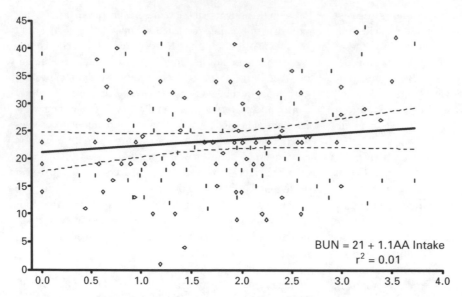

Figure 40.2. Blood urea nitrogen (BUN) across a range of amino acid intakes in infants with birth weight less than 1250 grams.

are essential components of cell membranes; they play a key role in normal brain and retinal development, and provide the substrate for synthesis of many hormones (eicosanoids). While much research is currently ongoing evaluating the nutritional requirements of the long-chain polyunsaturated essential fatty acids (arachadonic and docosahexaenoic acids) in the enterally fed infant,[33–36] the mainstay of fat intake in the parenterally nourished infant is intravenous lipid emulsions. Intravenous lipids are often provided as a 20% solution given its high caloric density and favorable phospholipid/triglyceride ratio.

A review of the metabolic milieu of the second and early third trimester fetus finds an intrauterine environment characterized by maternal – fetal amino acid transfer in excess of accretion needs, glucose transfer based on a facilitated transport system to meet needs, and minimal lipid transport/utilization. These findings are further supported when one considers the low levels of lipoprotein lipase and lecithin cholesterol acyl transferase present in the 20–28 week gestation fetus. It follows, therefore, that preterm infants of similar gestational age will have limited lipid tolerance, although this initial intolerance will improve as the infant matures.

While the lipid intake as a percentage of nonprotein caloric intake will be low initially, it is important that one consider not only the quantity, but the quality or composition of lipid as well. Preterm infants, and all humans for that matter, have specific lipid intake requirements to meet their essential fatty acid needs and can rapidly demonstrate a deficiency state if not exogenously provided. These infants require approximately 1–4% and 1% of their caloric intake to be in the form of linoleic and alpha-linolenic acid, respectively. Failing to provide these minimal intakes can result in an essential fatty acid deficiency state characterized by poor somatic, skin, and hair growth, impaired healing, and occasionally hematologic abnormalities. Providing approximately 0.5 g kg^{-1} day^{-1} of the current commercially available 20% intravenous lipid emulsion, a typical starting point in the smallest preterm infant, will meet these essential fatty acid requirements though higher intake will likely be required to optimize growth. While a host of lab studies has been described to monitor lipid tolerance, the most commonly assessed value is the triglyceride concentration. Since most neonatal intensive care units infuse the day's dose of lipids over 16–20 hours, serum triglyceride concentrations should be checked when the infant is not receiving lipid. Triglyceride concentrations should be measured once or twice weekly or following changes in intravenous lipid delivery. Triglyceride levels less than 150–200 mg dL^{-1} are typically considered evidence of tolerance. Typically, triglyceride concentrations are not measured in enterally fed infants.

Glucose

Glucose is an important nutrient in fetal as well as neonatal life where it serves as a metabolic fuel and provides a carbon supply for accretion. Throughout pregnancy there exists a materno – fetal gradient down which glucose transport is facilitated from mother to fetus. Cordocentesis studies

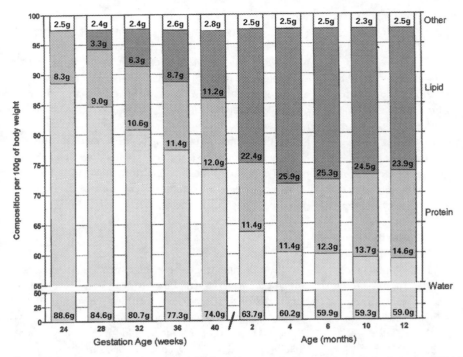

Figure 40.3. Changes in body composition from the second trimester through the first year of life. (Adapted from refs. 116 and 117.)

have noted that fetal glucose concentration is a function of gestational age and maternal glucose concentration, and that following week 20 of gestation the fetal glucose concentration is rarely below ~3 mmol L^{-1} (54 mg dL^{-1}).[37] At birth the umbilical venous glucose concentration has been shown to be 60%–80% of maternal venous concentrations. In the normal neonate, metabolic adaptation occurs over the first few hours of life resulting in a steady state blood glucose concentration whereby hepatic glucose production is balanced with peripheral utilization. However, many neonates requiring intensive nutritional care will not be able to meet the demands of this metabolic adaptation following birth or periods of stress and therefore require blood glucose sampling and nutritional interventions.

The medical history will often suggest which infants require screening and more frequent blood glucose concentration determinations. Infants born to mothers with pregnancies complicated by diabetes mellitus or requiring beta-mimetic tocolysis and oral hypoglycemic agents are at risk for early hypoglycemia. Additionally, many neonatal factors have been associated with altered glucose control, including the following: infection, intrauterine growth restriction, small for gestational age, thermal stress, hormonal and inborn errors of metabolism, hyperviscosity, and asphyxia.

When determining whether a blood glucose concentration is high, low, or normal, one must consider the individual patient. While there exists a body of literature attempting to define plasma glucose concentrations which represent hypo- and hyperglycemic states, these numbers fail to be applicable to all patients. Specifically, each individual patient demonstrates a unique set of physiologic and pathologic factors which have an impact on their response to their physical and nutritional environment. A normal term neonate without symptoms will likely not require blood glucose measurements. Conversely, any neonate with symptoms potentially referable to a low blood glucose concentration should have their blood glucose concentration assessed immediately. Those infants with risk factors for an altered metabolic response to low blood glucose concentrations (e.g., preterm, infant of diabetic mother) should have these assessments done preemptively.

When evaluating glucose intake, it is of most value in the parenterally nourished neonate to consider this intake in terms of the glucose infusion rate (GIR) which is often expressed as quantity (milligrams) of glucose delivered per kilogram of bodyweight per unit time (minute). In the term neonate, the steady state glucose utilization rate has been shown to be between 4 and 6 mg kg^{-1} min^{-1}.[38] The GIR which will meet basal metabolic needs falls near the higher end of this range ~6 mg kg^{-1} min^{-1}. On top of this basal GIR, an additional 2 mg kg^{-1} min^{-1} of glucose delivery is required, per gram of amino acid intake, to support growth and protein accretion.

When considering a blood glucose level, one must consider the individual patient's current and previous nutrient intake. Additionally, monitoring for hyper- and hypoglycemia allows for modification of current glucose intake and may provide evidence of change in patient status (e.g., sepsis, necrotizing enterocolitis). Neonates in the first week of parenteral nutrition, on advancing parenteral nutrition, or who have rapidly changing clinical conditions will need glucose concentrations measured daily. Once the infant is clinically stable and on a set nutrient delivery system, serum glucose monitoring frequency can be diminished or discontinued. Infants with gestational conditions that predispose them to neonatal hypoglycemia (e.g., infant of diabetic mother, intrauterine growth retardation) need to be monitored typically for the first 3 postnatal days, although more severe cases may need to be followed for up to a week.

Vitamin A

Vitamin A (retinol), a fat-soluble vitamin, is actively involved in a variety of respiratory epithelial growth, development, and regeneration processes.[39] Vitamin A deficiency has been shown to be involved in the pathophysiology of bronchopulmonary dysplasia and supplementation studies have shown benefit in preterm infants.[40–42] In those infants at highest risk for bronchopulmonary dysplasia (birthweight <1250 g), assessment of serum retinol levels soon after birth may guide supplementation for those infants with levels < 20 μg dL^{-1}. When assessing these levels, one must consider the impact other therapies may have. Specifically, postnatal steroid administration has been shown to increase serum vitamin A levels.[43] If supplementation is elected, weekly vitamin A levels should be assessed.

Vitamin E

Vitamin E, a tocopherol, is also a fat-soluble vitamin and is involved in myriad cellular functions. Through its role as an antioxidant, vitamin E helps maintain the integrity of cell membranes. Supplementation of very low birth weight (VLBW) infants with vitamin E has been attempted for a variety of disease processes (e.g., retinopathy of prematurity, hemolytic anemia, bronchopulmonary dysplasia, and intracranial hemorrhage). While such supplementa-

tion was found to reduce the risk of intracranial hemorrhage and severe retinopathy of prematurity, the risk of sepsis and necrotizing enterocolitis was found to be increased, particularly with serum levels >3.5 mg dL^{-1}.[44–47] With reference to the VLBW infant, the current recommendation of the American Academy of Pediatrics Committee on the Fetus and Newborn is 2.8 IU kg^{-1} day^{-1} of vitamin E not to exceed 7 IU day^{-1}. Additionally, the Committee suggested the normal serum range of 1 to 2 mg dL^{-1}. Vitamin E levels should be assessed in patients receiving supplemental vitamin E following any dosage modification and in patients where fat-soluble vitamin absorption may be impaired (e.g., cystic fibrosis).

Carnitine

Carnitine, a nonstructural amino acid, is an essential cofactor in a variety of biochemical steps involved in lipid metabolism. Specifically, carnitine participates in the transfer of long-chain fatty acids across the inner mitochondrial membrane in preparation for their subsequent metabolism. Additionally, carnitine aids in the maintenance of normal free coenzyme A levels.[48] Carnitine is found in varying concentrations in breast milk and infant formulas. Unless intentionally supplemented, most parenteral nutrition solutions will be free of carnitine. As the preterm infant has limited stores of carnitine at birth and has a limited capacity for carnitine synthesis, many studies have examined the role of supplemental carnitine in the preterm infant. In these studies, early carnitine supplementation was not found to improve growth, to prevent hypoglycemia, or to prevent episodes of apnea in preterm and VLBW infants.[49–52] Should an infant remain on exclusive parenteral nutrition for longer than 2 weeks, plasma carnitine levels should be obtained, compared with age-appropriate norms, and supplementation considered. Finally, in patients where primary carnitine deficiency is suspected, plasma carnitine levels are often obtained prior to the initiation of carnitine supplementation.

Iron

Iron deficiency is the most common single nutrient deficiency worldwide and can have a negative impact on motor and mental development in infants.[53–57] The fetal iron stores are typically bolstered at the end of the third trimester and provide for growth and red cell mass expansion over the first months of life. Infants born preterm do not benefit from this third trimester maternal–fetal iron transfer and, although not "iron deficient" at birth, they are particularly prone to the development of iron deficiency. In addition to their limited iron stores at birth, the rapid expansion of their red cell mass with growth and erythropoietin administration can consume body iron stores.[58] Finally, red blood cell iron can be depleted through phlebotomy if not replaced with transfusions. In addition to preterm infants, a large percentage of infants of diabetic mothers and those with intrauterine growth restriction have been found to have low iron stores at birth as evidenced by low newborn serum ferritin concentrations.[59,60] Serum ferritin concentrations assessed soon after birth in infants born near term have been correlated with iron status later in the first year of life.[61,62] Ferritin, the soluble storage form of iron in tissue, is synthesized in the liver as a function of cellular iron content. Low iron stores are the main cause of a low serum ferritin concentration suggesting the benefit of ferritin determinations in the assessment of iron deficiency. While excessive iron stores (overload) result in increased ferritin concentrations, a variety of other factors may also be involved and complicate body iron status. Specifically, as ferritin is an acute phase reactant, infections and other inflammatory processes may lead to increased ferritin levels. Following multiple blood transfusions in VLBW infants, the assessment of iron overload can be accomplished through the measurement of serum ferritin concentrations. A low or normal serum ferritin suggests no evidence of iron overload, while a high ferritin may be indicative of iron overload, infection, or other inflammatory process.[63] When assessing ferritin levels one must consider these factors and their potential impact. The fifth percentile for serum ferritin in a newborn infant is 60 μg L^{-1}. Thus, a serum ferritin concentration less than 60 μg L^{-1} is taken as evidence of iron deficiency until 40 weeks postconceptional age in a preterm infant. Thereafter, the levels normally decrease to the more standard definition of a ferritin <10 μg L^{-1} in the 9-month-old infant. The specific standard for post 40-week ferritin concentrations in preterm infants has not been well studied. When neonatal iron deficiency is suspected, particularly in those LBW infants cared for without receiving transfusion therapy, a serum ferritin concentration should be assessed as a low value may help direct iron supplementation and with determining the risk of iron deficiency in the follow-up period.

Visceral proteins

All body protein exists in a functional form, a situation quite different from that of body fats and carbohydrates, both of which can exist in functional and storage forms. Any change in body protein mass, therefore, represents a change in body function (e.g., loss of muscle protein mass results in decreased contractile strength). Monitoring the balance of protein synthesis has historically been accomplished through time-consuming nitrogen balance studies, often in conjunction with an ongoing clinical study. In routine clinical practice, however, serial assessments of a panel of serum visceral proteins have been shown to be a proxy for body protein synthesis trends and nitrogen balance.[64]

Visceral proteins are proteins measured in the serum and are contrasted to protein found in body organs which are termed somatic proteins. They are the product of visceral protein anabolism, with the major site of production residing in the liver. Each of the visceral proteins discussed here has one or more specific physiologic functions in the body. Prior to discussing the specific visceral proteins used in nutritional assessment, it is useful to review the characteristics of serum proteins that increase or decrease their usefulness as nutritional markers. The optimal serum protein being measured should have the following characteristics: a short biologic half-life, a rapid synthetic rate coupled with a constant catabolic rate, and a small body pool size (volume of distribution). The protein marker should be easily measured on available equipment and be relatively inexpensive. Additionally, alterations in body protein status should be reflected rapidly and result in measurable serum level changes of the marker being followed. Finally, this marker should only reflect changes in protein and energy status and preferably not act as a positive or negative acute phase reactant.[65,66] Albumin, transferrin, transthyretin, fibronectin, and 3-methyl histidine have all been employed in the nutritional assessment in neonates.

Albumin

Albumin is synthesized in the liver and is the most abundant plasma protein. Similar to the fetus, albumin concentrations are lower in preterm compared with term neonates and these levels increase with advancing gestational and chronologic age.[67] Once synthesized, approximately 40–50% of body albumin resides in the extravascular space with the balance being intravascular. Approximately 4% of total body albumin is broken down each day, yielding a relatively long half-life of 14–21 days. Given the wide volume of distribution and long half-life, albumin levels are slow to respond to changes in nutritional management or disease state. Albumin levels may also be influenced by changes in capillary permeability or large volume bodily fluid fluxes (e.g., volume resuscitation). These characteristics limit serum albumin's usefulness as a short-term marker of nutritional sufficiency. Conversely, albumin's characteristics support its use in longer-term assessments of nutritional status.

Transferrin

Similar to albumin, transferrin is synthesized in the liver and its serum concentration increases with increasing gestational and chronologic age. Transferrin serves as the major serum transport protein of ferric iron and its synthesis is tightly linked to the status of body iron stores. Transferrin serves as an early indicator of iron deficiency with levels increasing in relation to the severity of the deficiency. Compared with albumin, transferrin has a much smaller body pool size and biologic half-life (9 days). Despite these characteristics, its close association with iron status limits transferrin's usefulness as a marker of protein status in neonates. Indeed, elevated transferrin levels in the face of iron deficiency occur without regard to protein status.[68] A longitudinal study involving preterm infants found weekly transferrin levels to not be useful in monitoring their protein-energy status.[69] Finally, as a negative acute phase reactant, and similar to transthyretin, transferrin levels may be depressed in the face of infection and inflammatory stimuli.[70]

Transthyretin (prealbumin)

Transthyretin, along with retinol-binding protein, serves as the serum transport protein of both vitamin A and thryoxine. Transthyretin has a half-life of 2–3 days and responds to changes in nutrient balance within 7 days. Unlike serum transferrin and albumin concentrations, transthyretin in theory would seemingly be a better indicator of malnutrition because of its shorter half-life; no studies have shown prealbumin to be a more useful marker of nutritional status or predictor of outcome. Transthyretin has a high concentration of the amino acid tryptophan, and tryptophan has been shown to play a major role in the initiation of protein synthesis. It has one of the highest ratios of essential-to-nonessential amino acids of any protein in the body. Transthyretin has a low pool concentration in the serum, a half-life of 2 days, and a rapid response to lowered energy intake, even with 3 days of inadequate protein intake. Transthyretin concentrations do not appear to be influenced by fluctuations in hydration status. Transthyretin concentrations in the serum increase or decrease in relation to the severity or absence of energy deficits. The serum concentration of this protein increases when more than 55% of assessed protein and energy needs are met.[65] One study in a population of sick neonates showed transthyretin to be a highly accurate marker of nutritional adequacy.[71] However, transthyretin's usefulness is limited by its responsiveness to pre- and postnatal steroids. These agents can double the serum concentration of this protein and the elevation can persist for up to 2 weeks.[72,73]

Urinary 3-methylhistidine

3-Methylhistidine is a modified amino acid that is a component of the skeletal muscle proteins actin and myosin. As actin and myosin undergo routine turnover and are metabolized, 3-methylhistidine is liberated and subsequently excreted in the urine. Of interest, 3-methylhistidine does not participate in new protein formation, thus, the amount excreted relates directly to skeletal muscle turnover. The ratio of 3-methylhistidine to creatinine has been shown to be a useful marker for muscular protein turnover in LBW infants and is often cited in studies of the catabolic effects of surgery in this population.[74,75] It remains, however, a research technique and is not used in clinical settings.

Insulin-like growth factor (IGF) axis

The insulin-like growth factor axis consists of the two polypeptide IGFs, their six high affinity binding proteins (IGFBPs), and four recently described low affinity binding proteins.[76–80] The IGF axis has an important role in cellular differentiation and growth. The serum levels and functionality of the various IGF axis constituents have been shown to vary significantly from early embryonic development to adulthood.[81–83] IGF-1, IGFBP-2, and IGFBP-3 levels have been shown to be influenced by both gestational and chronologic age,[84–86] and many studies have shown their levels to be strongly influenced by nutritional status (Table 40.1). Animal studies have been important in guiding the design of human studies. One such study examined the effect of protein undernutrition and subsequent nutritional rehabilitation on IGF-1 and its binding proteins.[87] Following a period of protein undernutrition, where significant reductions in IGF-1 levels and the IGFBP-3/IGFBP-2 ratio were seen, nutritional rehabilitation, over a 10-day period, was associated with a significant elevation in IGF-1 levels and the IGFBP-3/IGFBP-2 ratio. These elevations were more pronounced at higher protein intakes. Another animal study evaluated the effect of fasting and re-feeding on IGFBP-2 mRNA levels and found significant and measurable changes as quickly as 2–6 hours after a nutritional modification.[88]

Human studies conducted by Smith *et al.* reported the use of IGF-1 and the IGFBs to monitor feeding among a group of preterm infants.[86] IGF-1 levels were found to correlate with caloric intake over the prior 3 days, with a more profound increase noted with increasing protein intake. IGFBP-3 levels were found to increase with increasing

Table 40.1. Insulin-like growth factor (IGF-1) and the insulin-like growth factor binding proteins' properties

IGF-1	Correlates strongly with length of gestation and days since birth. Levels increase with higher protein intakes; effect is more pronounced at higher gestational and chronologic ages. Levels increase with increasing caloric intake.
IGFBP-3	Correlates with length of gestation and length since birth. Levels only modestly affected by protein intake. Levels are more sensitive to changes in caloric intake.
IGFBP-2	Contrasts strongly with the regulation of IGF-1 and IGFBP-3. IGFBP-2 levels demonstrate an inverse correlation with advancing gestation and days since birth. Linear decrease in levels with increasing protein and caloric intake (protein effect stronger than caloric effect).

caloric intake alone. Finally, IGFBP-2 was found to vary inversely with dietary protein intake. In another study, these researchers found IGF-1, IGFBP-2, and IGFBP-3 to be regulated by dietary intake, with regulatory patterns similar to those found in older individuals. IGF-1 levels were found be most strongly correlated with protein intake, while IGFBP-3 levels were tied most closely to caloric intake.[89]

Assessment of IGF-1 and the IGFBPs may be useful in not only determining whether the absolute amount of each macronutrient is sufficient, but if the ratio/combination is optimal (calories and protein). It is clear that more research is needed to define the role of IGF-1 and its binding proteins as markers of nutrition before they enjoy widespread clinical use. One study recently showed that IGF-1, IGFBP-2, and IGFBP-3 could be followed using dried blood spots on filter paper.[85] This sampling technique has many benefits over standard sampling techniques, including increased stability and portability, and requiring only 50–75 μL of blood per sample. The current downside to using these tests clinically is their lack of rapid turn-around time from the laboratory.

In summary, serum albumin concentrations can be monitored as an indicator of protein status once or twice monthly in infants on prescribed protein diets (e.g., total parenteral nutrition). However, it is unclear whether the information gained adds much to what will be gleaned from anthropometric analysis. Serum transthyretin concentrations can be measured more frequently (e.g., weekly) because of the shorter half-life and can be useful in determining the prescription of macronutrients. A transthyretin concentration that decreases by more than 10% from the previous value suggests negative nitrogen balance and predicts poorer weight gain in preterm infants.

Anthropometrics

It is clear that the goal of nutritional management of all neonates should be to optimize quantitative and qualitative rates of growth to limit long-term morbidity and enhance long-term outcomes. The sufficiency of nutritional intake among infants is currently monitored by changes in weight gain, body length, and head circumference. Such measurements are easily made and have proven useful to track an infant's progress over time. Such measurements are post-hoc, with meaningful changes occurring days to weeks after the institution of a nutritional management plan. A recent study from the National Institutes of Child Health and Human Development Neonatal Network very low birth weight registry showed that while the survival in this population improved over the decade of the 1990s, the majority of these patients demonstrated poor postnatal growth.[90] Another report involving the Neonatal Network examined the longitudinal growth of VLBW infants (birth weight <1500 g) and found that once birth weight was regained their average daily weight gain was 14.4–16.1 g kg^{-1} day^{-1} (rate similar to reference intrauterine weight gain 15–18 g kg^{-1} day^{-1}).[22] Of note, in this study no specific nutritional management plans were followed. Pauls *et al.* however, reported postnatal growth curves for a population of extremely low birth weight (ELBW; birth weight <1000 g) infants receiving a standardized nutritional management plan and found mean daily weight gain of 15.7 g kg^{-1} day^{-1} once birth weight was regained.[91]

Taking the currently available fetal growth reference data and the information provided in these studies, most VLBW infants accrue a "weight deficit" of 198–335 g from birth until birth weight is regained.[92] While this "weight deficit" is the most obvious sign of poor postnatal growth, other parameters of growth have been found to suffer as well. A recent large multi-center retrospective review of the growth outcomes of neonates born between 23 and 34 weeks estimated gestational age found the incidence of extrauterine growth restriction to be 28%, 34%, and 16% for weight, length, and head circumference, respectively.[93] Further, despite achieving weight gain approximating that of intrauterine rates, the quality of this weight gain may be very different from that of the fetus (Figure 40.3). During late pregnancy the fetus typically gains 2 g kg^{-1} day^{-1} of body fat, whereas in rapidly growing premature infants, values as high as 5 g kg^{-1} day^{-1} have been reported.[94–96] The clinician requires tools to assess short- and longer-term changes in both quantitative and qualitative measures of growth. At present, techniques such as DEXA, Magnetic Resonance Imaging (MRI), and Total Body Electric Conductivity (TOBEC) have all been demonstrated to yield very accurate body composition data. These techniques, however, are limited in their wide-spread acceptance due to factors such as cost and patient logistics (e.g., movement of critically ill neonates to the scanner). Full discussions of these techniques and other methods of assessing body composition are found elsewhere in this text.

Anthropometric measurements

As previously stated, weight, length, and head circumference measurements are easily made, however, meaningful changes may significantly lag clinical nutrition decisions. When considering these measurements, it is important to ensure that each measurement is compared to an appropriate standard (growth chart/grid) and that one understands the limitations of the measurement technique.

Weight

Given a well-calibrated scale and close attention to technique, one can accurately determine an infant's weight. One must be aware of the various therapeutic devices an infant may have or have had during each weight determination. As an example, umbilical catheters (1 g) and pulse oximeter probes (23 g) by themselves weigh little, however, their percentage contribution to a daily weight could be significant in the smallest neonate.[97] Another factor to consider is the fluid balance from the prior to the current weight measurement. The sickest neonates may have significant fluid requirements, and may receive suboptimal nutritional intake, but may still demonstrate weight gain over time. Such weight gain may be a function of fluid balance and not nutritional management. Weight measurements should be made daily, if possible, around the same time.

Head circumference

Head or occipitofrontal circumference measurements in neonates can be accomplished without significant difficulty. One should use a measuring device that does not stretch such as a metal measuring tape. The circumference measurement should include the occiput and the most anterior portion of the frontal bone and the largest of multiple measurements should be recorded. Such longitudinal measurements have proven to be useful as a surrogate for growth of the underlying brain. Indeed, head circumference has been found to be proportional to brain weight and brain volume, particularly in infants and children.[98–100] Further, as postnatal brain growth is an important determinant of later cognitive function, longitudinal tracking of changes in head circumference is critical.[101] There are

limitations, however, to the usefulness of head circumference in the face of hydrocephalus and immediately after birth (molding and scalp edema). Furthermore, head circumference is poorly sensitive to malnutrition since the brain growth is spared at marginal caloric intakes that do not support linear growth and weight gain. Thus, the head circumference velocity will be the last to be affected during a period of malnutrition and the first to respond after re-institution of calories. Head circumference measurements should be made on postnatal day 3–5 and weekly thereafter. As predicted by third trimester fetal head circumference growth, the goal weekly head circumference change is 0.75 cm. However, after a period of no growth, the "catch-up" rate of weekly head growth can approach 2 cm. The head growth pattern of the typical premature infant is triphasic, with initial growth at less than expected rates while the infant is ill, followed by a period of rapid catch-up growth at greater than expected rates and finally ending with growth along the pre-designated percentile.[102]

Length

Length, when measured serially, is an excellent means of tracking longitudinal linear growth. Its measurement is the most accurate reflector of lean body mass when compared with weight or head circumference. Additionally, length measurements have proven useful as components of a variety of indicators which compare body weight/mass to length (ponderal index, body mass index). Length is often cited as the measurement most prone to error depending on the technique used. The use of a measuring tape by a single observer is likely to yield a very inaccurate measurement. In fact, a recent study suggested the use of a length-board or recumbent stadiometer is a more accurate means of assessing length.[103] As with head circumference, length measurements should be made and recorded on a weekly basis. As predicted by third trimester fetal weekly length change, the goal weekly length change is 0.75 cm.

Growth charts

A variety of growth charts exist which allows for comparison of an individual neonate's anthropometric measurements to a reference standard that is appropriate for one's patient population. A general understanding of how each growth chart was formulated and what limitations each may have is important. Two factors are of most importance: the population utilized and the time frame covered. Most widely used growth charts have a broad representation of the population, including a representative sample of most ethnicities and races. Additionally, these growth charts are often available for females and males. One limitation of most current growth charts is that they do not actually represent longitudinal measurements of individuals, rather age-specific measurements of large populations of individuals. The Lubchenco charts/curves were constructed from anthropometric data obtained at the time of birth and not from the longitudinal measurements of individual neonates.[104–106] In this regard, these charts might better be referred to as "size" charts. This fact, however, should not limit these charts usefulness when comparing a neonate to a reference population at each age point. A further issue to consider is the time frame from which the reference population data were taken. Growth charts representing contemporary population measurements are likely to be more representative when compared with charts formulated in the distant past. Differences may be due to changes in population nutritional practices, disease prevalence, and other environmental factors. As an example, by including a more appropriate sample of the population (better mix of breast and formula-fed infants), the 2000 Centers for Disease Control (CDC) growth charts were found to have noticeable differences from the previous 1977 National Center for Health Statistics growth charts. It is recommended to discontinue the use of the older charts.

When plotting a data point, one must ensure that the neonate's age is corrected if the chart does not compensate for preterm birth. Using the 2000 CDC charts requires one to determine each preterm neonate's gestationally corrected-age up through at least 24–36 months of age. On the other hand, the growth charts presented by Babson and Benda have a built-in correction for preterm birth and do not require gestational corrected-age determination.[107–109] As the infant transitions to discharge, he or she should be plotted on a curve adjusted for prematurity. The most specific curves for premature infants are the Infant Health and Development Program curves that have separate graphs for males and females and for VLBW and LBW infants.[110,111] Correction for prematurity typically continues in the follow-up period until 2 years of age.

Skinfold measurements

Measurement of skinfold thickness is an established means by which to assess the thickness of subcutaneous fat tissue in humans of all ages. Skinfold measurements are simple in concept and are easily performed on infants, which makes their use feasible in the clinical setting. Their use requires certain assumptions, one of which is that the thickness of the subcutaneous adipose tissue layer reflects total fat mass.[112] Recent studies in preterm infants using such techniques as TOBEC and isotopic dilution to validate skinfold measurements have shown that when total body fat exceeded 100 g (representing 5% of body weight), the proportion of total fat mass (TFM) that was subcutaneous fat mass was relatively constant at $34.6 \pm 9.8\%$.[113] Applying the techniques of Dauncey et al.[112] and McGowan[114] one is able to determine the absolute total fat mass in preterm infants weighing >2000 g.[115]

The actual calculation of total fat mass, using the Dauncey method, is based on the assumption that the body is composed of five cylinders: one trunk, two upper extremities, and two lower limbs. The volume of subcutaneous fat covering each cylinder is calculated as the product of length, circumference, and the thickness of the subcutaneous fat layer of each of the cylinders:

$$\text{Subcutaneous Fat Volume (SFV)}(\text{cm}^3) = L * T * (C - \pi T),$$

where L = Length (cm) and T = Thickness of the subcutaneous fat layer (half the skinfold thickness measurement less the thickness of the dermis layer) with the thickness of the dermis layer assumed to be 0.06 cm.[113] Trunk SFV: L = crown – rump length, C = mean of chest and abdominal circumferences, T = mean of subscapular and suprailiac skinfold thicknesses. Upper Extremity SFV: L = arm length, C = mid-arm circumference, T = triceps skinfold thickness. Lower Extremity SFV: L = leg length (crown-heel minus crown-rump length), C = mean of midthigh and midcalf circumferences, T = midthigh skinfold thickness.

The sum of all skinfold measurements (cm^3) is multiplied by the density of fat (0.9 g/cm^3) to determine the fat mass and subsequently the percentage of total body mass. Once applied, the skinfold calipers must be held in place until a stable measurement is made. In doing so, one can limit the impact fluctuations in tissue hydration can have on subcutaneous fat determinations. Serial measurements allow the determination of fat accretion over time and the comparison to that expected from fetal growth rates and reference fetal and infant data.[94,116–118] As with any patient measurement, every effort must be made to minimize measurement error. Again, length is often cited as the measurement most prone to error depending on the technique used. Skinfold measurements remain mostly research tools and are not routinely recommended in the clinical setting.

REFERENCES

1 Kashyap, S., Heird, W. Protein requirements of low birthweight, very low birthweight, and small for gestational age infants. In Raiha, N. ed. *Protein Metabolism during Infancy*. New York: Raven Press; 1993:133–51.

2 Rubecz, I., Mestyan, J., Varga, P., Klujber, L. Energy metabolism, substrate utilization, and nitrogen balance in parenterally fed postoperative neonates and infants. The effect of glucose, glucose + amino acids, lipid + amino acids infused in isocaloric amounts. *J. Pediatr.* 1981;**98**:42–6.

3 Zlotkin, S. H., Bryan, M. H., Anderson, G. H. Intravenous nitrogen and energy intakes required to duplicate in utero nitrogen accretion in prematurely born human infants. *J. Pediatr.* 1981;**99**:115–20.

4 Duffy, B., Gunn, T., Collinge, J., Pencharz, P. The effect of varying protein quality and energy intake on the nitrogen metabolism of parenterally fed very low birthweight (less than 1600 g) infants. *Pediatr. Res.* 1981;**15**:1040–4.

5 van Toledo-Eppinga, L., Kalhan, S. C., Kulik, W., Jakobs, C., Lafeber, H. N. Relative kinetics of phenylalanine and leucine in low birth weight infants during nutrient administration. *Pediatr. Res.* 1996;**40**:41–6.

6 Anderson, T. L., Muttart, C. R., Bieber, M. A., Nicholson, J. F., Heird, W. C. A controlled trial of glucose versus glucose and amino acids in premature infants. *J. Pediatr.* 1979;**94**:947–51.

7 Yu, V. Y., James, B., Hendry, P., MacMahon, R. A. Total parenteral nutrition in very low birthweight infants: a controlled trial. *Arch. Dis. Child.* 1979;**54**:653–61.

8 Saini, J., MacMahon, P., Morgan, J. B., Kovar, I. Z. Early parenteral feeding of amino acids. *Arch. Dis. Child.* 1989;**64**:1362–6.

9 van Lingen, R. A., van Goudoever, J. B., Luijendijk, I. H., Wattimena, J. L., Sauer, P. J. Effects of early amino acid administration during total parenteral nutrition on protein metabolism in pre-term infants. *Clin. Sci. (Lond).* 1992;**82**:199–203.

10 Rivera, A. Jr, Bell, E. F., Stegink, L. D., Ziegler, E. E. Plasma amino acid profiles during the first three days of life in infants with respiratory distress syndrome: effect of parenteral amino acid supplementation. *J. Pediatr.* 1989;**115**:465–8.

11 Van Goudoever, J. B., Colen, T., Wattimena, J. L. *et al.* Immediate commencement of amino acid supplementation in preterm infants: effect on serum amino acid concentrations and protein kinetics on the first day of life. *J. Pediatr.* 1995;**127**:458–65.

12 Thureen, P. J., Anderson, A. H., Baron, K. A. *et al.* Protein balance in the first week of life in ventilated neonates receiving parenteral nutrition. *Am. J. Clin. Nutr.* 1998;**68**:1128–35.

13 Rivera, A. Jr, Bell, E. F., Bier, D. M. Effect of intravenous amino acids on protein metabolism of preterm infants during the first three days of life. *Pediatr. Res.* 1993;**33**:106–11.

14 Denne, S. C., Karn, C. A., Ahlrichs, J. A. *et al.* Proteolysis and phenylalanine hydroxylation in response to parenteral nutrition in extremely premature and normal newborns. *J. Clin. Invest.* 1996;**97**:746–54.

15 Ziegler, E. E. Protein requirements of preterm infants. In Fomon, S. J., Heird, W. C. eds. *Energy and Protein Needs during Infancy.* New York: Academic Press; 1986.

16 Ziegler, E. E. Protein in premature feeding. *Nutrition* 1994;**10**:69–71.

17 Cairns, P. A., Stalker, D. J. Carnitine supplementation of parenterally fed neonates. *Cochrane Database Syst Rev.* 2000;**4**:CD000950.

18 Kanarek, K. S., Williams, P. R., Blair, C. Concurrent administration of albumin with total parenteral nutrition in sick newborn infants. *J. Parenter. Enteral Nutr.* 1992;**16**:49–53.

19 Ohls, R. K., Veerman, M. W., Christensen, R. D. Pharmacokinetics and effectiveness of recombinant erythropoietin administered to preterm infants by continuous infusion in total parenteral nutrition solution. *J. Pediatr.* 1996;**128**:518–23.

20 Kumpf, V. J. Parenteral iron supplementation. *Nutr. Clin. Pract.* 1996;**11**:139–46.

21 Go, W. Breastfeeding and the use of human milk. *Pediatrics* 1997;**100**:1035–9.

22 Ehrenkranz, R. A., Younes, N., Lemons, J. A. *et al.* Longitudinal growth of hospitalized very low birth weight infants. *Pediatrics* 1999;**104**:280–9.

23 Mukarram Ali Baig, M., Habibullah, C. M., Swamy, M. *et al.* Studies on urea cycle enzyme levels in the human fetal liver at different gestational ages. *Pediatr. Res.* 1992;**31**:143–5.

24 Raiha, N. C., Suihkonen, J. Development of urea-synthesizing enzymes in human liver. *Acta Paediatr. Scand.* 1968;**57**:121–4.

25 Wheeler, R. A., Jackson, A. A., Griffiths, D. M. Urea production and recycling in neonates. *J. Pediatr. Surg.* 1991;**26**:575–7.

26 Moran, B. J., Jackson, A. A. 15N-urea metabolism in the functioning human colon: luminal hydrolysis and mucosal permeability. *Gut* 1990;**31**:454–7.

27 Gresham, E. L., Simons, P. S., Battaglia, F. C. Maternal–fetal urea concentration difference in man: metabolic significance. *J. Pediatr.* 1971;**79**:809–11.

28 Thureen, P. J., Melara, D., Fennessey, P. V., Hay, W. W. Jr. Effect of low versus high intravenous amino acid intake on very low birth weight infants in the early neonatal period. *Pediatr. Res.* 2003;**53**:24–32.

29 Shiff, Y., Eliakim, A., Shainkin-Kestenbaum, R. *et al.* Measurements of bone turnover markers in premature infants. *J. Pediatr. Endocrinol. Metab.* 2001;**14**:389–95.

30 Koo, W. W. Laboratory assessment of nutritional metabolic bone disease in infants. *Clin. Biochem.* 1996;**29**:429–38.

31 Koo, W. W., Hammami, M., Hockman, E. M. Use of fan beam dual energy x-ray absorptiometry to measure body composition of piglets. *J. Nutr.* 2002;**132**:1380–3.

32 Gutcher, G., Cutz, E. Complications of parenteral nutrition. *Semin. Perinatol.* 1986;**10**:196–207.

33 Clandinin, M. T., Van Aerde, J. E., Parrott, A. *et al.* Assessment of feeding different amounts of arachidonic and docosahexaenoic acids in preterm infant formulas on the fatty acid content of lipoprotein lipids. *Acta Paediatr.* 1999;**88**:890–6.

34 Vanderhoof, J., Gross, S., Hegyi, T. *et al.* Evaluation of a long-chain polyunsaturated fatty acid supplemented formula on growth, tolerance, and plasma lipids in preterm infants up to 48 weeks postconceptional age. *J. Pediatr. Gastroenterol. Nutr.* 1999;**29**:318–26.

35 Clandinin, M. T., Claerhout, D. L., Lien, E. L. Docosahexaenoic acid increases thyroid-stimulating hormone concentration in male and adrenal corticotrophic hormone concentration in female weanling rats. *J. Nutr.* 1998;**128**:1257–61.

36 Clandinin, M. T., Van Aerde, J. E., Parrott, A. *et al.* Assessment of the efficacious dose of arachidonic and docosahexaenoic acids in preterm infant formulas: fatty acid composition of erythrocyte membrane lipids. *Pediatr. Res.* 1997;**42**:819–25.

37 Marconi, A. M., Paolini, C., Buscaglia, M. *et al.* The impact of gestational age and fetal growth on the maternal-fetal glucose concentration difference. *Obstet. Gynecol.* 1996;**87**:937–42.

38 Denne, S. C., Kalhan, S. C. Glucose carbon recycling and oxidation in human newborns. *Am. J. Physiol.* 1986;**251**:E71–7.

39 Biesalski, H. K., Nohr, D. Importance of vitamin-A for lung function and development. *Mol. Aspects Med.* 2003;**24**:431–40.

40 Shenai, J. P., Kennedy, K. A., Chytil, F., Stahlman, M. T. Clinical trial of vitamin A supplementation in infants susceptible to bronchopulmonary dysplasia. *J. Pediatr.* 1987;**111**:269–77.

41 Shenai, J. P., Chytil, F., Stahlman, M. T. Vitamin A status of neonates with bronchopulmonary dysplasia. *Pediatr. Res.* 1985;**19**:185–8.

42 Darlow, B. A., Graham, P. J. Vitamin A supplementation for preventing morbidity and mortality in very low birthweight infants. *Cochrane Database Syst. Rev.* 2002;**4**:CD000501.

43 Shenai, J. P., Mellen, B. G., Chytil, F. Vitamin A status and postnatal dexamethasone treatment in bronchopulmonary dysplasia. *Pediatrics* 2000;**106**:547–53.

44 Brion, L. P., Bell, E. F., Raghuveer, T. S. Vitamin E supplementation for prevention of morbidity and mortality in preterm infants. *Cochrane Database Syst. Rev.* 2003;**4**:CD003665.

45 Fish, W. H., Cohen, M., Franzek, D., Williams, J. M., Lemons, J. A. Effect of intramuscular vitamin E on mortality and intracranial hemorrhage in neonates of 1000 grams or less. *Pediatrics* 1990;**85**:578–84.

46 Johnson, L., Bowen, F. W. Jr, Abbasi, S. *et al.* Relationship of prolonged pharmacologic serum levels of vitamin E to incidence of sepsis and necrotizing enterocolitis in infants with birth weight 1,500 grams or less. *Pediatrics* 1985;**75**:619–38.

47 Brion, L. P., Bell, E. F., Raghuveer, T. S., Soghier, L. What is the appropriate intravenous dose of vitamin E for very-low-birthweight infants? *J. Perinatol.* 2004;**24**:205–7.

48 Scaglia, F., Longo, N. Primary and secondary alterations of neonatal carnitine metabolism. *Semin. Perinatol.* 1999;**23**:152–61.

49 Shortland, G. J., Walter, J. H., Stroud, C. *et al.* Randomised controlled trial of L-carnitine as a nutritional supplement in preterm infants. *Arch. Dis. Child Fetal Neonatal Ed.* 1998;**78**:F185–8.

50 Kumar, M., Kabra, N. S., Paes, B. Role of carnitine supplementation in apnea of prematurity: a systematic review. *J. Perinatol.* 2004;**24**:158–63.

51 O'Donnell, J., Finer, N. N., Rich, W., Barshop, B. A., Barrington, K. J. Role of L-carnitine in apnea of prematurity: a randomized, controlled trial. *Pediatrics* 2002;**109**:622–6.

52 Whitfield, J., Smith, T., Sollohub, H., Sweetman, L., Roe, C. R. Clinical effects of L-carnitine supplementation on apnea and growth in very low birth weight infants. *Pediatrics* 2003;**111**:477–82.

53 Lozoff, B., Jimenez, E., Wolf, A. W. Long-term developmental outcome of infants with iron deficiency. *N. Engl. J. Med.* 1991;**325**:687–94.

54 Lozoff, B., Wolf, A. W., Jimenez, E. Iron-deficiency anemia and infant development: effects of extended oral iron therapy. *J. Pediatr.* 1996;**129**:382–9.

55 Lozoff, B., Jimenez, E., Hagen, J., Mollen, E., Wolf, A. W. Poorer behavioral and developmental outcome more than 10 years after treatment for iron deficiency in infancy. *Pediatrics* 2000;**105**:E51.

56 Lozoff, B., Brittenham, G. M., Wolf, A. W. *et al.* Iron deficiency anemia and iron therapy effects on infant developmental test performance. *Pediatrics* 1987;**79**:981–95.

57 Deinard, A. S., List, A., Lindgren, B., Hunt, J. V., Chang, P. N. Cognitive deficits in iron-deficient and iron-deficient anemic children. *J. Pediatr.* 1986;**108**:681–9.

58 Rao, R., Georgieff, M. K. Neonatal iron nutrition. *Semin. Neonatol.* 2001;**6**:425–35.

59 Chockalingam, U. M., Murphy, E., Ophoven, J. C., Weisdorf, S. A., Georgieff, M. K. Cord transferrin and ferritin values in newborn infants at risk for prenatal uteroplacental insufficiency and chronic hypoxia. *J. Pediatr.* 1987;**111**:283–6.

60 Georgieff, M. K., Landon, M. B., Mills, M. M. *et al.* Abnormal iron distribution in infants of diabetic mothers: spectrum and maternal antecedents. *J. Pediatr.* 1990;**117**:455–61.

61 Morton, R. E., Nysenbaum, A., Price, K. Iron status in the first year of life. *J. Pediatr. Gastroenterol. Nutr.* 1988;**7**:707–12.

62 Georgieff, M. K., Wewerka, S. W., Nelson, C. A., Deregnier, R. A. Iron status at 9 months of infants with low iron stores at birth. *J. Pediatr.* 2002;**141**:405–9.

63 Ng, P. C., Lam, C. W., Lee, C. H. *et al.* Hepatic iron storage in very low birthweight infants after multiple blood transfusions. *Arch. Dis. Child. Fetal Neonatal Ed.* 2001;**84**:F101–5.

64 Clemmons, D. R., Klibanski A., Underwood, L. E. *et al.* Reduction of plasma immunoreactive somatomedin C during fasting in humans. *J. Clin. Endocrinol. Metab.* 1981;**53**:1247–50.

65 Spiekerman, A. M. Proteins used in nutritional assessment. *Clin. Lab. Med.* 1993;**13**:353–69.

66 Church, J. M., Hill, G. L. Assessing the efficacy of intravenous nutrition in general surgical patients: dynamic nutritional assessment with plasma proteins. *J. Parenter. Enteral Nutr.* 1987;**11**:135–9.

67 Reading, R. F., Ellis, R., Fleetwood, A. Plasma albumin and total protein in preterm babies from birth to eight weeks. *Early Hum. Dev.* 1990;**22**:81–7.

68 Morton, A. G., Tavill, A. S. The role of iron in the regulation of hepatic transferrin synthesis. *Br. J. Haematol.* 1977;**36**:383–94.

69 Georgieff, M. K., Amarnath, U. M., Murphy, E. L., Ophoven, J. J. Serum transferrin levels in the longitudinal assessment of

protein-energy status in preterm infants. *J. Pediatr. Gastroenterol. Nutr.* 1989;**8**:234–9.

70 Ritchie, R. F., Palomaki, G. E., Neveux, L. M., Navolotskaia, O. Reference distributions for the negative acute-phase proteins, albumin, transferrin, and transthyretin: a comparison of a large cohort to the world's literature. *J. Clin. Lab. Anal.* 1999;**13**:280–6.

71 Georgieff, M. K., Sasanow, S. R., Pereira, G. R. Serum transthyretin levels and protein intake as predictors of weight gain velocity in premature infants. *J. Pediatr. Gastroenterol. Nutr.* 1987;**6**:775–9.

72 Georgieff, M. K., Chockalingam, U. M., Sasanow, S. R. *et al.* The effect of antenatal betamethasone on cord blood concentrations of retinol-binding protein, transthyretin, transferrin, retinol, and vitamin E. *J. Pediatr. Gastroenterol. Nutr.* 1988;**7**:713–7.

73 Georgieff, M. K., Mammel, M. C., Mills, M. M. *et al.* Effect of postnatal steroid administration on serum vitamin A concentrations in newborn infants with respiratory compromise. *J. Pediatr.* 1989;**114**:301–4.

74 Gil, A., Faus, M. J., Robles, R. *et al.* Urinary 3-methylhistidine derivative as indicator of nutrients intake in low-birth-weight infants. *Horm. Metab. Res.* 1984;**16**:667–70.

75 Shew, S. B., Keshen, T. H., Glass, N. L., Jahoor, F., Jaksic, T. Ligation of a patent ductus arteriosus under fentanyl anesthesia improves protein metabolism in premature neonates. *J. Pediatr. Surg.* 2000;**35**:1277–81.

76 Clemmons, D. R., Busby, W. H., Arai, T. *et al.* Role of insulin-like growth factor binding proteins in the control of IGF actions. *Prog. Growth Factor Res.* 1995;**6**:357–66.

77 Firth, S. M., Baxter, R. C. Cellular actions of the insulin-like growth factor binding proteins. *Endocr. Rev.* 2002;**23**:824–54.

78 Baxter, R. C. Insulin-like growth factor (IGF)-binding proteins: interactions with IGFs and intrinsic bioactivities. *Am. J. Physiol. Endocrinol. Metab.* 2000;**278**:E967–76.

79 Hwa, V., Oh, Y., Rosenfeld, R. G. Insulin-like growth factor binding proteins: a proposed superfamily. *Acta Paediatr. Suppl.* 1999;**88**:37–45.

80 Hwa, V., Oh, Y., Rosenfeld, R. G. The insulin-like growth factor-binding protein (IGFBP) superfamily. *Endocr. Rev.* 1999;**20**:761–87.

81 D'Costa, A. P., Ingram, R. L., Lenham, J. E., Sonntag, W. E. The regulation and mechanisms of action of growth hormone and insulin-like growth factor 1 during normal ageing. *J. Reprod. Fertil. Suppl.* 1993;**46**:87–98.

82 Ghigo, E., Arvat, E., Gianotti, L. *et al.* Human aging and the GH-IGF-I axis. *J. Pediatr. Endocrinol. Metab.* 1996;**9**:271–8.

83 Ghigo, E., Arvat, E., Gianotti, L. *et al.* Hypothalamic growth hormone-insulin-like growth factor-I axis across the human life span. *J. Pediatr. Endocrinol. Metab.* 2000;**13** (Suppl. 6):1493–502.

84 Rajaram, S., Carlson, S. E., Koo, W. W., Rangachari A., Kelly, D. P. Insulin-like growth factor (IGF)-I and IGF-binding protein 3

during the first year in term and preterm infants. *Pediatr. Res.* 1995;**37**:581–5.

85 Schutt, B. S., Weber, K., Elmlinger, M. W., Ranke, M. B. Measuring IGF-I, IGFBP-2 and IGFBP-3 from dried blood spots on filter paper is not only practical but also reliable. *Growth Horm. IGF Res.* 2003;**13**:75–80.

86 Smith, W. J., Underwood, L. E., Keyes, L., Clemmons, D. R. Use of insulin-like growth factor I (IGF-I) and IGF-binding protein measurements to monitor feeding of premature infants. *J. Clin. Endocrinol. Metab.* 1997;**82**:3982–8.

87 Tovar, A. R., Halhali, A., Torres, N. Effect of nutritional rehabilitation of undernourished rats on serum insulin-like growth factor (IGF)-I and IGF-binding proteins. *Rev. Invest. Clin.* 1999;**51**:99–106.

88 Kita, K., Nagao, K., Taneda, N. *et al.* Insulin-like growth factor binding protein-2 gene expression can be regulated by diet manipulation in several tissues of young chickens. *J. Nutr.* 2002;**132**:145–51.

89 Smith, W. J., Nam, T. J., Underwood, L. E. *et al.* Use of insulin-like growth factor-binding protein-2 (IGFBP-2), IGFBP-3, and IGF-I for assessing growth hormone status in short children. *J. Clin. Endocrinol. Metab.* 1993;**77**:1294–9.

90 Lemons, J. A., Bauer, C. R., Oh, W. *et al.* Very low birth weight outcomes of the National Institute of Child Health and Human Development Neonatal Research Network, January 1995 through December 1996. NICHD Neonatal Research Network. *Pediatrics* 2001;**107**:E1.

91 Pauls, J., Bauer, K., Versmold, H. Postnatal body weight curves for infants below 1000 g birth weight receiving early enteral and parenteral nutrition. *Eur. J. Pediatr.* 1998;**157**:416–21.

92 Alexander, G. R., Himes, J. H., Kaufman, R. B., Mor, J., Kogan M. A United States national reference for fetal growth. *Obstet. Gynecol.* 1996;**87**:163–8.

93 Clark, R. H., Thomas, P., Peabody, J. Extrauterine growth restriction remains a serious problem in prematurely born neonates. *Pediatrics* 2003;**111**:986–90.

94 de Gamarra, M. E., Schutz, Y., Catzeflis, C. *et al.* Composition of weight gain during the neonatal period and longitudinal growth follow-up in premature babies. *Int. J. Vitam. Nutr. Res.* 1987;**57**:339.

95 Chessex, P., Reichman, B., Verellen, G. *et al.* Metabolic consequences of intrauterine growth retardation in very low birth-weight infants. *Pediatr. Res.* 1984;**18**:709–13.

96 Putet, G., Senterre, J., Rigo, J., Salle, B. Nutrient balance, energy utilization, and composition of weight gain in very-low-birth-weight infants fed pooled human milk or a preterm formula. *J. Pediatr.* 1984;**105**:79–85.

97 Hermansen, M. G., Hermansen, M. C. The influence of equipment weights on neonatal daily weight measurements. *Neonatal. Netw.* 1999;**18**:33–6.

98 Epstein, H. T., Epstein, E. B. The relationship between brain weight and head circumference from birth to age 18 years. *Am. J. Phys. Anthropol.* 1978;**48**:471–3.

99 Bartholomeusz, H. H., Courchesne, E., Karns, C. M. Relationship between head circumference and brain volume in

healthy normal toddlers, children, and adults. *Neuropediatrics* 2002;**33**:239–41.

100 Lindley, A. A., Benson, J. E., Grimes, C., Cole, T. M. 3rd, Herman, A. A. The relationship in neonates between clinically measured head circumference and brain volume estimated from head CT-scans. *Early Hum. Dev.* 1999;**56**:17–29.

101 Gale, C. R., O'Callaghan, F. J., Godfrey, K. M., Law, C. M., Martyn, C. N. Critical periods of brain growth and cognitive function in children. *Brain* 2004;**127**:321–9.

102 Georgieff, M. K., Hoffman, J. S., Pereira, G. R., Bernbaum, J. R., Hoffman-Williamson, M. Effect of neonatal caloric deprivation on head growth and 1-year developmental status in preterm infants. *J. Pediatr.* 1985;**107**:581–7.

103 Corkins, M. R., Lewis, P., Cruse, W., Gupta, S., Fitzgerald, J. Accuracy of infant admission lengths. *Pediatrics* 2002;**109**:1108–11.

104 Battaglia, F. C., Lubchenco, L. O. A practical classification of newborn infants by weight and gestational age. *J. Pediatr.* 1967;**71**:159–63.

105 Lubchenco, L. O., Hansman, C., Boyd, E. Intrauterine growth in length and head circumference as estimated from live births at gestational ages from 26 to 42 weeks. *Pediatrics* 1966;**37**:403–8.

106 Lubchenco, L. O., Hansman, C., Dressler, M., Boyd, E. Intrauterine growth as estimated from liveborn birth-weight data at 24 to 42 weeks of gestation. *Pediatrics* 1963;**32**:793–800.

107 Fenton, T. R. A new growth chart for preterm babies: Babson and Benda's chart updated with recent data and a new format. *BMC Pediatr.* 2003;**3**:13.

108 Babson, S. G., Benda, G. I. Growth graphs for the clinical assessment of infants of varying gestational age. *J. Pediatr.* 1976;**89**:814–20.

109 Sherry, B., Mei, Z., Grummer-Strawn, L., Dietz, W. H. Evaluation of and recommendations for growth references for very low birth weight (< or = 1500 grams) infants in the United States. *Pediatrics* 2003;**111**:750–8.

110 Guo, S. S., Roche, A. F., Chumlea, W. C., Casey, P. H., Moore, W. M. Growth in weight, recumbent length, and head circumference for preterm low-birthweight infants during the first three years of life using gestation-adjusted ages. *Early Hum. Dev.* 1997;**47**:305–25.

111 Gu, S. S., Wholihan, K., Roche, A. F., Chumlea, W. C., Casey, P. H. Weight-for-length reference data for preterm, low-birthweight infants. *Arch. Pediatr. Adolesc. Med.* 1996;**150**:964–70.

112 Dauncey, M. J., Gandy, G., Gairdner, D. Assessment of total body fat in infancy from skinfold thickness measurements. *Arch. Dis. Child.* 1977;**52**:223–7.

113 Sheng, H. P., Muthappa, P. B., Wong, W. W., Schanler, R. J. Pitfalls of body fat assessments in premature infants by anthropometry. *Biol. Neonate* 1993;**64**:279–86.

114 McGowan, A., Jordan, M., MacGregor, J. M. J. Skinfold thickness in neonates. *Biol. Neonate* 1974;**25**:66–84.

115 Catalano, P. M., Thomas, A. J., Avallone, D. A., Amini, S. B. Anthropometric estimation of neonatal body composition. *Am. J. Obstet. Gynecol.* 1995;**173**:1176–81.

116 Ziegler, E. E., O'Donnell, A. M., Nelson, S. E., Fomon, S. J. Body composition of the reference fetus. *Growth* 1976;**40**: 329–41.

117 Fomon, S. J., Nelson, S. E. Body composition of the male and female reference infants. *Annu. Rev. Nutr.* 2002;**22**:1–17.

118 Butte, N. F., Hopkinson, J. M., Wong, W. W., Smith, E. O., Ellis, K. J. Body composition during the first 2 years of life: an updated reference. *Pediatr. Res.* 2000;**47**:578–85.

41

Methods of measuring body composition

Kenneth J. Ellis

Baylor College of Medicine, and Body Composition Laboratory, USDA/ARS Children's Nutrition Research Center, Houston, TX

Introduction

There is increasing evidence that poor or excess nutrition during infancy and early childhood may be associated with increased risks for adverse health effects later in life. Postmenopausal osteoporosis, for example, can be viewed as a disease with a "pediatric origin" related to suboptimal mineralization of the skeleton during growth. Likewise, there is increasing interest in the association between body composition during infancy and the incidence of adolescent and adult obesity. For many years, the assessment of an infant's growth has been based on the measurement of body size (i.e., weight, length, body circumferences) and occasionally skinfold thicknesses. These indices have been very useful in our understanding of general growth on a population basis, but are usually too crude to distinguish significant changes in body composition for the individual infant except at the extremes of abnormal weight. Over the last several decades, a number of noninvasive techniques for the in vivo assessment of human body composition have been developed, and recently reviewed.[1] In most cases, the instruments used for these assays have been designed for use in adults, and it is only more recently that these technologies have been extended to the examination of pediatric populations.

The term "body composition" will have different meanings depending on one's own scientific background, experience, and interest. It can refer to the chemical makeup of specific tissues, organs, or the whole body, or it may be viewed from the prospective of physiological function or anatomical structure.[2] The simplest model divides body weight (Wt) into two compartments: fat mass (FM) and fat-free mass (FFM). More sophisticated models partition the FFM into its subcomponents, for example, water, protein, mineral, and glycogen. Alternately, the physiological model separates FFM into the body cell mass, defined as the active metabolizing tissues of the body,[3] and the remaining extracellular compartment consisting of water and solids. Body composition models can also reflect the development of measurement techniques. For example, a whole-body scan using dual-energy x-ray absorptiometry (DXA), can provide simultaneous estimates of the body's bone mineral mass, fat mass, and lean tissue mass.

The classic work of Fomon et al.[4,5] has led to the development of the reference fetus, reference infant, and reference child models of body composition. These models are based on body potassium (TBK), body water (TBW), and body calcium (TBCa) estimates collated from several different populations. The infant model was recently updated[6] using the same set of assays, but in a longitudinal study of contemporary children. Secondary assays, such as those based on the electrical properties of the body, have also been developed in recent years, but these have not been as widely accepted for use with infants. The following sections of this chapter describe the various measurement techniques that can be used and how they relate to the various body composition models.

Body water and electrolyte measurements

As noted previously, the basic two-compartment (2-C) model divides body weight into a FM and FFM compartment. In general, it is difficult to directly measure the FM compartment, however, the 2-C model is the basis for most assessments of body fatness (%FM), which is defined as the FM/Wt ratio expressed as a percent. The measurement of

Neonatal Nutrition and Metabolism. Second Edition, ed. P. Thureen and W. Hay. Published by Cambridge University Press.
© Cambridge University Press 2006.

the total FFM is equally difficult. Thus, it is calculated by extrapolation from the measurement of one or more of its subcompartments, such as total body water (TBW) or total body potassium (TBK). That is, FFM = k_1 × TBW or FFM = k_2 × TBK, and FM = Wt − FFM, where the values for k_1 and k_2 are assumed constant at a given age.

Natural potassium exists in several isotopic states, one being ^{40}K, which is radioactive. This isotope decays at a rate, such that one gram of K emits about 200 gammas of 1.46 MeV per minute. At this energy, most of the gammas will exit the body and can be detected using a whole-body counter.[7] For infants with normal body composition, it is assumed that the potassium content of the total FFM is relatively constant, thus the TBK value can be converted to a measure of FFM for infants.[8] Since this signal is natural, TBK measurements can be made as frequently as needed, and without risk to the infant. The in vivo assay of TBK has a precision of about ± 2–3% for infants.

The major component of the total FFM is body water. This compartment is measured by orally administering water labeled with a nonradioactive isotope of hydrogen or oxygen, and collecting plasma or urine samples for several hours afterwards from the infant. The samples must be processed before being assayed using isotope-ratio mass spectroscopy (MS) or Fourier-transformed infrared spectroscopy. Unlike TBK which is a natural assay, the dilution techniques for TBW require that an isotope be administered to the subject. Thus, some time interval is needed for the isotope to clear the body, or for it to return to its natural levels, before the assay can be repeated. In the case of infants, this is about 30 days for the deuterium dilution assay of TBW. An advantage of the TBW assay is that it can be performed in relatively remote geographical locations around the world, and the collected samples returned to a central laboratory for analysis. This can also be a disadvantage if the TBW results are of immediate interest, as might be in a clinical setting. The precision for the TBW assay in infants using D_2O dilution with MS analysis is reported at about ± 2%.

Bioelectrical techniques

Alternatives to the isotope dilution technique for the measurement of TBW have been developed. These are based on the general electrical properties of the body, presumably related to the FFM. The most common techniques are total body electrical conductivity (TOBEC), single-frequency bioelectrical impedance analysis (BIA), and multifrequency bioelectrical impedance spectroscopy (BIS). Each method relies on the electrical conductivity of the lean tissues in the body, which are influenced by their water and electrolyte content. For the TOBEC assay, the infant's body is placed in a very weak external electromagnetic field. When this is done, the free charge particles in the body will align with the magnetic field component of the external field causing a small perturbation in the current, which is measured. The procedure takes only a few minutes to perform, and can be repeated as frequently as needed without risk to the infant. TOBEC is a secondary assay, which means that the measured parameter (called the TOBEC number) must be calibrated using a more direct assay such as TBW or TBK. In terms of the size of the instrument, the infant TOBEC is comparable to that of an infant whole-body counter, thus making it not as portable as BIA or BIS.

The alternate electrical methods, BIA and BIS, are also based on the body's electrical properties. But in this case, electrodes are attached to the body, usually at the foot and hand, and a very weak alternating electrical current (800 μAmp) is passed through the body. For the BIA assay, the frequency is fixed at 50 kHz, while the BIS procedure varies the frequency from a few kHz to greater than 500 kHz. In both cases, the body's resistance (R) and reactance (Xc) to the electrical current are measured. This method has become popular, partly because the instruments are relatively inexpensive, easily portable, the measurement can be repeated frequently, and there are no measurable risks to the subject.[9] The basic model used to convert the R value, normalized for Ht^2, to an estimate of FFM has not been shown to be very applicable for infants.[1,10] Piccoli et al.[11] have proposed an alternative to the traditional BIA modeling, by using the R/Ht v. Xc/Ht relation to identify subjects with abnormal hydration. Extending this approach to infants needs clinical validation, but it is interesting because the assessment is made without knowledge of body weight.

Body volume measurements

The measurement of body volume can also be used to estimate body fatness if the densities of the FFM and FM are known. The classic technique is to measure body weight while the subject is totally submerged underwater, hence the name underwater weighing. In order for this technique to provide an accurate measure of %FM, the density of the FFM must be known very precisely, which can be difficult when working with infants where the hydration of the FFM can be changing rapidly during growth. Even so, the classic measurement technique, i.e., total submersion in water, completely rules out consideration of this assay for infants. However, an alternate methodology for measuring body volume, called air-displacement plethysmography (ADP), has been used successfully with older children and adults.[12] An infant-size instrument is still in the development phase[13] and holds promise for future studies in infants.

Bone mineral measurements

Single-photon absorptiometry was developed in the late 1960s for the measurement of bone density in the cortical region of the radius. This technology continued to improve, and the current technique is called dual-energy x-ray absorptiometry (DXA). As the name implies, x-rays are used to scan body regions for specific bone sites (lumbar spine, upper femur, radius) that are associated with increased risks of fractures. This assay has become the standard for the assessment of low bone mass in postmenopausal women. Most of the newest instruments can also be used to examine the whole body, the scan taking only a few minutes, and at a very low dose ($<10~\mu$Sv). In order to provide a quantitative measure of the body's bone mineral mass (BMC), the analysis also calculates the relative fat content of the soft tissues.[1] Thus, a whole-body DXA scan gives a 3-compartment (3-C) model of body weight: BMC, FM, and remaining non-bone, non-fat tissues, called LTM (lean tissue mass). Although the FM and LTM data are available, the commercial market for the sale of DXA instruments has remained focused on the measurement of bone in adults, mainly older females. As such, the design of most DXA scanners is not optimized for the measurement of infants or small children. Pediatric software is available as an option, but the manufacturers' technical support and continued development in this area have been slow, and will continue as such until a clearer market is identified.

Use of body composition data

Body composition data can be used in two ways. Firstly, it can be used to determine the relative status of the individual infant. That is, does the child have abnormal body composition, where normal can be defined relative to age, weight, or body size. Secondly, there may be the need to assess changes in body composition over time. For either application, it is known that there are gender differences in weight gain and relative composition during infancy.[14] Thus, the controls and study group should be matched for gender distribution (it is assumed that these groups will also

be matched for age). It may also be important to match for body length.

If the body compartment to be examined is bone mineral mass, then only the DXA assay can be used.[15] If it is FM or FFM, then several alternate methods can be used. However, whole-body DXA does give reasonably reliable estimates for FM and FFM, hence it may be the best overall method for use with infants. Furthermore, these instruments are probably the most frequently available in most clinical centers, although the instrument may need to be upgraded to include pediatric software. Compared with the alternate choices (TOBEC, TBK, TBW, BIA), DXA is most likely to become the reference method of pediatric body composition studies, as well as in the clinical setting. However, there is still the need for further development of the infant ADP method for the assessment of body fatness.[13] Likewise, there is the possibility that magnetic resonance techniques may be applied to body composition measurements in infants.

The excellent work by Pieltain et al.[16] shows that DXA has sufficient precision and sensitivity to detect differences in body composition between infant feeding groups after only 3 weeks, without using excessively large sample sizes. Gender differences in body composition at birth remain evident during the first 24 months of life.[6] What this does for a study with a mixed gender population is to increase the biological variability (SD) throughout the study period, requiring either larger sample sizes or longer time intervals to detect the same level of change if only one gender were used. I am not suggesting that only one gender be examined, but that investigators need to account for this effect when performing power calculations for sample size.

Selection of method for body composition assessment in infants

It is to be expected that any body composition assay should provide more information about the nutritional status of infants than that simply obtained using body weight. Furthermore, it is reasonable to assume that these body composition assays are reflective of the functional tissues in the body and energy stores.[17] A summary of the various body composition methods currently available for use in infants, along with their corresponding body composition compartment, and precision and accuracy is summarized in Table 41.1. In addition, the estimated minimal detectable changes (MDC) between two measurements that would be statistically significant for individual infants (clinical case) have been included. Smaller changes in body composition can be detected on a population basis.[16] Alternatively, if

Table 41.1. Precision and accuracy of different body composition methods and minimum detectable change for an infant

Body composition compartment	Methoda	Measurement precisionb (%)	Accuracyc (%)	Minimum detectable changed (3.5 kg infant)
TBW	D$_2$O dilution	1–2%	2–4%	100 ml (5%)
	BIA/BIS	2–4%	3–7%	200 ml (10%)
	TOBEC	2–3%	4–6%	150 ml (8%)
BCM	TBK	2–3%	3–5%	17 mEq (5%)
FFM	DXA	1.5%	1–4%	125 g (5%)
FM	DXA	2–3%	3–5%	40 g (8%)
BMC	DXA	<2%	3–5%	4 g (5%)

[a] BIA/BIS, bioelectrical impedance analysis and spectroscopy; DXA, dual-energy x-ray absorptiometry; TOBEC, total body electrical conductance; TBK, total body potassium (whole-body counting).

[b] Reproducibility for repeat measurements.

[c] Accuracy error for absolute mass.

[d] Values calculated for a 3.5 kg infant with 15% fat.

TBW, total body water; BMC, bone mineral mass; FFM, fat-free mass; FM, fat mass.

the measurement precision can be improved or the biological variability within the population reduced, this too will increase the probability of detecting smaller changes in body composition as significant. A second consideration (see following section) relates to the time interval between repeat measurements. This is crucial in the study of infants, where the accretion rates are changing rapidly. If the time interval between two measurements is too short, then the amount of change that would be needed to reach significance may not be physiologically possible (limited by the accretion rate). Likewise, if the time period between measurements becomes relatively long, then normal growth and physiological changes in body composition may mask the amplitude of the effect being studied, requiring larger sample sizes.

To assess the suitability of a body composition assay to detect longitudinal changes, the most important parameter is precision. The relation of MDC between two measurements (at 5% significance) and precision of the assay for an individual is given in Figure 41.1. If the precision is 1%, then MDC must be greater than 2.8%. If the precision is only 5%, then the MDC must be greater than 14%. That is, the poorer the precision, the greater must be the change in body composition to reach significance, which usually translates to a longer time interval between the two measurements. For population studies, the biological variability within the population will strongly influence the sample size.

Pieltain et al.[16] used whole-body DXA scans to examine changes in body composition of preterm infants fed either fortified human milk or a preterm infant formula. To detect a MDC after 3 weeks, at the 5% significance level, a

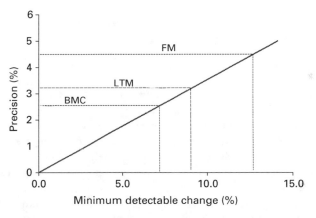

Figure 41.1. The relation between measurement precision and the minimum detectable change for an individual infant (5% significance level). The DXA precision for bone mineral content (BMC), fat mass (FM), and lean tissue mass (LTM) are shown.

sample size of 20–30 infants per group was sufficient. For this longitudinal study, the mean values of the minimal increases needed to reach statistical significance were 111 g for the lean tissue mass, 68 g for the fat mass, and 3.1 g for bone mineral content. To achieve statistical differences in each body composition compartment between the human milk and formula groups at discharge, the group differences would have to be greater than 160 g for lean tissue mass, 86 g for fat mass, and 4.1 g for bone mineral content, representing a total weight gain difference of at least 250 g. Wells[18] and Lapillonne et al.[17] have also reviewed the use of body composition assessment as an indicator of nutritional status in infancy, and these authors conclude that

Table 41.2. Body composition studies in infants

Longitudinal studies	Body composition assay	Time points	Reference
76 infants	TBW, TBK, TOBEC, DXA	0.5, 3, 6, 9, 12, 18, 24 months	6
48 healthy full term[28]	Whole-body DXA	1, 2, 3, 4, 5, 6 months	
34 healthy preterm[28]	Whole-body DXA	2, 4, 6 months	

Cross-sectional studies	Body composition assay	Age range	Reference
423 infants	TOBEC	2 weeks–12 months	20
163 healthy	BIA (phase angle)	1–7 days	11
28 infants	$H_2{}^{18}O$ dilution and BIA	<1 month	10
			14
64 infants	Whole-body DXA	birth – 18 month	14
106 healthy	whole-body DXA	1–2 months	23,24
214 infants	Whole-body DXA	birth – 12 months	21
153 SGA	Whole-body DXA	birth – 2 years	15

TBW, total body water; TBK, total body potassium; TOBEC, total body electrical content; DXA, dual-energy x-ray absorptiometry; BIA, bioelectrical impedance analysis; SGA, small-for-gestational age.

the DXA technique may offer the best examination of the composition of weight gain.

Reference body composition data for infancy

As previously noted, most instruments have not been developed for use with infants, thus the manufacturers do not routinely provide information such as reference data for infants. Most studies in infants provide only mean data, on a group basis at best. There are, however, several papers that do provide sufficiently detailed body composition information that these could be considered as references for infants.[6,17,19–24] These data have been derived using one or more of the assays previously described in this chapter. These include TBW by D_2O dilution, TBK by ^{40}K counting, TOBEC, BIA, and DXA. A summary of the studies with cross-sectional and longitudinal data is provided in Table 41.2. Of these assays, body composition data obtained using DXA has become the most widespread. Both cross-sectional and longitudinal data are available in these studies. The recent work by the Houston group[6,19] provides a contemporary update of the reference infant model of body composition, first established by the Iowa group.[5]

These studies provide sufficient information to derive reasonable estimates of the average rates of change (g day^{-1}) for the FM, FFM, and subcompartments of FFM. For example, the longitudinal body composition data reported by Butte *et al.*[6] can be used to derive age-specific accretion rates for Wt, FM, FFM, TBW, and BMC (see Figure 41.2).

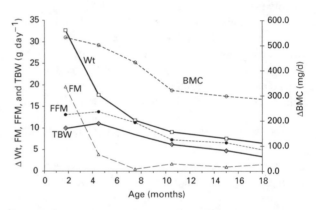

Figure 41.2. Average accretion rates for weight (Wt), fat mass (FM), fat-free mass (FFM), total body water (TBW), and bone mineral content (BMC) as a function of age for male infants.

As one would expect, accretion rates during the first weeks of life are higher than at later ages. The general pattern of accretion rates for infant girls were similar, although that for FM was slightly faster, while the FFM was slower. Thus, changes in body composition over a relatively short time interval can be expected to be gender-specific during infancy.

The ability to obtain multi-component composition data for infants is relatively new. As noted in the previous section, there are several studies that provide sufficient data to define a reference range for normal growth during infancy. When body composition information has been used with older children and adolescents, it has been customary to consider a value outside of ± 2.5 SD from the mean to be abnormal. It would seem reasonable to consider these limits for infants. However, the long-term health consequence of being outside of this range during infancy is not known. Thus, it is difficult to say with certainty that this represents a "significant" future risk, such that some form of intervention is immediately needed.

Infant studies using body composition

In the design of any infant study, there tend to be two areas of concern: selection of an appropriate control group, and the time duration of the study. A reference data set, if it is available, can be used as the control group. However, to insure that most external factors are controlled for, it may be better to simultaneously monitor changes in body composition using a control group concurrent with the "treated" group. When this is not practical or ethical, only then should an independent reference group be used for comparison. The established reference group, however, does provide the information that is often needed to calculate the appropriate sample size for a successful study. This of course leads to the question: "What is the appropriate reference population?" Many factors, such as whether the infants are preterm, full-term, appropriate-for-gestational age (AGA), or small-for-gestational age (SGA), will influence the decision for the appropriate "reference" group. Furthermore, the reference group may be defined by the target gains expected in body composition. For example, the NCHS/NHANES growth curves give national weight-for-age, height-for-age, and BMI-for-age percentiles for infants, but these are not true measures of body composition, but only body size.

The outcome variable of interest (FM, FFM, or BMC) will tend to dictate the choice of a body composition assay. This, in turn, will define the required length of the study period needed to achieve a statistically measurable difference between control and treated groups. During early infancy, the accretion rates (see Figure 41.2) are higher, thus a significant percentage change in mass will occur in a shorter time interval than if the study were started at an older age. Many infant feeding studies are started while the infant is still in the hospital awaiting discharge to take advantage of this effect. Therefore, caution must be used not to suggest the growth effects seen during the initial 3–6 weeks after birth will continue with equal intensity after hospital discharge because the accretion rates are dropping dramatically.

The expected changes in body composition will be dependent on both the age of the infants at the start of the study, and the length of time before the second measurement. These effects can be calculated from the table with the gender- and age-specific accretion rates calculated

by Butte et al.[6] Pieltain et al.,[16] for example, showed that whole-body DXA measurements in infants could detect significant differences in body composition between feeding groups after 3 weeks which corresponded to a weight difference of about 8%.

Summary

Each of the body composition methods presented in this chapter has its own set of advantages and disadvantages. For example, there are reasonably good FM and FFM reference percentile values as a function of age for TOBEC,[20] but this instrument is not widely available. Similar arguments can be easily made for whole-body counting of TBK and to a lesser extent for the deuterium dilution assay for TBW. The BIA technique is relatively easy to perform and has become widely available, but the body composition results for infants have been shown to be not much better than simply using weight and length measurements.[9] The DXA procedure is the only assay that provides a measure of bone mineralization for the whole body or a specific region such as the lumbar spine. Furthermore, a whole-body DXA scan also produces data for the relative fat and lean composition of the soft tissue mass. There are still sufficient differences among the various assays for the assessment of body fatness that it is recommended that only one method should be used for multi-site or longitudinal studies.[24] Even in these cases, there are other factors, such as geographical location, that may need to be considered when comparing differences in FM during infancy.[25]

If the outcome variable to be measured is the mineral compartment of bone, then the only technique currently available for use in infants is DXA. The manufacturers are providing better infant and pediatric software, but there is still room for continued improvement, especially when there is a transition between infant, pediatric, and adult software versions. DXA, however, is probably the technique that is most available to most pediatricians and investigators, as these instruments are located at most medical centers. A disadvantage of DXA, compared with the other techniques presented in this chapter, is that it requires the infant be exposed to a minimal x-ray dose (<10 μSv). This dose, however, is very small and is well within the natural variation of the radiation background levels in the USA and presents no measurable risk to the infant.

Accurate assessment of body composition in infancy and during early growth is relatively new. The relation between infant body composition and future health outcomes, except for extreme cases of malnutrition, remains unknown. Any extrapolation from infancy to childhood or adulthood should be done with caution. However, several retrospective studies have shown correlations between infant body size and early feeding mode with the risks for obesity, hypertension, and diabetes as adults.[26,27]

REFERENCES

1 Ellis, K. J. Human body composition: in vivo methods. *Physiolog. Rev.* 2000;**80**:649–80.

2 Wang, Z. R., Pierson, R. N. Jr, Heymsfield, S. B. The five-level model: a new approach to organizing body-composition research. *Am. J. Clin. Nutr.* 1992;**56**:19–28.

3 Moore, F. *The Body Cell Mass and Its Supporting Environment.* Philadelphia, PA: Saunders; 1963:22–6.

4 Ziegler, E. E., O'Donnell, A. M., Nelson, S. E., Fomon, S. J. Body composition of the reference fetus. *Growth* 1976;**40**:329–41.

5 Fomon, S. J., Haschke, F., Ziegler, E. E., Nelson, S. E. Body composition of reference children from birth to age 10 years. *Am. J. Clin. Nutr.* 1982;**35**:1169–75.

6 Butte, N. F., Hopkinson, J. M., Wong, W. W., Smith, E. O., Ellis, K. J. Body composition during the first 2 years of life: an updated reference. *Pediatr. Res.* 2000a;**47**:578–85.

7 Ellis, K. J., Shypailo, R. J. Whole body potassium measurements independent of body size. In Ellis, K. J., Eastman, J. D., eds. *Human Body Composition: In Vivo Methods, Models, and Assessment.* New York, NY: Plenum Press; 1993:371–6.

8 Burmeister, W., Romahn, A. Development of potassium content and energetics of body cell mass formation in premature infants. *Monatsschr Kinderheilkd.* 1971;**119**:307–9.

9 National Institutes of Health. Bioelectrical impedance analysis in body composition measurement: National Institutes of Health Technology Assessment Conference Statement. *Am. J. Clin. Nutr.* 1996;**64**:524S–32S.

10 Tang, W., Ridout, D., Modi, N. Assessment of total body water using bioelectrical impedance analysis in neonates receiving intensive care. *Arch. Dis. Child.* 1997;**77**:F123–6.

11 Piccoli, A., Fanos, V., Peruzzi, L. *et al.* Reference values of the bioelectrical impedance vector in neonates in the first week after birth. *Nutrition* 2002;**18**:383–7.

12 Fields, D. A., Goran, M. I., McCrory, M. A. Body composition assessment via air-displacement plethysmography in adults and children: a review. *Am. J. Clin. Nutr.* 2002;**75**:453–67.

13 Urlando, A., Dempster, P., Aitkens, S. A new air displacement plethsmograph for the measurement of body composition in infants. *Acta Diabetol.* 2002;**39**:154.

14 Rupich, R. C., Specker, B. L., Lieuw-A-Fa, M., Ho, M. Gender and race differences in bone mass during infancy. *Calcif. Tissue Int.* 1996;**58**:395–7.

15 Ichiba, H., Hirai, C., Fujimaru, M. *et al.* Measurement of bone mineral density of lumbar spine and whole body in low-birth-weight infants: comparison of two methods. *J. Bone Miner. Metab.* 2001;**19**:52–5.

16 Pieltain, C., De Curtis, M., Gerard, P., Rigo, J. Weight gain composition in preterm infants with dual-energy x-ray absorptiometry. *Ped. Res.* 2001;**49**:120–4.

17 Lapillonne, A., Salle, B. L. Methods for measuring body composition in newborns – a comparative analysis. *J. Ped. Endocr. Metab.* 1999;**12**:125–37.

18 Wells, J. C. K. A critique of the expression of paediatric body composition data. *Arch. Dis. Child.* 2001;**85**:67–72.

19 Butte, N. F., Wong, W. W., Hopkinson, J. M., Smith, E. O., Ellis, K. J. Infant feeding mode affects early growth and body composition. *Pediatrics* 2000b;**106**:1355–66.

20 de Bruin, N. C., van Velthoven, K. A. M., de Ridder, M. *et al.* Standards for total body fat and fat-free mass in infants. *Arch. Dis. Child.* 1996;**74**:386–99.

21 Koo, W. W. K., Walters, J. C., Hockman, E. M. Body composition in human infants at birth and postnatally. *J. Nutr.* 2000;**130**:2188–94.

22 Koo, B., Walters, J., Hockman, E., Koo, W. Body composition of newborn twins: intrapair differences. *J. Am. Coll. Nutr.* 2002;**21**:245–9.

23 Rigo, J., Nyamugabo, R. J., Picaud, J. C. *et al.* Reference values of body composition obtained by dual energy X-ray absorptiometry in preterm and term neonates. *J. Pediatr. Gastroenterol. Nutr.* 1998;**27**:184–90.

24 Butte, N., Heinz, C., Hopkinson, J. *et al.* Fat mass in infants and toddlers: comparability of total body water, total body potassium, total body electrical conductivity, and dual-energy X-ray absorptiometry. *J. Pediatr. Gastroenterol. Nutr.* 1999;**29**:184–9.

25 Galan, H. L., Rigano, S., Radaelli, T. *et al.* Reduction of subcutaneous mass, but not lean mass, in normal fetuses in Denver, Colorado. *Am. J. Obstet. Gynecol.* 2001;**185**:839–44.

26 Hediger, M. L., Overpeck, M. D., Kuczmarski, R. J., Ruan, W. J. Association between infant breast-feeding and overweight in young children. *J. Am. Med. Assoc.* 2001;**285**:2453–60.

27 Gillman, M. W., Rifas-Shiman, S. L., Camargo, C. A. Jr, *et al.* Risk of overweight among adolescents who were breast-fed as infants. *J. Am. Med. Assoc.* 2001;**285**:2461–7.

28 Avila-Diaz, M., Flores-Huerta, S., Martinez-Muniz, I., Amato, D. Increments in whole body bone mineral content associated with weight and length in pre-term and full-term infants during the first 6 months of life. *Arch Med. Res.* 2001:288–92.

42

Methods of measuring energy balance: calorimetry and doubly labeled water

Pieter J. J. Sauer

Department of Pediatrics, University Hospital Groningen, Groningen, The Netherlands

The energy balance is the equation relating the amount of energy taken up by an individual and the amount of energy used by the same individual. The difference between these two is the amount of energy stored, or lost by the body. In order to calculate the energy balance, one has to know the energy input into the infant, the amount of energy absorbed, the amount converted into heat for maintenance, activity, and thermoregulation, and the amount lost by the feces and in urine after metabolism of protein. The formulas for this are as follows:

$$\text{Energy}_{\text{intake}} = \text{energy}_{\text{maintenance}} + \text{energy}_{\text{activity}}$$
$$+ \text{energy}_{\text{thermoregulation}} + \text{energy}_{\text{growth}}$$
$$+ \text{energy}_{\text{urine+feces}}$$

How accurately all factors have to be known is dependent on the question raised. For example, if one is interested in growth over a prolonged period of time, differences of 3–4 kcal kg^{-1} day^{-1} in either the measurement of intake or expenditure might be important as 1–3 kcal kg^{-1} day^{-1} is needed for 1 g of growth.[1-3] To study the effect of physiologic or pharmacologic changes on energy expenditure, which might be more short-term effects, a difference in energy expenditure of 6–8 kcal kg^{-1} day^{-1} might be clinically relevant.[4]

In this chapter the different aspects of measuring the energy balance in preterm infants will be discussed.

Measuring energy intake

The measurement of energy intake might not be as simple as it appears. In formula-fed infants the actual amount of calories provided to the infant might not be the same as indicated by the manufacturer due to lack of solubility of fat, possibly bound to calcium. When the feeding is not vigorously shaken before administration or is left for some time in a horizontal setting, fat will precipitate and not be administered. In human milk the composition of milk is variable from feeding to feeding as well as during a single feeding. A real measurement of the composition of breast milk therefore is needed for determination of the energy balance. The measurements of spills and vomits, though hard to do, are nevertheless important.

The amount of nutrition taken up by the gastrointestinal tract is usually calculated as the difference between the enteral intake and losses in the feces. How long the feces should be collected in order to have a reliable estimate of the daily losses is not very well known. ElHennawy et al.[5] found a mean gastric time in preterm infants of approximately 16 days, and a mean transit time of 80 ± 50 hours. McClure and Newell[6] showed that the transit time is related to postnatal age and to the introduction of feeding after birth. Median transit time at 3 weeks of age was 32 hours for infants given early trophic feedings starting on the third day of life versus 49 hours in infants in whom enteral feedings were held until infants were off all respiratory support (mechanical ventilation and/or CPAP). In these same infants at 6 weeks of age, median transit time was 21 hours versus 33 hours in the early trophic versus delayed feeding groups, respectively. Moreover, they found a rather wide range in transit times, from 10–240 hours. A collection period of at least 3 days therefore seems needed in these infants.

In the feces, the amount of energy-containing substances (fat, carbohydrate, protein) can be measured separately or

Neonatal Nutrition and Metabolism. Second Edition, ed. P. Thureen and W. Hay. Published by Cambridge University Press.
© Cambridge University Press 2006.

the total energy content can be determined using bomb-calorimetry. One should realize that energy losses in the feces are not only due to nonabsorbed food, but also energy components may be excreted as bile or be excreted directly into the gastrointestinal tract. The magnitude of these last factors is unknown.

Methods to measure energy expenditure

Many rather diverse methods have been described to estimate the energy expenditure in newborn infants. On a theoretical basis, direct calorimetry is the gold standard. As direct calorimetry is expensive and difficult to perform, other methods have been sought. The most widely used method is indirect calorimetry; other methods include doubly labeled water, bicarbonate infusion, thermography, and heart rate variability.

Direct calorimetry

All energy used within the human body is given off as heat or spent as external work. Energy used for activity is also given off as heat. Energy absorbed, but not given off as heat is stored within the body. In human infants this is equivalent to growth. When body temperature is stable, heat production will be equal to heat loss and thereby energy expenditure of the infant. Heat is given off via radiation, convection, conduction, and evaporation. Radiation is the transfer of heat to surrounding surfaces. This heat loss can be important for infants in an open bed or single wall incubator placed in a rather cool room. Radiation can be reduced or reversed to warming under an overhead heater. Radiation is low in modern incubators, with a flow of heated air along the walls of the incubator. Convection is the heat loss due to airflow over the infant. This again can be important in an open bed, though in incubators with a low airflow it is limited. Conductive heat loss, due to direct heat transfer from the body, is low under almost all conditions. Evaporation is dependent on the absolute humidity of the environment and the airflow. Evaporation can be very important, especially in the very preterm infant in the first days of life in an environment with a low humidity. A direct calorimeter must measure all four methods of heat loss. Secondly, the temperature of the infant must be stable since a change in body temperature directly influences heat storage or heat loss. Studies using direct calorimetry in newborn infants are very limited.[2,7–9] Direct calorimetry requires sophisticated equipment with frequent calibration and limited access to the patients. One larger study on the metabolic rate

comparing direct and indirect calorimetry in preterm newborn infants has been done.[2] A scheme of the direct calorimeter used in that study is given in Figure 42.1. The results of both methods were very comparable. Therefore indirect calorimetry can be used to measure metabolic rate.

Indirect calorimetry

Indirect calorimetry is the most widely used method to measure energy expenditure in preterm and term infants. This method is considered to be rather simple and provides reliable results under appropriate conditions. Indirect calorimetry is based on the assumption that food-stuffs are oxidized in order to produce energy, consuming oxygen and producing carbon dioxide. By measuring these, and combined with the excretion of N_2 in urine (U_N) as an indicator of protein oxidation, the energy expenditure can be calculated. Different formulas have been proposed to calculate the energy expenditure from oxygen consumption and CO_2 production. The most widely used is the Weir's equation:

$$Energy\ expenditure = 3.941\ VO_2 + 1.106\ VCO_2$$
$$- 2.17\ U_N(10).$$

Weir showed that the error of neglecting the effect of protein oxidation (i.e., assuming $U_N = 0$) is negligible.[10] Energy expenditure therefore can be estimated from only the oxygen consumption and carbon dioxide production. Not only energy expenditure can be estimated from the oxygen consumption and carbon dioxide production; also the amount of carbohydrate and fat oxidized can be calculated. In all these calculations complete oxidation of all foodstuffs to CO_2 and H_2O is assumed.

Indirect calorimetry does have a number of theoretical and practical limitations.

Theoretical limitations

In indirect calorimetry it is assumed that all foodstuffs used are oxidized completely to CO_2 and H_2O, and that all CO_2 is immediately released by the body. Incomplete oxidation of foodstuffs therefore might influence results. The results are also influenced when one energy-containing substance (e.g., sugar) is converted in the body into another component (e.g., fat). In this process O_2 is consumed and CO_2 produced; however, in a different ratio compared to complete oxidation. This process will also influence the metabolic rate.

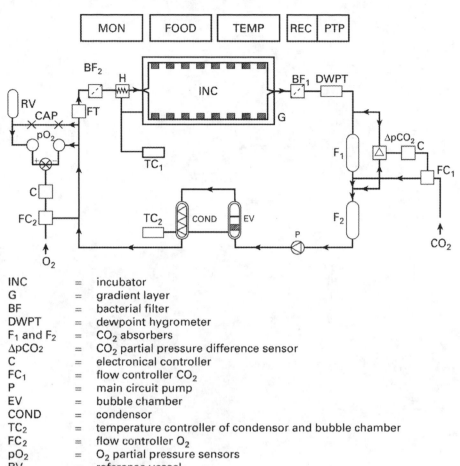

INC	=	incubator
G	=	gradient layer
BF	=	bacterial filter
DWPT	=	dewpoint hygrometer
F_1 and F_2	=	CO_2 absorbers
$\Delta pCO2$	=	CO_2 partial pressure difference sensor
C	=	electronical controller
FC_1	=	flow controller CO_2
P	=	main circuit pump
EV	=	bubble chamber
COND	=	condensor
TC_2	=	temperature controller of condensor and bubble chamber
FC_2	=	flow controller O_2
pO_2	=	O_2 partial pressure sensors
RV	=	reference vessel
CAP	=	capillary
FT	=	main circuit flow sensor
H	=	heat exchanger
TC_1	=	temperature controller of incubator and heat exchanger
MON	=	heart beat and apnea monitor
FOOD	=	feeding system
TEMP	=	thermometer system
REC	=	recorder
PTP	=	paper-tape puncher

Figure 42.1. Schematic diagram of a combined direct/indirect calorimeter.

Practical limitations

Practical problems are as important as the theoretical limitations of indirect calorimetry. Almost all systems for indirect calorimetry are based on the following principle: the concentration of oxygen and carbon dioxide is measured in the gas provided to the infant as well as the gas returned from the infant. From this difference in concentration, together with the flow rate of the gas, oxygen and carbon dioxide production can be calculated. Indirect calorimetry systems are either closed or open systems. In a closed system the whole body is included in the metabolic chamber.

The advantage of these systems is that the air entering into and leaving from the metabolic chamber can be very well controlled, thereby increasing precision. Negative aspects are that the infant has to breathe spontaneously and cannot be handled through the study. Although the closed system can be considered as the most reliable, due to the practical limitations, they are not popular. Most studies have used the open system where either a hood is placed over the infant or the infant is on CPAP or a ventilator.

Requirements for indirect calorimetry include the following:

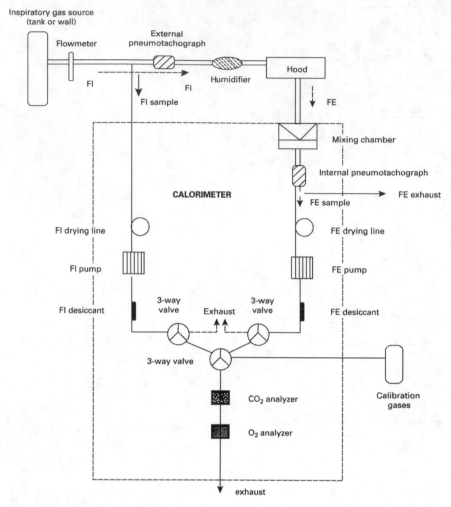

Figure 42.2. Schematic diagram of an indirect calorimeter.[11]

- The system can reliably and reproducibly measure very small differences in oxygen saturation and carbon dioxide production as well as gas flow rate.
- The inspiratory gas concentration is constant.
- There is a complete mixing of expired gas.

Considerations regarding the infant include the following:

- The infant needs to be in a stable situation, implying that the exhaled gas concentration reflects cell metabolism and is not affected by rapid changes, for instance as may occur with hyperventilation.
- Duration of measurement.
- Mode of respiration (spontaneous respiration, nasal CPAP, ventilation).
- Body weight.

The difference in oxygen and carbon dioxide concentration between the air to and from the calorimeter is usually in the order of 0.1%–0.2%.[11–17] A calorimeter must be able to

detect these small differences at a flow rate of 1–4 L min^{-1}. Also important is the stable concentration of oxygen and carbon dioxide of the air to the infant. Especially in tiny infants, this limits the use of compressed air from a standard source as well as from supplemental oxygen. Thureen *et al.*[11] showed that air from a wall source is too unstable to be used in a calorimeter. Behrens[12] showed that errors in measuring oxygen consumption increase with the percentage of oxygen in inspired air. For an accurate measurement the complete mixing of expired air is essential. Different systems therefore use a special mixing chamber in the system. An example of an indirect calorimeter system is given in Figure 42.2.

Reliable results are not only dependent on the characteristics of the apparatus, but also on the patients. The first assumption of indirect calorimetry is that the concentrations of CO_2 and oxygen in the body are constant. Increasing CO_2 production or oxygen consumption due to a higher metabolic rate must be translated into changes in the expired air. If a child starts crying during short periods of measurements, these requirements are not met, and results will not be correct. The required duration of a measurement is dependent on the question raised. Measurements of 10–15 minutes might be sufficient to show the effect of sleep states on metabolic rate.[18] However, if one is interested in 24-hour energy expenditure, the duration of the measurement must be longer. Bell et al.[19] and Schutze et al.[20] suggested that continuous measurements over 6 hours can predict 24 hours energy expenditure. This was recently supported by Perring.[21] Most studies on energy expenditure so far have been done in growing stable preterm infants. Studies in infants on ventilators as well as those in infants receiving supplemental oxygen are disputed.[22] In case of supplemental oxygen, errors are due to nonstable oxygen intake as well as to errors in the calculations used. In infants on continuous positive airway pressure (CPAP) and on ventilators leaks in the expired air become important, thereby making measurements potentially unreliable.[11,23–25] Bauer et al. described a method where all expired air was collected, including from air leaks around the tracheal tube and on nasal CPAP.[26]

Although this system might work in slightly older and bigger infants, it did not work in infants with a birth weight <1000g.[27] Moreover, it requires the continuous hand-held application of a collection chamber just above the infant, which is not very practical for measurements of 6 hours. Thureen et al.[11] recently described a system which makes it possible to perform indirect calorimetry in spontaneous breathing infants with supplemental oxygen up to 0.40 and in ventilated infants with an oxygen supply of up to 0.60. For the spontaneously breathing patients a hood within the hood system was used. By this system, both the air entering and leaving the hood is well-controlled. Although the system did not work with all ventilators, with certain ventilators reliable results were obtained. It is important to note that the authors only performed studies in infants with a tube leak of less than 5%. This again limits the applicability of this method, also as it is not easy to accurately define the tube leak. Most systems presently on the market are not designed for and cannot be used on infants of $<\sim$1000 g. Errors increase with a decrease in weight, due to the small volumes of O_2 consumed and CO_2 produced. Only closed systems and the system described by Thureen et al.[11] seem to be able to perform reliable measurements in infants up to 500 g.

Doubly labeled water

Another technique to estimate metabolic rate in the free-living individual is the use of doubly labeled water, $D_2{}^{18}O$. In

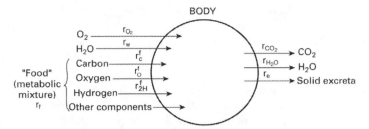

Figure 42.3. Principle of measuring energy expenditure with the double labeled water technique.

1955 Lifson et al.[28] described a method to calculate the CO_2 production from the difference in turnover rate between oxygen and hydrogen. This method is based on the principle that oxygen is lost via CO_2 and H_2O, whereas hydrogen is lost only via H_2O. The difference in turnover rate between oxygen and hydrogen is equal to CO_2 production (Figure 42.3). When a certain RQ is assumed, one can calculate the total energy expenditure. This method involves a number of assumptions as discussed recently.[29,30]

(1) The subject must be in a steady state of body composition, so total body water, solids, and weight must remain constant.

(2) All rates of intake and output of water and CO_2 remain constant.

(3) Water is the only form in which the hydrogen of body water is lost from the body, and water plus CO_2 are the only forms in which the oxygen of body water is lost.

(4) The enrichment of the hydrogen of water lost from the body is equal to that of the body water, and the enrichment of the oxygen of water and CO_2 lost from the body is equal to that of the body water.

(5) The normal abundance of isotopic oxygen and hydrogen is the same in all substances involved in the material balance.

(6) There is no isotopic re-entry into the body or entry into the body of isotopic water vapor or CO_2.

(7) The volume of distribution of labeled water is equal to the total body water (i.e., there is no incorporation of labeled hydrogen or oxygen of body water into other body constituents except in CO_2 in the case of O_2).

A number of these assumptions cannot be met, and corrections must be made. Firstly, the growing neonate is not in a steady state but increases body mass and body water over time. This problem can be overcome by measuring body composition at the beginning and the end of a 5-day period, the time period over which the turnover rate of oxygen and carbon dioxide is usually measured in the neonate. Secondly, the enrichment of all water lost by the body is not equal to the enrichment of body water. Specifically, the water lost by insensible water loss has an enrichment different from that of body water. For the different enrichments of water lost through the skin and via the lung, a correction factor has been introduced, as has a correction factor for the uptake of water through the skin and the lung.

The effects of fractionation are more important in the neonate compared with the adult owing to the high water turnover in the neonate relative to that in the adult. Finally, the precision by which the enrichment of body water can be measured is essential for this method. Fortunately, it has improved dramatically when using specially designed isotope ratio mass spectrometers with which enrichments as low as 0.0001% can be measured. Various studies have compared CO_2 production calculated from the doubly labeled method with CO_2 production and metabolic rate measured by indirect calorimetry. Studies in the adult showed a mean difference between the methods of 4–8%.[31,32]

A number of studies comparing indirect calorimetry with the $D_2{}^{18}O$ method were conducted in the preterm and term neonate. Roberts et al.[33] conducted a validation study in four preterm neonates. Indirect calorimetry was performed over most of 5 days with the decay curve of D_2O and $H_2{}^{18}O$ calculated from enrichment in urine. The mean difference between the methods of measuring CO_2 production was only 1.4% ± 4.8% (mean ± SD) and the difference in metabolic rate was 0.3% ± 2.6%. In this study a number of correction factors were used that have been debated by others.

Jones et al.[34] showed that a change in the composition of the feeding during a study may cause a shift in baseline enrichment, resulting in a major error in the estimation of CO_2 production. The doubly labeled water method can be regarded as a reliable method to measure total energy consumption in groups of individuals, including the preterm infant.[35] The results in the individual patient, however, show rather large differences between indirect calorimetry and the doubly labeled method, making this last method rather unreliable for individual measurements. It is uncertain if the method is accurate in the infant with changes in body water over the study period, such as infants with bronchopulmonary dysplasia (BPD). Leith et al.[36] studied infants with BPD while receiving dexamethasone. The metabolic rate observed in this study is rather surprisingly high, with a wide standard deviation. This might be due to changes in body water.

Labeled sodium bicarbonate

A recently described method to estimate the energy expenditure of preterm infants is the infusion of ^{13}C labeled

bicarbonate and the measurement of $^{13}CO_2$ in expired air.[37–39] The amount of CO_2 exhaled by the infant can be calculated from the percentage of infused tracer expired as $^{13}CO_2$. From the CO_2 production together with an estimated RQ, energy expenditure can be calculated. The method itself is simple and elegant, and can be used for instance in tiny infants on the ventilator. It does not require the collection of all expired air, and dilution of air does not influence the results. The only measurement needed is the ratio of $^{12}C/^{13}C$ in expired air at plateau, 2–3 hours after the start of a constant NaH-$^{13}CO_2$ infusion. Shew et al.[39] performed a study in spontaneously breathing postsurgical infants where they compared the results of NaH^{13}-CO_3 method with indirect calorimetry. Although there was a good correlation between both measurements, the $^{13}CO_2$ method showed a RaCO2 (turnover rate of CO_2) of 0.725 ± 0.021 mmol kg^{-1} day^{-1} compared with a CO_2 production of 0.489 ± 0.016 mmol kg^{-1} day^{-1} with indirect calorimetry, resulting in an energy expenditure of 89.5 ± 2.5 v. 60.2 ± 2.1 kcal kg^{-1} day^{-1}. This difference can be explained by the observation already made by Van Aerde et al. in 1985,[40] that part of the $^{13}CO_2$ liberated from bicarbonate might be trapped in slow turnover pools in the body (e.g., bones, tricarboxi-intermediates, etc). The unlabeled CO_2 production is in constant equilibration with these slow turnover pools and thereby reflects the real CO_2 production. Due to the trapping of labeled $^{13}CO_2$, which might be equilibrated only after a period of 12 or more hours, the $^{13}CO_2$ method overestimates the real CO_2 production. Van Aerde et al.[40] suggested the use of a correction factor based on energy intake of 0.7–0.9. When applying this correction factor, the method of labeled bicarbonate might be a very reasonable alternative to the doubly labeled water technique, as it is a rather cheap and simple method. As in the case with the doubly labeled water method, it only measures the CO_2 production, and energy expenditure measurement is based on an estimated RQ.

Infrared thermographic calorimetry

Recently infrared thermographic calorimetry was described as a new method to estimate total heat loss of newborn infants.[41] This method of direct calorimetry does not make use of specially designed incubators, but measures body surface temperature with infrared thermography together with estimations of evaporative water loss. The dry heat transfer of the body is calculated using standard equations for heat transfer. Body surface area and body surface temperature are measured by infrared thermography. In 10 infants with a mean birth weight of

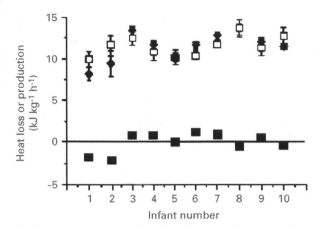

Figure 42.4. Mean (± SD) heat loss, as measured by infrared thermography (♦) and heat production as measured by indirect calorimetry (□). Difference between both methods n.

1.28 ± 0.47 kg this method was compared with indirect calorimetry. On average the results are in accordance, although some differences in individual patients exist (Figure 42.4). Further studies are needed to determine the minimum number of infrared thermographic calorimetry (ITC) pictures needed to qualify accurately the 24 hour energy expenditure in preterm infants. As ITC is a noninvasive method, it holds a promise for measuring energy expenditure, also in sick preterm infants.

Heart rate variability

Another noninvasive method of measuring energy expenditure in adolescents and adults is the measurement of the heart rate. Oxygen consumption shows a reasonable correlation with the heart rate in adults. Only one study is conducted in preterm infants. Chessex et al.[42] indicated a correlation between heart rate and oxygen consumption in preterm infants, suggesting that the heart rate might be used to estimate heat production. They showed that oxygen consumption increases when the heart rate increases over 160 beats min^{-1}. No correlation between heart rate and oxygen consumption was observed between 120 and 160 beats min^{-1}, while 80% of the time the heart rate of preterm infants is within this range. In preterm infants there is therefore no real correlation between heart rate and oxygen consumption, so this method cannot be used in these infants.

REFERENCES

1 Thureen, P. J. Measuring energy expenditure in preterm and unstable infants. *J. Pediatr.* 2003;**142**:366–7.

2 Sauer, P. J. J., Dane, J. H., Visser, H. K. A. Longitudinal studies on metabolic rate, heat production and energy cost of growth in low birth weight infants. *Pediatr. Res.* 1984;**18**:254–9.

3 Sauer, P. J. J. Neonatal energy metabolism. In Cowett, R. M. ed. *Principles of Perinatal–neonatal Metabolism.* New York: Springer Verlag; 1998:1001–25.

4 Carnielli, V. P., Verlato, G., Benini, F., Rossi, K. Metabolic and respiratory effects of theophylline in the preterm infant. *Arch. Dis. Child. Fetal Neonatal Edn.* 2000;**83**:F39–43.

5 ElHennawy, A. A., Sparks, J. W., Armentrout, D., Huseby, V., Berseth, C. L. Erythromycin fails to improve feeding outcome in feeding-intolerant preterm infants. *J. Pediatr. Gastroenterol. Nutr.* 2003;**37**:281–6.

6 McClure, R. J., Newell, S. J. Randomised controlled trial of trophic feeding and gut motility. *Arch. Dis. Child. Fetal Neonatal Edn.* 1999;**80**:F54–8.

7 Ryser, G., Jequier, E. Study by direct calorimetry of thermal balance on the first day of life. *Eur. J. Clin. Invest.* 1972;**2**:176–87.

8 Meis, S. J., Dove, E. L., Bell, E. F. *et al.* A gradient-layer calorimeter for measurement of energy expenditure of infants. *Am. J. Physiol.* 1994;**266**:R1052–60.

9 Dane, H. J., Holland, W. P. J., Sauer, P. J. J., Visser, H. K. A. A calorimetric system for metabolic studies of newborn infants. *Clin. Phys. Physiol. Meas.* 1985;**6**:36–46.

10 Weir, J. B. New methods for calculating metabolic rate with special reference to protein metabolism. *J. Physiol.* 1949;**109**:1.

11 Thureen, P. J., Phillips, R. E., DeMarie, M. P. *et al.* Technical and methodologic considerations for performance of indirect calorimetry in ventilated and non-ventilated preterm infants. *Crit. Care Med.* 1997;**25**:171–9.

12 Behrends, M., Kernbach, M., Bräuer, A. *et al.* In vitro validation of a metabolic monitor for gas exchange measurements in ventilated neonates. *Intens. Care Med.* 2001;**27**:228–35.

13 Marks, K. H., Coen, P., Kerrigan, J. R. *et al.* The accuracy and precision of an open-circuit system to measure oxygen consumption and carbon dioxide production in neonates. *Pediatr. Res.* 1987;**21**:58–65.

14 Handley, A. C., Spencer, S. A., Rakowski, S. Critical appraisal and further development of the methodology for open circuit calorimetry in neonates. *Early Hum. Dev.* 1991;**26**:167–76.

15 Ferrannini, E. The theoretical basis of indirect calorimetry: a review. *Metabolism* 1988;**37**:287–301.

16 Shortland, G. J., Fleming, P. J., Walter, J. H. Validation of a portable indirect calorimetry system for measurement of energy expenditure in sick preterm infants. *Arch. Dis. Child.* 1992;**67**:1207–11.

17 Ultman, J. S., Bursztein, S. Analysis of error in the determination of respiratory gas exchange at varying FIO_2. *J. Appl. Physiol.* 1981;**350**:210–16.

18 Dane, H. J., Sauer, P. J. J., Visser, H. K. A. Oxygen consumption and CO_2 production of low birthweight infants in two sleep states. *Biol. Neonate* 1985;**47**:205–10.

19 Bell, E. F., Rios, G. R., Wilmoth, P. K. Estimation of 24-hour energy expenditure from shorter measurement periods in preterm infants. *Pediatr. Res.* 1986;**20**:646–9.

20 Schulze, K., Stefanski, M., Masterson, J. An analysis of the variability in estimates of bioenergetic variables in preterm infants. *Pediatr. Res.* 1986;**20**:422–7.

21 Perring, J., Henderson, M., Cooke, R. J. Factors affecting the measurement of energy expenditure during energy balance studies in preterm infants. *Pediatr. Res.* 2000;**48**:518–23.

22 Kalhan, S. C., Denne, S. C. Energy consumption in infants with bronchopulmonary dysplasia. *J. Pediatr.* 1990;**116**:662–4.

23 Chwals, W. J., Laly, K. P., Woolley, M. M. Indirect calorimetry in mechanically ventilated infants and children: measurement accuracy with absence of audible airleak. *Crit. Care Med.* 1992;**20**:768–70.

24 Forsyth, J. S., Crighton, A. An indirect calorimetry system for ventilator dependent very low birthweight infants. *Arch. Dis. Child.* 1992;**67**:315–19.

25 Mayfield, S. R. Technical and clinical testing of a computerized indirect calorimeter for use in mechanically ventilated neonates. *Am. J. Clin. Nutr.* 1991;**54**:30–4.

26 Bauer, K., Ketteler, J., Laurenz, M., Versmold, H. In vitro validation and clinical testing of an indirect calorimetry system for ventilated preterm infants that is unaffected by endotracheal tube leaks and can be used during nasal continuous positive airway pressure. *Pediatr. Res.* 2001;**49**:394–401.

27 Bauer, K., Laurenz, M., Ketteler, J., Versmold, H. Longitudinal study of energy expenditure in preterm neonates <30 weeks gestation during the first three postnatal weeks. *J. Pediatr.* 2003;**142**:390–6.

28 Lifson, N., Gordon, G. B., McClintock, R. Measurements of total carbon dioxide production by means of $D_2{}^{18}O$. *J. Appl. Physiol.* 1955;**7**:704–10.

29 Ainslie, P. N., Reilly, T., Westerterp, K. R. Estimating human energy expenditure: a review of techniques with particular reference to doubly labeled water. *Sports Med.* 2003;**33**:683–98.

30 Wells, J. C. K. Energy metabolism in infants and children. *Nutrition* 1998;**14**:817–20.

31 Schoeller, D. A., Webb, P. Five-day comparison of the doubly labeled water method with respiratory gas exchange. *Am. J. Clin. Nutr.* 1984;**40**:153–8.

32 Klein, P. D., James, W. P. T., Wong, W. W. Calorimetric validation of the doubly labeled water method for determination of energy expenditure in man. *Hum. Nutr. Clin. Nutr.* 1984;**38C**:95–106.

33 Roberts, S. D., Coward, W. A., Schlingenseipen, K. H. Comparison of the doubly labeled water ($^2H_2{}^{18}O$) method with indirect calorimetry and a nutrient-balance study for simultaneous determination of energy expenditure, water intake and metabolizable energy intake in preterm infants. *Am. J. Clin. Nutr.* 1986;**44**:315–22.

34 Jones, P. J. H., Winthrop, A. L., Schoeller, D. A. Evaluation of doubly labeled water for measuring energy expenditure during changing nutrition. *Am. J. Clin. Nutr.* 1988;**47**:799–804.

35 Westerterp, K. R., Lafeber, H. N., Sulkers, E. J. Comparison of short term indirect calorimetry and doubly labeled water method for the assessment of energy expenditure in preterm infants. *Biol. Neonate* 1991;**60**:75–82.

36 Leith, C. A., Ahlrichs, J., Karn, C., Denne, S. C. Energy expenditure and energy intake during dexamethasone therapy for chronic lung disease. *Pediatr. Res.* 1999;**46**:109–13.

37 Sulkers, E. J., Van Goudoever, J. B., Leunisse, C. *et al.* Determination of carbon-labeled substrate oxidation rates. In Lafeber, H. N. ed. *Fetal and Neonatal Physiological Measurements.* Amsterdam: Excerpta Medica; 1991:297–304.

38 Kien, C. L. Isotopic dilution of CO_2 as an estimate of CO_2 production during substrate oxidation studies. *Am. J. Physiol.* 1989;**257**:E296–8.

39 Shew, S. B., Beckett, P. R., Keshen, T. H., Jahoor, F., Jaksic, T. Validation of a [^{13}C] bicarbonate tracer technique to measure neonatal energy expenditure. *Pediatr. Res.* 2000;**47**:787–91.

40 Van Aerde, J. E., Sauer, P. J. J., Pencharz, P. B. *et al.* The effect of energy intake and expenditure on the recovery of $^{13}CO_2$ in the parenterally fed neonate during a 4-hour period primed constant infusion of $NaH^{13}CO_3$. *Pediatr. Res.* 1985;**19**:806–10.

41 Adams, A. K., Nelson, R. A., Bell, E. F., Egoavil, C. A. Use of infrared thermographic calorimetry to determine energy expenditure in preterm infants. *Am. J. Clin. Nutr.* 2000;**71**:969–77.

42 Chessex, P., Reichman, B., Verellen, G. J. E. Relation between heart rate and energy expenditure in the newborn. *Pediatr. Res.* 1981;**15**:1071–82.

43

Methods of measuring nutrient substrate utilization using stable isotopes

Agneta L. Sunehag and Morey W. Haymond

Children's Nutrition Research Center, Baylor College of Medicine, Houston, TX

Introduction

During fetal life a continuous supply of nutrients is transferred to the fetus via the placenta. Transplacental transported glucose is the major energy substrate for the fetus, which has glucose demands of 4–8 mg kg^{-1} min^{-1}. The maternal–fetal transport of glucose occurs via passive diffusion facilitated by the glucose transporter system (specifically GLUT-1).[1,2,3] Amino acids are transferred by active transport,[1,2] and several classes of amino acid transporters have been identified in human placentas.[3] Transplacental transfer of fatty acids is small. It is regulated by maternal fatty acid concentrations and is mediated by a number of different proteins. At birth, the transplacental supply of nutrients is abruptly interrupted and the newborn infant must first mobilize its own substrate stores and then rapidly adjust to enteral feedings to meet the metabolic needs.

Glucose is the primary substrate for brain metabolism, and the brain utilizes about 20 times more glucose than muscle and fat per gram tissue. Infants have a large brain to body weight ratio (12% in infants v. 2% in an adult).[4] Thus, the glucose turnover rate on a per kg body weight basis in an infant is three times higher than that of an adult, ~30 μmol kg^{-1} min^{-1} (~6 mg kg^{-1} min^{-1}) v. 11 μmol kg^{-1} min^{-1} (~2 mg kg^{-1} min^{-1}). As a result, ~90% of total glucose utilization in an infant is by the brain. Following cessation of the transplacental flow of nutrients, most healthy term newborn infants promptly initiate hepatic glucose production to meet their high glucose demands and maintain normoglycemia. Since the hepatic glycogen content is limited, the neonate becomes dependent on gluconeogenesis as the primary mechanism to maintain euglycemia within a few hours of fasting.[5,6]

The rapid postnatal increase in plasma concentrations of glycerol and free fatty acids, high glycerol turnover rates and decreasing respiratory quotient indicate that lipolysis and lipid oxidation increase immediately following birth, thus demonstrating the importance of lipids as oxidative substrates.[7–14] Lipids also contribute to the maintenance of glucose homeostasis in infants in that hydrolysis of triglycerides generates glycerol, which is used directly for glucose production via gluconeogenesis,[10–14] and free fatty acids (FFA), which upon hepatic β-oxidation provide energy to drive the gluconeogenic process. FFA oxidation also generates ketone bodies (hydroxybutyric acid and acetoacetic acid). With the exception of the brain, plasma FFA and ketone bodies can be used as fuel by most body tissues, thus decreasing the demands of these tissues for glucose as an energy source. In the brain, ketone bodies, but not FFA, can cross the blood–brain barrier and partially supplant the need for glucose.[15] In addition, fatty acids are involved in the synthesis of phospholipids, biological membranes, myelin, gangliosides, glycolipids, and sphingolipids.

Endogenous as well as exogenous amino acids are of great importance in the rapidly growing neonate since they serve as the building blocks for the body proteins. Further, after deamination a number of amino acids are also utilized as oxidative fuel and gluconeogenic substrate.

Metabolic research in newborn infants is limited by several constraints. The studies must be minimally invasive, the blood samples very small, and each study must provide maximal information possible, because of the difficulty in recruiting newborns for studies. The use of compounds labeled with stable isotopes analyzed by gas chromatography-mass spectrometry (GCMS) or isotope ratio-mass spectrometry (IRMS) fulfill these requirements,

Neonatal Nutrition and Metabolism. Second Edition, ed. P. Thureen and W. Hay. Published by Cambridge University Press.
© Cambridge University Press 2006.

thus providing a very valuable tool for dynamic studies of neonatal metabolism.

Stable isotopes

Isotopes are chemically identical atoms with different atomic weights (masses) due to different numbers of neutrons in the shell, e.g., the carbon atom has 6 electrons and 6 protons. The most abundant carbon isotope is ^{12}C, which has 6 neutrons, whereas those containing 5, 7, or 8 neutrons are ^{11}C, ^{13}C, and ^{14}C. Some of these isotopes are radioactive and decay to other compounds while giving off radiation (e.g., ^{11}C and ^{14}C), while others do not and are, therefore, denoted stable (e.g., ^{12}C, ^{13}C). While radioactive isotopes cannot be used in infants and children for ethical reasons, stable isotopes are very useful since they are naturally occurring and nonradioactive. Therefore, compounds labeled with single or multiple stable isotopes or combinations of compounds labeled with stable isotopes can be used without risk regardless of age and size of the subjects.[16-20] Since substrates (glucose, amino acids, fatty acids etc.) labeled with stable isotopes are assumed to be metabolically equivalent to the corresponding unlabeled substrates, a specific labeled compound can be used to trace the metabolism of the corresponding unlabeled substrate in vivo.[16-20] A large number of substrates labeled with stable isotopes (e.g., ^{13}C, ^2H, ^{15}N) with high isotopic purity (98–99 atom%) are commercially available. Table 43.1 depicts examples of commonly used labeled substrates. For further information on available substrates labeled with stable isotopes see catalogues provided by the manufacturers. Gas chromatography–mass spectrometry (GC–MS), Gas chromatography–combustion–isotope ratio-mass spectrometry (GC–C–IRMS) and IRMS are commonly used to analyze compounds labeled with stable isotopes, although under selective circumstances, NMR is used. For the purpose of this chapter, we will focus exclusively on GC–MS, GC–C–IRMS and IRMS.

Gas chromatography (GC)–mass spectrometry (MS)

The sample to be analyzed is prepared for the GC–MS analysis by a procedure denoted "derivatization." Table 43.1 depicts examples of commonly used derivatization procedures.[21-25] The main purpose of this process is to lower the boiling point for the molecule to be analyzed, thus making it more volatile. The choice of derivatization procedure depends on the substrate to be analyzed, the mass spectrometry ionization mode (see below) and combination of tracers. The derivatized sample is injected at high temperature in the GC and carried through a capillary glass column by an inert gas, usually helium. In the column, the molecules to be analyzed (analyte) are separated from other components of the sample by a temperature-regulated interaction between the molecule in the carrier gas (the mobile phase) and the stationary phase coating the inner surface of the column.[17] Thus, at a specific time point, the analyte alone reaches the ion source of the mass spectrometer. The purpose of the mass spectrometer is to separate labeled from unlabeled molecules of the analyte. Briefly, the molecules enter the ion source of the mass spectrometer, where they are ionized either by direct bombardment of electrons (electron impact mode, EI) or after reacting with ions, generated by electron bombardment of a reactant gas (chemical ionization, CI). The most commonly used reactant gas is methane. Ions are separated based on their mass/charge (m/z) ratio by the mass analyzer. The signal is amplified in the electron multiplier, primarily based on the mass of the analyzed ion. Finally, a computer is interfaced with the mass spectrometer to collect and process the signal data. The data obtained give a ratio (mass to charge = m/z) between labeled and unlabeled ions. Irrespective of which compound is used, the data must be corrected for instrument deviations using standard curves prepared from standard solutions of carefully weighed mixtures of labeled (tracer) and unlabeled substrate (tracee). Using GC–MS, labeled and unlabeled molecules of, for example, glucose, amino acids, fatty acids, and glycerol can be analyzed.

Gas chromatography–combustion–mass spectrometry (GC–C–IRMS)

This technique measures the ratios of $^{13}CO_2$ and $^{12}CO_2$ or ^{15}N to ^{14}N in a sample. The GC principle is similar to that described above for GCMS, but the GC is not connected directly to the MS, but to a combustion oven, where the sample is oxidized at high temperature (940° for carbon and 980° for nitrogen) in the presence of a catalyst, resulting in CO_2, N_2, and H_2O. Following removal of H_2O, the CO_2, N_2, and H_2O are directed into the vacuum of the ion source via a dual inlet system with a switch valve that permits alternative inflow of the sample and the reference gas. Thus, the sample and the reference gas can be analyzed almost simultaneously. Since the mass spectrometer conditions are exactly the same during analysis of reference gas and sample, and the ratio between the $^{13}CO_2/^{12}CO_2$ and $^{15}N_2/^{14}N_2$ of the reference gases are known, the corresponding absolute ratios in the sample can be measured. This technique can be applied, for example, to glucose, amino acids, and fatty acids.

Table 43.1. Example of compounds labeled with stable isotopes

Labeled substrate	Derivative	Ionization mode	Column	Masses
[1-^{13}C]glucose	Penta-acetate (21)	PCI	17/1701	331; 332
		GC-C-IRMS	17/1701	$^{13}CO_2/^{12}CO_2$
[U-^{13}C]glucose	Penta-acetate (21)	PCI	17/1701	331–337
	Di-O-isopropylidene (22)	EI	17/1701/5	287–292
[6,6-^{2}H$_2$]glucose	Penta-acetate (21)	EI	17/1701	242–244
	Penta-acetate (21)	PCI	17/1701	331–333
	Di-O-isopropylidene (22)	EI	17/1701/5	287–289
[^{2}H$_3$]leucine	Heptafluorobutyric Anhydride (HFBA) (23)	NCI	5	349–352
[1-^{13}C]leucine	Heptafluorobutyric Anhydride (HFBA) (23)	NCI	5	349–350
[^{15}N$_2$]urea	2-Pyrimidinol-TBDMS (24)	EI	1701	153–155
[1-^{13}C]palmitate	Pentafluorobenzyl (PFBA) (25)	NCI	2330	255–256

Isotope ratio mass spectrometry (IRMS)

Breath samples can be directly injected in the mass spectrometer, and the $^{13}CO_2/^{12}CO_2$ ratio is analyzed using a reference gas as described above.

IRMS can also be used to measure the ratio of ^{2}H/^{1}H and ^{18}O/^{16}O in water derived from urine, plasma, or saliva. However, the sample must be converted to gaseous form. Several methods have been described for conversion of biological samples to ^{2}H/^{1}H.[26] In the most recent generation of IRMS instruments, the samples can be injected directly into a pyrolysis unit, in which the liquid sample is converted to ^{2}H/^{1}H gas at very high temperatures. The gas is subsequently forwarded online to the mass spectrometer and the ^{2}H/^{1}H ratio is measured. For measurement of ^{18}O, a water-CO$_2$ equilibration system is used. Briefly, CO$_2$ gas of known enrichment is placed in a vial with the water of interest. Following mechanical shaking for several hours, the oxygen in the water liberates into the CO$_2$ pool, the water vapor is eliminated using a cold trap[26] and the difference (delta) between the ^{18}O/^{16}O of CO$_2$ in the sample and that of the reference gas is measured by IRMS.[26] IRMS can, for example, be used in the analyses of substrate oxidation rates, energy expenditure using doubly labeled water (see below) and deuterium enrichment in body water (see below).

Analytical principles

Irrespective of the labeled compound used, the following dilution principles apply: when a stable labeled substrate is infused or ingested at a constant rate over time, labeled molecules (tracer) mix and eventually equilibrate with unlabeled molecules (tracee) in the plasma pool, and a condition of approximate steady state is reached. At steady state, substrate concentrations and the ratio between labeled and unlabeled molecules (i.e., tracer/tracee) in the mixing pool remain constant, i.e., the rate of entry (appearance rate, Ra) and loss of (disappearance rate, Rd) labeled and unlabeled substrates are equal. Since the infusion rate of the labeled substrate (tracer) is known, under fasting conditions i.e., no exogenous substrate is infused or ingested, Ra and Rd of the substrate can be calculated using the following equation:[16,18]

$$Ra = Rd = [(E_{infusate}/E_{plasma}) - 1] \times I$$
$$= [(E_{infusate}/E_{plasma}) \times I] - I \qquad (43.1)$$

where $E_{infusate}$ is the enrichment (tracer/(tracer+tracee)) of the infused tracer; E_{plasma} is the enrichment (tracer/(tracer + tracee)) above the naturally occurring enrichment of the tracer in plasma (mole percent excess, MPE%) at steady state and I the infusion rate of the tracer. In contrast to radioactive isotopes, stable isotopes are *not* mass less. Therefore, in the equation above, the infused tracer is subtracted i.e., Ra represents substrate produced endogenously. If any unlabeled substrate has been administered intravenously or orally, this must be subtracted as well. This model requires that the following assumptions be fulfilled:

(a) Sufficient infusion rate of the tracer to achieve tracer/tracee ratios which can be measured with high accuracy and precision i.e., for GCMS, tracer/tracee ratios should be $\geq$ 0.7–0.8%, for GC–C–IRMS $\geq$ 0.02%–0.05% (depending on number of labeled atoms) and for IRMS $\geq$ 0.01%.

(b) Sufficient duration of the isotope infusion to achieve equilibration of the tracer in the substrate pool.[27] Under conditions where a "true" isotopic steady state has not yet been fully achieved, the appearance (disappearance) rate of the substrate will be overestimated. The duration of tracer infusion required to reach tracer/tracee equilibrium is dependent on several factors, e.g., the turnover rate for the substrate – in a newborn infant the turnover rate for glucose is three times that of an adult. Thus, steady state for glucose is achieved faster in infants when compared to adults. By convention, most investigators use a priming dose of isotope to reach steady state faster. The priming dose is dependent on the size of the mixing pool. Usually a priming dose corresponding to 60–100 min of constant infusion is used. However, sometimes a larger prime is needed e.g., urea has a very large mixing pool, thus, a constant rate infusion of urea must be primed with a dose corresponding to 5–10 h of the constant infusion. Similarly, in hyperglycemic subjects, a larger glucose prime is required as compared with normoglycemic subjects.[28]

(c) No isotope effects i.e., the tracer and tracee are metabolically equivalent.

(d) No recycling of the tracer. Glucose can, for example, potentially recycle via glycogen storage and subsequent release or via the Cori cycle. Glucose recycling is dependent on the choice of glucose tracer. Thus, using glucose labeled with deuterium in the carbon 6 position ([6,6-^{2}H$_2$]glucose), the deuterium label is lost in the pyruvate-oxaloacetate and the malate-fumarate steps of the TCA cycle, and therefore, the [6,6-^{2}H$_2$]glucose can be regarded a non-recycling tracer (with regard to recycling in the Cori cycle). The [6,6-^{2}H$_2$]glucose tracer can, however, potentially recycle through glycogen. When [1-^{13}C]glucose is used, the ^{13}C label can recycle both via glycogen and the Cori cycle, resulting in a false increase in plasma ^{13}C enrichment and subsequently underestimation of glucose Ra.[29] Although the [U-^{13}C]glucose tracer is recycled via the Cori cycle, the likelihood that two uniformly labeled 3-carbon units will combine and form a new uniformly labeled glucose molecule is negligible and, thus, [U-^{13}C]glucose also can be regarded a non-recycling tracer.

Carbohydrate metabolism

In the fed state, the vast majority of plasma glucose is derived from the meal, while in the fasted state, glucose is produced from endogenous stores via glycogenolysis and gluconeogenesis. During infusion of glucose labeled with a stable isotope (^{13}C or ^{2}H), the tracer is diluted by unlabeled substrate (whether from feeding, an infusion of unlabeled glucose and/or from glucose produced via glycogenolysis and gluconeogenesis). When the tracer has equilibrated with unlabeled glucose (the tracee) and a condition of

approximate steady state is achieved, the appearance rate (Ra) and disappearance rate (Rd) of glucose (labeled and unlabeled) into (out of) the plasma pool can be calculated using equation 43.1 introduced above:[4,30]

$$\text{Glucose Ra} = \text{Rd} = [(E_{infusate}/E_{plasma}) - 1] \times I \quad (43.2)$$

where $E_{infusate}$ is the enrichment of the infused glucose tracer; E_{plasma} is the enrichment (MPE%) of this tracer in plasma at steady state and I the infusion rate of the glucose tracer. In this equation, the infused glucose tracer is subtracted. Thus, in the fasted state, glucose Ra represents glucose produced from the body stores (glucose production rate, GPR), i.e., from glycogenolysis and gluconeogenesis. If, however, unlabeled glucose is administered via feeding or IV infusion, this unlabeled glucose must also be subtracted, i.e.,

$$\text{GPR} = \text{Glucose Ra} - \text{exogenous unlabeled glucose} \quad (43.3)$$

If steady state cannot be achieved during a primed constant rate tracer infusion, glucose turnover can be calculated using non-steady state equations as described by Steele et al.[31] and modified by De Bodo et al.[32] This is a more complicated procedure involving assumptions about the volume of the mixing pool and whether a one, two, or multiple compartment model should be applied.

Using glucose labeled with ^{2}H and ^{13}C and the above described isotope dilution methods, we and others have demonstrated that (1) term healthy newborn infants produce glucose to maintain normoglycemia within a few hours of birth before any feedings[4,13,29] at rates (on a per kg body weight basis) about three times ($\sim$30 μmol kg^{-1} min^{-1}) those reported from normal adults after an overnight fast ($\sim$11 μmol kg^{-1} min^{-1});[4,33] (2) newborn infants of diabetic mothers studied within the first hours of life before any feedings had 20% lower glucose turnover rates (production and utilization) than those born to non-diabetic mothers;[34] (3) very premature infants, i.e., with gestational ages below 29 weeks can produce glucose at the same rate as term infants within the first day of life.[4,35–37] To our knowledge, there are no human data on fetal enzyme activities, but animal studies have demonstrated that at this gestational age (< 29 weeks), enzymes regulating glucose production are not activated. Thus, the reported results imply that the birth process itself activates these enzymes.

Although glucose turnover rates have been measured with high accuracy using isotope dilution methods for 30 years, estimating its two components gluconeogenesis and glycogenolysis has been a challenge for many investigators. This is because measures of gluconeogenesis are complicated by inflow, loss and exchange of carbons in the TCA cycle reactions. Thus, various approaches to measure gluconeogenesis using stable isotopes have been attempted in the past. Those pertinent to the pediatric population are discussed below.

(1) Estimates of the fraction of glucose production derived from a single substrate (tracing a labeled gluconeogenic precursor, e.g., glycerol, alanine, or lactate, to the product, glucose). Based on the appearance of ^{13}C in glucose following infusion of [2-^{13}C]glycerol, we and others[10–13] have demonstrated that in fasting term infants studied during the first day of life, glycerol accounted for about 10–20% of glucose production (measured by isotope dilution of [6,6-$^{2}H_2$]glucose). In addition, using the same study design, we demonstrated[14] that very premature infants (< 28 weeks) receiving only a small amount of intravenous glucose (one-third of their normal turnover rate) were capable of converting glycerol to glucose during the first day of life. Frazer et al.[38] showed in term AGA and SGA infants studied during their first 8 h of life, that about 10% of ^{13}C from infused [2,3-$^{13}C_2$]alanine appeared in blood glucose implying that newborn infants are capable of using amino acid carbon for glucose production in the immediate perinatal period. Further, Kalhan et al.[39] (using [$^{13}C_3$]lactate) reported that in newborn term infants lactate accounted for ~18% of glucose production. Collectively, these results clearly demonstrate that gluconeogenic key enzymes are activated at or within a few hours of birth independent of gestational age.

The use of a single tracer provides information only about the fraction contributed from this specific single gluconeogenic substrate and *not* the total fraction of glucose derived from gluconeogenesis. Further, this contribution from a single substrate is underestimated because tracer dilution due to inflow, loss and exchange of carbons in the TCA cycle is not taken into account.

(2) Estimates of total gluconeogenesis. Recently three new stable isotope methods with the potential to accurately measure total gluconeogenesis have been described. Each of them has both strengths and weaknesses. The three methods are: (1) Mass isotoper distribution analysis (MIDA) of plasma glucose during infusion of [U-^{13}C]glucose;[41,42] (2) MIDA during infusion of [2-^{13}C]glycerol;[42–44] (3) Ingestion (or infusion) of deuteriumoxide and measurement of deuterium enrichment in glucose carbon 5 or glucose carbon 6.[45–47] Because of the complexity of these models, we recommend the interested reader to carefully study the original publications for each of these models.

(3)[U-^{13}C]glucose MIDA (Figure 43.1).[40,41] This method was described by Katz and Tayek[40] but has been recently modified by Haymond and Sunehag.[41] Briefly, infused [U-$^{13}C_6$]glucose undergoes glycolysis and yields

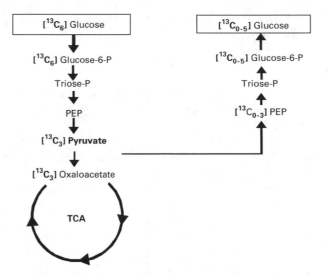

Figure 43.1. Endogenous and exogenous sources for plasma glucose. (From Sunehag, A. L., Haymond, M. W., Stable isotopes and gas chromatography-mass spectrometry in studies of glucose metabolism in children: in Stable Isotopes in Human Nutrition, Abrams, S. A. and Wong, W. W., eds, with permission)

[U-$^{13}C_3$]pyruvate, which in turn generates oxaloacetate labeled with ^{13}C in either C1-C3 or C2-C4. Oxaloacetate is subsequently converted to phosphoenolpyruvate (PEP) directly or following the reactions in the TCA cycle. As a result of the carbon fluxes and exchange in the TCA cycle, PEP will be labeled with ^{13}C in one, two, or three of its carbons. Thus, glucose generated from these singly, doubly, and triply labeled PEP molecules will be labeled by ^{13}C primarily in one (M + 1), two (M + 2), or three (M + 3) of its carbons, and to a very small extent in four (M + 4) or five carbons (M + 5). M + 1, M + 2, M + 3, M + 4, and M + 5 of glucose are labeled *isotopomers* of glucose, and can be generated only via the gluconeogenic pathway. Since the likelihood that [U-$^{13}C_6$]glucose (M + 6) will be formed by recombination of two M + 3 molecules is extraordinarily small, the M + 6 of glucose in the plasma space represents nonmetabolized labeled glucose. The isotopomer pattern of plasma glucose, i.e., the fraction of each isotopomer, is determined by gas chromatography-mass spectrometry after correction for natural abundance and contribution from the tracer.[48] It is of great importance that the infusion rate of the tracer is sufficient to achieve enrichments that can be measured with high accuracy by GCMS for each individual isotopomer (M + 1 through M + 6). Thus, at steady state, the enrichment of the largest isotopomer i.e., the M + 6, should not be below ~6–8%. The fraction of gluconeogenic molecules (% GNG molecules) can be calculated from the isotopomer pattern of plasma glucose using the following equation:

$$\% \text{ GNG molecules} = \sum_{1}^{5} M_i \Big/ \sum_{1}^{6} M_i \qquad (43.4)$$

where $\sum_{1}^{5} M_i$ is the labeled glucose molecules generated via gluconeogenesis (M1 through M5), and $\sum_{1}^{6} M_i$ is all labeled glucose molecules.

However, this would result in a significant underestimation of gluconeogenesis because of the tracer dilution (loss) in the TCA cycle. This dilution can be corrected by comparing the ^{13}C isotopomer pattern in lactate to that of glucose[40] or from the $^{12}C/^{13}C$ ratio in the labeled molecules of glucose.[41] Thus, gluconeogenesis as a fraction of glucose Ra is the product of gluconeogenic molecules and the dilution factor:

$$\text{Fractional GNG} = \underbrace{\sum_{1}^{5} M_i \Big/ \sum_{1}^{6} M_i}_{\text{Molecules via GNG}} \times \underbrace{\sum_{1}^{5} {}^{12}C_i \Big/ \sum_{1}^{5} {}^{13}C_i}_{\text{Tracer Dilution}} \qquad (43.5)$$

Glucose Ra is calculated from the [U-^{13}C]glucose enrichment (M + 6) using isotope dilution as described above. The rate of gluconeogenesis is then calculated from the product of fractional gluconeogenesis and glucose Ra.

(4) [2-^{13}C]glycerol MIDA (Figure 43.2).[42–44] This method was described by Hellerstein *et al.* [42,44] and by Neese *et al.*[43] Briefly, infused [2-^{13}C]glycerol is converted (in the liver) to dihydroxyacetone phosphate (which continuously is interconverted to glyceraldehyde–3-phosphate), thus providing a pool of singly labeled 3-carbon units at the triose phosphate level. As a result of combination of two 3-carbon units (i.e., two triose-phosphates) (precursor), the product, glucose, can be unlabeled, singly (M + 1), or doubly labeled (M + 2). The mass isotopomer distribution of M + 1 and M + 2 is dependent on the enrichment of the precursor pool according to the generic formula for the formation of a bio polymer, $(a+b) \times (a+b) = a^2 + 2ab + b^2$. In order to achieve reliable measures of gluconeogenesis using this method, the [2-^{13}C]glycerol tracer must be infused at a substrate rather than a tracer rate (25–50% of the glycerol turnover rate), which might have an impact on glucose metabolism. In addition, a second tracer is needed for measurement of glucose Ra, e.g., [U-^{13}C]glucose infused at a low rate i.e., ~0.1–0.4 μmol kg^{-1} min^{-1}, resulting in isotopic enrichments of 0.5–0.8% (depending on expected turnover rate). At this infusion rate, potential M + 1 and M + 2 generated by the [U-^{13}C]glucose tracer, which could interfere with those derived from the [2-^{13}C]glycerol tracer, are negligible.

(5) Deuterium oxide method with measures of the deuterium enrichment at glucose carbons 5 and 6 (Figure 43.3).[45–47] This method was described by Landau

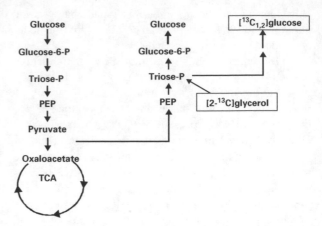

Figure 43.2. Schematic of the gluconeogenic pathway. (From Sunehag, A. L., Haymond, M. W., Stable isotopes and gas chromatography-mass spectrometry in studies of glucose metabolism in children: in *Stable Isotopes in Human Nutrition*, Abrams, S. A. and Wong, W. W., eds, with permission)

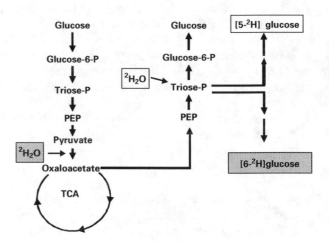

Figure 43.3. [U-^{13}C]glucose MIDA: Relation to the gluconeogenic pathway. (From Sunehag, A. L., Haymond, M. W., Stable isotopes and gas chromatography-mass spectrometry in studies of glucose metabolism in children: in *Stable Isotopes in Human Nutrition*, Abrams, S. A. and Wong, W. W., eds, with permission)

et al.[45,47] and Kalhan *et al.*[46] The principle of this model is that ingested (or infused) deuterium oxide equilibrates with the total body water pool. Subsequently, deuterium in body water exchanges with the hydrogens in intermediary compounds along the gluconeogenic pathway. Of particular interest for measurements of gluconeogenesis are the hydrogens at the methyl carbon of pyruvate (carbon 3) and the hydrogen at carbon 2 of glyceraldehyde-3-phosphate. When glucose is formed, pyruvate carbon

3 with its attached hydrogen/deuterium atoms becomes carbon 6 of glucose, while carbon 2 of glyceraldehyde-3-phosphate with its attached hydrogen/deuterium becomes carbon 5 of glucose. Thus, the deuterium enrichment in glucose carbon 6 represents gluconeogenesis from pyruvate and does not include the contribution from glycerol, while the deuterium enrichment at glucose carbon 5 is retained from the triose-phosphate level and is, therefore, purported to represent total gluconeogenesis i.e., including the contribution from glycerol.[47] Since the body water is the precursor pool for the hydrogen/deuterium, it can be measured in plasma or urine or from the deuterium enrichment at glucose carbon 2, since this is in total equilibration with body water.

To avoid potential side effects of deuterium oxide, only low doses (3–5 g kg^{-1} resulting in a body water enrichment of 0.3%–0.5%) are used in humans. A body water enrichment of this low magnitude would result in deuterium enrichment in glucose carbon 5 and 6 below the limit of accuracy for usual GCMS measurements. However, Landau et al.[45] and Kalhan et al.[46] have described a method to overcome this problem. Briefly, carbon 5 or 6 with their attached hydrogens/deuterium and hydroxyl group are cleaved off (using periodate),[45–47] thus generating formaldehyde. When formaldehyde is reacted with ammonium, hexamethylenetetramine (HMT), $C_6H_{12}N_4$, is formed. Each of the 6 carbons in HMT (with their attached hydrogens/deuterium) is derived from carbons 5 and 6 of glucose, respectively, resulting in HMT enrichments 6-fold higher than that in carbon 5 of glucose and 5-fold higher than that of glucose C6. The 5-fold increase instead of the theoretical 6-fold, is a result of incomplete proton exchange between body water and the methyl hydrogens of pyruvate. The HMT can be analyzed directly by GCMS without further derivatization. The HMT enrichments are converted to the corresponding glucose carbons 5 and 6 enrichments using standard curve prepared from [$^2H_7$]- or [5-$^2H_1$]glucose (glucose carbon 5) and [1-$^2H_1$]glucose converted to sorbitol for glucose carbon 6 measures.[45,46,49] Measurement of deuterium enrichment in glucose carbon 5 is an extremely tedious procedure requiring at least 0.5 mL plasma per sample,[47] while the glucose carbon 6 measures are simpler and require a smaller amount of plasma, but are less informative. HMT is analyzed by GCMS employing the EI mode. A non-polar GC column (No. 5) with thick film (1.0 μM) provides excellent chromatographic resolution. Gluconeogenesis as a fraction of glucose Ra can be calculated as follows:

$$\text{"Gluconeogenesis from pyruvate"} = (^2H_{C6}/2)/^2H_{body\,water}$$
(43.6)

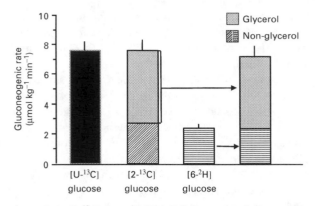

Figure 43.4. [2-^{13}C]glycerol MIDA: Relation to the gluconeogenic pathway. (From Sunehag, A. L., Haymond, M. W., Stable isotopes and gas chromatography-mass spectrometry in studies of glucose metabolism in children: in *Stable Isotopes in Human Nutrition*, Abrams, S. A. and Wong, W. W., eds, with permission)

where $^2H_{C6}$ is deuterium enrichment in glucose carbon 6 and $^2H_{body\,water}$ is deuterium enrichment in body water. The factor 2 is included because the 6th carbon of glucose has 2 covalently bound hydrogens.

$$\text{"Total gluconeogenesis"} = (^2H_{C5})/^2H_{body\,water}$$
(43.7)

where $^2H_{C5}$ is deuterium enrichment in glucose carbon 5.

Deuterium enrichment in plasma water or urine can be measured by IRMS (see above).

The [U-^{13}C]glucose MIDA, [2-^{13}C]glycerol MIDA, and the deuteriumoxide glucose C5 method are reported to reflect total gluconeogenesis, while the deuterium oxide glucose C6 method is thought to underestimate gluconeogenesis as a result of incomplete equilibration of the deuterium in body water and the hydrogens at pyruvate carbon 3, and because the contribution of glycerol is not included.

We have directly compared all three of these methods in infants and adults under identical conditions. The [U-^{13}C]glucose MIDA, [2-^{13}C]glycerol MIDA, and the deuteriumoxide glucose C6 methods were compared in three groups of prematurely born infants receiving total parenteral nutrition providing glucose at 17 μmol kg^{-1} min^{-1} (3 mg kg^{-1} min^{-1}) that is about one-half their normal glucose turnover rate.[50] Our results demonstrate that the [U-^{13}C]glucose and the [2-^{13}C]glycerol MIDA provide virtually identical estimates of gluconeogenesis accounting for about 70% of glucose production, while the deuteriumoxide glucose C6 estimate was significantly lower (Figure 43.4). Using [2-^{13}C]glycerol MIDA, the gluconeogenic contribution from glycerol and nonglycerol sources can be partitioned. We observed that the *nonglycerol contribution* measured by the [2-^{13}C]glycerol MIDA corresponded very well to the deuteriumoxide glucose C6 estimate (Figure 43.4). In conclusion, in infants receiving total parenteral nutrition, both [U-^{13}C]glucose and [2-^{13}C]glycerol MIDA are useful tools to measure total gluconeogenesis, while deuteriumoxide with measurements of the deuterium enrichment at glucose carbon 6 would underestimate gluconeogenesis by the contribution from glycerol. Unfortunately, the deuteriumoxide glucose carbon 5 method requires large blood sample volumes,[47] precluding its use in premature infants. We have, however, compared the [U-^{13}C]glucose MIDA with the deuteriumoxide glucose C5 methods in healthy young adults following a 66 h fast. Preliminary results demonstrate that the two methods estimate gluconeogenesis equally well.[51]

Although there are controversies regarding which of these methods provide most accurate estimates of gluconeogenesis, each of them may be uniquely useful depending on the study design and subject population e.g., (1) in infants and small children, the sample volume that can be withdrawn is limited; (2) a study including numerous samples requires simple sample preparation; and (3) use of multiple tracers in the same study may confuse the results. Recently, we have used the [U-^{13}C]glucose MIDA method in very premature infants receiving glucose alone at 17 μmol kg^{-1} min^{-1} (3 mg kg^{-1} min^{-1}) demonstrating that infusion of glycerol increased gluconeogenesis and prevented time-dependent decrease in hepatic glucose production.[52]

In a recent publication, Kalhan et al.[39] demonstrated that in 24–48 h old newborn term infants, gluconeogenesis from pyruvate (i.e., not including the contribution from glycerol) accounted for about 30% of glucose production using the deuteriumoxide glucose C6 method.

Protein metabolism

The newborn period has the highest growth rate of extrauterine life. Thus, it is important to determine the impact of nutritional interventions on neonatal protein metabolism i.e., proteolysis, protein oxidation, and protein synthesis. These parameters have been measured in newborn term and preterm infants under various nutritional conditions using infusion of individual or combined essential amino acids, e.g., leucine and phenylalanine labeled with stable isotopes (^{13}C or ^{2}H).

Leucine tracer

Leucine equilibrates rapidly with α-ketoisocaproic acid (αKIC) (the intracellular transamination product of

leucine).[53] Leucine labeled with ^{13}C, ^{2}H and ^{15}N is available, but here ^{13}C labeled leucine is used to exemplify the analytical principles. Thus, following infusion of [^{13}C]leucine, the ^{13}C isotopic enrichment of αKIC reflects dilution of the tracer in the intracellular space where protein and amino acid metabolism occur. From the enrichment of αKIC, the appearance rate of leucine (Leucine Ra) can be calculated as follows:

Leucine Ra (μmol kg^{-1}min^{-1})

$$= [(E_{infusate}/E_{plasma}) - 1] \times I \qquad (43.8)$$

where $E_{infusate}$ is the isotopic enrichment of the leucine tracer; E_{plasma} is the ^{13}C- enrichment (MPE%) of αKIC in plasma and I, the infusion rate of the leucine tracer (μmol kg^{-1} min^{-1}). In subjects fed enterally or parenterally, subtracting exogenously supplied leucine, Leucine Ra, is an indicator of proteolysis.

Leucine oxidation can be calculated from the enrichment of ^{13}CO$_2$ in breath samples obtained during the study using the following equation:

Leucine oxidation (μmol kg^{-1}min^{-1})

$$= (^{13}CO_2 \times V_{CO2})/(0.7 \times {}^{13}C_{\alpha KIC} \times 22.4 \times 1000 \times W) \qquad (43.9)$$

where ^{13}CO$_2$ is the ^{13}C enrichment in breath CO$_2$ (derived from the ^{13}C- leucine tracer); V_{CO2} is the total CO$_2$ production (measured by indirect calorimetry); $^{13}C_{\alpha KIC}$ is the ^{13}C enrichment in αKIC; 0.7 is the estimated fractional recovery of CO$_2$; 22.4 $\times$ 1000 converts mL of gas to μmol and W is the weight of the subject.

Nonoxidative disposal of leucine (NOLD) is an indicator of protein synthesis:

NOLD = Endogenous leucine Ra $-$ Leucine oxidation

$$(43.10)$$

Since the leucine content of 1 g of protein is 590 μmol,[54] the leucine data can be used to calculate proteolysis and protein synthesis.

Phenylalanine tracer

Estimates of proteolysis and protein synthesis can also be obtained using deuterated phenylalanine e.g., [^{2}H$_5$]phenylalanine and tyrosine (e.g., ^{2}H$_2$ tyrosine). Thus, phenylalanine and tyrosine appearance rates (Phe Ra and Tyr Ra), respectively, can be calculated using the same dilution equation as described above for leucine:

Phe Ra (μmol kg^{-1}min^{-1}) = [(E$_{infusate}$/E$_{plasma}$) $-$ 1] $\times$ I

$$(43.11)$$

where $E_{infusate}$ is the isotopic enrichment of the phenylalanine tracer; E_{plasma} is the $[^2H_5]$ enrichment of phenylalanine in plasma (MPE%) and I, the infusion rate of the phenylalanine tracer,

$$\text{Tyr Ra } (\mu\text{mol kg}^{-1}\text{min}^{-1}) = [(E_{infusate}/E_{plasma}) - 1] \times I$$

$$(43.12)$$

where $E_{infusate}$ is the isotopic enrichment of the tyrosine tracer; E_{plasma} is the $[^2H_2]$ enrichment of tyrosine in plasma (MPE%) and I, the infusion rate of the tyrosine tracer. Thus, in fed subjects, subtracting exogenously supplied phenylalanine provides a measure of endogenous phenylalanine Ra, an indicator of proteolysis. Hydroxylation of phenylalanine (Phe) to tyrosine (Tyr) (determined from the $^2H_4$ enrichment of tyrosine) provides a measure of irreversible loss of phenylalanine:

$$\text{Phe}_{\rightarrow \text{Tyr}} = \text{Tyr Ra} \times ([^2H_4] \text{ Tyr}/[^2H_5] \text{ Phe})$$
$$\times \text{Phe Ra}/(I_{Phe} + \text{Phe Ra}) \qquad (43.13)$$

where $^2H_4$ is the deuterium enrichment in tyrosine derived from Phenylalanine; I_{Phe} is the infusion rate of the phenylalanine tracer, and Phe Ra/$(I_{Phe} + \text{Phe Ra})$ corrects for the contribution from the phenylalanine tracer.

Nondisposable phenylalanine
(an indicator of protein synthesis) $= \text{Phe Ra} - \text{Phe}_{\rightarrow \text{Tyr}}$

$$(43.14)$$

Since the phenylalanine content of 1 g of protein is 280 μmol,[54] the phenylalanine data can be used to calculate proteolysis and protein synthesis.

Using these methods, it has been demonstrated that in term infants, parenteral amino acids suppressed proteolysis and increased protein oxidation, but had no impact on protein synthesis.[55] In contrast, in preterm infants parenteral amino acids did not suppress proteolysis, but increased protein synthesis.[56–58] These studies also clearly demonstrate that very premature infants can convert phenylalanine to tyrosine.[56,58] This is of significant importance, since most total parenteral nutrition solutions do not contain tyrosine. Van Goudoever et al.[59] showed that premature infants receiving parenteral amino acids from the first day of life had an improved leucine balance as a result of both increased estimates of protein synthesis and reduced proteolysis. In contrast, in response to feeding (following a 3–5 h fast), in premature infants proteolysis was suppressed while no change in protein synthesis was observed,[60] and in preterm infants fed protein-enriched human milk, protein turnover, but not protein disposition was correlated with protein intake.[61] In contrast to adults, parenteral glucose did not affect proteolysis in either term[62] or preterm

infants.[63] In addition, in very premature infants, a reduction of the glucose infusion rate to 17 μmol kg^{-1} min^{-1} (3 mg kg^{-1} min^{-1}) did not alter proteolysis.[50] Parenteral lipids have been reported to have no impact on proteolysis in healthy, term newborns.[62] In ill premature infants, amino acid but not glucose or lipid intake, was correlated with leucine oxidation and nonoxidative leucine disposal (an index of protein synthesis).[64] Liet et al.[65] investigated the effects of parenteral medium chain (MCT) v. long-chain tri-acylglycerol (LC) on leucine metabolism in preterm infants and reported that leucine oxidation was higher in infants receiving mixed MCT-LC when compared to those receiving only LC. However, no differences in leucine derived from protein break down or nonoxidative leucine disposal were observed. Thus, the resultant net leucine balance was less positive in the mixed MCT-LC group than in the LC group.

Urea tracer

Protein oxidation has also been estimated from the plasma appearance rate of urea during infusion of $[^{15}N_2]$urea in newborn infants using the following equation:[66]

$$\text{Protein}_{oxidation}(\text{mg kg}^{-1}\text{ min}^{-1}) = \text{Ra}_{urea} \cdot 0.47 \cdot 6.25$$

$$(43.15)$$

where Ra_{urea} is the rate of appearance of urea (mg kg^{-1} min^{-1}), 0.47 is the fraction of urea that is composed of nitrogen, and 6.25 is the inverse of the fraction of nitrogen in protein.[67] Under study conditions where ^{13}C labeled leucine is used in combination with other ^{13}C labeled tracers, and protein oxidation cannot be measured from the $^{13}CO_2$ enrichment, the $[^{15}N_2]$urea can be used to measure protein oxidation and the $[^{13}C]$leucine tracer to measure total leucine Ra.

Other amino acid tracers

Various other amino acids labeled with stable isotopes e.g., glutamine[68] and glycine[69] have been infused in newborn infants and their metabolic fate has been determined. In addition, [U-^{13}C]glucose (administered at rates resulting in $^{13}C_6$ enrichment of glucose of 60%) has been utilized to determine the capacity of premature infants to synthesize nonessential amino acids (glutamine, glycine, alanine, serine, aspartate, cysteine and proline) from glucose carbon,[70,71] demonstrating that premature infants have a reduced capacity to synthesize proline, aspartate, and cysteine. This would imply that these amino acids might be conditionally essential in infants born prematurely.[71]

Lipid metabolism

Glycerol and FFA metabolism

Lipids are important energy substrate providing over twice the calories of glucose or protein. Furthermore, hydrolysis of triglycerides (lipolysis) yields glycerol and free fatty acids (FFA). Glycerol is a potential gluconeogenic substrate, while the FFA upon hepatic β-oxidation provides energy to drive the gluconeogenic process as well as reducing equivalents crucial for many metabolic processes. Since glycerol is not re-esterified, plasma glycerol appearance rate (glycerol Ra) is a good indicator of lipolysis. Glycerol Ra can be measured using glycerol labeled with ^{13}C or ^{2}H using the same isotope dilution equations described above for glucose and amino acids.

Using a simultaneous infusion of [2-^{13}C]glycerol and [6,6-^{2}H$_2$] glucose, we and others have demonstrated that in healthy term infants, infants of diabetic mothers, growth-retarded infants and very premature infants, lipolysis was initiated in the immediate postnatal period at a rate 3 to 4 times that of a fasting adult. Further, 50%–90% of glycerol Ra was converted to glucose accounting for 10%–45% of glucose production in short-term fasted term and preterm infants.[10–12,13,50] Using ^{13}C labeled palmitate, Bougnères et al.[10] reported that mobilization of FFA from the triglyceride stores was a very active process during the first day of life in healthy newborn term, growth-retarded and slightly premature infants and that the FFA inflow was directly related to the length of the fasting period. The investigators also demonstrated a direct relationship between FFA flow and plasma palmitate concentrations, and between plasma concentrations of palmitate and β-hydroxybutyrate indicating that FFA oxidation is also active soon after birth.

Ketone body metabolism

Ketone body transport, β-hydroxybutyrate (3-OHB) + acetoacetate (AcAc) in neonates have been performed using D-3-hydroxy[4,4,4-^{2}H$_3$]butyrate.[72,73] Total ketone body appearance in plasma (Ra ketone bodies) was calculated using the following equations:

$$E\,KB = E\,OHB \times [OHB]/[OHB + AcAc]$$
$$+ EAcAc \times [AcAc]/[OHB + AcAc] \tag{43.16}$$

where EKB is total ketone body enrichment in plasma; E OHB and EAcAc are the plasma enrichments of β-hydroxybutyrate and acetoacetate, respectively; and [AcAc] and [OHB] are the plasma concentrations of β-hydroxybutyrate and acetoacetate, respectively.

$$Ra\,ketone\,bodies = [(E\,infusate/E\,plasma) - 1] \times I \tag{43.17}$$

where E infusate is the enrichment of the D-3-hydroxy[4,4,4-^{2}H$_3$]butyrate tracer; E plasma is the total ketone body enrichment (E KB). The results demonstrate that newborn term infants have an accelerated ketone body production and utilization even when fed every 4 hours.

Long chain FFA

Long-chain polyunsaturated fatty acids, particularly arachidonic acid (C20:4n-6) and docohexaenoic acid (C22:6n-3) are found in high concentrations in structural lipids of the CNS and are increased during growth. Animal studies have demonstrated that long-chain polyunsaturated FFA can be synthesized from linoleic acid (C18:3 n6) and linolenic acid (C18:3n-3). Using a continuous ingestion of formula labeled with [U-^{13}C]linoleic acid and [U-^{13}C]linolenic acid[74] or a single bolus dose of these tracers[75,76] it was demonstrated that both term and preterm infants are capable of synthesizing long-chain polyunsaturated FFA from linoleic and linolenic acid both via desaturation and elongation.

Other lipids

Lipids (phospholipids) are also important constituents of pulmonary surfactant. Surfactant reduces surface tension, thus facilitating alveolar expansion at the end of expiration. Lack of surfactant is a cause of respiratory distress syndrome in newborn infants. Bunt et al.[77] and Merchak et al.[78] studied surfactant synthesis and turnover in premature infants using [U-^{13}C]glucose as a precursor for palmitic acid in surfactant phosphatidylcholine. During intravenous infusion of [U-^{13}C]glucose (preceded by administration of exogenous surfactant via an endotracheal tube) a significant incorporation of ^{13}C from [U-^{13}C]glucose into palmitic acid in phosphatidyl choline in tracheal aspirate was observed. The fractional synthesis rate of surfactant phosphatidylcholine palmitic acid from glucose was 2.7% $\pm$ 1.3% per day[77] and 5.2% per day.[78] The metabolism of exogenous surfactant has also been investigated using surfactant labeled with ^{13}C-dipalmitoylphosphatidylcholine.[79]

Energy expenditure

Doubly labeled water, i.e., water in which the hydrogen and oxygen atoms are replaced by the stable isotopes ^2H and ^{18}O is a useful tool for measuring energy expenditure in free-living subjects. The principle is as follows: the subject receives a drink containing the mixed isotopes (^2H_2O and $H_2^{18}O$). Following an equilibration period of a few hours, urine and or saliva samples are obtained during the elimination period of the isotopes i.e., 5–8 days in infants and 14–21 days in adults. While the ^2H is eliminated only as water, the ^{18}O is eliminated both as water and CO_2. Thus, the CO_2 production rate (rCO_2) can be estimated from the difference in the elimination rates of ^2H and ^{18}O (measured by IRMS).[80-82]

$$rCO_2 = (N/2f_3)(k^{18}O - k^2H) - [(f_2 - f_1)/2f_3]rG \qquad (43.18)$$

where N is the total body water pool size (mol); $k^{18}O$ and k^2H are the elimination rates of ^{18}O and ^2H, respectively, per day; f_1 and f_2 are the fractionation factors for evaporative water loss of ^2H and ^{18}O, respectively, and f_3 is the fractionation factor for ^{18}O between CO_2 and H_2O.

Energy expenditure (EE) (KJ day^{-1}) is then calculated as follows:[83]

$$EE = 4.63\,CO_2 + 16.49\,(CO_2/RQ) \qquad (43.19)$$

Since the doubly labeled method does not measure O_2 consumption, RQ (respiratory quotient) is unknown. However, RQ can be replaced by FQ (food quotient), which can be estimated from the fractions of the dietary intake derived from protein, fat, carbohydrate, and alcohol.[83]

$$FQ = (p \times 0.81) + (f \times 0.71) + (c \times 1.0) + (a \times 0.67)$$
$$(43.20)$$

where p, f, c, and a are the fractions of the diet derived from protein, fat, carbohydrate, and alcohol, respectively. The constants are the values for FQ of the individual substrates.[84] It has been demonstrated that FQ is comparatively stable, ~0.85 in omnivorous adults and ~0.86–0.88 in vegetarians.[83] In breastfed infants, the FQ changes from ~0.84–0.87 during weaning. In bottle-fed infants the FQ ranged between 0.84–0.88.

The doubly labeled water method has been validated against the established indirect calorimetry method in adults[85] demonstrating good agreement between the methods. However, applying the doubly labeled water method to studies of newborn infants, particularly those born prematurely, may decrease its precision and accuracy because of their high growth rate, high body water content, high insensible water loss, and high water turnover compared to CO_2 production. Further, changes in body composition occurring during the study period may not be proportional to changes in the isotope dilution spaces. It may also be difficult to ascertain appropriate administration of the doubly labeled water. Roberts et al.[86] and Jensen et al.[87] compared the doubly labeled water method with indirect calorimetry over a 5-day period. The first study[86] included only four infants born after 27–34 weeks and studied at a postnatal age between 29 and 36 weeks. Only small differences were observed between the methods. However, there was a remarkably large variation in insensible water loss, 5.5%–32.9% of total water loss, and, surprisingly, the insensible water loss was not related to either gestational age or postnatal age. The second study[87] included 16 infants with a mean gestational age of 30 weeks at birth studied at a mean postnatal age of 30 days. The average energy expenditure agreed very well between the two methods, but there were large individual variations. It has to be noticed that in both studies, the majority of the infants were studied several weeks after birth. The potential analytical errors associated with the use of the doubly labeled water method in premature infants delineated above, are likely to be related to gestational as well as postnatal age.

Information about energy requirements in healthy and ill premature infants is much needed and the doubly labeled water method may provide a useful tool for addressing these issues. However, accurate estimates of energy expenditure in premature infants require measurement of (1) the total body water pool at beginning and end of the study period; and (2) intake and loss of water, and energy intake during the study period. Applying the doubly labeled water method to premature infants with chronic lung disease, demonstrated that dexamethasone did not affect energy expenditure.[88] De Meer et al.,[89] on the other hand, reported that premature infants with bronchopulmonary dysplasia (BPD) had increased energy expenditure compared with controls. A weakness of this study is that the controls were studied at a postnatal age of 1 month, while the BPD infants were studied at 2 months of age (gestational age and weight at birth were identical in the two groups). Finally, infants with congenital heart disease were shown to have increased energy expenditure.[90]

REFERENCES

1 Ogata, E. S. Carbohydrate metabolism in the fetus and neonate and altered neonatal glucoregulation. *Pediatr. Clin. N. Am.* 1986;**33**: 25–45.
2 Aynsley-Green, A. Metabolic and endocrine interrelations in the human fetus and neonate. *Am. J. Clin. Nutr.* 1985;**41** (Suppl. 2):399–417.

3 Knipp, G. T., Audus, K. L., Soares, M. J. Nutrient transport across the placenta. *Adv. Drug. Deliv. Rev.* 1999;**38**:41–58.

4 Bier, D. M., Leake, R. D., Haymond, M. W. *et al.* Measurement of "true" glucose production rates in infancy and childhood with 6,6-dideuteroglucose. *Diabetes* 1977;**26**:1016–23.

5 Gruenwald, P., Minh, H. N. Evaluation of body and organ weights in perinatal pathology. I. Normal standards derived from autopsies. *Am. J. Clin. Path.* 1960;**34**:247–53.

6 Shelley, H. J. Glycogen reserves and their changes at birth and in anoxia. *Br. Med. Bull.* 1961;**17**:137–43.

7 Persson, B., Gentz, J. The pattern of blood lipids, glycerol and ketone bodies during the neonatal period, infancy and childhood. *Acta Paediatr. Scand.* 1966;**55**:353–62.

8 Santerre, J., Karlberg, P. Respiratory quotient and metabolic rate in normal full-term and small-for-date newborn infants. *Acta Paediatr. Scand.* 1970;**59**:653–8.

9 Cross, K. W., Tizard, J. P. M., Trythall, D. A. H. The gaseous metabolism of the newborn infant. *Acta Paediatr. Scand.* 1957;**46**:265–85.

10 Bougnères, P. F., Karl, I. E., Hillman, L. S., Bier, D. M. Lipid transport in the human newborn. Palmitate and glycerol turnover and the contribution of glycerol to neonatal hepatic glucose output. *J. Clin. Invest.* 1982;**70**:262–70.

11 Fjeld, C. R., Cole, F. S., Bier, D. M. Energy expenditure, lipolysis, and glucose production in preterm infants treated with theophylline. *Pediatr. Res.* 1992;**32**:693–8.

12 Patel, D., Kalhan, S. Glycerol metabolism and triglyceride-fatty acid cycling in the newborn: effects of maternal diabetes and intrauterine growth retardation. *Pediatr. Res.* 1992;**31**:52–8.

13 Sunehag, A., Gustafsson, J., Ewald, U. Glycerol carbon contributes to hepatic glucose production during the first eight hours in healthy, term infants. *Acta Paediatr. Scand.* 1996;**85**:1339–43.

14 Sunehag, A., Ewald, U., Gustafsson, J. Extremely preterm infants (< 28 weeks) are capable of gluconeogenesis from glycerol on their first day of life. *Pediatr. Res.* 1996;**40**:553–7.

15 Cahill, G. F. Jr, Herrera, M. G., Morgan, A. P. *et al.* Hormone-fuel interrelationships during fasting. *J. Clin. Invest.* 1966;**45**:1751–69.

16 Bier, D. M. The use of stable isotopes in metabolic investigation. *Baillieres Clin. Endocrinol. Metab.* 1987;**1**:817–36.

17 Bier, D. M. Mass spectrometry and stable isotopes. In Sadubray, J. M., Tada, K., eds. *Inborn Metabolic Disease*. Berlin: Springer Verlag; 1990:45–53.

18 Bougneres, P. F. Stable isotope tracers and the determination of fuel fluxes in newborn infants. *Biol. Neonate* 1987;**52**:87–96.

19 Wolfe, R. R. Basic characteristics of isotope tracers. In Wolfe, R. R., ed. *Radioactive and Stable Isotope Tracers in Biomedicine. Principles and Practice of Kinetic Analyses*. New York, NY: Wiley-Liss Inc.; 1992:1–17.

20 De Meer, K., Roef, M. J., Kulik, W., Jakobs, C. *In vivo* research with stable isotopes in biochemistry, nutrition and clinical medicine: an overview. *Isotopes Environ. Health Stud.* 1999;**35**:19–37.

21 Argoud, G. M., Schade, D. S., Eaton, R. P. Underestimation of hepatic glucose production by radioactive and stable tracers. *Am. J. Phys.* 1987;**252**:E505–615.

22 Hachey, D. L., Parsons, W. R., McKay, S., Haymond, M. W. Quantitation of monosaccharide isotopic enrichment in physiologic fluids; by electron ionization or negative chemical ionization GC/MS using di-O-isopropylidene derivatives. *Anal. Chem.* 1999;**71**;4734–9.

23 Patterson, B. W., Hachey, D. L., Cook, G. L., Amann, J. M., Klein, P. D. Incorporation of a stable isotopically labeled amino acid into multiple human apolipoproteins. *J. Lipid Res.* 1991;**32**:1063–72.

24 Lee, B., Yu, H., Jahoor, F. *et al.* In vivo urea cycle flux distinguishes and correlates with phenotypic severity in disorder of the urea cycle. *Proc. Natl. Acad. Sci USA.* 2000;**5**:8021–6.

25 Hachey, D. L., Patterson, B. W., Reeds, P. J., Elsas, L. J. Isotopic determination of organic keto acid pentafluorobenzyl esters in biological fluids by negative chemical ionization gas chromatography/mass spectrometry. Analyt. Chem. 1991; **63**: 919–23.

26 Wong, W. W., Lee, L. S., Klein, P. D. Deuterium and oxygen-18 measurements on microliter samples of urine, plasma, saliva and human milk. *Am. J. Clin. Nutr.* 1987;**45**:905–13.

27 Tigas, S., Sunehag, A. L., Haymond, M. W. Impact of duration of infusion and choice of isotope label on isotope recycling in glucose homeostasis. *Diabetes* 2002;**51**:3170–5.

28 Heath, D. F. Errors inherent in the primed infusion method for the measurement of the rate of glucose appearance in man when uptake is not forced by glucose or insulin infusion. *Clin. Sci.* 1990;**79**:201–3.

29 Kalhan, S. C., Bier, D. M., Savin, S. M., Adam, P. A. J. Estimation of glucose turnover and ^{13}C recycling in the human newborn by simultaneous [1-^{13}C]glucose and [6,6-^{2}H$_2$]glucose tracers. *J. Clin. Endocrinol. Metab.* 1980;**50**:456–9.

30 Bier, D. M., Arnold, K. J., Sherman, W. R. *et al. In vivo* measurement of glucose and alanine metabolism with stable isotope tracers. *Diabetes* 1977;**26**:1005–15.

31 Steele, R., Wall, J. S., De-Bodo, R. C., Altzuler, N. Measurement of size and turnover rate of body glucose pool by the isotope dilution method. *Am. J. Physiol.* 1956;**187**:15–24.

32 De Bodo, R. C., Steele, R., Altszuler, N., Dunn, A., Bishop, J. S. On hormonal regulation of carbohydrate metabolism; studies with C^{14} glucose. *Recent Prog. Horm. Res.* 1963;**19**:445–88.

33 Haymond, M. W., Sunehag, A. L. Controlling the sugar bowl: regulation of glucose homeostasis in children. *Metab. Endocrinol. Clin. N. Am.* 1999;**28**:663–94.

34 Sunehag, A., Ewald, U., Larsson, A., Gustafsson, J. Attenuated hepatic glucose production but unimpaired lipolysis in newborn infants of mothers with diabetes. *Pediatr. Res.* 1997;**42**:492–97.

35 Sunehag, A., Ewald, U., Larsson, A., Gustafsson, J. Glucose production rate in extremely immature neonates (< 28 w) studied by use of deuterated glucose. *Pediatr. Res.* 1993;**33**:97–100.

36 Sunehag, A., Gustafsson, J., Ewald, U. Very immature infants (< 30 weeks) respond to glucose infusion with incomplete suppression of glucose production. *Pediatr. Res.* 1994;**36**:550–5.

37 Tyrala, E. E., Chen, X., Boden, G. Glucose metabolism in the infant weighing less than 1100 grams. *J. Pediatr.* 1994;**125**:283–7.

38 Frazer, T. E., Karl, I. E., Hillman, L. S., Bier, D. M. Direct measurement of gluconeogenesis from 2,3-^{13}C2 alanine in the human neonate. *Am. J. Physiol.* 1981;**240**:E615–21.

39 Kalhan, S. C., Parimi, P., Van Beek, R. *et al.* Estimation of gluconeogenesis in newborn infants. *Am. J. Physiol. Endocrinol. Metab.* 2001;**281**:E991–7.

40 Katz, J., Tayek, J. A. Gluconeogenesis and Cori cycle in 12, 20 and 40-hour fasted humans. *Am. J. Physiol.* 1998;**275**:E537–42.

41 Haymond, M. W., Sunehag, A. L. The reciprocal pool model for the measurement of gluconeogenesis using [U-^{13}C]glucose. *Am. J. Physiol.* 2000;**278**:E140–45.

42 Hellerstein, M. K., Neese, R. A. Mass isotopomer distribution analysis: a technique for measuring biosynthesis and turnover of polymers. *Am. J. Physiol.* 1992;**263**:E988–1001.

43 Neese, R. A., Schwartz, J-M., Faix, D. *et al.* Gluconeogenesis and intrahepatic triose phosphate flux in response to fasting or substrate loads. *J. Biol. Chem.* 1995;**270**:14452–66.

44 Hellerstein, M. K., Neese, R. A., Linfoot, P. *et al.* Hepatic gluconeogenic fluxes and glycogen turnover during fasting in humans. A stable isotope study. *J. Clin. Invest.* 1997;**100**:1305–19.

45 Landau, B. R., Wahren, J., Chandramouli, V. *et al.* Use of ^{2}H$_2$O for estimating rates of gluconeogenesis. *J. Clin. Invest.* 1995;**95**:172–8.

46 Kalhan, S. C., Trivedi, R., Singh, S. *et al.* A micromethod for the measurement of deuterium bound to carbon-6 of glucose to quantify gluconeogenesis in vivo. *J. Mass Spec.* 1995;**30**:1588–92.

47 Landau, B. R., Wahren, J., Chandramouli, V. *et al.* Contributions of gluconeogenesis to glucose production in the fasted state. *J. Clin. Invest.* 1996;**98**:378–85.

48 Fernandez, C. A., Des Rosiers, C., Previs, S. F., David, F., Brunengraber, H. Correction of 13C mass isotopomer distributions for natural stable isotope abundance. *J. Mass Spec.* 1996;**31**:255–62.

49 Muntz, J. A., Carrol, R. E. A method for converting glucose to fructose. *J. Biol. Chem.* 1960;**235**:1258–60.

50 Sunehag, A. L., Haymond, M. W., Schanler, R. J., Reeds, P. J., Bier, D. M. Gluconeogenesis in very low birth weight infants receiving total parenteral nutrition *Diabetes* 1999;**48**:791–800.

51 Sunehag, A. L., Clarke, L., Bier, D. M., Haymond, M. W. [U-^{13}C]glucose MIDA provides accurate measures of gluconeogenesis, is easy to perform and requires only small blood sample volumes. *Diabetes* 2001;**50** (Suppl. 2):A65.

52 Sunehag, A. L. Parenteral glycerol enhances gluconeogenesis in very premature infants. *Pediatr. Res.* 2003;**53**.

53 Schwenk, W. F., Beaufrere, B., Haymond, M. W. Use of reciprocal pool specific activity to model leucine metabolism in humans. *Am. J. Physiol.* 1985;**249**:E646–50.

54 Waterlow, J. C., Garlick, P. J., Millward, D. J. *Protein Turnover in Mammalian Tissue in the Whole Body.* Amsterdam: Elsevier North Holland; 1978:301–25.

55 Poindexter, B. B., Karn, C. A., Ahlrichs, J. A. *et al.* Amino acids suppress proteolysis independent of insulin throughout the neonatal period. *Am. J. Physiol.* 1997;**272**:E592–9.

56 Denne, S. C., Karn, C. A., Ahlrichs, J. A. *et al.* Proteolysis and phenylalanine hydroxylation in response to parenteral nutrition in extremely premature and normal newborns. *J. Clin. Invest.* 1996;**97**:746–54.

57 Rivera, A. Jr, Bell, E. F., Bier, D. M. Effect of intravenous amino acids on protein metabolism of preterm infants during the first three days of life. *Pediatr. Res.* 1993;**33**:106–11.

58 Pointdexter, B. B., Karn, C. A., Leitch, C. A., Liechty, E. A., Denne, S. C. Amino acids do not suppress proteolysis in premature neonates. *Am. J. Physiol. Endocrinol. Metab.* 2001;**281**:E472–8.

59 Van Goudoever, J. B., Colen, T., Wattimena, J. L. *et al.* Immediate commencement of amino acid supplementation in preterm infants: effect on serum amino acid concentrations and protein kinetics on the first day of life. *J. Pediatr.* 1995;**127**:458–65.

60 Denne, S. C., Karn, C. A., Liechty, E. A. Leucine kinetics after a brief fast and in response to feeding in premature infants. *Am. J. Clin. Nutr.* 1992;**56**:899–904.

61 Beaufrere, B., Putet, G., Pachiaudi, C., Salle, B. Whole body protein turnover measured with ^{13}C-leucine and energy expenditure in premature infants. *Pediatr. Res.* 1990;**28**:147–52.

62 Denne, S. C., Karn, C. A., Wang, J., Liechty, J. A. Effect of intravenous glucose and lipid on proteolysis and glucose production in normal newborns. *Am. J. Physiol.* 1995;**269**:E361–7.

63 Hertz, D. E., Karn, C. A., Liu, Y. M., Liecthy, E. A., Denne, S. C. Intravenous glucose suppresses glucose production but not proteolysis in extremely premature newborns. *J. Clin. Invest.* 1993;**92**:1752–8.

64 Thureen, P. J., Anderson, A. H., Baron, K. A. *et al.* Protein balance in the first week of life in ventilated neonates receiving parenteral nutrition. *Am. J. Clin. Nutr.* 1998;**68**:1128–35.

65 Liet, J. M., Piloquet, H, Marchini, J. S. *et al.* Leucine metabolism in preterm infants receiving parenteral nutrition with medium chain compared with long-chain triacylglycerol. *Am. J. Clin. Nutr.* 1999;**69**:539–43.

66 Kalhan, S. C. Rates of urea synthesis in the human newborn. Effect of maternal diabetes and small size for gestational age. *Pediatr. Res.* 1993;**34**:801–4.

67 Jequier, E., Acheson, K., Schutz, Y. Assessment of energy expenditure and fuel utilization in man. *Ann. Rev. Nutr.* 1987;**7**:187–208.

68 Darmaun, D., Roig, J. C., Auestad, N., Sager, B. K., Neu, J. Glutamine metabolism in very low birthweight infants. *Pediatr. Res.* 1997;**41**:391–6.

69 Amir, J., Reisner, S. H., Lapidot, A. Glycine turnover rates and pool sizes in neonates as determined by gas chromatography-mass spectrometry and nitrogen 15. *Pediatr. Res.* 1980;**14**:1238–44.

70 Miller, R. G., Jahoor, F., Reeds, P. J., Heird, W. C., Jaksic, T. A new stable isotope tracer technique to assess human neonatal amino acid synthesis. *J. Pediatr. Surg.* 1995;**30**: 1325–9.

71 Miller, R. G., Jahoor, F., Jaksic, T. Decreased cysteine and proline synthesis in parenterally fed, premature infants. *J. Pediatr. Surg.* 1995;**30**:953–7.

72 Bougneres, P. F., Lemmel, C., Ferre, P., Bier, D. M. Ketone body transportation in the human neonate and infant. *J. Clin. Invest.* 1986;**77**:42–8.

73 Bougneres, P. F., Balasse, E. O., Ferre, P., Bier, D. M. Determination of ketone body kinetics using a D-(-)-3-hydroxy[4,4,4–2H3]butyrate tracer. *J. Lipid Res.* 1986;**27**:215–20.

74 Sauerwald, T. U., Hachey, D. L., Jensen, C. L. *et al.* Effect of dietary alpha-linolenic acid intake on incorporation of docosahexaenoic and arachidonic acids into plasma phospholipids of term infants. *Lipids* 1996;**31** (Suppl.):S131–5.

75 Carnielli, V. P., Wattimena, D. J., Luijendijk, I. H. *et al.* The very low birth weight premature infant is capable of synthesizing arachidonic and docosahexaenoic acid from linoleic and linolenic acids. *Pediatr. Res.* 1996;**40**:169–74.

76 Sauerwald, T. U., Hachey, D. L., Jensen, C. L. *et al.* Intermediates in endogenous synthesis of C22:6 omega 3 and C20:4 omega 6 by term and preterm infants. *Pediatr. Res.* 1997;**41**: 183–7.

77 Bunt, J. E. H., Zimmerman, L. J., Wattimena, J. L. *et al.* Endogenous surfactant turnover in preterm infants measured with stable isotopes. *Am. J. Respir. Crit. Care Med.* 1998;**157**: 810–14.

78 Merchak, A., Patterson, B. W., Yarasheski, K. E., Hamvas, A. Use of stable isotope labeling technique and mass isotopomer distribution analysis of [13C]palmitate isolated from surfactant disaturated phospholipids to study surfactant *in vivo* kinetics in a premature infant. *J. Mass Spectrom.* 2000;**35**: 734–8.

79 Torresin, M., Zimmerman, L. J., Cogo, P. E. *et al.* Exogenous surfactant kinetics in infant respiratory distress syndrome: a novel method with stable isotopes. *Am. J. Respir. Crit. Care Med.* 2000;**161**:1584–9.

80 Lifson, N., Gordon, G. B., McClintock, R. Measurement of total carbon dioxide production by means of D_2O^{18}. *J. Appl. Physiol.* 1955;**7**:704–10.

81 Schoeller, D. A. Energy expenditure from doubly labeled water: some fundamental considerations in humans. *Am. J. Clin. Nutr.* 1983;**38**:999–1005.

82 Jones, R. H., Sonko, B. J., Miller, L. V., Thureen, P. J., Fennessey, P. V. Estimation of doubly labeled water energy expenditure with confidence intervals. *Am. J. Physiol. Endocrinol. Metab.* 2000;**278**:E383–9.

83 Black, A. E., Prentice, A. M., Coward, W. A. Use of food quotients to predict respiratory quotients for the doubly labeled water method of measuring energy expenditure. *Clin. Nutr.* 1986;**40C**:381–91.

84 Lusk, G. *The Elements of the Science of Nutrition.* New York, NY: Johnson Reprint Corp., 1976 (original version 1928).

85 Schoeller, D. A., Webb, P. Five-day comparison of the doubly labeled water method with respiratory gas exchange. *Am. J. Clin. Nutr.* 1984;**40**:153–8.

86 Roberts, B. R., Coward, W. A., Schlingenseipen, K.-H., Nohria, V., Lucas, A. Comparison of the doubly labeled water ($^2H_2{}^{18}O$) method with indirect calorimetry and a nutrient-balance study for simultaneous determination of energy expenditure, water intake, and metabolizable energy intake in preterm infants. *Am. J. Clin. Nutr.* 1986;**44**:315–22.

87 Jensen, C., Butte, N. F., Wong, W. W., Moon, J. K. Determining energy expenditure in preterm infants: comparison of $^2H_2{}^{18}O$ method and indirect calorimetry. *Am. J. Physiol.* 1992;**263**: R685–92.

88 Leitch, C. A., Alrichs, J., Karn, C., Denne, S. Energy expenditure and energy intake during dexamethasone therapy for chronic lung disease. *Pediatr. Res.* 1999;**46**:109–13.

89 de Meer, K., Westerterp, K. R., Houwen, R. H. J. *et al.* Total energy expenditure in infants with bronchopulmonary dysplasia is associated with respiratory status. *Eur. J. Pediatr.* 1997;**156**: 299–304.

90 Leitch, C. A., Karn, C. A., Peppard, R. J. *et al.* Increased energy expenditure in infants with cyanotic congenital heart disease. *J. Pediatr.* 1998;**133**:755–60.

44

Postnatal nutritional influences on subsequent health

Josef Neu[1], Amy Mackey[1], and Ying Huang[2]

[1]Department of Pediatrics, University of Florida, Gainesville, FL
[2]Children's Hospital of Fudan University, Shanghai, China

Introduction

It is clear that intrauterine undernutrition and subsequent low birth weight result in significant health problems during adult life. These include obesity, cardiovascular disease, hypertension, and Type 2 diabetes. Evidence for a relationship between early postnatal nutrition and the subsequent development of allergies, immune dysfunction, and autoimmune disorders such as Type 1 diabetes, is beginning to accumulate. Numerous questions about the effects of early postnatal nutrition on subsequent short as well as long-term health have been raised: What happens to infants born prematurely who are subjected to postnatal undernutrition for a "critical period" of rapid growth and development? Are these infants, if born appropriate for gestational age and subjected to nutritional stresses "programmed" for a greater susceptibility to chronic diseases such as obesity, Type 2 diabetes and hypertension, as are undernourished fetuses? Does it matter what infants are fed in terms of development of chronic diseases related to autoimmunity, such as Type 1 diabetes and asthma? Can under or overexposure to certain nutrients such as carbohydrates, lipids or proteins in early life have an effect on the development of chronic disease and can these effects be passed on to subsequent generations? In this chapter, we note that there are several remarkable similarities and differences between the chronic effects of pre- versus postnatal undernutrition. Some of the health consequences of early postnatal malnutrition and hypothetical mechanisms by which early nutrition "programs" the individual for long-term outcomes will be addressed.

Early feeding: growth, adiposity, and metabolism

Feeding volume and energy density

Several studies of postnatal nutritional deprivation suggest that different outcomes occur than if deprived prenatally. Epidemiological studies in humans show that nutritional deprivation in utero results in later obesity, hypertension, and Type 2 diabetes.[1] Similarly, in the laboratory, rats that have undergone undernutrition during fetal life have greater adiposity in adulthood.[2] These studies suggested that increased adiposity was due to increased adipocyte size and not number. Several studies evaluating the outcomes of postnatal nutrient restriction differ from those of prenatal nutrient restriction. The litter manipulation model in rodents has been used extensively to study the long-term effects of postnatal under- and overnutrition. In this model, pups are redistributed shortly after birth to either small or large litters, resulting in overnutrition or undernutrition during the suckling period, respectively. McCance[3] showed that rats undernourished during the suckling period followed a permanently diminished growth trajectory (Figure 44.1, top panel), whereas those undernourished after weaning compensated for the period of slowed growth and resumed the growth trajectory of their normally nourished littermates (Figure 44.1, bottom panel). Studies by others, using similar techniques, provided similar results.[4,5] However, the obesity in adult rats that were overnourished in infancy was due to increased adipocyte number, rather than size,[6] which is opposite from the increased size found in offspring of rats restricted during pregnancy.

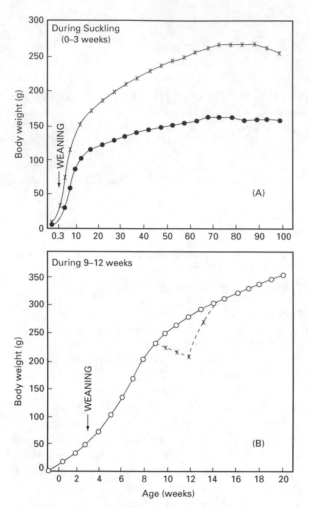

Figure 44.1. Effect of nutrient deprivation prior to weaning, Panel A and after weaning, panel B.[3] In panel A, litter size was manipulated in rats so that rats from large litter sizes (closed circles) received less milk than those from small litters (x) during the 21-day suckling period, by which time rats from large litters were substantially smaller than those from smaller litters. At this point both groups were fed normally, but the smaller animals (from large litters) continued to diverge in body size from the larger animals. Thus, 3 weeks of dietary intervention had resulted in a lifetime programming of growth trajectory. In panel B, equivalent dietary manipulation for a 3-week period a few weeks later had no lasting effect: the underfed animals (x) showed catch-up growth compared with the normally fed animals (circles) when they were re-fed; the critical window for growth programming by early nutrition had passed.

In a baboon model, the long-term effects of postnatal nutrition on later adiposity and adipocyte morphology were examined.[7] In this study, baboons were fed formulas of different energy densities throughout the suckling period. At 5-years of age, female baboons that were overnourished in the preweaning period were 40% heavier than their normally fed counterparts. The fat depots in the 5 year-old overnourished female baboons were five times that of the normally nourished females. In the males, no differences were seen in the body weights, but the overnourished males' adipose depots were three times greater than that of the control males.

Protein

The effects of dietary protein restriction in rats were examined during pregnancy, lactation, or both.[8,9] Lifetime effects on size were seen only in relation to postnatal nutritional manipulation. Animals fed by mothers that were fed a low protein diet during lactation were permanently smaller, whereas prenatal low protein diets fed to the mother had no long-term effect on the size of the offspring.

In another study designed to determine the effects of low protein diets on subsequent lipid metabolism in rats, plasma total cholesterol, HDL-cholesterol and triacylglycerol concentrations were all 20–50% lower in the 6-month-old offspring of rats exposed to the low protein diet during both gestation and suckling. Similar effects were found in the offspring of rats exposed to the low protein diet during suckling only. Only the decrease in plasma triacylglycerol concentration was significant in the group exposed to a low-protein diet during gestation only. These results are contrary to expectations based on the inverse relationship between birth weight and adult cardiovascular disease in humans, in whom restriction during gestation results in higher risk of cardiovascular disease.[1]

Lipids

In a study using rats, Reiser & Sidelman[10] varied dams' diets to affect milk cholesterol concentrations. At 32 weeks of age, the serum cholesterol concentration of male offspring that had consumed the highest concentrations of milk cholesterol during the suckling period was only 60% of that of control animals whose mothers had been fed a regular diet during lactation. This suggested that higher cholesterol feeding during infancy could result in decreased endogenous production of cholesterol in adulthood. A subsequent study of rats fed high fat and cholesterol diets from late gestation through lactation showed greater elevations in serum cholesterol in male offspring than controls.[11] However, in the former study,[10] the diets of the dams were varied during lactation only, thus the results may not be contradictory.

Hahn[12] studied the long-term effects of litter size in rodents on hepatic and adipose tissue enzyme activities. At 60 and 300 days of age, male rodents that were suckled in small litters had elevated plasma cholesterol concentrations and plasma insulin concentrations that were nearly twice as high as animals suckled in large litters of 18. The activity of hepatic beta-hydroxy-methylglutaryl-CoA (HMG-CoA) reductase (the rate-limiting enzyme in cholesterol biosynthesis) was 50% higher in the large litter than in the small litter animals at 60 but not at 240 days of age, suggesting a greater capability to synthesize cholesterol.

Mott *et al.*[13] examined the long-term effects of preweaning cholesterol intake on cholesterol homeostasis in baboons. In this model, infant baboons were either breast fed by their mothers or fed one of several formulas that varied in cholesterol concentration. After weaning, the animals were assigned to one of four diets that varied in cholesterol content and ratios of polyunsaturated to saturated fat. In adulthood, few differences were found in serum cholesterol concentration or metabolism among the groups fed different concentrations of cholesterol during infancy. The triacylglycerol and HDL-cholesterol concentrations in the adult baboons were 10%–15% lower in the mother-fed group than in all of the formula-fed groups. Also, animals fed by their mothers had a 15% higher ratio of VLDL + LDL to HDL (p = 0.08), which indicated a more atherogenic lipid profile. The breast-fed baboons on necropsy tended to have more extensive atherosclerotic lesions than did their formula-fed counterparts, but this trend was not statistically significant.

Overall, these results support the hypothesis that early postnatal nutrition has long-term effects on growth, adiposity, and lipid metabolism. However, the methodology used (litter expansion or contraction in rodents and/or the use of maternal milk versus artificial formula) may be flawed because the actual nutrient intake was difficult to determine. Better techniques need to be utilized to avoid confusion (see discussion of "pup in the cup" model in the "Carbohydrates" section).

Carbohydrates

Early studies of glucose metabolism in fasted rodents showed that rats suckled in small litters had a 2-fold higher insulin concentration in adulthood than those suckled in normal litters.[4] Also, glucose tolerance tests conducted at 18 weeks of age showed a hyper-insulinemic response in small-litter raised animals and a blunted insulin response in large-litter raised animals relative to controls suckled in normal size litters.[4] This early study suggested a long-term effect of early nutrition on carbohydrate metabolism in adulthood.

The litter alteration technique, although used in many rodent models, has significant shortcomings. Exact volume and nutrient composition that the pups are receiving are difficult to control and measure. Individual nutrients that the infants are receiving cannot be accurately altered. Experimental difficulties in rearing newborn pups with their dams thus limit investigation with nutritional modifications during the suckling period.

The artificial rearing technique, as described by Hall *et al.*, [14] sometimes called the "pup in the cup" model, partially circumvents this problem. This model involves placement of a soft catheter into the stomach using an esophageal approach and feeding the pups with a modified rat milk substitute formula, the components of which can be altered. Using this technique, feeding a high carbohydrate diet throughout the suckling period compared with a composition similar to that of rat milk, resulted in several alterations that were present not only short term, but persisted into adulthood and even the next generation of females.[15,16] The adaptations included a distinct leftward shift (increased sensitivity) in the insulin secretory capacity, increased hexokinase activity, increased gene expression of preproinsulin and related transcription factors and specific kinases in 12-day-old pancreatic islets isolated from the animals fed a high carbohydrate diet. These adaptations were also expressed into adulthood, sustaining the hyperinsulinemic condition in the postweaning period. At this time (100 days of postnatal age), high carbohydrate-fed rats also weighed approximately 140 g more than their mother fed controls. The high carbohydrate diet induced an upregulation of several clusters of genes including insulin, P13K, and GLUT-2 transporter.[15] The high carbohydrate-fed female rats also spontaneously transmitted the characteristics of chronic hyperinsulinemia and adult onset obesity to their progeny.[15] The plasma insulin levels of second generation rats were significantly increased (first observed on day 45), which may be aided by the basal hyperinsulinema demonstrated by islets isolated from 100-day-old rats. The growth of the second generation rats paralleled that of age-matched maternal fed rats up to postnatal Day 55, but there was in increase in the growth rate of these rats from Day 55 onward, with the onset of obesity by Day 100.

It was postulated that the mechanisms of this generation spanning effect might be due, in part, to epigenetic mechanisms. These can be triggered by changes in the environment and can occur in both somatic and germ cell lineage during development. Three phases of the programming elicited by feeding a high carbohydrate diet in infancy postulated by these investigators are described in Figure 44.2.[16] Histone deacetylation and DNA methylation may be potential mechanisms for these effects (this will be discussed in greater detail in the "Mechanisms of Programming" section).

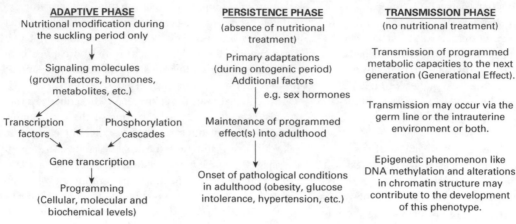

Figure 44.2.   Three phases of metabolic programming after feeding a high carbohydrate diet in the rat.[15,16] Possible mechanisms for the adaptations to the HC dietary intervention in the suckling period (Adaptive phase), the persistence into adulthood of these adaptations (Persistence phase), and for their transmission to the progeny (Transmission phase) are shown.

Early nutrition and Type I diabetes

A growing body of research suggests that infant feeding practices influence the risk for several chronic diseases of childhood and adolescence that are associated with autoimmunity including Type 1 diabetes, asthma, celiac disease, some childhood cancers, and inflammatory bowel disease. Artificial infant feeding and short-term (compared with long-term) breastfeeding have been associated with an increased risk for the development of Type 1 diabetes.[17,18]

A link between early introduction of cow's milk based formulas in infancy and an increased risk of Type 1 diabetes has been suggested.[17] Type 1 (insulin-dependent) diabetes mellitus, like other organ-specific autoimmune diseases, is thought to result from a disorder of immunoregulation. T cells specific for pancreatic islet beta cell constituents (autoantigens) exist normally, but are restrained by regulatory mechanisms (self-tolerant state). When regulation fails, beta cell-specific autoreactive T cells become activated and expand clonally. Current evidence indicates that islet beta cell-specific autoreactive T cells belong to a T helper 1 (Th1) subset, and these Th1 cells and their characteristic cytokine products, interferon gamma (IFN-γ) and interleukin 1 (IL-1), are believed to cause islet inflammation (insulitis) and beta cell destruction. Immune-mediated destruction of beta cells precedes hyperglycemia and clinical symptoms by many years because these become apparent only when most of the insulin-secreting beta cells have been destroyed. Therefore, several approaches are currently being tested or are under consideration for clinical trials to prevent or arrest autoimmune destruction of islet beta cells and insulin-dependent diabetes.

Removal of dietary antigens, specifically cow's milk proteins, from the diet of infants at risk for Type 1 diabetes is the basis of the currently ongoing Trial to Reduce Type 1 Diabetes in the Genetically at Risk (TRIGR). In this study, hydrolyzed protein formula is used during the first 6–8 months of life in infants at increased genetic risk for the development of diabetes. Preliminary results suggest that elimination of cow's milk proteins during infancy decreased the development of beta cell autoimmunity during the first years of life.[17] Other nutritional interventions that might downregulate the Th1 response include increasing the intake of omega-3 fatty acids in the diet[19] and prolonging the feeding of breast milk. Another approach to reduce beta cell autoimmunity is to increase the dietary intake of vitamin D. Vitamin D is an important steroid-like regulator of transcription, which might affect the expression of immunomodulatory genes. Preliminary studies of supplemental vitamin D intake suggest a decrease in the development of Type 1 diabetes.[20]

Other studies in diabetes-prone rats suggest that prior to the onset of diabetes they have an intestinal mucosal barrier that is more permeable than their nondiabetic counterparts.[21] Whether this "leakier" mucosal barrier plays a role in the pathogenesis of diabetes by allowing greater antigen penetration and imbalance of Th1/Th2 responses with resulting autoimmunity remains speculative. However, if a "leakier" intestinal barrier plays a role in the development of Type 1 diabetes, this suggests a role for nutritional interventions. These could include the use of protein hydrolysates[22] to decrease antigenic load, omega-3 fatty acids to decrease inflammation[23] and perhaps even short-chain fatty acids such as butyrate, that are known to affect intestinal intercellular barrier properties.[24]

Atopy, allergy and asthma

Allergic disease, a common cause of morbidity in young children, has increased in the last 20 years in most countries.[25] Although hereditary predisposition appears to be an important component for these diseases, the exposure of "allergenic" foods during infancy also appears to play a role. Whether only susceptible or all infants should receive exclusive breast feeding, and/or partially or extensively hydrolyzed protein formula for a finite period during infancy in order to prevent these diseases will require further study.[25]

Neurodevelopment

Several studies suggest that breast feeding promotes long-term neurodevelopment.[26] The evidence from studies in preterm infants is particularly strong. Human milk contains numerous factors such as hormones, free amino acids and preformed long-chain polyunsaturated fatty acids that may play a role in this effect. Whether the addition of certain human milk components such as long-chain polyunsaturated fatty acids to infant formulas result in improved neurodevelopmental outcome has been a topic of intense recent investigation,[27,28] and it is still unclear whether there are long-term benefits in terms of cognitive function.

Mechanisms of "programming" by early nutrition

As previously mentioned, some of the results of the postnatal nutritional deprivation studies differ somewhat from those of prenatal studies. However, it is clear that early postnatal undernutrition can have significant health effects that extend into adulthood. What are the mechanisms of some of these effects?

Our understanding of the biology underlying adaptations to critical events in early life that "memorize" them and facilitate alterations in later life under certain stimuli remains sparse. Terminology used to describe this phenomenon has been termed "programming"[26] and "metabolic imprinting".[29] Examples of critical windows wherein early exposure to a drug or hormone can result in life-long alterations include the effects of phenobarbital on cytochrome p450[30] and the effects of supraphysiologic concentrations of insulin causing a permanent defect in insulin binding to hepatic membrane receptors.[31] One dose of phenobarbital to a rat in early infancy can result in upregulation of p450 in adulthood.[30] Supraphysiologic concentrations of insulin during a critical period of infancy causes decreased binding of insulin to hepatic membranes during later life.[31]

Many of the previous studies of this "programming" have relied on retrospective epidemiologic studies, a few have been prospective clinical trials and others have been descriptive studies, none of which explain this phenomenon on a subcellular molecular level. Newly developed techniques in molecular biology and biochemistry, genomics and proteomics and epigenetics are likely to yield exciting new information in this area. Currently, most of this mechanistic work is in cell cultures, yeast and *Drosophila*, but is beginning to extend to mammals and humans. Several of the potential mechanisms for these effects are discussed in greater detail in other reviews.[26,29] We will briefly describe some of these putative mechanisms in this chapter.

Alterations in cell number

Decreases in cell number may be a potential mechanism for the changes observed in response to malnutrition. An example shown by Winick & Noble[32] is that severe malnutrition during the period of rapid cell division in the brain resulted in permanent deficits in brain cell number, whereas malnutrition in later periods of brain cell hypertrophy did not have permanent effects.

Clonal selection

Another example is clonal selection, which is comparable to Darwinian evolution operating at the cellular level. Clonal selection occurs when there is a disproportionate population growth of the most rapidly proliferating cells. For example, if the nutrient environment is deficient in structural fatty acids, cells with a slightly more efficient or more active lipogenic pathway could disproportionately populate a tissue and lead to permanent alterations in organ or tissue metabolism.

Metabolic differentiation

Another possible mechanism is that of metabolic differentiation. This is characterized by the ability of a cell to stably express a limited number of genes constitutively or in response to given stimuli. This stability is maintained through epigenetic mechanisms.[33,34] One of the most well-described molecular mechanisms that underlie epigenetic phenomena occurs when maternal or paternal alleles of specific genes are stably repressed on the inactive X chromosome.[35] It is likely that these same epigenetic mechanisms also contribute to metabolic differentiation. Three of these mechanisms include (1) regulation of DNA binding proteins, (2) modulation of chromatin structure, and (3) DNA methylation. These mechanisms likely function together to maintain the vast array of differentiated tissues that characterize higher organisms.[29]

Regulatory pattern of DNA binding proteins

Most genes are not regulated by a single transcription factor that binds to their promoter. Rather, a specific combination of transcription factors is frequently required to activate or repress transcription. Some of these transcription factors bind to their own promoters and to the promoters of other cell-specific transcription factor genes. This will cause a transcription factor, once expressed in a cell, to perpetuate its own transcription as well as related transcription factors for a particular cell type.

Alterations in chromatin structure

Chromatin is the combination of DNA packaged in a compact configuration with histone proteins and other DNA binding proteins. The fundamental unit of chromatin structure is the nucleosome, which consists of about 200 base pairs of DNA wrapped around a histone octamer.

Chromatin structure is highly correlated with gene expression during development. Tissue specific regulation of several genes has been correlated with alterations in local chromatin structure.[36] For chromatin to play a role in cell memory, and hence metabolic differentiation, the specific chromatin structure within a given region of DNA must be stably propagated from progenitor cells to progeny. For histones or other DNA binding proteins to be involved, they must detach from a region of DNA before the DNA polymerase can replicate it. One such model is based on histone modification. Amino acids on the histone tails may undergo several covalent post-translational modifications such as acetylation, ubiquitination, and phosphorylation. One of the best described histone modifications is hyperacetylation, which is associated with regions of open chromatin configuration.[36] The open hyperacetylated chromatin configuration (Figure 44.3) allows greater access of transcription factors to DNA, hence enhancing transcription.

For "memory" to occur, histone hyperacetylated regions of DNA need to be maintained in a transcriptionally active configuration. After replication, because histones remain in the vicinity of the replication fork (Figure 44.3), they could signal the acetylation of additional histones required for formation of complete nucleosomes. In this way, a specific chromatin configuration, altered by nutrition, could have a lasting effect on specific gene expression. One example of a nutrient known to affect histone acetylation is butyrate.[37]

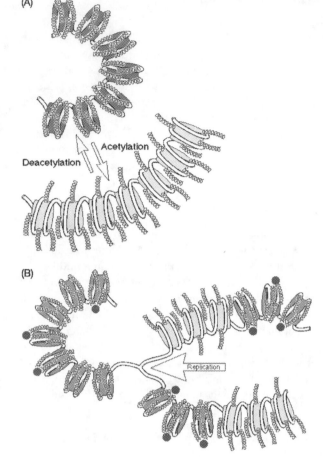

Figure 44.3. (A) Histone acetylation. When hyperacetylated, the chromatin configuration allows greater access of transcription factors to DNA, hence enhancing transcription.[36] (B) DNA replication-involvement of histone. For "memory" to occur, histone hyperacetylated regions of DNA need to be maintained in a transcriptionally active configuration. Histones remain in the vicinity of the replication fork and acetylation of additional histones is signaled. Thus, histone acetylation altered by nutrition could have a lasting, transgenerational effect.[37]

One interesting example of this phenomenon that is currently receiving considerable attention is the relationship between nutrition, histone hyperacetylation, and longevity. In this model, caloric restriction and three histone deacetylases modulate the expression of genes that affect the life span of yeast cells.[38] Elimination of nonessential amino acids from the growth medium potentiates processes that extend life span. Subsets of these processes are ones that limit glucose availability. The induction of these glucose-regulated processes is absolutely essential for the increased longevity afforded by caloric restriction.

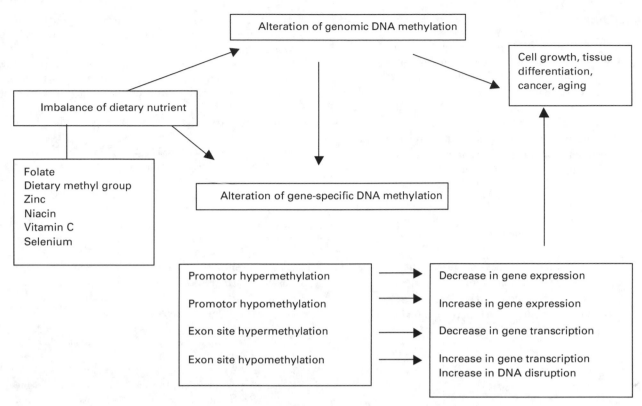

Figure 47.4. DNA methylation – relationships to nutrients. Imbalances of specific nutrients alter DNA methylation, which in turn can alter gene transcription and subsequent expression, resulting in aberrations in cell growth, differentiation, etc.[40]

Histone deacetylases have also been shown to modulate life span in *Drosophila*.[39] With knowledge of the mutual effects of caloric restriction and histone deacetylases in modulating life span, it should be possible to capitalize on these processes and pathways that are elicited by caloric restriction to better understand the processes of aging and its relationship to nutrition.

DNA methylation

Methylation of DNA is one mechanism by which mammals prevent the transcription initiation of certain genes. Nutrients such as vitamins B12, B6 and folate, ascorbic acid, amino acids such as methionine, and enzyme cofactors such as zinc and selenium are known to play a role in one carbon metabolism that contributes to methylation reactions (Figure 47.4). One well known effect is the relationship of neural tube defects and dietary folate insufficiency. However, mechanisms of vitamin deficiency or adequacy on DNA methylation and subsequent long-term outcome remain poorly understood. Methylation of DNA does not simply repress gene expression. Methylation changes how proteins interact with DNA, which leads to an increase or decrease in transcription and subsequent gene expression. Where the specific methylation sites are located plays a major role in their function.

The mechanism of DNA methylation relies on binding or nonbinding of methyl groups to cytosine p-guanine (CpG) aggregates, or "islands," which are frequently found in proximity to gene promoters, early exons, and in the 3' end of genes. Most of the cytosine nucleotides in the sequence CpG in mammalian DNA are methylated to 5-methyl-cytosine. The methylation pattern varies among cells in different tissues and is maintained through cycles of DNA replication by DNA methyltransferases that are highly selective for cytosines in the hemimethylated DNA generated when DNA methylated on both strands is replicated. Thus, this maintenance methylase activity allows a specific pattern of methylation to be transmitted to progeny cells, resulting in cell memory. Since early nutrition affects gene expression during differentiation, cell-specific DNA methylation may be changed, which might lead to persistent effects on the activity of the gene.

Conclusion

In this chapter, we have presented various aspects of post-natal nutrition and effects on subsequent health. Undernutrition and other nutritional perturbations in early postnatal life can have major consequences in later life. These include obesity, Types 1 and 2 diabetes, atherogenesis, allergic and atopic diseases, aging, and cognition. Some of the effects of postnatal undernutrition are similar and others differ from those of intrauterine undernutrition.

We are just beginning to learn about the mechanisms underlying some of these alterations. The information available on DNA methylation and histone acetylation only suggests possible cellular/molecular mechanisms for nutritional programming. It is likely that these do not function as single entities, but rather in concert with many other developmental processes. This may help explain the highly heterogeneous nature of why nutritional deprivation at one stage of life (prenatal) may cause completely different effects than a similar perturbation in later development (postnatal).

REFERENCES

1 Barker, D. J. P. Fetal nutrition and cardiovascular disease in adult life. *Lancet* 1993;**341**:938–41.

2 Jones, A. P., Friedman, M. I. Obesity and adipocyte abnormalities in offspring of rats undernourished during pregnancy. *Science* 1982;**215**:1518–19.

3 McCance, R. A. Food, growth and time. *Lancet* 1962;**2**:271–2.

4 Aubert, R., Suquet, J. P., Lemonnier, D. Long-term morphological and metabolic effects of early under- and over-nutrition in mice. *J. Nutr.* 1980;**110**:649–61.

5 Duff, D. A., Snell, K. Effect of altered neonatal nutrition on the development of enzymes of lipid and carbohydrate metabolism in the rat. *J. Nutr.* 1982;**112**:1057–66.

6 Faust, I. M., Miller, W. H. J. Effects of diet and environment on adipocyte development. *Int. J. Obes.* 1981;**5**:593–6.

7 Lewis, D. S., Bertrand, H. A., McMahan, C. A. *et al.* Preweaning food intake influences the adiposity of young adult baboons. *J. Clin. Invest.* 1986;**78**:899–905.

8 Desai, M., Crowther, N. J., Lucas, A., Hales, C. N. Organ-selective growth in the offspring of protein-restricted mothers. *Br. J. Nutr.* 1996;**76**:591–603.

9 Lucas, A., Baker, B. A., Desai, M., Hales, C. N. Nutrition in pregnant or lactating rats programs lipid metabolism in the offspring. *Br. J. Nutr.* 1996;**76**:605–12.

10 Reiser, R., Sidelman, Z. Control of serum cholesterol homeostasis by cholesterol in the milk of the suckling rat. *J. Nutr.* 1972;**102**:1009–16.

11 Kris-Etherton, P. M., Layman, D. K., York, P. V., Frantz, I. D. J. The influence of early nutrition on the serum cholesterol of the adult rat. *J. Nutr.* 1979;**109**:1244–57.

12 Hahn, P. Effect of litter size on plasma cholesterol and insulin and some liver and adipose tissue enzymes in adult rodents. *J. Nutr.* 1984;**114**:1231–4.

13 Mott, G. E., Jackson, E. M., DeLallo, L., Lewis, D. S., McMahan, C. A. Differences in cholesterol metabolism in juvenile baboons are programmed by breast- versus formula-feeding. *J. Lipid. Res.* 1995;**36**:299–307.

14 Hall, W. G. Weaning and growth of artificially-reared rats. *Science* 1975;**190**:1313–15.

15 Srinivasan, M., Laychock, S. G., Hill, D. J., Patel, M. S. Neonatal nutrition: metabolic programming of pancreatic islets and obesity. *Exp. Biol. Med.* 2003;**228**:15–23.

16 Patel, M. S., Srinivasan, M. Metabolic programming: causes and consequences. *J. Biol. Chem.* 2002;**277**:1629–32.

17 Åkerblom, H. K., Vaarala, O., Hyöty, H., Ilonen, J., Knip, M. Environmental factors in the etiology of type 1 diabetes. *Am. J. Med. Genet.* 2002;**115**:18–29.

18 Vaarala, O. Gut and the induction of immune tolerance in type 1 diabetes. *Diabetes Metab. Res. Rev.* 1999;**15**:353–61.

19 Krishna, M. I., Das, U. N. Prevention of chemically induced diabetes mellitus in experimental animals by polyunsaturated fatty acids. *Nutrition* 2001;**17**:126–51.

20 Zella, J. B., DeLuca, H. F. Vitamin D and autoimmune diabetes. *J. Cell Biochem.* 2003;**88**:216–22.

21 Meddings, J. B., Jarand, J., Urbanski, S. J., Hardin, J., Gall, D. G. Increased gastrointestinal permeability is an early lesion in the spontaneously diabetic BB rat. *Am. J. Physiol.* 1999;**276**:G951–7.

22 Scott, F. W., Rowsell, P., Wang, G. S. *et al.* Oral exposure to diabetes-promoting food or immunomodulators in neonates alters gut cytokines and diabetes. *Diabetes* 2002;**51**:73–8.

23 Calder, P. C. Can n-3 polyunsaturated fatty acids be used as immunomodulatory agents? *Biochem. Soc. Trans.* 1996;**24**:211–20.

24 Mariadason, J. M., Kilias, D., Catto-Smith, A., Gibson, P. R. Effect of butyrate on paracellular permeability in rat distal colonic mucosa ex vivo. *J. Gastroenterol. Hepatol.* 1999;**14**:873–9.

25 Chandra, R. K. Food hypersensitivity and allergic diseases. *Eur. J. Clin. Nutr.* 2002;**56**:S54–6.

26 Lucas, A. Programming by early nutrition: an experimental approach. *J. Nutr.* 1998;**128**:401S–6S.

27 Larque, E., Demmelmair, H., Koletzko, B. Perinatal supply and metabolism of long-chain polyunsaturated fatty acids: importance for the early development of the nervous system. *Ann. N. Y. Acad. Sci.* 2002;**967**:299–310.

28 Jensen, C. L., Heird, W. C. Lipids with an emphasis on long-chain polyunsaturated fatty acids. *Clin. Perinatol.* 2002;**29**:261–81.

29 Waterland, R. A., Garza, C. Potential mechanisms of metabolic imprinting that lead to chronic disease. *Am. J. Clin. Nutr.* 1999;**69**:179–97.

30 Bagley, D. M., Hayes, J. R. Neonatal phenobarbital imprinting of hepatic microsomal enzymes in adult rats: modulation by neonatal testosterone presence. *Toxicol. Appl. Pharmacol.* 1985;**79**:227–35.

31 Inczefi-Gonda, A., Csaba, G., Dobozy, O. Effect of neonatal insulin treatment on adult receptor binding capacity in rats. *Horm. Metab. Res.* 1982;**14**:221–2.

32 Winick, M., Noble, A. Cellular response in rats during malnutrition at various ages. *J. Nutr.* 1966;**89**:300–6.

33 Monk, M. Epigenetic programming of differential gene expression in development and evolution. *Dev. Genet.* 1995;**17**:188–97.

34 Barlow, D. P. Gametic imprinting in mammals. *Science* 1995;**270**:1610–13.

35 Jones, P. A., Takai, D. The role of DNA methylation in mammalian epigenetics. *Science* 2001;**293**:1068–70.

36 Turner, B. M. Cellular memory and the histone code. *Cell* 2002;**111**:285–91.

37 Sanderson, I. R., Naik, S. Dietary regulation of intestinal gene expression. *Ann. Rev. Nutr.* 2000;**20**:311–38.

38 Lin, S. J., Kaeberlein, M., Andalis, A. A. *et al.* Calorie restriction extends *Saccharomyces cerevisiae* lifespan by increasing respiration. *Nature* 2002;**418**:344–8.

39 Rogina, B., Helfand, S. L., Frankel, S. Longevity regulation by *Drosophila* Rpd3 deacetylase and caloric restriction. *Science* 2002;**298**:1745.

40 Friso, S., Choi, S. W. Gene-nutrient interactions and DNA methylation. *J. Nutr.* 2002;**132**:2382S–7S.

45

Growth outcomes of preterm and very low birth weight infants

Maureen Hack and Lydia Cartar

Department of Pediatrics, Case Western Reserve University, and Rainbow Babies and Children's Hospital, University Hospitals of Cleveland, Cleveland, OH

Despite advances in perinatal care and nutrition, growth failure remains a major problem for preterm infants who require neonatal intensive care.[1,2] This growth failure which occurs during the critical period of perinatal development has long-term implications for later growth attainment and for other aspects of health and development.[3–7]

Reports of perinatal growth failure and the potential for catch-up growth prior to the era of neonatal intensive care pertained mainly to low birth weight (LBW) infants, those weighing less than 2.5 kg.[8] More recent follow-up studies of children who experience intrauterine and/or neonatal growth failure pertain to preterm infants with very low birth weight (VLBW, less than 1500 g) or extremely low birth weight (ELBW, less than 1000 g). Initial reports following the introduction of neonatal intensive care in the 1970s described growth during infancy and childhood.[9–17] As the children have reached adolescence and young adulthood, information has been gained concerning final height attainment and other aspects of body growth.

This chapter will review the current knowledge concerning the growth outcomes of preterm infants and the correlates of these outcomes, and also summarize the results of a longitudinal study of the growth of a cohort of VLBW children born in Cleveland, Ohio and followed to 20 years of age.[18]

Definitions and review of methodology in studies of growth of preterm infants

The methodology used in the majority of studies has been to compare the mean growth measures of preterm infants, or rates of subnormal growth, to those of a term-born normal-birth-weight control population, or to national growth norms. Growth parameters examined have been body weight, length and head circumference, and to a lesser extent, body mass index (BMI) and skin-fold thickness. Most studies have reported findings according to birth-weight-specific subgroups rather than according to gestational age. This introduces bias since birth-weight-specific subgroups include children with intrauterine growth failure who are of a higher gestational age than children who have normal in-utero growth but are included in the sample because they fall below the selected birth-weight cut-off.[19] Examination of growth outcomes of VLBW populations has also been confounded by other aspects of population selection. Some studies have included only children who have normal intrauterine growth, i.e., are appropriate-for-gestational-age children (AGA) and excluded those born small-for-gestational-age (SGA) following intrauterine growth failure.[11,13] Some studies include only singleton births and exclude multiple births, many of whom are SGA. In some studies children with chronic illnesses, or those with neurologic impairments such as cerebral palsy, are excluded,[18,20–23] whereas in other studies such children are included.[11,16,24] Few have examined gender-specific growth outcomes [18,24,25] or considered parental size in their analyses. [16,18,24,26] There is also no consensus as to how long to correct for gestational age because of preterm birth. Some correct the children's ages into childhood [16] and even into adolescence.[26] Wang suggests correction to 3 years of age for VLBW children.[27] Elliman has shown that, for very immature infants, correction for gestational age makes a difference to the height z-score up to the age of 7 years. She has suggested that correction for gestational age should continue to age 3 years for children

Neonatal Nutrition and Metabolism. Second Edition, ed. P. Thureen and W. Hay. Published by Cambridge University Press.
© Cambridge University Press 2006.

born at 32 weeks gestation, to age 5 years for those born at 28 weeks gestation and to age 7 years for those born at 24 weeks gestation.[23]

Comparison between studies may also be confounded by the normative growth values used for evaluating in-utero and postnatal growth.[27] The use of regional specific norms is advisable, if available. Currently available normative values for in-utero growth are based on national birth records and pertain to birth weight only. Those most commonly used in the USA are by Alexander[28] and Zhang.[29] Kramer has published updated gender-specific Canadian norms for infants born between 1994 and 1996.[30] The only norms available for birth length and head circumference in North America are those of predominantly Caucasian infants from Montreal, Canada born in the years 1959–1963[31] and of predominantly African-American infants born in Detroit, USA in the years between 1984 and 1992.[32] Birth length of preterm infants is difficult to measure due to the difficulty in stretching out sick immature infants who are very often on ventilators.[18,22,33]

Most of the studies of VLBW growth in North America published prior to 2003 used the 1977 National Center for Health Statistics (NCHS) growth curves based on births in the years 1929–1975 and recognized by the World Health Organization for international use.[12,16,24,34] Updated growth curves were published by the Centers for Disease Control in 2000 based on births in the years 1966–1994.[35] They exclude VLBW children whereas the 1977 NCHS norms included all birth weight groups. The updated CDC growth curves extend from term birth to 20 years of age, include body mass index (BMI) for age charts and are considered to represent the combined size and growth patterns of breast- and formula-fed infants. The most recent British[21] and Australian[22,26] studies of VLBW outcomes have used the British Growth Reference of 1990 for comparative purposes.[36] These include weight and head circumference norms from 23 weeks gestation and length and BMI norms from 33 weeks gestation. The weight and length norms extend to age 22 years and the head circumference norms to age 18 years. Cole also recently published a British weight reference chart specifically for breast-fed babies who have different growth projectiles during the first year of life than formula-fed babies.[37] The British Growth Reference of 1990 and the updated CDC norms are sex-specific and have programs to convert growth measures to z or standard deviation (SD) scores. Z-scores provide a more sensitive measure of growth than percentile cut-offs. A z-score is calculated by subtracting the expected value for age and sex from the child's actual measurement and dividing the difference by the standard deviation for the measurement. A z-score of zero equals the median height or the

50th percentile. A z-score of −2 (−2 SDs) approximates the 2nd percentile.

It has been debated whether growth charts based on the growth of preterm LBW children[1,38,39] should be used for comparative purposes rather than those of normal birth weight term-born children.[40] We and others advocate the use of growth charts based on normal birth weight children since VLBW charts are based on the growth of preterm infants, many of whom are growth retarded at birth and/or have neonatal complications of prematurity and/or suboptimal postnatal nutrition.[1,20,38,41] Acceptance of the norms of such VLBW infants may lead to a complacency in efforts to maximize both neonatal and postdischarge growth.[42]

Examination of growth velocity is the best way to describe the dynamics of growth during infancy and childhood. However there are no growth velocity charts available which give normative values for growth velocity at various ages.[43] It is thus best to use a change in z (SD) scores or distance growth to measure the rate of growth over time.

There has been very little uniformity in the literature in the definition of subnormal growth attainment or catch-up growth. Subnormal growth attainment has been defined variously as less than the 10th percentile, less than the 5th percentile, less than the 3rd percentile or less than −2 standard deviations (the 2nd percentile) below normative growth.[30,44] "Catch-down growth" or "failure to thrive" has been defined as a decrease in growth velocity [41,45] or as evidenced by the crossing of percentiles on growth charts.[16] Ong has defined catch-down or catch-up growth between birth and 2 years of age as a fall-off or increase in weight or length of more than 0.67 standard deviations, which represents the width of each percentile band on standard growth charts, i.e., 2nd to 9th percentile, 9th to 25th percentile, 25th to 50th percentile and so on.[46]

Catch-up growth

The term "catch-up" growth was first introduced in 1963 by Prader to describe an increased velocity of growth which occurs after a temporary arrest of growth during infancy or early childhood: Prader defined catch-up growth as a return of the child's growth to its previous normal growth projectile.[47] The term "catch-up growth" currently pertains to an increased growth velocity following a period of growth retardation, even if this occurred in-utero. Catch-up growth has been variously defined as growth from below a defined subnormal range to above this range,[16,48] to the crossing of percentiles on normative growth charts, which is equivalent to an increase of more the 0.67 SD,[45,46] or to having achieved growth attainment similar to that of normal-birth-weight controls.[18]

In animal experiments of growth failure, the potential for catch-up growth is related to the age of onset, duration, and severity of the original growth failure. For example an animal will remain permanently stunted if the restriction of growth is prolonged, or if it is induced coincident with the timing of the species-specific growth spurt (i.e., during the pre-weaning period). If growth failure is induced during the subsequent body growth spurt, rapid catch-up is more likely.[49] Factors that affect the potential for catch-up or compensatory growth in animals include an increased appetite, tolerance for an increased quantity of nutrients, increased efficiency in the utilization of nutrients, increased rate of growth, and prolongation of the growth period.

Among humans catch-up growth is also probably dependent on the programming of appetite.[50] This is associated with high food intake, efficiency of food utilization and changes in body composition.[51,52] Among children born at term gestation who have suffered from intrauterine growth failure, catch-up growth is dependent on the cause and timing of the growth failure. Children born with major congenital malformations rarely demonstrate catch-up growth, but up to 85% of term-born children with growth failure resulting from placental or other undefined causes demonstrate catch-up growth to within the normal range. This usually occurs during infancy and early childhood.[48]

Catch-up growth following malnutrition during infancy may occur during childhood and adolescence,[53,54] although some report persistence of growth failure.[55] Many of these studies are confounded by the persistence of suboptimal nutrition and, in many cases, poor socio-environmental conditions. A remarkable catch-up of growth during late adolescence and early adulthood has been reported among slave populations.[56] In contrast to malnutrition that occurs during infancy and early childhood, the growth failure of preterm and VLBW infants occurs mainly during the critical period of perinatal brain growth.

Preterm and very low birth weight children

Early childhood growth outcomes of preterm and ELBW infants born in the 1990s

The majority of extremely premature and VLBW infants experience some degree of intrauterine and/or neonatal growth failure.[1,2,57] Despite advances in neonatal care and nutrition, many infants fail to grow adequately during the initial neonatal period with the result that the rates of subnormal weight, length and head circumference are much higher at the time of discharge home than at birth. Poor neonatal growth is most prevalent among the least mature and/or smallest infants, the majority of whom have high rates of neonatal morbidity and also tolerate feeds poorly.

With the exception of randomized controlled trials of nutritional and other therapeutic interventions,[58,59,60] there have been few reports of the post-discharge growth of very preterm and/or ELBW infants surviving in the 1990s and none concerning those born with birth weights of 1000–1500 grams.

Wood's report of the growth results of the Epicure study of infants born at less than 26 weeks' gestation in the UK in 1995 provides important information on the growth of very immature infants in the 1990s.[61] The population included 271 children who were followed to 30 months corrected age. At this age they were smaller on average when compared with the British Growth Reference Norms.[36] Their mean z-scores for weight were 0.27 at birth. Due to neonatal growth failure the mean z-scores dropped to -1.72 at the expected date of delivery (EDD) and then increased to -1.19 by 30 months corrected age. The mean z-scores for head circumference were 0.09 at birth, -0.86 at the EDD and -1.40 at 30 months corrected age, and the mean z-scores for length/height were -2.49 at the EDD and -0.70 SD at 30 months corrected age. At 30 months corrected age 25% of the children had subnormal weight (< -2 SD), 37% subnormal head circumference, 13% subnormal height, 24% subnormal BMI, and 7% a subnormal arm circumference. Eight percent of the children had a weight < -3 SD and 16% a head circumference < -3 SD. Significant correlates of poor growth included feeding problems, neurodevelopmental disability, severe chronic lung disease requiring home oxygen and postnatal steroid therapy.[61] Of note is the fact that the head circumference z-score decreased between the EDD and 30 months corrected age. Follow-up of this cohort to age 6 years revealed further catch-up in weight and height to mean z-scores of -1.21 and -0.97, respectively. There was also some catch-up in head circumference.[62]

Finnstrom reported on the outcomes of $367 \leq 1000$ g birth weight and ≥ 23 week gestation children born 1990–1992 in Sweden. At 36 months corrected age 24% of the children had subnormal (z-score < -2) weight, 17% subnormal height, and 10% subnormal head circumference, respectively.[63] O'Callahan reported similar results for an Australian cohort of $58 < 1000$ g birth-weight children born 1988–1990 of whom 17% had a weight below the 3rd percentile at age 2 years and 10% had a height below the 3rd percentile.[64]

The only recent reported growth outcomes of preterm children born in the USA pertains to an abstract describing the growth of 1136 500–1000 g birth-weight children included in the NICHD Multicenter Neonatal Research Network Follow-Up Program who were followed to 18 months corrected age. Seventeen percent of the children had a birth weight <10th percentile for gestational age. Because of neonatal growth failure, 99% were <10th percentile at 36 weeks corrected age (i.e., 4 weeks before the expected date of delivery). Some catch-up growth occurred during infancy. However, at 18 months corrected age 46% of children were still <10th percentile in weight, 43% < 10th percentile in length and 43% < 10th percentile in head circumference.[65]

The above review reveals that catch-up growth may occur during infancy and early childhood among ELBW and preterm infants, as evidenced by an increase in the z-scores and/or a decrease in the rates of subnormal growth with increasing age. However, as a group, the children remain significantly smaller in size during childhood than normal birth-weight controls or population norms. These results are similar to those described for very low and ELBW children born in the 1980s.[9–13,18,24,26] See also results of longitudinal studies below. Since there have been no recent studies, it is unknown whether VLBW children who have relatively low rates of neonatal morbidity, such as those with birth weights of 1000–1499 g, have better growth outcomes in the 1990's than those born before this time. For preterm children born at less than 32 weeks gestation in Switzerland, Bucher reported that at 2 years of age, when compared with term-born controls, the preterm population had significantly lower weights (−1.0 z-scores), shorter length (−1.23 z-scores) and smaller head circumference (−0.64 z-scores).[66]

Adolescent outcomes of VLBW children

Reported adolescent outcomes of VLBW and ELBW children pertain to births in the 1980s. Some of the studies report on growth at one point in time[21] and some report longitudinal growth.[22,24] The age of puberty is reported to be similar for VLBW and control subjects,[18,21,22,24,67] but examination of growth at fairly wide ages which span the pubertal growth spurt might confound comparisons between studies. The most recent reports are reviewed below.

Powls in the UK compared a cohort of 137 VLBW adolescents who had been treated at the Mercy Regional Neonatal Unit between 1980 and 1983 to school-mate controls. At age 11–13 years, 7% of the participants remained < the 3rd percentile and 23% <10th percentile in height. The mean difference in height, weight, and head circumference between the VLBW subjects and controls were 4.1 cm, 2.5 kg, and 0.89 cm, respectively.[21]

Ford in Australia compared the growth outcomes of two birth-weight-specific groups of neurologically normal VLBW infants born 1977–1982, and treated at a tertiary level referral hospital in Melbourne, to a normal-birth-weight comparison group.[22] The children were measured at ages 2, 5, 8, and 14 years old. At age 14 years the population included 73 < 1000 g birth-weight children, 92 children of 1000–1499 g birth weight, and 41 > 2499 g birth-weight children. The VLBW children had significantly lower weight, height, and head circumference z-scores than the normal birth weight group at all ages examined but the differences in weight and height decreased with increasing age, indicating continued catch-up growth up to age 14 years, such that there were no significant differences between the VLBW and NBW groups in the rates of subnormal (<−2 SD) weight or height at age 14 years (3% v. 0% and 4% v. 2%, respectively). The < 1000 g birth-weight subgroup had a significantly lower head circumference than the 1000–1499 g subgroup at all ages but by age 14 years they did not differ in mean weight or height z- scores. In an additional publication pertaining specifically to the <1000 g group, Doyle noted that catch-up growth occurred mainly between 8 and 14 years.[26]

Peralta-Carcelana in the USA compared 53 neurologically intact <1000 g birth-weight children born in Birmingham, Alabama with term-born controls at age 12–18 years. At this time the <1000 g birth weight group had significantly lower mean weight, height, and head circumference scores than the controls. Six percent had subnormal weight, 6% subnormal height, and 8% a subnormal head circumference. Body composition as measured by DEXA scans was similar between groups.[67]

Hirata, in San Francisco, USA followed 32 < 1000 g birth-weight infants born 1972–1981 to ages ranging from 12–18 years and reported catch-up of weight, height, and head circumference to the 50th percentile. Since only 31% of the subjects were followed, the results might not represent the whole cohort. Furthermore, the age span studied was very wide.[68]

Saigal in Canada compared 154 < 1000 g birth-weight children born 1977–1982 in a geographically defined region of Ontario (including those with neurologic impairments) with a normal-birth-weight control group.[24] At age 12–16 years the < 1000 g birth-weight group had a significantly lower mean weight, height, and head circumference and lower respective z-scores. Eight percent of the children were subnormal (<−2 SD) in height, 6% subnormal in weight, and 16% subnormal in head circumference. Males had higher rates of subnormal height and weight than females when compared with their sex-specific controls.

In a study of bone mineralization of VLBW adolescents, Weiler *et al.* reported that 25 VLBW subjects followed to age 17 years were significantly shorter than controls but that their bone age was appropriate for their body size.[69]

This review of adolescent growth attainment reveals that although catch-up growth occurs between childhood and adolescence, as a group the VLBW subjects remain significantly smaller than their normal birth weight controls in weight, height, and head circumference.

Correlates of growth and catch-up during childhood and adolescence among VLBW and preterm populations

Factors which may affect growth and catch-up after neonatal discharge include sociodemographic factors and ethnicity, pregnancy risk factors, infant birth data, measures of neonatal morbidity, the quality and quantity of neonatal nutrition, maternal behaviors, chronic illness of the infant during childhood, rehospitalizations, neurologic impairment, gender of the child and parental size.

Intrauterine growth failure is one of the major predictors of poor catch-up in growth. [11,14,15,16,21–24,33,41,67,70,71] When catch-up of VLBW SGA infants does occur, it occurs during infancy and early childhood whereas AGA children may demonstrate catch-up at later ages.[16] Low birth weight, irrespective of growth in-utero, is also a major determinant of poor catch-up growth following neonatal growth failure [12,14,15,16] as are low gestational age [14,15] and indices of neonatal morbidity.[11,14,15,70] Specific neonatal complications associated with poor growth and catch-up include necrotizing enterocolitis [61] and chronic lung disease or bronchopulmonary dysplasia.[12,61] Length of hospital stay, an index of many neonatal risk factors including extremely low birth weight, low gestational age and the severity of neonatal morbidity, is also associated with later growth and catch-up.[12,14,18,70,72] Rate of growth during infancy and early childhood and the size of the infant at each age also predicts growth attainment at later ages. Methods of neonatal nutrition have, as yet, not been shown to determine long-term growth attainment, although Fewtrell reported that the neonatal level of alkaline phosphatase, a measure of bone disease, predicted later height attainment at age 7 years.[33] Use of a postdischarge nutrient-enriched formula has been found to improve growth attainment at 18 months corrected age.[73,74]

Factors influencing growth during infancy and early childhood also include the persistence of chronic medical complications, mainly chronic lung disease,[14,61,75–77] rehospitalization during infancy,[14] neurologic impairment, mainly due to cerebral palsy,[11,12,16,41] feeding problems[61,78] and maternal caretaking behaviors[79] or disorders.[77]

Positive effects on growth of parental sociodemographic status, as measured by social class[12,80] and parental education[12] have been reported. In other studies these effects have varied.[11,13] In one study, black low birth weight children tended to put on more weight than white children.[81]

Poor growth and catch-up is more prevalent in male than female VLBW children.[13,20,24,33,63] This may be related to the fact that males have higher rates of neonatal morbidity.[82] Inferior growth attainment has also been reported for term-born SGA males compared with term SGA females.[48,83]

Genetic effect as measured by maternal or mid-parental height is also a major determinant of growth attainment among VLBW and preterm children.[12,13,16,21,26,33,67]

Failure to thrive, i.e., catch-down growth after the neonatal period, has not received much attention in the literature but may play an important role in the lack of ultimate catch-up growth seen among VLBW children. We previously reported that 16% of AGA VLBW children demonstrated failure to thrive as evidenced by a fall off in the growth percentiles to below the 3rd percentile between 40 weeks and 8 months corrected age. These children had higher rates of neurologic impairment and lower developmental scores than children who had a normal or accelerated growth velocity during infancy.[14] Casey and Kelleher reported failure to thrive in 20% of the Infant Health and Development Program low birth weight infant cohort.[41,45] Growth failure peaked at 8 months corrected age and was more common in children who were both SGA and very low birth weight, or who had an abnormal neurologic exam. Of interest is the fact that failure to thrive occurred equally among the children who received an intervention program and those who did not, and more often among infants of mothers with a college education.

Young adult growth outcomes of VLBW children

There have, to date, been only two reports of the adult growth attainment of VLBW infants. Ericson reported that 19-year-old male conscripts to the Swedish army were shorter and lighter than the rest of the Swedish population[84] and we have reported on the growth outcomes of 20-year VLBW men and women as compared with normal birth weight controls.[18] This study will be described in more detail.

20-year growth outcomes of VLBW men and women born 1977–1979 in Cleveland

As part of a comprehensive long-term study of VLBW outcomes, we examined gender-specific growth projectiles and correlates of growth from birth to age 20 years among a cohort of VLBW children born 1977–1979 in Cleveland, Ohio.[18,85]

Description of the population

The study population included 103 male and 92 female VLBW infants who had a mean birth weight of 1189 grams and mean gestational age of 29.8 weeks who were free of neurosensory impairment. Male VLBW had poorer health during infancy than female VLBW as evidenced by significantly higher rates of rehospitalization during the first year of life (39% v. 21%, p < 0.001). A population-based sample of 101 male and 107 female normal birth weight (NBW) subjects who had been selected at age 8 years served as controls.

Methods

Among the VLBW subjects, gender-specific longitudinal growth measures were examined at five points in time; at birth, at the expected term date (40 weeks corrected age), at 8 and 20 months, at 8 years corrected age, and at 20 years postnatal age. Weight and length z-scores were computed at birth and 40 weeks corrected age using the intrauterine growth standards of Usher.[31] Weight and height z-scores were computed at 8 and 20 months, and 8 and 20 years, from the revised CDC growth norms.[35] BMI z-scores were computed at 8 and 20 years. The results of the comparisons between the VLBW and NBW subjects were adjusted for maternal level of education and race via multiple linear regression analysis.

Results

Growth from birth to 20 years

Among the VLBW males, mean weight for age z-scores at birth, 40 weeks and 8 years were −0.7, −1.8, and −0.5; and height for age z-scores were −1.2, −2.8, and −0.5, respectively. For VLBW females, mean weight for age z-scores were −1.1, −2.0, and −0.2 and height for age z-scores were −1.2, −2.4, and −0.2, respectively (see Figure 45.1). At 8 years of age VLBW males had a significantly lower mean weight, height, and BMI than NBW controls whereas VLBW females differed significantly from their NBW controls in mean weight and BMI but not in height. Further catch-up growth in weight, height, and

BMI occurred between 8 and 20 years among VLBW females but not among VLBW males who remained significantly smaller than their controls at age 20 years (Figures 45.1, 45.2). At this time the mean weight of VLBW males was 69 kg v. 80 kg for controls (z-score −0.4 v. +0.5, p < 0.001); mean height was 174 cm v. 177 cm (z-score −0.4 v. +0.03, p < 0.01) and mean BMI was 23 v. 26, p < 0.001 respectively. For VLBW females mean weight was 65 kg v. 68 kg for controls (z-score +0.3 v. +0.5, NS), mean height was 162 versus 163 cm (z-score −0.3 v. −0.1, NS) and mean BMI was 25 v. 25 (NS), respectively. Rates of obesity (BMI > 30) for VLBW males were 7% compared with 15% for controls (p = 0.02) and for VLBW females 15% compared with 18% (p = 0.4) for controls.

There was a significant relationship between the maternal height z-score and that of her young adult child. The mothers of the VLBW males tended to be shorter than mothers of controls (mean height 161.6 v. 163.5 with z-scores of −0.26 and 0.02 respectively, p = 0.06) whereas the mean height of mothers of the VLBW females was similar to that of their control mothers (162.3 v. 163.1 cm with z-scores of −0.16 and −0.04 respectively, p = 0.48).

Nineteen (18%) male and 20 (22%) female VLBW subjects were born small for gestational age (SGA, weight < −2 SD for gestational age). The rates of subnormal growth attainment for the AGA and SGA children at the various time points of the study are presented in Figure 45.3. SGA females caught up to their AGA peers in height by 20 months and in weight by 8 years. At 20 years the rates of subnormal growth did not differ between AGA and SGA females. In contrast at age 20 years significantly more SGA than AGA VLBW males remained subnormal (< −2 SD) in weight (32% v. 6%, p < 0.005) and height (21% v. 4%, p < 0.02).

Correlates of growth among VLBW subjects

The multivariate correlates of weight and height attainment at the five time points of study are presented in Tables 45.1 and 45.2. Among VLBW males the birth-weight z-score, a measure of intrauterine growth, was significantly associated with weight attainment at 40 weeks, 8 and 20 months and 8 years, and with height at all five time points of study. Among females the birth-weight z-score was associated with weight at 40 weeks, 8 and 20 months and with height at 40 weeks, 8 months and 20 years. Among both males and females the neonatal hospital stay, used as a measure of neonatal illness, was associated with weight only at 40 weeks. It was more strongly associated with height and more so among males than among females. Among males the association between the neonatal hospital stay and height was significant at 40 weeks, 8 and 20 months and at 20 years, whereas among females the relationship

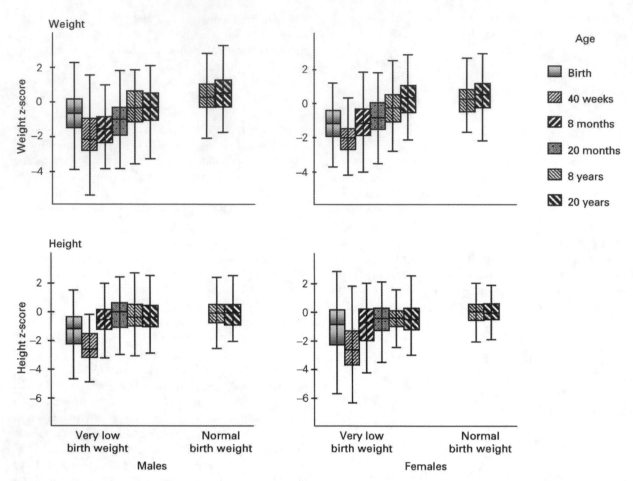

Figure 45.1. Weight and height z-scores at each age, contrasted between males and females. Box plots show median (solid line in box), the interquartile range (top and bottom of the box) and the range of the data.

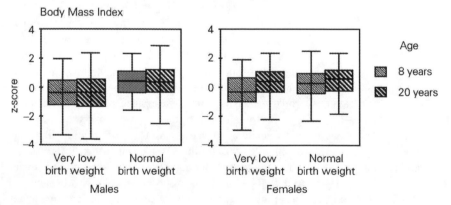

Figure 45.2. Body Mass Index z-scores at 8 and 20 years contrasted between males and females. Box plots show median (solid line in box), the interquartile range (top and bottom of box) and the range of the data.

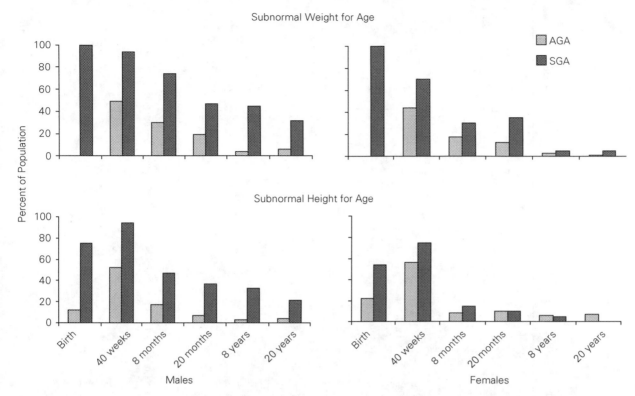

Figure 45.3. Percentage of very-low-birth-weight infants born appropriate (AGA) or small for gestational age (SGA)(<−2 SD) [31] with subnormal (<−2 SD)[35] weight or height for age at birth, 40 weeks, 8 months, 20 months, and 8 years corrected age and at 20 years postnatal age.

was significant only at 40 weeks. Maternal height was significantly related to VLBW height from 8 months among males and from 20 months among females. Among females black race and chronic illness, such as asthma, predicted 20-year weight, whereas no specific factor predicted the 20-year weight of the males.

Conclusion

The results of this study indicate that although male and female VLBW have similar rates of intrauterine and neonatal growth failure, VLBW females demonstrate greater catch-up in growth than males with the result that VLBW males remain significantly smaller than their NBW controls at age 20 years whereas VLBW females do not differ from their NBW controls. The effects of maternal height on child height were similar for males and females whereas intrauterine growth failure tended to play a greater role among males than among females. The negative effect of neonatal illness was greater among males whereas the positive effects of black race and chronic illness were greater among females.

Health implications of growth failure and catch-up growth

It has generally been felt that long-term beneficial effects will accrue from optimizing neonatal and postdischarge nutrition to prevent growth failure and/or accelerate catch-up growth during infancy. There is, however, growing evidence that children who grow rapidly during childhood are more likely to be obese as adults and at risk for metabolic disturbances such as insulin resistance. Based on epidemiologic evidence among predominantly term-born populations, it has been hypothesized that adaptations that the fetus and young infant make when undernourished induce alterations in metabolism, hormonal output and cardiac output which result in central obesity, diabetes and cardiovascular disease in middle age.[3,4,6,7] The subjects who grow rapidly i.e., those with catch-up in growth are at greatest risk for these sequelae.[4–7] Recent evidence from two studies from the Medical Research Council Childhood Nutrition Research Center in London, England suggests that similar effects may be seen among preterm survivors of neonatal intensive care.[86,87] Mortaz examined cholesterol

Table 45.1. Very low birth weight males and females. Multivariate analysis of correlates of weight z-score at 40 weeks, 8 and 20 months, and 8 and 20 years of age.

Independent variables	40 Weeks ß Coeff.[a]	95% CI	8 Months ß Coeff.	95% CI	20 Months ß Coeff.	95% CI	8 Years ß Coeff.	95% CI	20 Years ß Coeff.	95% CI
Males										
Education[b]										
< High school	−0.15	−0.72, 0.42	−0.30	−0.88, 0.27	−0.05	−0.64, 0.53	−0.52	−1.11, 0.07	−0.57	−1.16, 0.03
High school	−0.31	−1.25, 0.62	−0.93	−1.86, −0.01*	−0.94	−1.89, 0.02	−0.80	−1.76, 0.16	−0.32	−1.29, 0.66
Race (Black)[c]	0.40	−0.13, 0.93	0.12	−0.41, 0.66	0.24	−0.31, 0.79	0.42	−0.13, 0.97	0.35	−0.21, 0.92
Maternal height (cm)	−0.02	−0.06, 0.02	0.03	−0.01, 0.07	0.05	0.004, 0.09*	0.03	−0.02, 0.07	0.03	−0.01, 0.08
Birth weight z-score	0.47	0.28, 0.65***	0.44	0.26, 0.63***	0.40	0.21, 0.59***	0.22	0.03, 0.41*	0.10	−0.09, 0.30
Neonatal stay[d]	−0.97	−1.59, −0.35**	−0.38	−0.99, 0.24	−0.60	−1.24, 0.04	−0.09	−0.74, 0.55	−0.07	−0.72, 0.57
Chronic illness[e]	N/A	N/A	N/A	N/A	N/A	N/A	N/A	N/A	−0.43	−1.20, 0.33
R^2	0.37		0.35		0.34		0.18		0.13	
Females										
Education[b]										
< High school	0.16	−0.31, 0.63	0.63	−0.06, 1.31	0.38	−0.32, 1.08	−0.15	−0.76, 0.47	−0.10	−0.71, 0.52
High school	0.40	−0.24, 1.03	0.04	−0.89, 0.97	0.21	−0.74, 1.16	0.07	−0.74, 0.89	0.17	−0.66, 1.00
Race (Black)[c]	0.22	−0.18, 0.61	0.53	−0.05, 1.11	0.64	0.05, 1.23*	0.80	0.28, 1.32*	0.63	0.12, 1.14*
Maternal height (cm)	0.001	−0.03, 0.03	0.03	−0.01, 0.07	0.06	0.02, 0.10*	0.05	0.01, 0.08*	0.03	−0.01, 0.07
Birth weight z-score	0.53	0.36, 0.70***	0.41	0.16, 0.66**	0.27	0.01, 0.53*	0.17	−0.05, 0.40	0.12	−0.11, 0.34
Neonatal stay[d]	−0.61	−0.95, −0.26**	−0.20	−0.66, 0.26	0.30	−0.18, 0.77	0.08	−0.33, 0.49	0.07	−0.36, 0.49
Chronic illness[e]	N/A	N/A	N/A	N/A	N/A	N/A	N/A	N/A	0.85	0.22, 1.49**
R^2	0.43		0.26		0.24		0.22		0.23	

* $p < 0.05$; ** $p < 0.01$; *** $p < 0.001$.

[a] Refers to the coefficient of the independent variable in the linear regression model with weight z-score as the dependent variable and containing maternal education, race and height, birth weight z-score, neonatal hospital stay and chronic illness.

[b] At 8 years. Reference group consists of mothers with more than high school education.

[c] Maternal race used, coded as 1 Black, 0 White.

[d] Natural log of the length of the neonatal hospital stay (in days).

[e] At 20 years. Includes medical or psychiatric illness lasting 12 months or more.

Table 45.2. Very low birth weight males and females. Multivariate analysis of correlates of height z-scores at 40 weeks, 8 and 20 months, and 8 and 20 years of age.

Independent variables	40 Weeks		8 Months		20 Months		8 Years		20 Years	
	β Coeff.[a]	95% CI	β Coeff.	95% CI	β Coeff.	95% CI	β Coeff.	95% CI	β Coeff.	95% CI
Males										
Education[b]										
< High school	0.17	−0.61, 0.95	−0.06	−0.65, 0.54	0.18	−0.26, 0.62	−0.11	−0.52, 0.30	0.005	−0.43, 0.44
High school	0.28	−1.09, 1.64	−0.87	−1.82, 0.09	−0.64	−1.35, 0.08	−0.76	−1.42, −0.09*	−0.60	−1.31, 0.11
Race (Black)[c]	0.07	−0.66, 0.81	0.42	−0.13, 0.98	0.20	−0.21, 0.61	0.48	0.10, 0.86*	0.13	−0.28, 0.54
Maternal height (cm)	0.005	−0.05, 0.06	0.07	0.03, 0.11**	0.05	0.02, 0.08**	0.05	0.02, 0.08***	0.07	0.04, 0.10***
Birth weight z-score	0.73	0.47, 0.99***	0.41	0.22, 0.60***	0.37	0.23, 0.52***	0.26	0.12, 0.39***	0.18	0.04, 0.32*
Neonatal stay[d]	−1.86	−2.70, −1.01***	−1.01	−1.68, −0.33**	−0.71	−1.19, −0.24**	−0.33	−0.78, 0.11	−0.62	−1.09, −0.15*
Chronic illness[e]	N/A	N/A	N/A	N/A	N/A	N/A	N/A	N/A	0.08	−0.48, 0.64
R²		0.46		0.44		0.47		0.42		0.40
Females										
Education[b]										
< High school	0.19	−0.49, 0.88	0.53	−0.11, 1.16	0.14	−0.60, 0.87	0.08	−0.55, 0.70	−0.09	−0.66, 0.48
High school	0.64	−0.27, 1.55	0.50	−0.35, 1.35	0.18	−0.81, 1.17	0.24	−0.59, 1.06	−0.27	−1.03, 0.50
Race (Black)[c]	0.16	−0.41, 0.72	−0.001	−0.53, 0.53	0.81	0.20, 1.42*	0.67	0.15, 1.20*	0.24	−0.23, 0.71
Maternal height (cm)	−0.001	−0.04, 0.04	0.03	−0.001, 0.07	0.07	0.03, 0.11**	0.05	0.01, 0.08**	0.04	0.01, 0.08*
Birth weight z-score	0.67	0.42, 0.93***	0.27	0.04, 0.50*	0.21	−0.06, 0.48	0.08	−0.15, 0.31	0.21	0.004, 0.42*
Neonatal stay[d]	−1.10	−1.64, −0.55***	−0.29	−0.71, 0.14	−0.05	−0.54, 0.44	0.07	−0.35, 0.48	−0.09	−0.48, 0.31
Chronic illness[e]	N/A	N/A	N/A	N/A	N/A	N/A	N/A	N/A	−0.07	−0.65, 0.52
R²		0.45		0.19		0.22		0.18		0.16

$* p < 0.05; ** p < 0.01; *** p < 0.001.$

[a] Refers to the coefficient of the independent variable in the linear regression model with weight z-score as the dependent variable and containing maternal education, race and height, birth weight z-score, neonatal hospital stay and chronic illness.

[b] At 8 years. Reference group consists of mothers with more than high school education.

[c] Maternal race used, coded as 1 Black, 0 White.

[d] Natural log of the length of the neonatal hospital stay (in days).

[e] At 20 years. Includes medical or psychiatric illness lasting 12 months or more.

synthesis at age 8–12 years in a cohort of preterm children born 1982–1985 with birth weight <1750 g who had participated in a randomized trial of nutrition comparing lower nutrient diets of breast milk or term formula to a high nutrient preterm formula. Cholesterol synthesis was not affected by nutrition. However, children with lower birth-weight z-scores had lower predicted cholesterol absorption efficiency. Furthermore, predicted endogenous cholesterol synthesis was higher and cholesterol absorption efficiency was lower among children with the greatest catch-up growth between birth and follow-up, irrespective of growth in-utero.[86] Singhal followed this same population to adolescence and at age 13–16 years measured fasting 32–33 split proinsulin concentrations, a measure of insulin resistance. Only 216 of the original neonatal cohort of 926 subjects participated at this time, although the children followed did not differ in neonatal characteristics from those lost to follow up. The results indicated that the relative undernutrition among infants given the breast milk or term formula had possible beneficial effects on insulin resistance. Furthermore, greater weight gain in the first 2 weeks of life, irrespective of type of nutrition was associated with greater insulin resistance.[87] In this same population lower leptin levels were associated with breast milk feeding.[88]

These reports indicate that attempts to optimize neonatal nutrition and growth may possibly have long-term deleterious metabolic effects in preterm children. However, catch-up growth may also have beneficial effects. Positive short-term health benefits of early rapid growth have been reported among both SGA and AGA Brazilian children, as evidenced by lower rates of hospitalization during infancy and early childhood.[89,90] Rapid growth of preterm children during infancy, especially among those who failed to grow adequately in-utero or during the neonatal period, is regarded as a sign of health and resolution of chronic complications of prematurity. Catch-up of head size may also have beneficial effects on cognitive development. These positive effects of rapid growth need thus to be weighed against potential long-term deleterious metabolic effects. Based on information available at this time, there is not yet enough evidence to advocate a change in the current attempts to optimize growth of preterm infants both during the neonatal period and during infancy after discharge home.

Acknowledgments

Supported by grants (RO1 HD34177 and M01 RR00080, General Clinical Research Center) of the National Institutes of Health and in part by a grant (96–46) from the Genentech Foundation for Growth and Development.

REFERENCES

1 Ehrenkranz, R. A., Younes, N., Lemons, J. A. *et al.* Longitudinal growth of hospitalized very low birth weight infants. *Pediatrics* 1999;**104**:280–9.

2 Embleton, N. E., Pang, N., Cooke, R. J. Postnatal malnutrition and growth retardation: an inevitable consequence of current recommendations in preterm infants. *Pediatrics* 2001;**107**:270–3.

3 Barker, D. J. P. *Mothers, Babies and Health in Later Life.* Edinburgh: Churchill Livingston; 1998.

4 Forsen, T., Eriksson, J. G., Tuomilehto, J., Osmond, C., Barker, D. J. P. Growth in utero and during childhood among women who develop coronary heart disease: longitudinal study. *Br. Med. J.* 1999;**319**:1403–7.

5 Law, C. Adult obesity and growth in childhood. *Br. Med. J.* 2001;**323**:1320–1.

6 Cianfarani, S., Germani, D., Branca, F. Low birthweight and adult insulin resistance: the "catch-up growth" hypothesis. *Arch. Dis. Child. Fetal Neonatal Edn.* 1999;**81**:F71–3.

7 Fall, C. H. D., Osmond, C., Barker, D. J. P. *et al.* Fetal and infant growth and cardiovascular risk factors in women. *Br. Med. J.* 1995;**310**:428–32.

8 Douglas, J. W. B., Mogford, C. The results of a national inquiry into the growth of premature children from birth to 4 years. *Arch. Dis. Child.* 1953;**28**:436–45.

9 Ford, G., Rickards, A., Kitchen, W. H., Ryan, M. M., Lissenden, J. V. Relationship of growth and psychoneurologic status of 2-year-old children of birthweight 500–999 g. *Early Hum. Dev.* 1986;**13**:329–37.

10 Doyle, L. W., Ford, G. W., Abadilla, B., Warne, G. L., Callanan, C. Assessment of short stature in very low birthweight children. *J. Paediatr. Child Health* 1993;**29**:411–14.

11 Astbury, J., Orgill, A. A., Bajuk, B., Yu, V. Y. H. Sequelae of growth failure in appropriate for gestational age, very low-birthweight infants. *Dev. Med. Child Neurol.* 1986;**28**:472–9.

12 Ross, G., Lipper, E. G., Auld, P. A. M. Growth achievement of very low birth weight premature children at school age. *J. Pediatr.* 1990;**117**:307–9.

13 Qvigstad, E., Verloove-Vanhorick, S. P., Ens-Dokkum, M. H. *et al.* Prediction of height achievement at five years of age in children born very preterm or with very low birth weight: continuation of catch-up growth after two years of age. *Acta Pædiatr.* 1993;**82**:444–8.

14 Hack, M., Merkatz, I. R., Gordon, D., Jones, P. K., Fanaroff, A. A. The prognostic significance of postnatal growth in low birth weight infants. *Am. J. Obstet. Gynecol.* 1982;**143**:693–9.

15 Hack, M., Merkatz, I. R., McGrath, S. K., Jones, P. K., Fanaroff, A. A. Catch-up growth in very low birthweight infants: clinical correlates. *Am. J. Dis. Child.* 1984;**138**:370–5.

16 Hack, M., Weissman, B., Borawski-Clark, E. Catch-up growth during childhood among very-low-birth-weight children. *Arch Pediatr. Adolesc. Med.* 1996;**150**:1122–9.

17 Hack, M., Breslau, N., Weissman, B. *et al.* Effect of very low birth weight and subnormal head size on cognitive abilities at school age. *New Engl. J. Med.* 1991;**325**:231–7.

18 Hack, M., Schluchter, M., Cartar, L. *et al.* Growth of very low birthweight infants to age 20 years. *Pediatrics* [serial online]. 2003;**112**:e30–8. http://www.pediatrics.org/cgi/content/full/112/1/e30.

19 Arnold, C. C., Kramer, M. S., Hobbs, C. A., McLean, F. H., Usher, R. H. Very low birth-weight: a problematic cohort for epidemiologic studies of very small or immature neonates. *Am. J. Epidemiol.* 1991;**134**:604–13.

20 Casey, P. H., Kraemer, H. C., Bernbaum, J., Yogman, M. W., Sells, J. C. Growth status and growth rates of a varied sample of low birth weight, preterm infants: a longitudinal cohort from birth to three years of age. *J. Pediatr.* 1991;**119**:599–605.

21 Powls, A., Botting, N., Cooke, R. W. I., Pilling, D., Marlow, N. Growth impairment in very low birth weight children at 12 years: correlation with perinatal and outcome variables. *Arch. Dis. Child.* 1996;**75**:F152–7.

22 Ford, G. W., Doyle, L. W., Davis, N. M., Callanan, C. Very low birth weight and growth into adolescence. *Arch. Pediatr. Adolesc. Med.* 2000;**154**:778–84.

23 Elliman, A., Bryan, E., Walker, J., Harvey, D. The growth of low-birth-weight children. *Acta Pædiatr.* 1992;**81**:311–14.

24 Saigal, S., Stoskopf, B. L., Streiner, D. L., Burrows, E. Physical growth and current health status of infants who were of extremely low birth weight and controls at adolescence. *Pediatrics* 2001;**108**:407–15.

25 Finnström, O., Otterblad, P., Sedin, G. *et al.* Neurosensory outcome and growth at three years in extremely low birthweight infants: follow-up results from the Swedish national prospective study. *Acta Pædiatr.* 1998;**87**:1055–60.

26 Doyle, L. W. Growth and respiratory health in adolescence of the extremely low-birth weight survivor. *Clin. Perinatol.* 2000;**27**:421–32.

27 Wang, Z., Sauve, R. S. Assessment of postneonatal growth in VLBW infants: selection of growth references and age adjustment for prematurity. *Can. J. Public Health.* 1998;**89**:109–14.

28 Alexander, G. R., Himes, J. H., Kaufman, R. B., Mor, J., Kogan, M. A United States National Reference for fetal growth. *Obstet. Gynecol.* 1996;**87**:163–8.

29 Zhang, J., Bowes, W. A., Jr. Birth-weight-for-gestational-age patterns by race, sex, and parity in the United States population. *Obstet. Gynecol.* 1995;**86**:200–8.

30 Kramer, M. S., Platt, R. W., Wen, S. W. *et al.* A new and improved population-based Canadian reference for birth weight for gestational age. *Pediatrics* [serial online] 2001;**108**:1–7. http://www.pediatric.org/cig/content/full/108/2/e35.

31 Usher, R., McLean, F. Intrauterine growth of live-born Caucasian infants at sea level: standards obtained from measurements in 7 dimensions of infants born between 25 and 44 weeks of gestation. *Pediatrics* 1969;**74**:901–10.

32 Dombrowski, M. P., Wolfe, H. M., Brans, Y. W., Saleh, A. A. A., Sokol, R. J. Neonatal morphometry: relation to obstetric, pediatric, and menstrual estimates of gestational age. *Am. J. Dis. Child.* 1992;**146**:852–6.

33 Fewtrell, M. S., Cole, T. J., Bishop, N. J., Lucas, A. Neonatal factors predicting childhood height in preterm infants: evidence for a persisting effect of early metabolic bone disease. *J. Pediatr.* 2000;**137**:668–73.

34 Hamill, P. V., Drizd, T. A., Johnson, C. L. Physical growth: National Center for Health Statistics percentiles. *Am. J. Clin. Nutr.* 1979;**32**:607–29.

35 Kuczmarski, R. J., Ogden, C. L., Grummer-Strawn, L. M. *et al.* *CDC growth charts: United States Advance data from vital and health statistics.* No. 314. Hyattsville, MD: National Center for Health Statistics; 2000.

36 Cole, T. J., Freeman, J. V., Preece, M. A. British 1990 growth reference centiles for weight, height, body mass index and head circumference fitted by maximum penalized likelihood. *Stat. Med.* 1998;**17**:407–29.

37 Cole, T. J., Paul, A. A., Whitehead, R. G. Weight reference charts for British long-term breastfed infants. *Acta Pædiatr.* 2002;**91**:1296–300.

38 Casey, P. H., Kraemer, H. C., Bernbaum, J. *et al.* Growth patterns of low birth weight preterm infants: a longitudinal analysis of a large, varied sample. *J. Pediatr.* 1990;**117**:298–307.

39 Guo, S. S., Wholihan, K., Roche, A. F., Chumlea, W. C. Weight-for-length reference data for preterm, low-birth-weight infants. *Arch Pediatr. Adolesc. Med.* 1996;**150**:964–70.

40 Sherry, B., Mei, Z., Grummer-Strawn, L., Dietz, W. H. Evaluation of and recommendations for growth references for very low birth weight (<1500 grams) infants in the United States. *Pediatrics* 2003;**111**:750–8.

41 Kelleher, K. J., Casey, P. H., Bradley, R. H. *et al.* Risk factors and outcomes for failure to thrive in low birth weight preterm infants. *Pediatrics* 1993;**91**:941–8.

42 Atkinson, S. A., Brunton, J. A., Wauben, I. P. *et al.* Assessment of preterm infant's growth after term corrected age: should reference standards be based on growth of term or premature infants? *Pediatr. Res.* 1995;**37**:301A.

43 Cole, T. J. Presenting information on growth distance and conditional velocity in one chart: practical issues of chart design. *Stat. Med.* 1998;**17**:2697–707.

44 Goldenberg, R. L., Cliver, S. P. Small for gestational age and intrauterine growth restriction: definitions and standards. *Clin. Obstet. Gynecol.* 1997;**40**:704–14.

45 Casey, P. H., Kelleher, K. J., Bradley, R. H. *et al.* A multifaceted intervention for infants with failure to thrive. *Arch. Pediatr. Adolesc. Med.* 1994;**148**:1071–7.

46 Ong, K. K., Ahmed, M. L., Emmett, P. M. *et al.* Association between postnatal catch-up growth and obesity in childhood: prospective cohort study. *Br. Med. J.* 2000;**320**:967–71.

47 Prader, A., Tanner, J. M., von Harnack, G. A. Catch-up growth following illness or starvation: an example of developmental canalization in man. *J. Pediatr.* 1963;**62**:646–59.

48 Albertsson-Wikland, K., Wennergren, G., Wennergren, M., Vilbergsson, G., Rosberg, S. Longitudinal follow-up of growth in children born small for gestational age. *Acta Pædiatr.* 1993;**82**:438–43.

49 Wilson, P. N., Osbourne, D. F. Compensatory growth after undernutrition in mammals and birds. *Biol. Rev.* 1959;**35**:324–63.

50 Ong, K. K. L., Preece, M. A., Emmett, P. M., Ahmed, M. L., Dunger, D. B. Size at birth and early childhood growth in relation to maternal smoking, parity and infant breast-feeding: longitudinal birth cohort study and analysis. *Pediatr. Res.* 2002;**52**:863–7.

51 Ashworth, A. Growth rates in children recovering from protein-calorie malnutrition. *Br. J. Nutr.* 1969;**23**:835–45.

52 Ounsted, M., Sleigh, G. The infant's self-regulation of food intake and weight gain. Difference in metabolic balance after growth constraint or acceleration in utero. *Lancet* 1975;**1**:1393–7.

53 Dreizen, S., Spirakis, C. N., Stone, R. E. A comparison of skeletal growth and maturation in undernourished and well-nourished girls before and after menarche. *J. Pediatr.* 1967;**70**:256–63.

54 Galler, J. R., Ramsey, F., Solimano, G. A follow-up study of the effects of early malnutrition on subsequent development. I. Physical growth and sexual maturation during adolescence. *Pediatr. Res.* 1985;**19**:518–23.

55 Stoch, M. B., Smyth, P. M. 15-year developmental study on effects of severe undernutrition during infancy on subsequent physical growth and intellectual functioning. *Arch. Dis. Child.* 1976;**51**:327–36.

56 Steckel, R. H. The remarkable catch-up growth of American slaves. *Ann. Hum. Biol.* 1987;**14**:111–32.

57 Bukowski, R., Gahn, D., Denning, J., Saade, G. Impairment of growth in fetuses destined to deliver preterm. *Am. J. Obstet. Gynecol.* 2001;**185**:463–7.

58 Fewtrell, M. S., Morley, R., Abbott, R. A. *et al.* Double-blind, randomized trial of long-chain polyunsaturated fatty acid supplementation in formula fed to preterm infants. *Pediatrics* 2002;**110**:73–82.

59 O'Connor, D. L., Hall, R., Adamkin, D. *et al.* Growth and development in preterm infants fed long chain polyunsaturated fatty acids: a prospective, randomized controlled trial. *Pediatrics* 2001;**108**:359–71.

60 Yeh, T. F., Lin, Y. J., Huang, C. C. *et al.* Early dexamethasone therapy in preterm infants: a follow-up study. *Pediatrics* [serial online]. 1998;**101**:1–8. http://www.pediatrics.org/cgi/content/full/101/5/e7.

61 Wood, N. S., Costeloe, K., Gibson, A. T. *et al.* The EPICure Study: Growth and associated problems in children born at 25 weeks or less gestational age. *Arch. Dis. Child.* 2003;**88**:F492–500.

62 Bracewell, M. A., Marlow, N., Wolke, D. Catch-up growth in extremely preterm children at 6 years. *Pediatr. Res.* 2003;**53**:352A.

63 Finnström, O., Otterblad, P., Sedin, G. *et al.* Neurosensory outcome and growth at three years in extremely low birthweight infants: follow-up results from the Swedish national prospective study. *Acta Pædiatr.* 1998;**87**:1055–60.

64 O'Callaghan, M. J., Burns, Y., Gray, P. *et al.* Extremely low birth weight and control infants at 2 years corrected age: a comparison of intellectual abilities, motor performance, growth and health. *Early Hum. Dev.* 1995;**40**:115–25.

65 Dusick, A., Vohr, B., Steichen, J., Wright, L., Mele, L. Factors affecting growth outcome at 18 months in extremely low birthweight (ELBW) infants. *Pediatr. Res.* 1998;**43**:213A.

66 Bucher, H. U., Killer, C., Ochsner, Y., Vaihinger, S., Fauchere, J. Growth, developmental milestones and health problems in the first 2 years in very preterm infants compared with term infants: a population based study. *Eur. J. Pediatr.* 2002;**161**:151–6.

67 Peralta-Carcelen, M., Jackson, D. S., Goran, M. I. *et al.* Growth of adolescents who were born at extremely low birth weight without major disability. *J. Pediatr.* 2000;**136**:633–40.

68 Hirata, T., Bosque, E. When they grow up: the growth of extremely low birth weight (≤1000 gm) infants at adolescence. *J. Pediatr.* 1998;**132**:1033–5.

69 Weiler, H. A., Yuen, C. K., Seshia, M. M. Growth and bone mineralization of young adults weighing less than 1500 g at birth. *Early Hum. Dev.* 2002;**67**:101–12.

70 Ross, G., Krauss, A. N., Auld, P. A. M. Growth achievement in low-birth-weight premature infants: relationship to neurobehavioral outcome at one year. *J. Pediatr.* 1983;**103**:105–8.

71 Amin, H., Singhal, N., Sauve, R. S. Impact of intrauterine growth restriction on neurodevelopmental and growth outcomes in very low birthweight infants. *Acta Pædiatr.* 1997;**86**:306–14.

72 Sauve, R. S., Geggie, J. H. Growth and dietary status of preterm and term infants during the first two years of life. *Can. J. Public Health* 1991;**82**:95–100.

73 Lucas, A., Fewtrell, M. S., Morley, R. *et al.* Randomized trial of nutrient-enriched formula versus standard formula for post-discharge preterm infants. *Pediatrics* 2001;**107**:703–11.

74 Cooke, R. J., Embleton, N. D., Griffin, I. J., Wells, J. C., McCormick, K. P. Feeding preterm infants after hospital discharge: growth and development at 18 months of age. *Pediatr. Res.* 2001;**49**:719–22.

75 Markestad, T., Fitzhardinge, P. Growth and development in children recovering from bronchopulmonary dysplasia. *J. Pediatr.* 1981;**98**:597–602.

76 Yu, V., Orgill, A., Lim, S. Growth and development of very low-birth-weight infants recovering from bronchopulmonary dysplasia. *Arch. Dis. Child.* 1983;**58**:791–4.

77 Tudehope, D. I., Burns, Y., O'Callaghan, M., Mohay, H., Silcock, A. The relationship between intrauterine and postnatal growth on the subsequent psychomotor development of very low birthweight (VLBW) infants. *Aust. Paediatr. J.* 1983;**19**:3–8.

78 Lemons, P. K., Lemons, J. A. Transition to breast/bottle feedings: the premature infant. *J. Am. Coll. Nutr.* 1996;**15**:126–35.

79 DeWitt, S. J., Sparks, J. W., Swank, P. B. *et al.* Physical growth of low birthweight infants in the first year of life: impact of maternal behaviors. *Early Hum. Dev.* 1997;**47**:19–34.

80 Teranishi, H., Nakagawa, H., Marmot, M. Social class difference in catch up growth in a national British cohort. *Arch. Dis. Child.* 2001;**84**:218–21.

81 Seed, P. T., Ogundipe, E. M., Wolfe, C. D. A. Ethnic differences in the growth of low-birthweight infants. *Paediatr. Perinat. Epidemiol.* 2000;**14**:4–13.

82 Stevenson, D. K., Verter, J., Fanaroff, A. A. *et al.* Sex differences in outcomes of very low birthweight infants: the newborn male disadvantage. *Arch. Dis. Child. Fetal Neonatal Edn.* 2000;**83**:F182–5.

83 Paz, I., Seidman, D. S., Danon, Y. L. *et al.* Are children born small for gestational age at increased risk of short stature? *Am. J. Dis. Child.* 1993;**147**:337–9.

84 Ericson, A., Kallen, B. Very low birthweight boys at the age of 19. *Arch. Dis. Child. Fetal Neonatal Edn.* 1998;**78**:F171–4.

85 Hack, M., Flannery, D.J., Schluchter, M. *et al.* Outcomes in young adulthood for very-low birth weight infants. *New Engl. J. Med.* 2002;**346**:149–57.

86 Mortaz, M., Fewtrell, M. S., Cole, T. J., Lucas, A. Birth weight, subsequent growth, and cholesterol metabolism in children 8–12 years old born preterm. *Arch. Dis. Child.* 2001;**84**:212–17.

87 Singhal, A., Fewtrell, M., Cole, T. J., Lucas, A. Low nutrient intake and early growth for later insulin resistance in adolescents born preterm. *Lancet* 2003;**361**:1089–97.

88 Singhal, A., Farooqi, I. S., O'Rahilly, S. *et al.* Early nutrition and leptin concentrations in later life. *Am. J. Clin. Nutr.* 2002;**75**:993–9.

89 Victora, C. G., Barros, F. C., Horta, B. L., Martorell, R. Short-term benefits of catch-up growth for small-for-gestational-age infants. *Int. J. Epidemiol.* 2001;**30**:1325–30.

90 Eriksson, J. Commentary: early 'catch-up' growth is good for later health. *Int. J. Epidemiol.* 2001;**30**:1330–1.

46

Post-hospital nutrition of the preterm infant

Diane M. Anderson[1] and Richard J. Schanler[2]

[1] Department of Pediatrics, Baylor College of Medicine, Houston, TX
[2] Schneider Children's Hospital at North Shore, North Shore University Hospital, Manhasset, NY and
Albert Einstein College of Medicine, Bronx, NY

Post-hospital nutrition of the preterm infant

Precise nutrient requirements and achievable growth remain to be defined for the premature infant post-hospital discharge. While fetal growth serves as the standard for the infant less than 37 weeks gestation and breastfeeding meets the needs of the healthy term infant, neither goal meets the needs of the premie graduate. The graduate of the newborn intensive care unit (NICU) frequently enters into the home setting at a physical size which is significantly less than that of the fetus of the same postmenstrual age.[1] Nutrient need may be further altered by gender, ethnicity, hospital course and post hospital clinical status.[2,3]

The limited number of investigations on nutrition post-hospital discharge differ in their infant population, study diet, duration of study diet, and final results. Post discharge formulas have recently been developed and may meet the nutrient demands for selected premature infants. Continued monitoring of the infant's dietary intake, anthropometric measurements, and clinical status will help to determine if the infant's needs are met or if nutrient supplementation is indicated.

Growth

Premature infants can grow at the fetal growth rate of at least $15\,g\,kg^{-1}day^{-1}$ in the NICU.[4] This rate results in growth that parallels fetal growth, but because adequate weight gain commences only after 1–2 weeks it does not result in catch-up growth during the hospital stay.[4,5] Although most premature infants begin life appropriately grown, they are frequently discharged at a weight less than the 10th percentile for age.[6] This smaller size may be related to deficient nutrient intakes as well as clinical complications which have heightened nutrient demand and/or interfere with nutritional intake.[4,7] Illnesses such as chronic lung disease, late onset sepsis, necrotizing enterocolitis, and severe intraventricular hemorrhage have been associated with lower rates of growth compared with infants not manifesting these conditions.[4]

To achieve catch-up growth, premature infants must grow at a rate greater than what the term infant achieves.[1] As a group, low birth weight premature infants remain smaller than term infants for the first 3 years of corrected age.[8] At 8 years of age, very low birth weight (VLBW) infants are reported to remain smaller in all growth measurements than term infants.[9] During adolescence, there have been reports of VLBW infants catching up in physical growth.[10,11] By 20 years of age female infants have demonstrated catch-up growth in their weight, length, and body mass index, and male infants remain smaller in all three parameters as compared to term infants.[12] The small-for-gestational-age (SGA) male infant has a greater incidence of remaining small in weight and height at 20 years of age. These studies demonstrate that catch-up physical growth can occur beyond the first 3 years of life.[12] However, at 20 years of age, premature infants remain at high risk for neurodevelopmental problems including low cognitive and achievement scores and failure to complete secondary education.[10] Poor head growth as defined by a head circumference 2 SD below the mean at 8 months of age has been linked to poor neurodevelopment at 8 years of age.[13] To what degree appropriate nutrition during infancy affects ideal brain growth and adult neurodevelopment is unknown.

Neonatal Nutrition and Metabolism. Second Edition, ed. P. Thureen and W. Hay. Published by Cambridge University Press.
© Cambridge University Press 2006.

Table 46.1. Selected nutrient comparison of human milk and US infant formulas per liter

Nutrient	Human milk	Standard term formula	Enriched, postdischarge formula	Premature infant formula
Energy (kcal)	670	670	730	810
Protein (g)	10	14	21	24
Fat (g)	35	36	40	43
Carbohydrate (g)	70	73	76	87
Calcium (mg)	280	530	835	1400
Phosphorus (mg)	147	320	475	740
Sodium (mmol)	8	8	11	18
Iron (mg)	0.4	12.2	13.3	14.6
Zinc (mg)	1.2	6	9	12.2
Vitamin A (mg)	0.7	0.6	1	3.0
Vitamin D (μg)	0.5	10	14	40

In many of these studies, the nutrient intake of the infants was not explored. This important link of dietary intake may shed light on the growth and developmental outcomes. Clinical management including nutrition support has changed in the NICU and may be reflected in the outcomes of the present premature infants.

Studies of formula-fed infants

Postdischarge nutrition has been studied in randomized trials of formula-fed infants. Occasional studies have included a breastfeeding reference group. Postdischarge, premature infants have been fed premature infant formula (PTF), premature discharge formula (PDF), or standard-term formula and the outcomes of physical growth and neurological development have been examined.[14–16] The PDFs have a nutrient composition that is between that of standard infant formula and the PTFs, and PDFs are available for use in the home setting. The PDF formula provides increased amounts of energy, protein, calcium, phosphorus, magnesium, and vitamin D. See Table 46.1 for nutrient comparison. Investigations have varied in the study population, study milk, length of time that the study milk was consumed, and the infant's age that growth and development was assessed.

In a preliminary study done in England, a PDF was fed to 32 formula-fed infants postdischarge.[17] Infants who had a birth weight less than 1850 g were recruited from one NICU and they were discharged home feeding either a standard term formula or a PDF. The formulas were fed in the NICU beginning at approximately 37 weeks' gestation and continued to 9 months corrected age (CA). The infants fed the PDF displayed greater weight and length gain at 9 months of CA. On entry, both groups had a mean weight between the 3rd and 10th percentile. The infants fed the term formula remained at the lower percentile at 9 months CA, whereas the weight of infants fed PDF was closer to the 25th percentile for age. At study entry the mean length in both groups was near the 25th percentile, and at 9 months CA the infants fed term formula remained at the 25th percentile, but the length of the infants fed PDF was closer to the 50th percentile. No differences were observed between the two groups regarding head circumference growth, subscapular and triceps skinfold thicknesses, feeding tolerance, or milk consumption. Also, at 9 months CA infants fed the PDF formula demonstrated greater bone mineralization and skeletal growth (bone width).[18] Metabolic bone disease during the neonatal period may lead to shorter stature at 18 months and continue to be a factor for linear growth through 12 years of age.[2,19] It is unknown if the use of PDF in the postdischarge period can enhance height growth for the infant who suffered from osteopenia in the NICU. Neurodevelopmental outcomes were not assessed in this investigation.[17]

Lucas *et al.* expanded their 1992 investigation by conducting a randomized trial of standard formula or PDF in a large sample (n = 284) of infants from 5 NICUs and evaluated the outcomes of physical growth and neurodevelopment at 9 and 18 months of age.[16] Entry criteria included a birth weight of less than 1750 g and gestational age of less than 37 weeks. Standard term formula or PDF was begun around 36 weeks gestation in the NICU and continued until 9 months CA. Infants who were fed the PDF were larger in weight and length at 9 months CA. At 18 months there were no differences in attained weight and length, but the z-score for length was significantly closer to the 50th percentile in the PDF group. When examined by gender, male infants demonstrated a greater difference between the two formula-fed groups for differences in weight and length at 9 and 18 month CA. As reported before, head circumference, mid arm circumference and skinfold thickness did not differ between the two groups. The incidence of illness and feeding tolerance did not vary between the two groups. Neurodevelopment was assessed at 9 and 18 months CA using the Bayley Scales of Infant Development II and the Knobloch, Passamanick, and Sherrards' Developmental Screening Inventory. There were no differences between groups for any of these tests.

In addition to the two formula-fed groups in the above study, 65 breastfed infants were followed for the first 9 months of CA to serve as a reference group.[16] This group of infants was supplemented with standard term formula when breast milk was not available. The breastfed group differed from the other groups in that the mothers were older, had more education, were of a higher social economic group, and breastfed for a minimum of 6 weeks. The breastfed infants were significantly smaller by weight and length than both formula groups at 6, 12, and 26 weeks, but at 9 months CA the breastfed groups' body weight only differed from the PDF group. At enrollment into the study the breast-fed group had significantly smaller mid upper arm circumferences (MUAC) and triceps and subscapular skinfold thickness and weight standard deviation scores. At 9 months CA the breastfed group remained smaller in MUAC and triceps measurement. The breastfed group was not followed beyond 9 months. Intake of solid foods was significantly less for the breastfed group than the formula-fed groups at 12 and 26 weeks CA. Although this decrease in size suggests that the breastfed premature infant may need nutrient supplementation postdischarge,[16] the lesser rate of growth of the human milk-fed premature infant has been associated with better health and shorter hospital stay than those fed formula.[20]

One study in the US evaluated infants with a birth weight $\leq$ 1800 g from six cities.[14] Study infants were not breastfed and were enrolled into a randomized trial of feeding a standard term formula or PDF for 12 months CA. Study formula was initiated 2 to 4 days prior to discharge. Infants fed the PDF displayed greater body weight at 1 and 2 months CA. This trend continued to 6 months CA for infants whose birth weight was less than 1250 g, but disappeared at 3 months CA for larger premature infants. For male infants fed PDF whose birth weight was less than 1250 g, weight gain was greater from study day one to term and total body weight was greater at 12 months CA than for infants fed standard formula. Length was also greater at 3 and 6 month CA for

the infants fed PDF. Head circumference was greater in the PDF group who were less than 1250 g birth weight at term, 1, 3, 6, and 12 months of CA. Here again improved growth was more pronounced with male infants. Dietary intakes were examined. For the PDF group, milk intakes were less in the first month, and protein intakes were greater at term, 2, and 3 months compared with the standard formula group.

Biochemically, the group fed PDF had higher blood levels of prealbumin, retinol binding protein, and urea nitrogen at term and 9 months CA. No difference was noted between the two groups for their blood albumin and hemoglobin levels. Noteworthy in this study is that only 53 (42%) of the 125 study infants completed the study at 12 months CA. In summary, it appears that for male infants with a birth weight < 1250 g feeding PDF confers an advantage for physical growth during the first 6 months of CA compared with standard term formula. Thus, the results do not provide clear guidelines for postdischarge feeding.

A study in Newcastle, England, compared the nutrient intake, physical growth, biochemical parameters, body composition, and neurological development of premature infants fed one of three different discharge diets.[3,15,21] At discharge, group one was fed PTF until 6 months CA, group 2 was fed PTF until term age and then switched to term infant formula and the third group was fed standard term formula. In this study, the infants had a birth weight $\leq$ 1750 g, birth gestation was $\leq$ 34 weeks and growth was occurring at $\geq$ 25 g day^{-1} at discharge. The period of intervention was 6 months, with follow up at 12 and 18 months.

Milk intakes were greater for the groups fed standard term formula versus those fed the premature infant formula, but energy intakes remained equal, suggesting dietary intake adjusted to meeting energy needs.[15] Since the PTF is more nutrient dense, the nutrient intakes were higher for infants fed premature infant formula.[15,22,23] Girls had greater milk intakes than boys from discharge to 6 months CA, but no difference in energy or nutrient intakes were reported.[15] Milk intakes decreased from term to 6 months CA for both boys and girls.[15] The timing of solid food introduction did not vary by gender or formula group, and was generally introduced around 7 weeks CA.[15]

The results of this study identified male gender and PTF as major factors affecting outcome. At 6 months CA, weight and length were greater for boys fed the PTF until 6 months CA than boys fed the standard term formula or those fed PTF until term. At 18 months CA boys who had been fed the PTF until 6 months CA continued to be larger (1.0 kg in weight, 2 cm in length, and 1 cm in head circumference) than boys fed standard term formula.[3] Boys fed the PTF were larger than girls fed the premature infant formula at all ages.[15]

With increasing age, serum total protein, albumin, and blood urea nitrogen (BUN) levels increased.[15] No differences were noted by gender in BUN, or serum total protein, albumin, or calcium levels.[15] BUN was higher in those infants fed the premature infant formulas which provided greater protein intakes.[15] Girls had higher serum phosphorus levels and lower serum alkaline phosphatase levels than boys.[15]

Body composition in the Newcastle study was described by the use of dual energy x-ray absorptiometry at discharge, term and CA of 12 weeks, 6 months, and 12 months.[21] Between discharge and term, gains in weight, lean body mass, fat mass, and bone mineral mass were similar for the groups receiving PTF. From term to 12 months of age, the groups receiving standard term formula were similar in gains of weight, lean body mass, fat mass, and bone mineral mass. Girls displayed no difference in growth velocity by formula group, but boys gain more weight, lean body mass, and fat mass if fed PTF. With time, weight, lean body mass, and fat mass increased in all infants significantly.[21] The percent fat mass increased from discharge to 6 months CA, but the percentage decreased from 6 to 12 months CA. In girls fed the PTF, increased weight and lean mass were demonstrated, but not percent fat mass from term to 12 weeks CA. These differences were not noted in girls at either 6 or 12 months CA by diet. At 12 months CA, boys fed preterm formula for 6 months CA were larger in weight, lean body mass, fat mass, but not percent of fat mass. Bone area and bone mineral mass was greater in girls fed preterm infant formula at term and 12 weeks CA, but this difference was not seen at 6 and 12 months CA. Bone mineral density never varied by diet in the girls. For the first 12 months of CA with boys fed the premature infant formula bone area and, bone mineral mass were greater than those fed standard term formula.[21] The percent fat mass was always larger in girls although the absolute fat mass did not differ from boys.[15] No differences were noted between girls or boys fed the PTF in gains of bone area, bone mineral mass, bone area or, bone mineral density.[21]

The investigators noted that boys and girls fed the PTF had the same intakes of energy, protein, calcium, and phosphorus, but yet they displayed differences in weight gain, lean body mass gain, weight, and lean body mass. This suggests that gender may influence nutrient utilization and/or need during infancy. Boys fed the PTF displayed an increase in body weight which was reflected by an increase in lean body mass and fat mass without an increase in the percent of fat mass.[15] The PTF-fed infants received greater nutrient intake without an increase in energy intake, which may more closely meet the needs of the premature infant. Not only were differences noted between the use of PTF versus the use of term formula, but gender differences were present. For male infants, premature infant formula fed to 6 months CA resulted in differences in physical size and growth composition.

At 18 months CA, the Bayley Scales of Infant Development II was used to assess mental and psychomotor development.[3] Diet had no effect on the test scores among the males or between male and female infants fed PTF until 6 months CA.[3] However, when all infants were compared by gender, females displayed a higher mental development index.[3] This difference is due to the lower developmental scores displayed by male infants fed term formula.[3]

The most noteworthy finding in the Newcastle studies is that the small differences attributed to PTF at 6 months persisted well beyond the period of dietary intervention, with continuing advantages at 12 and 18 months. This observation suggests that if intervention is planned, it should continue for at least 6 months if a beneficial outcome is desired. The study also presents data on gender differences which need to be explored further. Whether an enriched diet, such as fed in the other studies of Carver et al. and Lucas et al.[14,16] would provide the same benefits as a PTF is not known. Use of premature formula designed for use in the nursery has not been recommended as a formula for postdischarge.[24] The high mineral and vitamin content may be excessive for the infant who weighs more than 2500 g and is not fluid restricted. However, it should be noted that PTF used in the studies in England differs markedly from the PTF used in the USA. The English PTF more closely resembles the American PDF formula. Thus, these data may be interpreted overall as showing marginal benefit for an enriched diet in the postdischarge period.

Studies of breastfed infants

The provision of human milk postdischarge has received limited study. No randomized trials have been conducted on former premature infants breastfed in the postdischarge period. Chan followed 43 formula-fed and 16 breastfed infants up to 16 weeks postdischarge.[25] The formula-fed infants received either standard, premature, or low birth weight formulas for 8 weeks postdischarge and the breastfed infants received a 400 IU supplement of vitamin D per day. From 8 weeks to 16 weeks, all formula fed infants received standard infant formula. The formula-fed infants always weighed more than the breast-fed infants. Head circumferences and body length did not differ among the groups, but the infants fed premature or low birth weight formulas displayed a greater rate of growth in these parameters from discharge to 16 weeks than the breast-fed infants.

Biochemically, serum calcium and 25-hydroxy vitamin D levels did not vary among groups, but the breastfed group displayed lower serum phosphorus levels at 8 weeks postdischarge and higher serum alkaline phosphatase levels at 8, and 16 weeks postdischarge. Bone mineral content was lower in breastfed infants at discharge, 2, 8, and 16 weeks postdischarge. At 8 weeks postdischarge bone mineral content was greater in the infants fed PTF than those fed term formula, but the difference was not present at 16 weeks postdischarge. Although these observations were not derived from randomized studies, clinicians should be aware of a potential problem with growth of the premature breastfed infant in the postdischarge period. Furthermore, the data support the need to have standards of growth and nutrient intakes in the postdischarge period.

Studies in small for gestational age infants

There is one report of SGA term infants who experience improved growth with the use of the PDF in place of standard term formula for the first 9 months of life.[26] Length was greater at 1 cm at 9 months of age and remained greater by 0.9 cm at 18 months. Growth parameters of weight, head circumference, and skinfold measurements did not differ between groups. At 9 months of age the infants fed PDF had a lower developmental quotient of 99.5 versus the infants fed term formula at 102.[27] When analyzed by gender, the difference was only noted for female infants. By 18 months of life, this difference disappeared. At present, the use of PDF for the growth-restricted, term infant is not recommended.[27] Additional long-term developmental follow-up is indicated.

In this investigation, a group of breastfed, SGA infants were followed for 18 months of age to assess growth.[26] At 9 months, the breastfed infants had greater gain in head circumference than the infants fed term formula. At 18 months, the breastfed infants had larger weights, lengths, and head circumferences than infants fed term formula and were longer than those infants fed PDF. However there were no differences between the growth of breastfed and formula fed SGA infants when the factors of social class, maternal education, parental size, infant gender, size at enrollment, age at follow-up, and birth order were controlled.[26] The mothers in the breastfed group were older, had more education, were of a higher social class, were taller and the head circumferences of both mothers and fathers were greater for the breastfed group as compared with the parents of the formula-fed infants.[26,27] Most important, the breastfed group had higher developmental scores than both formula-fed groups at 18 months.[27] Human milk does offer the SGA

infant the advantages of greater developmental outcomes and physical growth that is equaled by formula-fed infants.

Goals for discharge

Before discharge the infant should have an established pattern of weight gain while consuming the diet for discharge. Physiologically the infant should be able to breast or bottle feed without cardio-respiratory compromise. Nutritional risks should be assessed and the appropriate therapies and dietary modification should be made. Parents should demonstrate the ability to feed their infant by breast, bottle, or alternative methods if indicated. In addition, they should demonstrate correct formula preparation and supplement dosage.

The American Academy of Pediatrics, Committee on Fetus and Newborn has provided goals to be achieved for the infant to have a successful transition home from the hospital.[28] These goals include that the infant is physiologically stable, the family is prepared to provide care, the primary care physician is established, support services are established in the community and medical specialists are linked as indicated. An appointment within the first week of discharge to ensure early and appropriate follow-up care is indicated.

Multidisciplinary support of the family is an ongoing process and continues after discharge. Additional resources may include, but are not limited to: the NICU developmental follow-up clinics, pulmonary clinics, feeding clinics and community support programs which often provide home visitation programs by healthcare professionals. These community programs may include Children's Rehabilitative Services, Children with Special Health Care Needs, Special Supplemental Nutrition Program for Women Infants and Children (WIC), and Early Intervention Programs. The primary physician needs to receive follow-up information from the hospital personnel as well as the community setting personnel to ensure coordination of the infant's care.

Suggested approach for post-discharge nutrition

There are several options for milk selection and supplementation at discharge, but the appropriate selection remains controversial because of the lack of data to support one recommendation over another.[29] An individual approach is indicated.

Table 46.2. Selected nutrient comparison of post-discharge formula, human milk, and milk combinations per liter

Nutrient	Enriched or post-discharge formula (PDF)	Human milk (HM)	Human milk + PDF powder = 24 kcal per oz	6 feeds of HM + 2 feeds of PDF 22 kcal per oz
Energy (kcal)	730	670	810	686
Protein (g)	21	10	12.5	12.8
Calcium (mg)	835	280	424	419
Phosphorus (mg)	475	147	228	229
Iron (mg)	13.3	0.4	2.7	3.6
Zinc (mg)	9	1.2	2.7	3.2
Vitamin D (mcg)	14	0.5	3.0	1.2

Breastfeeding premature infants

Strategies to support breastfeeding success and professional and parent breastfeeding resources need to be identified.[30] Prior to discharge, it must be determined if the infant can breastfeed successfully and continue to grow at an adequate rate. If the infant is breastfeeding well, weight gain is adequate (more than 20 g day^{-1}), and there are no persisting abnormal nutritional biochemical measures, then the postdischarge diet should include exclusive breastfeeding. In this scenario, the infant also should receive a multivitamin and an iron supplement. Follow-up weight checks at 1 week, and serially thereafter, must be encouraged. Measurement of biochemical indices (serum alkaline phosphatase, phosphorus, albumin, BUN) may be helpful.

If the infant has a rate of growth less than 20 g day^{-1}, is unable to consume ad libitum quantities of breast milk (more than 180 ml kg^{-1}day^{-1}), or has persistent biochemical abnormalities (elevated alkaline phosphatase and/or low serum phosphorous, albumin, and BUN), then supplemental nutrition must be provided in addition to breastfeeding. The supplemental nutrition usually is in the form of commercially prepared formula. The enriched PDFs have been used for this purpose because the nutrient density is greater than that of term formula, and there are powdered preparations that can be mixed to whatever strength is desirable/needed. Mothers may express milk and add the powdered supplement to breast milk, or breastfeed and provide 2–3 feedings of PDF each day. The PDF can be used in the standard 22 kcal per oz strength or concentrated as needed. For the infant who requires fluid restriction, breastfeeding may be possible if the powdered formula is used as a supplement. When breastfeeding and supplemental PDF are used, the infant's vitamin and iron status should be considered. Vitamin supplements are needed. Iron at 2 mg kg^{-1} day^{-1} should be given unless $\geq$ 90 ml kg^{-1} day^{-1} of PDF is consumed; then 1 mg kg^{-1} day^{-1} of iron is indicated. See Table 46.2 for nutrient comparison.

Formula feeding premature infants

For the formula-fed premature infant the same criteria should be considered: infants who are unable to ingest quantities of milk in excess of 180 ml kg^{-1} day^{-1}, have rates of weight gain less than 20 g day^{-1}, or have persisting biochemical abnormalities should be given PDF near discharge. In general, these infants tend to have birth weights < 1250 g, restricted milk intake, and/or biochemical evidence of rickets or hypoproteinemia. If the exclusive diet is PDF, then no additional vitamins or iron are required. If term formula is fed, the infant should be given iron-fortified formula. If term formula is fed, the infant also should be given multivitamins for about 2 months.

Duration of feeding postdischarge diets

When supplemented, specialized postdischarge nutrition is provided it should be continued for 6 months or to approximately 9 months CA.[24,31] Iron supplements at 2 mg kg^{-1} day^{-1} for the exclusive breastfed infant should be provided for the first year of life.[23] Only iron-fortified formulas should be given and, if used, no additional iron supplementation is indicated. Multivitamins are needed to provide 200 IU per day of vitamin D for the breastfed infant.[32] Multivitamins are not indicated for infants receiving PDF, and those premature infants who have achieved 3 kilograms of weight and are consuming standard term formula.[24] The introduction of solid foods should be when the infant is at the corrected developmental age such that this skill can be accomplished.[33]

Monitoring

The frequency of office or home visits will be determined by the clinical condition of the infant. Infants who have had concerns about milk intake, growth or abnormal biochemical indices should be seen more frequently, beginning at 1 week postdischarge. Infants who have active chronic

Table 46.3. Growth velocities for corrected gestational age

Age	Weight (g day^{-1})^{29,37}	Length (cm week^{-1})^{29,37}	Head circumference (cm month^{-1} (age))^{33}
0–3 months	25–30	0.7–1.0	1.6–2.5 (1 month)
3–12 months	10–15	0.4–0.6	0.8–1.4 (4 months)
			0.3–0.8 (8 months)
			0.2–0.4 (12 months)

lung disease and are discharged home on oxygen and/or mechanical support requiring fluid restriction will need frequent assessments to ensure that nutrition provided meets the needs of the individual infant. Within the first week of discharge, weekly and then monthly visits become appropriate as the infant demonstrates growth.

When plotting growth parameters of the premature infant, corrected age should be used for the first 3 years of life.[34] Without adjusting for prematurity, the use of chronological age leads to a significant increased number of infants labeled as having poor weight or length growth.

There are two types of growth charts that can be utilized to monitor the growth of premature infants postdischarge. This first type is based on the actual growth of premature infants.[8] On these charts, the infant's growth can be compared with the growth of other premature infants. The plotted premature infant should grow as well as, if not greater than, the growth curves since they are based on the growth of premature infants. However, growing well on these charts does not signify that catch-up growth has occurred since the growth of term infants is not included in these charts.

The second type of chart is the 2000 Centers for Disease Control and Prevention (CDC) growth charts based on the growth of infants who weighed ≥ 1500 g at birth.[35] Plotting onto the CDC charts will allow the assessment that catch-up growth has occurred.[36]

Growth velocity can be utilized to monitor growth. Weekly weight trends are helpful to assess the infant who is demonstrating poor growth and requires diet manipulations. See Table 46.3 for growth rates.

Laboratory assessment for mineral status should include serum alkaline phosphatase activity levels, serum calcium, and serum phosphorus for infants who have a history of osteopenia or are considered at risk for this disease due to poor calcium and phosphorus intakes while in the NICU. For protein status, albumin, and BUN can be followed. When growth is poor or laboratory values are abnormal the diet should be reevaluated. Increased concentration of a PDF or additional formula feedings per day for the breastfed infant are possible considerations.

Summary

There is little evidence to support strong recommendations for nutrition management of the postdischarge premature infant. Suggested guidelines are provided, but it is expected that research will continue to elucidate more clearly the specific nutrient needs of this high-risk infant population.

The goal is to provide nutrition to facilitate optimal growth and development for premature infants. Continued evaluation of growth and development must take place to ensure the best outcome for these small infants. Early detection of problems can facilitate a quick change in nutritional management as indicated. Since the nutrition required to achieve this goal remains unknown, constant monitoring must occur to ensure the health of each child.

REFERENCES

1 Heird, W. C. Determination of nutritional requirements in preterm infants, with special reference to "catch-up" growth. *Semin. Neonatal.* 2001;**6**:365–75.
2 Klein, C. J. Nutrient requirements for preterm infant formulas. *J. Nutr.* 2002;**132**:1395S–577S.
3 Cooke, R. J., Embleton, N. D., Griffin, I. J., Wells, J. C., McCormick, K. P. Feeding preterm infants after hospital discharge: growth and development at 18 months of age. *Pediatr. Res.* 2001;**49**:719–22.
4 Ehrenkranz, R. A., Younes, N., Lemons, J. A. *et al.* Longitudinal growth of hospitalized very low birth weight infants. *Pediatrics* 1999;**104**:280–9.
5 Fenton, T. R. A new growth chart for preterm infants: Babson and Benda's chart updated with recent data and a new format. *BMC Pediatrics* 2003;**3**:13.
6 Cazacu, A., Fraley, J. K., Schanler, R. J. We are inadequately nourishing healthy low birth weight infants. *Pediatr. Res.* 2001;**49**:343A.
7 Embleton, N. E., Pang, N., Cooke, R. J. Postnatal malnutrition and growth retardation: an inevitable consequence of current recommendations in preterm infants? *Pediatrics* 2001;**107**:270–3.
8 Casey, P. H., Kraemer, H. C., Bernbaum, J., Yogman, M. W., Sells, J. C. Growth status and growth rates of a varied sample of low

birth weight, preterm infants: a longitudinal cohort from birth to three years of age. *J. Pediatr.* 1991;**119**:599–605.

9 Hack, M., Weissman, B., Breslau, N. *et al.* Health of very low birth weight children during their first eight years. *J. Pediatr.* 1993;**122**:887–92.

10 Hack, M., Flannery, D. J., Schluchter, M. *et al.* Outcomes in young adulthood for very-low-birth-weight infants. *New Engl. J. Med.* 2002;**346**:149–57.

11 Hirata, T., Bosque, E. When they grow up: the growth of extremely low birth weight (≤1000 gm) infants at adolescence. *J. Pediatr.* 1998;**132**:1033–5.

12 Hack, M., Schluchter, M., Cartar, L. *et al.*. Growth of very low birth weight infants to age 20 years. *Pediatrics* 2003;**112**: e30–8.

13 Hack, M., Breslau, N., Weissman, B. *et al.*. Effect of very low birthweight and subnormal head size on cognitive abilities at school age. *New Engl. J. Med.* 1991;**325**:231–7.

14 Carver, J. D., Wu, P. Y. K., Hall, R. T. *et al.* Growth of preterm infants fed nutrient-enriched or term formula after hospital discharge. *Pediatrics* 2001;**107**:683–9.

15 Cooke, R. J., Griffin, I. J., McCormick, K. *et al.* Feeding preterm infants after hospital discharge: Effect of dietary manipulation on nutrient intake and growth. *Pediatr. Res.* 1998;**43**:355–60.

16 Lucas, A., Fewtrell, M. S., Morley, R. *et al.* Randomized trial of nutrient-enriched formula versus standard formula for post-discharge preterm infants. *Pediatrics* 2001;**108**:703–11.

17 Lucas, A., Bishop, N. J., King, F. J., Cole, T. J. Randomised trial of nutrition for preterm infants after discharge. *Arch. Dis. Child.* 1992;**67**:324–7.

18 Bishop, N. J., King, F. J., Lucas, A. Increased bone mineral content of preterm infants fed with a nutrient enriched formula after discharge from hospital. *Arch. Dis. Child.* 1993; **68**: 573–8.

19 Fewtrell, M. S., Cole, T. J., Bishop, N. J., Lucas, A. Neonatal factors predicting childhood height in preterm infants: Evidence for a persisting effect of early metabolic bone disease? *J. Pediatr.* 2000;**137**:668–73.

20 Schanler, R. J., Shulman, R. J., Lau, C. Feeding strategies for premature infants: beneficial outcomes of feeding fortified human milk versus preterm formula. *Pediatrics* 1999;**103**:1150–7.

21 Cooke, R. J., McCormick, K., Griffin, I. J. *et al.* Feeding preterm infants after hospital discharge: Effect of diet on body composition. *Pediatr. Res.* 1999;**46**:461–4.

22 Griffin, I. J. Postdischarge nutrition for high risk neonates. *Clin. Perinatol.* 2002;**29**:327–44.

23 Griffin, I. J. and Abrams, S. A. Iron and breastfeeding. *Pediatr. Clin. N. Am.* 2001;**48**:401–13.

24 American Academy of Pediatrics, Committee on Nutrition. Nutritional needs of the preterm infant. In Kleinman, R. E., ed. *Pediatric Nutrition Handbook.* 5th edn. American Academy of Pediatrics; 2004;23–54.

25 Chan, G. M. Growth and bone mineral status of discharged very low birth weight infants fed different formulas or human milk. *J. Pediatr.* 1993;**123**:439–43.

26 Fewtrell, M. S., Morley, R., Abbott, R. A. *et al.* Catch-up growth in small-for-gestational-age term infants: a randomized trial. *Am. J. Clin. Nutr.* 2001;**74**:516–23.

27 Morley, R., Fewtrell, M. S., Abbott, R. A. Neurodevelopment in children born small for gestational age: a randomized trial of nutrient-enriched versus standard formula and comparison with a reference breastfed group. *Pediatrics* 2004;**113**:515–21.

28 American Academy of Pediatrics, Committee on Fetus and Newborn. Hospital discharge of the high-risk neonate: proposed guidelines. *Pediatrics* 1998;**102**:411–17.

29 Hall, R. T. (2001) Nutritional follow-up of the breastfeeding premature infant after hospital discharge. *Pediatr. Clin. N. Am.* 2001;**48**:453–60.

30 Cox, J. H., Doorlag, D. Nutritional care at transfer and discharge. In S. Groh-Wargo, M. Thompson, J. Cox, eds. *Nutritional Care for High-Risk Newborns.* Rev. 3rd edn. Chicago: Precept Press, Inc.;2000:549–65.

31 Dusick, A. M., Poindexter, B. B., Ehrenkranz, E. A., Lemons, J. A. Growth failure in the preterm infant: can we catch up? *Semin. Perinatol.* 2003;**27**:302–10.

32 American Academy of Pediatrics, Committee on Nutrition. Breastfeeding. In R. E. Kleinman ed. *Pediatric Nutrition Handbook* 5th edn. American Academy of Pediatrics;2004:55–85.

33 Theriot, L. (2000). Routine nutrition care during follow-up. In S. Groh-Wargo, M. Thompson, and J. Cox eds. *Nutritional Care for High-Risk Newborns.* Rev. 3rd. Chicago: Precept Press, Inc.;2000:567–83.

34 Wang, Z., Sauve, R. S. Assessment of postneonatal growth in VLBW infants: selection of growth references and age adjustment for prematurity. *Can. J. Pub. Health.* 1998;**89**:109–14.

35 Odgen, C. L., Kuczmarski, R. J., Flegal, K. M. *et al.* Centers for disease control and prevention 2000 growth charts for the United States: Improvements to the 1977 National Center for Health Statistics Version. *Pediatrics* 2002;**109**:45–60.

36 Sherry, B., Mei, A., Grummer-Strawn, L., Dietz, W. H. Evaluation of and recommendations for growth references for very low birth weight (≤1500 g) infants in the United States. *Pediatrics* 2003;**111**:750–8.

37 Fomon, S. J., Nelson, S. E. In ed. S. J. Fomon Nutrition of Normal Infants. St. Louis: Mosby;1993:36–84.

Index